The Science of Sleep

The Science of Sleep

BENJAMIN RUSAK, PhD, FRSC
DISTINGUISHED RESEARCH PROFESSOR EMERITUS
DEPARTMENTS OF PSYCHIATRY AND PSYCHOLOGY & NEUROSCIENCE
DALHOUSIE UNIVERSITY, HALIFAX, CANADA

OXFORD
UNIVERSITY PRESS

OXFORD
UNIVERSITY PRESS

Oxford University Press is a department of the University of Oxford. It furthers the University's objective of excellence in research, scholarship, and education by publishing worldwide. Oxford is a registered trade mark of Oxford University Press in the UK and in certain other countries.

Published in the United States of America by Oxford University Press
198 Madison Avenue, New York, NY 10016, United States of America.

Library of Congress Cataloging-in-Publication Data
Names: Rusak, Benjamin author
Title: The science of sleep / Benjamin Rusak.
Description: New York, NY : Oxford University Press, [2025] |
Includes bibliographical references. |
Identifiers: LCCN 2025023538 | ISBN 9781605352978 hardback |
ISBN 9780197828397 | ISBN 9781605357874 epub | ISBN 9780197828526
Subjects: LCSH: Sleep—Research
Classification: LCC RA786 .R87 2025
LC record available at https://lccn.loc.gov/2025023538

DOI: 10.1093/med/9781605352978.001.0001

Printed by Integrated Books International, United States of America

MIX
Paper
FSC FSC® C183721

The manufacturer's authorized representative in the EU for product safety is
Oxford University Press España S.A., Parque Empresarial San Fernando de Henares,
Avenida de Castilla, 2 – 28830 Madrid (www.oup.es/en or product.safety@oup.com).
OUP España S.A. also acts as importer into Spain of products made by the manufacturer.

This volume is dedicated to the memory of my late father and mother, Jacob and Gusta, and my oldest brother, Henry, who struggled against terrible odds during World War II but survived and brought me and my brother Sheldon to a new world. It is also dedicated to the generations that have followed, including the newest addition, Robin Elliot.

Contents

D. IMPACTS OF SLEEP DURATION & QUALITY

E. FUNCTIONS OF SLEEP

Preface

This volume grew out of my teaching interests related to sleep and circadian rhythms. It was developed based on lectures for an introductory, one-semester course called "The Science of Sleep" that I offered starting in 2011 to undergraduate science students at Dalhousie University, mostly students majoring in psychology, neuroscience, or medical sciences.

Students taking the course were interested in sleep for a variety of reasons, including having their own sleep problems, having family members with sleep disorders, their experience working shifts during summer jobs, or curiosity about dreams and sleep in general. By the time they had reached the third year of their undergraduate science studies, however, they typically had acquired very little knowledge about the basic science of sleep that could serve as a framework within which we could begin to address their questions. The goal of the course (and this volume) was to introduce students to aspects of basic research related to sleep.

This book is not a review of clinical sleep medicine, for which there are many available resources. It is intended to provide a broad introduction to what we have learned from scientific research into the mechanisms producing the phenomena of sleep, the systems that regulate sleep, and what its functions are. Clinical conditions are addressed in some cases, however, because they inform our understanding of the physiology of sleep regulation. In other cases, they are discussed because knowledge of the mechanisms regulating sleep and circadian rhythms has important implications for understanding and treating clinical conditions. Although the volume is focused primarily on sleep in people, it discusses research on other species when it informs our understanding of the mechanisms of sleep or sets the boundaries and context for discussions of the functions of sleep.

The amount of material included in this volume exceeds what I could review in a one-semester course, especially for students with a minimal neuroscience background. I would typically include the first seven chapters and one or two related to sleep and health or sleep and cognition/shift work. The chapters related to physiological regulation of sleep and its features are more heavily neuroscience-based than others. I used these as resources for senior-level seminars for neuroscience majors. Colleagues have used draft sections of the book along with selected readings to create their own structure for courses taught in other institutions.

The selection of topics covered is somewhat idiosyncratic, driven by my own background and interests, which include circadian physiology, psychiatric illnesses, and learning and memory. I also tried to extend my coverage to areas with which I was unfamiliar, but which I felt were essential to addressing the larger picture of the scientific study of sleep. This goal led me to read the literature on many new topics related to sleep science, from which I learned a great deal.

I recognize that this volume is not comprehensive in its coverage of either the background or the current status of any of the topics included. A complete review of some of these individual subjects could fill a volume this size on its own. Nor can I pretend that the coverage in any topic area is completely up to date, as I am reminded on an almost daily basis via emails announcing the contents of upcoming publications. I tried to follow these updates until the end of 2022 and partway through 2023 and into 2024, but I had to accept that any review of a rapidly growing research field is necessarily out of date by the time it is published. My hope is that the broad principles identified in relation to the nature of sleep, its regulation, and its functions will remain valid in the face of onrushing torrents of new data or, at least, provide a context for understanding and integrating these new findings.

The book is divided into five parts. Part A provides some general background and a brief overview of research methods and of the historical development of scientific research related to sleep and to circadian rhythms.

Part B covers factors that regulate or influence sleep. These include how sleep is controlled by homeostatic and circadian mechanisms, how it changes over the human lifespan, how cultural and environmental influences modify sleep, and how it is expressed in species other than humans.

Part C covers the physiological regulation of sleep, including the influence of circadian mechanisms, the pineal gland and melatonin, brainstem and forebrain mechanisms (including the neurotransmitter systems that are key to the regulation of sleep), and thalamocortical mechanisms that produce the electrophysiological features of sleep and influence conscious awareness across the stages of sleep.

Part D addresses several aspects of how adequate and inadequate sleep affect people. It includes a review of how sleep and sleep loss affect human performance and cognition, how shift work and jet lag affect sleep, and the resulting consequences for human health. It discusses the effects of experimental sleep restriction and of spontaneous short and long sleep on several aspects of health, including metabolism, weight regulation, vascular function, the immune system, and pain perception.

It also reviews the complex relations between sleep and major psychiatric disorders, including anxiety disorders, depression, bipolar illness, and schizophrenia as well as the relations between sleep and Alzheimer's disease.

Part E addresses the functions of sleep. It provides a brief overview of different ideas about how we can explain the existence of sleep and its features, and discusses some of the strengths and weaknesses of several hypotheses about why we sleep. Two chapters then review one of the most active areas of current sleep research, namely, the functions of sleep in memory and the physiological mechanisms that are involved in these functions. A brief final chapter summarizes some of the evidence related to plasticity and the functions of sleep.

There are also four appendices. Appendix A deals with dreaming and its mechanisms in REM and NREM sleep. Including this topic in the text, which introduces REM sleep and the early work linking it to dreaming, distracted from the main themes of that chapter, so it was included as an appendix for interested readers.

Appendix B deals with the topic that is the most common focus of clinical sleep laboratories, namely, sleep disordered breathing—in particular, sleep apnea. The wealth of basic and clinical research on this topic is far beyond what could be addressed within the framework of this volume. But the existence of often-undetected sleep apnea in large segments of the population can have a significant impact on the outcomes of population-based studies that relate sleep amounts and quality to other health conditions. This short appendix is intended to acknowledge the importance of this condition, to give readers a brief introduction to some basic facts about it, and to provide references that could serve as entry points into the literature.

Appendix C is intended for readers who are less familiar with the tools of neuroscience that are used to study the physiological mechanisms of sleep. It provides brief, nontechnical descriptions of some of the major techniques used and a few words about the strengths and limitations of these methods. Appendix D deals with a side issue related to narcolepsy and the immune system that involves some technical aspects related to immunization that may not be of interest to most readers but provides some insights into the mechanisms that regulate REM sleep and can trigger narcolepsy.

Some of the studies reviewed in this volume included findings of differences between male and female participants (e.g., in sleep features, timing, or health consequences of altered sleep). These results are discussed as gender, rather than sex, differences. This terminology reflects the fact that participants who are recruited to laboratory or survey studies typically self-identify as being male or female. Very few studies include additional measures of genetic or hormonal features related to biological sex. Thus, the observed differences are most appropriately attributed to self-identified gender.

Covering the broad range of topics in this volume, many of which fall outside my own direct research experience, risks introducing errors of fact or interpretation. Despite reviews of these chapters by experts on most of these topics, and their many helpful clarifications and corrections, it is likely that some errors remain or have since crept into the text. The responsibility for these lies entirely with me and not with the reviewers. I hope the errors are few, but I apologize for any that remain, and I welcome readers' input and corrections.

Acknowledgments

Many friends and colleagues helped with the production of this volume over the (many) years that I worked on it. I am especially grateful to those who read and provided feedback on multiple chapters and on specific issues throughout the process: Samuel Deurveilher, Kazue Semba, and Ralph Mistlberger. I am also grateful to those who provided helpful criticisms and suggestions on individual chapters, including Martin Alda, Alex Borbély, Julie Carrier and Thaïna Rosinvil, Kimberly Cote, Mary Ganguli, and Mary Harrington.

Other colleagues answered questions and helped clarify aspects of their own work: Isabel Arnulf, Derk-Jan Dijk, Gabriella Gobbi, Steven Pan, Henning Tiemeier, and Hans Van Dongen. Many thanks to all of you. Special thanks to Meeok (Ella) Kim for her untiring efforts in producing dozens of figures. I also thank Kenneth Catania, Vincent Cassone, Gail Eskes, Laura Lewis, Steven Lockley, Antonia Scholz, Melissa Vollrath, Marilyn & Sarah Klein, Nellie, Gus, and Marcus for their figure contributions. Other colleagues gave their approval for reuse of figures, for which I am grateful; these are acknowledged in the figure legends.

During the development of this book, the publisher obtained reviews and suggestions from other experts, many of which were anonymous; so I thank them, collectively and anonymously, for their efforts. These generous reviewers corrected errors and directed my attention to significant related topics and publications. Their feedback was enormously helpful to me, and the most critical among them were probably the most helpful.

The history of this book began with my interest in teaching about aspects of the science of sleep and my difficulty in finding a textbook that covered the topics of interest. Since then, more than a decade of Dalhousie students have gone through the resulting class and provided feedback that helped shape its content. Mary Harrington and Kimberly Cote also used draft portions of some chapters in their own teaching and gathered more feedback from students at Smith College and Brock University. Thanks to all of them.

This book was originally intended to be published by Sinauer Associates, and an editor at Sinauer, Sydney Carroll, provided support and guidance through the difficult early stages of development of the book, which was planned to include seven chapters. After 2017, Sinauer became an imprint of Oxford University Press, and the editorial role changed. Craig Panner, Emily Yu, and Janine Fisher at OUP took over the task of guiding me through the even more difficult, later stages of the process, as the volume evolved into 19 chapters. It is hard to judge whether I was more surprised by the arcane complexity of the book development and publishing process or whether the editors were more surprised by my naiveté. In any case, I thank them for their efforts and guidance.

Finally, I am grateful to family and friends for their support, as well as for their discretion in gradually starting to avoid the subject of progress on the book as the years passed. I am especially grateful to Gail for her patience and support, and for—usually—managing to maintain her composure on learning that I was back to editing something in Chapter 1.

Abbreviations

5-HT	5-hydroxytryptamine (serotonin)
AAD	auto-activation deficit
AAP	American Association of Pediatrics
Aβ	amyloid β (beta)
ACh	acetylcholine
AChE	acetylcholinesterase
AD	Alzheimer's disease
ADHD	attention deficit hyperactivity disorder
ADP	adenosine diphosphate
ARAS	ascending reticular activating system
AS	active sleep
ASD	autism spectrum disorder
ATP	adenosine triphosphate
BBB	blood-brain barrier
BDNF	brain-derived neurotrophic factor
BF	basal forebrain nuclei
BMI	body-mass index
BRAC	basic rest–activity cycle
BSWS	bihemispheric slow-wave sleep
Ca^{2+}	calcium ion
cAMP	cyclic adenosine monophosphate
CBT-I	Cognitive Behavioral Therapy for Insomnia
CCTT-2	Children's Color Trails Test 2
CeA	central nucleus of the amygdala
CRP	C-reactive protein
CSF	cerebrospinal fluid
CT	circadian time
DA	dopamine
DBP	diastolic blood pressure
DLMO	dim-light melatonin onset
DMH	dorsomedial hypothalamic nucleus
DMN	default mode network
DNA	deoxyribonucleic acid
DOW	disk-over-water
DRN	dorsal raphe nucleus
DSPS	delayed sleep phase syndrome
EDS	excessive daytime sleepiness
EEG	electroencephalogram
EMG	electromyogram
EOG	electrooculogram
EPSP	excitatory postsynaptic potential
ERP	event-related potential
FFI	fatal familial insomnia
fMRI	functional magnetic resonance imaging
FSH	follicle stimulating hormone
GABA	γ-gamma aminobutyric acid
GAD	generalized anxiety disorder
GFAP	glial fibrillary acidic protein
GHB	γ-gamma hydroxybutyrate
GRP	gastrin-releasing peptide
HA	histamine
HCRTR	hypocretin receptor
HDL	high-density lipoprotein
HLA	human leukocyte antigen
HOMA	Homeostatic Model Assessment
HPA	hypothalamic-pituitary-adrenal
HRT	hormone replacement therapy
IL	interleukin
IPSP	inhibitory postsynaptic potential
ir	immunoreactive
ISI	Insomnia Severity Index
LAN	light at night
L-DOPA	levodopa
LD	light-dark
LDL	low-density lipoprotein
LC	locus coeruleus
LDT	laterodorsal tegmental nucleus
LGN	lateral geniculate nucleus
LH	lateral hypothalamic area
LPO	lateral preoptic area
LTD	long-term depression
LTP	long-term potentiation
M1	primary motor area
MAP	mean arterial pressure
M/E	morningness/eveningness
MCH	melanin concentrating hormone
MCI	mild cognitive impairment
MCTQ	Munich ChronoType Questionnaire
MEG	magnetoencephalography
MFB	medial forebrain bundle
MGN	medial geniculate nucleus
MnPO	median preoptic nucleus
MR	Mendelian randomization
mRNA	messenger ribonucleic acid
MSL	motor sequence learning
MSLT	Multiple Sleep Latency Test
MTL	medial temporal lobe
MTR	magnetization transfer ratio
MWT	Maintenance of Wakefulness Test
N1	NREM stage 1 sleep

N2	NREM stage 2 sleep
N3	NREM stage 3 sleep (slow-wave sleep)
NE	norepinephrine
NMDA	N-methyl-D-aspartate
NMS	neuromedin S
NO	nitric oxide
NREM	non-rapid eye movement (sleep)
ORP	odds ratio product
OSA	obstructive sleep apnea
OTC	over-the-counter
PCPA	para-chlorophenylalanine
PD	Parkinson's disease
PD	panic disorder
PET	positron emission tomography
PFC	prefrontal cortex
pfLH	perifornical lateral hypothalamus
PG	prostaglandin
PGO	ponto-geniculo-occipital
PH	posterior hypothalamus
PHI	peptide histidine isoleucine
PK2	prokineticin 2
PKA	cyclic AMP-dependent protein kinase
PLM	periodic limb movement
PMDD	premenstrual dysphoric disorder
PPI	prepulse inhibition
PPT	pedunculopontine tegmental nucleus
PRC	phase response curve
PRF	pontine reticular formation
PS	paradoxical sleep
PSG	polysomnogram
PSP	postsynaptic potential
PSQI	Pittsburgh Sleep Quality Index
P-tau	hyperphosphorylated tau protein
PTSD	post-traumatic stress disorder
PVN	paraventricular hypothalamic nucleus
PVT	Psychomotor Vigilance Test
QS	quiet sleep
REM	rapid eye movement
REMBD	REM sleep behavior disorder
RHT	retinohypothalamic tract
RLS	restless legs syndrome
RNA	ribonucleic acid
ROS	reactive oxygen species
SAD	seasonal affective disorder
SBP	systolic blood pressure
SCG	superior cervical ganglion
SCN	suprachiasmatic nucleus
SDB	sleep-disordered breathing
SIDS	sudden infant death syndrome
SLD	sublaterodorsal tegmental nucleus
SMA	supplementary motor area
SOL	sleep onset latency
SO	slow oscillation
SPZ	subparaventricular zone
SRTT	Serial Reaction Time Task
SSRI	selective serotonin reuptake inhibitor
SWA	slow-wave activity
SWE	slow-wave energy
SWR	sharp-wave ripple
SWS	slow-wave sleep
T1D	type 1 diabetes
T2D	type 2 diabetes
tACS	transcranial alternating current stimulation
tDCS	transcranial direct current stimulation
TES	transcranial electrical stimulation
TH	tyrosine hydroxylase
TIB	time in bed
TMN	tuberomammillary nucleus
TMR	targeted memory reactivation
TMS	transcranial magnetic stimulation
TNFα	tumor necrosis factor α (alpha)
TPJ	temporoparietal junction
TRN	thalamic reticular nucleus
TTFL	transcription/translation feedback loop
USWS	unihemispheric slow-wave sleep
VIP	vasoactive intestinal peptide
vlPAG	ventrolateral periaqueductal gray
VLPO	ventrolateral preoptic nucleus
vmPFC	ventromedial prefrontal cortex
VP	vasopressin
vPAG	ventral periaqueductal gray
VTA	ventral tegmental area
VTD	visual texture discrimination
WASO	wake after sleep onset

A.

History & Methods

CHAPTER 1

Introduction to Sleep Research

1.1 OVERVIEW

This chapter starts with a discussion of ideas about the nature of sleep and its role in our lives. It then reviews the historical development of the scientific study of sleep, including early observational and experimental studies and the invention of technologies that allowed the development of the modern science of sleep. It discusses early views about dreaming and the later discovery of rapid eye movement (REM) sleep, with its important implications for understanding the nature of sleep and the mechanisms regulating it.

1.2 Why sleep?

A quick look through virtually any archive of human literature, mythology, or art reveals many references to sleep. This is not surprising, since sleep is a universal feature of every person's life, occupying close to a third of each 24 h period; over a lifetime of, for example, 85 years, we spend >25 of those years asleep. Sleep is also a compelling drive that cannot be resisted for very long; thus, it is both a familiar companion and an irresistible compulsion. Yet it is also steeped in mystery because, for most of human history, we understood so little about it. As a result, this powerful, puzzling drive has figured prominently in human thought, writing, and other creative arts throughout history.

The presence of sleep as a universal feature of human life raises a fundamental question: Why do we do it? Other behaviors that we are driven to perform, and that occupy far fewer hours of our lives—eating, drinking, having sex—have an obvious impact either on our short-term survival or on our long-term reproductive success. From an evolutionary perspective, the time we commit to these activities seems well justified; we know why we do them. But sleep remains a mystery because we understand little about the function of this (in)activity that occupies such a large proportion of our lives.

Indeed, our society's prevailing attitude seems to be that sleep has little or no functional importance. Consider, for example, the advertising campaign slogan for one high-caffeine drink intended to promote activity and prevent sleep: "No one ever wishes they'd slept more through college"; or the comment attributed to the late British prime minister Margaret Thatcher that "sleep is for wimps." In contrast to these views, however, there is considerable scientific evidence for specific functions served by sleep and even more evidence demonstrating the harmful effects of not getting enough sleep, as reviewed in Chapters 13–18.

The mystery of why we sleep deepens further when we consider one of its characteristic features, namely, the loss of conscious awareness of the external world. Unlike while we are awake, we can spend hours of time asleep without awareness of the passage of time nor of anything that happens in our surroundings. For early humans, living in environments in which they were often at risk of attack by predators or by other humans, the loss of awareness of the outside world must have been potentially dangerous. Even today, while most of us live in more secure environments, we often hear about deaths and injuries during the night when people failed to detect the outbreak of a fire until it had progressed to a dangerous state. The fact that we sleep despite the risks associated with unconsciousness reinforces the idea that sleep is somehow important but without providing much of an indication of why. What benefits does sleep bring that can compensate for the increased risks associated with loss of awareness of one's surroundings?

Another kind of risk associated with sleep is what economists call opportunity cost, that is, the cost of giving up other potential opportunities to engage in a particular activity. If early humans were anything like modern humans, they would have felt that there were not enough hours in the day to engage in life's serious business of improving reproductive fitness by securing food, mates, territory, social status, knowledge, and other useful resources as well as raising children, painting, writing, making music, and dancing ... and generally enjoying oneself. Humans must often have wondered what benefit sleep conferred that could offset both its increased risks and the costs of giving up other potential benefits.

Adding even further to the mystery of sleep is that, when we wake up, we often retain memories of fantastic mental activities that we experienced during sleep. Sleep interrupts the continuous internal monologue that characterizes human consciousness during waking and substitutes the often-bizarre narratives of half-remembered dreams. As a result, people have also often reflected on and written about the causes, nature, and meaning of the altered mental activities, or states of consciousness, that characterize sleep.

The writings of the Greek philosopher Aristotle (ca. 350 BCE) had a centuries-long influence on European ideas about science, nature, and physiology. His discussion of why we sleep centered on the issue of the loss of consciousness, which he saw as being the defining characteristic of sleeping organisms. He argued that we know someone is awake because of their ability to perceive their environment and to perceive their own consciousness. The flip side of that argument was that we know someone is asleep by the loss of those abilities; sleep was therefore explicitly defined as the *absence* of the core features of waking.

His account of the cause of sleep was that it results from the need for the organ of sense perception in humans and animals to periodically take a break from its ongoing activity. Thus, all animals sleep to allow the organ of perception (not the sensory organs, but a central "perceiver" —located in the chest, in his view) to recuperate from its activities. Because he believed that plants do not perceive, they were assumed to neither need nor have the capacity for sleep (Aristotle, 350 BCE).

The idea that sleep serves a restorative function is an obvious intuition; people typically feel bad when they have not had a chance to sleep and feel better after sleeping. But this logical deduction does not tell us much about the mechanisms responsible for the need for sleep nor about the process of recuperation. Which aspects of our physiology require sleep for us to function well, and how does sleep achieve the needed recovery?

Another interpretation of sleep that is common in our myths and literature relates to its superficial resemblance to death, because both involve the loss of consciousness and of the ability to act in the world. It was probably a common view in many cultures that the presumed seat of consciousness and motivator of action, the soul or spirit, departs the body at death. The apparently similar, but only temporary, loss of both voluntary activity and consciousness during sleep could be seen as a reversible form of the same process. It is probably because of this linkage that in one version of Greek mythology, the goddess Nyx (Night) has twin sons: Thanatos (Death) and Hypnos (Sleep).

In many cultures, this association is reflected in stories about those whose sleep closely resembles death, as in Washington Irving's familiar tale of Rip van Winkle, who "slept" for 20 years; or the Brothers Grimm version of the German folk tale of Snow White, whose poisoned sleep so resembled death that she was encased in a glass coffin while awaiting her rescue by Prince Charming. The idea of a motivating soul leaving the body during sleep, and the fear that it may not return, is reflected in an ancient Hebrew prayer that is recited on awakening, in which a person gives thanks to the Lord for restoring the soul to the body. Similarly, an 18th-century English prayer runs, "Now I lay me down to sleep, I pray the Lord my soul to keep. If I die before I wake, I pray the Lord my soul to take." Other acknowledgments of the parallels between sleep and death are woven into the fabric of English literature. Shakespeare's Macbeth describes sleep as "the death of each day's life," and says of the recently murdered King Duncan: "after life's fitful fever he sleeps well," while Hamlet ponders, "in that sleep of death, what dreams may come?"

This somewhat morbid association of sleep with death is offset by the equally common view in literature of its restful and restorative properties, echoing Aristotle's view that sleep serves the need for rest and recovery. Shakespeare's Macbeth also says that sleep "knits up the ravell'd sleeve of care," while in his Sonnet 73, he refers to sleep as "death's second self that seals up all in rest." This last quote links these two aspects of sleep that have echoed through human literature: the potentially dangerous flight of the soul and loss of consciousness, simulating death, alongside the restful, beneficial effects of sleep. Together, these views reflect the common-sense understanding that sleep is a costly, and possibly risky, break in activity and awareness as well as a welcome opportunity for the body and mind, weakened somehow by the day's activities, to rest and to be restored to a state of strength and health.

These commonly held ideas preceded the scientific study of sleep, which began in the late 19th and early 20th century. As in many other areas of human understanding, the results of scientific investigations of sleep revealed that common-sense views can include both accurate insights and mistaken ideas.

1.2.1 Summary

Sleep is universally present in peoples' lives, but it is a state that people have long regarded with mixed feelings. These include positive feelings about the rest and recovery that sleep provides, feelings of anxiety and vulnerability related to the experience of loss of consciousness, and resentment about the time taken away from waking activities. Overlying these feelings is a sense of mystery about sleep related to several features: our loss of awareness of the external world and of the passage of time; the experience of often bizarre and sometimes frightening dreams, the meaning of which is unknown; the strength of the compulsion to sleep; and our lack of understanding of what functions sleep serves that justify the years of our lives devoted to it.

1.3 Early research on sleep

Any brief history of a scientific discipline is bound to be incomplete; a variety of small and large contributions often combine to create new insights and knowledge, some of which are well remembered and documented, and others largely forgotten. In addition, new types of research made possible by technical advances are often conducted by several people at roughly the same time. What follows, therefore, is a selective history highlighting some important developments, which is based in part on more detailed summaries of the early development of the field provided by the late American physician and sleep researcher William Dement, himself one of the modern pioneers of the field (Dement, 2005).

One early idea about why organisms sleep came from studies conducted in the early 20th century by several researchers, including Ishimori in Japan and Legendre & Piéron in France (for a summary, see Kubota, 1989). They deprived dogs of sleep for long periods of time, and then injected either brain extracts or cerebrospinal fluid from these dogs into others that had not been sleep deprived. The observation that recipient dogs then became sleepy, but that similar extracts from non-sleep-deprived dogs were ineffective, led to the conclusion that a chemical agent that promotes sleep builds up in the brain during prolonged waking. A corollary of this idea was that the presumed toxin must normally be eliminated by processes that occur during sleep. The idea that sleep reverses the accumulation of a toxic change in the brain or body that happens while awake has recurred throughout the history of sleep research; some findings related to this idea are discussed later in this volume (see Sections 11.6 and 15.5.3).

Other early research on sleep depended on the invention of methods to record the electrical activity of the brain [for references to this early work, see (Ahmed & Cash, 2013; Pelayo & Dement, 2017; Stone & Hughes, 2013)]. Conceptual and technological developments in the late 19th century led to the conclusion that neuronal activity is electrical. They also provided methods for recording the brain's electrical activity from electrodes that were either inserted into the brain or attached to the scalp. These methods depended on the development of amplifiers that could turn the tiny voltage changes detected by these electrodes into electrical signals large enough to drive electromechanical recorders, which could generate permanent records of the brain's electrical activity.

Richard Caton in Liverpool, England (1875) (Ormerod, 2006) and Adolf Beck in Krakow, Poland (1891) independently demonstrated that the patterns of electrical activity recorded from the brains of animals changed as they cycled among the behavioral states of quiet waking, high arousal, and sleep. Beck observed that during sleep the brain's electrical activity showed slow rhythms with high amplitudes (large voltage changes). Sensory stimulation that woke an animal triggered a switch to faster rhythms with lower amplitudes.

The German psychiatrist, Hans Berger, published a series of papers beginning in 1929 on the effects of a variety of stimuli and events on recordings of the human brain's electrical activity, which he made using surface electrodes on the scalp. He referred to these recordings as electroencephalograms (EEGs), a term that combines the words for electricity, the brain, and writing, that is, written records of the electrical activity of the brain (largely the electrical activity of the cortex). Berger's publications included a detailed and accurate description of the electrical patterns associated with sleep and waking in people.

Although there was skepticism at first that the tiny voltage changes occurring in the brain could be detected from outside the skull, several laboratories demonstrated that this was possible, and EEG recordings came to play a central role in the development of sleep research. These studies confirmed the key EEG features that distinguished sleep from waking. Sleep was characterized by high-amplitude slow waves but also by bursts of faster activity called "sleep spindles" (see Chapter 2 for details). During waking, the EEG showed low-amplitude, faster waves.

Nathaniel Kleitman (1895–1999), a physiologist at the University of Chicago, was a critical contributor to the development of human sleep research during this period. Starting as a refugee who landed in New York City, he moved to Chicago where he rapidly earned a PhD and then established the world's preeminent sleep laboratory. Kleitman made many important contributions to the experimental study of sleep (and daily rhythms), which are discussed throughout this volume. Among his accomplishments, he published a major compendium of available sleep research in 1939, which he later updated (Kleitman, 1963). One of his fundamental contributions to sleep research will be reviewed in detail in Section 1.4.3).

An early insight into the neural mechanisms regulating sleep emerged from a devastating influenza pandemic that swept through the world beginning in 1918 and killed an estimated 40 million people in the years following the end of the First World War (Taubenberger, 2006; Triarhou, 2006; von Economo, 1930). Many who survived the viral infection developed a mysterious medical condition, *encephalitis lethargica* (inflammation of the brain with sleepiness). Patients suffered from various sleep-related symptoms, but especially from either an inability to sleep (insomnia[1]) or extreme sleepiness (somnolence). Later stages of the illness in those who survived longer term also included other severe neurological and psychiatric

[1] Literally, "not sleeping." This term is used informally in this chapter to refer to "great difficulty sleeping." This is different from the clinical definition of chronic insomnia, as presented in **Box 4.3** (Section 4.4.5).

symptoms.[2] Constantin von Economo, a neurologist at the University of Vienna, investigated the anatomical correlates of the sleep-related symptoms by studying the pathological changes in the brains of patients who had died. He discovered that the type of sleep disturbance observed was related to the location of the brain damage that followed the viral infection.

He concluded that the diencephalon (a region of the forebrain), near the third ventricle, includes structures that both promote sleep (in the anterior part of the hypothalamus) and inhibit sleep (in the posterior hypothalamus) (Triarhou, 2006; von Economo, 1930). Because the viral infection (or the immune system's responses to infection … it is not clear which caused the damage) resulted in varying amounts of brain damage, he was only able to point to the involvement of relatively broad hypothalamic/preoptic regions. Von Economo argued that the neural regions that he had identified acted on the cortex to periodically generate sleep (anterior hypothalamus) and wakefulness (posterior hypothalamus).

This novel idea of localized, subcortical mechanisms that triggered or suppressed cortical signs of sleep contrasted to the popular belief at the time that sleep resulted from a global reduction in neural activity or of blood supply throughout the brain (von Economo, 1930). von Economo's ideas were prescient; it was many years later that his hypothesis of localized subcortical regulators of sleep and waking, and even the proposed hypothalamic locations of some of the centers involved, were confirmed by experimental research in animal models (see Chapter 11).

In the laboratory of Alfred Loomis[3] at Princeton University in the 1930s, EEG recordings were made from people while both awake and asleep, including continuous overnight recordings. Loomis and his colleagues followed up on Berger's human sleep recordings by experimenting with light and sound to study the effects of sensory stimulation during sleep on both the EEG and behavior. In order to compare the EEG patterns of sleep and waking without the confounding effects of darkness during sleep and light while awake, they recorded the EEG of some participants while they were either asleep or lying awake in the dark.[4]

Using specially designed amplifiers and automatic recording systems, Loomis and colleagues made a particular study of the "alpha rythm" (as they spelled it) and how it changed from waking to sleep. They noted that individuals typically transitioned during the night through different stages of sleep, characterized by different EEG patterns, which they labeled A–E. They also published records of these sleep stages and their transitions during the night that look quite similar to more modern hypnograms (literally, "sleep writing/drawing") (Loomis et al., 1937). The alpha pattern was characteristic of the A state, during which people were awake or drowsy, while sleep onset was followed by transition to a low-voltage B state which lacked alpha rhythms. The C state included sleep spindles, while the D state included spindles mixed with what they called "random" waves (large, slow waves of 0.5–3 cycles per second [Hz]), and the E state was dominated by these high-amplitude slow waves.

They noted the difficulty of waking people from stages D and E, suggesting a deeper stage of sleep, and presented some evidence that dreams were associated with the low-voltage B state. The idea of multiple sleep stages with different EEG patterns was consistent with evidence published by others during this period, including Herbert Jasper and Nathaniel Kleitman. Many of these observations, such as the association of sleep spindles with an early phase of sleep, the links between a low-amplitude EEG and dreams, and between large-amplitude EEG waves and a deep stage of sleep were confirmed by subsequent studies. The formal classification system for sleep staging based on EEG recordings, which was developed later and remains in use today (see Section 2.3) echoes some aspects of Loomis' system.

At about the same time, the Belgian electrophysiologist Frédéric Bremer conducted research involving surgical manipulations in animals to study the neural mechanisms involved in switching among states of arousal. This research went beyond the correlational studies that reported associations between different electrical patterns and different states of consciousness, or those between different locations of brain damage and specific sleep disorders. He published the results of experiments in which he transected the brainstems of cats, either at the level of the lower medulla (called an encéphale isolé) or more rostrally at the level of the midbrain (cerveau isolé), and then studied the resulting cortical EEG patterns; for a summary of his work, see (Kerkhofs & Lavie, 2000).

Recordings from the cortex of cats with a midbrain transection (cerveau isolé) revealed cortical electrical patterns that resembled those of sleep, from which they did not regain the electrical signs of waking (Bremer, 1935). Those with a lower, medullary transection (encéphale isolé) continued to go through alternating cycles of electrical activity that resembled those seen during periods of sleep and waking in intact

[2] During and following the COVID-19 pandemic (2020–2023), there was accumulating evidence of long-lasting neurological symptoms in some patients after recovery from the acute phase of illness, the extent of which remains to be determined.

[3] Loomis was a remarkable figure. He was a lawyer, soldier, wealthy financier, and amateur scientist. He contributed administratively and scientifically to many areas, including to the development of naval navigation systems, radar, and nuclear physics. Despite being a non-scientist by training, he was elected to the US National Academy of Sciences (Alvarez, 1980).

[4] This approach created the need to keep waking participants from falling asleep while lying down in darkness for hours. So the experimenters had them recite poetry or listen to music, including Ravel's dramatic *Bolero* (Loomis et al., 1937)—not a typical procedure in modern sleep laboratories.

animals. The cortex of a cerveau isolé cat could receive sensory input only from the olfactory and optic nerves, which enter the brain from the front. It could not receive input from other cranial nerves (about half of which are sensory), which enter below the level of the cut in the medulla. In the encéphale isolé preparation, however, these cranial nerves were intact and could provide sensory input that would ultimately reach the cortex.

Because only the cortices of encéphale isolé cats were able to generate the electrical patterns associated with waking, the results suggested that sensory input arising from most of the cranial nerves was needed to arouse the brain and maintain wakefulness. In contrast, the interruption of most sensory input to the brain in the cerveau isolé preparation produced a continuous, sleep-like EEG pattern. This interpretation of Bremer's results was consistent with the general view at the time (and going back to Aristotle and beyond) that sleep is a passive condition resulting from the global withdrawal or cessation of arousing sensory input (see Dement, 2005; von Economo, 1930).

Subsequent to Bremer's work, Horace Magoun and his colleagues Giuseppe Moruzzi and Donald Lindsley published the results of critical studies related to the physiology of arousal and the role of sensory input (Lindsley et al., 1949; Moruzzi & Magoun, 1949). They showed that cats with a transection at the level of the medulla-spinal cord junction (encéphale isolé) could be aroused to sustained cortical wakefulness by electrical stimulation of a core region of the brainstem (the reticular formation), which they called the ascending reticular activating system (ARAS). Relatively brief, natural sensory stimulation could also cause sustained cortical activation, but only in animals with an intact ARAS. If the reticular formation was damaged by lesions, sensory stimulation would cause transient cortical arousal during the stimulation, but it did not trigger the sustained cortical arousal seen in animals with an intact reticular formation.

In contrast to these results, direct electrical stimulation of the reticular formation was able to trigger sustained cortical activation regardless of whether the primary sensory input pathways were intact or interrupted. Thus, an intact ARAS was *necessary* for sensory stimuli to produce sustained activation of the cortex. In addition, stimulation of the ARAS was *sufficient* on its own to produce cortical arousal, even if the primary sensory projections to the cortex were absent. These results challenged the idea that input from the principal sensory projections was critical to sustaining cortical arousal (Lindsley et al., 1949).

Magoun's group concluded that the ARAS mediates arousal to external stimuli because it is innervated by collateral fibers branching off from the principal pathways that carry specific sensory information to the thalamus (e.g., auditory and somatosensory projections) (Starzl et al., 1951) (**Figure 1.1**). They proposed that the ARAS is activated by this blended collateral input, and its output to the forebrain, rather than activity in the primary sensory pathways, is

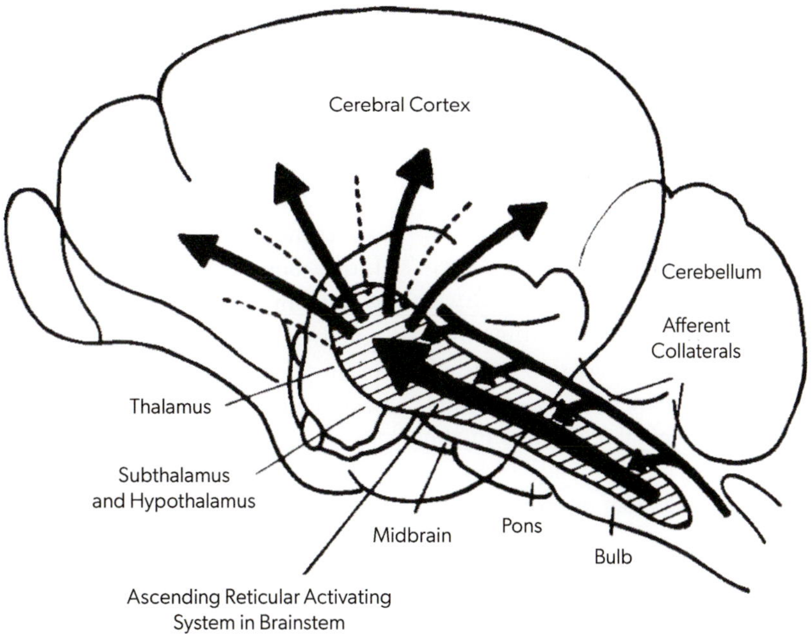

Figure 1.1 An early diagram showing the general location of the ascending reticular activating system (ARAS; corresponding to the brainstem reticular formation in the cat). The key elements are the afferent collaterals (small arrows) that project into the ARAS from primary sensory pathways. The ARAS projections reach the thalamus (large arrow), which in turn projects to many regions of the cerebral cortex (medium arrows). Reprinted with permission of the American Physiological Society © 1951, from Starzl, T. E. et al. (1951). Collateral afferent excitation of the reticular formation of the brain stem. *J Neurophysiol* 14:479–496. © American Physiological Society (1951); permission conveyed through Copyright Clearance Center, Inc. doi: 10.1152/jn.1951.14.6.479.

responsible for sustaining cortical arousal and wakefulness. This conclusion differed from the earlier view of Bremer, who attributed the lack of waking in his cerveau isolé preparation to the lack of direct sensory input to forebrain structures. The concept of the ARAS has since been refined through the identification of specific neurotransmitter projections in the brainstem and forebrain that contribute to the arousal system; see, e.g., (Brown et al., 2012). The roles of the neurotransmitters in these projections are discussed in Chapters 10 and 11.

The existence of a specialized, arousal-promoting system in the brainstem indirectly suggested an explanation for how an anterior hypothalamic system could promote sleep as von Economo had proposed. Studies involving stimulation of the preoptic/anterior hypothalamic region showed that activation of this region blocked the wake-promoting activity of the reticular formation (Sterman & Clemente, 1962). The combination of these results suggested that the onset of sleep was triggered by a hypothalamic mechanism that inhibited the arousing input from the ARAS to the cortex. Although it included the active involvement of hypothalamic activity, this model of sleep regulation could still preserve the historical view that sleep was a response to a reduction in arousing input to the cortex. A different set of observations that came from studies of eye movements during sleep, and were related to the phenomenon of dreaming, led to a different view of the nature of sleep and how it is related to cortical activation.

1.3.1 Summary

Early thinking about sleep focused on its role in recovering from the exertions of waking activities and saw it as the passive result of the withdrawal of arousing stimulation. When new technologies permitted experimental studies of the brain during waking and sleep, the results indicated that the behavioral states of sleep and waking are correlated with different patterns of electrical activity in the brain. Low-amplitude, fast EEG rhythms were recorded during waking; and high-amplitude, slow rhythms were recorded during sleep. Results obtained by Loomis and colleagues also demonstrated more complex changes in the EEG over the course of a night's sleep.

Bremer's experimental work showed that interrupting the route to the cortex from sensory projections that enter through the brainstem prevented the cortex from producing the electrical pattern of waking and led to a permanent sleep-like state. These findings were consistent with the view that sleep was a passive response to the loss of sufficient sensory stimulation to rouse the cortex to wakefulness.

Magoun and colleagues showed instead that, in an encéphale isolé preparation, sustained cortical activation required the activity of a specialized arousal system (the ARAS) in the core of the brainstem that received collateral input from sensory systems. In the absence of the ARAS, direct sensory input alone could trigger only transient cortical activation. This novel mechanism was an important breakthrough in identifying the neural basis of wakefulness, but it did not fundamentally change the standard view at the time that sleep is the result of the absence of sufficient sensory stimulation (direct or indirect) to sustain waking.

Despite von Economo's earlier proposal that a localized center in the rostral hypothalamus promoted sleep, the ancient idea that sleep is a state of quiet rest remained the dominant view into the middle of the 20th century. It would require other observations to trigger the important conceptual shift to thinking about sleep as a complex, instinctive behavior that is actively organized and generated by the nervous system. These observations linked EEG features to dreaming, a topic that had been largely untouched by physiological investigations.

1.4 Dreams and REM sleep

1.4.1 Thinking about dreaming

Ancient texts from different cultures indicate that people have always been interested in the nocturnal mental experiences we call dreams and developed ideas about their origins and meaning. The loss of waking consciousness during sleep suggested that the engine of thought (the "soul") had fled the body. That belief led logically to the conclusion that the thoughts that occurred during sleep must come from an external source, but one that is not visible. As a result, people interpreted dreams as communications to the sleeper from supernatural beings. These messages from gods or spirits were sometimes thought to provide useful advice or to predict the future, but they could also be deceptive and potentially dangerous. In Homer's *Iliad* (Book 2), for example, Zeus deliberately sends a false dream to trick Agamemnon, the leader of the Greek armies. The dream convinced him that the gods would aid his troops in battle and that the besieged city of Troy would fall quickly to their attack. Instead, the assault on the city was disastrous for his troops.

Dreams, even *true* dreams, were seen to be disguised so that their real meaning was hidden in cryptic metaphors or symbolic representations. Thus, there was often a need for a skilled interpreter to uncover the hidden meaning beneath the surface content of the dream. One example is in the biblical book of Genesis, in which Joseph interprets his own and others' dreams and, most critically for the narrative, is brought from prison to interpret the dreams of Egypt's Pharaoh. These dreams included images of seven fat cattle and seven lean cattle, with the lean ones devouring the fat cattle. Joseph's interpretation was that the dream forecast seven years of abundant crops followed by seven years of famine. Based on his interpretation (and on his skills in organizing extensive food storage during the years of abundance), Joseph ensured the survival of the Egyptians during the famine that followed the prophetic dream and was richly rewarded for his insights. The biblical book of Daniel similarly contains numerous descriptions of dreams that are disguised predictions of the future, requiring Daniel's skill for their interpretation.

1.4.2 Freud, dreams, and sleep

A quite different theory of the origin of dreams emerged during the 19th century, when many medical practitioners had a clinical interest in dreams and their interpretation. This interest was shared by Sigmund Freud, the Viennese physician whose psychological theories exerted a profound influence on Western culture throughout the 20th century (and beyond). The interpretation of dreams was a topic that was central to his theories as well as being the title of his first book, published originally in German in 1900 (Freud, 1913). His view was that dream interpretation was "the royal road to knowledge of the unconscious activities of the mind." Freud believed that dreams represented the (often disguised) discharge of hidden instinctual desires and that they expressed a form of wish fulfillment. The structure of dreams, and their often-bizarre narrative content, were ways of expressing powerful instinctual drives (often sexual in nature) in a safe manner, without causing the dreamer the anxiety prompted by acknowledging these drives and without allowing their associated arousal and distress to disrupt sleep.

This view of dreams echoed the ancient idea of hidden messages being conveyed to the dreamer, and, as in many biblical and other tales, the services of a skilled dream interpreter were required to extract the meaning of the messages. But Freud believed that the source of the dream content was the internal psychic activity of the dreamer—his or her suppressed instinctual needs—not an external, supernatural being. The qualified interpreter was therefore a psychoanalyst rather than a soothsayer. The goal of dream interpretation was not prediction of the future, but analysis of the underlying drives and suppressed motives that the dream expressed in hidden form. Freud used his method of dream interpretation and the resulting insights it provided to treat the psychological problems (neuroses) of his patients, which he believed arose from suppression of instinctual drives.

Through his writings and those of both his admirers and his critics, Freud's concepts pervaded and shaped psychological and psychiatric theory and practice for decades. Even more remarkable is the degree to which versions of concepts he introduced or popularized (e.g., dream interpretation itself, Oedipus complex, ego, superego, id, repression, the subconscious, etc.) have diffused throughout popular culture, affecting literature, drama, art, films, and other media. His belief that dreams represented disguised messages (albeit messages to and from oneself) was consistent with ancient beliefs, but he added the idea that the function of the disguise was to prevent anxiety and arousal that could disrupt sleep (see **Box 1.1**).

BOX 1.1 Freud's View of Sleep and Dreams

Freud did not discuss sleep very much in *The Interpretation of Dreams* (Freud, 1913). He wrote: "I have had little occasion to concern myself with the problem of sleep, as this is essentially a physiological problem .... The literature of sleep will therefore not be considered here" (Chapter 1, p. 4). Thus, he distinguished the physiological processes of sleep from the psychological processes of dreams. But he also emphasized the importance of the individual's drive to sleep as a critical factor in the generation of dreams: "The wish to sleep which ... represents the ego's contribution to the dream, must thus always be taken into account as a motive of dream-formation, and every successful dream is a fulfillment of this wish" (Chapter 4, p. 198). By "successful" he meant that the dream expressed the hidden psychological drive, while still allowing physiological sleep. He noted that dreams were important for preserving sleep continuity: "There is no doubt that they [memories of daytime events] are the actual disturbers of sleep, and not the dream, which, on the contrary, strives to guard sleep" (Chapter 7, p. 445).

The clear implication of these statements is that the "physiological" process of sleep has valuable recuperative properties that must be preserved. The mind of the sleeper must, therefore, go to great lengths in dream formation to disguise instinctual drives and memories of disturbing daytime experiences to avoid disrupting sleep and losing its physiological benefits.

It is important to remember that when Freud wrote about the nature of dreams and their role in sleep at the end of the 19th century, there was little knowledge of sleep physiology, and there was nothing known about the physiology of dreaming. It would be decades before the first publications that described the electrophysiology of the sleeping human brain and a half century before the first studies linked the physiology of sleep to the experience of dreaming.

1.4.3 The discovery of REM sleep

Early research on the physiology of dreaming marked a critical break point in thinking about the mechanisms underlying the regulation of sleep. For that development, we return to the work of Nathaniel Kleitman in Chicago and a summary of that work by William Dement (Dement, 2005). Kleitman felt that sleep had an intensity dimension—that it could be either lighter or deeper (as Loomis had also proposed for his sleep stages). He was interested in assessing eye movements as a possible marker for the depth of sleep, in part because he had noted that the slow, rolling eye movements in a drowsy individual signaled the imminent onset of sleep, then diminished during the early phase of sleep. These slow eye movements were particularly obvious in infants, so a graduate student in his laboratory, Eugene Aserinsky, undertook to watch infants as they slept to document their eye movement patterns. Later studies were conducted with adults.

In addition to periodic visual observations, Aserinsky and Kleitman recorded the electrical activity of eye muscles automatically using electrodes attached near the eyes. The resulting recordings (electrooculograms or EOGs) reflected the patterns of eye movements. Initially, they saved recording paper (and the time required to analyze the recordings), by sampling EOG and EEG activity only periodically. Each 30 sec period of recording generated a foot of recording paper, so an 8 h sleep session would produce nearly 1,000 feet (292 m) of paper. They later expanded recordings to full nights, which revealed previously undocumented cycles of eye movements recurring throughout the night, initially during a recording session involving Aserinsky's 8-year-old son (Brown, 2003).

Aserinsky and Kleitman reported that the slow, rolling eye movements associated with drowsiness stopped shortly after changes in the EEG pattern indicated sleep onset (**Figure 1.2**). During the night, however, bursts of rapid, jerky, bilaterally symmetrical eye movements emerged, which were different from those that preceded sleep onset. These rapid eye movements (REMs) (**Figure 1.3**) were associated with an apparent "lightening" of sleep, along with the appearance of more rapid breathing and heart rates, consistent with autonomic arousal.

The most surprising finding, however, was that sleep periods with high numbers of REMs were accompanied by cortical EEG patterns with rapid, low-amplitude activity, resembling that of waking (Aserinsky & Kleitman, 1953). These wake-like EEG recordings from people who were clearly asleep were quite different from the slow, high-amplitude EEG waves that had previously been reported to characterize sleep in most studies.

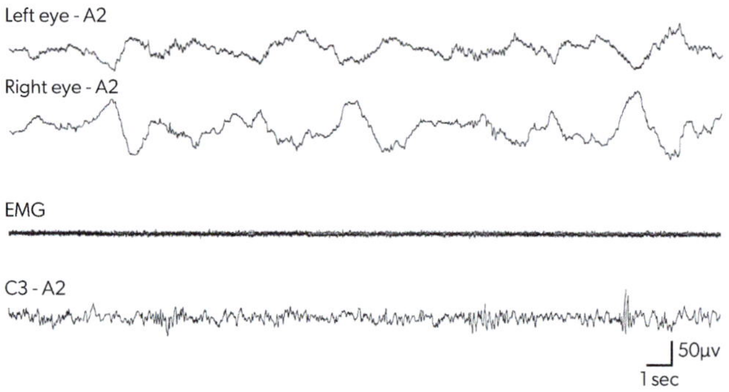

Figure 1.2 Electrooculograms (EOGs; recordings of eye movements), recorded from an individual who is falling asleep, are shown in the top two channels. Below them are the electromyogram (EMG; chin muscle recording) and a single channel of the electroencephalogram (C3-A2, indicating an electrode that is placed on the left side near the center of the head (C3), referenced to an electrode on the earlobe (A2); see **Figure 2-1** for details). This person has transitioned from quiet waking into non-REM (NREM) Stage 1 sleep (N1). The EOG channels show slow rolling movements of both eyes. These occur in people when they are very drowsy and about to fall sleep and can persist into the early part of N1 sleep. The EMG shows a low level of muscle tone, and the EEG shows a relatively low-voltage pattern with only scattered alpha activity, an indication that the individual has fallen asleep. The higher amplitude event near the end of the EEG record is a vertex sharp wave, characteristic of early sleep. Calibration lines show 50 µV and 1 s. Reprinted from Rechtschaffen, A. & Kales, A. (Eds.). (1968). *A Manual of Standardized Techniques and Scoring System for Sleep Stages in Human Subjects*. Washington, DC: NIH Publication No. 204, US Government Printing Office.

The sleep episodes with REMs appeared in adults after an initial period of sleep without significant eye movements, and then recurred periodically every 2 h or less, three or four times during the night. The length of these episodes varied during the night but averaged about 20 min. A critical observation was that when people were awakened during periods of sleep with large numbers of REMs, they were much more likely to report recent dream content than when awakened from sleep without REMs. Their publication (Aserinsky & Kleitman, 1953) established the robust association between what came to be called REM sleep and the subjective experience, and overt reporting, of dreams.

Dement conducted studies to further describe the overnight patterns of EOG and EEG changes in both humans and cats. He and Kleitman obtained continuous overnight records from people and staged the paper records in 30 sec segments (i.e., assigned a stage label to each segment) to determine the pattern

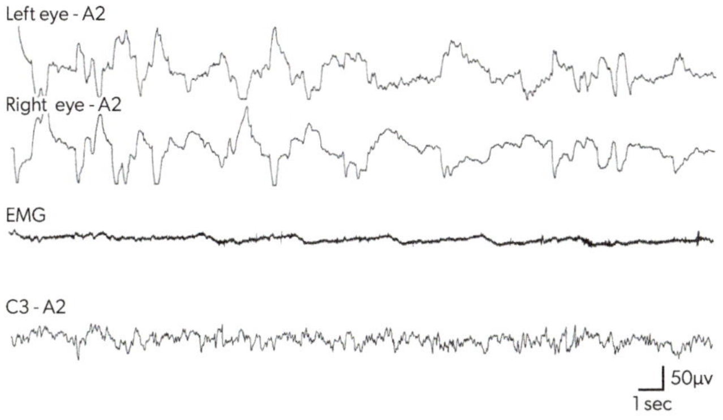

Figure 1.3 EOG, EMG, and EEG recordings during rapid eye movement (REM) sleep. The EOG channels (top two lines) show the characteristic bursts of rapid, high-amplitude, conjugate eye movements that give this sleep stage its name. Each recording is made from an electrode attached near the outside edge of one eye. As a result, a synchronous movement of both eyes toward the right would involve an outward movement of the right eye (away from the nose) and an inward movement of the left eye (toward the nose), generating electrical signatures with opposite signs. The EMG shows virtually no electrical activity (atonia), while the EEG from a central scalp placement (bottom line) shows the low-voltage, fast oscillations typical of this stage. This EEG record would be difficult to distinguish from a waking EEG without the evidence contained in the EOG and EMG records. The fluctuations in the EMG channel may represent slight jaw movements related to respiration. See Figure 1.2 for other labels. Calibration lines show 50 µV and 1 s. Reprinted from Rechtschaffen, A. & Kales, A. (Eds.). (1968). *A Manual of Standardized Techniques and Scoring System for Sleep Stages in Human Subjects.* Washington, DC: NIH Publication No. 204, US Government Printing Office.

of changes that occurred throughout the night (see Chapter 2). They reported that soon after falling asleep people "descended" from wakefulness through a series of progressively deeper non-REM (NREM) sleep stages (1–4, with Stage 4 having the largest number of slow waves). The first REM sleep period occurred an hour or more after sleep onset and was labeled "emergent Stage 1" (i.e., Stage 1 during emergence from deeper sleep), in contrast to descending Stage 1 (while initially falling asleep) (**Figure 1.4**). Participants went through alternating REM and NREM sleep periods in cycles averaging just over 90 min in length during the whole sleep period (Dement & Kleitman, 1957).

REM sleep occupied approximately 20–25% of the night's sleep, with longer REM sleep episodes occurring later, so that most REM sleep was concentrated in the second half of the night. Dement and Kleitman also confirmed the strong positive correlation between REM sleep and reports of dreaming, and even that the amount of dream recall was related to how long a participant had been in the REM sleep stage before being awakened. They noted that those awakened from sleep that included large, slow waves (typically Stage 4 NREM sleep) tended not to report a coherent dream narrative and were often "somewhat bewildered," though they might report a vague thought or feeling (Dement & Kleitman, 1957). Dement also reported similar patterns of EEG activity in sleeping cats, and noted a surprisingly high arousal threshold (i.e., resistance to waking) during REM sleep, despite the activated, wake-like cortical EEG during this stage (Dement, 1958).

Michel Jouvet and colleagues in Lyon, France studied the same phenomenon in cats, but they referred to it as paradoxical sleep (PS).[5] The "paradox" referred to the discrepancy between an EEG with an activated pattern and the apparent state of deep sleep, from which it was difficult to wake the cat. Jouvet's group reported the cyclic appearance in cats of PS in 5–10 min bouts that began only after an initial period of slow-wave sleep and recurred periodically during a 4 h recording session, closely paralleling the general structure of sleep in people.

During PS, cats showed a complete, sustained loss of postural muscle tone (atonia), despite the occurrence of phasic twitching of the eyes (REMs), and of other peripheral structures (e.g., ears and feet) as well as changes in autonomic system function. They attributed the loss of postural muscle tone to descending inhibition of spinal motor systems by a region of the pons (Jouvet et al., 1959). These observations set the stage for decades of subsequent research on the motor aspects of PS/REM sleep and on the mechanisms in the pons involved in regulating this sleep stage (see Chapter 10).

These studies in both humans and cats confirmed several consistent features of REM sleep. First, the cortical EEG recorded during REM sleep resembled the pattern seen in an awake, aroused organism, in contrast to the patterns seen during the NREM sleep stages that dominated the early part of sleep. Cortical EEGs during waking and REM sleep were especially similar in cats; but even in humans, EEG samples from these stages were not reliably distinguishable on their own. Second, the threshold for awakening from REM sleep was quite high, which was inconsistent with an EEG pattern that appeared to reflect light sleep or arousal and with signs of physiological activation. As assessed by the awakening threshold, REM sleep was a very deep stage of sleep, despite the EEG and respiratory features that were more characteristic of waking.

Third, NREM sleep and REM sleep alternated rhythmically throughout the sleep phase, but with different periodicities in cats and humans (discussed further in Chapter 7). Finally, the self-reported mental activity of people changed profoundly during the night. Periods of dreaming during

[5] Dement reported that he preferred "REM sleep" as the name for this stage because both the expanded version of that abbreviation and Jouvet's "paradoxical sleep" were too long to generate repeatedly on a typewriter when writing a manuscript. But, he suggested, if word processors had existed then, he might have used the term that Jouvet preferred (Dement & Pelayo, 2018).

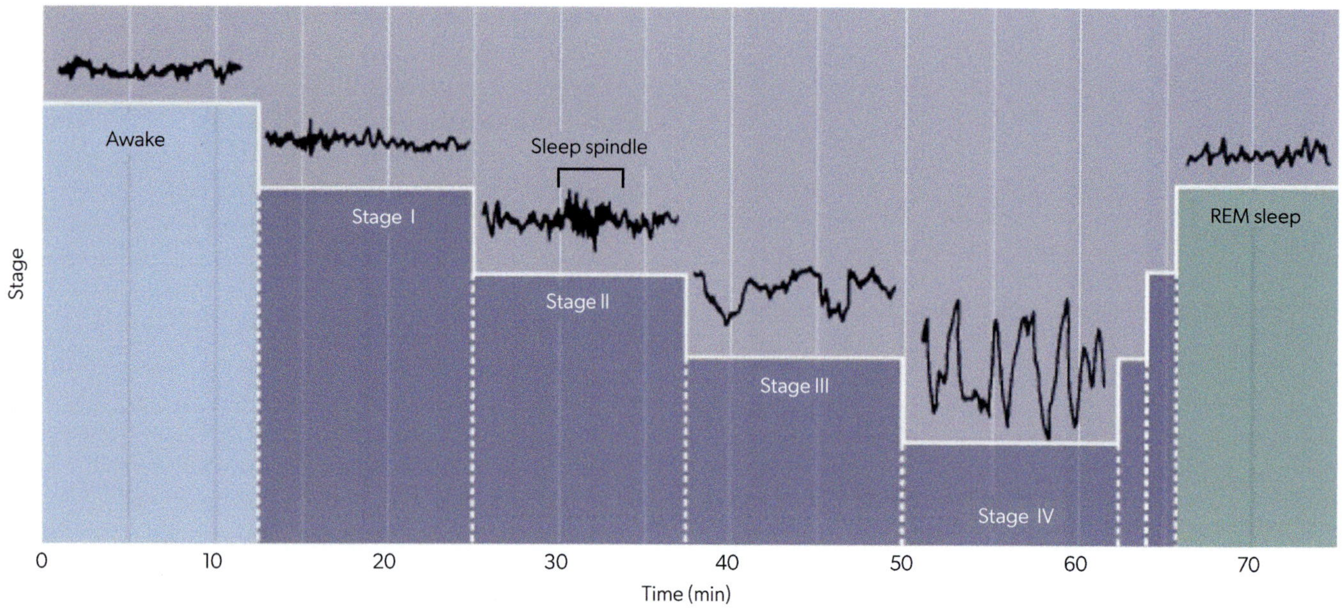

Figure 1.4 EEG patterns during the stages of human sleep, labeled here using Roman numerals. The awake EEG shows low-amplitude (~30 µV), fast oscillations, including alpha activity, which begin to slow in Stage 1 (N1), and slow further in Stage 2 (N2). Stage 2 is characterized by the presence of sleep spindles (see Chapter 2), which are bursts of higher-frequency activity against a background of slower waves. Stages 3 and 4 (together = N3) involve increasing amplitude and further slowing of EEG waves which, in the deepest sleep stages, range up to 200 µV in amplitude. During REM sleep, there is an abrupt change to low-amplitude, fast EEG oscillations that resemble those of waking or Stage 1 sleep. Reprinted with permission from Purves D. et al. (Eds.). (2012). *Neuroscience* 5th ed. Sunderland, MA: Sinauer Associates, © Oxford University Press (2012); permission conveyed through Copyright Clearance Center, Inc.

REM sleep were often characterized by bizarre and illogical content, visual imagery, and strong emotional content as well as a lack of insight into the unreality of these experiences while they occurred. These episodes alternated with NREM sleep periods during which awakened participants reported a relative lack of mental activity. See Appendix A for more discussion of the complex relations between sleep states and dreaming.

1.4.4 A different model of sleep

The evidence for an activated cortical state occurring during a deep stage of sleep in both cats and humans, and the rhythmic alternation between NREM and REM sleep stages, required a new model of the nature of sleep. These findings were inconsistent with the idea that sleep is a uniform, passive state of rest, characterized by reduced cortical activation because of a withdrawal of arousing input to the cortex.

The key feature of this model is that sleep is seen as a physiological process that is actively generated by the nervous system. This conclusion is consistent with von Economo's proposal that there are separate subcortical mechanisms responsible for promoting and inhibiting sleep. The concept that there are neural mechanisms that initiate sleep and rhythmically modify its features during the night was not readily accepted in the 1950s, and it took considerable effort to get the early results related to REM sleep published (Dement, 2005). But this view of sleep as an actively generated product of the brain is now universally accepted.

These early studies of REM sleep led to the conclusion that mammals regularly generate at least three distinct states of consciousness over a 24 h day, accompanied by equally distinct physiological characteristics: waking, NREM sleep, and REM sleep. The fact that the two types of sleep cycle regularly during a sleep period with a species-characteristic periodicity also implied that the generation of these states was an active process, regulated by internal mechanisms that differed among species. The idea of sleep as an actively generated set of brain states was a radical departure from the accepted view of the passive nature of sleep that harkened back at least to Aristotle in western philosophy and science.[6]

[6] Most cultures developed views about the meaning and nature of sleep, in many cases within a religious or spiritual context (Bulkeley, 1996). In some cultures, the three states of consciousness (waking, deep sleep, and dreaming sleep) were recognized and named, although their physiological correlates were unknown. See, for example, the states of consciousness described in the first chapter of the sacred Hindu text called the Mandukya Upanishad (https://tinyurl.com/3wsv5vnf; verses 3-5, downloaded May 6, 2025).

1.4.5 Summary

In many cultures, dreams were attributed to external, supernatural sources and were often believed to foretell future events. In 19th-century Europe, dreams were instead seen as a source of insight into the workings of the human mind. Sigmund Freud saw dreams as the product of attempts to both discharge the energies associated with suppressed instinctual drives and to disguise the actual underlying motivation to avoid stressing and waking the sleeper. Thus, dreams served in part as a psychological mechanism to preserve the continuity of sleep, which was seen as a physiological necessity.

Research in the laboratories of Kleitman, Dement, and Jouvet in the 1950s in people and cats showed that the slow, high-amplitude EEG waves seen shortly after sleep onset were followed by periods of fast, low-amplitude EEG activity, like that of waking. These states of cortical arousal were accompanied by bouts of rapid eye movements, postural atonia, and signs of physiological arousal, while the individual remained soundly asleep. When people were awakened during these REM sleep episodes, they were likely to report elaborate, often fantastic dream content. Those awakened from periods of slow EEG activity tended instead to report little mental activity and felt sluggish and confused. Bouts of REM sleep alternated cyclically with periods of NREM sleep, and the length of these cycles was shorter in cats than in people.

These results were inconsistent with the view of sleep as a passive state of rest resulting from loss of activating input to the cortex. In fact, cortical activation was a defining characteristic of the newly described REM sleep stage. Despite early resistance to accepting this evidence, it led eventually to the current view of mammalian sleep as an actively generated, rhythmically expressed set of species-typical brain states, including both NREM and REM sleep stages. It also led to the view that elaborate dream experiences are a product of the specific patterns of neural activity that characterize REM sleep episodes (but see Appendix A).

This review summarizes three different perspectives on the nature of sleep. From a behavioral viewpoint, common experience that was also reflected in the writings of philosophers and poets emphasized sleep as a period of disengagement from the environment, permitting rest and recovery from the rigors of waking life. From a subjective perspective, sleep involved the loss of conscious awareness of the external world, as well as anxieties about the risks associated with the apparent loss of contact with the outside world. It also involved the experience of mysterious and sometimes frightening images and narratives during dreams.

But the physiological studies of the 20th century in a few mammalian species, including people, yielded a new perspective on sleep. The picture that emerged was that of a rhythmically changing state generated by the brain with a species-typical temporal structure that correlated with these subjective experiences. These components of the definition of sleep will be revisited in Chapter 7 in the context of studies of sleep in an array of species beyond those contributing to the early studies of sleep physiology.

Literature cited

Ahmed, O. J., & Cash, S. S. (2013). Finding synchrony in the desynchronized EEG: The history and interpretation of gamma rhythms. *Front Integr Neurosci, 7*, 58. doi: 10.3389/fnint.2013.00058

Alvarez, L. W. (1980). Alfred Lee Loomis 1887–1975 *Biographical Memoirs* (Vol. **51**, pp. 308–341). Washington, DC: National Academy of Sciences.

Aristotle. (350 BCE). On sleep and sleeplessness (J. I. Beare, Trans.). http://tinyurl.com/yxqw5qda

Aserinsky, E., & Kleitman, N. (1953). Regularly occurring periods of eye motility, and concomitant phenomena, during sleep. *Science, 118*(3062), 273–274.

Bremer, F. (1935). Cerveau <<isolé>> et physiologie du sommeil. *C R Seances Soc Biol Fil, 118*, 1235–1241.

Brown, C. (2003). The stubborn scientist who unraveled a mystery of the night. *Smithsonian Magazine*, October, 2003.

Brown, R. E., Basheer, R., McKenna, J. T., Strecker, R. E., & McCarley, R. W. (2012). Control of sleep and wakefulness. *Physiol Rev, 92*(3), 1087–1187. doi: 10.1152/physrev.00032.2011

Bulkeley, K. (1996). Dreaming as a spiritual practice. *Anthropol Conscious, 7*(2), 1–15.

Dement, W., & Kleitman, N. (1957). The relation of eye movements during sleep to dream activity: An objective method for the study of dreaming. *J Exp Psychol, 53*(5), 339–346.

Dement, W. C. (1958). The occurrence of low voltage, fast, electroencephalogram patterns during behavioral sleep in the cat. *Electroencephalogr Clin Neurophysiol, 10*(2), 291–296.

Dement, W. C. (2005). History of sleep physiology and medicine. In M. H. Kryger, T. Roth, & W. C. Dement (Eds.), *Principles and Practice of Sleep Medicine* (5th ed., pp. 1–15). St. Louis: Elsevier.

Dement, W. C., & Pelayo, R. (2018). Reminiscences of Michel Jouvet. *Sleep Med, 49*, 78–80. doi: 10.1016/j.sleep.2018.05.035

Freud, S. (1913). *The Interpretation of Dreams* (A. A. Brill, Trans. 3rd ed.). New York: MacMillan.

Jouvet, M., Michel, F., & Courjon, J. (1959). Sur un stade d'activité cérébrale rapide au cours du sommeil physiologique. *C R Séances Soc Biologie Fil, 153*, 1024–1028.

Kerkhofs, M., & Lavie, P. (2000). Frédéric Bremer 1892–1982: A pioneer in sleep research. *Sleep Med Rev, 4*(5), 505–514. doi: 10.1053/smrv.2000.0112

Kleitman, N. (1963). *Sleep and Wakefulness*. Chicago, IL: University of Chicago Press.

Kubota, K. (1989). Kuniomi Ishimori and the first discovery of sleep-inducing substances in the brain. *Neurosci Res, 6*, 497–518.

Lindsley, D. B., Bowden, J. W., & Magoun, H. W. (1949). Effect upon the EEG of acute injury to the brain stem activating system. *Electroencephalogr Clin Neurophysiol, 1*(4), 475–486.

Loomis, A. L., Harvey, E. N., & Hobart III, G. A. (1937). Cerebral states during sleep, as studied by human brain potentials. *J Exp Psychol, 21*(2), 127–144.

Moruzzi, G., & Magoun, H. (1949). The brain stem reticular formation and activation of the EEG. *Electroencephalogr Clin Neurophysiol, 1*(4), 455–473.

Ormerod, W. (2006). Richard Caton (1842–1926): Pioneer electrophysiologist and cardiologist. *J Med Biogr, 14*, 30–35.

Pelayo, R., & Dement, W. C. (2017). History of sleep physiology and medicine. In M. H. Kryger, T. Roth, & W. C. Dement (Eds.), *Principles and Practice of Sleep Medicine* (6th ed., pp. 3–14). St. Louis: Elsevier.

Starzl, T. E., Taylor, C. W., & Magoun, H. W. (1951). Collateral afferent excitation of the reticular formation of the brain stem. *J Neurophysiol, 14*(6), 479–496.

Sterman, M., & Clemente, C. (1962). Forebrain inhibitory mechanisms: cortical synchronization induced by basal forebrain stimulation. *Exp Neurol, 6*, 91–102.

Stone, J. L., & Hughes, J. R. (2013). Early history of electroencephalography and establishment of the American Clinical Neurophysiology Society. *J Clin Neurophysiol, 30*, 28–44.

Taubenberger, J. K. (2006). The origin and virulence of the 1918 "Spanish" influenza virus. *Proc Am Philosoph Soc, 150*(1), 86–112.

Triarhou, L. C. (2006). The percipient observations of Constantin von Economo on encephalitis lethargica and sleep disruption and their lasting impact on contemporary sleep research. *Brain Res Bull, 69*, 244–258. doi: 0.1016/j.brainresbull.2006.02.002

von Economo, C. (1930). Sleep as a problem of localization. *J Nerv Ment Dis, 71*(3), 249–259.

CHAPTER 2

Methods for Sleep Research

2.1 OVERVIEW

This chapter discusses the standard electrophysiological tools used to study sleep, introduces the concept of sleep staging, and reviews the physiological correlates of different sleep stages. It discusses the underlying mechanisms that contribute to the characteristic features of different EEG patterns, describes the rhythmic nature of sleep, and discusses the strengths and weaknesses of the standard methods used for studying sleep. It describes some alternative methods for studying sleep that are not based on electrophysiological recordings and introduces some specialized methods used to evaluate the effects of sleep loss.

2.2 Measuring sleep

2.2.1 Electrophysiological recordings

Before EEG recordings were developed, deciding whether a person or animal was asleep depended on observing their behavior, and behavioral criteria are still useful in some situations. The formal, behavioral criteria for defining sleep as a species-typical state and an instinctive drive are discussed in detail in Section 7.2.2 (Campbell & Tobler, 1984); they are summarized here briefly.

People and animals entering sleep usually adopt a characteristic sleep posture and location, become immobile, and stop engaging with the environment. They also show an elevated threshold to respond to environmental stimuli but can be awakened with a sufficiently strong stimulus. Most critically for distinguishing sleep from other states of immobility, sleep is homeostatically regulated: Deprivation of the opportunity to sleep leads to a rebound increase in the motivation to sleep and to a later increase in sleep (see Chapter 5).

Watching a person sleep can be a boring activity, since sleeping people don't usually do any of the interesting things they might do while awake. But sleepers do periodically make postural adjustments, change their breathing patterns, and as discussed in Chapter 1, generate rapid eye movements (REMs) beneath closed eyelids. Less frequently, they may also produce more elaborate behaviors, including kicking, walking, and talking (see Section 10.7). These behaviors hint at what EEG recordings also reveal—that there is much more going on in the sleeping brain than casual observation (or introspection) reveals.

As discussed in Chapter 1, our first insights into the hidden complexities of sleep resulted from the development over the last century of EEG methods that permitted observation of the electrical activity of the brain. In contrast to the early simple dichotomy that waking brains produce low-voltage, fast EEG rhythms, and sleeping brains produce high-voltage, slow rhythms, there are specific EEG features that allow us to distinguish several stages of sleep. The EEG is therefore key to identifying sleep stages as well as detecting neurological symptoms, such as sleep-related seizure activity, that may be relevant to clinical diagnoses.

The EEG, however, cannot provide all the information needed to characterize the several stages of sleep or to diagnosis many sleep-related disorders. For example, the EEG during REM sleep can be very difficult to distinguish from that seen while awake or shortly after sleep onset (see **Figure 1.4**). Identifying REM sleep therefore depends on recording the rapid eye movements and loss of muscle tone that are unique to this stage. The minimal assessment tools needed to study sleep stages, therefore, include the EEG, the electrooculogram (EOG), and recordings of the electrical activity of muscles (typically chin muscles in people)—the electromyogram (EMG) (**Figure 2.1**).

Other physiological measures that are usually obtained in clinical sleep settings, and in many research laboratories, include recordings of heart rate, oxygen saturation of the blood, air flow through the nostrils, respiratory effort measured from the chest and abdomen, and leg movements. These measures are critical for diagnosing sleep-related breathing disorders (see Appendix B) and motor disorders. Together, these measures contribute to producing a polysomnogram (PSG), which

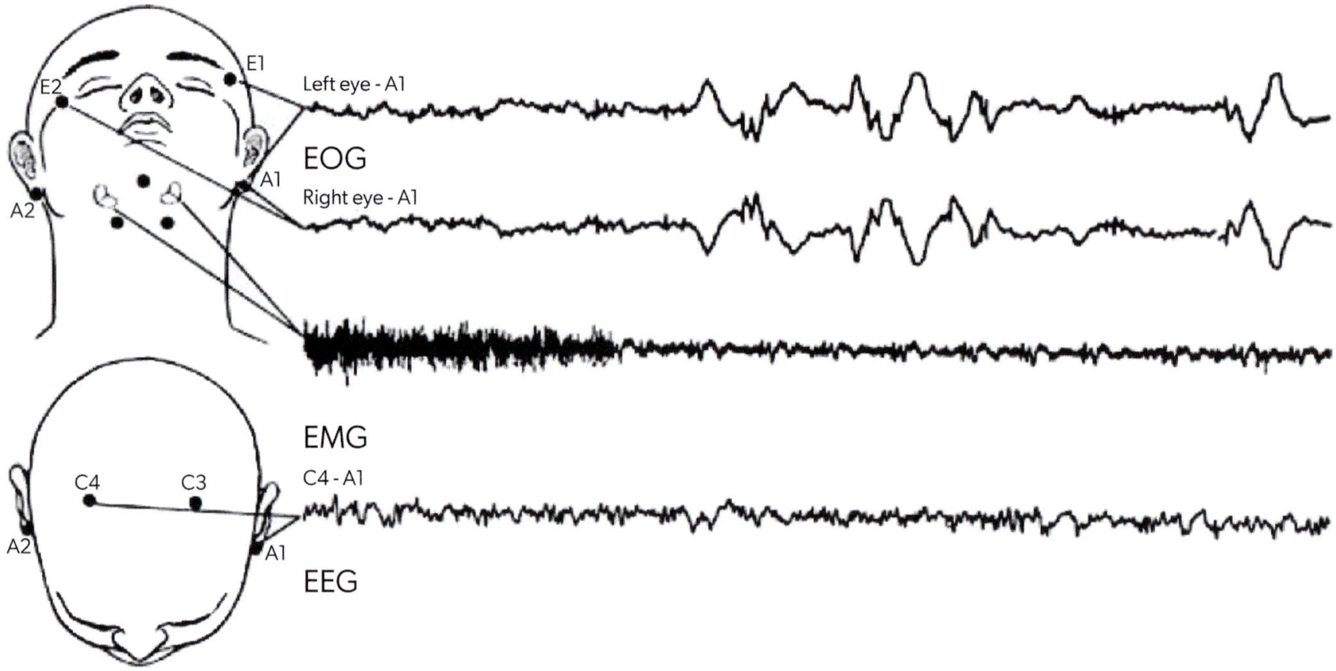

Figure 2.1 This figure illustrates the minimal components that are required to distinguish sleep stages. Electrooculogram (EOG) electrodes are attached to the skin over muscles outside the left and right eyes (E1, E2; top two lines), referenced to an electrode on the left earlobe (A1). Electromyogram (EMG) electrodes are attached to record electrical activity from chin muscles, (mental and submental muscles: from *mentum*, chin in Latin), in this case showing a gradual decline in the amplitude of muscle tone from high to low levels (going from left to right). The electroencephalogram (EEG) electrodes in this illustration are positioned to record from a central brain region (C2, C3), and are also referenced to the electrode at A1. Standard polysomnogram (PSG) recordings would include many more EEG electrodes positioned over different brain regions. The low-voltage EEG signal, combined with strongly reduced muscle tone and rapid, conjugate eye movements (EOG traces) in the right half of the illustration, indicate that this segment of the recording represents a transition into REM sleep. Reprinted from Rechtschaffen, A. & Kales, A. (Eds.) (1968) *A Manual of Standardized Techniques and Scoring System for Sleep Stages in Human Subjects*. Washington, DC: NIH Publication No. 204, US Government Printing Office.

provides a comprehensive picture of the physiology of a sleeping person.

An EEG record is produced by amplifying and recording tiny electrical signals that result from the activity of neurons within the brain. These signals are usually acquired using surface electrodes attached to the scalp in people, or from depth electrodes inserted into the brain itself in animal studies (and sometimes in people during clinical evaluations related to diagnosis and treatment of epilepsy). In human sleep studies, multiple electrodes are usually attached to specific sites on the scalp using a standardized placement system (the "10/20 system"). Appropriately secured electrodes can detect neural activity from underlying brain structures stably for many hours. Because the human neocortex (which we will usually abbreviate as "cortex")[1] is very large and lies immediately below the skull and scalp, its electrical activity dominates the human EEG. As discoveries in the 20th century demonstrated, the EEG changes recorded from the surface of the scalp are highly correlated with a person's stages of sleep and waking, their cognitive activity, and their awareness of the environment.

2.2.2 Describing the EEG

We have referred to fast EEG rhythms, that are characteristic of waking and REM sleep, and slow EEG rhythms that are seen in NREM sleep. We can attach some numbers to these descriptions by applying a mathematical tool to identify the oscillation frequencies that contribute to these EEG patterns (Fourier analysis).[2] EEGs are complex wave forms that include a mixture of frequencies. Fourier analysis identifies the component

[1] The human cortex is composed principally of 6-layered neocortex (also called isocortex), but olfactory cortical structures and the hippocampus have simpler structures (3–5 layered) and are usually called paleocortex (Aboitiz et al., 2002).

[2] The method is named in honor of Jean-Baptiste Joseph Fourier, an 18th-century French mathematician who is credited with contributing to this insight while working on the problem of heat transfer in solids. He did this along with fighting in the French revolution, serving Napoleon Bonaparte in European wars, founding the Cairo Institute in Egypt, working as a professor in France and England, and serving under Napoleon as the Prefect of a Département in France (state governor). He was honored as one of 72 people whose names were inscribed on the Eiffel Tower in Paris (https://en.wikipedia.org/wiki/Joseph_Fourier).

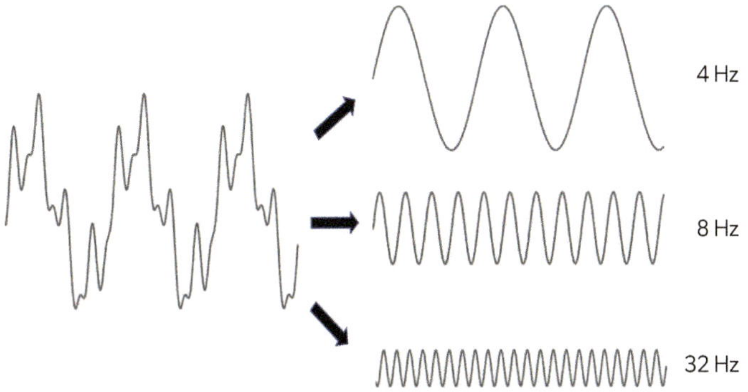

Figure 2.2 The left side shows a complex waveform within which one can detect visually an irregular, slow oscillation (the human visual system is an excellent Fourier analyzer, which can detect rhythmic patterns within noisy signals). The lines on the right side represent the results of a Fourier analysis of this waveform, that is, its decomposition into a set of pure sine waves. The 4 Hz (cycles/second) sine wave represents the frequency that dominates the complex waveform. The 8 and 32 Hz sine waves represent components that modify the basic 4 Hz rhythm to generate the complex waveform. When summed together with appropriate weightings (amplitudes), the component frequencies derived from a Fourier analysis would reproduce the complex waveform. Reprinted from Yuan, I. et al. (2020) Using electroencephalography (EEG) to guide propofol and sevoflurane dosing in pediatric anesthesia. *Anesthesiology Clin* 38:709–725. © Elsevier (2020). doi: 10.1016/j.anclin.2020.06.007.

frequencies that contribute to producing these complex patterns (**Figure 2.2**). This analysis is based on the mathematical insight that any complex waveform can be decomposed into a series of pure sine waves of different frequencies that are weighted differently, depending on how strongly each frequency is represented in that waveform. Thus, a waveform with any arbitrary shape (like an EEG record) can be decomposed into a series of pure sine waves of different frequencies, each with a different weighting. Conversely, the appropriately weighted addition of this sine wave series can reconstruct the original waveform.

Fourier analysis yields a power spectrum, which plots how much power (weighting) is associated with each pure sine-wave frequency that contributes to a given waveform. In the example shown in **Figure 2.3**, the EEG sample in panel **A** has been analyzed using a Fourier analysis to generate the power spectrum in panel **B**. The large peak on the left side of the spectrum indicates that the waveform is characterized by a dominant frequency (given in cycles per second or Hertz [Hz]) of ~11 Hz. Another way of saying this is that a pure sine wave with a frequency of 11 Hz is a very good fit to the overall shape of this waveform.

Other frequencies modify the shape of the basic 11 Hz waveform, as shown by the lower peaks to the right of the largest peak in the spectrum. The contributions of these additional frequencies (modeled as higher frequency sine waves) are what give the waveform its complex shape and make it look different from a pure 11 Hz sine wave. By applying Fourier analysis, we can describe the stages of sleep in terms of the EEG frequencies that dominate each stage. These frequency ranges are designated using Greek letters, although the exact values represented by each letter have varied among researchers and clinicians. Typical (approximate), dominant frequencies relevant to staging sleep/arousal states are the following:

β: beta: >12 Hz
α: alpha: 8–12 Hz
θ: theta: 4–8 Hz
δ: delta: <4 Hz

The open-ended beta range is also often divided into low-frequency beta (e.g., 12–20 or 30 Hz), also called sigma (σ), and high-frequency beta (20 or 30–60 Hz), also called gamma (γ). However, the term "sigma" is also often used to refer only to the bottom of this range (12–16 Hz). The terminology used for frequencies below 4 (sometimes 4.5) Hz is not consistent across studies. Some reports refer to all EEG frequencies below 4 Hz as slow waves. In this volume, we will divide slow EEG rhythms into two frequency/amplitude ranges: Waveforms with frequencies greater than 1 Hz (i.e., 1–4 Hz) with a voltage amplitude of 75–140 μV (microvolts) are called delta or slow waves. Those with very low frequencies (<1 Hz; usually 0.5–1.0 Hz) and very high amplitudes (>140 μV) are called slow oscillations (SOs) (Massimini et al., 2004; Steriade, 1994; Steriade et al., 1993b). This distinction between slow (delta) waves and slow oscillations is based on physiological evidence that is reviewed in Section 12.2.5.

2.2.3 Summary

The human EEG, usually measured from surface electrodes on the scalp, provides the key evidence that allows discrimination of waking and of several sleep stages, supplemented by information from EOG and EMG recordings. EEG patterns can be

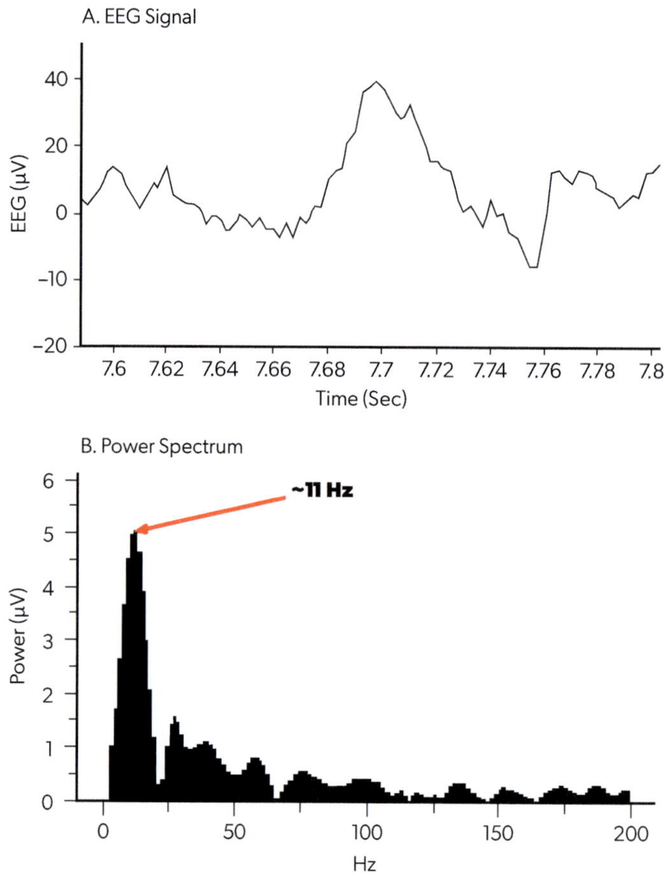

Figure 2.3 The top panel shows a sample of an EEG signal that has been subjected to a Fourier analysis. The results of the analysis are plotted as a power spectrum shown in the lower panel. Frequencies are plotted from low to high (left to right) along the X axis in cycles per second (Hz). The height of the plotted values indicates the power (in microvolts, μV) with which each frequency of sine wave contributes to the waveform shown above. The highest peak (arrow at ~11 Hz) indicates that a sine wave with that frequency accounts for the basic shape of the waveform, while higher frequencies contribute to the shape of the waveform in proportion to the power plotted at each frequency. Despite the presence of many other frequencies, EEG segments are often described with reference to the dominant frequency (i.e., the one contributing the greatest power); therefore, this could be referred to as an 11 Hz waveform or a sample of alpha activity (i.e., a rhythm falling in the 8–12 Hz range). Adapted with permission from http://www.medicine.mcgill.ca/physio/vlab/biomed_signals/signals.htm, courtesy of Dr. Melissa Vollrath, McGill University.

analyzed using a mathematical tool, called Fourier analysis, to identify the dominant frequencies present. These frequencies are divided into ranges labeled with Greek letters that are characteristic of different stages of sleep and waking.

2.3 Stages of sleep

2.3.1 Transition to sleep

The EEG features recorded during different sleep stages differ somewhat depending on the locations of recording electrodes (e.g., above the frontal vs. occipital cortical regions; see Chapter 12). The features described below are those most commonly observed and used to distinguish among sleep stages in healthy, young adult people (Carskadon & Dement, 2011).

Adult humans, when fully awake and engaged with the environment (eyes open), show a low-amplitude, desynchronized EEG pattern dominated by high frequencies in the beta range, with some alpha activity (see **Figure 1.4**). If they relax, especially with eyes closed, the EEG shifts in most people toward a slower pattern dominated by alpha waves (8–12 Hz), especially in more caudal (posterior) brain regions. If, in this state of relaxed wakefulness, individuals open their eyes and attend to their surroundings, they typically revert to a higher frequency pattern with more beta-range EEG activity.

While awake, eye movements recorded by the EOG are voluntary and task-related, and the EMG shows high muscle tone. In the seconds or minutes before falling asleep, slow, involuntary, rolling eye movements occur, which may also persist into the first stage of sleep (see **Figure 1.2**). These eye movements gradually cease as the individual falls asleep.

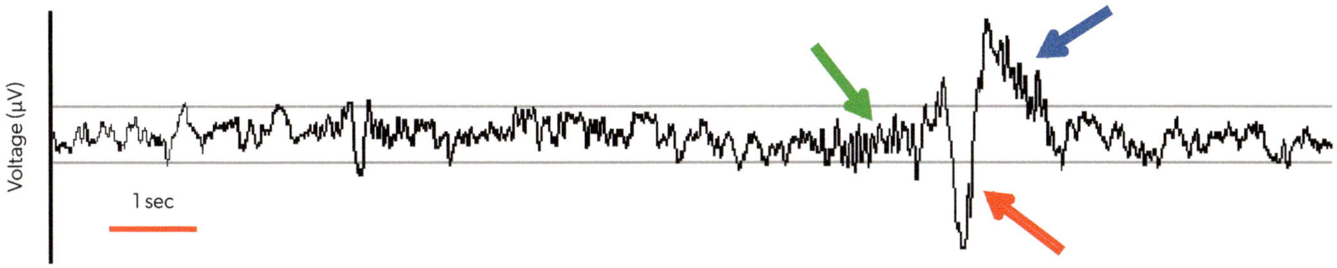

Figure 2.4 Examples of electrical features during Stage 2 sleep. The figure shows a 15 sec segment of EEG recording (negative plotted downward) from a central electrode placement that shows a sleep spindle (green arrow) and a K complex (red arrow). The K complex is characterized by a sharp negative half-wave, followed by a broader positive half-wave. There is likely a second sleep spindle (blue arrow), which appears during the K complex, making it more difficult to detect. The horizontal grey lines enclose a 75 µv window, and the calibration bar equals 1 sec. Note that sleep EEG recordings are often shown with negative plotted upward rather than downward. Negative limbs of K complexes and of slow waves are associated with local inhibition of neural activity and are referred to as "down-states" or "Off-states," reflecting hyperpolarized local field potentials. It therefore seems more consistent with this terminology, and less confusing, to show negative changes as downward deflections. Image courtesy of Antonia Scholz, Sleep Disorders Laboratory, Nova Scotia Health, Halifax, Nova Scotia.

2.3.2 NREM sleep stages

Sleep begins with a transition stage called NREM Stage 1 sleep (or N1 sleep); see **Figure 1.4**). This stage is characterized by some slowing of the EEG, resulting in decreasing beta power and increasing delta power (Merica & Gaillard, 1992), loss of the alpha rhythm, and a fairly low voltage, mixed-frequency pattern, often with strong power in the theta band. The EMG maintains stable, moderately low activity, and respiration and heart rate start to slow. In N1, people lose awareness of their surroundings, but even weak external stimuli can cause a rapid return to full wakefulness, sometimes accompanied by a denial of having been asleep. N1 sleep is usually a brief transition stage between waking and later sleep stages in healthy, young adults, although it often intrudes into later parts of sleep in older people; see Chapter 4.

From N1 sleep, a person enters NREM Stage 2 sleep (or N2 sleep), which is usually considered the first true sleep stage. During N2, physiological functions, such as heart rate and breathing, slow; responsiveness to the environment decreases (i.e., arousal thresholds increase); EMG tone declines somewhat; and the EEG shows mixed frequencies that tend to be slower than in N1, including theta in more frontal regions. The onset of N2 sleep is also marked by the first appearance of sleep spindles and K complexes (**Figure 2.4**).

Sleep spindles[3] are defined as periodic bursts of rapid EEG activity lasting 0.5–1.5 sec. The EEG frequencies within spindles are usually in the range of ~12–16 Hz, with that range divided into slow (12–14 Hz) and fast (14–16 Hz) spindles.[4] Sleep spindles appear during N2 sleep at a rate of 3–8 per minute, and they also occur during NREM Stage 3 sleep (or N3 sleep) but may be more difficult to detect amid the very large, slow waves characteristic of that stage (Cox et al., 2017).

Sleep spindles are often closely associated with K complexes during N2 sleep. Typical K complexes recorded from either a scalp or intracranial electrode last longer than 0.5 sec and occur at a rate of 1–3 per minute; they are most common in recordings from frontal cortical regions (McCormick et al., 1997). They include a high-amplitude, negative half-wave "down-state" (or Off), often—but not always—followed by a slower positive half-wave "up-state" (or On) (**Figure 2.4**). This terminology refers to whether neurons contributing to this waveform are being hyperpolarized (inhibited, during an Off state) or depolarized (excited, during an On state).

In intracortical recordings from the brains of epilepsy patients being studied in preparation for surgery, K complexes were usually detected as isolated negative Off states, with limited evidence for positive On states. During these intracortical recordings, local field potentials (measured with a large macroelectrode) that were identified as K complexes were accompanied by reduced firing of nearby single, cortical neurons (recorded with microelectrodes). These results are consistent with the interpretation that many K complexes represent a transient, local region of cortical hyperpolarization (Off state) (Cash et al., 2009; Gonzalez et al., 2018; Mak-McCully et al., 2015).

K complexes appear spontaneously, but they can also be evoked by introducing auditory or other sensory stimulation

[3] The name "sleep spindle" refers to an initial increase in EEG amplitude followed by a gradual decrease during the event, producing a characteristic voltage envelope that, with some imagination, can be seen as roughly spindle-shaped.

[4] Other definitions for the spindle range (also referred to as "sigma") have also been used (Cox et al., 2017), including, for example, 7–14 Hz (Steriade et al., 1993a), 9–15 Hz (Mölle et al., 2011) and 11–16 Hz (Schabus et al., 2006), with correspondingly different definitions of slow and fast spindles within those ranges.

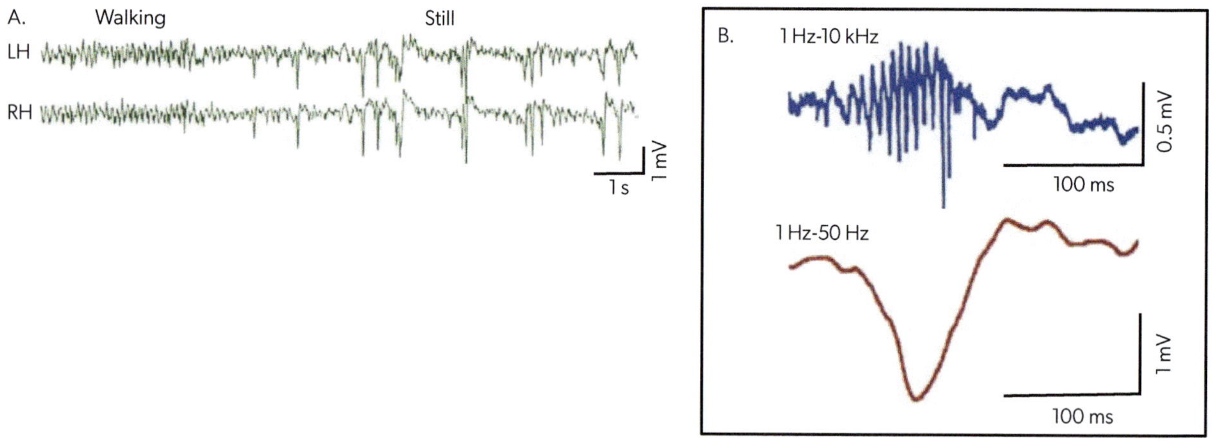

Figure 2.5 A. Recordings from the left and right hippocampus (LH, RH) of a rat show theta activity during walking that is replaced by synchronous high-amplitude negative waves (sharp-waves) when the rat stops moving (still). **B.** On an expanded time scale (see the calibration bars), a recording of the hippocampal local field potential (red) shows the large-amplitude sharp wave, and a recording from the hippocampal pyramidal cell layer (blue) shows a burst of high-frequency firing (ripple) that accompanies the sharp wave. Adapted with permission of John Wiley & Sons from Buzsáki, G. (2015) Hippocampal sharp wave-ripple: a cognitive biomarker for episodic memory and planning. *Hippocampus* 25:1073–1188. © The Authors (2015), published by Wiley Periodicals, Inc.; permission conveyed through Copyright Clearance Center, Inc. doi: 10.1002/hipo.22488.

during sleep (Cash et al., 2009; Halász, 2005). They are considered to be closely related to the slow oscillations seen in N3 sleep (see next paragraph), but they occur as isolated events during N2 sleep (as in **Figure 2.4**), while slow oscillations usually occur in a continuous series during N3 sleep (as in **Figure 1.4**) (Amzica & Steriade, 1997); see below and Chapter 12.

As sleep continues, N2 is followed by what were traditionally scored as NREM Stages 3 and 4. These stages are characterized by further slowing of breathing and heart rate, with maintained low EMG activity and no significant EOG activity. The EEG changes that define these stages include continued frequency slowing and the appearance of distinct, high-amplitude delta or slow waves (1–4 Hz, 75–140 μV). Stages 3 and 4 were distinguished based on whether a scoring epoch (typically 30 sec in duration) included 20–50% delta waves (Stage 3), or >50% delta waves (Stage 4). This distinction was removed from standard clinical scoring procedures by the American Academy of Sleep Medicine (Silber et al., 2007), so these stages are now usually scored together in clinical studies as NREM sleep Stage 3 (N3), which is also called slow-wave sleep (SWS).

Note that SWS in people refers only to N3 sleep (i.e., Stages 3 and 4) and should not be used to refer to either N1 or N2 sleep, which contain few, if any, slow waves. In this volume, we refer to Stages 3 and 4 separately when discussing research in which those stages were distinguished; otherwise, we refer jointly to these stages as N3 sleep or SWS. N3 sleep is defined by the presence in a scoring epoch of at least 20% delta/slow waves (1–4 Hz), while excluding the 0.5–1.0 Hz range, which we call slow oscillations (SOs) (Steriade et al., 1993b). Although some researchers include 0.5–1.0 Hz rhythms as part of the definition of SWS, there is physiological and functional evidence supporting the distinction between slow waves and SOs (see Section 12.2.5).[5]

The hippocampus of all mammals produces electrical patterns called sharp-wave ripples (SWRs) that are most frequent during N3 sleep but may also occur in rats during periods of quiet waking and while eating or drinking (Buzsáki, 2015; Wilson & McNaughton, 1994). These electrical features include a large negative-going field potential 40–100 ms long (the sharp wave) that occurs bilaterally and is accompanied by rapid oscillatory activity (110–200 Hz or higher; the "ripple") in the hippocampal pyramidal cell layer (**Figure 2.5**) (Buzsáki, 2015).

Sharp waves represent highly synchronous bursts of activity in hippocampal pyramidal neurons, which often coincide with the occurrence of sleep spindles in the cortex (Siapas & Wilson, 1998). Buzsáki proposed that cortical sleep spindles trigger hippocampal SWRs and that these, in turn, continue the hippocampal–cortical "dialogue" by enhancing and prolonging spindles, resulting in their frequent simultaneous occurrence (Buzsáki, 2015). SWRs and their interaction with cortical features have been implicated in sleep-dependent brain plasticity (Buzsáki, 1998), which is discussed in Chapter 18.

2.3.3 Depth of sleep

In discussing sleep stages, we sometimes refer to them as being "deeper" or "lighter," although the meaning of those terms is often

[5] A different way of categorizing low-frequency EEG waves during sleep has been proposed, based on a computerized classification of waveforms (Siclari et al., 2014). The benefit of this alternative approach remains to be established in future studies.

not clear. In fact, "depth of sleep" does not have a single meaning but can be discussed only in relation to the results of specific tests (Williams et al., 1964). Many different measures have been used to assess sleep depth. These include how difficult it is to wake someone from that stage, e.g., Loomis's stages D and E were distinguished this way (see Chapter 1) or the degree of either EEG or behavioral responsiveness to external stimuli during that stage. Sleep depth could also be reflected in the degree of physiological arousal or type of mental activity (e.g., dreaming or not) that occurs during that stage. Other indices could include the degree of drowsiness that follows awakening from a sleep stage, or the capacity of that stage to serve a restorative or recovery function.

Another proposed measure of sleep depth is based on the ratio of power in different EEG frequency bands, for example, odds ratio product (ORP). Very low ORP values in a 30 s sleep interval robustly predicted continued sleep during the next 30 s, suggesting deep, stable sleep; very high values reliably predicted waking in the next 30 s (Younes et al., 2015). High ORP values during NREM sleep were also associated with self-reported, poor sleep quality in a large cohort of men and women, perhaps reflecting increased cortical activation during sleep (Lechat et al., 2022).

Applying the criterion of how intense a stimulus is needed to wake someone, N3 would be considered a very deep sleep stage, because responsiveness to external stimuli is minimal. Consistent with this view is the fact that the highly synchronized, delta-dominated EEG of N3 is very distinct from the activated, beta-dominated EEG of alert wakefulness, when responsiveness is maximal.[6] Probably as a result of the EEG characteristics of people in N3 sleep, those awakened from it are often groggy and disoriented, requiring some time to become fully alert and able to perform normally (Dement & Kleitman, 1957). Drowsiness during the period immediately after waking from N3 sleep is accompanied by persistent higher levels of delta waves and less beta-frequency activity (Gorgoni et al., 2015); see **Box 2.1**.

BOX 2.1 Sleep Inertia

Persistent reduced alertness and impaired cognitive performance, despite having crossed the threshold into wakefulness, is called sleep inertia. The duration of sleep inertia depends on several factors. One of these is the stage of sleep from which one wakens, with considerable inertia when waking from N3 sleep and less when waking from other NREM stages or some phases of REM sleep (Broughton, 1968; Dement & Kleitman, 1957; Tassi & Muzet, 2000). There is also increased inertia at the trough of the circadian body temperature cycle (Scheer et al., 2008), after longer vs. shorter daytime naps (Brooks & Lack, 2006; Trotti, 2017), when waking is imposed rather than spontaneous (Ikeda & Hayashi, 2010), and if there had been prior sleep deprivation (Gorgoni et al., 2015; McHill et al., 2019). The amount of sleep inertia identified is also influenced by the measures of alertness or cognitive performance that are used to assess it.

These factors interact with each other; e.g., prior sleep deprivation results in more N3 sleep during recovery sleep (see Chapter 5) and more persistent sleep inertia when the individual is woken. These interactions are important for situations in which shift workers (e.g., in health care, protection services, the military, or industry) lose sleep and attempt to compensate using naps. The degree of sleep inertia they suffer may be critically important if they need to perform effectively shortly after they are forced to wake up from a nap because of a crisis (see Chapter 13). For reviews related to sleep inertia, see (Hilditch & McHill, 2019; Tassi & Muzet, 2000; Trotti, 2017).

2.3.4 REM sleep

REM sleep typically emerges out of N2 sleep. The EEG amplitude in REM sleep is low, with mixed frequencies in the theta range as well as some alpha; as a result, the EEG is difficult to distinguish from that of waking or N1 sleep (**Figures 1.3 and 1.4**). The onset of REM sleep, however, is heralded by the sudden loss of skeletal muscle tone, especially in postural muscles, as shown by the flattening of the EMG (atonia). Simultaneously, the EOG begins to show bursts of REMs that give this stage its usual name. Eye movements are conjugate (both eyes moving together in the same direction) and occur under closed eyelids (see **Figure 1.3**). REMs and atonia do not normally occur during other sleep stages or while awake, so the occurrence of these motor features distinguishes REM sleep from waking, despite the similarity of the EEG patterns.

In animal studies using electrodes implanted in the brain, REM sleep also includes the presence of very prominent, regular, theta-frequency rhythms in the hippocampus, and the presence of ponto-geniculo-occipital (PGO) spikes (or waves). These are large-amplitude waveforms detected sequentially in the brainstem pons (which plays a critical role in the generation of the features of REM sleep, including atonia; see Chapter 10) and in two important structures in the mammalian visual system: the lateral geniculate nuclei of the thalamus and the occipital cortex (Datta, 1997; Nelson et al., 1983). These PGO waves appear in other mammalian species (Gott et al., 2017), but these features are difficult to detect in people using scalp electrodes, presumably because of the volume of the overlying cortex. Depth recordings directly from the human brain

[6] This account does not explain why there is also a high threshold for arousal during some parts of REM sleep episodes, when the EEG resembles that of waking. This issue is discussed further in Chapter 12.

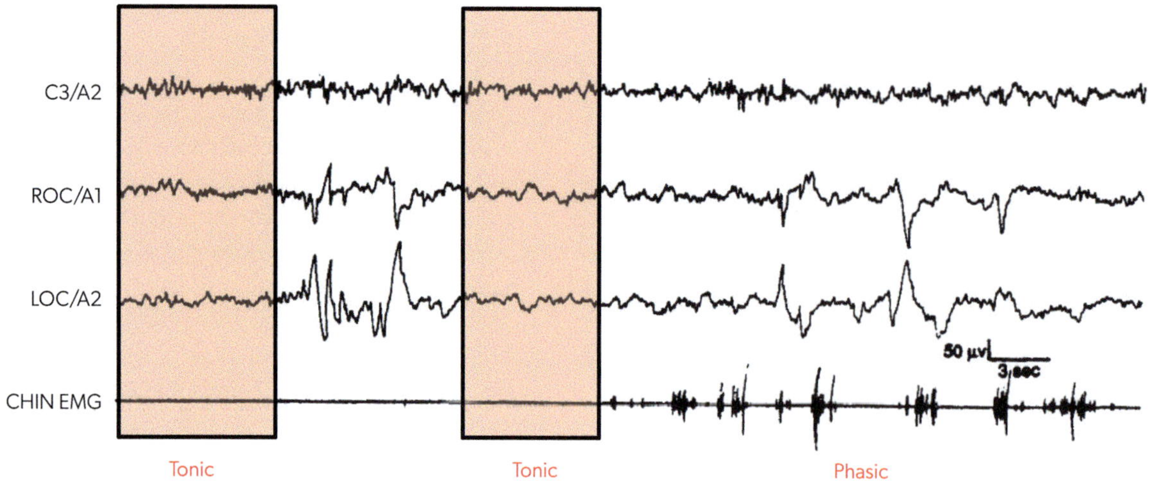

Figure 2.6 An example of cortical EEG, EOG, and chin EMG channels recorded during REM sleep. The EEG (C3/A2) shows a low-voltage, activated pattern; the right and left electrooculogram channels (ROC/A1, LOC/A2) show conjugate eye movements, and the Chin EMG record shows atonia with superimposed bursts of twitching activity. The segments of the recordings in red boxes can be described as tonic REM sleep, showing only the sustained features of cortical activation and muscle atonia. The rest of the figure can be described as phasic REM sleep, in which irregular events like muscle twitches and jerky, conjugate eye movements occur. ROC/LOC refers to the right/left outer canthus, the lateral point at which the upper and lower eyelids meet where these electrodes are placed. Calibration bars show 50 µV and 3 s. Adapted with permission of Elsevier, Ltd. from Carskadon, M. A. & Dement, W.C. (2000) Normal human sleep: an overview. In: M. H. Kryger et al. (Eds.), *Principles and Practice of Sleep Medicine* (3rd edition, pp. 15–25). Philadelphia. © Elsevier, 2000.

obtained during surgical procedures, however, indicated that pontine waves (usually referred to as P-waves in rats and people) also occur in human REM sleep, often—but not always—in association with REMs (Lim et al., 2007); see discussion in Section 12.2.6.

REM sleep is also accompanied by somewhat chaotic changes in several aspects of physiological regulation. In parallel to the occurrence of REMs, there are bursts of phasic motor activity in other small, peripheral muscles, such as those in the hands, feet, and face, while postural muscles remain paralyzed. The normal mechanisms of homeothermic body temperature regulation which function in SWS become disabled in REM sleep (Glotzbach & Heller, 1976; Jouvet et al., 1959; Martelli et al., 2014), and brain temperature shows sustained increases in cats and rabbits (Csernai et al., 2019; Parmeggiani, 2007). Respiratory and vascular functions become erratic, with rapid or irregular breathing and heart rate, changes in blood pressure regulation, and the presence of penile erection in men and vaginal signs linked to sexual arousal in women[7] (Fisher et al., 1983; Fisher et al., 1965).

[7] Whether knowledge of the signs of physiological and apparent sexual arousal during dreams contributed to Freud's view that dreams are related to repressed drives, especially sexual drives, is unclear. A historical review indicated that sleep-related penile erections were referred to in documents dating back centuries, long before REM sleep was identified, and were sometimes linked to dreams with sexual content (van Driel, 2014). However, erections occur in 80–90% of REM sleep episodes, while erotic content of dreams is reported to be relatively rare, so these features do not appear to be causally linked (Hirshkowitz & Schmidt, 2005).

The characteristics of REM sleep can be grouped as either tonic (sustained) or phasic (varying) features. Tonic features include postural muscle paralysis, low-voltage cortical EEG, and disrupted temperature regulation. Phasic features include REMs and peripheral muscle twitches (**Figure 2.6**). Although the usual scoring methods for sleep studies consider these features together in identifying REM sleep, the distinction between tonic and phasic aspects of REM sleep may be functionally important.

The label "paradoxical" that Jouvet applied to this sleep stage relates to the discrepancy between a sleeping person's behavior and physiology. During REM sleep, a person remains soundly asleep, immobile with respect to postural muscles, and generally unaware of the environment. Despite cortical EEG patterns and autonomic disturbances consistent with a high level of arousal, there is a very high threshold for awakening in response to external stimuli during REM sleep, similar to that of N3 sleep (Williams et al., 1964). However, response thresholds depend on whether stimuli occur during phasic or tonic REM sleep (Ermis et al., 2010; Price & Kremen, 1980) (see discussion in Section 12.3.3).

Awakenings from REM sleep generate reports of dreaming about 80% of the time (Foulkes, 1962; Nielsen, 1999), often including bizarre and irrational narrative and visual elements as well as sometimes strong emotional content. During dreams, the sleeper typically lacks awareness that the experience is a dream and lacks insight into the physically impossible characteristics of the dream narrative (except in the case of lucid dreaming; see Appendix A). The desynchronized/low voltage EEG resembling that of waking is consistent with the experience of mental activity in the form of dreams but inconsistent with other signs of sleep, including reduced awareness of the environment.

The decades since the discovery of REM sleep, its cyclic expression during the night, and its strong correlation with reported dreams, witnessed several important developments. The REM sleep stage became an important research focus for psychologists and psychiatrists interested in dreaming, who now had an objective, neurophysiologically defined target to study in addition to the self-reported data that had comprised dreaming research previously.

A second trend, however, was the regular observation that people waking out of NREM sleep, especially N1 and N2 sleep, also sometimes reported experiencing mental activity, although not as frequently as out of REM sleep (Chellappa et al., 2011; Foulkes, 1962; Hobson et al., 2000; Nielsen, 2000). This development led to debates about the extent to which dreaming is linked specifically to REM sleep, and about whether the quality of mental activity during REM sleep differs from that during NREM sleep (Hobson et al., 2000; Nielsen, 2000; Smith et al., 2004; Takeuchi et al., 2001). Because this is a relatively specialized issue and requires some background information related to the neural control of sleep that is reviewed in later chapters, this topic is addressed in more detail in Appendix A.

2.3.5 Summary

Sleep in healthy, adult humans passes through several distinct stages, which are marked by changes in the dominant EEG frequencies shown and by the appearance of specific EEG features. Gradual slowing of the EEG from N1 to N3 sleep is accompanied by increasing parasympathetic dominance, as indicated by slowing of heart rate and breathing, reduced body temperature, and reductions in muscle tone. N2 sleep is marked by the appearance of sleep spindles and K complexes, while the EEG in N3 sleep is dominated by slow waves and even slower, larger slow oscillations. During N3 sleep, the hippocampus also generates distinctive electrical patterns called sharp-wave ripples.

These NREM sleep stages alternate during the night with periods of REM sleep, which is characterized by low-voltage EEG activity, postural muscle atonia, rapid eye movements, twitching of small peripheral muscles, autonomic arousal, and loss of normal temperature regulation. PGO waves (also called P-waves) are closely associated with REMs in some species. Similar waveforms have been recorded from the human pons during REM sleep, but they are less closely linked to eye movements.

REM sleep is remarkable in part because people report dreams with high reliability when awakened from this stage but less often from other sleep stages. There is debate over the extent to which there are differences in the reported irrational content and emotional intensity of mental activity associated with REM sleep and with lighter NREM sleep stages. But differences in reported mental activity between REM sleep and N3 sleep are very marked. Awakening from N3 sleep produces few reports of cognitive activity and is associated with more sleep inertia, a period of reduced alertness and cognitive slowing after waking.

2.4 Sources of EEG patterns

The electrical features recorded by EEG electrodes attached to the scalp represent the summation of minute electrical signals from many thousands, if not millions, of neurons in the cortical regions underlying the electrodes. When recorded from the scalp surface, these summed signals typically fall in the microvolt (μV) range (1 μV = 1 millionth of a volt). The EEG reflects principally the sum of slow, graded excitatory (depolarizing) and inhibitory (hyperpolarizing) postsynaptic potentials (EPSPs and IPSPs) that are generated in the soma and dendrites of neurons.

In the brain, these postsynaptic potentials are the result of a neuron receiving and summing many excitatory and inhibitory synaptic inputs from other neurons, which modify its membrane potential and, therefore, the probability that it will generate action potentials (neuronal "firing"). Action potentials themselves probably contribute relatively little to the EEG because these all-or-none depolarizations are very brief (1–2 ms) relative to the graded PSPs, which last for much longer. The major contributors to mammalian EEG recordings are postsynaptic potentials occurring in large pyramidal neurons with somata located in layer 5 of the 6-layered neocortex. These neurons are arranged in dense, parallel arrays, perpendicular to the cortical surface, an arrangement that is favorable for generating voltage differences that can be detected by surface electrodes (Kirschstein & Köhling, 2009); **Figure 2.7**.

Low-voltage, fast EEG patterns are characteristic of an awake, alert brain. Understanding why low-voltage EEG patterns occur in the waking cortex depends on understanding how populations of cortical neurons function in this state. When a single surface electrode records the activity of a large population of neurons consisting of some that are being excited and others inhibited at the same time, largely independently of each other, the resulting electrical pattern is described as desynchronized. If, at one time point, about half of a population of neurons contributing to that electrode's recording are being depolarized (i.e., their electrical potential is becoming more positive) and half hyperpolarized (electrical potential becoming more negative), the algebraic sum of their electrical potentials will be close to 0 volts (referenced to a common

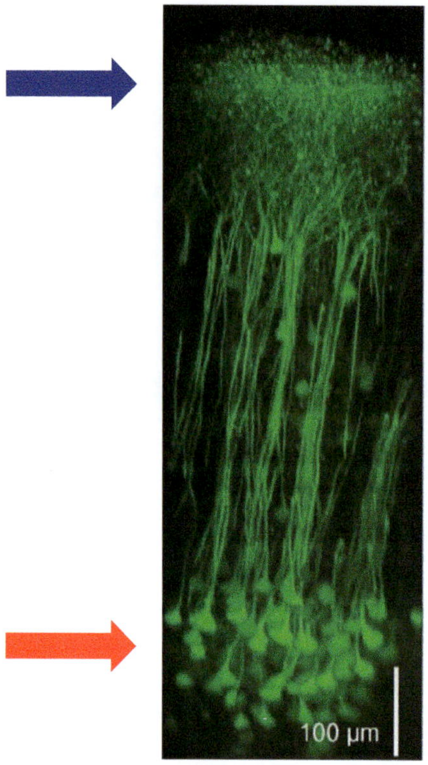

Figure 2.7 An image based on two-photon excitation showing the typical orientation of clusters of cortical pyramidal cells in the mouse somatosensory cortex. Cell bodies are packed into layer 5, deep in the cortex (red arrow), and their apical (emerging from the apex or top) dendrites stretch toward the superficial layers of the cortex where they branch into large dendritic fields (blue arrow). This layered arrangement creates an electrical voltage difference between the depth and surface of the cortex (a "dipole") which facilitates measurement of electrical signals by electrodes on the surface of the scalp. Adapted with permission of Dr. Bert Sakmann and SfN from Krieger, P. et al. (2007). Synaptic connections between layer 5B pyramidal neurons in mouse somatosensory cortex are independent of apical dendrite bundling. *J Neurosci* 27(43):11473–11482. Copyright © 2007, Society for Neuroscience. doi: 10.1523/JNEUROSCI.1182-07.2007.

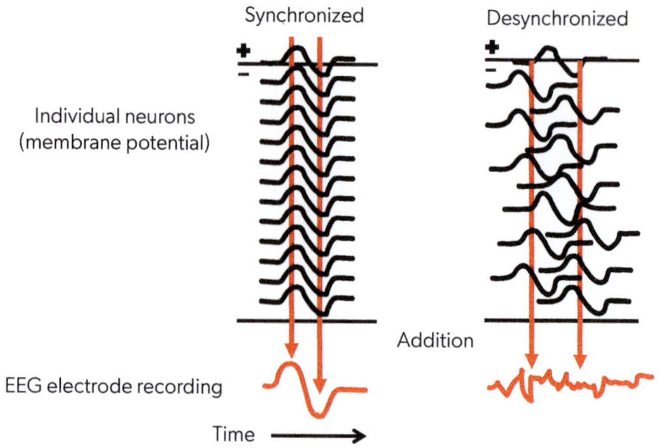

Figure 2.8 Models illustrating an intuitive idea of how activity in a population of neurons can give rise to either high-voltage (large amplitude), slow waves or low-voltage, fast waves in EEG recordings. Each black line represents the changing voltage (membrane potential) of an individual neuron over time as its membrane becomes more depolarized (+) and then more hyperpolarized (–). On the left, all neurons that are being recorded by a single EEG electrode attached to the scalp are doing the same thing at the same time—their activity is synchronous. Voltage changes at all time points are summed algebraically across nine neurons to produce the bottom waveform, as illustrated by the vertical red arrows at two time points. The result is that the coordinated voltage changes in all neurons add up to a large-amplitude wave of similar shape in the recording made by an EEG electrode on the scalp (bottom left), characteristic of the slow EEG activity of N3 sleep. On the right, each model neuron shows identical voltage changes but out of synchrony with other neurons. As a result, the algebraic sum of their activity, recorded from an EEG electrode at any time point reflects both hyperpolarizations and depolarizations in different neurons. These values average out (red arrows) to near zero, with very small, irregular voltage changes around that value (bottom right). Slight changes in the balance of activity among many neurons will generate only small negative or positive voltages that will change quickly, which is typical of an EEG recording made using a scalp electrode during waking.

ground, which is usually an electrode attached to an earlobe in human studies).

Small, irregular shifts in the balance of depolarizing and hyperpolarizing inputs to individual cells will cause the voltage averaged across this large cell population to fluctuate rapidly between slightly positive and negative values near 0 volts. As a result, the peak-to-trough amplitude of the summed potential changes recorded by an EEG electrode will be small. A desynchronized neural population therefore generates EEG recordings showing unstable, low-voltage, fast oscillations (**Figure 2.8, right**).

One interpretation of why an alert cortex would show this pattern is that when a neuron is processing information, it is receiving input continuously from hundreds of other neurons. Its moment-to-moment shifts in membrane potential will be somewhat different from those of a neighboring neuron that may be receiving input from an overlapping, but partly different, set of input neurons, and performing a different function. If, for example, a neuron in the auditory cortex responds most robustly to a 900 Hz tone at a particular volume, while its neighbor is more strongly tuned to a 1000 Hz tone, they will become maximally activated (depolarized) at slightly different times while a person listens to a piece of music or to someone speaking. As a result, these neurons will not be synchronous in their activity. This lack of synchrony will be multiplied across many thousands of neurons contributing to a recording from a single surface electrode, each processing different inputs and performing different functions.

Mircea Steriade noted, however, that the so-called desynchronized EEG actually contains high-frequency oscillations (in the beta and gamma frequency ranges) that are synchronous across spatially restricted, functionally related cortical and thalamic networks (Ahmed & Cash, 2013; Steriade et al., 1996). He therefore recommended the use of the term "activated" rather than "desynchronized" in describing low-voltage, rapid oscillations in EEG recordings.[8]

During deep NREM sleep stages, EEG patterns include high-voltage, slow waves (**Figure 2.8, left**). These larger, slower waves reflect increased synchrony in the population, that is, more of the neurons recorded by a single surface electrode become depolarized and hyperpolarized at the same time. Summed across a large cell population, this will result in larger average voltage changes, producing high amplitude waves in the EEG that reverse polarity slowly.

In the mammalian cortex, slow rhythms result from two processes. First, during NREM sleep, there is a reduction in several types of excitatory input to the thalamus and cortex and an increase in levels of the inhibitory neurotransmitter GABA (γ-aminobutyric acid) (see Chapters 10 and 11). The resulting hyperpolarization causes both cortical and thalamic neurons to spontaneously generate slow waves with large amplitudes. Second, the slow waves in cortex are synchronized in part because they receive a common, slow oscillating input from the thalamus that modulates their membrane potentials at the same time and in the same direction (Steriade, 1994).

When cortical neurons are being driven to generate slower oscillations in this synchronous mode during sleep, they are no longer processing information in the same independent, selective mode in which they normally operate during waking. More details concerning the generation of low-frequency EEG rhythms and the implications of this interpretation for information processing during sleep are reviewed in Chapter 12.

During REM sleep, there is cortical activation that is superficially similar to that of an alert, waking person, even though the individual is not attending to external environmental stimuli or engaging in other typical waking activities. As discussed in more detail in Chapters 10 and 11, this cortical activation depends on the release in the cortex of one excitatory neurotransmitter, acetylcholine, while other excitatory inputs remain suppressed. The activated cortical pattern likely depends on this input and on interactions among cortical regions, rather than input from external sources. The frequent report of elaborate dreams on waking from REM sleep indicates that this pattern of cortical activation facilitates (or permits) dream production.

[8] Since any measurable rhythmicity in the EEG (e.g., an alpha rhythm in a low-voltage recording) implies at least a degree of synchronization among a subset of neurons, the use of "activated" to describe these patterns is more accurate. However, the term "desynchronized" is still used commonly, probably because it implies an intuitive explanation for the visible differences between rapid, low-voltage and slow, high-voltage oscillations.

2.4.1 Summary

The EEG recorded from scalp electrodes reflects primarily the postsynaptic potentials generated by very dense arrays of large cortical pyramidal neurons. Slow, high-amplitude EEG oscillations reflect the synchronous activity of many thousands of neurons being recorded by each electrode. These oscillations result from both the intrinsic activity of cortical neurons when they are hyperpolarized and the impact of similar synchronizing inputs received from the thalamus. The high degree of synchronous activity in the cortex during N3 sleep is associated with relatively little experience of cognition during this stage.

Low-amplitude, activated EEG patterns during waking reflect more independent information processing by individual neurons within the cortex while contributing to perception, motor activity, cognition, etc. Similar low-amplitude cortical EEG activity during REM sleep depends primarily on activation by acetylcholine and interactions within the cortex and is associated with frequent reports of elaborate dream activity.

2.5 The rhythms of sleep

2.5.1 Sleep distribution during the night

The structure and features of sleep depend on the characteristics of the individual being studied. Sleep patterns differ among species (see Chapter 7), but even among people, sleep patterns differ depending on age, mental and physical health status, previous sleep history, cultural background, gender, and time of day at which sleep is recorded. The standard description offered below of a "normal" sleep pattern is, therefore, valid only for an idealized, healthy, young-adult human from an industrialized society, who has stable, habitual sleep patterns, has not consumed sleep-modifying drugs, and is sleeping at their usual time of night. If any of these modifiers is changed (e.g., health status, age, time of day, etc.), aspects of the sleep recorded will also be different (Carskadon & Dement, 2011).

In describing this normal night's sleep, we will refer to the stages of sleep defined earlier and to the characteristic physiological features of these stages. It is important to note, however, that the transitions among NREM sleep stages may be gradual, and that elements characteristic of one stage can appear briefly in other stages. The boundaries between sleep stages are not absolute, but sleep staging is a vital tool for describing, comparing, and analyzing sleep patterns and for clinical evaluation of sleep disorders.

A normal night of sleep in a young adult person (**Figure 2.9**) begins with a gradual fall from alertness to N1 sleep, which is maintained for very few minutes. This transition stage is followed by N2 sleep (lasting ~10–25 min) and marked by the appearance of sleep spindles and K complexes along with progressive slowing of EEG rhythms. The proportion of delta waves in the EEG increases gradually until they occupy at least 20% of 30 sec scoring epochs, which defines the onset of N3 (including NREM stages 3 and 4). The first N3 episode typically lasts ~25–45 min. After this period of N3, body movements often signal a gradual lightening of sleep toward N2 again, from which, after a few minutes, the sleeper enters REM sleep, generally for only a brief period (~5 min). As a result, the first REM sleep episode of the night does not usually appear until after 60–90 min of NREM sleep (including N3) has occurred.

The sleeper will then pass through several more NREM–REM cycles, with cycle lengths averaging 90–110 min over the course of the night (measured, e.g., from one REM sleep onset to the next) (**Figure 2.9**). The second and subsequent cycles will include smaller amounts of N3 during the NREM sleep episodes (often disappearing completely after the second cycle), and increased lengths of REM sleep. During later cycles of the night, the NREM sleep phase consists almost exclusively of N2 sleep, which is why this stage occupies most of a night's total sleep duration (45–55%), while N3 sleep comprises 13–23%. Sometimes associated with stage transitions, and especially with REM sleep bouts, sleep may be interrupted by brief arousals to EEG-defined wakefulness (<5% of the night), of which people usually have little or no memory in the morning. People pass through 4–6 NREM–REM sleep cycles before waking spontaneously in the morning, typically out of a REM sleep episode. If, instead, a person is woken by an alarm in the morning, arousal might occur from either REM or NREM (likely N2) sleep, since the timing of waking would be unrelated to the physiology of the sleeper.

REM sleep occupies 20–25% of the sleep period, and it is concentrated in the second half; N3 occupies 13–23% of the sleep period, and it is concentrated in the first half (**Figure 2.9**). The roughly symmetrical, but opposite, distributions of these sleep stages might suggest that there is a single control mechanism that switches between promoting first NREM and then REM sleep during the night. In fact, that is not the case; the principal mechanisms that regulate the timing of N3 and REM sleep are different and, largely, but not completely, independent of each other.

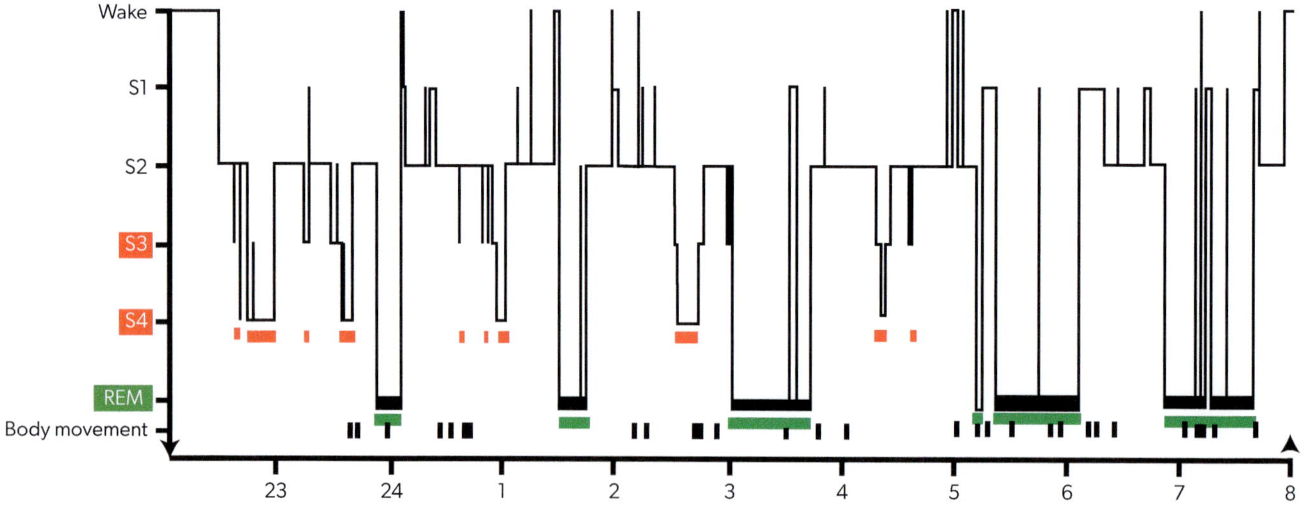

Figure 2.9 A hypnogram recorded from a healthy 14-year-old girl. The hours of sleep are shown on the X axis and the sleep stages on the Y axis. The period in bed is indicated between the small, down- and up-pointing black arrowheads. In this older slide, NREM stages S3 and S4 (now often called N3) are plotted separately. Episodes of N3 sleep are marked with red bars and REM sleep is marked with green bars. The figure illustrates the alternation between NREM and REM sleep, and the gradual reduction in N3 and increase in REM sleep during the night. Body movements often associated with REM sleep or light N1 sleep are shown as black marks above the X axis. Adapted with permission of Elsevier, Ltd. from Carskadon, M. A. & Dement, W.C. (1989). Normal human sleep: an overview. In: M. H. Kryger et al. (Eds.), *Principles and Practice of Sleep Medicine* (1st edition, pp. 3–13). Philadelphia. © Elsevier (1989).

As we will discuss in more detail in Chapter 5, the pressure to generate N3 sleep is related to the duration of prior waking (i.e., the length of time since an individual last slept and produced NREM sleep = "sleep debt") (Webb & Agnew, 1971). REM sleep, on the other hand, is strongly affected by the circadian system, the internal mechanism that imposes daily rhythmicity on many aspects of our physiology (Carskadon & Dement, 1980; Czeisler, Zimmerman, et al., 1980; Wurts & Edgar, 2000); see Chapter 3.

These influences were illustrated in a study in which young men took naps at one of several times of day after either their usual nocturnal sleep or after a night of total sleep deprivation (Endo et al., 1981). Their sleep at night showed the usual pattern of high N3 and low REM sleep amounts early in the night, which switched to the opposite pattern later in the night (**Figure 2.10, A**). During naps at different daytime phases after a night's sleep, REM sleep amounts were high in the morning but low later in the day, while N3 sleep amounts were low in the morning and increased across the day. Thus, N3 sleep during a nap increased as the length of prior waking increased, while REM sleep amounts fell over the same period. REM sleep amounts were also negatively correlated with the daily body temperature rhythm, which is tightly linked to the circadian system.

When participants were first sleep deprived overnight and then given nap opportunities at three times of day on different occasions, they showed increasing amounts of N3 sleep later in the day (dashed line ['SWS'] in **Figure 2.10, B**), consistent with the idea that the longer they were awake before napping, the greater was the pressure to generate N3 sleep. However, the probability of REM sleep (solid line in **Figure 2.10, B**) followed its usual circadian pattern and *decreased* during naps later in the day, despite participants having been awake for longer at the later nap times. The decline in REM sleep amounts later in the day was not the result of N3 sleep taking up all the scheduled nap opportunity; N3 sleep never occupied more than 50% of the total nap opportunity (Endo et al., 1981).

The high probability of entering REM sleep during the second half of the night continued during the early morning after waking up and decreased during the afternoon and evening until it was very low at usual bedtime (**Figure 2.10**) (Czeisler, Zimmerman, et al., 1980; Dinges, 1986). We cannot normally detect this daily rhythm of REM sleep probability since we do not normally sleep during the daytime. The daily rhythm is revealed, however, under experimental conditions that require individuals to sleep at unusual circadian phases. These include: having scheduled daytime nap opportunities (as in **Figure 2-10**); having participants live without access to time-of-day information, during which spontaneous sleep timing can become desynchronized from the circadian cycle (Czeisler, Weitzman, et al., 1980) (see Section 3.5.1); and scheduling participants in time-free environments to sleep at unusual circadian phases "forced desynchronization") (Dijk & Czeisler, 1995); see Section 3.5.2 and Chapter 8.

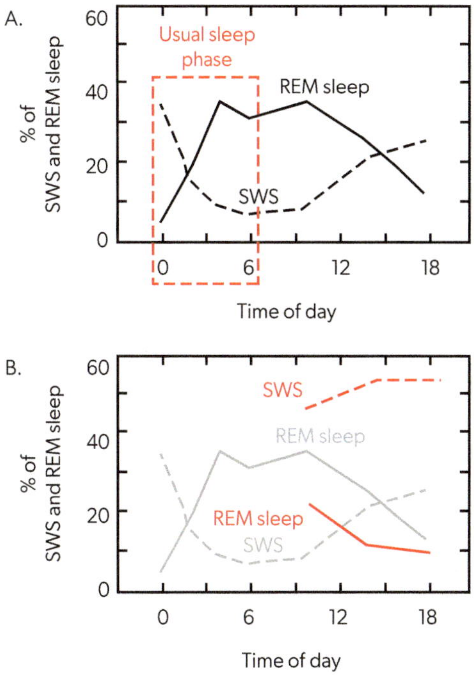

Figure 2.10 **A.** The proportions of REM sleep (solid black line) and SWS (N3, dashed black line) during the usual sleep phase (red outline) and during naps taken on different days at different times of day (X axis): in the morning (09:00–12:00), afternoon (13:00–16:00) and evening (17:00–20:00). There was a high proportion of SWS early in the nighttime sleep phase (i.e., near midnight, or 0 h) and a decrease during the sleep phase. There was a low amount of REM sleep at sleep onset, which increased during the second half of the sleep phase. During daytime naps there were high REM sleep amounts in the morning and decreasing amounts in the afternoon and evening, while SWS amounts increased across the day toward the usual early-night, peak levels. **B.** Sleep data from panel A are reprinted as light gray lines. The red lines show the amounts of SWS (dashed) and REM sleep (solid) during naps in the morning, afternoon, and evening, on different days, after nights of total sleep deprivation. During morning naps, SWS amounts were highly elevated relative to baseline values at that time (see panel A) because participants had accumulated a high level of sleep debt. Amounts continued to increase in the afternoon and evening as sleep deprivation lengthened. REM sleep amounts were high in the morning but declined during the day, roughly in parallel to the decline after a full night's sleep, despite continuing sleep deprivation. This effect is the result of strong regulation of REM sleep amounts by a circadian mechanism that promotes REM sleep in the late night and early morning and not in the late day and early night. Adapted with permission of Oxford University Press and the Sleep Research Society from Endo, S. et al. (1981) Persistence of the circadian rhythm of REM sleep: a variety of experimental manipulations of the sleep-wake cycle. *Sleep* 4:319–328. © Sleep Research Society (1981). doi: 10.1093/sleep/4.3.319.

2.5.2 NREM–REM sleep cycle

Based on observing the self-selected feeding cycles of infants, Kleitman proposed that humans have a "basic rest–activity cycle" (BRAC) that is reflected in the 90–110 min NREM–REM sleep cycle of adults (Kleitman, 1982). He proposed that the BRAC influences physiological and mental functions during the day and is expressed in the form of NREM–REM cycles during sleep at night. Some studies have reported cyclic changes with approximately this periodicity in behavioral, cognitive, and physiological measures as well as in EEG asymmetries between left and right hemispheres while awake (Klein & Armitage, 1979; Lavie, 1980; Oswald et al., 1970; Shannahof-Khalsa et al., 2001). Despite some evidence suggesting that the mechanism timing REM sleep may continue to run during the daytime (see Section 5.6) (Schulz et al., 1975), it remains unclear whether the more subtle cycles detected during the day are continuous with the NREM–REM cycles of sleep.

The BRAC identified by Kleitman in infants had a much shorter period than the adult NREM–REM cycle. In newborn humans, the NREM–REM cycle (also called the Quiet-Active sleep cycle) is 40–50 min long; it lengthens gradually over the course of childhood to 90–110 min. As discussed in Chapter 4, this cycle lengthening is one of many changes in sleep that occur between birth and adulthood. These changes are part of broader changes in brain anatomy and function that occur over the course of development. It is not clear, however, which (if any) of these developmental changes contribute to the lengthening of the NREM–REM cycle.

One idea is that longer NREM–REM cycles may be linked to larger body sizes. Cycle length is 90–110 min in adult humans, ~85 min in chimpanzees, 40–50 min in newborn humans, ~28 min in cats, and 10–12 min in rats and hamsters. However, not all species follow this proposed relationship to body size. The estimated cycle length in elephants (based on observations, not EEG recordings) was reported to be ~72 min, which falls far short of the value predicted by the relationship observed in other species (Tobler, 1995). Other herbivorous ungulates (goats, horses, and cows) also show shorter cycle lengths than predicted by their body sizes (Dallaire et al., 1974). Since these related species have similar cycle lengths despite body size differences, one possibility is that their phylogenetic relatedness or their similar ecological niches influence their cycle lengths.

Other factors that have been proposed to affect NREM–REM cyclicity include metabolic rate (which is linked to body size), and neural features such brain size or the ratio of cortical volume to that of the rest of the brain (i.e., the degree of encephalization) (Dallaire et al., 1974). See Section 7.4.3 for a discussion of this topic. There is no agreement about what determines differences in NREM–REM sleep cycle lengths, but there appears to be a role for body size, other physiological/anatomical characteristics as well as ecological and phylogenetic factors.

2.5.3 Summary

N3 sleep is most common in the first half of the night, while REM sleep and N2 dominate the second half. NREM and REM sleep are regulated by different mechanisms: The amount of N3 sleep shown is determined by the buildup of sleep debt while awake, but REM sleep expression is strongly regulated by circadian phase. When people nap during the day, the rhythm of REM sleep probability and its link to circadian time can be observed.

There are typically 4–6 NREM–REM cycles during the night in adult humans who are allowed to sleep at will, averaging 90–110 min each. Infants start with much shorter cycles, which lengthen as they mature through childhood. Similarly, smaller mammalian species tend to have shorter NREM–REM cycles. But this generalization related to body size appears to be modified by other characteristics, such as relative brain size, phylogenetic relatedness, and ecological factors.

2.6 Issues related to laboratory sleep studies

2.6.1 Impacts of sleep staging

Laboratory sleep studies use standardized definitions for each sleep stage and a scoring method that is based on detailed descriptions of each EEG, EOG, and EMG feature that contributes to identifying these stages. A manualized method for visually scoring sleep records was provided in a publication edited by Rechtschaffen and Kales (Rechtschaffen & Kales, 1968, often referred to as 'R & K'). With subsequent modifications (e.g., Stages 3 and 4 being collapsed into N3 sleep for clinical studies), this approach remains the standard method for scoring sleep studies (Keenan & Hirshkowitz, 2005; Silber et al., 2007). There have been publications describing computer-automated and computer-assisted scoring methods, but none has been accepted as a substitute for the R & K manual.

Note that these criteria are applicable to adult human sleep recorded under carefully prescribed conditions. Sleep in other species and in humans at different developmental stages differs to varying degrees from that of adult humans, and modified staging criteria may be applied (Grigg-Damberger et al., 2007).

The standard names for sleep stages (e.g., "non-REM" or NREM sleep) label most of sleep by exclusion; this tends to suggest a special importance for REM sleep. The use of "N1–N3" (although it derives from the same terminology) reduces this implied emphasis. NREM sleep stages share some characteristics (similar body posture, loss of conscious awareness, and progressively reduced responsiveness to external events), and there is continuity in mechanisms that regulate them. Physiological activation decreases gradually across NREM stages, with falling body temperature and slowing heart rate and breathing, as parasympathetic dominance increases. There is also progressive slowing of EEG rhythms across NREM sleep stages, reflecting a gradual increase in hyperpolarization of thalamic and cortical neurons (see Chapter 12).

But NREM sleep stages are also defined by their distinctive features: Sleep spindles and K complexes first appear in N2, while slow oscillations and delta waves dominate N3. Dream reports from N1 occur more frequently than from other NREM sleep stages (see Appendix A). These features are not, however, exclusive to each NREM stage. K complexes in N2 are thought to be closely related to the slow oscillations of N3, and sleep spindles are present in N3, but harder to detect against its high-amplitude background EEG (see Chapter 12).

The boundaries between sleep stages are not absolute, and one cannot assume that all sleep episodes that meet the definition of a particular sleep stage are physiologically identical (Schulz, 2008). For example, we noted that REM sleep can be further divided into phasic and tonic substages, which may be functionally different. The defining characteristics of one sleep stage can also appear in other stages. Thus, delta-frequency EEG activity can intrude briefly during waking and in sleep stages other than N3 (Bernardi et al., 2019). For example, "micro-sleeps" with delta waves occur with increasing frequency during prolonged waking. Similarly, very brief episodes of EEG-defined waking ("micro-arousals") can occur during all sleep stages (Mathur & Douglas, 1995). There may also be mixed or transition episodes that combine elements normally associated with different sleep or waking states. Some of these atypical features may indicate state instability related to an underlying clinical condition, but most appear to be normal, moment-to-moment variations in brain function that occur in healthy individuals.

REM sleep, however, involves a clear discontinuity in regulation from NREM stages, with a relatively abrupt transition to a very different cluster of EEG and other physiological characteristics. In addition, distinct regulatory mechanisms control the expression of REM and NREM sleep (see Section 2.5.1 and Chapters 10–12).

Sleep staging provides clinicians and researchers with a common vocabulary for summarizing the nature and quality of a person's sleep. This vocabulary facilitates describing how sleep changes during early development, during aging, or because of illness. For example, sleep staging allows documentation of a gradual decline in the amount of N3 sleep during adolescence and again during aging, when there is also an increase in N1 sleep; see Chapter 4. Changes in sleep stages may also be characteristic of some clinical conditions. For example, there is an increase in REM sleep amounts and a decrease in latency to the first REM sleep episode in patients with depression (Kupfer, 1976) (see Chapter 15), and there is disruption of the organization and regulation of REM sleep in the sleep disorder narcolepsy (Broughton et al., 1986; Sorensen et al., 2013); see Chapter 11.

2.6.2 Sleep environments

Both clinical and research studies of sleep are typically conducted in a hospital-based or stand-alone sleep laboratory under highly controlled conditions. These conditions include isolating an individual in a very quiet, darkened bedroom in an environment that is new to them, and attaching them to an array of unfamiliar electrical and mechanical sensors, some of which may not be very comfortable. These are not the conditions under which most people typically sleep. People usually sleep in familiar surroundings in their own homes and without physiological monitoring, often with a bed partner. Home environments are also likely to be noisier, brighter, more social, and more inconsistent over time than the sleep laboratory environment.

The use of highly standardized conditions in a controlled environment is essential for diagnosing intrinsic sleep disorders in individuals suspected of having one of these conditions. If the goal is to identify physiological causes of sleep disruption and to accurately measure their consequences for sleep quality and duration, patients must be isolated from any potential external sources of sleep disturbance (e.g., loud noises, bright lights, interactions with pets or other people). Similarly, sleep researchers must control their study participants' environment so that effects of experimental manipulations can be attributed reliably and unquestionably to only those manipulations and not to unrelated events that occur unpredictably and inconsistently among research participants.

It does not follow, however, that individuals studied under controlled laboratory conditions are showing their usual sleep patterns. In fact, there is a well-recognized phenomenon in sleep laboratories that many people also experience during temporary overnight stays in other new places, for example, when traveling and staying in a hotel. This "first-night effect" refers to the disrupted sleep experienced by many people during their first night of trying to sleep in unfamiliar surroundings (Agnew et al., 1966). This disruption is reflected in longer latencies to enter deeper sleep stages and persistence of alpha activity later into the sleep phase (Tamaki et al., 2005).

The first-night effect is also expressed asymmetrically in the two hemispheres, with signs of increased vigilance and reduced SWS intensity primarily in the left hemisphere during the night (Tamaki et al., 2016). This finding is discussed in

Sections 7.5.3 and 12.3.2. In some studies, researchers use an adaptation night to familiarize participants with the novel environment and then collect the actual experimental data on a second night, when the novelty effect is absent or at least minimized (Tamaki et al., 2005).

The opposite effect may also occur; sleep problems that patients experience in their home environments cannot always be reproduced in the laboratory. In these cases, the combination of isolation, quiet, and dark may promote better sleep in the laboratory than patients experience in what may be a less ideal sleep environment at home.

In many clinical and research settings, regularly absorbing the additional cost of an adaptation night may not be possible. There is therefore, increasing interest in finding ways to accurately measure sleep and related physiological processes in people in their usual home environments, using a minimum of instrumentation. The development of increasingly more compact and portable computers and sleep recording devices permits such studies in the home, at least for basic diagnostic tests. In addition to portable versions of traditional laboratory EEG-recording systems sold to clinicians and researchers, devices are being developed for the home consumer market, and this trend is likely to grow. One compact, home-based recording device, for example, combines several EEG placements and sensors for movement and heart-rate/respiration to achieve good concordance with PSG and sleep technician staging (Arnal et al., 2020).

While the approach of using home-based monitoring in some form can address issues such the first-night effect, it also has potential shortcomings. These include the absence of an attending sleep technologist to troubleshoot problems with data acquisition or recording quality during the night, the lack of complete physiological monitoring that is necessary for the identification of some sleep disorders and neurological conditions, and the risk that uncontrolled conditions in the home environment may affect the results. Thus, there is a trade-off between the benefits and limitations of studies conducted in naturalistic, but relatively uncontrolled, conditions in a familiar home environment and those conducted in the standardized and controlled, but unfamiliar, environment of a sleep laboratory.

2.6.3 Summary

Sleep staging emphasizes the distinct features of different parts of sleep periods and it serves important functions in communications about sleep among researchers and clinicians, and in the diagnosis of sleep disorders. There is a degree of continuity among NREM sleep stages, but each also has its distinct features. There is, however, a sharp discontinuity between NREM stages and REM sleep in both physiological features and regulatory mechanisms.

The combination of laboratory sleep studies and sleep staging in highly controlled environments is essential for the analysis of human sleep for clinical diagnostic purposes and for research studies. However, there are also limitations to this approach. The laboratory environment is very different from that in which patients and research participants normally sleep. As a result, the sleep quality observed may be either worse (e.g., first-night effect) or better (for those who normally sleep in suboptimal environments) than their habitual sleep. Home-based monitoring of sleep is one approach to addressing these issues but carries its own limitations.

2.7 Other methods of studying sleep

The use of a full PSG system to assess sleep in a laboratory remains the reference method for measuring sleep and is the only effective way to diagnose many sleep disorders (the gold standard method, as it is often described, even though gold is no longer a monetary standard). Another method that has been used extensively to estimate basic sleep parameters is actigraphy. This approach uses a small electronic device (an actigraph), typically shaped like a wristwatch and worn on the nondominant wrist (or elsewhere), to measure activity patterns using miniature accelerometers, which are sensitive to the acceleration associated with movement.

Movement data are downloaded to a computer, and software is used to estimate parameters such as time of sleep onset, sleep end, total sleep duration, and degree of sleep disruption. Actigraphy alone, however, is generally not useful for distinguishing sleep stages since gross motor pattern alone cannot discriminate all sleep stages, nor can it be used to detect symptoms of most sleep disorders.

There are several brands of research-quality actigraphs that use different proprietary software and hardware configurations, so each needs to be validated against PSG to determine how well it estimates sleep variables. Different methods of analyzing actigraphy data can generate systematically different results (e.g., Schoch et al., 2019). In addition, actigraphic analysis needs to be validated for each population being studied, because its validity may vary with age, medical conditions, and treatments. For example, actigraphy results correlated better with PSG measures in children with attention-deficit/hyperactivity disorder during treatment with methylphenidate than when they were unmedicated (Waldon et al., 2016).

Studies have found robust correlations between results obtained between specific actigraphs and PSG in estimating basic sleep parameters in healthy people (Ancoli-Israel et al., 2003), in people with sleep disorders (Littner et al., 2003),

BOX 2.2 Consumer Actigraphy

There has been a rapid proliferation of activity-based devices aimed at the consumer market (consumer wearables) that use proprietary (undisclosed) algorithms to assess sleep amounts and quality, and to try to measure sleep stages. Comparisons of results from PSG and several consumer wearables found discrepancies for some measures, but fairly good correlations for others; e.g., (de Zambotti et al., 2017; Mantua et al., 2016; Shambroom et al., 2012).

These devices are attractive in part because their wide distribution permits collection of massive amounts of home-based sleep data. Fitbit reported in 2018 on the sleep patterns of Americans which were determined using six *billion* sleep nights, based on activity data and other physiological measures (https://tinyurl.com/yskzz7r4). But as with other activity-based devices, there are limitations to the accuracy of such estimates (Meltzer et al., 2015). Developments such as the availability of a publicly accessible algorithm used to identify sleep stages (based on combining actigraphy, heart rate, and other data from an Apple Watch) could be advantageous in facilitating validation and comparison studies across laboratories and devices (Walch et al., 2019). A recent review discussed progress in the application of artificial intelligence to measure sleep recorded with consumer wearables (Djanian et al., 2022).

in patients with bipolar disorder (Kaplan et al., 2012), and in a mixed group of healthy controls and those with insomnia (see Section 4.4.5 for a definition of insomnia) (Marino et al., 2013). But studies also reported that actigraphy overestimated sleep duration and sleep efficiency (time spent asleep as a percentage of time in bed) in healthy adults and in children. Actigraphs are generally good at detecting sleep but are less accurate at identifying wake during the sleep period. Depending on the amount and pattern of activity shown during sleep in different populations, actigraphy may over- or underestimate wake episodes during sleep (Meltzer, Montgomery-Downs, et al., 2012; Meltzer, Walsh, et al., 2012; Pollak et al., 2001; Sitnick et al., 2008). Other measures, such as peripheral (wrist) temperature and body position, have been added to motion detection to improve correlations with PSG recordings (Ortiz-Tudela et al., 2014); see **Box 2.2**.

Actigraphy is a generally valid way to measure a limited number of sleep parameters, and it has many advantages, including low cost (relative to PSG studies), no first-night effect, feasibility of recording continuously over weeks, and the fact that recordings can be made in the usual sleep environment of the participant (Ancoli-Israel et al., 2003). Actigraphy is useful clinically for detecting abnormal timing of daily sleep periods and circadian rhythm abnormalities that can contribute to sleep problems. Actigraphy is also used in research studies to confirm stable baseline sleep timing for days before research participants enter a study, for which standard PSG recordings would not be feasible or affordable.

Another important tool used in many studies related to sleep is the Multiple Sleep Latency Test (MSLT). In this test, individuals first undergo a PSG study overnight. During the next day, they are tested 4 or 5 times at 2 h intervals to measure their latency to fall asleep. During each test, participants lie in a quiet, darkened bedroom for a maximum of 20 min while PSG is recorded. Participants are instructed to try to fall asleep or to not resist falling asleep. The latency to fall asleep during these tests reflects the degree of sleep drive: unusually short latencies are considered a sign of excess sleepiness, caused by a specific sleep disorder or by insufficient prior sleep (Carskadon et al., 1986; Sullivan & Kushida, 2008); see Section 13.2.2. For example, rapid sleep onset accompanied by short-latency entry into REM sleep are characteristic of patients with narcolepsy; see Section 11.3.2.

Adults with no sleep problems typically show average latencies to sleep onset of 10–20 min. Latencies of <5 min are associated with excessive daytime sleepiness and cognitive performance deficits, and latencies of 5–9 min are considered ambiguous. Onset latencies vary with age in healthy controls (Levine et al., 1988; Roehrs & Roth, 1992) and with age and gender in those being assessed clinically for excess sleepiness (Cairns et al., 2019). As for most physiological processes, sleep onset latency is also affected by the time of day at which naps are evaluated, with the shortest latencies observed in mid-afternoon (**Figure 2.11**) (Carskadon & Dement, 1992; Philip et al., 2012), a time corresponding roughly to the "post-lunch dip," during which adults in some societies nap spontaneously; see Sections 4.3 and 6.2.

A different approach to assessing daytime sleepiness is the Maintenance of Wakefulness Test, which measures how long people can *resist* falling asleep in a sleep-compatible environment over four spaced trials, rather than how quickly people can fall asleep when encouraged to do so (as in the MSLT) (Sullivan & Kushida, 2008).

2.7.1 Summary

Laboratory-based PSG studies do not allow assessment of sleep over long periods of time and during ordinary daily life. Actigraphy is a method based on motion detection that allows

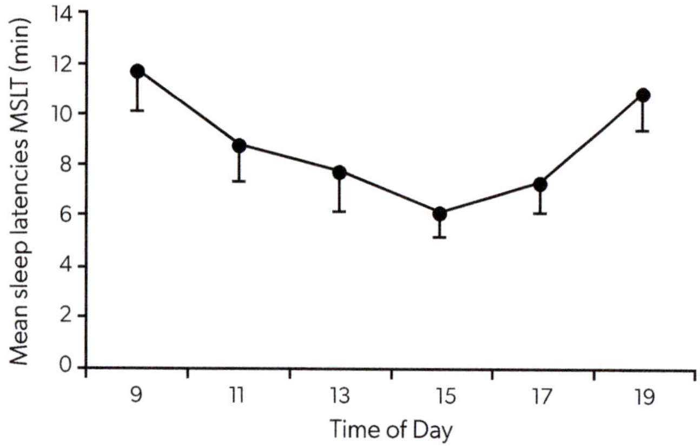

Figure 2.11 Healthy men aged 46–55 years were allowed a baseline sleep night with 8 h of time in bed (23:00–07:00). The next day they were tested for latency to fall asleep every 2 h after initial waking (Multiple Sleep Latency Tests; (MSLTs). The shortest sleep-onset latencies (Y axis) occurred at 15:00, indicating maximal daytime sleepiness at that phase. The increased alertness in the evening (19:00) would likely continue into the later "wake maintenance zone"; see Section 5.7.3.Reprinted with permission of Oxford University Press and the Sleep Research Society from Philip, P. et al. (2012) Acute versus chronic partial sleep deprivation in middle-aged people: differential effect on performance and sleepiness. *Sleep* 35:997–1002. © Sleep Research Society (2012). doi: 10.5665/sleep.1968.

continuous measurement in a noninvasive way for days or weeks at a time. Software programs are used to convert activity measures into estimates of sleep parameters, such as timing of sleep onset and end, total sleep duration, and stability of sleep. These estimates correspond well, but not perfectly, to those obtained by PSG, but the analysis methods need to be validated against PSG measurement for each type of device and for each population studied.

Actigraphy alone is not useful for sleep staging, but new methods involving additional measures, such as heart rate, body temperature, and heart-rate variability that can be obtained simultaneously, may allow such analyses in the future. Actigraphy is useful for obtaining estimates of major sleep parameters at low cost and over long periods of time, for diagnosing circadian rhythm abnormalities that affect sleep, and for documenting the baseline sleep patterns of patients or research participants before they are studied in the laboratory.

Other frequently used laboratory tests are the Multiple Sleep Latency Test and Maintenance of Wakefulness Test. These tests are used to detect abnormally short sleep onset latencies during the day, which may reflect a sleep disorder or habitual inadequate sleep.

Literature cited

Aboitiz, F., Montiel, J., Morales, D., & Concha, M. (2002). Evolutionary divergence of the reptilian and the mammalian brains: considerations on connectivity and development. *Brain Res Rev, 39*, 141–153.

Agnew, H. W., Webb, W. B., & Williams, R. L. (1966). The first night effect: an EEG study of sleep. *Psychophysiology, 2*(3), 263–266.

Ahmed, O. J., & Cash, S. S. (2013). Finding synchrony in the desynchronized EEG: the history and interpretation of gamma rhythms. *Front Integr Neurosci, 7*, 58. doi: 10.3389/fnint.2013.00058

Amzica, F., & Steriade, M. (1997). The K-complex: its slow (<1-Hz) rhythmicity and relation to delta waves. *Neurology, 49*(4), 952–959. doi: 10.1212/WNL.49.4.952

Ancoli-Israel, S., Cole, R., Alessi, C., Chambers, M., Moorcroft, W., & Pollak, C. P. (2003). The role of actigraphy in the study of sleep and circadian rhythms. *Sleep, 26*(3), 342–392.

Arnal, P. J., Thorey, V., Debellemaniere, E., Ballard, M. E., Bou Hernandez, A., Guillot, A., … Sauvet, F. (2020). The Dreem Headband compared to polysomnography for electroencephalographic signal acquisition and sleep staging. *Sleep, 43*(11), zsaa097. doi:10.1093/sleep/zsaa097

Bernardi, G., Betta, M., Ricciardi, E., Pietrini, P., Tononi, G., & Siclari, F. (2019). Regional delta waves In human rapid eye movement sleep. *J Neurosci, 39*(14), 2686–2697.

Brooks, A., & Lack, L. (2006). A brief afternoon nap following nocturnal sleep restriction: Which nap duration is most recuperative? *Sleep, 29*(6), 831–840.

Broughton, R. (1968). Sleep disorders: disorders of arousal? *Science, 159*(3819), 1070–1078.

Broughton, R., Valley, V., Aguirre, M., Roberts, J., Suwalski, W., & Dunham, W. (1986). Excessive daytime sleepiness and the pathophysiology of narcolepsy-cataplexy: a laboratory perspective. *Sleep, 9*(1), 205–215.

Buzsáki, G. (1998). Memory consolidation during sleep: a neurophysiological perspective. *J Sleep Res, 7*(Supplement 1), 17–23.

Buzsáki, G. (2015). Hippocampal sharp wave-ripple: a cognitive biomarker for episodic memory and planning. *Hippocampus, 25*, 1073–1188. doi: 0.1002/hipo.22488

Cairns, A., Trotti, L. M., & Bogan, R. (2019). Demographic and nap-related variance of the MSLT: results from 2,498 suspected hypersomnia patients. *Sleep Med, 55*, 115–123. doi: 10.1016/j.sleep.2018.12.013

Campbell, S. S., & Tobler, I. (1984). Animal sleep: a review of sleep duration across phylogeny. *Neurosci Biobehav Rev, 8*, 269–300.

Carskadon, M., & Dement, W. (1980). Distribution of REM sleep on a 90 minute sleep-wake schedule. *Sleep, 2*(3), 309–317.

Carskadon, M. A., & Dement, W. C. (1992). Multiple sleep latency tests during the constant routine. *Sleep, 15*, 396–399.

Carskadon, M. A., & Dement, W. C. (2011). Normal human sleep: an overview. In M. H. Kryger, T. Roth, & W. C. Dement (Eds.), *Principles and Practice of Sleep Medicine* (5th ed., pp. 16–26). St. Louis: Elsevier.

Carskadon, M. A., Dement, W. C., Mitler, M. M., Roth, T., Westbrook, P. R., & Keenan, S. (1986). Guidelines for the Multiple Sleep Latency Test (MSLT): a standard measure of sleepiness. *Sleep, 9*(4), 519–524.

Cash, S. S., Halgren, E., Dehghani, N., Rossetti, A. O., Thesen, T., Wang, C., … Ulbert, I. (2009). The human K-complex represents an isolated cortical down-state. *Science, 324*(5930), 1084–1087. doi: 10.1126/science.1169626

Chellappa, S. L., Frey, S., Knoblauch, V., & Cajochen, C. (2011). Cortical activation patterns herald successful dream recall after NREM and REM sleep. *Biol Psychol, 87*(2), 251–256. doi: 10.1016/j.biopsycho.2011.03.004

Cox, R., Schapiro, A. C., Manoach, D. S., & Stickgold, R. (2017). Individual differences in frequency and topography of slow and fast sleep spindles. *Front Hum Neurosci, 11*, 433. doi: 10.3389/fnhum.2017.00433

Csernai, M., Borbély, S., Kocsis, K., Burka, D., Fekete, Z., Balogh, V., … Barthó, P. (2019). Dynamics of sleep oscillations is coupled to brain temperature on multiple scales. *J Physiol, 597*(15), 4069–4086. doi: 10.1113/JP277664

Czeisler, C. A., Weitzman, E. D., Moore-Ede, M. C., Zimmerman, J. C., & Knauer, R. S. (1980). Human sleep: its duration and organization depend on its circadian phase. *Science, 210*, 1264–1267.

Czeisler, C. A., Zimmerman, J. C., Ronda, J. M., Moore-Ede, M. C., & Weitzman, E. D. (1980). Timing of REM sleep is coupled to the circadian rhythm of body temperature in man. *Sleep, 2*, 329–346.

Dallaire, A., Toutain, P.-L., & Ruckebusch, Y. (1974). Sur la périodicité du sommeil paradoxal: faits et hypothèses. *Physiol Behav, 13*, 395–400.

Datta, S. (1997). Cellular basis of pontine ponto-geniculo-occipital wave generation and modulation. *Cell Mol Neurobiol, 17*(3), 341–365.

Dement, W., & Kleitman, N. (1957). The relation of eye movements during sleep to dream activity: an objective method for the study of dreaming. *J Exp Psychol, 53*(5), 339–346.

de Zambotti, M., Rosas, L., Colrain, I. M., & Baker, F. C. (2017). The sleep of the ring: comparison of the OURA sleep tracker against polysomnography. *Behav Sleep Med, 17*(2), 124–136. doi: 10.1080/15402002.2017.1300587

Dijk, D. J., & Czeisler, C. A. (1995). Contribution of the circadian pacemaker and the sleep homeostat to sleep propensity, sleep structure, electroencephalographic slow waves, and sleep spindle activity in humans. *J Neurosci, 15*, 3526–3538.

Dinges, D. F. (1986). Differential effects of prior wakefulness and circadian phase on nap sleep. *Electroencephalogr Clin Neurophysiol, 64*(3), 224–227.

Djanian, S., Bruun, A., & Nielsen, T. D. (2022). Sleep classification using consumer sleep technologies and AI: a review of the current landscape. *Sleep Med, 100*, 390–403. doi: 10.1016/j.sleep.2022.09.004

Endo, S., Kobayashi, T., Yamamoto, T., Fukuda, H., Sasaki, M., & Ohta, T. (1981). Persistence of the circadian rhythm of REM sleep: a variety of experimental manipulations of the sleep-wake cycle. *Sleep, 4*(3), 319–328.

Ermis, U., Krakow, K., & Voss, U. (2010). Arousal thresholds during human tonic and phasic REM sleep. *J Sleep Res, 19*(3), 400–406. doi: 10.1111/j.1365-2869.2010.00831.x

Fisher, C., Cohen, H. D., Schiavi, R. C., Davis, D., Furman, B., Ward, K., ... Cunningham, J. (1983). Patterns of female sexual arousal during sleep and waking: vaginal thermo-conductance studies. *Arch Sex Behav, 12*(2), 97–122.

Fisher, C., Gross, J., & Zuch, J. (1965). Cycle of penile erection synchronous with dreaming (REM) sleep. *Arch Gen Psychiatr, 12*(1), 29–45.

Foulkes, W. D. (1962). Dream reports from different stages of sleep. *J Abnorm Soc Psychol, 65*(1), 14–25.

Glotzbach, S. F., & Heller, H. (1976). Central nervous regulation of body temperature during sleep. *Science, 194*(4264), 537–539.

Gonzalez, C. E., Mak-McCully, R. A., Rosen, B. Q., Cash, S. S., Chauvel, P. Y., Bastuji, H., ... Halgren, E. (2018). Theta bursts precede, and spindles follow, cortical and thalamic downstates in human NREM sleep. *J Neurosci, 38*(46), 9989–10001. doi: 10.1523/JNEUROSCI.0476-18.2018

Gorgoni, M., Ferrara, M., D'Atri, A., Lauri, G., Scarpelli, S., Truglia, I., & De Gennaro, L. (2015). EEG topography during sleep inertia upon awakening after a period of increased homeostatic sleep pressure. *Sleep Med, 16*(7), 883–890. doi: 10.1016/j.sleep.2015.03.009

Gott, J. A., Liley, D. T., & Hobson, J. A. (2017). Towards a functional understanding of PGO waves. *Front Hum Neurosci, 11*, 89. doi: 10.3389/fnhum.2017.00089

Grigg-Damberger, M. M., Gozal, D., Marcus, C. L., Quan, S. F., Rosen, C. L., Chervin, R. D., ... Iber, C. (2007). The visual scoring of sleep and arousal in infants and children. *J Clin Sleep Med, 3*(2), 201–240.

Halász, P. (2005). K-complex, a reactive EEG graphoelement of NREM sleep: an old chap in a new garment. *Sleep Med Rev, 9*(5), 391–412. doi: 10.1016/j.smrv.2005.04.003

Hilditch, C. J., & McHill, A. W. (2019). Sleep inertia: current insights. *Nat Sci Sleep, 11*, 155–165. doi: 10.2147/nss.S188911

Hirshkowitz, M., & Schmidt, M. H. (2005). Sleep-related erections: clinical perspectives and neural mechanisms. *Sleep Med Rev, 9*(4), 311–329. doi: 10.1016/j.smrv.2005.03.001

Hobson, J. A., Pace-Schott, E. F., & Stickgold, R. (2000). Dreaming and the brain: toward a cognitive neuroscience of conscious states. *Behav Brain Sci, 23*, 793–842.

Ikeda, H., & Hayashi, M. (2010). The effect of self-awakening from nocturnal sleep on sleep inertia. *Biol Psychol, 83*(1), 15–19. doi: 10.1016/j.biopsycho.2009.09.008

Jouvet, M., Michel, F., & Courjon, J. (1959). Sur un stade d'activité cérébrale rapide au cours du sommeil physiologique. *C R Séances Soc Biologie Fil, 153*, 1024–1028.

Kaplan, K. A., Talbot, L. S., Gruber, J., & Harvey, A. G. (2012). Evaluating sleep in bipolar disorder: comparison between actigraphy, polysomnography, and sleep diary. *Bipolar Disord, 14*(8), 870–879. doi: 10.1111/bdi.12021

Keenan, S., & Hirshkowitz, M. (2005). Monitoring and staging human sleep. In M. H. Kryger, T. Roth, & W. C. Dement (Eds.), *Principles and Practice of Sleep Medicine* (5th ed., pp. 1602–1609). St. Louis: Elsevier.

Kirschstein, T., & Köhling, R. (2009). What is the source of the EEG? *Clin EEG Neurosci, 40*(3), 146–149.

Klein, R., & Armitage, R. (1979). Rhythms in human performance: 11/2-hour oscillations in cognitive style. *Science, 204*, 1326–1328.

Kleitman, N. (1982). Basic rest-activity cycle–22 years later. *Sleep, 5*(4), 311–317.

Kupfer, D. J. (1976). REM latency: a psychobiologic marker for primary depressive disease. *Biol Psychiatry, 11*, 159–174.

Lavie, P. (1980). Ultradian rhythmicity (circa 90 min) in physiologic processes–evidence for multioscillatory phenomena. *J Interdiscipl Cycle Res, 11*, 171–177.

Lechat, B., Hirotsu, C., Appleton, S., Younes, M., Adams, R. J., Vakulin, A., ... Eckert, D. J. (2022). A novel EEG marker predicts perceived sleepiness and poor sleep quality. *Sleep, 45*(5), zsac051. doi:10.1093/sleep/zsac051

Levine, B., Roehrs, T., Zorick, F., & Roth, T. (1988). Daytime sleepiness in young adults. *Sleep, 11*(1), 39–46.

Lim, A., Lozano, A., Moro, E., Hamani, C., Hutchison, W., Dostrovsky, J., ... Murray, B. (2007). Characterization of REM-sleep associated ponto-geniculo-occipital waves in the human pons. *Sleep, 30*(7), 823–827.

Littner, M. R., Kushida, C. A., Anderson, W. M., Bailey, D., Berry, R. B., Davila, D. G., ... Johnson, S. F. (2003). Practice parameters for the role of actigraphy in the study of sleep and circadian rhythms: an update for 2002. *Sleep, 26*(3), 337–341.

Mak-McCully, R. A., Rosen, B. Q., Rolland, M., Regis, J., Bartolomei, F., Rey, M., ... Halgren, E. (2015). Distribution, amplitude, incidence, co-occurrence, and propagation of human K-complexes in focal transcortical recordings. *eNeuro, 2*(4). doi: 10.1523/ENEURO.0028-15.2015

Mantua, J., Gravel, N., & Spencer, R. M. (2016). Reliability of sleep measures from four personal health monitoring devices compared to research-based actigraphy and polysomnography. *Sensors (Basel), 16*(5), 646. doi: 10.3390/s16050646

Marino, M., Li, Y., Rueschman, M. N., Winkelman, J. W., Ellenbogen, J. M., Solet, J. M., ... Buxton, O. M. (2013). Measuring sleep: accuracy, sensitivity, and specificity of wrist actigraphy compared to polysomnography. *Sleep, 36*(11), 1747–1755. doi: 10.5665/sleep.3142

Martelli, D., Luppi, M., Cerri, M., Tupone, D., Mastrotto, M., Perez, E., ... Amici, R. (2014). The direct cooling of the preoptic-hypothalamic area elicits the release of thyroid stimulating hormone during wakefulness but not during REM sleep. *PLoS One, 9*(2), e87793. doi: 10.1371/journal.pone.0087793

Massimini, M., Huber, R., Ferrarelli, F., Hill, S., & Tononi, G. (2004). The sleep slow oscillation as a traveling wave. *J Neurosci, 24*(31), 6862–6870. doi: 10.1523/JNEUROSCI.1318-04.2004

Mathur, R., & Douglas, N. J. (1995). Frequency of EEG arousals from nocturnal sleep in normal subjects. *Sleep, 18*(5), 330–333.

McCormick, L., Nielsen, T., Nicolas, A., Ptito, M., & Montplaisir, J. (1997). Topographical distribution of spindles and K-complexes in normal subjects. *Sleep, 20*(11), 939–941.

McHill, A. W., Hull, J. T., Cohen, D. A., Wang, W., Czeisler, C. A., & Klerman, E. B. (2019). Chronic sleep restriction greatly magnifies performance decrements immediately after awakening. *Sleep, 42*(5), zsz032. doi: 10.1093/sleep/zsz032

Meltzer, L. J., Hiruma, L. S., Avis, K., Montgomery-Downs, H., & Valentin, J. (2015). Comparison of a commercial accelerometer with polysomnography and actigraphy in children and adolescents. *Sleep, 38*(8), 1323–1330. doi: 10.5665/sleep.4918

Meltzer, L. J., Montgomery-Downs, H. E., Insana, S. P., & Walsh, C. M. (2012). Use of actigraphy for assessment in pediatric sleep research. *Sleep Med Rev, 16*(5), 463–475. doi: 10.1016/j.smrv.2011.10.002

Meltzer, L. J., Walsh, C. M., Traylor, J., & Westin, A. M. (2012). Direct comparison of two new actigraphs and polysomnography in children and adolescents. *Sleep, 35*(1), 159–166. doi: 10.5665/sleep.1608

Merica, H., & Gaillard, J.-M. (1992). The EEG of the sleep onset period in insomnia: a discriminant analysis. *Physiol Behav, 52*, 199–204.

Mölle, M., Bergmann, T. O., Marshall, L., & Born, J. (2011). Fast and slow spindles during the sleep slow oscillation: disparate coalescence and engagement in memory processing. *Sleep, 34*(10), 1411–1421.

Nelson, J. P., McCarley, R. W., & Hobson, J. A. (1983). REM sleep burst neurons, PGO waves, and eye movement information. *J Neurophysiol, 50*, 784–797.

Nielsen, T. A. (1999). Mentation during sleep: the NREM/REM distinction. In R. Lydic & H. A. Baghdoyan (Eds.), *Handbook of Behavioral State Control: Cellular and Molecular Mechanisms* (pp. 101–128). Boca Raton: CRC Press.

Nielsen, T. A. (2000). A review of mentation in REM and NREM sleep: "covert" REM sleep as a possible reconciliation of two opposing models. *Behav Brain Sci, 23*(6), 851–866. doi: 10.1017/s0140525x0000399x

Ortiz-Tudela, E., Martinez-Nicolas, A., Albares, J., Segarra, F., Campos, M., Estivill, E., ... Madrid, J. A. (2014). Ambulatory circadian monitoring (ACM) based on thermometry, motor activity and body position (TAP): a comparison with polysomnography. *Physiol Behav, 126*, 30–38. doi: 10.1016/j.physbeh.2013.12.009

Oswald, I., Merrington, J., & Lewis, H. (1970). Cyclic "on demand" oral intake by adults. *Nature, 225*, 959–960.

Parmeggiani, P. L. (2007). REM sleep related increase in brain temperature: a physiologic problem. *Arch Ital Biol, 145,* 13–21.

Philip, P., Sagaspe, P., Prague, M., Tassi, P., Capelli, A., Bioulac, B., ... Taillard, J. (2012). Acute versus chronic partial sleep deprivation in middle-aged people: differential effect on performance and sleepiness. *Sleep, 35*(7), 997–1002. doi: 10.5665/sleep.1968

Pollak, C. P., Tryon, W. W., Nagaraja, H., & Dzwonczyk, R. (2001). How accurately does wrist actigraphy identify the states of sleep and wakefulness? *Sleep, 24*(8), 957–965.

Price, L. J., & Kremen, I. (1980). Variations in behavioral response threshold within the REM period of human sleep. *Psychophysiology, 17,* 133–140.

Rechtschaffen, A., & Kales, A. (Eds.). (1968). *A Manual of Standardized Terminology, Techniques and Scoring System for Sleep Stages of Human Subjects.* Washington, DC: Public Health Service, US Government Printing Office, National Institutes of Health Publication No. 204.

Roehrs, T., & Roth, T. (1992). Multiple Sleep Latency Test: technical aspects and normal values. *J Clin Neurophysiol,* 9(1), 63–67.

Schabus, M., Hödlmoser, K., Gruber, G., Sauter, C., Anderer, P., Klösch, G., ... Zeitlhofer, J. (2006). Sleep spindle-related activity in the human EEG and its relation to general cognitive and learning abilities. *Eur J Neurosci, 23*(7), 1738–1746. doi: 10.1111/j.1460-9568.2006.04694.x

Scheer, F. A., Shea, T. J., Hilton, M. F., & Shea, S. A. (2008). An endogenous circadian rhythm in sleep inertia results in greatest cognitive impairment upon awakening during the biological night. *J Biol Rhythms, 23*(4), 353–361. doi: 10.1177/0748730408318081

Schoch, S. F., Jenni, O. G., Kohler, M., & Kurth, S. (2019). Actimetry in infant sleep research: an approach to facilitate comparability. *Sleep, 42*(7), zsz083. doi:10.1093/sleep/zsz083

Schulz, H. (2008). Rethinking sleep analysis. *J Clin Sleep Med, 4*(2), 99–103.

Schulz, H., Dirlich, G., & Zulley, J. (1975). Phase shift in the REM sleep rhythm. *Pflügers Archiv, 358,* 203–212.

Shambroom, J. R., Fabregas, S. E., & Johnstone, J. (2012). Validation of an automated wireless system to monitor sleep in healthy adults. *J Sleep Res, 21*(2), 221–230. doi: 10.1111/j.1365-2869.2011.00944.x

Shannahof-Khalsa, D. S., Gillin, J. C., Yates, F. E., Schlosser, A., & Zawadzki, E. M. (2001). Ultradian rhythms of alternating cerebral hemispheric EEG dominance are coupled to rapid eye movement and non-rapid eye movement stage 4 sleep in humans. *Sleep Med, 2,* 333–346.

Siapas, A., & Wilson, M. (1998). Coordinated interactions between hippocampal ripples and cortical spindles during slow-wave sleep. *Neuron, 21,* 1123–1128.

Siclari, F., Bernardi, G., Riedner, B. A., LaRocque, J. J., Benca, R. M., & Tononi, G. (2014). Two distinct synchronization processes in the transition to sleep: a high-density electroencephalographic study. *Sleep, 37*(10), 1621–1637. doi: 10.5665/sleep.4070

Silber, M. H., Ancoli-Israel, S., Bonnet, M. H., Chokroverty, S., Grigg-Damberger, M. M., Hirshkowitz, M., ... Iber, C. (2007). The visual scoring of sleep in adults. *J Clin Sleep Med, 3*(2), 121–131.

Sitnick, S. L., Goodlin-Jones, B. L., & Anders, T. F. (2008). The use of actigraphy to study sleep disorders in preschoolers: some concerns about detection of nighttime awakenings. *Sleep 31*(3), 395–401.

Smith, M. R., Antrobus, J. S., Gordon, E., Tucker, M. A., Hirota, Y., Wamsley, E. J., ... Emery, R. N. (2004). Motivation and affect in REM sleep and the mentation reporting process. *Conscious Cogn, 13*(3), 501–511. doi: 10.1016/j.concog.2004.03.002

Sorensen, G. L., Knudsen, S., & Jennum, P. (2013). Sleep transitions in hypocretin-deficient narcolepsy. *Sleep, 36*(8), 1173–1177. doi: 10.5665/sleep.2880

Steriade, M. (1994). Sleep oscillations and their blockage by activating systems. *J Psychiatr Neurosci, 19*(5), 354–358.

Steriade, M., Amzica, F., & Contreras, D. (1996). Synchronization of fast (30–40 Hz) spontaneous cortical rhythms during brain activation. *J Neurosci, 16,* 392–417.

Steriade, M., Nuñez, A., & Amzica, F. (1993a). Intracellular analysis of relations between the slow (<1 Hz) neocortical oscillation and other sleep rhythms of the electroencephalogram. *J Neurosci, 13*(8), 3266–3283.

Steriade, M., Nuñez, A., & Amzica, F. (1993b). A novel slow (<1 Hz) oscillation of neocortical neurons in vivo: depolarizing and hyperpolarizing components. *J Neurosci, 13*(8), 3252–3265.

Sullivan, S. S., & Kushida, C. A. (2008). Multiple Sleep Latency Test and Maintenance of Wakefulness Test. *Chest, 134*(4), 854–861. doi: 10.1378/chest.08-0822

Takeuchi, T., Miyasita, A., Inugami, M., & Yamamoto, Y. (2001). Intrinsic dreams are not produced without REM sleep mechanisms: evidence through elicitation of sleep onset REM periods. *J Sleep Res, 10,* 43–52.

Tamaki, M., Bang, J. W., Watanabe, T., & Sasaki, Y. (2016). Night watch in one brain hemisphere during sleep associated with the first-night effect in humans. *Curr Biol, 26*(9), 1190–1194. doi: 10.1016/j.cub.2016.02.063

Tamaki, M., Nittono, H., Hayashi, M., & Hori, T. (2005). Examination of the first-night effect during the sleep-onset period. *Sleep, 28*(2), 195–202.

Tassi, P., & Muzet, A. (2000). Sleep inertia. *Sleep Med Rev, 4*(4), 341–353. doi: 10.1053/smrv.2000.0098

Tobler, I. (1995). Is sleep fundamentally different between mammalian species? *Behav Brain Res, 69*(1–2), 35–41.

Trotti, L. M. (2017). Waking up is the hardest thing I do all day: sleep inertia and sleep drunkenness. *Sleep Med Rev, 35,* 76–84. doi: 10.1016/j.smrv.2016.08.005

van Driel, M. F. (2014). Sleep-related erections throughout the ages. *J Sex Med, 11*(7), 1867–1875. doi: 10.1111/jsm.12557

Walch, O., Huang, Y., Forger, D., & Goldstein, C. (2019). Sleep stage prediction with raw acceleration and photoplethysmography heart rate data derived from a consumer wearable device. *Sleep, 42*(12), 1–19. doi: 10.1093/sleep/zsz180/5549536

Waldon, J., Begum, E., Gendron, M., Rusak, B., Andreou, P., Rajda, M., & Corkum, P. (2016). Concordance of actigraphy with polysomnography in children with and without attention-deficit/hyperactivity disorder. *J Sleep Res, 25*(5), 524–533. doi: 10.1111/jsr.12402

Webb, W. B., & Agnew, H. W., Jr. (1971). Stage 4 sleep: Influence of time course variables. *Science, 174*(4016), 1354–1356.

Williams, H. L., Hammack, J. T., Daly, R. L., Dement, W. C., & Lubin, A. (1964). Responses to auditory stimulation, sleep loss and the EEG stages of sleep. *Electroencephalogr Clin Neurophysiol, 16,* 269–279.

Wilson, M. A., & McNaughton, B. L. (1994). Reactivation of hippocampal ensemble memories during sleep. *Science, 265,* 676–679.

Wurts, S. W., & Edgar, D. M. (2000). Circadian and homeostatic control of rapid eye movement (REM) sleep: promotion of REM tendency by the suprachiasmatic nucleus. *J Neurosci, 20*(11), 4300–4310.

Younes, M., Ostrowski, M., Soiferman, M., Younes, H., Younes, M., Raneri, J., & Hanly, P. (2015). Odds ratio product of sleep EEG as a continuous measure of sleep state. *Sleep, 38*(4), 641–654. doi: 10.5665/sleep.4588

CHAPTER 3

History and Methods of Circadian Rhythms Research

3.1 OVERVIEW

Daily (circadian) rhythms play several important roles in the regulation of sleep and waking. This chapter introduces the core historical observations that led to an understanding of the mechanisms that produce daily rhythms. It also introduces the laboratory methods that are used currently in circadian rhythms research, with a focus on those that are relevant to understanding how circadian rhythms influence human sleep. Finally, it discusses the impact of laboratory conditions on the expression of circadian rhythms.

3.2 A short history of circadian rhythms research

3.2.1 External vs. internal sources of rhythms

For as long as humans have been aware of their own sleep-wake cycles, they have also been aware of other daily rhythms in their behavior and in the behavior of other organisms. For example, Psalm 104 in the King James version of the Bible, written several millennia ago and attributed to the Hebrew king David, refers to daily rhythms in both animals and people. It describes how nightfall triggers the beasts of the forest to emerge and actively seek their prey, but when the sun rises, "they gather themselves together, and lay them down in their dens. Man goeth forth unto his work and to his labor until the evening."

This short passage reflects an awareness of several essential facts: that animals and people show daily rhythms in behavior; that some species are day-active (diurnal) and others night-active (nocturnal); and that these rhythms are linked to, and triggered by, the cycle of day and night. As discussed in more detail in Chapters 5, 8, and 9, the mechanisms that regulate the daily behavioral rhythms described in this psalm also play a key role in regulating sleep. It was many centuries after these verses were written, however, before the first steps were taken that led to an understanding of the sources of daily rhythms and how they are connected to the cycle of day and night.

The first report usually cited as opening the way to scientific research on daily rhythms involved a study of what were then called the "sleep movements" of plants. These rhythmic, daily leaf movements are readily observed in many plants, including the common household "prayer plant" (*Maranta leuconeura*), which flattens its leaves during the day to face toward the sun and folds them closed during the night (https://vimeo.com/5460429).

Research related to these movements in another species, the "sensitive plant" (*Mimosa pudica*) provided the first evidence that led to identifying one of the two principal regulatory mechanisms that control human sleep. Jean-Jacques d'Ortous de Mairan, a French astronomer, reported in 1729 to the *Académie française* the results of a study in which he placed these plants in a darkened location for an extended period without access to external lighting and looked in periodically to determine the position of the leaves. He reported that the leaves continued to move up and down in synchrony with the external day–night cycle, to which the plants were not exposed. de Mairan concluded (in translation) that the sensitive plant "senses the sun without seeing it in any way" (de Mairan, 1729).

This conclusion implied that the plants retained the ability to track the time of day and the sun's daily cycles without being exposed to the lighting changes that occur during day and night. This was a revolutionary idea, since people had assumed that it was the cycle of light and dark that cued the daily rhythms shown by people, animals, and plants. Yet de Mairan's observation suggested that these plants could sense, and be synchronized by, a different, unknown correlate of the day–night cycle.

This phenomenon was studied by others, and about a century later Augustin Pyramus de Candolle, a Swiss botanist, repeated de Mairan's study while maintaining the mimosa plants in constant light, rather than constant darkness. He confirmed that daily leaf movements continued rhythmically without exposure to an external light-dark cycle. But he found that the rhythm of these leaf movements had changed so that the cycle length (period) was not 24 h, but about 2 h shorter. Although the cycles of leaf movements continued, they drifted out of synchrony with the (unseen) external cycle of day and night because of their non-24 h periods (de Candolle, 1832).

This finding could not be explained by the ability of plants to detect the sun's cycles using a subtle, non-light cue, as de Mairan's conclusion implied ("sensing the unseen sun"). The plants' non-24 h rhythms were clearly no longer linked to the 24 h solar-day cycle, yet they persisted.

By the early 20th century, plant biologists demonstrated conclusively that plants generated near-24 h rhythms in the absence of external time cues and that these rhythms did not depend on subtle environmental cycles (Bünning, 1960). Since the periodicity of the leaf movements corresponded neither to the day–night cycle nor to any other external cycle, the only possible source for these rhythms was the internal physiology of the plants.

Studies of animal daily rhythms in the early 20th century led to the same conclusion. The American psychologist Curt Richter recorded the rhythms of rats using an automated running-wheel apparatus. He demonstrated robust activity rhythms in blinded rats that continued for months in the absence of external time cues, even though they were not synchronized to any external cycle (see e.g., Richter, 1971). The German scientists Hans Kalmus and Erwin Bünning demonstrated in 1935 that the daily emergence rhythms of adult fruit flies from their pupae persisted under constant environmental conditions with periods that deviated from 24 h (for these results and related references, see Bünning, 1960).

Maynard Johnson, an American studying the behavior of white-footed mice (*Peromyscus leucopus*), observed that the period of the activity rhythms generated by these mice changed systematically in response to changes in the intensity of the constant lighting to which they were exposed. These results hinted at the mechanism by which these rhythms can become linked to the day–night cycle (see Chapter 8). He concluded that "the animal has an exceptionally substantial and durable self-winding and self-regulating physiological clock, the mechanism of which remains to be worked out" (Johnson, 1939, p. 326).

3.2.2 Circadian rhythms

The Romanian physician and chronobiologist (a term he coined, meaning "time biologist") Franz Halberg later gave the output of this physiological clock the name by which it is now commonly known. He joined the Latin words for about (*circa*) and a day (*dies*) to generate the word "circadian" to describe rhythms that express periods *near* 24 h in length in the absence of external time cues (Halberg et al., 1959). The accumulated evidence demonstrated clearly that animals, plants, and other organisms generate circadian rhythms internally, using one or more physiological clocks (also called circadian oscillators; **Figure 3.1**).

After the rather slow accumulation of knowledge of circadian rhythms from the 18th to the early 20th century, research on these rhythms accelerated in the 1950s and led to the development of a body of knowledge describing the fundamental principles on which circadian clocks operate; these were summarized, for example, in a landmark meeting, the proceedings of which were published in 1960 (Chovnick, 1960).

This growth accelerated even more during the 1970s, in association with the explosive growth of the fields of neuroscience and molecular biology that began then and continues today. The tools and concepts developed in these fields strongly influenced research on circadian rhythms. There was a focus on identifying and analyzing the neural structures in animals

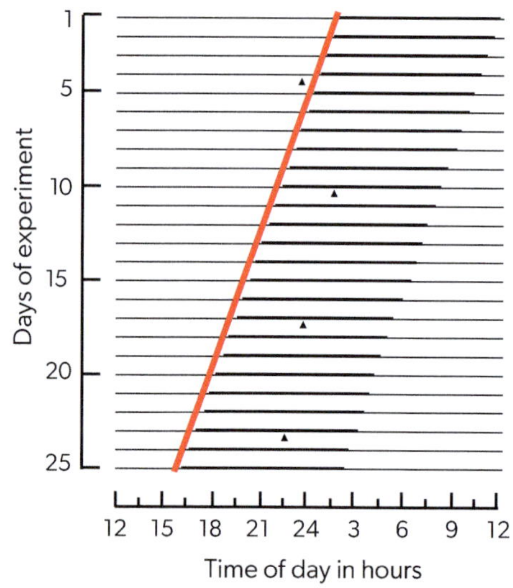

Figure 3.1 A. A record of the free-running activity rhythm of a Northern flying squirrel (*Glaucomys volans*) over 25 days in constant darkness. Each 24 h period (12:00–12:00) is plotted below the previous 24 h period (Y axis). The thick dark lines represent pen movements caused by the rotation of an activity wheel, and the red line represents an estimate of the free-running period based on the timing of successive activity onsets. The squirrel free-ran with a period that was slightly shorter than 24.0 h, so it began activity earlier every day, relative to external time of day (X axis). Adapted with permission from DeCoursey, P. J. (1960) Phase control of activity in a rodent. In: A. Chovnick (Ed.), *Biological Clocks, Cold Spring Harbor Symposia on Quantitative Biology*, Vol. XXV, pp. 49–55. Cold Spring Harbor. © Cold Spring Harbor Laboratory Press (1960).

that are responsible for generating circadian rhythms (Rusak & Zucker, 1979) as well as identifying the genetic and molecular mechanisms that are involved in making the internal circadian clock tick (Takahashi, 1995).[1]

The study of circadian physiology is now an active and diverse field of research, only a portion of which touches on the regulation of sleep. Although research on circadian rhythms began with investigations into "sleep" movements in plants, the fields of (mammalian) sleep and circadian rhythms research evolved relatively independently of each other at first (with several important exceptions, such as Jürgen Aschoff; see Section 3.5). But there are now large areas of intellectual overlap between these fields. There is increasing recognition that a full understanding of the regulation and physiology of both human sleep and circadian rhythms requires knowledge of at least the fundamental principles and core information in both fields. For example, in recent years, the US-based Sleep Research Society added the phrase "*Advancing Sleep and Circadian Science*" to its logo.

The connections between mechanisms that regulate sleep and circadian rhythms are reflected in many parts of this volume, but several chapters address circadian rhythms in more detail. Chapter 5 reviews evidence for the important role of circadian rhythms in the regulation of sleep, arousal, and performance. Chapter 8 discusses the involvement of the principal mammalian circadian clock, the suprachiasmatic nucleus (SCN), in the physiology of sleep-wake regulation, especially as it changes during aging. Chapter 9 discusses the involvement in sleep regulation of other components of the vertebrate circadian system; namely, the pineal gland and its hormone product melatonin, which are closely tied to the SCN.

3.2.3 Summary

Early references to daily rhythms in animals and people implied that the rising and setting of the sun triggered the behavioral changes that produced diurnal and nocturnal activity patterns in different species. In the 18th and 19th centuries, studies of plants demonstrated, however, that they did not rely on external lighting cycles, but generated rhythms internally that became desynchronized from the day–night cycle when they were housed under constant lighting conditions.

Later research confirmed these findings in species ranging from single-celled organisms to multicellular plants, fungi, animals, and people. Daily rhythms in the physiology and behavior of most living organisms were shown to be organized by internal circadian clocks that generate stable, near-24 h rhythms in the absence of rhythmic cues in the environment. The circadian system plays important roles in the regulation of several aspects of sleep, which are discussed in later chapters.

[1] Molecular and genetic research on circadian mechanisms led to a Nobel Prize being awarded to Jeff Hall, Michael Rosbash, and Michael Young in 2017 for their discovery of the basic molecular components inside cells that are responsible for circadian rhythm generation (see **Box 8.1** in Section 8.2.2).

3.3 Studying circadian rhythms

Many different methods are used to study circadian rhythms because they are found in virtually every measurable physiological and behavioral parameter and in species as different as single-celled plants and humans. Historically, methods used to study rhythms in vertebrates included recording rhythms of locomotor activity (e.g., wheel-running in rodents, perch-hopping in small birds, actigraphy in people), food or water intake, body temperature, and sleep-wake cycles.

Newer methods include molecular-based techniques for the measurement of rhythms in various plant or animal tissues. For example, organisms can be genetically engineered to link a circadian clock gene to activation of a fluorescent reporter protein or an enzyme, and light detectors can then be used to study rhythmic expression of that gene in tissues in vitro or even in a freely moving intact animal (Yamaguchi et al., 2016). The following summary is limited to reviewing the basic principles of conducting research on circadian rhythms, and the methods used in studies that are most closely related to the regulation of sleep in people.

3.3.1 Free-running and entrained rhythms

Circadian rhythms are endogenously (internally) generated cycles of behavior and physiology that express periods in constant conditions (i.e., in the absence of external time cues) near 24 h. In constant conditions, these rhythms are described as free-running (DeCoursey, 1960). Circadian rhythm periods measured in constant conditions vary among species, among individuals within a species, and systematically at different constant light intensity levels, but they remain clustered near 24 h. The fact that these rhythms persist in the absence of environmental time cues is the key evidence that there is an internal clock capable of keeping track of near-24 h time for living organisms.

In the presence of external time cues, any daily rhythm observed might be the product of an internal clock or it might be a direct response to environmental stimuli. In laboratories in which the circadian rhythms of plants, fungi, animals, or people are studied, environmental controls are quite strict, with external light completely excluded, temperature kept stable, and other factors (e.g., humidity) held within narrow limits. Only under such conditions can the function of the internal clock be studied independently of external cycles and without disturbance from unpredictable environmental events. The resulting isolation also permits controlled studies of the effects of external inputs on the circadian system. For example, laboratory studies of how light affects the internal clock can include manipulating the timing, intensity, wavelength, and duration of acute light exposure against a background of continuous darkness.

As suggested by the previously quoted psalm, however, daily rhythms in the natural world do not normally free-run with a near-24 h periodicity. Internal clocks are usually synchronized to the external 24 h cycle of day and night, the most obvious feature of which is the change in light availability and intensity. Expressing physiological and behavioral rhythms that are appropriately timed relative to the day–night cycle thus depends on two distinct steps: the internal generation of an approximately 24 h rhythm and the synchronization of that rhythm to an external cycle. By analogy with the term used in physics to describe the synchronization of two physical oscillators, the latter process is called *entrainment*. In biology, this term refers to control by an external cycle of both the period and the phase of an endogenously generated rhythm. The entraining cycle is usually referred to as a *zeitgeber*, a German word meaning "time giver."

The period control component of the definition of entrainment is demonstrated when the free-running (non-24 h) period of the internal clock is changed in the presence of an external cycle to match the period of that cycle. The external cycle has a period of 24 h in the natural world but may be any similar value (e.g., 23.0 or 24.5 h) in a laboratory in which artificial lighting cycles can be produced with different period lengths. Phase control is demonstrated by the circadian rhythm adopting and then maintaining a stable timing relation to the zeitgeber cycle (e.g., awakening daily at a consistent phase of the lighting cycle) (**Figure 3.2, top**).

The term "entrainment" implies more than simple synchrony between two rhythms. To test whether an external cycle is entraining an organism's rhythm, it is important to first check whether the free-running period happens to be identical to that of the imposed cycle. For example, the free-running period of the activity rhythm shown by the flying squirrel in **Figure 3.1** was ~23.6 h, but the sample of squirrels studied included the range of 22.96 to 24.35 h periods, so some might produce rhythms indistinguishable from 24.0 h. An animal with an exact 24.0 h rhythm could, in principle, maintain synchrony with a fixed 24.0 h external cycle without being entrained by it. Another potential issue is that an animal might appear to be entrained to an imposed lighting cycle but might actually be responding to a different stimulus in the environment, for example, disturbance resulting from a person entering the room or giving it access to food at the same time every day.

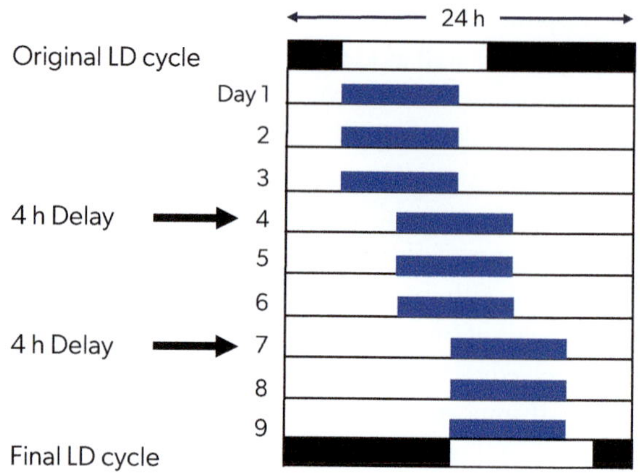

Figure 3.2 This model of re-entrainment shows the daily activity rhythm of a diurnal animal as a blue rectangle during a series of nine 24 h periods (Y axis) running from top to bottom. The daily light phase is shown as a white bar in the original light–dark (LD) cycle at the top of the figure. The animal's activity shows a 24 h rhythm with onset shortly after the beginning of the light phase, illustrating period control by the lighting cycle. On Day 4, the timing of the light phase is delayed by 4 h, and is delayed again by 4 h on Day 7, resulting in the final LD cycle shown at the bottom of the figure. After each shift of the lighting cycle, the animal becomes resynchronized to the new LD cycle and reestablishes the original phase relation to it. These results illustrate that both the period and phase of the animal's activity rhythm are being controlled by the 24 h lighting cycle, which meets the definition of entrainment. As illustrated in **Figure 3.3**, phase shifts may be either immediate, as shown here, or may involve one or more transient cycles before the phase shift is completed.

The simplest way to determine whether an external lighting cycle is entraining an animal in the laboratory is to shift the timing of that cycle by several hours (phase shift) while holding everything else constant. If the rhythm's stable phase relation to the lighting cycle were coincidental or caused by another cue, a change in the lighting cycle should have no effect on the rhythm. In almost all cases, however, a shift in the lighting cycle is followed by a corresponding shift in the entrained rhythm, which then reestablishes its previous phase relation to the lighting cycle (i.e., it re-entrains) (**Figure 3.2**).

A phase shift of the zeitgeber cycle followed by re-entrainment of the animal's rhythm shows that the external cycle controlled the phase of the internally generated rhythm. This kind of study is analogous to a person traveling rapidly across multiple time zones and experiencing a new lighting cycle. The advance shift shown at the bottom of **Figure 3.3** illustrates that re-entrainment can be gradual, so a jet traveler might experience the uncomfortable symptoms of jet lag for several days while they gradually re-entrain their behavior and physiology to the shifted time cues present in the new location (for more on jet lag, see Section 13.10).

3.3.2 Mechanisms of entrainment

Our understanding of the mechanisms responsible for entrainment developed from studies that modeled the effects of light on circadian rhythms in different species. This approach involved housing animals in constant darkness (in which their rhythms would free-run) and occasionally interrupting the darkness with short periods of light (e.g., 5–60 min in length) to assess the effects on the timing of their circadian rhythms.

Studies of this type were conducted, for example, by Patricia DeCoursey on activity rhythms in Syrian hamsters (*Mesocricetus auratus*) and Northern flying squirrels (*Glaucomys volans*) (DeCoursey, 1961), and by Colin Pittendrigh and colleagues, on eclosion rhythms in fruit flies (*Drosophila* sp.) and activity rhythms in hamsters (Daan & Pittendrigh, 1976; Pittendrigh, 1960). They found that brief light pulses affected circadian rhythms in a way that can account for rhythm entrainment to cycles of light exposure. Depending on the phase of the free- running rhythm at which they occurred, light pulses caused a phase delay shift (lengthening of the period for at least one cycle), a phase advance shift (shortening of the period for at least one cycle), or no shift (**Figure 3.3**).

Note that under constant free-running conditions in a laboratory, there is no external day or night, but organisms still show physiological and behavioral cycles like those shown in a real, day–night cycle. In other words, they function based on internal circadian time (= subjective time) in the absence of an external time frame. The principal divisions of these internally generated cycles are referred to as the subjective day and subjective night. These are defined as the phases when an organism behaves in constant conditions as it would during a real day or night, respectively.

Thus, under constant environmental conditions, the subjective day for a diurnal species, such as a human, is the time during which the individual is awake and active. For a nocturnal rodent, like a hamster, however, the subjective day is the period during which it is most likely to be asleep in a burrow and disengaged from its environment, as it would be during a real day. Similarly, the subjective night for people includes their usual sleep period, but it is the most active daily phase for a nocturnal hamster.

A phase response curve (PRC) is a critical tool used in the analysis of entrainment. It is a plot of the size and direction of phase shifts produced by brief light pulses (or other stimuli) against the circadian/subjective times at which the light pulses were presented (**Figures 3.3** and **3.4**) (Daan & Pittendrigh, 1976). The PRC is a uniquely useful tool for understanding how an external zeitgeber affects the underlying clock and for predicting how different organisms will entrain to a zeitgeber, such as a light-dark cycle.

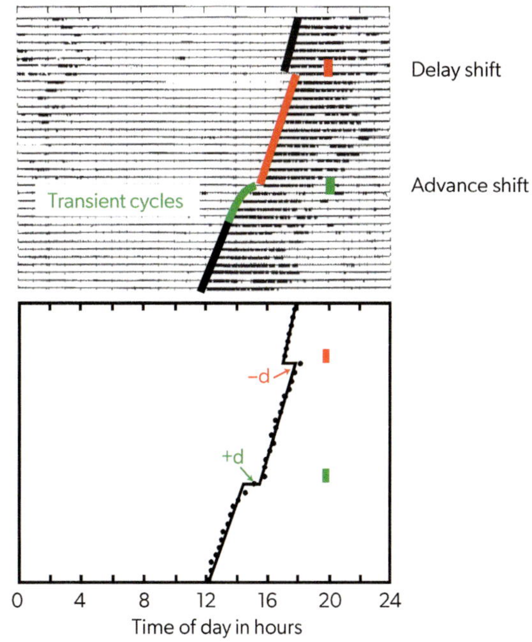

Figure 3.3 Illustrations of the phase shifts induced by brief light pulses delivered to a golden hamster (*Mesocricetus auratus*) housed otherwise in continuous darkness in an activity wheel. **Top**: The activity rhythm (black marks) free-ran with a period slightly less than 24 h (black diagonal line, top) until the hamster was exposed to a 15 min light pulse (red symbol) early in its active phase. The result was an abrupt delay of its next expected activity onset, followed by a free-run beginning at the delayed phase (straight red line). A second light pulse (green symbol) was given late in its active phase; it caused a phase advance of the free-running rhythm. The full advance occurred over several advancing cycles (Transient cycles; curved green line) before a stable free-running rhythm was reestablished (black line, bottom). Transients are often observed after light pulses that cause advance shifts. **Bottom:** The same data were replotted showing only the onsets of daily activity as a series of dots. This figure illustrates how the size and direction of the phase shifts are calculated by determining the difference (d) (e.g., in minutes) between the predicted timing of activity onsets, based on the previous free-running rhythm, and the actual timing of activity onsets on the days after the light pulses. The notations (−d and +d) represent the amount and direction of the phase shifts (delay [−] or advance [+]) caused by the light pulses. Adapted with permission from Daan, S. & Pittendrigh, C. S. (1976) A functional analysis of circadian pacemakers in nocturnal rodents. II. The variability of phase response curves. *J Comp Physiol* 106:253–266. © Springer-Verlag (1976). doi: 10.1007/BF01417857.

The details of PRC shape and amplitude differ among species and individuals as well as in relation to the strength of the zeitgeber signal (e.g., light intensity), but PRCs have several common features. These include: a phase during which the circadian clock is relatively unaffected by the stimulus (the so-called dead zone; **A** in **Figure 3.4**), which falls during the subjective day; a phase during which it causes delay shifts of different sizes (the early

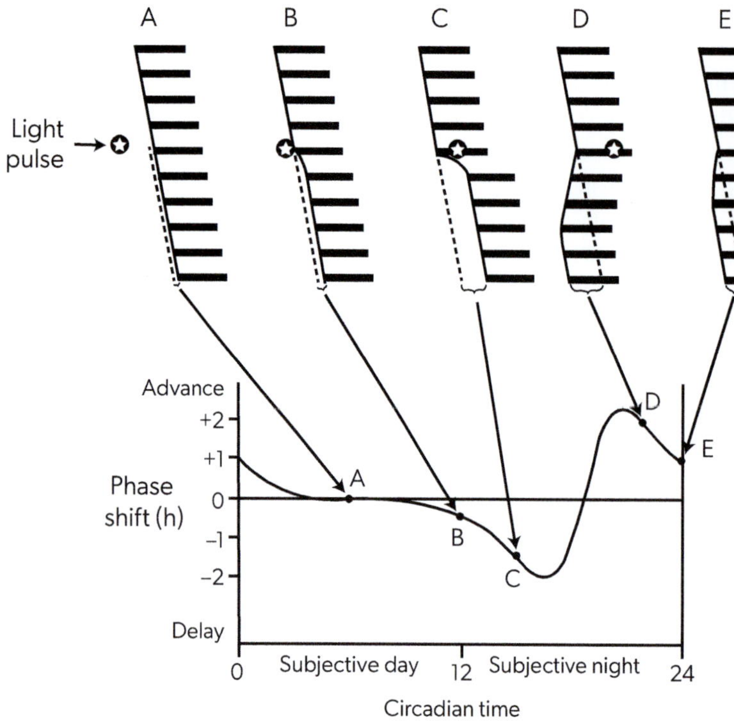

Figure 3.4 An illustration of how phase response curves (PRCs) are generated. Free-running organisms, typically in constant darkness, are exposed to a brief light pulse at various circadian phases (= subjective or circadian time). The phase-shifting effect of the light pulse on the rhythm is calculated (see **Figure 3-3**) and plotted against the circadian time at which the light pulse was given. For a nocturnal animal, the time of activity onset is considered equivalent to circadian time (CT) 12, the beginning of the subjective night, and the phase of each light pulse is calculated relative to this anchor phase. Note that the X axis is plotted as 24 circadian hours, which are not equivalent to 60 min hours. Rather each circadian hour is 1/24 of a circadian cycle. Thus, a circadian hour will be >60 min for organisms with a free-running period longer than 24 h and <60 min for those with circadian periods less than 24 h. The **top portion** shows the effects on activity rhythms of light pulses given at different circadian phases. During the subjective day (A), there is no resulting phase shift. During the early subjective night there are small and large phase delays (B, C), depending on timing, and during the late subjective night, light causes large and small phase advances (D, E). The **bottom portion** shows the plotted PRC made up of data points from many phase-shift experiments, plotted in hours of advance or delay shifts on the Y axis against circadian time on the X axis. By convention, advance shifts (+) are plotted above and delay shifts (−) below the zero line. Adapted with permission of Dr. Martin C. Moore-Ede from Moore-Ede, M. C., Sulzman, F. M. & Fuller, C. A. (1982). *The Clocks That Time Us*. Cambridge: Harvard University Press. © Dr. Martin C. Moore-Ede (1982).

subjective night; **Figure 3.4, B & C**); and a phase during which it causes advance shifts of different sizes (late subjective night; **Figure 3.4, D & E**). Note that this means that diurnal humans and nocturnal hamsters are both maximally sensitive to the phase-shifting effects of light during the subjective night, regardless of whether the night is their rest or active phase.

Information about how brief light pulses affect free-running rhythms, as represented in PRCs, allowed the development of models of the entrainment process. These demonstrated how natural lighting cycles could modify non-24 h, internally generated, free-running rhythms by causing phase shifts that lengthen or shorten their periods to match the 24.0 h periods of natural days (Pittendrigh & Daan, 1976). The sensitivity to phase-shifting effects of light is largely confined to the interval between dusk and dawn (**Figure 3.4**). Natural lighting cycles exert their entraining effects principally at the margins of this sensitive zone around dusk and dawn.

Some diurnally active species, however, entrain without exposure to light at these transition phases because they stay in darkened underground burrows except during the middle of the day (Hut et al., 1999). Entrainment in these species may result from the lighting cycle continuously altering the period of the circadian system, a so-called parametric effect[2] of light on period, rather than only through abrupt shifts of the phase of the rhythm (Beersma et al., 1999; Hut et al., 1999). Both mechanisms may operate in natural environments and may be relevant to entrainment in people. But the general principle remains that repeated exposures to daily lighting cycles reset the timing of the internal clock by lengthening or shortening endogenously generated circadian periods to match the period of the external cycle.

[2] This term refers to the fact that period and amplitude are parameters of an oscillation. Abrupt phase-shifting effects, as illustrated in **Figure 3.3**, are instead usually referred to as "non-parametric" effects.

Lighting cycles are considered the universal zeitgeber for circadian systems, but other environmental factors can serve similar functions, depending on the species. Daily temperature cycles, for example, can have entraining effects in some species, and a variety of other stimuli may also act as zeitgebers or can have important modulating effects on circadian rhythm entrainment (Mistlberger & Rusak, 2010).

Through the process of entrainment, each internally generated circadian rhythm adopts a 24.0 h period and establishes a stable unique position (is phase relation) relative to the zeitgeber cycle, which is typically a light-dark cycle. Because of the mechanics of entrainment, clocks with naturally short, free-running periods become stably entrained at an early phase relative to the external cycle (phase lead), while long-period clocks become entrained at a later phase of the zeitgeber cycle (phase lag) (**Figure 3.5**).

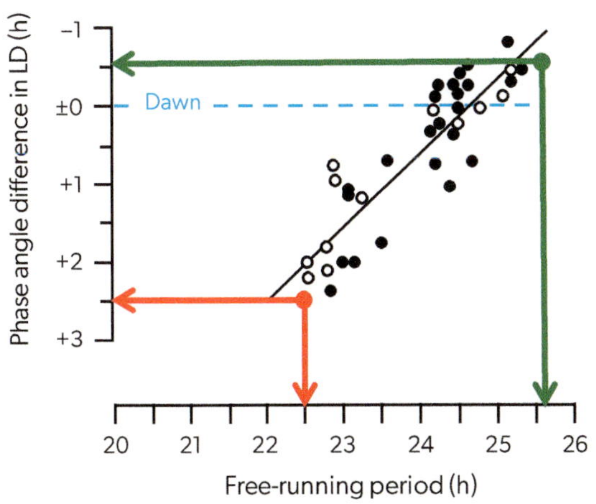

Figure 3.5 Illustration in songbirds (chaffinches, *Fringilla coelebs*) of how the period of the free-running rhythm, generated by an internal oscillator, relates to the entrained phase of that rhythm when exposed to a 24 h light-dark cycle. The Y axis shows the time of activity onset for individual birds relative to the onset of light (dawn, dashed blue line) when entrained to the 24 h light-dark cycle (+ indicates a phase lead: onset occurs before dawn; and - a phase lag: onset occurs after dawn). This is usually referred to as the "phase angle." Each bird's entrained phase is plotted against the free-running period of its activity rhythm in dim constant illumination on the X axis. The fitted diagonal line illustrates the systematic, linear relation between the length of an oscillator's spontaneous period and the phase it adopts relative to an external cycle when it becomes entrained. The arrows indicate that individual birds with different natural periods entrained at very different phases relative to the external cycle. A bird with a short-period rhythm (22.5 h; red dot and arrows) entrained with activity onset leading light onset by ~2.5 h, while a bird with a long-period rhythm (25.6 h; green dot and arrows) entrained with activity onset lagging light onset by ~0.5 h. Adapted with permission of Elsevier, Ltd. from Aschoff, J. & Wever, R. (1966) Circadian period and phase-angle difference in chaffinches (*Fringilla coelebs* L.). *Comp Biochem Physiol* 18:397–404. © Elsevier (1966). doi: 10.1016/0010-406x(66)90197-6.

Thus, when two day-active birds with different natural periods in constant light were exposed to the same 24.0 h lighting cycle, both became entrained and expressed 24.0 h rhythms. But the bird with a natural circadian period of 22.5 h in constant light became active every day more than 2 h before dawn (phase lead), while the bird with a 25.0 h circadian period became active ~0.5 h after dawn (phase lag) (**Figure 3.5**) (Aschoff & Wever, 1966). This feature of circadian rhythm entrainment has important implications for understanding aspects of human sleep. Differences in circadian period among people lead to the expression of "early-bird" and "night-owl" phenotypes—those who spontaneously prefer to go to bed early and to rise early (showing a phase lead), versus those who prefer to stay up late and sleep late (showing a phase lag), relative to external time.

A study that assessed the intrinsic circadian periods of adult men and women using a forced-desynchronization protocol (see Section 3.5.2) found a small but significant gender difference in average period, with women showing a ~6 min shorter period than men (24.09 vs. 24.19 h, based on body temperature rhythms). More women than men also had circadian periods shorter than 24.0 h (Duffy et al., 2011), which would predict more advanced phases of entrainment on average in women. Gender differences in human preferences for times of waking and sleep onset are discussed further in Section 4.4.2.

3.3.3 Summary

Circadian clocks can be entrained by exposing them to 24 h or near-24 h light-dark (and some other) cycles (zeitgebers), which act by changing the period of the internal clock to match the period of the zeitgeber. The process of entrainment to a daily zeitgeber can be modeled as a series of phase shifts each cycle that are induced in the clock's endogenous circadian rhythm by exposure to light or other zeitgebers. But in some circumstances, entrainment may involve both such abrupt phase shifts and gradual parametric effects of light on the period of the oscillator.

Circadian systems re-entrain gradually through a series of transient cycles after significant changes in the timing of a zeitgeber cycle, such as occurs following jet travel across multiple time zones. The resulting disturbances of sleep, alertness, and digestion persist while the circadian clock and the rhythms it regulates gradually resynchronize to the external cycles in their new environment.

PRCs represent the phase-shifting sensitivity of circadian clocks to light (or to other cues), and variations in their structure and in the free-running circadian period can explain why individuals entrain differently to the same external cycles. Thus, people with short-period circadian clocks prefer an advanced phase of both sleep and wake onset relative to external time, and those with long-period clocks prefer a delayed phase relative to the same external cues.

3.4 Masking effects

Since we cannot easily measure the phase of the circadian clock itself in an intact organism, especially a person, researchers use behavioral or physiological processes (e.g., activity, body temperature) that are driven by the clock as an index of its phase. But uncontrolled external events (e.g., noise, temperature changes, meals) can affect these measures directly, complicating interpretation of the data and potentially resulting in incorrect inferences about the behavior of the circadian clock.

Thus, a sudden noise during the day might cause a sleeping mouse to wake up to investigate, thus becoming active and raising its body temperature during its rest phase. During its daily active phase, a loud noise might instead cause it to stop its usual activity and freeze in fear. These effects of external stimuli that are exerted directly on behavior or physiology are called *masking effects*. This term refers to the idea that external stimuli that modify behavior or physiology directly, rather than by acting through the circadian system, can mask or obscure the actual state of the circadian system at that time (Aschoff & von Goetz, 1989; Mrosovsky, 1999). While potentially interfering with measurement of circadian rhythms in the laboratory, masking effects in the natural world can also be seen as adaptive responses to environmental events that may either reinforce or inhibit behavior dictated by the circadian system, depending on circumstances (Gall & Shuboni-Mulligan, 2022; Mrosovsky, 1999).

In the case of a sleeping mouse disturbed by a noise, activity stimulated by an external event makes it active when its circadian clock is dictating rest. This is an example of positive masking, provoking a behavior at an inappropriate circadian phase. An environmental change that instead inhibits behaviors that would normally occur at that time exerts a negative masking effect—for example, putting a dark cover over a canary's cage during the day so that it stops hopping on its perches and singing.

Masking can also interfere with tests of whether an external cycle can entrain a circadian rhythm. Masking effects can mimic entrainment by altering behavior directly—stimulating activity during one part of the day or inhibiting it at another time. Masking stimuli may thereby synchronize behavior without entraining the internal clock.

To take a familiar example, an alarm clock can wake you up at 06:30 daily, but that does not necessarily mean that the alarm has entrained your circadian system to wake you at that time of day. (As discussed in Chapter 4, for many young people, 06:30 may be several hours before their internal clocks would trigger waking.) A stringent test is needed to determine whether observed synchronization (alarm clock and waking occurring at the same time) results from masking of behavior or entrainment of a circadian clock.

The test for entrainment illustrated in **Figure 3.6** is based on an important principle: the phase of a free-running rhythm under constant environmental conditions (when no masking or entraining effects are possible) must reflect the timing of the underlying internal clock. As a result, after a possible entraining cycle is removed, the initial phase from which the rhythm begins to free-run in constant conditions reveals whether behavioral synchronization, observed while the cycle was present, involved entrainment or masking. Details of the methods and interpretation of the test results are shown in the legend to **Figure 3.6**.

The most extreme case of masking would involve the expression of a robust rhythm when an external cycle is present, but complete loss of rhythmicity when the organism is studied under constant conditions. That result would imply that the rhythm was not controlled by a circadian clock and that the external cycle acted directly on behavior or physiology. In that hypothetical case, shifting the external cycle would shift the organism's rhythm immediately to any arbitrary phase one chose.

We can illustrate the consequences of not having a circadian clock by using a thought experiment involving transporting such a hypothetical individual instantaneously from Halifax to Beijing (using a Star Trek transporter, perhaps). The local lighting cycle in Beijing would immediately impose its rhythm on the physiology of the individual, who would be instantly adapted to local time, 12 h out of phase with Halifax time.

But, as mentioned in Section 3.3, that does not happen. The fact that daily rhythms are the product of entrainment by an external cycle of a robust, internal clock makes it difficult to shift rhythms substantially from their current timing. A large shift in the timing of a zeitgeber eventually causes a parallel shift in the timing of an entrained circadian system, but it usually occurs through a series of transient cycles (as illustrated for a single stimulus in **Figure 3.3**). This tendency of circadian clocks to maintain their internal timing and to adjust only slowly to substantial changes in external time cues is important for understanding the impact of jet travel and of shift work on circadian rhythms and sleep (see Chapter 13).

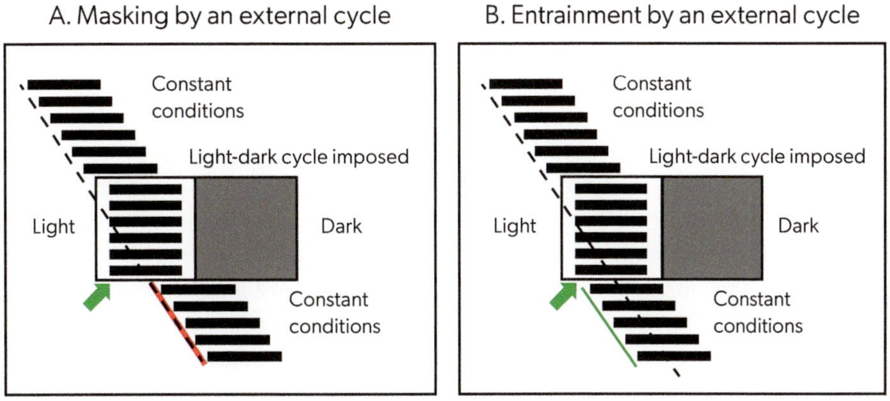

Figure 3.6 **A.** An activity rhythm (black bars) free-runs in continuous darkness (Constant conditions) over several days. The dashed line indicates the onset of activity over those days; it reflects the period and phase of the underlying oscillator driving the rhythm. In the presence of a daily light-dark cycle, activity becomes stably synchronized to the start of the daily light phase, looking like stable entrainment of the underlying oscillator by the lighting cycle. Once released to constant conditions again, however, the rhythm free-runs (red line) starting at a point predicted by extrapolation of the phase of the prior free-run (black dashed line), not from the time of apparent entrainment at the beginning of the light phase. If this were entrainment, the free-run would have begun at the point indicated by the green arrow. This is an example of masking by an external cycle. The external cycle affected only the overt behavior not the underlying circadian oscillator. This outcome is unlikely in the case of a 24 h lighting cycle unless the animal were blind, since animals almost universally entrain to lighting cycles, but it could arise when testing other cyclic environmental factors (e.g., daily alarm clock signals or temperature cycles) for their capacity to entrain a circadian rhythm. **B.** As in panel **A**, activity free-runs under constant conditions and becomes synchronized to the external light-dark cycle. However, when released to constant conditions again, the free-run (green line) starts from a phase (green arrow) dictated by the previously imposed external cycle rather than from a phase dictated by the prior free-running rhythm (black dashed line). This finding demonstrates that the underlying circadian oscillator that drives the activity rhythm was entrained by the external cycle. The synchronization observed while the light-dark cycle was present was the result of entrainment, not masking.

3.4.1 Summary

Masking refers to effects of environmental cues that influence physiology or behavior directly rather than by acting through the circadian clock. These effects can induce immediate changes in physiology or behavior that are inconsistent with the dictates of the internal clock. Because physiological and behavioral rhythms are used to infer the phase of the underlying circadian system, masking effects can obscure the actual phase of the clock and lead to incorrect interpretations. It is, therefore, critical to distinguish between masking and entraining effects of external stimuli using appropriate studies.

A hypothetical organism that does not have an internal circadian clock could be synchronized by external masking cues so that it behaves as if it is being entrained. A large shift in the external cycle could determine whether the process is masking or entrainment. A clockless organism would become synchronized immediately to a shift in external cycles, adapting instantly to the newly imposed timing. That is not what happens to real animals or to people. They have internal circadian systems that resist large phase shifts and adapt only slowly to newly imposed external cycles through the process of circadian re-entrainment.

3.5 Studying human circadian rhythms

3.5.1 Effects of isolation from zeitgebers

In studies of human circadian rhythms, as for other species, it is critical to exclude any possible uncontrolled influence of external stimuli. Some of the first studies of people in constant environments involved living in underground caves for weeks or months and recording their sleep-wake and other rhythms. Deep caves offer the benefits of constant temperatures as well as total darkness, but they lack the precise control of experimental conditions that is possible in a laboratory setting. Well-publicized examples include Nathaniel Kleitman and Bruce Richardson living in Kentucky's Mammoth Cave for 32 days in 1938 (Siegel, 2001) and repeated multi-week stays in caverns and underground glaciers by Michel Siffre, starting in 1962 (Chouvet et al., 1974).

A different approach to studying human circadian rhythms and sleep in temporal isolation was developed in laboratory settings, including pioneering work by Jürgen Aschoff and Rütger Wever in Andechs, Germany beginning in the 1950s.

They developed isolated laboratories in an underground bunker which allowed one or more people to be studied while they lived in time-free environments. Participants remained inside the laboratory for weeks without any direct contact with the outside world (except by intercom communication with technicians) and without access to information about external time. Students studying for examinations or working on their theses were reportedly happy to have the time to do so without the usual distractions of life in the outside world; very few found the isolation disturbing and asked to be released early.

Aschoff and Wever reported that some participants developed a strong interest in guessing what time it was in the external world and used relatively subtle cues to try to guess. For example, participants were in contact periodically through intercoms with research assistants who scheduled cognitive and other tests. Some participants attempted to guess, based on the voice of the assistant, whether they were hearing from the day crew or the night crew. The assistants had to start working on irregularly staggered schedules to conceal information about time of day.

Other laboratories also used time-free environments to study human rhythms, including that of John Mills and colleagues at the University of Manchester, in the UK, and that of Charles Czeisler at Harvard University in the United States. Even modern, purpose-built laboratories may provide study participants with unintended hints about time of day. When temporal isolation laboratories were built inside hospitals or university buildings, participants could pay attention to the vibrations generated by nearby elevators moving in their shafts. Knowing the usual work habits of people, they could try to guess when the typical workday started or ended based on these vibrations. Some facilities, like that at Harvard, went to great lengths to isolate the laboratory structurally from contact with its surrounding building that could transmit vibrations or noise.

Aschoff and Wever reported that individuals rapidly lost track of external time in the absence of any relevant cues. Their meal patterns, body temperature, and sleep-wake cycles began to free-run with periods different from 24 h. Some participants also showed dissociations in period between different rhythms. In particular, their self-selected sleep-wake cycles could run at periods very different from 24 h (either much longer or somewhat shorter), while their body temperature rhythms free-ran with periods that stayed close to 24 h (Aschoff & Wever, 1976). Siffre's cave studies had also reported sleep-wake cycle lengths stretching up to 50 h in some cases, with body temperature rhythms staying in the circadian range (Chouvet et al., 1974; Colin et al., 1968). This phenomenon of different rhythms running with different periods is referred to as spontaneous *internal desynchronization*. It provided early evidence suggesting that there is more than one internal timing mechanism contributing to the regulation of human daily rhythms. However, the nature of the timing mechanisms involved is uncertain, and several possibilities have been discussed (Aschoff & Wever, 1976; Eastman, 1982; Kronauer et al., 1982).

One interpretation of this phenomenon derives from evidence that the expression of sleep-wake cycles with very short or long periods was associated with other behavioral and physiological changes. Average hourly activity levels were lower in those with very long wake lengths and higher in those with short wake lengths so that total activity amounts were similar during wake phases of very different lengths (Aschoff, 1993; Aschoff et al., 1986). In parallel to these changes, those with long subjective days ate meals at longer intervals and estimated an hour as being longer than did those with short subjective days (Aschoff, 1993; Aschoff et al., 1986). Those with very short sleep-wake cycles during desynchronization also had higher average body temperatures than those with very long cycles, suggesting that they had higher metabolic rates (Daan et al., 2013).

Taken together, these results suggest that individual differences in metabolic rates during internal desynchronization contributed to the observed differences in time estimation, meal timing, activity levels, and total lengths of wake and sleep periods (Aschoff, 1993; Aschoff et al., 1986; Daan et al., 2013). These changes occurred, however, while the principal circadian pacemaker driving body temperature rhythms continued to run with a near-24 h periodicity. These spontaneous changes prompted the development of an important experimental method for studying how circadian systems influence sleep (*forced* desynchronization), as described in Section 3.5.2.

3.5.2 Other methods for studying human rhythms

Even in complete temporal isolation, with no external disturbances, people are exposed to events that can affect the measurement of rhythms that are used to index the state of the circadian clock. Rhythms in core body temperature and secretion of the pineal hormone melatonin (see Chapter 9) are closely tied to the central circadian clock and are used to assay its current state (Shanahan & Czeisler, 1991). But these rhythms are also subject to masking effects.

For example, large meals can modify body temperature and increase sleepiness, so participants' self-selected meal patterns could alter these measures. Body temperature and some hormone levels, including melatonin levels, change depending on whether a person is lying down, standing, or sitting (Deacon & Arendt, 1994). Temperature also increases during exercise and falls during sleep in both people and animals (Franken et al., 1992). As a result, a person's self-selected mealtimes, body position, and sleep timing in a temporal isolation environment can influence key measures of the phase of the circadian system.

These effects can be seen as forms of *internal masking*. This term refers to changes in the value of a target measure that result from the participant's own behavior rather than from either an external disturbance or the dictates of the circadian clock. Thus, to get a pure measure of the state of the underlying circadian clock using the body temperature or melatonin rhythm as an index, one must eliminate any potential impact of the individual's own self-selected activities.

One method of addressing these issues is to study participants' rhythms using what is called a constant routine. In this procedure, a participant maintains an unchanging posture (often semi-recumbent on a reclining chair), is kept awake, and consumes identical, isocaloric mini-meals at frequent intervals (e.g., every 2 h) throughout a 36–48 h period in constant, very dim illumination. This approach allows assessment of circadian rhythms that are uncontaminated by the impact of either environmental events or behavioral changes that can modify the measures being recorded (Duffy & Dijk, 2002).

However, there is also a risk that the measures used to prevent both internal and external masking effects might themselves affect circadian rhythm measurement. Thus, lack of sleep and of postural change during a constant routine might have subtle effects on circadian rhythms, even if they are successful in preventing the more pronounced effects of allowing participants to eat, sleep, and move at will. In an animal model, for example, sleep deprivation itself (one component of a 36–48 h constant routine in people) can cause shifts in circadian rhythms (Antle & Mistlberger, 2000).

Another method used in human circadian research that is especially relevant to studies of sleep is forced desynchronization. This approach imposes unusual sleep-wake patterns that mimic the pattern of spontaneous desynchronization generated by some people during long-term, temporal isolation. This technique depends on the fact that circadian clocks cannot be synchronized to external cycles that differ very much from the intrinsic, free-running period of the clock. Thus, if a participant in a time-free environment is permitted to sleep starting every 21 or 28 h, the circadian pacemaker responsible for generating temperature and melatonin rhythms does not entrain to these cycles. Instead, the circadian system free-runs with a period near 24 h, while sleep opportunities occur at 21 or 28 h intervals.

As a result, over the course of ~30 sleep-wake cycles with periods of 21 h or 28 h (i.e., occurring over 26 or 35 "real", 24 h days), sleep episodes necessarily coincide with all possible phases of a person's internally generated circadian cycle. In contrast, in the usual 24 h environment, sleep typically occurs only during the circadian night phase. This protocol allows experimenters to measure whether, and how, the circadian system affects many features of sleep, such as sleep onset latency, sleep duration, sleep spindle production, and REM or N3 sleep probability, independently of other factors that could affect these measures (Dijk & Czeisler, 1995; Mills et al., 1977). The results of these studies demonstrate a critical role for the circadian system in regulating sleep, which will be discussed in several later chapters, especially in Chapter 8.

3.5.3 Summary

Studies of people living in time-free environments showed that they continued to express internally generated circadian rhythms, as other species do. However, even under these conditions, peoples' rhythms could still be influenced by the effects of internal masking. This refers to the impact of the person's own behavior (choice of mealtimes, exercise, body position, or sleep) on markers of the circadian system. The constant routine method prevents people from producing these interfering influences, but at the cost of studying them under highly constrained and unusual conditions, including a lack of sleep over 36–48 h.

In some people living in constant conditions, daily rhythms dissociated to produce a state of internal desynchronization. Body temperature and melatonin rhythms continued to free-run with a circadian period, while sleep-wake and other behavioral rhythms would express quite different periods, either much longer or shorter than the circadian cycle. The direction of these effects appears to be related to metabolic rates, with faster metabolic rates being related to shorter self-selected sleep and wake durations.

These observations prompted the use of forced internal desynchronization to study how the circadian system influences sleep. People in time-free environments were scheduled to sleep at non-circadian intervals over many days, while their circadian system continued to free-run. This approach ensured that sleep occurred at all possible circadian phases over a period of about a month. It allowed detection of the impact of the circadian system on many aspects of sleep-wake regulation that cannot be readily observed under normal living conditions.

3.6 Impacts of laboratory environments

As discussed earlier in relation to sleep studies, there is also an unavoidable tension in circadian rhythm research between the need for rigid environmental control and the resulting loss of information about factors operating in more naturalistic settings. Controlled environments allow researchers to replicate identical conditions among individual participants and across laboratories. By reducing interference from unplanned disturbances, they also permit precise analysis of the effects of experimental manipulations on behavioral and physiological rhythms.

But these controlled environments necessarily eliminate some factors that may have important effects in natural environments. There are many anecdotal reports and some experimental results showing that external events that are usually excluded from laboratory environments (including weather changes, twilight transitions, moonlight cycles, the presence of other species, and social interactions) can affect the expression of daily rhythms (Fuchikawa et al., 2016; Mistlberger & Rusak, 2010; Rusak, 1981).

There is substantial evidence, for example, that the timing of daily rhythms is altered by predation pressures and by resource competition within and between species.

For example, of two related species of spiny mice (*Acomys* sp.) with overlapping habitats in a desert region in Israel, one species showed minimal foraging activity at night when members of the other, more aggressive species, were present. But their activity became mostly nocturnal when the other species was excluded (Shkolnik, 1971). A study of groups of Norway rats (*Rattus norvegicus*) living in a semi-natural enclosure found that social dominance and competition determined the daily timing of feeding by non-dominant individuals (Calhoun, 1962). The daily activity and feeding patterns of desert hamsters (*Phodopus roborovskii*) studied in the Mongolian desert in China were altered by the presence of more aggressive rodent competitors (Scheibler et al., 2013). Sleep timing also differed between two closely related sloth species (*Bradypus* sp.) that were exposed to different predation pressures in their natural habitats (Voirin et al., 2014).

Few well-controlled studies have made direct comparisons of rhythms obtained in laboratories to those in natural environments. The circadian rhythms of golden hamsters (*Mesocricetus auratus*) are often the subject of laboratory studies because of their precise, strongly nocturnal activity rhythms. But a population of hamsters studied in their natural environment expressed quite different rhythms, perhaps in response to local predation pressure from nocturnal species (Gattermann et al., 2008). Another study demonstrated that the feeding rhythms of house mice (*Mus musculus*), which are nocturnal in the laboratory, can be relatively arrhythmic or primarily diurnal in semi-natural external enclosures, depending on season, snow cover, and other, unknown factors (Daan et al., 2011).

The daily activity rhythms of fruit flies (*Drosophila melanogaster*) studied in the laboratory under a fixed light-dark cycle and controlled temperature were dramatically different from those recorded from flies under one set of field conditions (Vanin et al., 2012) (**Figure 3.7**). High-amplitude temperature cycles and gradual twilight transitions at dawn and dusk during the field study appeared to be particularly important

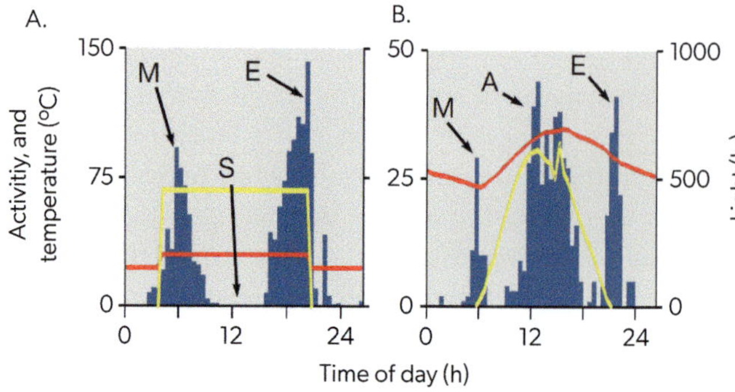

Figure 3.7 **A.** Daily activity patterns (left Y axis) of a single male fruit fly in a laboratory setting under a typical light-dark cycle (yellow line shows light intensity; right Y axis in B) and very low amplitude temperature cycle (red line; left Y axis). There are peaks of activity in the morning (M) and evening (E), and a midday quiescent period ("siesta": S). **B.** An activity recording from another male fruit fly in the field under natural lighting and temperature conditions (a summer day in Treviso, Italy), showing the light intensity (yellow line), temperature (red line), and a very different activity pattern, including small M and E components and a very prominent afternoon peak of activity (A). Reprinted with permission from Vanin, S. et al. (2012) Unexpected features of Drosophila circadian behavioural rhythms under natural conditions. *Nature* 484:371–375. © Springer:Nature (2012). doi: 10.1038/nature10991.

influences. This conclusion is consistent with evidence that introducing gradual twilight transitions to a lighting cycle altered entrainment of hamsters in a laboratory (Boulos et al., 1996).

Controlled laboratory environments are essential for studying endogenous circadian mechanisms and for the precise analysis of how environmental stimuli affect the circadian system. But some factors that vary in the field and are usually kept constant in the laboratory have a significant impact on the expression of rhythmicity. Field studies contribute to a better understanding of how the regulatory systems analyzed in laboratory studies respond to the much greater complexities of real-world environments.

3.6.1 Summary

The highly controlled laboratory environments that permit precise analyses of circadian mechanisms necessarily exclude many factors that can affect the expression of daily rhythms in natural environments. These factors include physical variables, such as the gradual changes in temperature, humidity, and light during a day in the natural world as well as biological factors, such as the presence of conspecifics, competitors, prey, and predators. There is evidence that all these factors modify the expression of daily rhythms in the natural world, although the mechanisms involved in many of these effects are not well understood.

Literature cited

Antle, M., & Mistlberger, R. (2000). Circadian clock resetting by sleep deprivation without exercise in the Syrian hamster. *J Neurosci, 20*(24), 9326–9332.

Aschoff, J. (1993). On the relationship between motor activity and the sleep-wake cycle in humans during temporal isolation. *J Biol Rhythms, 8*(1), 33–46.

Aschoff, J., & von Goetz, C. (1989). Masking of circadian activity rhythms in canaries by light and dark. *J Biol Rhythms, 4*(1), 29–38.

Aschoff, J., von Goetz, C., Wildgruber, C., & Wever, R. A. (1986). Meal timing in humans during isolation without time cues. *J Biol Rhythms, 1*, 151–162.

Aschoff, J., & Wever, R. (1966). Circadian period and phase-angle difference in chaffinches (*Fringilla coelebs* L.). *Comp Biochem Physiol, 18*, 397–404.

Aschoff, J., & Wever, R. (1976). Human circadian rhythms: A multioscillatory system. *Fed Proc, 35*, 2326–2332.

Beersma, D. G. M., Daan, S., & Hut, R. A. (1999). Accuracy of circadian entrainment under fluctuating light conditions: Contributions of phase and period responses. *J Biol Rhythms, 14*(4), 320–329.

Boulos, Z., Macchi, M., Houpt, T. A., & Terman, M. (1996). Photic entrainment in hamsters: Effects of simulated twilights and nest box availability. *J Biol Rhythms, 11*, 216–233.

Bünning, E. (1960). Opening address. In A. Chovnick (Ed.), *Biological Clocks* (Vol. **XXV**, pp. 1–9). Cold Spring Harbor: The Biological Laboratory.

Calhoun, J. B. (1962). *The Ecology and Sociology of the Norway Rat* (Public Health Service Publication No. 1008). Bethesda: US Department of Health, Education and Welfare.

Chouvet, G., Mouret, J., Coindet, J., Siffre, M., & Jouvet, M. (1974). Périodicité, bicircadienne du cycle veille-sommeil dans des conditions hors du temps. Étude polygraphique. *Electroencephalogr Clin Neurophysiol, 37*(4), 367–380.

Chovnick, A. (Ed.) (1960). *Biological Clocks, Cold Spring Harbor Symposia on Quantitaive Biology*, Vol. XXV. Cold Spring Harbor: The Biological Laboratory.

Colin, J., Timbal, J., Boutelier, C., Houdas, Y., & Siffre, M. (1968). Rhythm of the rectal temperature during a 6-month free-running experiment. *J Appl Physiol, 25*(2), 170–176.

Daan, S., Honma, S., & Honma, K. (2013). Body temperature predicts the direction of internal desynchronization in humans isolated from time cues. *J Biol Rhythms, 28*(6), 403–411. doi: 10.1177/0748730413514357

Daan, S., & Pittendrigh, C. S. (1976). A functional analysis of circadian pacemakers in nocturnal rodents. II. The variability of phase response curves. *J Comp Physiol A, 106*, 253–266.

Daan, S., Spoelstra, K., Albrecht, U., Schmutz, I., Daan, M., Daan, B., ... Lipp, H. P. (2011). Lab mice in the field: unorthodox daily activity and effects of a dysfunctional circadian clock allele. *J Biol Rhythms, 26*(2), 118–129. doi: 10.1177/0748730410397645

Deacon, S., & Arendt, J. (1994). Posture influences melatonin concentrations in plasma and saliva in humans. *Neurosci Lett, 167*, 191–194.

de Candolle, A.-P. (1832). Physiologie végétale, deuxieme tome, pp. 860–861. Retrieved July 26, 2022, from https://gallica.bnf.fr/ark:/12148/bpt6k97954584/f415.item.texteImage

DeCoursey, P. J. (1960). Phase control of activity in a rodent. In A. Chovnick (Ed.), *Biological Clocks, Cold Spring Harbor Symposia on Quantitaive Biology*, Vol. XXV, pp. 49–55. Cold Spring Harbor: The Biological Laboratory.

DeCoursey, P. J. (1961). Effect of light on the circadian activity rhythm of the flying squirrel, Glaucomys volans. *Z Vergleich Physiol, 44*, 331–354.

de Mairan, J. J. O. (1729). Observation botanique. *Hist Acad Roy Sci, Paris*, 35.

Dijk, D. J., & Czeisler, C. A. (1995). Contribution of the circadian pacemaker and the sleep homeostat to sleep propensity, sleep structure, electroencephalographic slow waves, and sleep spindle activity in humans. *J Neurosci, 15*, 3526–3538.

Duffy, J. F., Cain, S. W., Chang, A. M., Phillips, A. J., Munch, M. Y., Gronfier, C., ... Czeisler, C. A. (2011). Sex difference in the near-24-hour intrinsic period of the human circadian timing system. *Proc Natl Acad Sci (USA), 108*(Suppl 3), 15602–15608. doi: 10.1073/pnas.1010666108

Duffy, J. F., & Dijk, D.-J. (2002). Getting through to circadian oscillators: Why use constant routines? *J Biol Rhythms, 17*(1), 4–13.

Eastman, C. (1982). The phase-shift model of spontaneous internal desynchronization in humans. In J. Aschoff, S. Daan, & G. Groos (Eds.), *Vertebrate Circadian Systems* (pp. 262–267). Heidelberg: Springer-Verlag.

Franken, P., Tobler, I., & Borbély, A. A. (1992). Sleep and waking have a major effect on the 24-hr rhythm of cortical temperature in the rat. *J Biol Rhythms, 7*, 341–352.

Fuchikawa, T., Eban-Rothschild, A., Nagari, M., Shemesh, Y., & Bloch, G. (2016). Potent social synchronization can override photic entrainment of circadian rhythms. *Nat Commun, 7*, 11662. doi: 10.1038/ncomms11662

Gall, A. J., & Shuboni-Mulligan, D. D. (2022). Keep your mask on: the benefits of masking for behavior and the contributions of aging and disease on dysfunctional masking pathways. *Front Neurosci, 16*. doi:10.3389/fnins.2022.911153

Gattermann, R., Johnston, R. E., Yigit, N., Fritzsche, P., Larimer, S., Ozkurt, S., ... McPhee, M. E. (2008). Golden hamsters are nocturnal in captivity but diurnal in nature. *Biol Lett, 4*(3), 253–255. doi: 10.1098/rsbl.2008.0066

Halberg, F., Halberg, E., Barnum, C. P., & Bittner, J. J. (1959). Physiologic 24-hour periodicity in human beings and mice, the lighting regime and daily routine. In R. B. Withrow (Ed.), *Photoperiodism and Related Phenomena in Plants and Animals* (pp. 803–878). Washington, DC: American Association for the Advancement of Science.

Hut, R. A., van Oort, B. E. H., & Daan, S. (1999). Natural entrainment without dawn and dusk: the case of the European ground squirrel (*Spermophilus citellus*). *J Biol Rhythms, 14*(4), 290–299.

Johnson, M. S. (1939). Effect of continuous light on periodic spontaneous activity of white-footed mice (Peromyscus). *J Exp Zool, 82*, 315–328.

Kronauer, R. E., Czeisler, C. A., Pilato, S. F., Moore-Ede, M. C., & Weitzman, E. D. (1982). Mathematical model of the human circadian system with two interacting oscillators. *Am J Physiol, 242*, R3–R17.

Mills, J. N., Minors, D. S., & Waterhouse, J. M. (1977). The physiological rhythms of subjects living on a day of abnormal length. *J Physiol, 268*, 803–826.

Mistlberger, R. E., & Rusak, B. (2010). Circadian rhythms in mammals: Formal properties and environmental influences. In M. H. Kryger, T. Roth, & W. C. Dement (Eds.), *Principles and Practice of Sleep Medicine* (5th ed., pp. 363–375). St. Louis: Elsevier.

Mrosovsky, N. (1999). Masking: history, definitions, and measurement. *Chronobiol Int, 16*(4), 415–429. doi: 10.3109/07420529908998717

Pittendrigh, C. S. (1960). Circadian rhythms and the circadian organization of living systems. In A. Chovnick (Ed.), *Biological Clocks, Cold Spring Harbor Symposia on Quantitaive Biology*, Vol. XXV, pp. 159–184. Cold Spring Harbor: The Biological Laboratory.

Pittendrigh, C. S., & Daan, S. (1976). A functional analysis of circadian pacemakers in nocturnal rodents. IV. Entrainment: Pacemaker as clock. *J Comp Physiol A, 106*, 291–331.

Richter, C. P. (1971). Inborn nature of the rat's 24-hour clock. *J Comp Physiol Psych, 75*(1), 1–4.

Rusak, B. (1981). Vertebrate behavioral rhythms. In J. Aschoff (Ed.), *Biological Rhythms* (pp. 183–205). New York: Plenum Press.

Rusak, B., & Zucker, I. (1979). Neural regulation of circadian rhythms. *Physiol Rev, 59*(3), 449–526. doi: 10.1152/physrev.1979.59.3.449

Scheibler, E., Wollnik, F., Brodbeck, D., Hummel, E., Yuan, S., Zhang, F.-S., ... Wu, X.-D. (2013). Species composition and interspecific behavior affects activity pattern of free-living desert hamsters in the Alashan Desert. *J Mammal, 94*(2), 448–458. doi: 10.1644/12-mamm-a-115.1

Shanahan, T. L., & Czeisler, C. A. (1991). Light exposure induces equivalent phase shifts of the endogenous circadian rhythms of circulating plasma melatonin and core body temperature in men. *J Clin Endocr Metab, 73*, 227–235.

Shkolnik, A. (1971). Diurnal activity in a small desert rodent. *Int J Biometerol, 15*(2-4), 115–120.

Siegel, J. M. (2001). A tribute to Nathaniel Kleitman. *Arch Ital Biol, 139*, 3–10.

Takahashi, J. S. (1995). Molecular neurobiology and genetics of circadian rhythms in mammals. *Ann Rev Neurosci, 18*, 531–553.

Vanin, S., Bhutani, S., Montelli, S., Menegazzi, P., Green, E. W., Pegoraro, M., ... Kyriacou, C. P. (2012). Unexpected features of Drosophila circadian behavioural rhythms under natural conditions. *Nature, 484*, 371–375. doi: 10.1038/nature10991

Voirin, B., Scriba, M. F., Martinez-Gonzalez, D., Vyssotski, A. L., Wikelski, M., & Rattenborg, N. C. (2014). Ecology and neurophysiology of sleep in two wild sloth species. *Sleep, 37*(4), 753–761. doi: 0.5665/sleep.3584

Yamaguchi, Y., Okada, K., Mizuno, T., Ota, T., Yamada, H., Doi, M., Kobayashi, M., Tei, H., ... Okamura, H. (2016). Real-time recording of circadian *Per1* and *Per2* expression in the suprachiasmatic nucleus of freely moving rats. *J Biol Rhythms, 31*(1), 108–111. doi: 10.1177/0748730415621412

B.

Factors Affecting Sleep

CHAPTER 4

Sleep Across the Human Lifespan

4.1 OVERVIEW

Sleep is a dynamic process that changes across developmental stages from birth to old age, with the most dramatic changes occurring early in development. In reviewing the typical patterns of these lifespan changes in sleep, it is important to recognize that physiological age does not map perfectly onto chronological age. For example, early developmental markers, including sitting up, sleeping through the night, first tooth eruption, first step, etc. occur at somewhat different chronological ages among "typically developing" infants (i.e., those with no chronic illness or global developmental delay). Similarly, people age physiologically at different rates, so physical fitness and cognitive functions may be better preserved in some 80-year-olds than in some 60-year-olds. Thus, attributing sleep characteristics to specific ages should be seen as stating only a rough average around which there is substantial variation.

This chapter reviews the changes in the types and amounts of sleep shown over the course of development and during maturity and aging. It discusses the ambiguity of sleep states in early infancy, uncertainty as to their continuity with adult sleep stages, and evidence for early circadian regulation of sleep before entrainment to external cycles. This chapter reviews changes in sleep quality and patterns associated with major life transitions, including puberty, pregnancy, and menopause. It discusses the impact of puberty and aging on preferred sleep-wake timing (chronotype), and the negative consequences for adolescents of disconnects between delays in chronotype and scheduling of school attendance. It also explores the difficult issue of trying to determine which alterations in sleep features during development and aging are attributable to changes in internal sleep-regulatory mechanisms and which are attributable to other internal or external influences.

4.2 Sleep in infants

4.2.1 Development of daily rhythms

As new parents know, or soon learn to their regret, the sleep pattern described in Chapter 2 for a healthy young adult is typical only of this age group, and very different from that of newborn infants. As will be discussed later in this chapter, this lesson gets reinforced years later when their infant has grown into an adolescent and again displays sleep patterns different from those of the idealized young adult.

Newborn human infants show little if any circadian modulation of their sleep–wake cycles, with relatively brief sleep episodes occurring throughout the day and night (a polyphasic pattern, i.e., multiple sleep–wake cycles per day). The patterns of sleep and waking change rapidly during the first year of life, but it is not clear to what extent these changes result from physiological maturation of the infant or from the behavioral and other interventions attempted by sometimes desperate, sleep-deprived parents.

A classic study of infants during the first 6 months of life described the development of a generally nocturnal sleep pattern by 12–14 weeks (~3–4 months) of age in most infants (Kleitman & Engelmann, 1953). A more recent study that involved parents recording sleep diaries for their infants for 6 days each month from birth to 1 year of age found similar results. There was a rapid increase in the proportion of infants sleeping through the night during months 2 and 3 of life, and by 6 months of age >50% met the criterion of being asleep regularly between 22:00 and 06:00 (Henderson et al., 2010).

The record of sleep patterns of one infant girl ("4F") in the older study provides some fascinating insights into the maturation of the underlying mechanisms involved (**Figure 4.1**) (Kleitman & Engelmann, 1953). This infant's parents indulged her by allowing feeding and sleep on demand, and they indulged the experimenters by the remarkable feat of

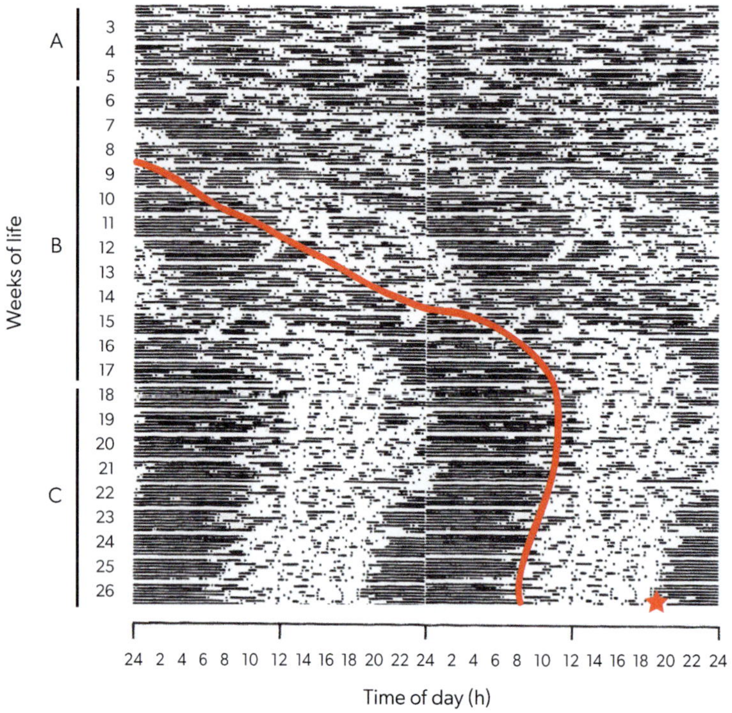

Figure 4.1 The self-selected sleep (black horizontal lines), wake (white areas) and feeding (black dots) of an infant girl (4F) from about the first week of life until 6 months of age. Weeks of age are numbered from top to bottom on the Y axis and time of day is shown on the X axis. The data are double-plotted to show continuous 48 h periods across the record from left to right. This plot makes the continuity of the emerging sleep–wake rhythm easier to detect visually. The apparently arrhythmic pattern shown at first (**A**) is followed by the emergence of an unstable rhythm with a period greater than 24 h that slants across the record from left to right (**B**) until about 16–18 weeks of age. The red line shows an estimate of the average daily times of onset of the major active phase as rhythmicity begins to emerge starting about weeks 6–9. About weeks 16–18, the period of the rhythm starts to gradually shorten until it is less than 24 h (**C**). By the end of the record, the rhythm appears to have become aligned with the 24 h day, with waking at ~06:00–08:00 and overnight sleep starting ~18:00–19:00 (red star). Adapted with permission of the American Physiological Society from Kleitman, N. & Engelmann, T. J. (1953) Sleep characteristics of infants. *J Appl Physiol* 6:269–282. © American Physiological Society (1953); permission conveyed through Copyright Clearance Center, Inc. doi: 10.1152/jappl.1953.6.5.269.

recording the timing of each feeding and sleep event from day 11 to day 182 of life.[1] Because feeding and sleep occurred on demand, the course of her development provides an opportunity to observe the maturation of sleep and circadian regulatory systems longitudinally and in the absence of deliberately imposed parental influences.

The resulting record of 4F's sleep and waking indicates that the first few weeks of life were quite chaotic (**Figure 4.1 A**), with no obvious daily structure to the timing of sleep, waking, or feeding. By about the 6th week of life, waking began to consolidate somewhat, but the relatively consolidated wake episode began to scan across the 24 h day with a period of ~25 h (**Figure 4.1 B**). Consolidation increased over the following weeks, and the period of the rhythm then shortened gradually toward 24 h, while continuing to cross all phases of the parents' 24 h day. By about 18 weeks of age, the infant showed a robust daily rhythm with sustained waking starting about 10:00 and a major sleep period beginning ~22:00–24:00. The length of the daily rhythm then shortened to slightly less than 24 h (**Figure 4.1 C**), gradually shifting the infant's principal sleep and wake phases earlier, until she settled on a bedtime of ~19:00 by 24 weeks of age.

Despite a handful of subsequent studies of individual infants, the record of 4F remains the most striking example of the apparent expression early in human life of a free-running circadian rhythm of sleep and wake (with a period >24 h) that only gradually becomes entrained to a 24 h cycle. One interpretation of these results is that the internal circadian clock that controls sleep cyclicity (and other rhythms) matures very early in development and is only later entrained to the day–night cycle. The idea that the circadian clock develops very early, and before external entrainment is possible, is supported by evidence suggesting the presence of a functioning circadian clock

[1] This would have been done with paper and pencil records. There are now devices and apps being sold that continuously monitor infants' activity, body temperature, respiration, sounds produced, and even the state of their diapers, among other measures.

prenatally in golden hamsters (*Mesocricetus auratus*), despite this species having the shortest gestation period among placental mammals (16 days) (Davis & Gorski, 1988; Viswanathan & Davis, 1997).

It is unknown which factors determined the age at which 4F became entrained to a 24 h schedule. It is possible that exposure to daily lighting cycles was involved. It is also possible that social cues played a role, despite the infant being allowed to choose her own feeding and sleep times. Parental responses to the infant's social interactions at different times of day and night, depending on their own states of alertness, would likely have been different, which might have contributed to the process of synchronization.

In a later study of a single male infant from birth to 6 months of age, entrainment of sleep and wake to a 24 h rhythm appeared much earlier than for 4F (about day 30 vs. day 120). The male infant was also on a self-selected schedule, but the family involved maintained its own rigid daily schedule, and the infant slept in the parents' bedroom. The parents also regularly measured the infant's melatonin and body temperature rhythms and ensured that he was exposed to natural light every day and was not exposed to any artificial light between sunset and sunrise. The earlier emergence of 24 h rhythmicity in this infant has tentatively been attributed to the natural light exposure during the day and the lack of artificial illumination at night (McGraw et al., 1999).

Since lighting conditions were not documented in earlier studies, we do not know to what extent differences in exposure to lighting cycles were important. In uncontrolled studies with single participants, different outcomes could be related to individual characteristics of the infants studied rather than to different external conditions.

Some naturalistic studies of infants in their home environments used actigraphy to monitor activity periodically during the first year. There was already a clear difference between day and night activity levels at 3 months of age, which became more clearly defined by 6 and 9 months (Rojo-Wissar et al., 2022; Sadeh et al., 1995). It remains unclear which factors determine the pattern of emergence of robust day–night rhythms in human infants. Brain maturation, parental scheduling, social interactions, and lighting conditions could all influence the development of sleep–wake regulatory systems and of circadian rhythm entrainment.

4.2.2 Early development of sleep architecture

Many aspects of a human neonate's physiology are initially immature and undergo major developmental changes in early life (Stern et al., 1969). Changes in brain organization are especially rapid during the first years of life, making it difficult to compare infant EEG features to those of adults. Infant sleep may not show all the features of adult sleep stages discussed in Chapter 2, or may show mixed characteristics that are difficult to classify. As a result, human infant sleep states are often labeled as active sleep (AS; resembling REM sleep) and quiet sleep (QS; resembling NREM sleep), with some sleep classified as "indeterminate" or "transitional" (Heraghty et al., 2008; Stern et al., 1969). In other mammalian species, which are born at earlier stages of development (e.g., rats or hamsters), the characteristics of sleep may be even more difficult to match to adult sleep stages.

There is much debate about whether the different sleep states observed in infants are functionally equivalent to adult sleep stages and whether they are developmentally continuous with them (Blumberg et al., 2005; Heller & Frank, 2009). It is not clear at what developmental stage the term "active sleep," for example, should be replaced by "REM sleep." Therefore, we will generally refer to the development of sleep in infants using the adult terminology while acknowledging that these states may not be strictly equivalent to adult sleep stages.

Over a 24 h period, a full-term, newborn human (i.e., 38–40 weeks gestational age, depending on starting point) typically sleeps ~16–18 h daily, broken up into 2–4 h sleep periods scattered across the day and night. The infant in **Figure 4.1**, for example, starts off sleeping a little over 15 h daily. REM sleep occupies ~50% (8–9 h) of sleep time (compared to ~20% in young adults) and alternates with NREM sleep in ~50–60 min cycles. States resembling REM and NREM sleep are also detectable in premature infants, possibly as early as 30 weeks of gestation. Those at a gestational age of 34 weeks show ~60% REM-like sleep, and those born at earlier developmental stages show increasingly higher proportions of this stage during ~1 h samples recorded during daytime (Georgoulas et al., 2021) (**Figure 4.2**).

One hypothesis is that high levels of REM (active) sleep in early development promote the crucial growth of neural connectivity during this period. REM sleep may selectively enhance projections that are functionally useful (e.g., within the motor system) while helping to eliminate connections that do not contribute to efficient motor patterns (see Sections 18.4.2 and 18.10). There is a significant positive correlation between the amount of REM sleep over several days (determined by a machine-learning algorithm derived from direct observation) in premature infants in a neonatal intensive care unit and the volume of brain white matter assessed at an age equivalent to full-term (Wang et al., 2024). These results are consistent with a role for REM sleep in increasing neural connectivity. They are also consistent with evidence of plasticity-related activity in sensorimotor systems of infant rats during twitching movements characteristic of REM sleep (Blumberg et al., 2020).

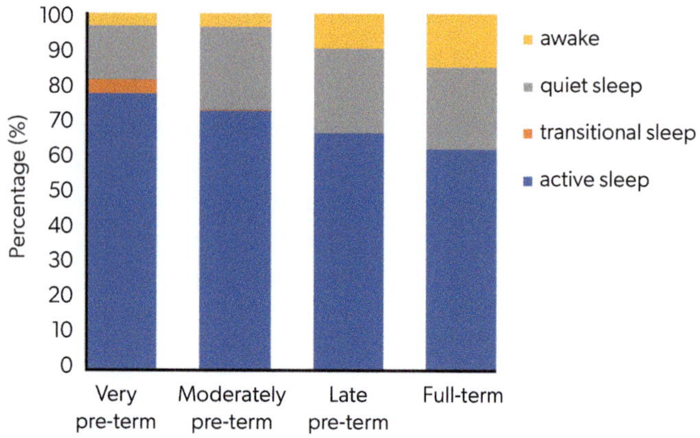

Figure 4.2 Sleep was recorded using EEG and behavioral measures in infants of different degrees of prematurity, and in full-term infants. The duration of active sleep (blue)—the infant analog of REM sleep—took up a larger proportion of the day in more premature infants, confirming the idea that this stage decreases developmentally *in utero*, as it continues to do after birth. Very preterm: ~28–32 weeks; Moderately preterm: ~32–34 weeks; Late preterm: ~34–37 weeks; Full term: ~37–40 weeks. Reprinted with permission of Oxford University Press and the Sleep Research Society under Creative Commons Attribution License (http://creativecommons.org/licenses/by/4.0/) from Georgoulas, A. et al. (2021) Sleep-wake regulation in preterm and term infants. *Sleep* 44:1-10. © Sleep Research Society (2020). doi: 10.1093/sleep/zsaa148.

Very early in postnatal development, newborns fall directly into REM sleep at sleep onset, which would be abnormal in healthy adults sleeping at night. By 3 months of age, total sleep time decreases, and there is more NREM sleep and more waking. REM sleep occurs later in each sleep episode, which begins to mimic the distribution of these stages across nocturnal sleep in adults. This shift may reflect maturation of homeostatic control of sleep. Lengthening waking episodes would cause an increased drive to express NREM sleep, which would tend to occur shortly after sleep onset, thereby delaying REM sleep to later in the episode (see Chapter 5).

By 6 months of age, the typical adult pattern has been established with NREM sleep regularly occurring at sleep onset. Since the circadian system is a critical regulator of the timing of REM sleep (see Section 2.5), the maturation of circadian control of sleep physiology during the first months of life (see **Figure 4.1**) likely contributes to this shift. By 6 months, the REM sleep proportion has fallen to ~25%, not far from adult values, reflecting a corresponding increase in time awake (Coons & Guilleminault, 1982).

These sleep patterns in the early postnatal period appear to be related to the fact that human infants share some features with mammals that are altricial (literally, "needing nourishment"), a term that refers to mammals like mice, rats, and cats, that are completely dependent on their parents at birth (**Figure 4.3 B**). Altricial mammalian young are born with no fur, with eyes and ears sealed shut, only partially formed limbs, and an immature sleep-wake pattern consistent with their early developmental stage.

Precocial mammalian species, like guinea pigs, deer, or horses, have young that are born at a much more mature developmental stage: fully furred, eyes open, able to walk, and looking and acting much like small adults (**Figure 4.3 A**). Precocial neonates show essentially adult-like EEG sleep patterns by 1 week after birth (Ibuka, 1984). They do, however, show higher levels of REM sleep prenatally, a stage at which both their sleep and anatomy more closely resemble those of altricial neonates.

Human neonates are unusual in showing a mixture of altricial and precocial characteristics at birth. They have

A. Precocial B. Altricial

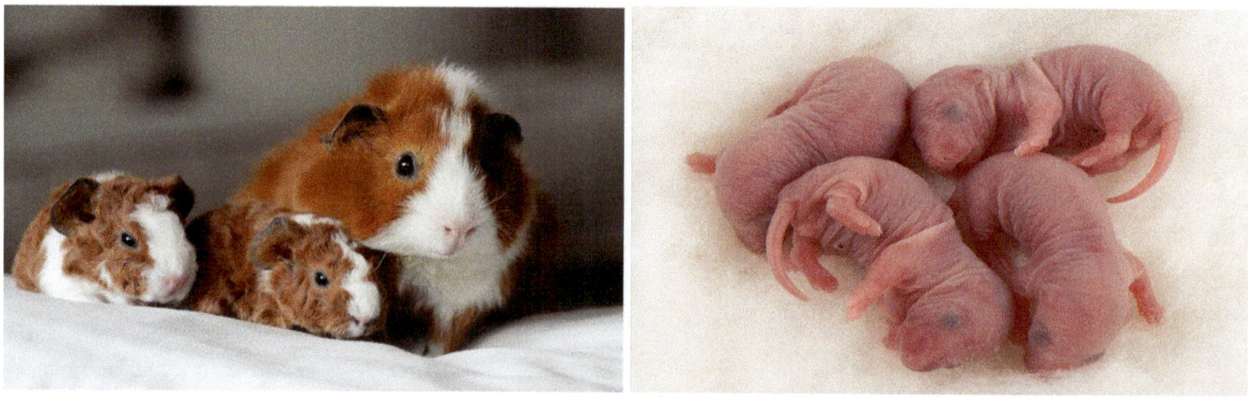

Figure 4.3 Differences between precocial and altricial newborn mammals. **A.** The guinea pig mother (*Cavia porcellus*) is accompanied by two newborn, precocial offspring, which are fully furred, capable of walking, and equipped with open eyes and ears, looking much like miniature adults. Naomi Marcin/Shutterstock. **B.** The altricial, newborn mice (*Mus musculus*) have no fur, their eyes are sealed over, ears closed and adhering to the head, and their digits are only partially formed. Kungfu01/Shutterstock.

well-formed digits and well-developed visual and auditory functions, as do the precocial neonates of other primates and of species like deer and horses. But their initial sleep patterns are more similar to those of altricial species, which is consistent with some of their other characteristics: they cannot stand, move about independently, or cling to their mothers as other primate neonates can do.

4.2.3 Summary

Sleep changes dramatically during maturation of human infants from birth through the first few months of life. Full-term, human neonates show a predominance of REM-like (active) sleep, which often occurs at sleep onset, and an irregular polyphasic sleep and waking pattern. With increasing amounts of NREM sleep and waking during the first year of life, NREM sleep begins to occur more frequently at sleep onset, perhaps reflecting maturation of homeostatic regulatory mechanisms.

There is evidence suggesting that the human circadian clock begins functioning and affecting the timing of sleep and waking early during the first year of life, before sleep becomes consolidated and entrained to the external 24 h cycle. As circadian control is imposed, the scattered sleep bouts of neonates gradually coalesce into a major sleep episode during the night and one or more shorter daytime naps. It is unclear to what extent maturation, exposure to lighting cycles, social interactions, or other cues contribute to this process.

Whether the active and quiet states of sleep in infants are functionally equivalent to REM and NREM sleep stages in adults is uncertain. Human infants show a mixture of altricial and precocial features at birth. They have some features that are characteristic of precocial species, including the degree of maturity of their auditory and visual functions. But the large amount of REM-like sleep that they show initially is consistent with their other altricial characteristics, such as lack of independent locomotion. Even more REM-like sleep is seen in premature human infants and prenatally in precocial mammals, while fully precocial species show adult-like sleep patterns shortly after birth. REM-like sleep may be important during early development for experience-dependent growth and selective strengthening of neural projections that are functionally useful, for example, in relation to their rapidly developing motor systems.

4.3 Sleep in childhood

Parents are often interested in learning what the appropriate sleep durations are for children as they grow and mature. One approach to answering this question is to consult population-based surveys of average sleep durations at different ages. Survey results, however, do not necessarily reflect what is developmentally "normal" nor how much sleep children need. This raises the question of how we can determine sleep need, which is discussed below and in Chapter 13, but is difficult to answer conclusively.

From the earliest stages of development, parental beliefs, attitudes, and behaviors related to children's sleep influence the durations and patterns of sleep shown (Sadeh et al., 2010). These influences differ among societies, change over the years, and vary among cultural subgroups within a society. Survey results inevitably reflect the current norms in the particular cultural environment(s) being studied. In industrial societies, changes in family lifestyles and in related cultural norms over recent decades have changed what parents consider to be the sleep needs of their children; these issues are discussed further in Chapter 6.

A study of reported sleep patterns in young children conducted across 13 countries reported large differences in the regular use of bedtime routines. The presence of a consistent parent–child bedtime routine was associated with children having earlier bedtimes, longer sleep durations, and fewer reported sleep problems (Mindell, Li, et al., 2015). In studies combining actigraphy with parental reports of sleep routines and timing in infants, earlier bedtimes and more consistent nightly routines were also associated with longer sleep durations (Adams et al., 2020; Tsai et al., 2022).

However, there are also exceptions to these findings, as summarized in a recent meta-analysis. It noted that among several studies that reported on patterns of parental involvement with the sleep of children aged 1–3 years, and on the impacts of children's sleep locations, there were exceptional findings that were inconsistent with the most common observations. It also highlighted the difficulty of summarizing across studies, given differences in terminology used, inconsistencies in parental behaviors over time, and potential impacts of cultural differences among study participants (Cook et al., 2023).

Reports of observed sleep durations in children are also influenced by the different methods used to assess sleep, which include polysomnography (PSG) in a laboratory setting or at home, actigraphy, parental reports, self-reports (in older children), and sleep diaries. Parental reports were shown to overestimate sleep durations relative to actigraphy at 6 months of age, especially for long- and short-sleeping infants (Quante et al., 2021). Studies of older children also observed significant differences between parental reports and actigraphy, especially for total sleep duration and nighttime waking (Kushnir & Sadeh, 2013; Werner et al., 2008).

Similarly, some reports indicated that by 12 months of age children's sleep is reduced to 14–15 h daily, including one major consolidated sleep period and 1–2 naps (Heraghty et al., 2008; Iglowstein et al., 2003). However, a study that used actigraphy found that children slept only about 11 h daily at 12 months of age, and it noted the very high variability in sleep durations among children at any one chronological age (Acebo et al., 2005).

An American study reported a gradual decline in the total number of hours of sleep daily after 1 year of age, reaching 9–9.5 h by age 5 (Acebo et al., 2005) (**Figure 4.4**). This value included both night sleep and daytime naps, the number and length of which decreased up to about age 5. A meta-analysis of sleep stages and overall duration reported a continuing decrease in total sleep duration, especially in the amount of N3 sleep, from age 5 into adolescence/young adulthood (Ohayon et al., 2004) (**Figure 4.5**). There was also an increase in N2 sleep over this period and, because the absolute duration of REM sleep was relatively stable while total sleep time decreased, there was a modest increase in the percentage of REM sleep.

In some countries, daytime naps are much reduced or lost by school age, but in other societies afternoon naps ("siestas") are considered normal among both children and adults (see Chapter 6). People living in societies in which afternoon naps are uncommon, and often frowned upon, still tend to become less alert at this time of day during a so-called post-lunch dip (see **Figure 2.11**). This label refers only to timing of naps or sleepiness, since the dip occurs even if one does not eat lunch.

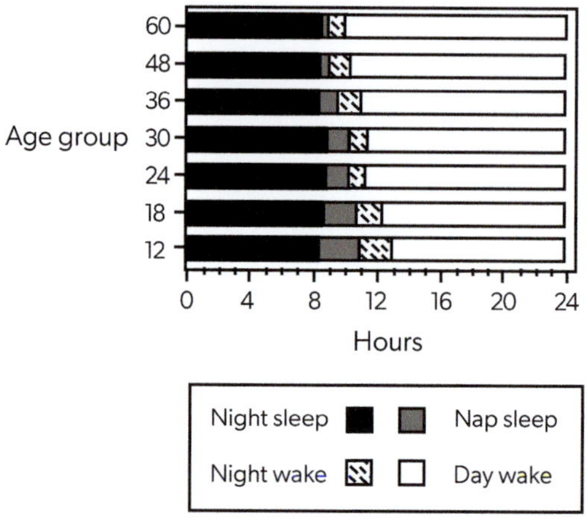

Figure 4.4 Changes in the durations of night sleep (black), nap sleep (grey), wakefulness at night (stippled), and waking during the day (white) from 12 to 60 months of age (Y axis, bottom to top). Total sleep duration (night and naps) falls over this period, sleep becomes more consolidated during the night with less night waking, and waking becomes more consolidated during the day as daytime napping decreases. Reprinted with permission of Oxford University Press and the Sleep Research Society from Acebo, C. et al. (2005) Sleep/wake patterns derived from activity monitoring and maternal report for healthy 1- to 5-year-old children. *Sleep* 28:1568–1577. © Sleep Research Society (2005). doi: 10.1093/sleep/28.12.1568.

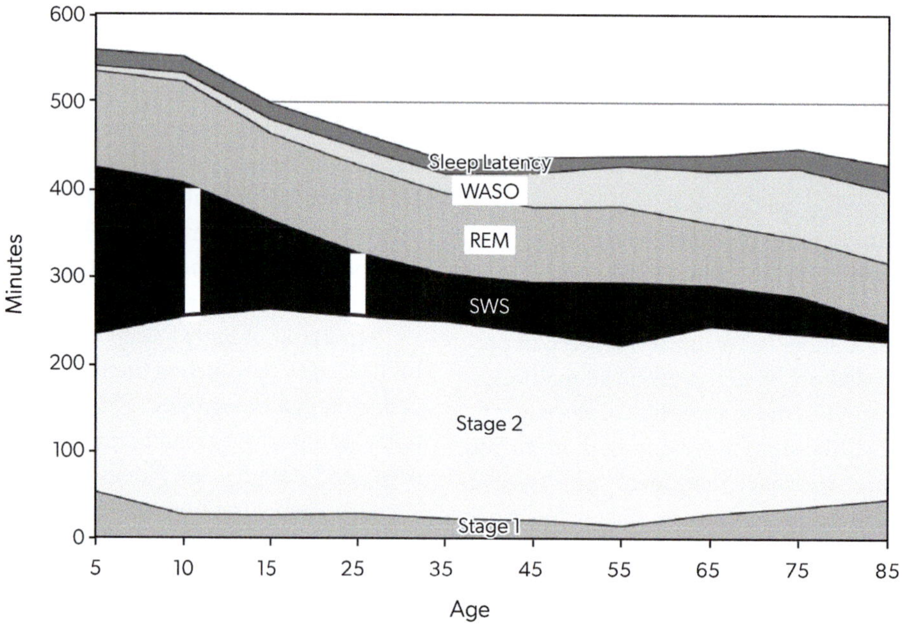

Figure 4.5 A summary of the results of a meta-analysis of studies of sleep at different ages, showing the changes in total sleep duration (minutes on the Y axis), proportions of sleep stages, wake after sleep onset (WASO) and sleep onset latency from age 5 to 85 years. The vertical white bars inserted at ages 10 and 25 in the SWS section illustrate the dramatic decrease in SWS amounts during adolescence and young adulthood. There is another decline in SWS during aging (mostly in men; see text and **Figure 4.15**) along with increases in N1 (Stage 1) sleep, sleep onset latency, and WASO, starting during middle age and continuing into older age groups. Adapted with permission of Oxford University Press and the Sleep Research Society from Ohayon, M. M. et al. (2004) Meta-analysis of quantitative sleep parameters from childhood to old age in healthy individuals: developing normative sleep values across the human lifespan. *Sleep* 27:1255–1273. © Sleep Research Society (2004). doi: 10.1093/sleep/27.7.1255.

Evidence suggests that a tendency to nap after midday may be biologically ancient (and even occurs in monkeys; see **Figure 8.11 C**), but is subject to cultural modification (Strogatz et al., 1987); for a review, see Monk, 2005. Some adults in "non-siesta" societies may schedule naps for this time if their daily schedules allow, and others may simply increase their stimulant intake (e.g., caffeine) to counteract the effects of the dip. Attitudes toward daytime naps appear, however, to be changing in some historically non-siesta societies (see Section 6.2).

Changing cultural trends over time affect the sleep of young children, as demonstrated in a longitudinal study of sleep in Switzerland. The study involved three cohorts of children born, respectively, in 1974, 1979, and 1986, each of which were followed until they were 16 years old. As expected, there was a gradual decrease in sleep duration over development, but there was also a systematic decrease in sleep duration across successive cohorts. This change was especially pronounced in the first years of life. Sleep durations at 1 year of age had decreased by almost an hour between the first and last cohorts (12 years apart), largely because of progressively later sleep onset times (Iglowstein et al., 2003). Given the very high degree of parental control over children's sleep timing at 1 year of age, this observation implies a rapidly emerging cultural trend toward permitting later sleep onsets and shorter durations for very young children.

Other studies also point to how parental attitudes influence sleep durations of their children. A population-based study in Portugal documented the gradual decline of sleep duration with later bedtimes and fixed wake times on school nights for children aged 4–11. Sleep durations were longer, however, on nights before "free days" (no morning obligations) because both bedtimes and wake-up times were delayed (Clara & Allen Gomes, 2019). Similarly, a Canadian study reported a delay in the timing of sleep onset in later childhood that occurred selectively on weekends. This outcome was apparently the result of parents relaxing their enforcement of bedtimes for older children on weekend nights but not on school nights (Touchette et al., 2008).

These reports of how much sleep children get (and those related to adolescents in the next section) return us to the question of how much sleep children and adolescents actually need. One approach used to address this question was to base an answer on the published literature related to the effects of inadequate sleep durations. The resulting review synthesized the outcomes of more than 850 published reports on negative health and cognitive consequences of inadequate sleep amounts in children and adolescents (see Chapters 13–15). Acknowledging that there are also individual differences in sleep need, the resulting recommendations included ranges of sleep duration required to promote optimal development and health (i.e., to avoid the observed negative effects of short sleep) in children aged 4 months to 18 years (Paruthi et al., 2016). Their recommendations are summarized in **Box 4.1**.

BOX 4.1 Recommended Sleep Durations for Children

- Infants 4–12 months old: 12–16 h per 24 h (including naps)
- Children 1–2 years old: 11–14 h per 24 h (including naps)
- Children 3–5 years old: 10–13 h per 24 h (including naps)
- Children 6–12 years old: 9–12 h per 24 h
- Teenagers 13–18 years old: 8–10 h per 24 h

Adapted from Paruthi, S., Brooks, L. J., D'Ambrosio, C., Hall, W. A., Kotagal, S., Lloyd, R. M., ... Wise, M. S. (2016). Recommended amount of sleep for pediatric populations: a consensus statement of the American Academy of Sleep Medicine. *J Clin Sleep Med*, *12*(6), 785–786. doi: 10.5664/jcsm.5866

4.3.1 Summary

There is a gradual decline in the amount of N3 sleep, an increase in N2 sleep, and stable amounts of REM sleep over childhood. Total sleep time also decreases over the years of childhood, and its timing becomes gradually more delayed. This developmental sequence is a product of both physiological maturation and parental and cultural influences. Culturally determined parental behavior related to bedtime routines and beliefs about the sleep needs of their children influence the length and timing of children's sleep and how it is modified by expectations of next-day activities.

There is a gradual decline in the length and frequency of daytime naps during early childhood, and their elimination by school age in some societies. But in other societies, daytime sleep is preserved into adulthood for many people in the form of siestas. The weaning of children from daytime naps is, in part, a preparation for school attendance in societies where this occurs beginning about age 5. There are, however, ongoing cultural changes in both siesta and non-siesta societies in relation to the acceptability of daytime sleep in both children and adults (see Chapter 6).

Given the cultural and social influences on the length and pattern of children's sleep, as well as the impact of individual differences, it is difficult to determine how much sleep individual children need at different ages. One approach to developing guidelines for lengths of sleep children need considered the negative consequences of short sleep durations on cognition and health in children. The resulting guidelines indicate ranges for the lengths of sleep children and adolescents of different ages need for optimal health and developmental outcomes.

4.4 Sleep in adolescence

4.4.1 Sleep EEG changes

Adolescence is a period marked by major changes in endocrine function, secondary sexual characteristics, body size, and social roles (including increasing autonomy and responsibility), many of which are linked to sexual maturation (Patton & Viner, 2007). Physiological and social changes occurring during adolescence affect the timing and organization of sleep, as they do most other aspects of life.

Several features of sleep physiology, including total sleep duration (see **Figure 4.5**), change during the period beginning with the onset of puberty and extending through adolescence. One longitudinal study described a steep decline at about the age of puberty in EEG delta power density during NREM sleep. This is a measure of the amount of power per unit time in the delta frequency band as assessed using Fourier analysis (see Chapter 2). Although it was stable during ages 9–11 years, delta power density declined steeply in adolescents aged 12–14 years (Feinberg et al., 2006). The decline in delta power density began about 1 year earlier in girls than in boys, which correlates with differences in the timing of onset of both sexual maturation and changes in cortical organization.

When studied into adolescence (up to 16.5 years old), the decline in delta-band power continued and was matched by a steep decline in cortical theta power that had begun earlier (between 6 and 9 years) (Campbell & Feinberg, 2009). A large study of adolescents from 12–21 years of age found a decline in N3 sleep and delta power over that age range, with somewhat larger changes in males than females during later adolescence (i.e., after all had gone through puberty) (Baker et al., 2016).

One interpretation of the reduced power in slow EEG frequencies during adolescence is that it results from a reduction in cortical synaptic connectivity and gray matter volume that occurs during that period (Buchmann et al., 2011). These changes might result in a reduced potential for local neural synchrony, and therefore a reduction in the amplitude of EEG waveforms in the theta and delta ranges during both waking (Whitford et al., 2007) and sleep (Feinberg et al., 2006) (see **Figure 2.8**). Reduced slow-wave activity in older people has also been attributed to a reduction in connectivity in frontal cortical regions, and a resulting reduction in local neural synchrony (Carrier et al., 2011; Chylinski et al., 2022).

The reduction in synapse numbers during adolescence is related to rapid growth in the number of synapses during early childhood (before age 5), followed by experience-dependent pruning of synapses that is most intense in early adolescence (**Figure 4.6**), resulting in a refined pattern of neural connectivity (Huttenlocher, 1979; Marin, 2016; Whitford et al., 2007).

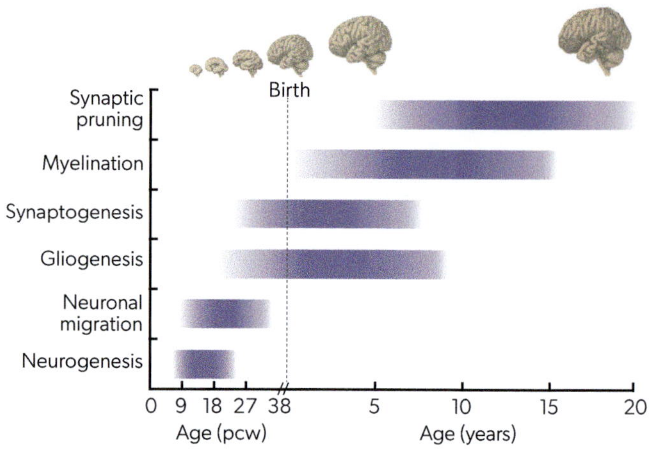

Figure 4.6 An approximate timeline of different aspects of human brain development. The darker parts of each bar represent the ages at which there is the greatest intensity of the process indicated on the Y axis. Age on the X axis is shown as post-conception weeks [Age (pcw)] and as years after birth [Age (years)]. The images at the top of the figure illustrate the relative sizes of the brain at different ages and the changes in gross anatomical features. Genesis of new synapses peaks before age 5, and the rate of synaptic pruning is highest in early adolescence. Reprinted with permission from Marin, O. (2016) Developmental timing and critical windows for the treatment of psychiatric disorders. *Nat Med* 22:1229–1238. © Springer: Nature (2016). doi: 10.1038/nm.4225.

The extent of synaptic pruning during adolescence was quantified in the results of a study of one small cortical region (primary visual cortex) in macaque monkeys (*Macaca mulatta*). It found that synapse numbers in this region fell by 45% starting about the time of puberty. That reduction over <2.5 years corresponded to losing synapses at a remarkable average rate of 5,000/second over that period in this one cortical region (Bourgeois & Rakic, 1993).

Pruning of synaptic connections after a period of exuberant synapse formation in early childhood may be critically important for the normal development of adult brain functions (Boksa, 2012; Feinberg, 1983). Adolescence is a period marked by the emergence of major psychiatric disorders (Paus et al., 2008), which may be linked to altered patterns of synaptic pruning during this period. For example, the presence of a genetic feature that promotes overly aggressive pruning of connections in the prefrontal cortex was linked to an increased probability of developing schizophrenia (Sekar et al., 2016). The establishment of distinctive, stable patterns of connectivity in brain circuits (the "connectome") was found to be delayed in the brains of adolescents with developing psychiatric symptoms, compared to those of healthy controls, which may be related to altered pruning patterns (Kaufmann et al., 2017).

BOX 4.2 Mechanisms of Gray Matter Reduction in Adolescent Brains

Cortical tissue is divided into gray matter, made up mostly of cell bodies, and white matter, made up mostly of myelinated fiber tracts (the myelin coating on axons providing the white color), and a small volume of cerebrospinal fluid. During adolescence, there is a reduction in the ratio of the volume of gray matter to that of white matter, which could represent absolute decreases in gray matter and/or increases in white matter.

One change that could be responsible for an increase in white matter volume is an increase in myelination. An imaging method that detects myelination (mean-centered MTR) showed that a modest rate of increase in white matter volume in female adolescents (**Figure 4.7A, left**) can be accounted for by a parallel increase in the rate of myelination (**Figure 4.7B, left**). However, in male adolescents during the same period, there were steeply *opposite* changes in white matter volume (increasing; **Figure 4.7A, right**) and in this measure of myelination (decreasing; **Figure 4.7B, right**).

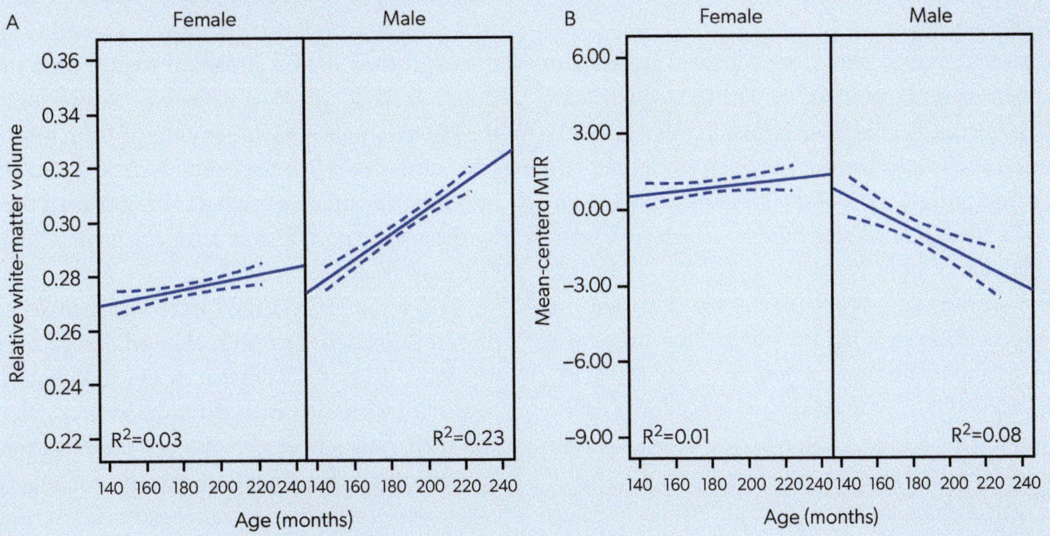

Figure 4.7 **A.** The Y axis shows changes in the relative volume of white matter (i.e., relative to gray matter volume) in human brains across adolescence (~12–20 years of age, shown as months on the X axis). Relative volumes of white matter increased in both females and males but more steeply in males. The solid lines show the average changes in these measures as a function of age and the dashed lines enclose error estimates around these mean values. The R^2 values indicate the proportion of variation in these measures that is accounted for by age. These values show that relative white matter volume is strongly age-dependent in males (age accounts for 23% of the variation) but less so in females (3%). **B.** Changes in mean-centered magnetization transfer ratio (MTR, a magnetic resonance imaging-based indirect measure of myelination) during the same period. The age-related changes in females parallel those in relative white matter volume, suggesting that increasing myelination can account for the small change in the proportion of white matter in the brain. The steep decline in mean-centered MTR in males is opposite to the change in relative white matter volume, indicating that something other than increasing myelination must account for the relative changes in white matter volume in males. Reprinted with permission from Paus, T. et al. (2008). Why do many psychiatric disorders emerge during adolescence? *Nat Rev Neurosci* 9:947–957. © Springer: Nature (2008). doi: 10.1038/nrn2513.

Thus, the modest increases in the ratio of white to gray matter seen in adolescent females can be accounted for by increased myelination, while the more dramatic increases in this ratio in adolescent males do not appear to be related to increased myelination (Paus et al., 2008). There is evidence that suggests instead that the steep increase in white matter signal in adolescent males may be related to testosterone-dependent increases in the diameter of axons (Pesaresi et al., 2015).

Brain changes observed during adolescence vary across regions of cortex and differ between males and females; they are complex, dependent on the measurement method used, and sometimes difficult to interpret (Kaufmann et al., 2017; Paus et al., 2008; Sowell et al., 2003); see **Box 4.2**. Much remains to be learned about how male and female brains change during adolescent development and how these modifications are linked to changes in EEG parameters, sleep, and risks of mental illness.

4.4.2 Adolescent sleep delay

The most obvious changes in sleep patterns shown by adolescents are a delay in the timing of sleep onset and a gradual reduction in total sleep time, often below recommended amounts, and especially on school nights. Reduced sleep durations result from delayed sleep onsets combined with fixed waking times that are set by school schedules. On weekends or holidays, during which wake times are not determined by external factors (free days), onset of both sleep and waking are typically delayed in adolescents. As a result, sleep duration on those nights can lengthen even beyond recommended levels as a rebound response to previous school-night sleep deprivation (Andrade et al., 1993; Carskadon, 2004; Crowley et al., 2007; Wolfson & Carskadon, 1998).

Young children tend to show early phase preferences (e.g., waking their parents at 06:00 or earlier) which start to delay as they approach puberty (Carskadon et al., 1993). The adolescent delay in sleep timing has been attributed to a change in the underlying period of the circadian clock regulating sleep–wake timing or to a change in sensitivity to the phase-shifting effects of light (Crowley et al., 2007; Micic et al., 2016). There is some support for increased sensitivity to the delaying effects of evening light exposure, but only early in adolescence, at about the time of puberty (Crowley et al., 2015). There is also evidence supporting a lengthening of the circadian period during adolescence, which is seen in people as well as in several other species, presumably as a result of hormonal and neural changes (Crowley et al., 2018). Based on oscillator theory, a longer circadian period predicts a delay in preferred timing of sleep onset and end, while a shorter circadian period predicts an advanced phase preference (see Chapter 3 and **Figure 3.5**).

Different preferences for timing of sleep, waking and other activities represent different chronotypes (e.g., "night-owl," or evening type vs. "lark," or morning type). One way of assessing these tendencies is by using a self-report questionnaire that asks about preferred times for sleep, waking, and specific activities (e.g., taking an examination or engaging in an athletic competition), such as the original Horne-Östberg Morningness-Eveningness Questionnaire (Horne & Östberg, 1976), or one of several similar survey tools that have been developed (Smith et al., 1989).

One of these questionnaires, the Munich ChronoType Questionnaire (MCTQ) (Zavada et al., 2009), was made available to a large number of participants through a web-based link. It was used to collect chronotype data from ~25,000 participants (up to 2004) across a broad age range, mostly from Germany and Switzerland. The target measure used to represent chronotype (and therefore apparent phase of entrainment) was the timing of the midpoint of the sleep period on free days. This measure showed a gradual shift toward a more delayed chronotype beginning about the age of puberty and peaking at about age 20, then a slower drift back toward an earlier phase preference throughout adulthood (**Figure 4.8, A**) (Roenneberg et al., 2004). A recent meta-analysis of studies that used actigraphy reported effects of age on sleep duration and efficiency, but especially strong effects on the timing of sleep. It confirmed a gradual delay of sleep timing up to age 21, and a gradual advance of sleep timing beginning about age 22 (Evans et al., 2021).

The pattern of change in MCTQ scores and in sleep onset is closely matched to the timing of the onset of melatonin secretion in the evening under circadian clock control. The dim-light melatonin onset (DLMO)[2] marks the time at which melatonin levels rise above a threshold value marking the beginning of the circadian night phase (see Section 9.4) (Lewy & Sack, 1989). A review of studies of DLMOs across the lifespan found a similar change from advanced phases in early childhood to a maximal delay at about age 20, followed by a slow advance through adulthood until the average phase in the oldest people was similar to that of young children (Kennaway, 2023).

When the MCTQ data were analyzed separately by (self-reported) gender, the results showed that young girls started to develop a delayed preference earlier than boys (**Figure 4.8 B**), consistent with their earlier decline in sleep delta power density and their typically earlier onset of puberty. Young men, however, eventually became more extreme evening types, and their chronotypes remained significantly delayed relative to those of women throughout young adulthood and into middle age. This difference was lost before age 45, corresponding roughly to the typical timing of onset of the menopause transition in women.

The rather abrupt reversal in trend from increasing to decreasing delay preference also occurred at an earlier average age in women (~19.5) than in men (~20.9). This age of reversal of the adolescent chronotype tendency was proposed to represent a biological marker for the end of adolescence (Roenneberg et al., 2004). A large school-based survey of children and adolescents confirmed the more delayed phase in male than female adolescents but reported a somewhat earlier loss of the delaying tendency, closer to age 17–18, depending on the statistical model used (Randler et al., 2019).

The standard deviations around the averages in **Figure 4.8** indicate the extent of variation among individuals. While most of these individual differences are unexplained, there is evidence supporting an endocrine basis for chronotype variation

[2] Dim light at the time of sampling is important because melatonin production is very sensitive to light exposure, so even moderately bright evening light can suppress its rise. See Chapter 9 for details about the regulation of melatonin production and the use of DLMO as a marker of circadian phase.

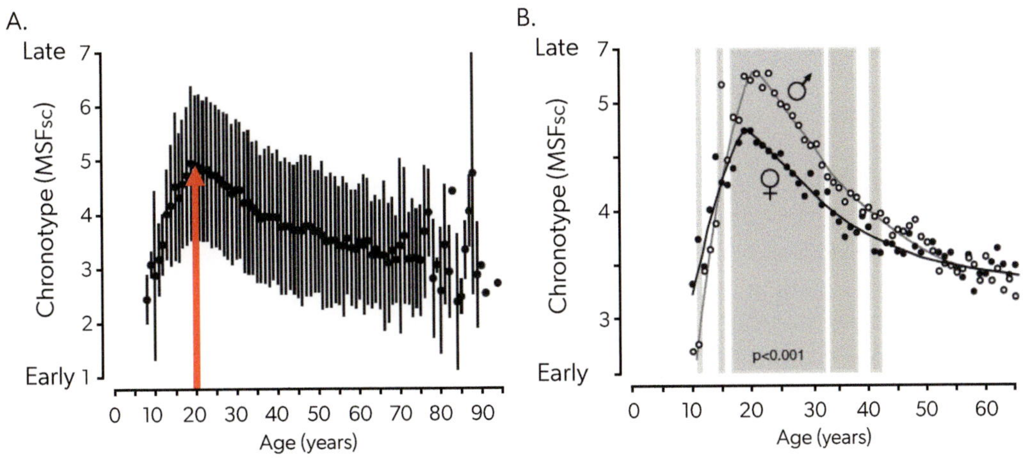

Figure 4.8 Chronotypes of ~25,000 participants from a web-based survey. **A.** Chronotypes are defined in relation to the midpoint of the sleep phase on days with no constraints on sleep timing (MSFsc; Y axis), with evening-type (Late) preference at the top and morning-type (Early) preference at the bottom. Children under 10 had a strong morning/early chronotype, and this shifted toward an evening/late chronotype over adolescence until about age 20 (red arrow). At that point, phase preference started to reverse back toward earlier phases through adulthood and into old age. Mean values in the oldest groups (>75 years) are probably not reliable, given the small number of participants in those age categories, leading to high variability. Values shown are means (black dots) ± standard deviations. **B.** The same data as in **A** were replotted separately for males and females. Females (♀) started to shift to a later phase preference at a younger age than males (♂), consistent with an earlier onset of puberty in girls than in boys, but males developed more extreme eveningness. Females started to reverse toward an earlier phase preference just before age 20, and males started to reverse around age 21. The inflection point at which phase preference starts to reverse has been proposed to represent a biological marker for the end of physiological adolescence and beginning of adulthood. Males had a consistently more delayed chronotype than females throughout adulthood until about age 45, when the two curves converged. Ages at which gender differences were statistically significantly different at $p<0.001$ are marked with gray areas. Adapted with permission of Elsevier, Ltd. from Roenneberg, T. et al. (2004) A marker for the end of adolescence. *Curr Biol* 14:R1038–1039. © (2004) Elsevier. doi: 10.1016/j.cub.2004.11.039

among young men. Young-adult men with higher levels of testosterone, sampled either in the morning (in saliva samples) or cumulatively over several months (in hair samples), were positively correlated with more extreme evening chronotype scores (Jankowski et al., 2019; Randler et al., 2012).

Several features of these data are consistent with an influence on chronotype of changes in sex hormone levels:

- the delaying tendency began around puberty onset and differed between males and females in parallel to differences in the timing of puberty;
- the age of reversal from delaying to advancing phase preferences differed in young men and women;
- there was a gender difference in phase preference during most of young adulthood and early middle age;
- this gender difference was lost at about the beginning of menopause;
- young men with higher testosterone levels had more delayed rhythms.

The idea that sex hormones acting on the period of the circadian clock are responsible for these phase preference changes is consistent with evidence from animal studies that both estrogen and testosterone can affect aspects of circadian organization, including circadian period (Daan et al., 1975; Morin, Fitzgerald, & Zucker, 1977).

Findings related to other brain functions support a role for testosterone during puberty in reorganizing neural systems. For example, performing a task involving emotional regulation strongly activated the thalamus and amygdala in children and the prefrontal cortex in adults. In a study of 14-year-olds performing this task, those with higher testosterone levels among both boys (from testes and adrenal glands) and girls (from ovaries and adrenals) showed a more adult-like pattern of activation (Tyborowska et al., 2016).

4.4.3 Other influences on chronotype

Although most people shift their preferred wake and sleep phases to later times during adolescence, there is variability within any population. Thus, a small number of people retain a childhood preference for early awakening and bedtimes throughout their lives. These preferences have been shown to have a genetic basis in some cases. Studies of lineages in which many members are extreme morning types throughout life (Familial Advanced Sleep Phase Syndrome) demonstrated a role for a mutation in a gene (*CASEIN KINASE Iδ*) that influences expression of a circadian clock gene (*PER2*), thereby shortening circadian rhythm periods and leading to advanced phase preferences (Toh et al., 2001; Xu et al., 2005). (See **Figure 8.8 B** and **Box 8.1** for an introduction to circadian clock genes.)

Polymorphisms in other genes that influence circadian periodicity have instead been linked to extreme delayed phase preferences. These genes include the circadian clock genes *PER3*, *CLOCK*, and *CRY1* (Patke et al., 2017; Zhang & Kay, 2010). Another factor that affects sleep timing is sensitivity of the specialized retinal mechanism that is involved in entrainment (see Section 8.2.4). Increased sensitivity to light in the evening would promote larger circadian phase delays, resulting in later preferred sleep and wake timing.

These results indicate that there are genetic factors that contribute to some people having a characteristic circadian entrainment pattern that is either more advanced or delayed than that of most of the population. Similarly, individuals of other species can differ from their species-typical pattern in circadian rhythm entrainment and in the timing of seasonal reproduction (often based on circadian mechanisms) (Johnston & Zucker, 1983; Prendergast et al., 2001).

Thus, "species-typical" timing patterns are not necessarily universal among members of a species. Humans are a typically diurnal species, but they also show significant chronotype variation, including some having relatively more nocturnal phase preferences. There are probably advantages for a small number of individuals in a population to differ from the species-typical activity/rest pattern (either lifelong or at certain life stages) because this allows them to fill temporal niches (ecological niches in time rather than in space) for which most of the population is not well suited.

In addition to physiological mechanisms, there are also strong social factors operating that encourage progressively later bedtimes during adolescence. Setting the bedtimes of children is a role for parents in many societies (but not all; see Chapter 6), and this child-rearing function is usually relinquished gradually during adolescence. During the transition from complete parental control to complete autonomy, bedtime is often a battleground that serves as a proxy for a host of other issues related to the emerging independence of teens. Control of bedtime not only marks a stage of development but also signals the acquisition of a privilege previously reserved for parents and older siblings. In addition, late evenings are often when social interactions occur beyond parental control. The attractions of peer interactions and the associated peer pressures undoubtedly play a role in further encouraging many adolescents to adopt later bedtimes. Thus, both physiological and social factors conspire to encourage delay of the sleep phase among adolescents (Crowley et al., 2018).

Combined with fixed school start times (see next section), this delaying tendency results in adolescents getting considerably less sleep than recommended for either teenagers (8–10 h) or adults (7–9 h). A survey of American university students (17–24 years old) found that 25% reported getting less than 6.5 h of sleep per night, 20% had missed an entire night of sleep during the previous month, 35% reported staying up until 03:00 at least once per week, and 15% reported falling asleep in class at least once per week (Lund et al., 2010).

4.4.4 School start times and social jetlag

The gradual decline in overall sleep duration during adolescence (see **Figure 4.5**) masks the fact that sleep durations are often much shorter on nights preceding school attendance than on weekend or vacation nights (**Figure 4.9**). Larger differences between weekend and school-night sleep durations predicted worse academic performance in a study we conducted involving >1,700 grade 7–12 students in Halifax County, Nova Scotia (LeBlanc et al., 1997, unpublished data).

In some jurisdictions, school start times for teenagers may be as early as 07:15, and lengthy commutes can require waking up 1–2 h earlier. A survey reported that in 2011–2012, the average start time for American middle and secondary schools was ~08:00, and ~8% had start times before 07:30. Despite the known progressive delay in chronotype later in adolescence, secondary school start times were paradoxically earlier than those for middle schools (Wheaton et al., 2015) (**Figure 4.10**). A recent issue of the journal *Sleep Health* included a series of

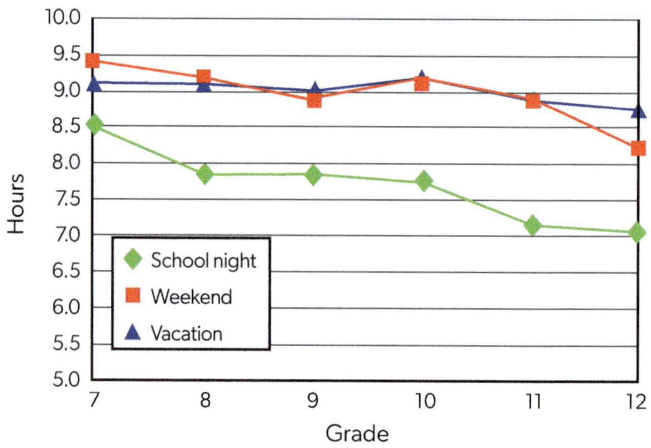

Figure 4.9 Hours of self-reported sleep from >1,700 students in grades 7–12 from a randomized survey of schools in Halifax County, Nova Scotia in 1998. The hours of sleep (Y axis) are shown separately for periods of vacation (blue), weekend nights (red), and school nights (green). Sleep durations declined with age (from grade 7 to 12), but there was a large gap between sleep durations on school nights and on weekend and vacation nights across age groups. Data from Leblanc, J., Rusak, B. et al., unpublished (1997).

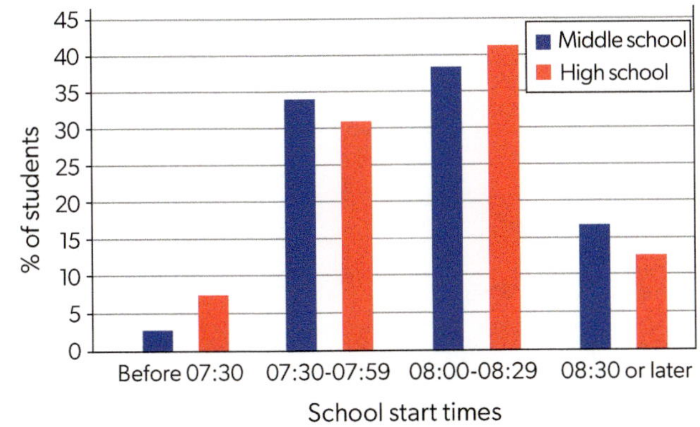

Figure 4.10 Results of a survey of school start times in the USA in 2011–2012. The Y axis shows the percentage of students in middle school (blue) and high school (red) attending schools with the start times shown on the X axis. Note that although most students develop a more delayed chronotype later in adolescence, there was a higher percentage of high-school than middle-school students with school start times before 07:30, and a smaller percentage with start times after 08:30. Source: Data from Wheaton, A. G. et al. (2015) School start times for middle school and high school students — United States, 2011–12 school year. *Morbidity and Mortality Weekly Reports* 64(30):809–813. Centers for Disease Control and Prevention; U.S. Department of Health and Human Services.

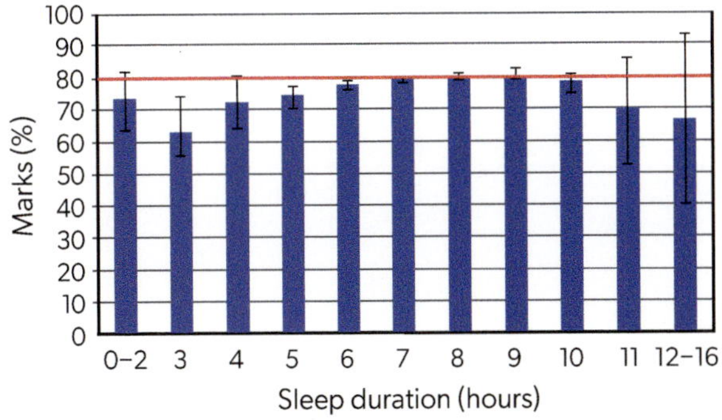

Figure 4.11 The self-reported average school marks (with 95% confidence intervals; Y axis) of students (grades 7–12) in Halifax County, Nova Scotia, whose sleep durations are shown in **Figure 4.9**. Their average self-reported, school-night sleep durations are shown on the X axis. Note that those reporting 7–9 h sleep nightly reported higher marks on average (horizontal red line) than those with shorter average sleep times. The average values reported for long (11–16 h) and very short (0–2 h) sleep durations are probably unreliable because they are based on very few students, resulting in high variability. Data from Leblanc, J., Rusak, B. et al., unpublished (1997).

articles providing updated reviews on several aspects of the relations between school start times and students' academic performance and health (Troxel & Hale, 2022).

A study that used actigraphy found that students with school start times before 08:30 had shorter sleep durations than those with later start times (Nahmod et al., 2019), and self-reports among 16/17 year-olds in Norway also showed longer school-night sleep durations in those with later school start times (Evanger et al., 2023). School start times probably contribute significantly to the fact that over the last 20 years, sleep durations have been getting shorter for teenagers, with 15-year-olds showing the largest increase in the proportion getting <7 h sleep nightly. In addition, students from racial and ethnic minority groups and those in lower socioeconomic groups were less likely than others to get at least 7 h sleep nightly (Keyes et al., 2015) (see Chapter 6 for further discussion).

The effects of short sleep during the school year were reflected in the relation between self-reported grades and average sleep durations on school nights among grade 7–12 students (**Figure 4.11**). The best grades were reported by those who slept ~7–9 h nightly, with worse grades reported for those with shorter or (perhaps) longer sleep durations (LeBlanc et al., 1997, unpublished data). This result is very similar to the curvilinear relationship reported for scores on standardized achievement tests among South Korean grade 9 students, with highest achievement scores for those sleeping 8.5 h (Chan et al., 2023).

Problems associated with early school start times and short sleep on school nights go far beyond poor academic performance and daytime sleepiness. Those with short sleep on school days showed more depressed moods, reported more risk-taking behaviors (O'Brien & Mindell, 2005) and engaged in more self-harming behaviors (Hysing et al., 2015). Youth aged 11–20 who met recommended durations for three measures (physical activity, screen time, and sleep) had lower levels of both depressive and anxiety symptoms. Meeting recommended durations of sleep on its own was strongly related to reduced levels of depressive and anxiety symptoms (Sampasa-Kanyinga et al., 2021). Students attending high schools in a Virginia county with early start times (~07:20) had increased risks of automobile accidents during commutes compared to those in a very similar county with later start times (~08:45) (Vorona et al., 2014; Vorona et al., 2011) (**Figure 4.12**). Adults in the same counties did not differ in accident rates.

Remote online schooling adopted by many jurisdictions during the first phase of the COVID-19 pandemic presented the opportunity to assess the impact of morning commute times on adolescent sleep while schools' virtual start times remained constant. Without the requirement for morning commutes, students attending online classes had a significant increase in total sleep time measured by actigraphy, and they self-reported reduced sleepiness and anxiety (Stone et al., 2021).

Several school districts have tested the effects of delaying school start times to allow more time for adolescents to sleep during the school week. These changes resulted in increased sleep durations, improved daytime alertness, reduced fatigue, and reduced depressive mood (Lo et al., 2018; Owens et al.,

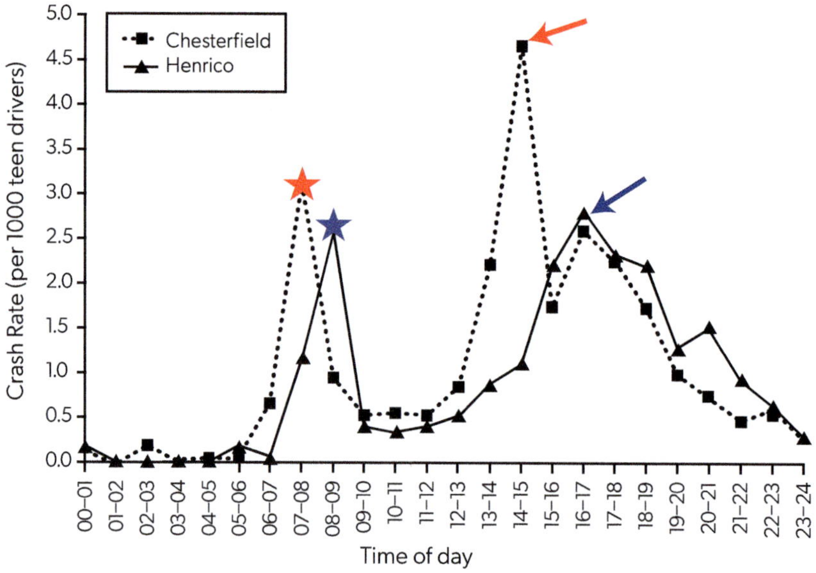

Figure 4.12 Automobile crash rates in two otherwise similar Virginia counties with different school start times for teenagers. Those in Chesterfield County with an earlier start time had an earlier peak of accidents (red star) occurring during the commute to school at 07:00-08:00 (7-8 a.m.) than those in Henrico County, whose commute time was at 08:00-09:00 (8-9 a.m.) (blue star). Note that although the peak morning crash rate was only slightly higher in the county with earlier school start times, it was more dramatically different during the afternoon commute after school. The presumably more sleep-deprived students in Chesterfield County showed a very sharp accident peak after school dismissal at 14:00-15:00 (2-3 p.m., red arrow), while the Henrico teens had a smaller peak after their dismissal time at 16:00-17:00 (4-5 p.m., blue arrow). Adapted with permission of AASM from Vorona, R. D. et al. (2014) Adolescent crash rates and school start times in two central Virginia counties, 2009-2011: a follow-up study to a southeastern Virginia study, 2007-2008. *J Clin Sleep Med* 10:1169-1177. Permission conveyed through Copyright Clearance Center, Inc. Copyright © American Academy of Sleep Medicine (2014). doi: 10.5664/jcsm.4192.

2014; Owens et al., 2010; Wahlstrom, 2002). Instituting a 30 min delay in start times at a high school in one study reduced the percentage of students getting <7 h of sleep by >79% and increased the percentage getting >8 h sleep from 16.4% to 54.7% (Owens et al., 2010). A working group of the American Academy of Pediatrics recommended that schools adopt similar measures in order to permit adolescents to get 8.5–9.5 h of sleep during the school week (Owens et al., 2014).

People with physiologically delayed rhythms who are required to attend school or work early in the morning are considered to suffer from "social jet lag" (Wittmann et al., 2006)—a mismatch between external societal demands and internal temporal physiology. This condition is labeled by analogy with the effects on physiology of jet lag caused by rapidly crossing multiple time zones (see Section 13.9). Social jet lag is typically measured as the difference between the time of the mid-sleep phase on free days (with no early work or social obligations) and the mid-sleep phase on school or workdays. For those with delayed chronotypes, the timing of morning obligations determines when they wake up rather than the dictates of their own physiology. Their physiological rhythms also promote late sleep onset, which combines with early waking to produce habitual short sleep on work/school days (Wolfson & Carskadon, 1998), as illustrated by the three curves in **Figure 4.9**. Reverting to their preferred sleep/wake timing and generating make-up sleep on weekends produces instability of sleep–wake and other cycles over the week, which may have other negative health effects, as discussed in Section 14.6.1.

Social jet lag has been linked to poorer academic performance in high school and university students (LeBlanc et al. 1997, unpublished data) (Haraszti et al., 2014), inadequate control of glucose levels in adults with Type 1 diabetes (Larcher et al., 2016), increased cardiovascular risk in adult shift workers (Madeira et al., 2021), and higher body-mass indices in preteen girls (Higgins et al., 2021).

Chronotype affects school performance by influencing the timing of daytime alertness and cognitive functioning as well as by effects on sleep duration and timing. Those with a strong evening preference tend to perform poorly in the early morning—their "wrong" time of day. Young adolescents (11–14 years old) classified as having either morning or evening preferences were tested on several executive function tasks either in the morning or in the early afternoon. Those with a morning chronotype performed better during tests in the morning and, conversely, those with an evening chronotype performed better later in the day, independently of preceding sleep durations (Hahn et al., 2012).

Chronotype and sleep duration, however, can act together to produce morning performance deficits. Secondary-school students with an evening chronotype were most likely to also have short sleep on school nights. They performed poorly on tests in the morning relative to those with morning chronotypes. On afternoon tests, performance was similar regardless of chronotype (van der Vinne et al., 2015). Similar interactions between chronotype, time of day of testing, and sleep duration were described for university students. Morning types performed better or worse than evening types, depending on the timing of their class and, therefore, of their in-class tests, while they were on a fixed class schedule. However, this difference disappeared during an examination period. Without regular class schedules and wakeup times, students with both chronotypes presumably had the flexibility to get adequate sleep before examinations (Haraszti et al., 2014).

4.4.5 Delayed sleep phase syndrome (DSPS)

While some adolescents cope with the impacts of their delayed sleep preferences, for others the timing of sleep becomes a very significant problem. In its most extreme form, this is recognized as a circadian-rhythm disorder, delayed sleep phase syndrome (DSPS) (also called delayed sleep–wake phase disorder), which may persist into adulthood (**Figure 4.13**). A diagnosis of DSPS usually requires not only an extreme preference for delayed sleep and wake timing but also the persistence of delayed timing despite the individual's best efforts to achieve an earlier bedtime. These best efforts would include maintaining a stable sleep–wake schedule; avoiding light exposure during the evening (which would cause phase delays); and encouraging bright light exposure in the early morning to target the phase advance portion of the PRC (see **Figure 3.4**).

As previously discussed, there are several mechanisms that could contribute to a preference for very delayed sleep onset and wake times. These include having a circadian pacemaker with a longer free-running period (see **Figure 3.5**); altered light sensitivity or phase-shifting capacity resulting in inadequate phase advances; or psychological factors. There is evidence in some people that DSPS is associated with longer free-running periods of melatonin and body temperature rhythms (Micic et al., 2016) (**Figure 4.14**). Other patients with DSPS have been shown to have increased sensitivity to the delaying effects of light in the evening, reflected in both greater light suppression of melatonin levels (see Section 9.2.2) and larger phase shifts of the melatonin rhythm by light exposure (Aoki et al., 2009; Watson et al., 2018). A delayed phase of sleep onset could expose people to more light late in the evening, which would prompt even more strongly delayed sleep–wake rhythms, especially in those with increased phase-shifting sensitivity to light.

Those with even longer circadian periods than DSPS patients (**Figure 4.14**) may fail to entrain at all, resulting in highly disruptive, free-running, sleep–wake rhythms in the presence of 24 h day–night cues (non-24 h sleep–wake disorder). The existence of free-running rhythms in normal lighting environments has been documented in small numbers of both blind and sighted people (Hayakawa et al., 2005; Klein et al.,

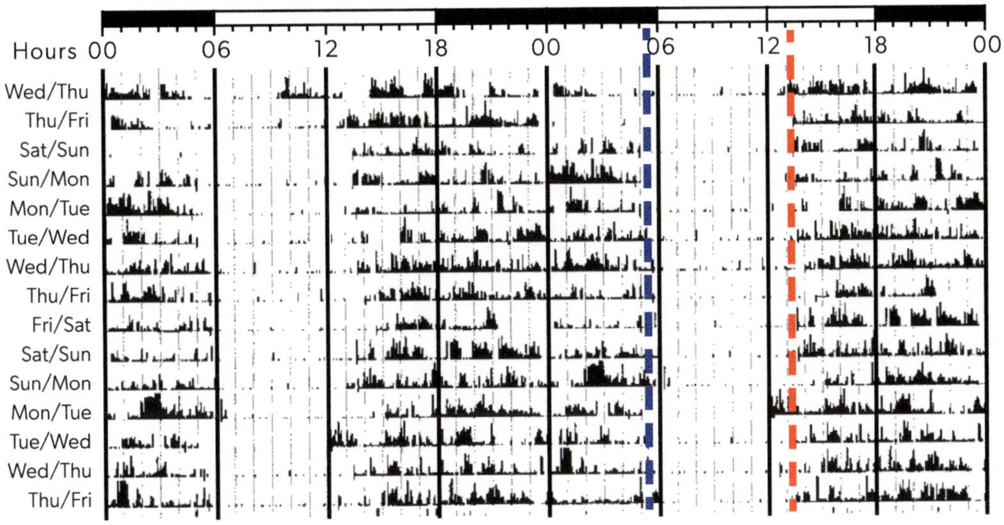

Figure 4.13 Two weeks of actigraphic recordings from an individual with delayed sleep phase syndrome. Successive days are shown on the Y axis and time of day on the X axis (double-plotted, showing 48 h). The white bars at the top indicate the day phase (06:00–18:00). The dashed red line indicates the approximate typical phase of activity onset (~13:00) for this individual. Sleep onset was variable but typically occurred near 05:00 (blue dashed line). Adapted with permission from Reid, K. J. & Zee, P. C. (2004) Circadian rhythm disorders. *Semin Neurol* 24(3):315–325. © Thieme Medical Publishers Inc (2004). doi: 10.1055/s-2004-835063.

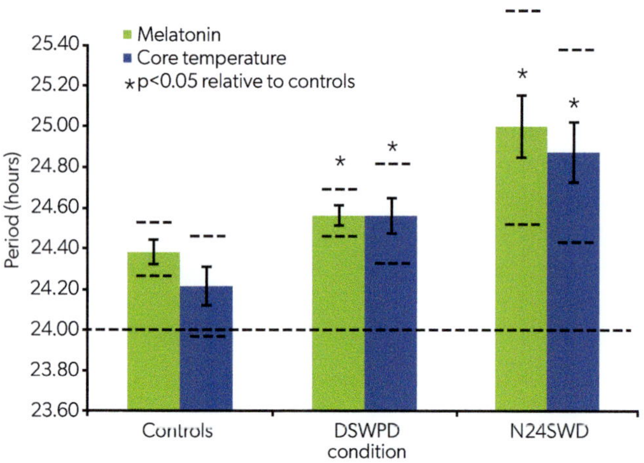

Figure 4.14 Estimates of the periods of free-running circadian rhythms of melatonin levels (green columns) and of body temperature (blue columns) measured under an 80-h modified ultradian constant routine. Young adult participants had 20 min sleep opportunities during each hour. Participants were controls, patients with delayed sleep-wake phase disorder (DSWPD), and patients with non-24 h sleep-wake disorder (N24SWD), who tend to free-run even under normal day-night conditions. The values shown are the mean free-running periods ± SEM (vertical lines) and ± 95% confidence intervals (dashed lines) for each measure. Significant differences ($p<0.05$) between controls and the clinical groups are indicated by *. Reprinted with permission of Dr. Gorica Micic from Micic, G. et al. (2016) Circadian melatonin and temperature taus in delayed sleep-wake phase disorder and non-24-hour sleep-wake rhythm disorder patients: an ultradian constant routine study. *J Biol Rhythms* 31:387–405. © Sage Publications, Inc. (2016). doi: 10.1177/0748730416650069.

1993; McArthur et al., 1996; Miles et al., 1977) (see **Figure 9.5** and Section 9.4).

However, only about half of patients with DSPS in one study showed the delayed timing of the onset of melatonin secretion that would be expected if the circadian system were delayed, either because of a long natural period or an excess of delaying over advancing shifts (or both) (Murray et al., 2017). This evidence suggests that there may be two types of superficially similar delayed sleep phase disorders, one of which is more attributable to psychological and environmental factors (Abbott et al., 2023).

Delayed timing of sleep onset may reflect a willful desire to stay up and sleep late, or a sleep disorder, such as sleep-onset insomnia (inability to fall asleep at a person's desired bedtime; see **Box 4.3**). This is a very common condition among adolescents, which may be related to anxiety about school attendance/academic performance or social relations. Distinguishing these conditions is important because treatments aimed at insomnia or anxiety will likely be ineffective if the underlying cause is a circadian entrainment disorder. Similarly, those with sleep-onset insomnia related to other causes would not benefit from treatments aimed at altering their phase of circadian rhythm entrainment.

A useful test is assessing sleep timing and quality on free days when there is no externally set wake time. If the individual regularly falls asleep quickly at their preferred phase under those conditions, sleeps an adequate duration (even if it is during 04:00–12:00), and enjoys refreshing sleep without daytime sleepiness, it is unlikely to be related to other causes and more likely that a circadian mechanism is involved.

Because it typically arises in childhood or adolescence, DSPS can have lifelong consequences by disrupting school attendance and limiting academic achievement. A mature undergraduate student spoke to me once about his circadian pattern. He had an extremely delayed preference during his teen years and dropped out of university because he was unable to get to daytime classes regularly. While working for years at

BOX 4.3 Insomnia

We will use the term "insomnia" throughout this volume. Its literal meaning is "lack" or "absence" of sleep, but the term is usually used clinically to refer to occasional difficulty getting to sleep or staying asleep. "Chronic insomnia" is a major clinical condition that has been defined in somewhat different ways but includes several core elements. These are: complaints of chronic (>3 months) difficulty initiating or maintaining sleep; early awakening; interrupted or non-restorative sleep, resulting in clinically significant distress or impairment in social, occupational, educational, academic, behavioral, or other important areas of functioning. For reviews, see (Bastien, 2011; Riemann et al., 2022).

These symptoms are obtained by self-report from an individual. Objectively determined short sleep duration is not a necessary element for the clinical diagnosis of chronic insomnia. Objective measures show that some insomnia patients have sleep durations that fall within normal limits, but others have reduced sleep amounts. As discussed in Section 14.8, some researchers and clinicians distinguish these groups as having "insomnia" versus "insomnia with objectively determined short sleep." The role of objective sleep measures in assessing insomnia disorder patients was recently reviewed (Frase et al., 2023).

Insomnia has also been traditionally categorized as either "primary" or "secondary," with the latter category including insomnia symptoms that are assumed to be the product of a variety of other underlying conditions. The basis for, and validity of, these distinctions, as well as proposed multidimensional approaches to assessing insomnia, have been reviewed recently (Nyhuis & Fernandez-Mendoza, 2023).

a number of jobs more suited to his preferred schedule (e.g., night watchman), he also wrote (at night) and published science fiction stories.

At the time I met him, he was returning to university to get a degree. While he still found it difficult to get to daytime classes, his delayed phase preference was no longer as strong as it had been a few years earlier, and he was coping. Presumably he had passed beyond the peak of delay tendency illustrated in **Figure 4.8**. It is likely that others with strongly delayed circadian systems gravitate toward occupations that allow them more flexibility to match their sleep–wake and work schedules to their physiology (e.g., writers, artists, bartenders, musicians).[3]

Treatments for DSPS are limited, and some are not very practical. These include rigid sleep scheduling, avoiding evening light exposure, and using evening melatonin and early morning light exposure to phase advance the clock (see Chapter 9). These approaches are likely to be effective only in moderate cases. The amount of phase advance that was achieved by a single administration of appropriately timed melatonin combined with 3 h of early morning bright light was less than 1 h (Burke et al., 2013). This combination might help those with small rhythm delays but not people with more extreme delays and presumably only those with adequate circadian sensitivity to phase-advancing light cues.

Light treatment combined with coaching was implemented for teens with chronically delayed bedtimes who slept less than ~7 h on weeknights and showed extended sleep on weekends. The treatment included a single weekend of early-morning, bright light exposure (2.5 h) in a laboratory to advance the circadian systems of the most-delayed teens. In addition, participants received coaching to develop individualized time-management plans that were implemented over 2 weeks. These were designed to facilitate scheduling their own activities in order to allow them to go to sleep up to 2 h earlier than usual. This combined motivational and light-treatment approach produced substantial advances in sleep onset time (~1.5 h) and increases in total sleep time (~1.0 h) as well as improving daytime alertness (Crowley et al., 2023).

A method that was attempted in a small number of individuals with DSPS was called chronotherapy. Because they could not advance their sleep to an earlier phase, experimenters got them to delay their sleep by 2–3 h daily around the clock until they reached a more suitable bedtime (e.g., midnight). While this approach produced at least temporary improvements in some individuals (Czeisler et al., 1981), it was disruptive and needed rigid adherence to the new sleep phase. Because they could not advance their rhythms, even small delays were not corrected, so they would tend to drift toward a more delayed phase. In addition, this approach is risky because a few treated individuals reportedly continued delaying rather than stabilizing (i.e., they developed free-running rhythms).

4.4.6 Summary

A physiological tendency to lengthen circadian periods combined with social factors that promote late-night activity result in a delayed chronotype, including late preferred sleep and wake times, beginning around the time of puberty and extending through adolescence. A role for changes in sex hormones that are known to influence circadian rhythms is suggested by several findings: the delaying tendency emerges earlier in females, who typically have earlier puberty onsets; males become more delayed than females, and this difference persists through middle age; there is a larger delay in males with higher testosterone levels; and the gender difference is reduced starting about the time of menopause.

Sleep durations and SWS amounts decrease across childhood and these changes continue during adolescence. Combining these changes with a tendency toward sleep delay and very early scheduling of school start times in many jurisdictions leads to shortened sleep, poor school attendance and performance as well as mood, anxiety, and behavioral problems in those most strongly affected. Delaying school start times can lengthen sleep durations and improve adolescents' daytime functioning, mental health, and safety.

The combination of a delayed phase of circadian rhythm entrainment and fixed early-morning obligations result in social jet lag in many adolescents, which has similar effects as actual jet lag in reducing sleep amounts and impairing health and performance. A delayed chronotype also selectively impairs test performance in the morning, which is layered onto the effects on performance of inadequate amounts of sleep.

Extreme forms of a delayed chronotype may be diagnosed as DSPS, which can limit school achievement and career potential. Several genes involved in circadian rhythm regulation have been implicated in this syndrome, while other genes are linked to Advanced Sleep Phase Syndrome. More extreme lengthening of circadian period can result in free-running or unstably entrained rhythms (non-24 h sleep–wake disorder), despite exposure to 24 h light-dark cycles.

[3] Lewis Carroll, the author of *Alice's Adventures in Wonderland* and *Through the Looking-Glass*, may have been familiar with this condition. In his mock-epic poem, *The Hunting of the Snark* (1876), published by Macmillan & Co. (CC-BY-SA4.0), he described the distinctive characteristics of the mythical "snark" as including an extremely delayed daily rhythm:

"Its habit of getting up late you'll agree
That it carries too far, when I say
That it frequently breakfasts at five-o'clock tea,
And dines on the following day."

(Lewis Carroll, *The Hunting of the Snark [An Agony in Eight Fits], Fit the Second, The Bellman's Speech*)

Rigid sleep scheduling combined with appropriately timed daily light exposure and melatonin treatments to advance rhythms can reduce symptoms in those with moderate amounts of sleep–wake delay but are unlikely to be effective in the most extreme cases. Combining motivational approaches with more limited weekend light treatments can reduce the burdens associated with other treatments and can be effective for teenagers with moderately delayed sleep timing and shortened habitual sleep durations.

4.5 Sleep in adult women

Most studies of sleep in adults have focused on older people, who report sleep problems most frequently, with less research directed at young and middle-aged adults. Men do not undergo major, rapid physiological changes as adults that could affect sleep, similar to those occurring during puberty. Adult women, however, may undergo significant physiological changes associated with menstrual cycles,[4] pregnancy, and menopause, which can affect sleep. Both genders are also affected, though not necessarily to the same extent, by sleep disruption associated with caring for a newborn, which occurs mostly in this age group. The following two sections review some sleep changes related to menstrual cycles and during pregnancy; issues related to menopause are discussed in Section 4.6.

4.5.1 Menstrual cycle effects on sleep

Many studies of sleep have been conducted in relation to menstrual cycles, but few have followed individuals through full cycles. Most have sampled sleep at distinct cycle phases, often mid-follicular and mid- or late-luteal phases. Some of these studies were conducted in healthy controls along with women with a diagnosis of premenstrual dysphoric disorder (PMDD).[5]

Studies of women without health complaints reported differences in sleep between follicular and luteal phases. For example, women showed decreased REM sleep amounts/percentages and delayed REM sleep onset during the luteal relative to the follicular phase (Parry et al., 1999; Shechter et al., 2010). Another study observed small decreases in REM sleep and increases in power in the EEG spindle frequency band during the luteal phase (Driver et al., 1996); for reviews, see (Baker & Driver, 2007; Carrier et al., 2017).

Increased sleep spindle numbers and increased fast spindle density were also reported during sleep in the luteal compared to follicular phase after a learning experience (Genzel et al., 2012; Plamberger et al., 2021). Spindles (in particular, fast spindles) are known to be involved in strengthening memory consolidation (see Section 18.6.2). These studies also confirmed that post-sleep memory performance was relatively enhanced in the luteal vs. follicular phase, consistent with the observed differences in sleep spindle numbers during the post-learning consolidation period.

These results suggest that elevated progesterone levels during the luteal phase are responsible for the increase in sleep spindles. This hypothesis was supported by evidence that there is a positive correlation between individual progesterone levels and spindle density in the luteal phase. In addition, women taking oral contraceptives that contained potent synthetic progestins showed changes in spindles and memory performance similar to those of women in the luteal phase of spontaneous menstrual cycles (Plamberger et al., 2021).

Responses to sleep loss also differed across menstrual phases. In a constant routine, vigilance task performance was relatively protected from the effects of sleep loss during the luteal compared to the follicular phase (Vidafar et al., 2018). Women in the luteal phase were also partially protected from the effects of overnight sleep restriction on daily rhythms of cortisol secretion, compared to women in the follicular phase (LeRoux et al., 2014).

Animal models confirmed a role for female sex hormones in modifying both spontaneous sleep and recovery sleep after sleep loss. Female rodents that undergo spontaneous 4 or 5 day estrous cycles showed reduced sleep and increased activity that is phase-advanced on the night of proestrus, as estrogen levels rise to their peak values, followed by increased rebound sleep on the next day (Morin, Fitzgerald, Rusak, et al., 1977; Swift et al., 2020). Despite the reduced amounts of NREM and REM sleep, rats in proestrus also showed higher power in the delta range (0.5–4.0 Hz) and in the gamma range (30–60 Hz) during NREM sleep and increased theta power (5–9 Hz) during REM sleep (Swift et al., 2020).

The influence of female sex hormones on sleep were confirmed in ovariectomized rats that were treated with one or both principal female sex hormones at physiological levels. High doses of an estrogen (17β estradiol) that mimicked proestrus levels reduced both NREM and REM sleep

[4] Human menstrual cycles average ~28 days (with variation among women and in some women across cycles). Menstrual cycles include a follicular phase during which an ovum develops in response to rising estrogen levels, leading to ovulation and a subsequent decrease in estrogen. Following ovulation, the luteal phase occurs, during which the corpus luteum produces increasing amounts of progesterone. In the absence of pregnancy, after about 2 weeks the corpus luteum degenerates and both progesterone and estrogen levels fall. This is followed by the next follicular phase, starting with the onset of menses as a result of shedding of uterine tissue and followed by gradually increasing estrogen levels (Fritz & Speroff, 1982).

[5] Some women have mild premenstrual (late-luteal) physical or emotional symptoms, without significant functional consequences. PMDD is a diagnosis reserved for a small proportion (~3–8%) of women who regularly have severe physical, emotional, or cognitive symptoms that interfere with their ability to function in the late luteal phase but that remit soon after onset of menses (Steiner, 2000).

and increased wake periods that interrupted sleep. During recovery sleep after deprivation, high estradiol levels produced larger increases in REM sleep but not NREM sleep (Deurveilher et al., 2009).

Sleep patterns across the menstrual cycle have also been studied in patients with severe depressive symptoms in the premenstrual phase along with controls. Both groups showed similar, small differences across the menstrual cycle in Stage 3 sleep and in wake episodes during sleep. Patients with premenstrual depression differed from controls in having more Stage 2 sleep and less REM sleep, but these differences were not related to menstrual cycle phase (Parry et al., 1989). A later study of patients with a diagnosis of PMDD did not replicate these few group differences, but found that both controls and patients showed REM sleep decreases and delayed REM sleep latencies during the luteal phase (Parry et al., 1999).

Another study included women with both PMDD and late-luteal phase insomnia symptoms, along with controls. It reported increased body temperatures, increased Stage 2 sleep, and decreased REM sleep during the luteal phase, relative to the follicular phase, but these changes occurred in both groups. The only group differences observed were increased SWS and decreased melatonin levels in PMDD/insomnia patients relative to controls (Shechter et al., 2012).

Several of these studies reported reduced amounts of REM sleep in women during the luteal phase, but PMDD patients showed few differences from controls. Heterogeneity among participants in these relatively small studies and differences in late-luteal symptom profiles in patient groups probably contributed to some inconsistent findings. These observations support the conclusion that altered sleep responses to late-luteal hormonal changes are unlikely to be related to the development of PMDD.

4.5.2 Pregnancy and sleep

During pregnancy, high proportions of people report inadequate sleep, insomnia, night awakenings, and daytime sleepiness, especially as pregnancy progresses (Hedman et al., 2002; Mindell, Cook, et al., 2015; Okun et al., 2015). Total sleep time (including naps) may actually increase in the first trimester, perhaps in response to increased progesterone levels. However, even at this early stage, those with significant nausea, urinary frequency, and backache can have disturbed sleep with reduced amounts of N3 and REM sleep.

Although symptoms may start in the first trimester, many increase progressively into the third trimester in response to weight gain, joint pain, and other physical changes. These symptoms are often related to difficulty finding a comfortable sleep position, backache, contraction pains, heartburn, and frequent urination (Baratte-Beebe & Lee, 1999; Hedman et al., 2002). In addition, there are reports of progressive increases in the frequency of sleep-related disorders, including restless legs syndrome, breathing disorders, and snoring (Hedman et al., 2002; Mindell, Cook, et al., 2015; Pien & Schwab, 2004). Self-reported shorter sleep and poor sleep quality during pregnancy were more common among African American women than in other racial/ethnic groups, even after accounting for maternal education level and socioeconomic status (Lucchini et al., 2022).

Pregnant people often report anxiety related to their own health, childbirth, or the health of their child as well as rumination and depression that may be related to these issues (Geissbuehler & Eberhard, 2002; Kalmbach et al., 2020). The first few months after giving birth are characterized by very large decreases in total sleep time, undoubtedly in part because of infant-related sleep disruption, but post-pregnancy endocrine changes may also be involved (Hedman et al., 2002; Lee et al., 2000).

Several reviews have evaluated the connections between sleep problems during pregnancy and both fetal and maternal outcomes. One report concluded that poor sleep quality, insomnia, and short duration sleep were linked to adverse pregnancy outcomes, including depression, gestational diabetes, hypertension, risk of caesarean deliveries, and preterm births. These outcomes were proposed to be linked to sleep problems through stress and its effects on the immune and hypothalamic-pituitary-adrenal (HPA) systems (Palagini et al., 2014). Short sleep, whether maintained or further shortened in the course of pregnancy, as well as long reported sleep, were also associated with apparent increased risk of developmental delay in offspring (Li et al., 2023).

Inflammation can influence birth timing through several routes and has been implicated in causing preterm births (Challis et al., 2009). In pregnant women with depression, short and disturbed sleep were associated with increased pro-inflammatory cytokines (markers of immune system activation; see Section 14.9). Changes in some cytokines were weakly associated with several negative infant outcomes (preterm birth, low birth weight) (Okun et al., 2013). One study concluded that immune system activation associated with poor sleep during pregnancy was linked to increased risk of preterm births in African American women but not in European American women in their sample (Blair et al., 2015).

It is difficult, however, to draw strong conclusions about the extent to which these associations indicate a causal role for inadequate sleep in relation to poor outcomes for maternal health and infant development (Chang et al., 2010). An important issue is that most studies do not have relevant information about preexisting stress, immune system function, and sleep quality before pregnancy, which might contribute to these outcomes. Many studies also involved small numbers of participants, and there are few longitudinal studies that could trace potential causal links among these variables.

One longitudinal study that did obtain sleep recordings before pregnancy and followed participants during pregnancy reported substantial declines in total sleep, REM sleep, sleep efficiency, and N3 sleep through all of pregnancy, relative to a follicular phase baseline.[6] The changes in several measures were larger for those experiencing their first pregnancies (Lee et al., 2000). Based on other evidence that these changes in sleep increase stress and immune system activation (see Section 14.9), these results strengthen the likelihood that these sleep changes during pregnancy are one factor that contributes to increased risks for negative maternal and infant outcomes.

4.5.3 Summary

Women undergoing spontaneous menstrual cycles showed decreased REM sleep amounts during the luteal phase, and some studies also reported decreases in N2 sleep and increased sleep spindle activity. There were no dramatic differences in sleep features between those with PMDD and controls. The luteal phase was also marked by increased numbers of fast spindles during sleep after a learning experience and better subsequent memory performance, which were related to the levels of progesterone. Artificial progestins in oral contraceptives had similar effects on both spindles and memory.

Studies in animal models also implicate changes in hormone levels during spontaneous estrous cycles in affecting sleep and activity levels. Female rodents showed phase advances and increased levels of activity, along with reduced sleep, during the proestrus day when estrogen levels peaked. They also showed higher delta power during NREM sleep and more theta power during REM sleep at that time. Hormone replacement studies in ovariectomized rats confirmed that increased estrogen levels reduced both NREM and REM sleep.

Pregnancy is associated with changes in several aspects of sleep, including difficulty initiating or maintaining sleep, insomnia complaints, and daytime sleepiness. The factors contributing to these changes include physical discomfort, frequent urination, pain, heartburn, sleep apnea, anxiety, restless legs symptoms, and snoring. Some studies reported that total sleep duration (including naps) increased during the first trimester but decreased subsequently. In general, sleep problems got worse as pregnancy progressed, and large decreases in sleep amounts also occurred in the weeks after giving birth.

Studies have shown associations between poor sleep quality and increased risk of complications during pregnancy, including depression, gestational diabetes, hypertension, risk of caesarean deliveries, and preterm births. Some of these conditions are also linked to postnatal developmental delay in their infants. These conditions have been proposed to be linked to short and disrupted sleep through stress-related changes in immune system and HPA function, especially in some minority groups.

A difficulty with attributing some of these conditions to sleep loss and quality during pregnancy is that few studies have baseline data on sleep, stress, and other health conditions before pregnancy. One longitudinal study did compare baseline follicular phase sleep to sleep throughout pregnancy and reported progressive decreases in total, N3, and REM sleep, and in sleep efficiency—especially in first pregnancies. This evidence supports the interpretation that pregnancy produces changes in key sleep features that are linked to health problems in other circumstances, and that have the potential to contribute to negative maternal and infant outcomes.

4.6 Sleep in adulthood and aging

4.6.1 Sleep changes in older people

Both self-reports and objective studies indicate that adults show progressive changes in sleep beginning in middle-age and continuing into older age groups. Relative to younger people, these changes include shorter sleep; decreases in slow wave activity (SWA) and REM sleep percentages; increases in higher-frequency EEG bands (more N1 sleep); a reduction in sleep efficiency (i.e., increased WASO, especially late in the night); and more tendency to nap during the day (Buysse et al., 2005; Buysse et al., 1992; Carrier et al., 2001; Carrier et al., 1997; Espiritu, 2008; Foley et al., 1995). These results are consistent with a gradual reduction across adulthood in the capacity (or need) to generate slower EEG frequencies as well as an increased tendency toward EEG signs of arousal during sleep (Carrier et al., 2001) (see **Figure 4.5**).[7]

It is not clear, however, which of these differences are caused by aging-related changes in sleep mechanisms and which are secondary consequences of other age-related changes. Sleep changes in older adults can result from altered work patterns (more flexible schedules after retirement) (Borbély et al., 2017; Hagen et al., 2016), increases in primary sleep disorders, or

[6] Both pregnancy and the follicular phase are characterized by elevated progesterone levels.

[7] Analyses of one American survey found that people over 65 self-reported *longer* sleep durations than younger groups, based on responses to a single question about usual nightly sleep length. The authors noted, however, the risk that respondents might have based their answers on time spent in bed rather than on actual sleep time (Jean-Louis et al., 2021).

increases in physical or psychiatric health conditions that indirectly affect sleep quality.

Primary sleep disorders that become more frequent during aging can severely disrupt sleep, including sleep apnea (interruptions in breathing; see Appendix B), periodic limb movements (rhythmic kicking during sleep), and restless legs syndrome (unpleasant, sometimes painful sensations in the legs, with an irresistible feeling of needing to move).

Other medical conditions that can disturb sleep include joint inflammation and pain (e.g., arthritis), other pain syndromes, and frequent urination (from prostate growth in men or from reduction of bladder elasticity in both men and women), all of which increase in frequency during adulthood and aging. Medications are often prescribed for these conditions, as well as for psychiatric conditions and sleep disorders, so polypharmacy (treatment with multiple drugs) is more the norm than the exception among older people. Many commonly used drugs (both prescription and nonprescription) can either cause sedation or increase insomnia, disrupt sleep continuity, and reduce its quality or exacerbate symptoms of existing sleep disorders (Barczi & Teodorescu, 2011).

All of these factors that are secondary consequences of aging can obscure the impact of aging on the systems that regulate sleep. A meta-analysis of a large number of sleep studies conducted on people of different ages based its conclusions on the strength of the data and on the degree to which each study controlled for possible confounding factors (Ohayon et al., 2004) (see **Figure 4.5**). In particular, the authors tried to separate effects of older age from effects of illnesses that increase during aging. They concluded that the most robust and reliable changes in sleep parameters that occurred from adolescence through adulthood and into older age groups were the following:

- Increased latencies to fall asleep;
- Increased percentage of WASO, and a (probably related) decrease in total sleep time;
- Increased percentages of both N1 and N2 sleep;
- Decreased percentage of REM sleep after childhood (but relatively stable after age 60), with a small decrease in REM sleep latency;
- Decreased percentage of N3 and SWA.

The impact of aging on the circadian system is another factor that influences both the timing of sleep and, indirectly, some sleep parameters. Beginning with the most delayed morningness/eveningness (M/E) preference around age 20 (see Section 4.4.2 and **Figure 4.8**), there is a gradual increase in morningness during the middle and later years of life, reflecting an advance in the circadian phase of entrainment.

A study of people aged 20–59 noted that differences in M/E scores among participants predicted many of the same sleep features as did differences in age, suggesting that these changes may be linked. It assessed the extent to which increased morningness could account for changes in sleep parameters across middle age. Mediation analyses showed that differences in M/E scores were responsible for all of the variance associated with age in relation to habitual bedtime, alertness after waking, and percentages of REM sleep and N1 sleep. In addition, M/E scores accounted for ~50% of the variance associated with age for total sleep time, amount of sleep in the last 2 h of a sleep period, and amount of REM sleep and rapid eye movement activity (Carrier et al., 1997).

Increased morningness during aging is linked to a phase advance of the circadian system, as indicated by measures such as the body temperature minimum and the onset of melatonin secretion (DLMO), so that these occurred at earlier clock times than in younger people (Duffy et al., 1999; Kerkhof, 1991). However, wake timing in older people (64–80 years) occurred even earlier than predicted by their degree of circadian phase advance (i.e., sooner after their body temperature minimum). These results suggested that another influence on the timing of waking was that older people could not sustain sleep for as long after their (advanced) body temperature minimum as younger people. This change contributed to lighter sleep and more wake episodes late in the sleep phase, followed by an earlier final waking (Carrier et al., 1997; Duffy et al., 1999).[8]

4.6.2 Gender differences in sleep EEG features

Although the age-related changes discussed above appear in mixed-gender groups of older people, some sleep features are affected differently by aging in men and women. During adolescence, N3 sleep amounts decrease in both males and females (see Section 4.4.1), but males show a higher rate of reduction over adolescence, and older male adolescents also show increases in WASO and lower sleep efficiency, while older female adolescents do not (Baker et al., 2016). Another study found that even women in their 20s showed more power in low frequency EEG bands than men during NREM sleep. This finding was tentatively attributed to differences in skull characteristics (Dijk et al., 1989), a factor which is discussed further in the next section.

A study of young adults in a narrow age range (31–40 years) found no statistically significant gender difference in

[8] Another effect of aging is a reduction in the amplitude of circadian rhythms, which probably contributes to these effects. This is a complex issue that is addressed in detail in Section 8.4.

N3 sleep but reported that men had quantitatively less N3 sleep and also showed more N1 sleep and lower sleep efficiency than women (Roehrs et al., 2006). A study of 20–60 year-old adults reported a significant gender difference with women showing more power density in lower EEG frequency bands (up to ~10 Hz as well as around 14–15 Hz) than men (Carrier et al., 2001).

The tendency for men to show more pronounced changes in sleep features as they age has been confirmed in numerous studies. A study involving nearly 2700 people aged 37 to 92 reported a strong decline in N3 and a parallel increase in N1 sleep during aging in men (consistent with the summary that included both genders in **Figure 4.5**) but little change in women over this age range (Redline et al., 2004). Others have also reported well-preserved N3 sleep in middle-aged and older women, but not men, and increased N1 sleep in men (Unruh et al., 2008) (**Figure 4.15**). Taken together, these results indicate that there is a decline in N3 sleep and an increase in N1 sleep in men beginning as early as adolescence and accelerating into older age groups, but that the changes during aging are small or undetectable in older women.

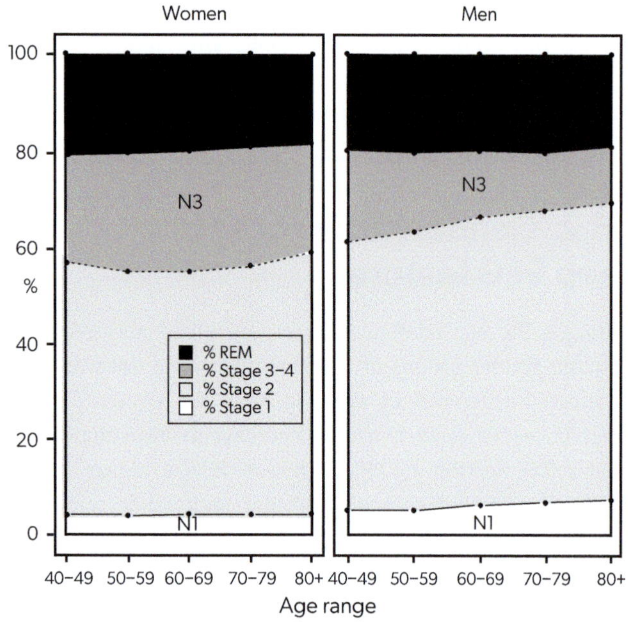

Figure 4.15 Sleep stage percentage changes from age 40 to 80+ years in women (left panel) and men (right panel). Men showed a steep decrease in % N3 sleep (dark gray) and an increase in % N1 sleep (white, at the bottom) and % N2 sleep (light gray). Women showed very small decreases in % REM sleep (black, top) but no systematic changes in N1 or N3 sleep. Reprinted with permission of John Wiley and Sons, Ltd. from Unruh, M. L. et al. (2008) Subjective and objective sleep quality and aging in the Sleep Heart Health Study. *J Am Geriatr Soc* 56:1218–1227. Copyright © The Authors, Journal compilation © 2008, The American Geriatrics Society. doi: 10.1111/j.1532-5415.2008.01755.x.

4.6.3 Impact of age and gender on EEG features

These conclusions raise questions about the mechanisms that result in these sleep changes in older men and what accounts for the differential effects in men and women. One technical issue that could affect the assessment of N3 sleep during aging is that there is a decrease in the size of delta-frequency waves in EEG recordings from older people, which may be as dramatic as 50–75% decreases (Zepelin, 1983). This amplitude change reduces the number of EEG waves that meet both the frequency criterion for delta waves (i.e., they are slow) and the amplitude criterion (at least 75 μV). As a result, there are fewer EEG features that can contribute to meeting the usual criteria for identifying N3 sleep. This loss of amplitude could result in scoring less N3 and more N2 sleep amounts in older people, especially men (Bliwise, 2000; Rosenberg et al., 1979); see **Figure 4.15**.

One likely contributor to the smaller size of slow waves in older people is a reduction in cortical thickness in key brain regions, probably reflecting a general loss of neuron numbers during aging (Dubé et al., 2015). A lower density of neurons and, as a consequence, a reduction in connectivity in a cortical region will result in a smaller number of synchronized neurons contributing to the production of each low-frequency wave at that location and therefore a smaller signal recorded from the scalp (Chylinski et al., 2022).

Another result of cortical shrinkage during aging would be that recording electrodes on the scalp would be further from the underlying current sources in the cortex, which would also result in recording smaller voltage changes. Similarly, the gender differences observed might be related to the fact that men on average have thicker skulls, which would produce a larger gap between EEG current sources and recording electrodes. There is indirect support for this hypothesis from a study showing that the size of event-related potentials (ERPs) recorded from the scalp depended on the thickness of the skull and the resulting distance between a scalp electrode and the underlying cortex (Pfefferbaum & Rosenbloom, 1987).

Regardless of the causes of EEG changes, the decline in measurable slow waves during aging (primarily in men) results in part from applying a standard amplitude criterion across all ages (Muehlroth & Werkle-Bergner, 2020). In one study, counting all EEG waves, regardless of amplitude, that met a frequency criterion of 0.5–3.0 Hz in men (50–60 years), generated a similar SWS percentage as in younger men (Webb & Dreblow, 1982). The implications of this analysis, however, would depend on determining whether all low-frequency EEG waves are functionally similar regardless of amplitude.

A different approach to this issue involved establishing group-specific criteria for detecting slow waves in four groups, composed of young (~20–30 years) and older (~50–70 years) men and women. An algorithm used a signal-to-noise ratio specific to each of the four groups to establish minimal amplitude criteria that allowed exhaustive, automatic detection of slow waves while applying group-specific amplitude thresholds. The resulting data indicated no gender difference in the density of these normalized slow waves in either age cohort, although the average amplitude of slow waves was higher in women. With respect to age, however, the results still showed a robust decline in the number of slow waves in the older groups of both genders (Rosinvil et al., 2021).

These results suggest that the age-related decrease in the number of slow waves results from changes in the mechanisms involved in their generation, such as reductions in neuron numbers and cortical thickness. Differences between men and women in the number of slow waves detected appear instead to be related to EEG amplitude differences that could result from gender differences in skull thickness, as previously suggested for younger people (Dijk et al., 1989).

It is unclear, however, what the functional implications are of applying the same or different amplitude criteria to different groups. If smaller, slow EEG waves serve the same function in older people as larger waves do in young people, then the observed amplitude reduction in older men would be functionally irrelevant. It is therefore important to understand whether or not the changes seen in delta-band EEG activity in older people have functional consequences.

Many studies have shown that SWS and delta-range EEG activity during sleep after acquiring new information are related to the success of memory consolidation (see Chapters 17 and 18). The relevance of delta power to this function was supported by evidence that the extent of reduction in EEG delta and theta power in older people (average age in mid-70s) was correlated with the reduction in benefits of overnight sleep for memory performance (Westerberg et al., 2012).

Another study found that poor memory performance in older people was associated with prefrontal cortical atrophy; this relationship was mediated by reductions in SWA during N3 sleep (Mander et al., 2013). A study of older adults (average age 67) found that reduced prefrontal EEG power in the "slow delta range" (0.5–1.0 Hz, also called "slow oscillations") during the first nocturnal N3 period was linked to poorer performance on executive cognitive tasks (Anderson & Horne, 2003). These results support the idea that low-frequency EEG activity during sleep is important for some cognitive functions in older people, but it is unclear whether and how the amplitude of slow waves contributes to these functions.

Complicating this issue is evidence that the positive correlation seen in young people between the amount of SWS and the strength of memory consolidation is reported inconsistently in older people. Similarly, sleep deprivation that affected memory consolidation in young people did not do so consistently in older people (Scullin, 2013; Scullin & Bliwise, 2015). These results have been interpreted to indicate that there are developmental changes in how sleep mechanisms affect memory functions, which reduce the relevance of SWS to memory consolidation in older people (Scullin et al., 2019). This interpretation further complicates the analysis of whether the reduced amplitude of slow waves in aging (men) is functionally important.

REM sleep has also been implicated in some forms of memory consolidation in both people and animals (see Chapters 17 and 18. Regulation of REM sleep differs between younger and older adults. A study compared young people (average age ~21, all male) to older people (average age ~82, 2/3 female). The older group did not show an early-night peak in N3 sleep and showed a flat distribution of REM sleep episode lengths across the night, in contrast to the late-night increase in REM sleep seen in young adults (Hayashi & Endo, 1982) (**Figure 4.16**; compare to Figures 2.9 and 2.10). The lack of competition from N3 sleep early in the night in the older group might have contributed to an increased proportion of REM sleep at that phase. The strong imbalance in gender between groups complicates interpretation of these results.

However, a study in which there were no significant age differences in the duration of N3 or total NREM sleep during the first half of the night also reported a flattened temporal distribution of REM sleep among older, compared to younger, participants. The total amount of REM sleep was very similar in the two age groups, but it was concentrated in the second half of the night in young people (78% of the total) and less so in older people (58% of the total) (Sonni & Spencer, 2015). A likely explanation relates to the strong impact of circadian regulation on the expression of REM sleep (see Chapter 5). A reduction in circadian rhythm amplitude during aging, for which there is considerable supporting evidence (see Chapter 8), would reduce the circadian impact on REM sleep expression and allow it to occur more equally through the night. It is not known whether the redistribution of REM sleep during the night in older people has any functional implications.

4.6.4 Menopause and subjective sleep quality

Several lines of evidence indicate that N3 sleep is a priority during recovery sleep after deprivation and contributes to some of the health benefits of sleep (see Chapters 5, 14, and 15). These results suggest that older men with reduced N3 sleep might be more likely to complain about their sleep quality than older women with better-preserved N3 sleep. Nevertheless, older women have a higher incidence of insomnia complaints. This difference persists even after controlling for gender differences

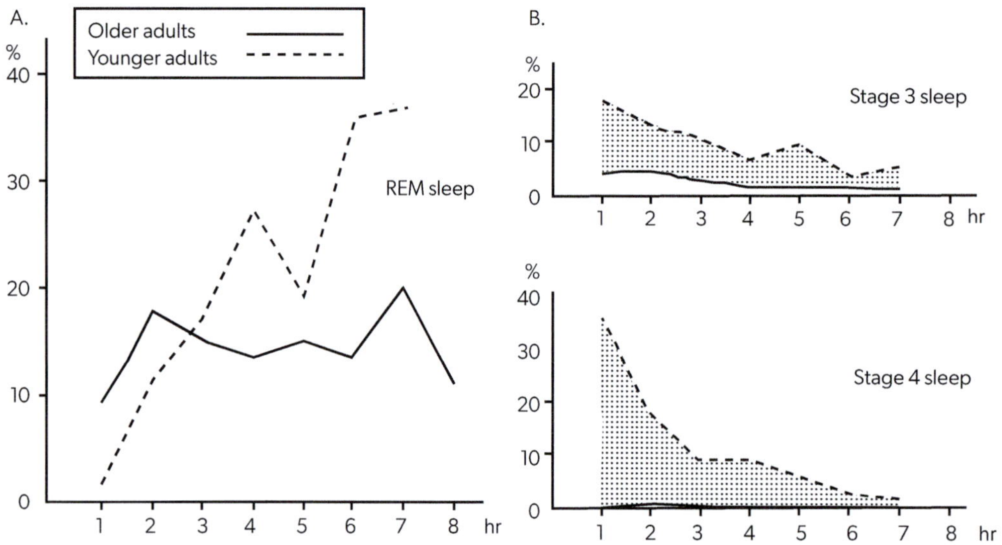

Figure 4.16 **A.** The hourly percentage of REM sleep (Y axis) across a night's sleep (X axis) for older (solid line) and younger participants (dashed line). The typical pattern in young adults of showing little REM sleep early during the night and high levels later was not seen in the older participants. **B.** The percentage of SWS (Stages 3 and 4) across the hours of sleep (X axis) in younger and older participants. Amounts of Stage 3 sleep were much lower in the older participants (solid line; top panel) than the younger participants (dashed line), and Stage 4 sleep was essentially absent in the older group (solid line; bottom panel). The stippled area indicates the difference in the percentage of Stage 3 or 4 sleep between younger and older participants across a night's sleep. Note that the older group included both male (5) and female (10) participants, while the younger group included 13 males. Reprinted with permission of Oxford University Press and the Sleep Research Society from Hayashi, Y. & Endo, S. (1982) All-night sleep polygraphic recordings of healthy aged persons: REM and Slow-Wave Sleep. *Sleep* 5(3):277–283. © Sleep Research Society (1982). doi: 10.1093/sleep/5.3.277.

in the prevalence of anxiety and depression, both of which can disturb sleep (Unruh et al., 2008; Zhang & Wing, 2006).

One possibility is that the observed gender difference in reporting sleep problems in older people is related to the onset of menopause in women (usually around age 45–50, but sometimes earlier). Menopause is a process that occurs over a period of years, involving cessation of ovulation, reduction in levels of estrogen and progesterone, and increases in levels of follicle stimulating hormone (FSH). Discussions of how menopause influences women's sleep may focus on either changes that occur during the lengthy peri-menopausal transition or those that characterize women in their post-menopausal years.

Reviews have concluded that peri- and post-menopausal women (including younger women who undergo menopause as a result of surgical removal of ovaries to treat cancer) report more sleep problems than pre-menopausal women, although these effects are not uniform across ethnic groups (Baker et al., 2018; Brown & Gervais, 2020; Xu & Lang, 2014). In trying to understand the basis for complaints of poor sleep, it is important to distinguish clinical populations (those seeking medical treatment) from the general population. Most studies of women from the general population confirmed self-reports of reduced sleep quality during and after menopause but did not find objective evidence using PSG that sleep was disturbed relative to younger women (Unruh et al., 2008; Young et al., 2003).

Some women, however, do show objective sleep disturbances during the menopausal transition. Studies have reported more total wake time and reduced sleep efficiency (time asleep as a proportion of time in bed) in menopausal women (Xu et al., 2011), and an increased incidence of apnea symptoms (periodic breathing cessations), even in those with no reported sleep complaints (Block et al., 1980). In some women, a relatively rapid reduction of reproductive hormone levels (especially estrogen) during menopause results in frequent hot flashes (sudden sensations of heat, sometimes with sweating), which can greatly disrupt sleep (Baker et al., 2018; Brown & Gervais, 2020).

There are inconsistent findings about whether hot flashes contribute to self-reported sleep disturbances, but the largest study that used objective recordings of both hot flashes and sleep (using actigraphy) found strong temporal associations between hot flashes and waking during sleep (Thurston et al., 2019). One study of peri-menopausal women controlled for the presence of hot flashes and depressive symptoms, which are also linked to sleep problems. It found that the number of self-reported awakenings was associated with reduced estrogen levels and increased FSH levels, a marker of a later stage of the menopausal transition (Coborn et al., 2022). Thus, both hormonal changes and the presence of hot flashes appear to contribute independently to sleep disruption for some women during the menopausal transition.

Another possible contributor to reports of poor sleep quality in women during menopause relates to changes in EEG characteristics during sleep. A cross-sectional study comparing women at different stages of the menopausal transition found increased high-frequency (beta range) EEG activity during NREM and REM sleep in women who were post-menopausal compared to those who were pre- or early peri-menopausal. The study also found an association between increased EEG beta power and self-reports of hot flashes (Campbell et al., 2011).

A subsequent study (3.5 years later) involved participants from the same cohort who had not yet passed through menopause in the first study. It confirmed that those who had become post-menopausal between these studies had increased power in the beta-frequency band during NREM sleep compared to those who still remained pre- or early peri-menopausal, although no association with hot flashes was found (Matthews et al., 2021). The finding of increased beta power was associated with the transition to post-menopause and not with age. This increase reflects lighter sleep in post-menopausal women, which could contribute to a perception of poorer sleep quality. Lighter sleep might also increase the probability that both environmental and physiological stimuli (e.g., hot flashes, night sweats) could disturb sleep and trigger arousals.

Another longitudinal PSG study involved women who were studied at baseline (average age 46 years) and ~10 years later, spanning the menopausal transition, so that all were post-menopausal at the 10-year evaluation, as assessed by high FSH levels. This study reported that there were different changes in sleep characteristics related to changes in levels of FSH (progression of the menopausal transition) and to the passage of 10 years (aging). For example, higher FSH levels were weakly associated with longer sleep onset latencies, while aging had a stronger effect in shortening onset latencies. Although participants showed higher amounts of hot flashes and more sleep disturbances than 10 years earlier, they also showed increased amounts of N3 sleep as a function of age, consistent with other findings of robust preservation of N3 sleep in older women (Kalleinen et al., 2021).

This study also found higher amounts of N1 sleep in post-menopausal women, relative to their values 10 years earlier (Kalleinen et al., 2021), which is consistent with the observation of increased EEG beta power in post-menopausal women (Matthews et al., 2021). The difference between these studies in attributing some sleep changes to aging versus menopausal status could be related to studying women over different age ranges (3.5 vs. 10 years) and using different measures to assess menopausal status.

If the endocrine changes associated with menopause trigger sleep problems, hormone replacement therapy (HRT) might be expected to improve these symptoms. Some studies reported that HRT reduced menopausal sleep symptoms by reducing hot flashes, other somatic symptoms, and mood disturbances (Polo-Kantola et al., 1998), while others noted no differences between female insomnia patients related to whether they were undergoing HRT or not (Xu et al., 2011). These differences may be related to the observation that the largest effects of HRT were seen in those with the most severe insomnia symptoms (Polo-Kantola et al., 1998), and may also be influenced by differences in the hormones used during treatment (Brown & Gervais, 2020) and by the type of clinical population studied.

Despite the possible influence of menopause-related symptoms on sleep, older women have objectively better sleep quality (i.e., more N3 and less N1) than older men but report more sleep complaints. One study attempted to reconcile this apparent contradiction by examining the ratio of delta-band EEG activity during NREM sleep to the "background" level of delta activity during REM sleep (Latta et al., 2005). The assumption underlying this approach was that NREM delta activity reflects homeostatic sleep regulation and the recuperative functions of sleep. In contrast, the low level of delta power during REM sleep is unrelated to the recovery function of sleep. See Chapter 5 for a discussion of delta power homeostasis.

This interpretation was based on evidence that REM sleep delta-band power does not change across successive REM sleep episodes during the night. Delta-band power in NREM sleep, however, is homeostatically regulated. It decreases across NREM sleep episodes during the night because generating NREM delta rhythms gradually reduces the accumulated homeostatic sleep need. The results of this analysis showed that older men had *higher* ratios of NREM to REM sleep delta activity than older women. This finding was interpreted as reflecting better homeostatic regulation of sleep need, even though men's raw NREM delta-band power was lower than that of women (Latta et al., 2005).

If this interpretation were correct, a higher frequency of sleep complaints among older women could be accounted for by sleep being less effective in satisfying their homeostatic sleep needs compared to either older men or younger women. This conclusion might be related to a finding in younger people using a more typical assay of homeostasis. Young women showed a larger increase in the amount of SWA than young men during recovery sleep after sleep deprivation (Armitage et al., 2001). If this result reflects a greater need in women for increased sleep after sleep loss, less effective homeostatic regulation in older women might further increase their dissatisfaction with their sleep quality.

Other factors may contribute to gender differences in both objective and subjective sleep quality during aging. These could include how easily sleep is disturbed by internal and external stimuli (see Chapter 12), as well as the expectations people have of their sleep during aging, and how their subjective experience of sleep matches up to these expectations.

4.6.5 Summary

Sleep quality is usually reported to deteriorate with age; the changes contributing to this outcome may begin quite early in middle age. In addition to any direct effects of aging on sleep regulation, other factors likely influence the quality of sleep in the general population of older people. These include changes in the phase of circadian entrainment and the timing of sleep within the circadian night phase; inability to sustain sleep throughout the latter part of the sleep phase; increases in primary sleep disorders; increases in physical and psychiatric health conditions that affect sleep indirectly; and in some cases, the effects of drug treatments for these conditions.

There is consistent evidence that sleep EEG characteristics change during aging, particularly in men. These changes include reductions in N3 sleep (defined using standard criteria for amplitude and frequency), increases in N1 sleep, increased WASO, reduced REM sleep percentage, and redistribution of REM sleep more evenly across the night. A reduction in circadian rhythm amplitude may account for the altered timing of REM sleep, which is strongly influenced by the circadian system.

Loss of cortical neurons and connectivity, as well as cortical shrinkage, likely contribute to the reduced amplitude of slow waves in older men, which in turn contributes to reduced amounts of N3 sleep, based on the usual scoring criteria. Reduced N3 sleep has been linked to impairment in a number of cognitive and other functions, including memory consolidation. It is not known whether there are any functional consequences of the flattened distribution of REM sleep expression in older people, but the reduced percentage of REM sleep may also have consequences for some aspects of memory consolidation.

Older women tend to report more sleep problems than older men, despite having better preserved N3 sleep and less increase in N1 sleep. Several factors may contribute to this finding, including menopause-related hot flashes and night sweats, reduced hormone levels, increased sensitivity to environmental stimuli, and more high-frequency EEG activity during sleep. Some of these effects may be characteristic only of the menopausal transition, but others may persist into the post-menopausal phase. However, there are conflicting accounts as to whether specific sleep changes in older women are attributable to age versus their menopausal transition.

One attempt to account for the gender difference in sleep complaints relates to apparently less complete sleep homeostasis in older women than men. This idea is based on a model of homeostasis that incorporates the ratio of delta-band activity during NREM sleep to background delta-band activity (during REM sleep), which does not appear to be homeostatically regulated. The validity of this measure of homeostatic regulation remains to be evaluated.

4.7 Challenges in studying aging effects on sleep

4.7.1 Cross-sectional comparisons

As discussed above, older people have more disrupted sleep at night and take more naps during the day than younger people (Espiritu, 2008), but the causes of these differences are not well understood. An ideal study of age-related changes in sleep would track sleep longitudinally over the full lifespan of individuals who remain healthy and live under similar circumstances throughout their lives. No such study can be done, although some partial longitudinal information is available. Most studies on this topic have instead been cross-sectional (comparing people from different age groups at a single time point). Cross-sectional comparisons between groups show differences in sleep at different ages, but for reasons discussed below, they cannot determine whether these differences result from the effects of aging on sleep-regulatory mechanisms.

One interpretational problem is that older participants will have had many more opportunities than young comparison groups to experience life events that could affect their sleep in addition to any potential effects of aging. These life experiences could include different, and more varied, histories of light exposure, diet, shift work, transmeridian flights, use of medications, drugs or alcohol, and current or past physical or psychiatric illnesses.

It is not possible to equate such life experiences, so the alternative is to use statistical methods to try to exclude these potential influences. These methods, however, can only control for variables for which there is information about exposure history and that are recognized ahead of time as likely to influence sleep or daily rhythms.

One example of a factor that would not usually be considered in this context relates to the effects of different histories of light exposure. Short-term adaptation to different light intensities can change responses of the human circadian/pineal system to light (Chang et al., 2011; Hébert et al., 2002; Smith et al., 2004), which is the principal zeitgeber for daily rhythms. The impacts of long-term differences in the history of light exposure on light sensitivity and the rhythms entrained by light are unknown.

Another issue that can affect comparisons between different age groups is the possibility of survivor effects. This term refers to the fact that any sample of older participants is drawn from a pool of survivors of a larger age cohort that inevitably got

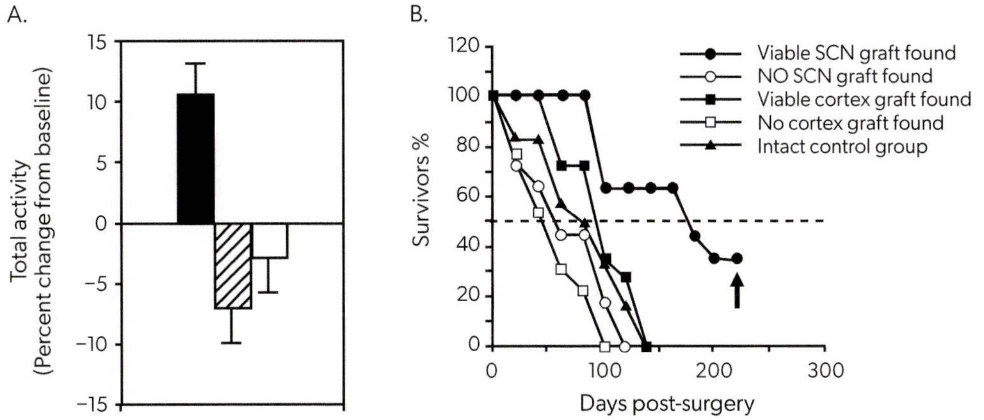

Figure 4.17 Adult golden hamsters were implanted with a fetal suprachiasmatic nucleus (SCN, the principal circadian pacemaker), or with a cortex tissue graft, or were left intact. SCN transplants are known to restore circadian rhythms in animals with disrupted rhythms (see Chapter 8 & **Figure 8.9**). **A.** Those with a viable SCN graft showed increased activity levels (black column) compared to those with a cortical graft (hatched column) or intact controls (white column). **B.** All groups except those with a viable SCN graft died at a similar rate over the following months, while those with a viable SCN graft survived much longer (black circles). The black arrow indicates when the study was ended, with ~35% of the group with viable SCN grafts still alive. The increased longevity may be a consequence of restoration of circadian rhythmicity or may be a result of their increased activity levels or other, unknown consequences of receiving a fetal SCN graft. Reprinted with permission of Dr. Martin Ralph from Hurd, M. W. & Ralph, M. R. (1998) The significance of circadian organization for longevity in the golden hamster. *J Biol Rhythms* 13:4340–4436. © Sage Publications, Inc. (1998). doi: 10.1177/074873098129000255.

smaller with the passage of time. According to statistics from the US Center for Disease Control in 2009 (http://tinyurl.com/k3z6a9g), only ~50% of those born in that year are expected to survive to ~age 82, while about 98% of that birth cohort will survive to their early 20s. The very low risk of young people dying (after age 1) increases steadily with age. As a result, a sample of people in their 80s will be drawn from a birth cohort that is only ~50% of its starting size, while a sample of those in their 20s will come from a largely intact birth cohort.

80-year-olds recruited for a hypothetical comparison study represent a subpopulation whose genetic, physiological, life history, and other characteristics allowed them to survive longer than half their birth cohort. That is predictably not the case for about half of the younger group to which they will be compared, who will lack some undetermined features (e.g., genetic makeup) associated with surviving to their 80s. It is therefore difficult to attribute differences in sleep between the groups solely to the impacts of 60 additional years of aging.

The significance of this theoretical issue is reinforced by evidence that better quality sleep and preserved daily rhythms are correlated with healthier aging and longer survival, as reviewed in Chapters 14 and 15 (Lim et al., 2013; Sterniczuk et al., 2013; Tranah et al., 2011; Zuurbier et al., 2015). Thus, people who live into their 80s are likely to have more of the characteristics that preserve sleep and circadian rhythm quality than others in their full birth cohort, while those in their 20s would be a mixed group.

Complementing these observational findings in people is evidence from hamsters carrying a genetic mutation that disrupted daily rhythmicity; these hamsters had shorter lifespans than wild-type hamsters. Restoration of normal rhythmicity by implanting a wild-type suprachiasmatic nucleus[9] into hamsters that carried this mutation restored circadian rhythmicity and lengthened survival (Hurd & Ralph, 1998) (**Figure 4.17**).

4.7.2 Representativeness of older research participants

Another issue that can affect interpretation of age-group comparisons in experimental laboratory studies is the degree to which those engaged in a study are representative of their age cohort.

A study of activity levels of people from different age groups found that those who participated in research studies were generally healthier and more vigorous than the general population they represented. This finding probably reflects the fact that research participation would be more challenging for people with poor health or chronic medical conditions. Most relevant to this discussion, older research participants differed even more from the general population that they represented than did younger participants (Golomb et al., 2012). This result is not surprising because most common, chronic medical conditions increase in frequency with age. Thus, results from participants in laboratory studies, especially those in older

[9] The suprachiasmatic nucleus (SCN) is the principal pacemaker of the mammalian circadian system. A fetal SCN can survive transplantation into the brain of an adult animal with disrupted rhythms and can restore circadian rhythmicity; see Chapter 8.

groups, likely overestimate the quality of health in the general age group from which they were sampled.

Participants are recruited to research studies based on both inclusion criteria (e.g., being in a particular age group) and exclusion criteria. For studies of "normal" sleep, exclusion criteria typically include medical conditions or current treatments that are likely to affect participants' sleep. As an example, a study of daytime sleepiness and performance compared a sample of people undergoing "healthy aging" (average age ~83 years) to younger participants (average age ~25 years). This publication was unusual in reporting on how the application of exclusion criteria influenced recruitment to the study. The result was that older potential participants were excluded primarily for medical problems, whereas younger potential participants were excluded for "personality disorders, substance abuse, obesity, and family history of depression" (Hoch et al., 1992).

Because potentially relevant conditions occur with different frequencies in different age groups, applying the same exclusion criteria to all groups inevitably results in excluding people for different reasons in younger and older groups. In this study, even after excluding those with conditions or treatments that would likely affect sleep, 19 out of 23 older participants had stable medical conditions for which they were receiving drug treatments (e.g., heart disease, hypertension, thyroid disease, arthritis), while none of the 30 younger participants in the study had chronic medical conditions. The older group also had predictably earlier habitual wake times and more regular daily schedules than those in their 20s (Hoch et al., 1992).

These observations indicate how difficult it is to evaluate effects of aging on sleep mechanisms independently of the impact of health changes that accompany aging and may indirectly affect sleep. The requirements of research, especially those of demanding laboratory studies, also ensure that those participating will be a hardy subset of the population that they represent. The differences observed between younger and older participants in EEG features, sleep organization, and sleep timing have important implications for understanding sleep problems during aging. But laboratory studies of sleep in older people probably underestimate the extent of sleep changes present in this age group in the general population, where more than 80% of surveyed participants over age 65 report sleep problems. Other issues related to sleep in older people are reviewed in Chapter 8.

4.7.3 Summary

Controlled longitudinal studies of sleep in individuals over the entire lifespan are not feasible, so cross-sectional comparisons among age groups are used to assess how sleep mechanisms change with age. These studies have several limitations. Older participants have typically had a wider range of experiences that could have effects on sleep than younger people (shiftwork, light exposure changes, transmeridian travel, illnesses, etc.). It is unclear to what extent sleep features in older people are a product of age-related changes in sleep-regulatory (or circadian) mechanisms or of individuals' life histories.

In addition, older people are survivors of larger cohorts that shrank with time, so those available for recruitment to research in their 80s, for example, represent ~50% of their birth cohort. Participants in their 20s are, in contrast, drawn from a near-complete birth cohort and will inevitably have a more varied makeup with respect to any features that can potentially influence lifespan. There is evidence that better sleep quality and more robust circadian functions are associated with increased longevity. As a result, the genetic and physiological characteristics that promote more robust sleep and circadian functions will likely be represented more strongly in the older age group.

Research participants are also typically healthier and more vigorous than the population from which they are sampled, and that is especially true of older groups. As a result, the observed differences between older and younger people in EEG features, sleep timing, continuity, and organization probably do not represent the full extent to which sleep differs between age cohorts in the general population.

Because of the challenges in interpreting comparisons between samples drawn from different age cohorts, it is difficult to conclude which sleep changes during aging result from primary changes in sleep and circadian regulatory mechanisms (see Chapter 8) and which arise secondarily from factors such as life experiences, illnesses, and genetic differences that influence longevity. What is clear is that the differences in sleep features observed in laboratory studies of older people (especially men) probably underestimate the extent of sleep changes in that age group in the general population.

Literature cited

Abbott, S. M., Phillips, A. J., Reid, K. J., Cain, S. W., & Zee, P. C. (2023). What's in a name? delayed by any other name is still a circadian disorder: a call for improved nomenclature for delayed sleep-wake phase disorder subtypes. *Sleep, 46*(11), zsad222. doi:10.1093/sleep/zsad222

Acebo, C., Sadeh, A., Seifer, R., Tzischinsky, O., Hafer, A., & Carskadon, M. A. (2005). Sleep/wake patterns derived from activity monitoring and maternal report for healthy 1- to 5-year-old children. *Sleep, 28*(12), 1568–1577.

Adams, E. L., Savage, J. S., Master, L., & Buxton, O. M. (2020). Time for bed! Earlier sleep onset is associated with longer nighttime sleep duration during infancy. *Sleep Med, 73*, 238–245. doi: 10.1016/j.sleep.2020.07.003

Anderson, C., & Horne, J. A. (2003). Prefrontal cortex: links between low frequency delta EEG in sleep and neuropsychological performance in healthy, older people. *Psychophysiology, 40*, 349–357.

Andrade, M. M., Benedito-Silva, A. A., Domenice, S., Arnhold, I. J., & Menna-Barreto, L. (1993). Sleep characteristics of adolescents: a longitudinal study. *J Adolesc Health, 14*(5), 401–406.

Aoki, H., Ozeki, Y., & Yamada, N. (2009). Hypersensitivity of melatonin suppression in response to light in patients with delayed sleep phase syndrome. *Chronobiol Int, 18*(2), 263–271. doi: 10.1081/cbi-100103190

Armitage, R., Smith, C., Thompson, S., & Hoffman, R. (2001). Sex differences in slow-wave activity in response to sleep deprivation. *Sleep Research Online, 4*(1), 33–41.

Baker, F., & Driver, H. (2007). Circadian rhythms, sleep, and the menstrual cycle. *Sleep Med, 8*(6), 613–622. doi: 10.1016/j.sleep.2006.09.011

Baker, F. C., de Zambotti, M., Colrain, I. M., & Bei, B. (2018). Sleep problems during the menopausal transition: prevalence, impact, and management challenges. *Nat Sci Sleep, 10*, 73–95. doi: 10.2147/NSS.S125807

Baker, F. C., Willoughby, A. R., de Zambotti, M., Franzen, P. L., Prouty, D., Javitz, H., … Colrain, I. M. (2016). Age-related differences in sleep architecture and electroencephalogram in adolescents in the National Consortium on Alcohol and Neurodevelopment in Adolescence sample. *Sleep, 39*(7), 1429–1439. doi: 0.5665/sleep.5978

Baratte-Beebe, K. R., & Lee, K. (1999). Sources of midsleep awakenings in childbearing women. *Clinical Nursing Research, 8*(4), 386–397.

Barczi, S. R., & Teodorescu, M. (2011). Medical and psychiatric dsorders and the medications used to treat them. In M. H. Kryger, T. Roth, & W. C. Dement (Eds.), *Principles and Practice of Sleep Medicine* (pp. 1524–1535). St. Louis: Saunders.

Bastien, C. H. (2011). Insomnia: neurophysiological and neuropsychological approaches. *Neuropsychol Rev, 21*(1), 22–40. doi: 10.1007/s11065-011-9160-3

Blair, L. M., Porter, K., Leblebicioglu, B., & Christian, L. M. (2015). Poor sleep quality and associated inflammation predict preterm birth: heightened risk among African Americans. *Sleep, 38*(8), 1259–1267. doi: 10.5665/sleep.4904

Bliwise, D. L. (2000). Normal aging. In M. H. Kryger, T. Roth, & W. C. Dement (Eds.), *Principles and Practice of Sleep Medicine* (3rd ed., pp. 26–42). Philadelphia: Saunders.

Block, A. J., Wynne, J. W., & Boysen, P. G. (1980). Sleep-disordered breathing and nocturnal oxygen desaturation in postmenopausal women. *Am J Med, 69*(1), 75–79.

Blumberg, M. S., Dooley, J. C., & Sokoloff, G. (2020). The developing brain revealed during sleep. *Curr Opin Physiol, 15*, 14–22. doi: 10.1016/j.cophys.2019.11.002

Blumberg, M. S., Karlsson, K. A. E., Seelke, A. M. H., & Mohns, E. J. (2005). The ontogeny of infant sleep: a response to Frank and Heller (2003). *J Sleep Res, 14*(1), 91–98. doi: 10.1111/j.1365-2869.2004.00

Boksa, P. (2012). Abnormal synaptic pruning in schizophrenia: urban myth or reality? *J Psychiatry Neurosci, 37*(2), 75–77. doi: 10.1503/jpn.120007

Borbély, A. A., Rusterholz, T., & Achermann, P. (2017). Three decades of continuous wrist-activity recording: analysis of sleep duration. *J Sleep Res, 26*(2), 188–194. doi: 10.1111/jsr.12492

Bourgeois, J.-P., & Rakic, P. (1993). Changes of synaptic density in the primary visual cortex of the macaque monkey from fetal to adult stage. *J Neurosci, 13*(7), 2801–2820.

Brown, A. M. C., & Gervais, N. J. (2020). Role of ovarian hormones in the modulation of sleep in females across the adult lifespan. *Endocrinology, 161*(9), bqaa128. doi:10.1210/endocr/bqaa128

Buchmann, A., Ringli, M., Kurth, S., Schaerer, M., Geiger, A., Jenni, O. G., & Huber, R. (2011). EEG sleep slow-wave activity as a mirror of cortical maturation. *Cereb Cortex, 21*(3), 607–615. doi: 10.1093/cercor/bhq129

Burke, T. M., Markwald, R. R., Chinoy, E. D., Snider, J. A., Bessman, S. C., Jung, C. M., & Wright, K. P., Jr. (2013). Combination of light and melatonin time cues for phase advancing the human circadian clock. *Sleep, 36*(11), 1617–1624. doi: 10.5665/sleep.3110

Buysse, D., Monk, T., Carrier, J., & Begley, A. (2005). Circadian patterns of sleep, sleepiness and performance in older and younger adults. *Sleep, 28*(11), 1365–1376.

Buysse, D. J., Browman, K. E., Monk, T. H., Reynolds Iii, C. F., Fasiczka, A. L., & Kupfer, D. J. (1992). Napping and 24-hour sleep/wake patterns in healthy elderly and young adults. *J Am Geriatr Soc, 40*, 779–786.

Campbell, I. G., Bromberger, J. T., Buysse, D. J., Hall, M. H., Hardin, K. A., Kravitz, H. M., … Gold, E. (2011). Evaluation of the association of menopausal status with delta and beta EEG activity during sleep. *Sleep, 34*(11), 1561–1568. doi: 10.5665/sleep.1398

Campbell, I. G., & Feinberg, I. (2009). Longitudinal trajectories of non-rapid eye movement delta and theta EEG as indicators of adolescent brain maturation. *Proc Natl Acad Sci USA, 106*(13), 5177–5180. doi: 10.1073 pnas.0812947106

Carrier, J., Land, S., Buysse, D. J., Kupfer, D. J., & Monk, T. H. (2001). The effects of age and gender on sleep EEG power spectral density in the middle years of life (ages 20–60 years old). *Psychophysiology, 38*(2), 232–242.

Carrier, J., Monk, T. H., Buysse, D. J., & Kupfer, D. J. (1997). Sleep and morningness-eveningness in the 'middle' years of life (20–59 y). *J Sleep Res, 6*(4), 230–237. doi: 10.1111/j.1365-2869.1997.00230.x

Carrier, J., Semba, K., Deurveilher, S., Drogos, L., Cyr-Cronier, J., Lord, C., & Sekerovick, Z. (2017). Sex differences in age-related changes in the sleep-wake cycle. *Front Neuroendocrinol, 47*, 66–85. doi: 10.1016/j.yfrne.2017.07.004

Carrier, J., Viens, I., Poirier, G., Robillard, R., Lafortune, M., Vandewalle, G., … Filipini, D. (2011). Sleep slow wave changes during the middle years of life. *Eur J Neurosci, 33*(4), 758–766. doi: 10.1111/j.1460-9568.2010.07543.x

Carskadon, M. (2004). Sleep deprivation: health consequences and societal impact. *Med Clin N Am, 88*(3), 767–776. doi: 10.1016/j.mcna.2004.03.001

Carskadon, M., Vieira, C., & Acebo, C. (1993). Association between puberty and delayed phase preference. *Sleep, 16*(3), 258–262.

Challis, J. R., Lockwood, C. J., Myatt, L., Norman, J. E., Strauss, J. F., 3rd, & Petraglia, F. (2009). Inflammation and pregnancy. *Reprod Sci, 16*(2), 206–215. doi: 10.1177/1933719108329095

Chan, N. Y., Wu, W. J., Chan, J. W. Y., Chan, K. C. C., Li, A. M., Man Chan, S. S., … Wing, Y. K. (2023). Sleep and academic performance among students in Hong Kong: curvilinear relationship suggesting an optimal amount of sleep. *Sleep Med, 106*, 97–105. doi: 10.1016/j.sleep.2023.04.001

Chang, A. M., Scheer, F. A., & Czeisler, C. A. (2011). The human circadian system adapts to prior photic history. *J Physiol, 589*(Pt 5), 1095–1102. doi: 10.1113/jphysiol.2010.201194

Chang, J. J., Pien, G. W., Duntley, S. P., & Macones, G. A. (2010). Sleep deprivation during pregnancy and maternal and fetal outcomes: is there a relationship? *Sleep Med Rev, 14*(2), 107–114. doi: 10.1016/j.smrv.2009.05.001

Chylinski, D., Narbutas, J., Balteau, E., Collette, F., Bastin, C., Berthomier, C., … Van Egroo, M. (2022). Frontal grey matter microstructure is associated with sleep slow waves characteristics in late midlife. *Sleep, 45*(11), zsac178. doi:10.1093/sleep/zsac178

Clara, M. I., & Allen Gomes, A. (2019). An epidemiological study of sleep-wake timings in school children from 4 to 11 years old: insights on the sleep phase shift and implications for the school starting times' debate. *Sleep Med, 66*, 51–60. doi: 10.1016/j.sleep.2019.06.024

Coborn, J., de Wit, A., Crawford, S., Nathan, M., Rahman, S., Finkelstein, L., … Joffe, H. (2022). Disruption of sleep continuity during the perimenopause: associations with female reproductive hormone profiles. *J Clin Endocrinol Metab, 107*(10), e4144–e4153. doi:10.1210/clinem/dgac447

Cook, G., Carter, B., Wiggs, L., & Southam, S. (2023). Parental sleep-related practices and sleep in children aged 1–3 years: a systematic review. *J Sleep Res, 22*, e14120. doi:10.1111/jsr.14120

Coons, S., & Guilleminault, C. (1982). Development of sleep-wake patterns and non-rapid eye movement sleep stages during the first six months of life in normal infants. *Pediatrics, 69*(6), 793–798.

Crowley, S., Acebo, C., & Carskadon, M. (2007). Sleep, circadian rhythms, and delayed phase in adolescence. *Sleep Med, 8*(6), 602–612. doi: 10.1016/j.sleep.2006.12.002

Crowley, S. J., Cain, S. W., Burns, A. C., Acebo, C., & Carskadon, M. A. (2015). Increased sensitivity of the circadian system to light in early/mid-puberty. *J Clin Endocrinol Metab, 100*(11), 4067–4073. doi: 10.1210/jc.2015-2775

Crowley, S. J., Velez, S. L., Killen, L. G., Cvengros, J. A., Fogg, L. F., & Eastman, C. I. (2023). Extending weeknight sleep of delayed adolescents using weekend morning bright light and evening time management. *Sleep, 46*(1), zsac202. doi:10.1093/sleep/zsac202

Crowley, S. J., Wolfson, A. R., Tarokh, L., & Carskadon, M. A. (2018). An update on adolescent sleep: new evidence informing the perfect storm model. *J Adolesc, 67*, 55–65. doi: 10.1016/j.adolescence.2018.06.001

Czeisler, C. A., Richardson, G. S., Coleman, R. M., Zimmerman, J. C., Moore-Ede, M. C., Dement, W. C., & Weitzman, E. D. (1981). Chronotherapy: resetting the circadian clocks of patients with delayed sleep phase insomnia. *Sleep, 4*, 1–21.

Daan, S., Damassa, D., Pittendrigh, C. S., & Smith, E. R. (1975). An effect of castration and testosterone replacement on a circadian pacemaker in mice (Mus musculus). *Proc Natl Acad Sci USA, 72*, 3744–3747.

Davis, F. C., & Gorski, R. A. (1988). Development of hamster circadian rhythms: role of the maternal suprachiasmatic nucleus. *J Comp Physiol A, 162*, 601–610.

Deurveilher, S., Rusak, B., & Semba, K. (2009). Estradiol and progesterone modulate spontaneous sleep patterns and recovery from sleep deprivation in ovariectomized rats. *Sleep, 32*(7), 865–877.

Dijk, D. J., Beersma, D. G. M., & Bloem, G. M. (1989). Sex differences in the sleep EEG of young adults: visual scoring and spectral analysis. *Sleep, 12*(6), 500–507.

Driver, H. S., Dijk, D. J., Werth, E., Biedermann, K., & Borbély, A. A. (1996). Sleep and the sleep electroencephalogram across the menstrual cycle in young healthy women. *J Clin Endocr Metab, 81*, 728–735.

Dubé, J., Lafortune, M., Bedetti, C., Bouchard, M., Gagnon, J. F., Doyon, J., ... Carrier, J. (2015). Cortical thinning explains changes in sleep slow waves during adulthood. *J Neurosci*, *35*(20), 7795–7807. doi: 10.1523/JNEUROSCI.3956-14.2015

Duffy, J. F., Dijk, D.-J., Hall, E. F., & Czeisler, C. A. (1999). Relationship of endogenous circadian melatonin and temperature rhythms to self-reported preference for morning or evening activity in young and older people. *J Investig Med*, *47*(3), 141–150.

Espiritu, J. R. D. (2008). Aging-related sleep changes. *Clin Geriatr Med*, *24*(1), 1–14, v. doi: 10.1016/j.cger.2007.08.007

Evanger, L. N., Bjorvatn, B., Pallesen, S., Hysing, M., Sivertsen, B., & Saxvig, I. W. (2023). Later school start time is associated with longer school day sleep duration and less social jetlag among Norwegian high school students: results from a large-scale, cross-sectional study. *J Sleep Res*, *32*(4), e13840. doi:10.1111/jsr.13840

Evans, M. A., Buysse, D. J., Marsland, A. L., Wright, A. G. C., Foust, J., Carroll, L. W., ... Hall, M. H. (2021). Meta-analysis of age and actigraphy assessed sleep characteristics across the lifespan. *Sleep*, *44*(9), zsab088. doi:10.1093/sleep/zsab088

Feinberg, I. (1983). Schizophrenia: caused by a fault in programmed synaptic elimination during adolescence? *J Psychiatr Res*, *17*(4), 319–334.

Feinberg, I., Higgins, L. M., Khaw, W. Y., & Campbell, I. G. (2006). The adolescent decline of NREM delta, an indicator of brain maturation, is linked to age and sex but not to pubertal stage. *Am J Physiol*, *291*(6), R1724–R1729. doi: 10.1152/ajpregu.00293.2006

Foley, D. J., Monjan, A. A., Brown, S. L., Simonsick, E. M., Wallace, R. B., & Blazer, D. G. (1995). Sleep complaints among elderly persons: an epidemiologic study of three communities. *Sleep*, *18*, 425–432.

Frase, L., Nissen, C., Spiegelhalder, K., & Feige, B. (2023). The importance and limitations of polysomnography in insomnia disorder-a critical appraisal. *J Sleep Res*, *32*(6), e14036. doi: 10.1111/jsr.14036

Fritz, M. A., & Speroff, L. (1982). The endocrinology of the menstrual cycle: the interaction of folliculogenesis and neuroendocrine mechanisms. *Fertil Steril*, *38*(5), 509–529. doi: 10.1016/s0015-0282(16)46628-8

Geissbuehler, V., & Eberhard, J. (2002). Fear of childbirth during pregnancy: a study of more than 8000 pregnant women. *J Psychosom Obstet Gynaecol*, *23*(4), 229–235. doi: 10.3109/01674820209074677

Genzel, L., Kiefer, T., Renner, L., Wehrle, R., Kluge, M., Grozinger, M., ... Dresler, M. (2012). Sex and modulatory menstrual cycle effects on sleep related memory consolidation. *Psychoneuroendocrinology*, *37*(7), 987–998. doi: 10.1016/j.psyneuen.2011.11.006

Georgoulas, A., Jones, L., Laudiano-Dray, M. P., Meek, J., Fabrizi, L., & Whitehead, K. (2021). Sleep-wake regulation in preterm and term infants. *Sleep*, *44*(1), zsaa148. doi:10.1093/sleep/zsaa148

Golomb, B. A., Chan, V. T., Evans, M. A., Koperski, S., White, H. L., & Criqui, M. H. (2012). The older the better: are elderly study participants more non-representative? A cross-sectional analysis of clinical trial and observational study samples. *Br Med J Open*, *2*, 6. doi: 10.1136/bmjopen-2012-000833

Hagen, E. W., Barnet, J. H., Hale, L., & Peppard, P. E. (2016). Changes in sleep duration and sleep timing associated with retirement transitions. *Sleep*, *39*(3), 665–673. doi: 10.5665/sleep.5548

Hahn, C., Cowell, J. M., Wiprzycka, U. J., Goldstein, D., Ralph, M., Hasher, L., & Zelazo, P. D. (2012). Circadian rhythms in executive function during the transition to adolescence: the effect of synchrony between chronotype and time of day. *Dev Sci*, *15*(3), 408–416. doi: 10.1111/j.1467-7687.2012.01137.x

Haraszti, R. A., Ella, K., Gyongyosi, N., Roenneberg, T., & Kaldi, K. (2014). Social jetlag negatively correlates with academic performance in undergraduates. *Chronobiol Int*, *31*(5), 603–612. doi: 10.3109/07420528.2013.879164

Hayakawa, T., Uchiyama, M., Kamei, Y., Shibui, K., Tagaya, H., Asada, T., ... Takahashi, K. (2005). Clinical analyses of sighted patients with non-24-hour sleep-wake syndrome: a study of 57 consecutively diagnosed cases. *Sleep*, *28*(8), 945–952.

Hayashi, Y., & Endo, S. (1982). All-night sleep polygraphic recordings of healthy aged persons: REM and Slow-Wave Sleep. *Sleep*, *5*(3), 277–283.

Hébert, M., Martin, S. K., Lee, C., & Eastman, C. I. (2002). The effects of prior light history on the suppression of melatonin by light in humans. *J Pineal Res*, *33*(4), 198–203.

Hedman, C., Pohjasvaara, T., Tolonen, U., Suhonen-Malm, A. S., & Myllylä, V. V. (2002). Effects of pregnancy on mother's sleep. *Sleep Med*, *3*, 37–42.

Heller, H. C., & Frank, M. G. (2009). Sleep: development and circadian control. In L. R. Squire (Ed.), *Encyclopedia of Neuroscience* (pp. 1049–1053). Cambridge: Academic Press.

Henderson, J. M. T., France, K. G., Owens, J. L., & Blampied, N. M. (2010). Sleeping through the night: the consolidation of self-regulated sleep across the first year of life. *Pediatrics*, *126*(5), e1081–e1087. doi: 10.1542/peds.2010-0976

Heraghty, J. L., Hilliard, T. N., Henderson, A. J., & Fleming, P. J. (2008). The physiology of sleep in infants. *Arch Dis Child*, *93*(11), 982–985. doi: 10.1136/adc.2006.113290

Higgins, S., Stoner, L., Black, K., Wong, J. E., Quigg, R., Meredith-Jones, K., & Skidmore, P. M. (2021). Social jetlag is associated with obesity-related outcomes in 9-11-year-old children, independent of other sleep characteristics. *Sleep Med*, *84*, 294–302. doi: 10.1016/j.sleep.2021.06.014

Hoch, C. C., Reynolds III, C. F., Jennings, R., Monk, T., Buysse, D., Machen, M., & Kupfer, D. (1992). Daytime sleepiness and performance among healthy 80 and 20 year olds. *Neurobiol Aging*, *13*(2), 353–356.

Horne, J. A., & Östberg, O. (1976). A self-assessment questionnaire to determine morningness-eveningness in human circadian rhythms. *Int J Chronobiol*, *4*(2), 97–110.

Hurd, M. W., & Ralph, M. R. (1998). The significance of circadian organization for longevity in the golden hamster. *J Biol Rhythms*, *13*(5), 430–436.

Huttenlocher, P. R. (1979). Synaptic density in human frontal cortex – developmental changes and effects of aging. *Brain Res*, *163*, 195–205.

Hysing, M., Sivertsen, B., Stormark, K. M., & O'Connor, R. C. (2015). Sleep problems and self-harm in adolescence. *Br J Psychiatry*, *207*(4), 306–312. doi: 10.1192/bjp.bp.114.146514

Ibuka, N. (1984). Ontogenesis of circadian sleep-wakefulness rhythms and developmental changes of sleep in the altricial rat and in the precocial guinea pig. *Behav Brain Res*, *11*, 185–196.

Iglowstein, I., Jenni, O. G., Molinari, L., & Largo, R. H. (2003). Sleep duration from infancy to adolescence: reference values and generational trends. *Pediatrics*, *111*(2), 302–307. doi: 10.1542/peds.111.2.302

Jankowski, K. S., Fajkowska, M., Domaradzka, E., & Wytykowska, A. (2019). Chronotype, social jetlag and sleep loss in relation to sex steroids. *Psychoneuroendocrinology*, *108*, 87–93. doi: 10.1016/j.psyneuen.2019.05.027

Jean-Louis, G., Shochat, T., Youngstedt, S. D., Briggs, A. Q., Williams, E. T., Jin, P., ... Seixas, A. A. (2021). Age-associated differences in sleep duration in the US population: potential effects of disease burden. *Sleep Med*, *87*, 168–173. doi: 10.1016/j.sleep.2021.09.004

Johnston, P. G., & Zucker, I. (1983). Lability and diversity of circadian rhythms of cotton rats Sigmodon hispidus. *Am J Physiol*, *244*, R338–R346.

Kalleinen, N., Aittokallio, J., Lampio, L., Kaisti, M., Polo-Kantola, P., Polo, O., ... Saaresranta, T. (2021). Sleep during menopausal transition: a 10-year follow-up. *Sleep*, *44*(6), zsaa283. doi: 10.1093/sleep/zsaa283

Kalmbach, D. A., Cheng, P., Ong, J. C., Ciesla, J. A., Kingsberg, S. A., Sangha, R., ... Drake, C. L. (2020). Depression and suicidal ideation in pregnancy: exploring relationships with insomnia, short sleep, and nocturnal rumination. *Sleep Med*, *65*, 62–73. doi: 10.1016/j.sleep.2019.07.010

Kaufmann, T., Alnaes, D., Doan, N. T., Brandt, C. L., Andreassen, O. A., & Westlye, L. T. (2017). Delayed stabilization and individualization in connectome development are related to psychiatric disorders. *Nat Neurosci*, *20*(4), 513–515. doi: 10.1038/nn.4511

Kennaway, D. J. (2023). The dim light melatonin onset (DLMO) across ages, methodologies and sex and its relationship with morningness/eveningness. *Sleep*, *46*(5), zsad033. doi:10.1093/sleep/zsad033

Kerkhof, G. A. (1991). Differences between morning-types and evening-types in the dynamics of EEG slow wave activity during night sleep. *Electroencephalogr Clin Neurophysiol*, *78*, 197–202.

Keyes, K. M., Maslowsky, J., Hamilton, A., & Schulenberg, J. (2015). The great sleep recession: changes in sleep duration among US adolescents, 1991-2012. *Pediatrics*, *135*(3), 460–468. doi: 10.1542/peds.2014-2707

Klein, T., Martens, H., Dijk, D. J., Kronauer, R. E., Seely, E. W., & Czeisler, C. A. (1993). Circadian sleep regulation in the absence of light perception: Chronic non-24-hour circadian rhythm sleep disorder in a blind man with a regular 24-hour sleep-wake schedule. *Sleep*, *16*, 333–343.

Kleitman, N., & Engelmann, T. G. (1953). Sleep characteristics of infants. *J Appl Physiol*, *6*(5), 269–282.

Kushnir, J., & Sadeh, A. (2013). Correspondence between reported and actigraphic sleep measures in preschool children: the role of a clinical context. *J Clin Sleep Med*, *9*(11), 1147–1151. doi: 10.5664/jcsm.3154

Larcher, S., Gauchez, A. S., Lablanche, S., Pepin, J. L., Benhamou, P. Y., & Borel, A. L. (2016). Impact of sleep behavior on glycemic control in type 1 diabetes: the role of social jetlag. *Eur J Endocrinol*, *175*(5), 411–419. doi: 10.1530/EJE-16-0188

Latta, F., Leproult, R., Tasali, E., Hofmann, E., & Van Cauter, E. (2005). Sex differences in delta and alpha EEG activities in healthy older adults. *Sleep*, *28*(12), 1525–1534.

Lee, K. A., Zaffke, M. E., & McEnany, G. (2000). Parity and sleep patterns during and after pregnancy. *Obstet Gynecol*, *95*, 14–28.

LeRoux, A., Wright, L., Perrot, T., & Rusak, B. (2014). Impact of menstrual cycle phase on endocrine effects of partial sleep restriction in healthy women. *Psychoneuroendocrinology, 49*, 34–46. doi: 10.1016/j.psyneuen.2014.06.002

Lewy, A. J., & Sack, R. L. (1989). The dim light melatonin onset as a marker for circadian phase position. *Chronobiol Int, 6*(1), 93–102.

Li, Y.-S., Lee, H.-C., Huang, J.-P., Lin, Y.-Z., Au, H.-K., Lo, Y.-C., … Chen, Y.-H. (2023). Adverse effects of inadequate sleep duration patterns during pregnancy on toddlers suspected developmental delay: a longitudinal study. *Sleep Med, 105*, 68–77. doi: 10.1016/j.sleep.2023.02.022

Lim, A. S., Kowgier, M., Yu, L., Buchman, A. S., & Bennett, D. A. (2013). Sleep fragmentation and the risk of incident Alzheimer's disease and cognitive decline in older persons. *Sleep, 36*(7), 1027–1032. doi: 10.5665/sleep.2802

Lo, J. C., Lee, S. M., Lee, X. K., Sasmita, K., Chee, N., Tandi, J., … Chee, M. W. L. (2018). Sustained benefits of delaying school start time on adolescent sleep and well-being. *Sleep, 41*(6), zsy052. doi:10.1093/sleep/zsy052

Lucchini, M., O'Brien, L. M., Kahn, L. G., Brennan, P. A., Glazer Baron, K., Knapp, E. A., … Environmental Influences on Child Health Organization. (2022). Racial/ethnic disparities in subjective sleep duration, sleep quality, and sleep disturbances during pregnancy: an ECHO study. *Sleep, 45*(9), zsac075. doi: 10.1093/sleep/zsac075

Lund, H. G., Reider, B. D., Whiting, A. B., & Prichard, J. R. (2010). Sleep patterns and predictors of disturbed sleep in a large population of college students. *J Adolesc Health, 46*(2), 124–132. doi: 10.1016/j.jadohealth.2009.06.016

Madeira, S. G., Reis, C., Paiva, T., Moreira, C. S., Nogueira, P., & Roenneberg, T. (2021). Social jetlag, a novel predictor for high cardiovascular risk in blue-collar workers following permanent atypical work schedules. *J Sleep Res, 30*(6), e13380. doi:10.1111/jsr.13380

Mander, B. A., Rao, V., Lu, B., Saletin, J. M., Lindquist, J. R., Ancoli-Israel, S., … Walker, M. P. (2013). Prefrontal atrophy, disrupted NREM slow waves and impaired hippocampal-dependent memory in aging. *Nat Neurosci, 16*(3), 357–364. doi: 0.1038/nn.3324

Marin, O. (2016). Developmental timing and critical windows for the treatment of psychiatric disorders. *Nat Med, 22*(11), 1229–1238. doi: 10.1038/nm.4225

Matthews, K. A., Lee, L., Kravitz, H. M., Joffe, H., Neal-Perry, G., Swanson, L., … Hall, M. H. (2021). Influence of the menopausal transition on polysomnographic sleep characteristics: a longitudinal analysis. *Sleep, 44*(11), zsab139. doi:10.1093/sleep/zsab139

McArthur, A. J., Lewy, A. J., & Sack, R. L. (1996). Non-24-hour sleep-wake syndrome in a sighted man: circadian rhythm studies and efficacy of melatonin treatment. *Sleep, 19*(7), 544–553.

McGraw, K., Hoffmann, R., Harker, C., & Herman, J. H. (1999). The development of circadian rhythms in a human infant. *Sleep, 22*(3), 303–310.

Micic, G., Lovato, N., Gradisar, M., Burgess, H. J., Ferguson, S. A., & Lack, L. (2016). Circadian melatonin and temperature taus in delayed sleep-wake phase disorder and non-24-hour sleep-wake rhythm disorder patients: an ultradian constant routine study. *J Biol Rhythms, 31*(4), 387–405. doi: 10.1177/0748730416650069

Miles, L. E. M., Raynal, D. M., & Wilson, M. A. (1977). Blind man living in normal society has circadian rhythms of 24.9 hours. *Science, 198*, 421–423.

Mindell, J. A., Cook, R. A., & Nikolovski, J. (2015). Sleep patterns and sleep disturbances across pregnancy. *Sleep Med, 16*(4), 483–488. doi: 10.1016/j.sleep.2014.12.006

Mindell, J. A., Li, A. M., Sadeh, A., Kwon, R., & Goh, D. Y. (2015). Bedtime routines for young children: a dose-dependent association with sleep outcomes. *Sleep, 38*(5), 717–722. doi: 10.5665/sleep.4662

Monk, T. H. (2005). The post-lunch dip in performance. *Clin Sports Med, 24*(2), e15–e23. doi: 10.1016/j.csm.2004.12.002

Morin, L. P., Fitzgerald, K. M., Rusak, B., & Zucker, I. (1977). Circadian organization and neural mediation of hamster reproductive rhythms. *Psychoneuroendocrinology, 2*, 73–98.

Morin, L. P., Fitzgerald, K. M., & Zucker, I. (1977). Estradiol shortens the period of hamster circadian rhythms. *Science, 196*, 305–307.

Muehlroth, B. E., & Werkle-Bergner, M. (2020). Understanding the interplay of sleep and aging: methodological challenges. *Psychophysiology, 57*(3), e13523. doi: 10.1111/psyp.13523

Murray, J. M., Sletten, T. L., Magee, M., Gordon, C., Lovato, N., Bartlett, D. J., … Delayed Sleep on Melatonin Study Group. (2017). Prevalence of circadian misalignment and its association with depressive symptoms in delayed sleep phase disorder. *Sleep, 40*(1), zsw002. doi: 10.1093/sleep/zsw002

Nahmod, N. G., Lee, S., Master, L., Chang, A. M., Hale, L., & Buxton, O. M. (2019). Later high school start times associated with longer actigraphic sleep duration in adolescents. *Sleep, 42*(2), zsy212. doi:10.1093/sleep/zsy212

Nyhuis, C. C., & Fernandez-Mendoza, J. (2023). Insomnia nosology: a systematic review and critical appraisal of historical diagnostic categories and current phenotypes. *J Sleep Res, 32*(6), e13910. doi:10.1111/jsr.13910

O'Brien, E. M., & Mindell, J. A. (2005). Sleep and risk-taking behavior in adolescents. *Behav Sleep Med, 3*(3), 113–133.

Ohayon, M. M., Carskadon, M. A., Guilleminault, C., & Vitiello, M. V. (2004). Meta-analysis of quantitative sleep parameters from childhood to old age in healthy individuals: developing normative sleep values across the human lifespan. *Sleep, 27*(7), 1255–1273.

Okun, M. L., Buysse, D. J., & Hall, M. H. (2015). Identifying insomnia in early pregnancy: validation of the Insomnia Symptoms Questionnaire (ISQ) in pregnant women. *J Clin Sleep Med, 11*(6), 645–654. doi: 10.5664/jcsm.4776

Okun, M. L., Luther, J. F., Wisniewski, S. R., & Wisner, K. L. (2013). Disturbed sleep and inflammatory cytokines in depressed and nondepressed pregnant women: an exploratory analysis of pregnancy outcomes. *Psychosom Med, 75*(7), 670–681. doi: 10.1097/PSY.0b013e31829cc3e7

Owens, J., Adolescent Sleep Working Group, & Committee on Adolescence. (2014). Insufficient sleep in adolescents and young adults: an update on causes and consequences. *Pediatrics, 134*(3), e921–932. doi: 10.1542/peds.2014-1696

Owens, J. A., Belon, K., & Moss, P. (2010). Impact of delaying school start time on adolescent sleep, mood and behavior. *Arch Pediatr Adolesc Med, 164*(7), 608–614.

Palagini, L., Gemignani, A., Banti, S., Manconi, M., Mauri, M., & Riemann, D. (2014). Chronic sleep loss during pregnancy as a determinant of stress: impact on pregnancy outcome. *Sleep Med, 15*(8), 853–859. doi: 10.1016/j.sleep.2014.02.013

Parry, B. L., Mendelson, W. B., Duncan, W. C., Sack, D. A., & Wehr, T. A. (1989). Longitudinal sleep EEG, temperature, and activity measurements across the menstrual cycle in patients with premenstrual depression and age-matched controls. *Psychiatry Res, 30*, 285–303.

Parry, B. L., Mostofi, N., LeVeau, B., Nahum, H. C., Golshan, S., Laughlin, G. A., & Gillin, J. C. (1999). Sleep EEG studies during early and late partial sleep deprivation in premenstrual dysphoric disorder and normal control subjects. *Psychiatry Res, 85*, 127–143.

Paruthi, S., Brooks, L. J., D'Ambrosio, C., Hall, W. A., Kotagal, S., Lloyd, R. M., … Wise, M. S. (2016). Recommended amount of sleep for pediatric populations: a consensus statement of the American Academy of Sleep Medicine. *J Clin Sleep Med, 12*(6), 785–786. doi: 10.5664/jcsm.5866

Patke, A., Murphy, P. J., Onat, O. E., Krieger, A. C., Ozcelik, T., Campbell, S. S., & Young, M. W. (2017). Mutation of the human circadian clock gene *CRY1* in familial delayed sleep phase disorder. *Cell, 169*(2), 203–215 e213. doi: 10.1016/j.cell.2017.03.027

Patton, G. C., & Viner, R. (2007). Pubertal transitions in health. *Lancet, 369*, 1130–1139. doi: 0.1016/S0140-6736(07)60366-3

Paus, T., Keshavan, M., & Giedd, J. N. (2008). Why do many psychiatric disorders emerge during adolescence? *Nat Rev Neurosci, 9*(12), 947–957. doi: 10.1038/nrn2513

Pesaresi, M., Soon-Shiong, R., French, L., Kaplan, D. R., Miller, F. D., & Paus, T. (2015). Axon diameter and axonal transport: in vivo and in vitro effects of androgens. *Neuroimage, 115*, 191–201. doi: 10.1016/j.neuroimage.2015.04.048

Pfefferbaum, A., & Rosenbloom, M. (1987). Skull thickness influences P3 amplitude. *Psychopharmacol Bull, 23*(3), 493–496.

Pien, G. W., & Schwab, R. J. (2004). Sleep disorders in pregnancy. *Sleep, 27*(7), 1405–1417.

Plamberger, C. P., Van Wijk, H. E., Kerschbaum, H., Pletzer, B. A., Gruber, G., Oberascher, K., … Hoedlmoser, K. (2021). Impact of menstrual cycle phase and oral contraceptives on sleep and overnight memory consolidation. *J Sleep Res, 30*(4), e13239. doi: 10.1111/jsr.13239

Polo-Kantola, P., Erkkola, R., Helenius, H., Irjala, K., & Polo, O. (1998). When does estrogen replacement therapy improve sleep quality? *Am J Obstetr Gynecol, 178*, 1002–1009.

Prendergast, B. J., Kriegsfeld, L. J., & Nelson, R. J. (2001). Photoperiodic polyphenisms in rodents: neuroendocrine mechanisms, costs, and functions. *Quart Rev Biol, 76*(3), 293–325.

Quante, M., Hong, B., von Ash, T., Yu, X., Kaplan, E. R., Rueschman, M., … Redline, S. (2021). Associations between subjectively and objectively measured sleep duration and timing in infants at age 6 months. *Sleep, 44*(4), zsaa217. doi: 10.1093/sleep/zsaa217

Randler, C., Ebenhöh, N., Fischer, A., Höchel, S., Schroff, C., Stoll, J. C., & Vollmer, C. (2012). Chronotype but not sleep length is related to salivary testosterone in young adult men. *Psychoneuroendocrinology, 37*, 1740–1744. doi: 0.1016/j.psyneuen.2012.02.008

Randler, C., Vollmer, C., Kalb, N., & Itzek-Greulich, H. (2019). Breakpoints of time in bed, midpoint of sleep, and social jetlag from infancy to early adulthood. *Sleep Med, 57*, 80–86. doi: 10.1016/j.sleep.2019.01.023

Redline, S., Kirchner, H. L., Quan, S. F., Gottlieb, D. J., Kapur, V., & Newman, A. (2004). The effects of age, sex, ethnicity, and sleep-disordered breathing on sleep architecture. *Arch Intern Med, 164*, 406–418.

Riemann, D., Benz, F., Dressle, R. J., Espie, C. A., Johann, A. F., Blanken, T. F., … Van Someren, E. J. W. (2022). Insomnia disorder: state of the science and challenges for the future. *J Sleep Res*, *31*(4), e13604. doi:10.1111/jsr.13604

Roehrs, T., Kapke, A., Roth, T., & Breslau, N. (2006). Sex differences in the polysomnographic sleep of young adults: a community-based study. *Sleep Med*, *7*(1), 49–53. doi: 10.1016/j.sleep.2005.05.008

Roenneberg, T., Kuehnle, T., Pramstaller, P. P., Ricken, J., Havel, M., Guth, A., & Merrow, M. (2004). A marker for the end of adolescence. *Curr Biol*, *14*(24), R1038–R1039. doi: 10.1016/j.cub.2004.11.039

Rojo-Wissar, D. M., Bai, J., Benjamin-Neelon, S. E., Wolfson, A. R., & Spira, A. P. (2022). Development of circadian rest-activity rhythms during the first year of life in a racially diverse cohort. *Sleep*, *45*(6), zsac078. doi: 10.1093/sleep/zsac078

Rosenberg, R. S., Zepelin, H., & Rechtschaffen, A. (1979). Sleep in young and old rats. *J Gerontol*, *34*(4), 525–532.

Rosinvil, T., Bouvier, J., Dubé, J., Lafrenière, A., Bouchard, M., Cronier, J., … Lina, J. M. (2021). Are age and sex effects on sleep slow waves only a matter of EEG amplitude? *Sleep*, *44*(3), zsaa186. doi:10.1093/sleep/zsaa186

Sadeh, A., Acebo, C., Aytur, S., & Carskadon, M. A. (1995). Activity-based assessment of sleep-wake patterns during the 1st year of life. *Infant Behavior and Development*, *18*, 329–337.

Sadeh, A., Tikotzky, L., & Scher, A. (2010). Parenting and infant sleep. *Sleep Med Rev*, *14*(2), 89–96. doi: 10.1016/j.smrv.2009.05.003

Sampasa-Kanyinga, H., Chaput, J. P., Goldfield, G. S., Janssen, I., Wang, J., Hamilton, H. A., … Colman, I. (2021). The Canadian 24-hour movement guidelines and psychological distress among adolescents: les directives canadiennes en matiere de mouvement sur 24 heures et la detresse psychologique chez les adolescents. *Can J Psychiatry*, *66*(7), 624–633. doi: 10.1177/0706743720970863

Scullin, M. K. (2013). Sleep, memory, and aging: the link between slow-wave sleep and episodic memory changes from younger to older adults. *Psychol Aging*, *28*(1), 105–114. doi: 10.1037/a0028830

Scullin, M. K., & Bliwise, D. L. (2015). Sleep, cognition, and normal aging: integrating a half century of multidisciplinary research. *Perspect Psychol Sci*, *10*(1), 97–137.

Scullin, M. K., Gao, C., Fillmore, P., Roberts, R. L., Pruett, N., & Bliwise, D. L. (2019). REM sleep mediates age-related decline in prospective memory consolidation. *Sleep*, *42*(6), zsz055. doi:10.1093/sleep/zsz055

Sekar, A., Bialas, A. R., de Rivera, H., Davis, A., Hammond, T. R., Kamitaki, N., … McCarroll, S. A. (2016). Schizophrenia risk from complex variation of complement component 4. *Nature*, *530*(7589), 177–183. doi: 10.1038/nature16549

Shechter, A., Lesperance, P., Ng Ying Kin, N. M., & Boivin, D. B. (2012). Nocturnal polysomnographic sleep across the menstrual cycle in premenstrual dysphoric disorder. *Sleep Med*, *13*(8), 1071–1078. doi: 10.1016/j.sleep.2012.05.012

Shechter, A., Varin, F., & Boivin, D. B. (2010). Circadian variation of sleep during the follicular and luteal phases of the menstrual cycle. *Sleep*, *33*(5), 647–656.

Smith, C., Reilly, C., & Midkiff, K. (1989). Evaluation of three circadian rhythm questionnaires with suggestions for an improved measure of morningness. *J Appl Psychol*, *74*(5), 728–738.

Smith, K. A., Schoen, M. W., & Czeisler, C. A. (2004). Adaptation of human pineal melatonin suppression by recent photic history. *J Clin Endocrinol Metab*, *89*(7), 3610–3614. doi: 10.1210/jc.2003-032100

Sonni, A., & Spencer, R. M. C. (2015). Sleep protects memories from interference in older adults. *Neurobiol Aging*, *36*(7), 2272–2281. doi: 10.1016/j.neurobiolaging.2015.03.010

Sowell, E. R., Peterson, B. S., Thompson, P. M., Welcome, S. E., Henkenius, A. L., & Toga, A. W. (2003). Mapping cortical change across the human life span. *Nat Neurosci*, *6*(3), 309–315. doi: 10.1038/nn1008

Steiner, M. (2000). Premenstrual syndrome and premenstrual dysphoric disorder: guidelines for management. *J Psychiatr Neurosci*, *25*(5), 459–468.

Stern, E., Parmalee, A. H., Akiyama, Y., Schultz, M. A., & Wenner, W. H. (1969). Sleep cycle characteristics in infants. *Pediatrics*, *43*, 65–70.

Sterniczuk, R., Theo, O., Rusak, B., & Rockwood, K. (2013). Sleep disturbance is associated with incident dementia and mortality. *Curr Alzheimer Res*, *10*(7), 767–775. doi: 10.2174/15672050113109990134

Stone, J. E., Phillips, A. J. K., Chachos, E., Hand, A. J., Lu, S., Carskadon, M. A., … Team, C. S. (2021). In-person vs home schooling during the COVID-19 pandemic: differences in sleep, circadian timing, and mood in early adolescence. *J Pineal Res*, 1–12. doi: 10.1111/jpi.12757

Strogatz, S. H., Kronauer, R. E., & Czeisler, C. A. (1987). Circadian pacemaker interferes with sleep onset at specific times each day: role in insomnia. *Am J Physiol*, *253*, R172–R178.

Swift, K. M., Keus, K., Echeverria, C. G., Cabrera, Y., Jimenez, J., Holloway, J., … Poe, G. R. (2020). Sex differences within sleep in gonadally-intact rats. *Sleep*, *43*(5), zsz289. doi:10.1093/sleep/zsz289

Thurston, R. C., Chang, Y., Buysse, D. J., Hall, M. H., & Matthews, K. A. (2019). Hot flashes and awakenings among midlife women. *Sleep*, *42*(9), zsz131. doi:10.1093/sleep/zsz131

Toh, K. L., Jones, C. R., He, Y., Eide, E. J., Hinz, W. A., Virshup, D. M., … Fu, Y.-H. (2001). An hPer2 phosphorylation site mutation in familial advanced sleep phase syndrome. *Science*, *291*(5506), 1040–1043. doi: 10.1126/science.1057499

Touchette, É., Mongrain, V., Petit, D., Tremblay, R. E., & Montplaisir, J. Y. (2008). Development of sleep-wake schedules during childhood and relationship with sleep duration. *Arch Pediatr Adolesc Med*, *162*(4), 343–349.

Tranah, G. J., Blackwell, T., Stone, K. L., Ancoli-Israel, S., Paudel, M. L., Ensrud, K. E., … Group, S. O. F. R. (2011). Circadian activity rhythms and risk of incident dementia and mild cognitive impairment in older women. *Ann Neurol*, *70*(5), 722–732. doi: 10.1002/ana.22468

Troxel, W. M., & Hale, L. (2022). Virtual special issue: updates on school start times and adolescent sleep health. *Sleep Health*, *8*(6), 567–568. doi: 10.1016/j.sleh.2022.09.001

Tsai, S. Y., Lee, C. C., Tsai, H. Y., & Tung, Y. C. (2022). Bedtime routines and objectively assessed sleep in infants. *J Adv Nurs*, *78*(1), 154–164. doi: 10.1111/jan.14968

Tyborowska, A., Volman, I., Smeekens, S., Toni, I., & Roelofs, K. (2016). Testosterone during puberty shifts emotional control from pulvinar to anterior prefrontal cortex. *J Neurosci*, *36*(23), 6156–6164. doi: 10.1523/JNEUROSCI.3874-15.2016

Unruh, M. L., Redline, S., An, M. W., Buysse, D. J., Nieto, F. J., Yeh, J. L., & Newman, A. B. (2008). Subjective and objective sleep quality and aging in the Sleep Heart Health Study. *J Am Geriatr Soc*, *56*(7), 1218–1227. doi: 10.1111/j.1532-5415.2008.01755.x

van der Vinne, V., Zerbini, G., Siersema, A., Pieper, A., Merrow, M., Hut, R. A., … Kantermann, T. (2015). Timing of examinations affects school performance differently in early and late chronotypes. *J Biol Rhythms*, *30*(1), 53–60. doi: 10.1177/0748730414564786

Vidafar, P., Gooley, J. J., Burns, A. C., Rajaratnam, S. M. W., Rueger, M., Van Reen, E., … Cain, S. W. (2018). Increased vulnerability to attentional failure during acute sleep deprivation in women depends on menstrual phase. *Sleep*, *41*(8), zsy098. doi:10.1093/sleep/zsy098

Viswanathan, N., & Davis, F. C. (1997). Single prenatal injections of melatonin or the D1-dopamine receptor agonist SKF 38393 to pregnant hamsters sets the offsprings' circadian rhythms to phases 180 degrees apart. *J Comp Physiol*, *180*, 339–346.

Vorona, R. D., Szklo-Coxe, M., Lamichhane, R., Ware, J. C., McNallen, A., & Leszczyszyn, D. (2014). Adolescent crash rates and school start times in two central Virginia counties, 2009–2011: a follow-up study to a southeastern Virginia study, 2007–2008. *J Clin Sleep Med*, *10*(11), 1169–1177. doi: 10.5664/jcsm.4192

Vorona, R. D., Szklo-Coxe, M., Wu, A., Dubik, M., Zhao, Y., & Ware, J. C. (2011). Dissimilar teen crash rates in two neighboring southeastern Virginia cities with different high school start times. *J Clin Sleep Med*, *7*(2), 145–151.

Wahlstrom, K. (2002). Changing times: findings from the first longitudinal study of later high school start times. NASSP Bulletin (Vol. 86, pp. 3–21): National Association of Secondary School Principals.

Wang, X., de Groot, E. R., Tataranno, M. L., van Baar, A., Lammertink, F., Alderliesten, T., … Dudink, J. (2024). Machine learning-derived active sleep as an early predictor of white matter development in preterm infants. *J Neurosci*, *44*(5), e1024232023. doi: 10.1523/JNEUROSCI.1024-23.2023

Watson, L. A., Phillips, A. J. K., Hosken, I. T., McGlashan, E. M., Anderson, C., Lack, L. C., … Cain, S. W. (2018). Increased sensitivity of the circadian system to light in delayed sleep-wake phase disorder. *J Physiol*, *596*(24), 6249–6261. doi: 10.1113/JP275917

Webb, W. B., & Dreblow, L. M. (1982). A modified method for scoring slow wave sleep of older subjects. *Sleep*, *5*(2), 195–199.

Werner, H., Molinari, L., Guyer, C., & Jenni, O. (2008). Agreement rates between actigraphy, diary, and questionnaire for children's sleep patterns. *Arch Pediatr Adolesc Med*, *162*(4), 350–358. doi: 10.1001/archpedi.162.4.350

Westerberg, C. E., Mander, B. A., Florczak, S. M., Weintraub, S., Mesulam, M.-M., Zee, P. C., & Paller, K. A. (2012). Concurrent impairments in sleep and memory in amnestic mild cognitive impairment. *J Int Neuropsych Soc*, *18*(3), 490–500. doi: 0.1017/S135561771200001X

Wheaton, A. G., Ferro, G. A., & Croft, J. B. (2015). School start times for middle school and high school students – United States, 2011–12 school year. Morbidity and Mortality Weekly Report, *64*, 809–835.

Whitford, T. J., Rennie, C. J., Grieve, S. M., Clark, C. R., Gordon, E., & Williams, L. M. (2007). Brain maturation in adolescence: concurrent changes in neuroanatomy and neurophysiology. *Hum Brain Mapp*, *28*(3), 228–237. doi: 10.1002/hbm.20273

Wittmann, M., Dinich, J., Merrow, M., & Roenneberg, T. (2006). Social jetlag: misalignment of biological and social time. *Chronobiol Int*, *23*(1–2), 497–509. doi: 10.1080/07420520500545979

Wolfson, A., & Carskadon, M. (1998). Sleep schedules and daytime functioning in adolescents. *Child Dev*, *69*(4), 875–887.

Xu, M., Belanger, L., Ivers, H., Guay, B., Zhang, J., & Morin, C. M. (2011). Comparison of subjective and objective sleep quality in menopausal and non-menopausal women with insomnia. *Sleep Med*, *12*(1), 65–69. doi: 10.1016/j.sleep.2010.09.003

Xu, Q., & Lang, C. P. (2014). Examining the relationship between subjective sleep disturbance and menopause: a systematic review and meta-analysis. *Menopause*, *21*(12), 1301–1318. doi: 10.1097/GME.0000000000000240

Xu, Y., Padiath, Q. S., Shapiro, R. E., Jones, C. R., Wu, S. C., Saigoh, N., ... Ptáček, L. J., & Fu, Y.-H. (2005). Functional consequences of a CKIδ mutation causing familial advanced sleep phase syndrome. *Nature*, *434*, 640–644.

Young, T., Rabago, D., Zgierska, A., Austin, D., & Finn, L. (2003). Objective and subjective sleep quality in premenopausal, perimenopausal, and postmenopausal women in the Wisconsin Sleep Cohort Study. *Sleep*, *26*(6), 667–672.

Zavada, A., Gordijn, M. C. M., Beersma, D. G. M., Daan, S., & Roenneberg, T. (2009). Comparison of the Munich ChronoType Questionnaire with the Horne-Östberg's Morningness-Eveningness score. *Chronobiol Int*, *22*(2), 267–278. doi: 10.1081/cbi-200053536

Zepelin, H. (1983). Normal age related changes in sleep. In M. H. Chase & E. D. Weitzman (Eds.), *Sleep Disorders: Basic and Clinical Research* (Vol. 4, pp. 431–444). New York: Spectrum Publications.

Zhang, B., & Wing, Y.-K. (2006). Sex differences in insomnia: a meta-analysis. *Sleep*, *29*(1), 85–93.

Zhang, E. E., & Kay, S. A. (2010). Clocks not winding down: unravelling circadian networks. *Nat Rev Mol Cell Biol*, *11*(11), 764–776. doi: 10.1038/nrm2995

Zuurbier, L. A., Luik, A. I., Hofman, A., Franco, O. H., Van Someren, E. J., & Tiemeier, H. (2015). Fragmentation and stability of circadian activity rhythms predict mortality: the Rotterdam study. *Am J Epidemiol*, *181*(1), 54–63. doi: 10.1093/aje/kwu245

CHAPTER 5

Homeostatic and Circadian Regulation of Sleep

5.1 OVERVIEW

Sleep is regulated principally by the interaction of two mechanisms: a homeostatic regulator and a circadian clock. This chapter discusses the nature of homeostasis and reviews evidence related to homeostatic regulation of total sleep amounts, NREM sleep and its features, and REM sleep. It discusses evidence that other mechanisms may be activated when homeostatic mechanisms are unable to compensate for lost sleep. It describes the potent effects of the circadian system on the timing of REM sleep and its minimal effect on NREM sleep regulation. This chapter also reviews several competing models that have been proposed to be involved in the regulation of REM sleep and of the alternation between NREM and REM sleep.

The final section of this chapter reviews a widely accepted model of how homeostatic and circadian mechanisms interact to shape the patterns of sleep observed, called the two-process model. It also discusses the functional significance of this dual regulatory mechanism for sleep and for other motivated behaviors.

5.2 Homeostasis

5.2.1 An early study of effects of sleep loss

In 1887, George T. W. Patrick was appointed head of the Department of Mental and Moral Science and Didactics at the State University of Iowa, where he established one of the earliest psychology laboratories in the United States. A few years later, he and his assistant, J. Allen Gilbert, published what was apparently the first scientific report on the effects of extended sleep deprivation on cognition and on subsequent sleep (Patrick & Gilbert, 1896).

They kept three healthy young men awake for periods of ~90 h (3¾ days) and studied their cognitive and motor functions as well as observing how long they slept when later allowed to do so. Their publication included both interesting observations and prescient speculations, which are discussed below in Section 5.3.1. Among their observations were that sleep deprivation led to a progressive increase in the tendency to sleep; one participant became so sleepy during the final 24 h of the study that he had to be monitored continuously to keep him awake. They also observed that there was an increase in the amount of sleep shown after the deprivation period. The three participants slept 10.5–15.5 h during the night after sleep deprivation ended and felt fully refreshed afterwards. This amounted to recovering 16–35.5% of the sleep they had lost during their extended wake period, based on their reports of their usual sleep habits.

The most obvious and consistently observed consequence of sleep deprivation is a compelling drive to fall asleep. Even the most willing human experimental participant who is deprived of sleep for many hours will experience an increasingly irresistible tendency to fall asleep, eventually even while sitting up and in mid-conversation. Many pilots, drivers, air traffic controllers, and medical personnel have also had the experience of a compelling need to sleep when their jobs kept them awake through their normal sleep phase, despite their strong motivation to stay awake, and despite the disastrous consequences that could follow if they fell asleep (see Chapter 13).

5.2.2 The nature of homeostasis

An increasing drive to do something after being deprived of the opportunity to do it is characteristic of motivational systems that are regulated homeostatically. The term homeostasis (from the Greek *omoios* [similar], and *stasis* [state maintenance]) was coined by the American physiologist Walter Cannon (Cannon, 1929) to capture the essence of ideas advanced earlier by the

19th century French physiologist Claude Bernard (see Gross, 1998). Bernard had noted that most of the physiological processes of organisms tend to maintain a constant—presumably optimal—state of the "milieu intérieur" (internal environment), despite continually changing external conditions.

Homeostasis is, therefore, the mechanism by which organisms respond to spontaneous or externally induced changes in their internal environments by corrective actions that restore the initial condition, thus allowing their internal state to be largely independent of environmental variations. Such homeostatic mechanisms in mammals regulate, for example, body temperature, the concentration of carbon dioxide and oxygen in the blood as well as energy and fluid balance. Cannon saw these mechanisms as the product of evolutionary processes that by trial and error arrived at an array of optimal settings for each species' physiological parameters. He called these defended physiological values "the wisdom of the body," which was also the title of a popular book he published in 1932.

To achieve stable homeostasis, organisms must have internal mechanisms that are sensitive to physiological parameters (e.g., carbon dioxide concentration, body temperature), and that can trigger corrective responses when the current values shift outside appropriate limits (see, e.g., Prabhakar & Semenza, 2015). Borrowing from the terminology of engineering, these mechanisms can be modeled as regulators, each of which has a set point that indicates the optimal level for the parameter it measures. The regulator detects deviations from that set point (errors). If a deviation is large enough, the regulator triggers processes that correct the error, such as shivering to generate heat, sweating to cool off, or faster breathing to blow off excess carbon dioxide.

This model of how physiological parameters are regulated is analogous to the way a thermostat works to regulate temperature in a house. It measures the current temperature in a room and, if it deviates more than a threshold amount from the set point, turns on a heating or cooling system. As a result, the room heats up or cools down until the difference between the current temperature and the set point is eliminated, at which time the thermostat turns the heating/cooling system off again.

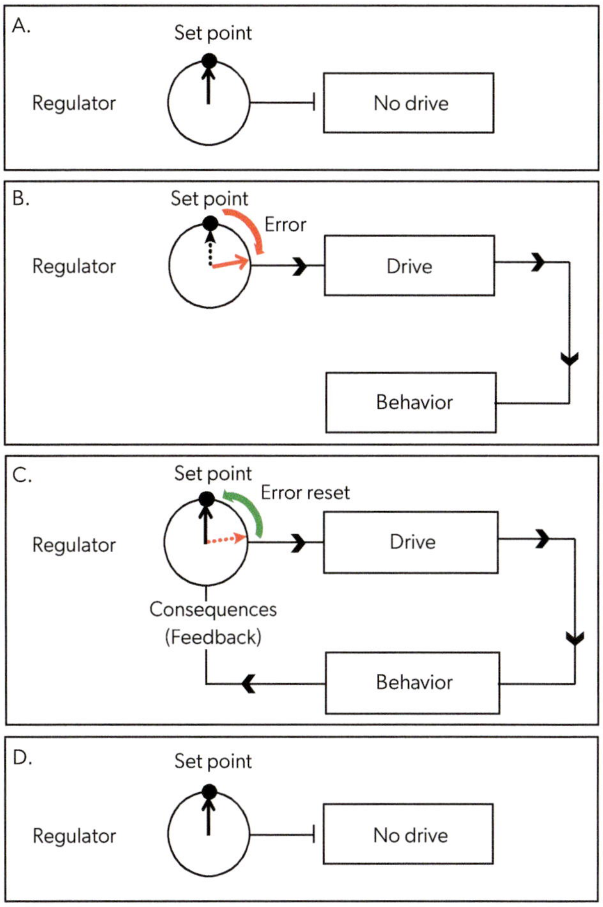

Figure 5.1 **A.** A control-system model illustrating the operation of a homeostatically regulated mechanism that controls the expression of a drive state (e.g., hunger, thirst). The key element is a regulator that senses the state of a critical variable (black arrow). The regulator has a set point (black circle) that represents the optimal value for that variable. When the current measure of the variable is near the set point, there is no drive activated. **B.** When the current measure of the variable (red arrow) deviates significantly from the ideal value at the set point (dotted black arrow), an error signal (error; curved red arrow) is generated. If the deviation is large enough, the regulator triggers a drive state that leads the organism to engage in behaviors that could satisfy the related drive (e.g., eating, drinking). **C.** When the behaviors triggered by the drive state are successful, the physiological consequences of the behavior provide a feedback signal to the regulator that resets (green arrow) the current reading back to the set point. **D.** Once the homeostatic drive has been satisfied, the homeostatic regulatory system comes back to rest, with no related drive being activated.

5.2.3 Homeostasis of sleep

We can apply a similar homeostatic model to the regulation of, for example, body weight or fluid balance. A hypothetical regulator for each of these parameters would have a set point reflecting the ideal value that is appropriate for each organism. Deviations from the set point generate signals that trigger behaviors aimed at correcting the errors. In this case, the signal takes the form of a changed motivational state or drive; namely, increased hunger or thirst, rather than a physiological response like sweating or faster breathing (**Figure 5.1 A, B**). Engaging in the behavior linked to that motivational state (finding food or water and consuming it) satisfies the drive. Feedback signals from the results of the corrective action reach the regulator, eliminate the error signal, and cancel the drive. As a result, the system comes back to rest in its ideal state (**Figure 5.1 C, D**).

Evidence that sleep is regulated in the same way, that is, that deprivation of sleep (creating a deviation from the set point)

BOX 5.1 Set Points, Settling Points, and the Regulation of Body Weight

There have been arguments raised against trying to apply a simple set-point model derived from physiological regulation to more complex physiological/behavioral systems, the focus of which has been the regulation of body weight/energy balance. An alternative proposal for body-weight regulation, for example, is based on the idea that an animal or person has several mechanisms that promote energy expenditure and others that promote energy intake. These opposing systems are activated by many different inputs to perform their independent functions. As a result, they achieve a balance between energy intake and expenditure that determines the organism's body weight.

This weight is considered a settling point (i.e., the compromise value on which the two competing regulatory systems "settle" as a result of their opposing actions), rather than a predetermined set point (Wirtshafter & Davis, 1977). In contrast to the set-point model, there is no proposed single regulatory mechanism that is genetically programmed to sense and defend a target body weight. Instead, the "wisdom of the body" results from the balance achieved by the dynamic interplay of opposing regulatory systems that respond to many inputs. (A settling-point model for sleep regulation has also been discussed, see Stephenson et al., 2015.)

Regardless of whether the system regulating body weight involves a set-point or a settling-point mechanism, animal and human studies consistently show that body weight is homeostatically regulated. Manipulations that lower or raise body weight result in compensatory physiological changes that bring body weight back toward baseline values over the long term; for a review, see Speakman et al., 2011.

One unique study examined the body weight and metabolic changes that occurred in a group of 14 contestants on the reality TV program, *The Biggest Loser*. The goal of the program was for overweight participants to compete to lose the most weight. Contestants lost large amounts of weight (mostly body fat) very quickly during the weeks of the program. They lost an impressive average of 58.3 kg (128.5 lb) by the end of the series. But they also developed dramatically *lower* resting metabolic rates, an apparent physiological response to weight loss that would reduce energy expenditure and therefore promote weight gain.

Six years later, their average body weights were only 17.3 kg (38.1 lb) lower than at baseline, having regained 41.0 kg (90.4 lb), or >70% of the average weight lost. Remarkably, their resting metabolic rates were even lower than at the end of the series, as if their bodies were still working hard to recover the lost weight by further reducing energy expenditure (Fothergill et al., 2016) (http://tinyurl.com/hb22smb). These findings demonstrate the difficulty of maintaining body weight losses in the face of homeostatic responses to weight loss that oppose the changes.

leads to a later increase in the drive to sleep and in the amount of sleep, is a central argument in favor of the idea that sleeping, like consuming water or food, satisfies an essential physiological need. Some have questioned whether regulators and set points for motivated behaviors are real physiological mechanisms or only metaphors (see **Box 5.1**) and have proposed alternative models (e.g., Speakman et al., 2011). But for the purpose of discussing the physiological importance of sleep, we can ask whether there is evidence of homeostatic regulation, that is, whether the sleep regulatory system acts *as if* a set-point regulatory mechanism were operating as in **Figure 5.1**.

5.2.4 Summary

The first published study of long-term sleep loss in humans found that participants developed a progressively increased drive to sleep and later increased their sleep durations during a single recovery night, relative to their baseline sleep durations. This evidence indicated that the amount of sleep is regulated homeostatically: Lost sleep increases the drive to sleep and is, at least in part, compensated for by increasing sleep amounts. Regulation of sleep was therefore similar to the regulation of other important physiological functions (energy or water balance) that respond to deficits by triggering drives and increasing compensatory behaviors.

There are different views as to whether the homeostatic mechanisms regulating complex behavioral/physiological processes involve a genetically determined set point or a settling point representing the compromise value of opposing regulatory systems. Regardless of the underlying mechanism involved, this initial evidence indicated that sleep, like other critical physiological functions, is homeostatically regulated.

5.3 Homeostatic regulation of sleep and slow-wave activity

5.3.1 Effects of sleep loss on subsequent sleep

An important observation in the report by Patrick and Gilbert was that sleep deprivation led to an immediate increase in sleep duration during a recovery period, as predicted by a homeostatic model. But the increase did not correspond 1:1 to the duration of sleep lost; the three participants averaged only about a 25% increase over their usual sleep durations during a single recovery night (Patrick & Gilbert, 1896).

The authors discussed several possible explanations for the lack of complete compensation for lost sleep. They suspected, for example, that despite the strong motivation of the participants to stay awake, and the constant attention of a "watcher" who prodded them awake at the first overt signs of sleep, participants might have experienced very short sleep episodes ("short and, perhaps, refreshing nap[s]") during the study. They inferred that short sleep episodes had intruded into waking, based also on their observations of brief lapses of attention during behavioral testing, and on the need for repeated interventions to keep the participants awake. But the total duration of these brief episodes would not have been enough to account for all of the lost sleep that was not compensated for during the recovery night.

Patrick & Gilbert also noted that the depth of recovery sleep in one participant (measured as the intensity of a somatosensory stimulus needed to wake him) indicated that recovery sleep was "deeper" and, they presumed, more efficient than usual sleep. Finally, they speculated that some of the recuperative effects of sleep might also have been achieved in weaker form during periods of quiet waking. These ideas were based solely on behavioral observations, since their study was conducted decades before EEG recording methods were developed. But research over the next century has supported and extended several of their observations and speculations:

- After sleep deprivation, there is a rebound increase in the duration of recovery sleep compared to baseline sleep durations, but it is not enough to make up for all of the hours of lost sleep time.
- During sleep deprivation, people can show very brief sleep episodes ("microsleeps"), reflected in brief lapses of attention (and slow EEG oscillations), even while appearing awake.
- Recovery sleep is "deeper" after deprivation, and this change may allow more complete recovery than suggested by its limited duration.
- Some of the benefits of sleep may be achieved in weaker form during quiet, waking rest.

Later studies documented that the duration of recovery sleep after sleep deprivation, verified by EEG and including several subsequent recovery nights, does not equal the duration of sleep lost. A particularly dramatic example was that of a 17-year-old (Randy Gardner) who voluntarily deprived himself of sleep for 264 h (11 days) in order to set a world record. He slept only ~15 h during his first recovery night (and ~10 and 9 h on the two following nights) (Gulevich et al., 1966; Ross, 1965); see Section 14.3.2 for a discussion of Gardner's experience. No baseline sleep recordings were made before his deprivation period, but if one assumes that his recorded sleep a few weeks later was typical, he would have averaged ~6.7 h sleep/night, and therefore would have lost ~74 h of sleep over 11 nights. He did not appear to be on his way to recovering this lost sleep, since he had made up only ~14 h of additional sleep during the three recovery nights (<20% of lost sleep).

Before trying to interpret this result and the similar findings by Patrick & Gilbert (1896), it is useful to think about whether sleep duration, a common-sense measure of the extent of recovery, is the right measure to use. Asking a similar question with respect to another motivated behavior, food intake, can help clarify the issue. For the purpose of this analysis, we can make the simplifying assumption that the motivation to eat is related only to maintaining energy balance (i.e., a stable balance of energy intake and expenditure).[1] When people do not eat for an extended period, they do not take in their usual amount of food energy, and as a result develop a negative energy balance relative to a baseline period. Homeostatic mechanisms are activated to compensate for the lost intake of calories.

Achieving homeostatic regulation of energy balance does not, however, depend on making up for the total number of minutes of lost food intake; there are other options to achieve homeostasis. These include reducing usual activity levels and thereby lowering energy expenditure; reducing body temperature and metabolic rate (see **Box 5.1** for the opposite phenomenon), both of which also reduce energy expenditure; and when recovery feeding occurs, eating more quickly, or choosing foods with higher caloric content to increase energy intake. Thus, energy balance could, in principle, be restored without much, if any, increase in the number of minutes spent eating, nor necessarily even in the amount of food consumed.

The goal of homeostasis in this case is to restore energy balance, not to replace the time usually spent eating. In other words, the hypothetical homeostatic regulator has a set point for energy balance, not for the length of time spent eating. Similarly, when intense exercise increases the concentration of carbon dioxide in the blood, breathing rates increase to eliminate the excess carbon dioxide and bring in needed oxygen. Breathing rate is not the target of homeostatic regulation; it is the mechanism that helps to restore an appropriate blood gas concentration, which is the actual target of regulation.

Each of these examples shows the important distinction between the *targets* of homeostatic regulation (energy balance or blood gas composition) and the *mechanisms* (e.g., calorie

[1] What actually contributes to our motivation to eat is obviously more complicated and would include factors such as the incentive properties of the food, learned habits, social interactions, etc.

intake/lowered metabolic rate or breathing rate change) that achieve the regulation (Beersma & Daan, 2015).

Turning to sleep regulation, we can ask the same question. Is there homeostatic regulation of sleep duration? Based on the studies we have discussed, the answer is that the duration of sleep increases somewhat after sleep loss, but there does not appear to be complete compensation for the hours of sleep lost. Thus, the length of sleep does not appear to be the target of homeostatic regulation. Sleep is a mechanism that facilitates homeostatic regulation of a physiological target, just as rapid breathing and increased food intake are examples of mechanisms that facilitate regulation of blood gases and energy balance (Beersma & Daan, 2015).

If sleep is the regulatory mechanism involved, the obvious next question is what is the target function that is being regulated by the mechanism of sleeping, and that results in the negative effects of not sleeping. The assumption of most researchers is that the target(s) of homeostatic regulation are one or more changes in brain function that occur during extended waking and need to be reversed during recovery sleep. Some suggestions about the nature of these changes are discussed below and in Section 11.6. In our relative ignorance of the function(s) of sleep, we turn to sleep duration as a convenient marker, and we attribute our daytime sleepiness and cognitive impairment today to not getting enough hours of sleep last night. While this is superficially correct, it puts the focus on the reduced length of sleep (a measure of the activity of a regulatory mechanism) rather than on the physiological changes (the targets of regulation) that occurred during extended waking and led to the daytime deficits.

We do not yet know all of the physiological changes that are caused by extended waking and reversed by sleep, which might be the actual targets of homeostatic regulation (see Chapter 16). Identifying these targets could be facilitated by finding measures of sleep that are regulated more completely than duration. One suggestion made by Patrick & Gilbert was that sleep had an intensity dimension, and that a greater "depth" of recovery sleep might help compensate for the effects of extended waking. Later research identified a feature of sleep that appears to reflect its intensity and is a better indicator of sleep need and of recovery processes during sleep than duration alone, which is the topic of the next section.

5.3.2 Slow-wave activity (SWA) and homeostasis

Evidence from electrophysiological recordings that were not available to Patrick and Gilbert strongly reinforces one of their conclusions: Recovery sleep is not only longer than usual but also has EEG features indicating that it is deeper than baseline sleep. This research has focused primarily on the low-frequency EEG activity that characterizes N3 sleep.

To review the terminology introduced in Chapter 2, N3 sleep (SWS) is defined as epochs of sleep occupied by at least 20% delta waves. Delta waves themselves are typically defined as having frequencies of 1–4.5 Hz with an amplitude of 75–140 μV. A consistent finding in human studies is that recovery sleep after a night of sleep deprivation includes more N3 sleep than a normal baseline night. In particular, there is an increase in the amount of N3 sleep early in the night, beyond the already high levels normally shown at that time (**Figure 5.2**) (Borbély et al., 1981; Carskadon & Dement, 2011). Randy Gardner also showed increased SWS during recovery nights after being awake for 11 days (Gulevich et al., 1966).[2]

As described in Chapter 2, Fourier analysis is used to characterize the frequencies expressed in the EEG. Fourier analysis yields a power spectrum indicating the extent to which different frequencies are represented in an EEG sample (see **Figures 2.2** and **2.3**). The amount of delta-band power shown during N3 sleep, however, does not represent all of the power in this frequency band during sleep. These low frequencies are present to a lesser extent in EEG recordings from other sleep stages and even during waking. For example, EEG segments that do not contain enough delta waves to be labeled N3 are labeled N2 sleep, but they could potentially include up to 20% delta waves.

Spectral power in a broader EEG frequency band (0.5 or 0.75–4.5 Hz is referred to as slow-wave activity (SWA). This measure includes both the traditional delta range (1.0–4.5 Hz) and the range of slow oscillations (0.5–1.0 Hz); see Section 12.2.5. Fourier analysis shows that SWA is present in the EEG throughout the night, but to different extents during different sleep stages (Achermann et al., 1993). Not surprisingly, the greatest amount of SWA is found early in the night when most N3 sleep occurs (**Figure 5.3**), but it is also present in other NREM sleep stages and to a minor extent in REM sleep and waking.

The amount of SWA reflects the degree of accumulated sleep need or sleep debt, which is another way of saying "how long an individual has been awake." In adult humans who have been awake all day, the amount of SWA produced is high immediately after they fall asleep and decreases over the

[2] Note that rats who have undergone lengthy periods of sleep loss do not show immediate increases in NREM sleep but show increased REM sleep amounts. However, after relatively short, complete loss of all sleep (6 h), they do show immediate increases in NREM sleep and SWA (Tobler & Borbély, 1990; Wang et al., 2023). For a discussion of the likely mechanisms that account for these differences, see Section 5.5.2.

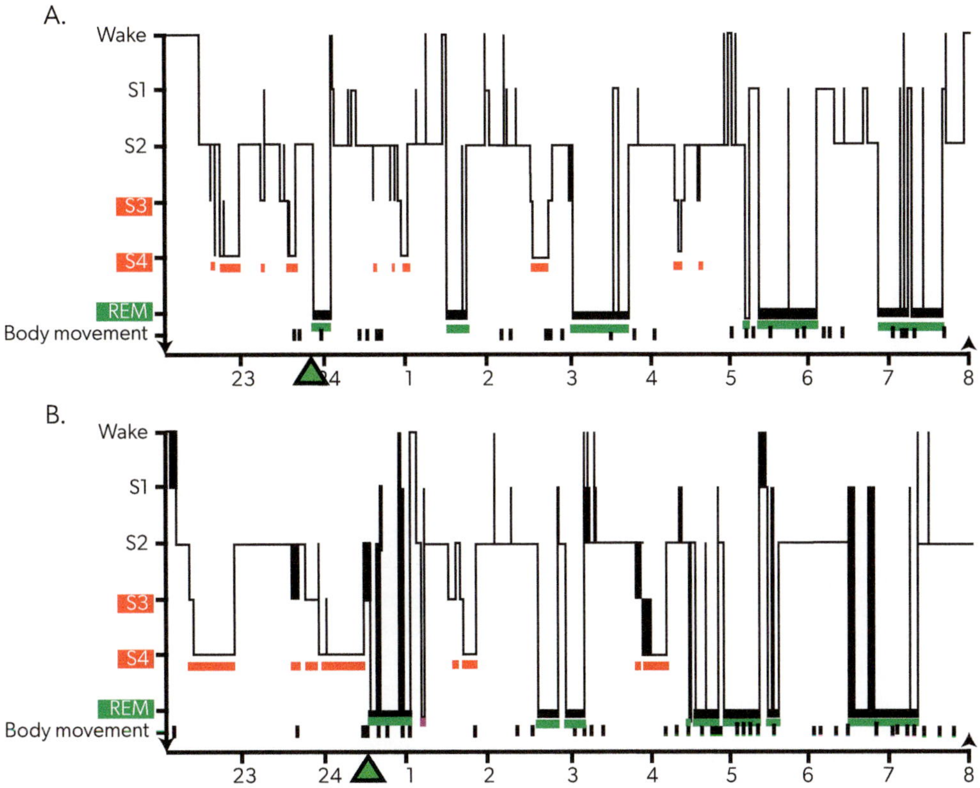

Figure 5.2 Hypnograms illustrating the sleep stages expressed during a baseline night of sleep (**A**) and during a night following overnight sleep deprivation (**B**) in a 14-year-old girl. The X axes show clock time, with time in bed indicated by a small black arrowhead pointing down at 22:00 h and an upward-pointing arrowhead at wake-up time (08:00). Episodes of N3 or slow-wave sleep (Stages 3 & 4 combined) are underlined in red and REM sleep in green. The baseline night (**A**) shows the typical pattern in a young person, with N3 sleep concentrated early in the night and REM sleep late in the night. There was a first brief REM sleep period starting about 1.5 h after sleep onset (green triangle). During the recovery night after 38 h of waking, (**B**) sleep onset was much faster, there was more sustained N3 sleep early in the night, and there were increased amounts over the first 6 h of sleep. The first REM sleep episode during recovery sleep was delayed relative to the baseline night and occurred about 2.25 h after sleep onset (green triangle). The homeostatic drive to generate N3 sleep after deprivation resulted in a large increase as soon as sleep was allowed, which appeared to delay onset of the first REM sleep episode. Black marks below the records indicate body movements. Adapted with permission of Elsevier, Ltd. from Carskadon, M. A. & Dement, W. C. (1989) Normal human sleep: an overview. In: M. H. Kryger, et al. (Eds.), *Principles and Practice of Sleep Medicine* (1st edition, pp. 3–13). Philadelphia. © Elsevier Ltd. (1989).

course of a night's sleep as they generate SWA and satisfy their sleep need (**Figures 5.3 A**). If a person also stays awake overnight, sleep need is increased further and SWA is even higher when they are allowed to fall asleep the next morning (**Figure 5.3 B**). The amount of SWA shown is strongly determined by the length of prior waking and, during a sleep episode, by the amount of preceding sleep that included SWA. But there is only minor modulation of SWA by the circadian system, as demonstrated in studies of people using the forced desynchronization method (Dijk, 2009; Dijk & Czeisler, 1995) (**Figure 5.4**).

Other evidence strongly supports the idea that the amount of SWA produced during sleep reflects a homeostatic response to accumulated time spent awake. When people took naps at different times during the day, the amount of SWA was higher during naps taken late in the day (after a longer time awake) than during naps taken early in the day, consistent with the idea that the length of prior waking determined the accumulated sleep need (Endo et al., 1981); see Section 2.5.1, **Figure 2.10**.

Even more striking evidence of homeostatic regulation was the finding that the amount of SWA (and of SWS) produced during a daytime nap reduced the amount shown during the next night's sleep. Paying down part of an accumulated SWS/SWA debt during a daytime nap reduced the amount still "owed" and therefore the amount produced during sleep at night (Borbély et al., 1981; Feinberg et al., 1992; Werth et al., 1996) (**Figure 5.5**). Afternoon naps that included N3 sleep strongly reduced SWS the next night, even

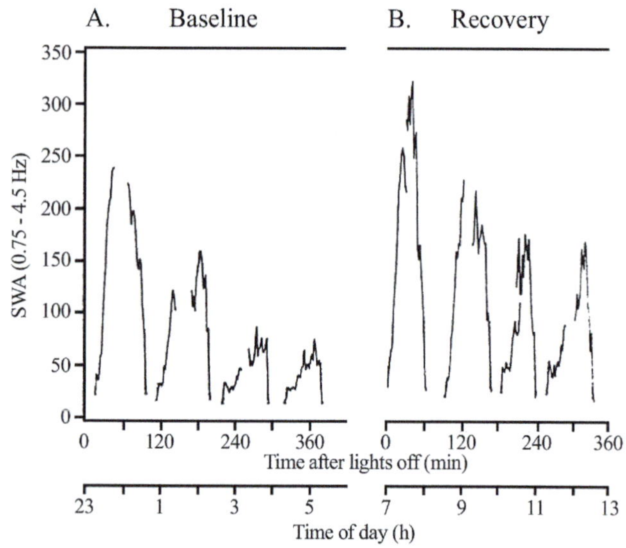

Figure 5.3 Analysis of the effects of sleep deprivation on slow-wave activity (SWA) during morning recovery sleep, plotted as percentage amounts relative to the average SWA in NREM sleep during the baseline night (= 100%, Y axis). **A.** The rise and fall of SWA associated with each bout of NREM sleep during a baseline night of EEG recording. **B.** SWA during a recovery sleep opportunity the morning after total overnight sleep deprivation. There are similar patterns of declining SWA levels across the sleep periods in both panels, reflecting the operation of homeostatic mechanisms within a sleep period. Producing SWA early in the sleep period reduced the drive to express SWA (i.e., sleep debt was partially paid off). The overall higher level of SWA throughout all episodes during recovery sleep in **B**, however, also demonstrates that the drive to express SWA increased after overnight sleep deprivation. Homeostatic regulation of SWA operates both within a sleep period, as well as over longer time periods. Reprinted with permission of Elsevier, Ltd. from Dijk, D. -J. et al. (1991) EEG power density during recovery sleep in the morning. *Electroencephalogr Clin Neurophysiol* 78(3):203–214. © Elsevier (1991). doi: 10.1016/0013-4694(91)90034-2.

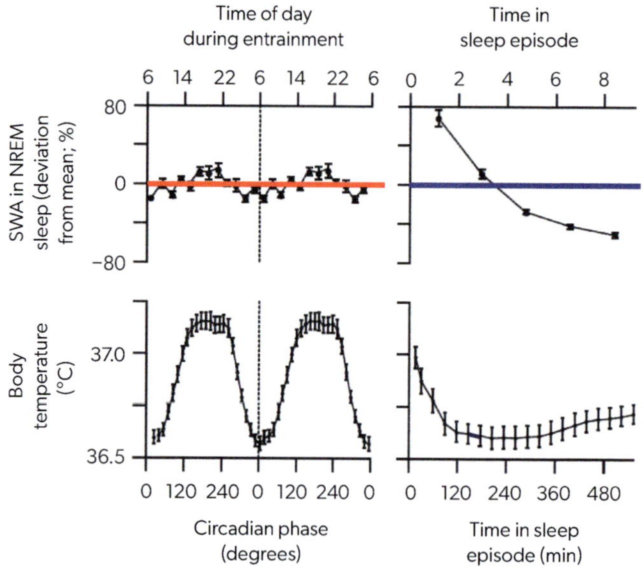

Figure 5.4 **Left Panel:** Derived waveform of the circadian variation in slow-wave activity (SWA) (0.75–4.5 Hz) during NREM sleep (Y axis in upper graph) and circadian variation in core body temperature in degrees Celsius (lower graph) from people in a forced-desynchronization protocol living in temporal isolation. SWA values are plotted against circadian phase (lower X axis) and against the equivalent time of day when entrained normally to a 24 h day (upper X axis). The Y axis shows SWA % deviations from the daily mean amount of SWA activity, indicated by the horizontal red line. Body temperature is plotted with the low point of body temperature set at circadian phase 0. Values are double-plotted across 48 circadian hours. Body temperature shows a clear circadian variation, and SWS shows only a minor circadian modulation, with a small increase in the mid-afternoon and early evening. **Right Panel**: The upper graph shows the average SWA in NREM sleep plotted against time since the start of a sleep episode, shown in hours (upper X axis). SWA is plotted as the % deviation from the daily mean (blue line). Amounts of SWA declined steeply as a function of time during a sleep period (as in **Figure 5.3**), indicating strong homeostatic regulation of SWA amounts during sleep episodes. The lower graph shows average body temperature plotted in degrees Celsius against time during sleep (lower X axis). Body temperature follows a different pattern from SWA. It first falls steeply at the beginning of the sleep period and then rises gradually later during sleep, under circadian clock control. Adapted with permission from Dijk, D.-J. & Czeisler, C. A. (1995) Contribution of the circadian pacemaker and the sleep homeostat to sleep propensity, sleep structure, electroencephalographic slow waves, and sleep spindle activity in humans. *J Neurosci* 15:3526–3538. © Society for Neuroscience (1995). doi: 10.1523/JNEUROSCI.15-05-03526.1995.

though total sleep length was only slightly reduced (Campbell et al., 2005). As a result, the total amount of SWS during a 24 h period was homeostatically defended. Thus, the amount of SWS or SWA produced reflects how much sleep drive has accumulated as a result of being awake, minus how much of the drive has already been satisfied by producing SWS/SWA during earlier naps.

In studies in which people were encouraged to sleep for very long durations, some participants showed small increases in SWA or SWS late in the lengthy (~15 h) sleep phase (Christ et al., 1996; Dijk, Cajochen, et al., 1991). Despite scattered, brief wake episodes late in their sleep periods, it is unlikely these were long enough to increase homeostatic sleep need. It is more likely that the small increase in SWA was a response to circadian influences. With sleep onset around midnight, the increases occurred near the afternoon "post-lunch dip" or siesta time in some cultures (see Section 4.3; **Figures 2.11** and **8.11 C**). The timing of these small increases is consistent with evidence for a weak circadian influence that decreases wakefulness and promotes expression of sleep and SWA in the afternoon (Dijk, 2009), as illustrated in **Figure 5.4**.

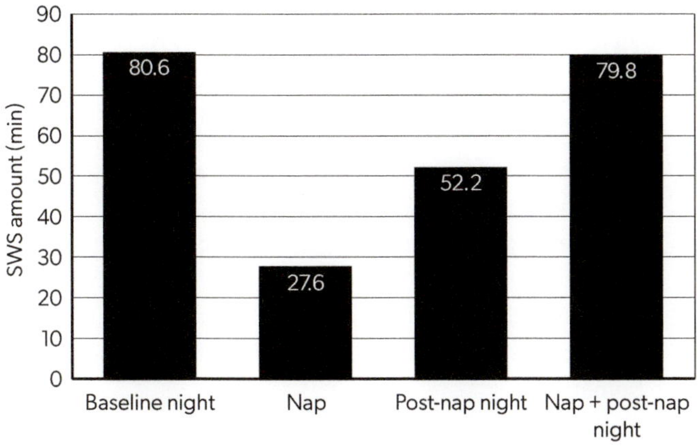

Figure 5.5 Duration of slow wave sleep (SWS) in men during a baseline night of sleep (1st column), during a nap on the following day (2nd column; starting at 18:00 h; ~2 h sleep opportunity), and during the following night after the nap (3rd column). The 4th column on the right is the total of the amounts of SWS shown during the nap and during the following night's sleep, which is essentially equal to the amount shown during the baseline night. When a person naps, the amount of SWS produced is effectively "subtracted" from the total amount required (i.e., baseline night amount), so only the difference between the amount shown during the baseline night and the amount produced during a nap is produced during the next night. Source: data from Werth, E. et al. (1996) Dynamics of the sleep EEG after an early evening nap: experimental data and simulations. *Am J Physiol* 271:R501–R510. © American Physiological Society (1996). doi: 10.1152/ajpregu.1996.271.3.R501.

5.3.3 Process S and Process C

Despite this minor influence of circadian phase, the principal regulator of the amount of SWA in people is homeostasis.[3] As deprivation of SWA lengthens during waking, the pressure to express it increases; generating SWA reduces that pressure. This process of accumulating and satisfying the need for SWA has been called Process S (Borbély, 1982b). This concept emerged out of studies of recovery from sleep deprivation conducted in relation to circadian regulation of sleep (referred to as Process C), initially in rats and later in people.

A key observation in the early rat studies was that when they were sleep deprived and then allowed to sleep during the daily light phase (when they would normally show their main sleep episodes), rats showed minimal changes in total sleep amounts, but large increases in SWA (Borbély, 2022; Borbély & Neuhaus, 1979). However, when deprivation ended at the start of the daily dark (active) phase, rats showed a biphasic change in sleep, with only a small increase in SWA early in the dark phase and a later large increase during the following light phase. The competing drive to be awake and active early in the dark phase (reflecting the influence of Process C) reduced the amount of SWA produced, but the pressure to produce SWA was expressed later as a result of increased homeostatic pressure (Process S). These observations led to the development of a model of sleep regulation in which the homeostatic sleep regulator (Process S) interacted with the circadian regulator of sleep (Process C), to control the expression of sleep, its timing, and its composition.

In models of SWA regulation, the level of Process S at any time point reflects the degree of physiological need for sleep. That has a dual meaning: The level of Process S corresponds to the current degree of sleepiness (the strength of the drive to fall asleep), and it also predicts the amount of SWA that will be generated when sleep occurs. The timing of sleep, however, is a function of the circadian influence represented by Process C. Mathematical models of sleep regulation have been developed that use the observed dynamics of increases and decreases in Process S and its interaction with Process C to successfully model and predict patterns of sleep in both people and animals under a variety of experimental conditions (Borbély, 2022; Borbély et al., 2016; Daan et al., 1984; Franken et al., 1991). This model is discussed in more detail in Section 5.7.

5.3.4 The target(s) of regulation

In the standard model, process S represents the accumulation during waking of something in the brain (sometimes facetiously called "sleep stuff") that is reversed by periods of sleep that include SWA. It is easiest to think of "sleep stuff" as an actual chemical product of wakefulness that accumulates in brain tissue and needs to be metabolized or otherwise eliminated by sleeping. There is at least one possible neurochemical candidate for this role (adenosine) that is discussed in Section 11.6. But it could also represent a process rather than a chemical (e.g., gradual changes in synaptic function, cellular metabolism, or other neural mechanisms that occur during waking and are reversed during sleep).

It is clear that sleep is homeostatically regulated, and there is especially robust homeostatic regulation of SWA. However, this evidence does not prove that generating SWA is itself an essential component of the underlying restorative process—the target of sleep. Some have raised questions about whether the available evidence requires the existence of a sleep "homeostat" (Frank, 2021). Others have questioned which features of SWA and its time course after sleep loss reflect homeostatic responses, and how these are dynamically regulated (Hubbard et al., 2020). Without knowing precisely which wake- and sleep-related changes are

[3] There may be species differences in the relative roles of homeostatic and circadian mechanisms. In a study of squirrel monkeys (*Saimiri sciurus*), there were only modest homeostatic increases in sleep duration and in delta power after sleep loss; but, unlike in people, these measures were strongly affected by circadian phase (Klerman et al., 1999).

being regulated during SWA, it is uncertain whether the production of slow, high-amplitude EEG rhythms is part of the brain's recovery process, or whether it is only a (normally) reliable physiological correlate of an unidentified process. There is evidence supporting the second idea.

Benzodiazepines and related drugs that act on brain $GABA_A$ receptors suppress both delta- and theta-band activity and reduce SWS but are still able to promote restorative sleep acutely in patients with insomnia.[4] It is not known why sleep with pharmacologically reduced SWS can still be restorative, but it may be related to the expression of increased amounts of N2 sleep or of lower-amplitude, slow EEG rhythms that do not meet the criteria defining SWS (Borbély et al., 1991; Brunner et al., 1991; Feinberg et al., 1977).

There are a variety of cellular changes that have been documented during sleep loss which could be the targets of repair mechanisms that operate during SWA. For example, changes in the structure and function of mitochondria and the Golgi apparatus, and in the activity of enzymes regulating DNA functions, have been documented after sleep loss in mice and fruit flies (Wang & Aton, 2022). There is also evidence that DNA damage accumulates during waking (Zada et al., 2021).

Sleep loss has also been shown to increase levels of amyloid beta (Aβ) in the brains of mice and people (Kang et al., 2009; Ooms et al., 2014; Xie et al., 2013), which is linked to increased risk of developing neurodegenerative conditions such as Alzheimer's disease (AD). SWA reduces levels of Aβ in the cerebrospinal fluid (Ju et al., 2017; Varga et al., 2016), which may reduce the risk of neurodegenerative changes. These findings suggest that SWA helps clear potentially toxic substances from the brain (see Section 15.5 for more details). Another potential role for SWA is repairing damage to neuronal connectivity. An extreme example of a condition that may induce such damage is maintaining the brain at low temperatures; see **Box 5.2**.

At a molecular level, sleep and waking have been linked to changes in ion concentrations in the brain, which may also be the targets of homeostatic processes, or part of the mechanisms implementing homeostasis. Levels of extracellular potassium ions (K^+) in the cortex of mice rise during waking and fall during sleep, while levels of calcium (Ca^{2+}) and magnesium (Mg^{2+}) ions do the opposite. Infusing artificial cerebrospinal fluid that mimicked an extracellular "wake-type" ion profile locally onto the cortex resulted in a decrease in local 1–4 Hz

---

[4] The immediate benefits, however, often wane over time, as tolerance can develop. In addition, with chronic use, there are risks of daytime sleepiness, cognitive and motor impairment, drug misuse, rebound insomnia after discontinuation, and the development of physiological and/or psychological dependence (Brandt & Leong, 2017; Schifano et al., 2019). As a result, benzodiazepines and related drugs are usually recommended only for short courses of treatment for acute insomnia symptoms. See **Box 11.3** in Section 11.3.4 for more discussion of insomnia treatments and benzodiazepines.

BOX 5.2 SWA Homeostasis in Hibernation?

The operation of sleep homeostasis was proposed to explain a surprising fact about hibernation: When some rodents emerge from hibernation, the first thing they do is sleep. A possible homeostatic explanation for this priority is that the lack of sleep during weeks of hibernation was compensated by sleeping immediately when they came out of hibernation.

Small mammals that hibernate in winter retreat to an insulated shelter and drop their body and brain temperatures profoundly, so that these approach environmental temperatures. During these periods of sometimes extreme hypothermia, brain activity is minimal, with the cortex profoundly silent and only a few brain structures (including the suprachiasmatic nuclei; see Chapter 8) continuing to show low levels of metabolic activity (Kilduff et al., 1982). These metabolic reductions are critical to saving energy because brain activity is responsible for large proportions of the body's total energy usage. To cite what is probably an extreme mammalian example, the activity of the human brain accounts for 20–25% of the body's total energy usage at rest (Herculano-Houzel, 2012).

Arctic ground squirrels (*Spermophilus perryii*) are classic winter hibernators, dropping their body and brain temperatures to near 0° C for days or weeks at a time. After each period of hypothermia, they expend a great deal of energy to warm themselves back to euthermic temperatures (i.e., high body temperatures normally shown in the active season). After some hours of euthermia, they again cool down and reenter hibernation for days or weeks (Daan et al., 1991; Strijkstra & Daan, 1998). The process of repeatedly rewarming and then maintaining euthermic temperatures for several hours can consume 70–90% of the stored energy that the animals use during the entire, several months-long hibernation period (Thomas et al., 1990; Wang, 1979).

During the hours of euthermia, squirrels typically sleep, generating a long bout of SWA immediately after becoming euthermic. The amount of SWA is positively correlated with the length of the preceding period of hypothermia. Although this looks like a homeostatic response to the lack of sleep during hypothermia, that turns out not to be a likely interpretation. When squirrels are prevented from sleeping early in their euthermic period, a homeostatic explanation would predict that they would then show an even larger increase in SWA since the duration without sleep would have been further extended. In contrast to that prediction, when sleep was allowed only late in the euthermic period, squirrels produced only low amounts of SWA, similar to what they would normally

BOX 5.2 Continued

produce at that phase of their rewarming cycle (Larkin & Heller, 1999; Strijkstra & Daan, 1998).

An alternative explanation is that long periods without neural activity during hypothermia cause a gradual withdrawal and reduction of neuronal synapses and dendrites (Popov & Bocharova, 1992). Euthermia occurs periodically to permit neural activity that rapidly restores synaptic connections that have been weakened (Larkin & Heller, 1999; Strijkstra & Daan, 1998). Generating SWA may be the preferred and most efficient way to engage in this form of neuronal repair, but the process can apparently also occur at euthermic temperatures while awake. This conclusion echoes the early intuition that some of the restorative benefits of sleep can also be achieved in weaker form during quiet waking (Patrick & Gilbert, 1896).

Unlike in ground squirrels, another species, the Djungarian hamster (*Phodopus sungorus*), shows periods of reduced brain/body temperature each day under some conditions (daily torpor). After a period of torpor, these hamsters showed immediate increases in SWA, which were augmented if they were also sleep deprived after arousal from torpor, consistent with a robust homeostatic response to sleep loss during torpor. However, daily torpor bouts in this species last only a few hours, and brain temperature is generally maintained at >20° C (Deboer & Tobler, 2000). These short hypothermic bouts at elevated temperatures are unlikely to result in the presumed loss of neuronal connectivity that occurs during hibernation by ground squirrels over days or weeks at near 0° C brain temperatures.

activity, while infusing a "sleep-type" ion profile increased 1–4 Hz activity. These results indicate that different patterns of extracellular ion concentrations are not only correlates of local EEG patterns, but can actually regulate the appearance of SWA (Ding et al., 2016).

Consistent with this conclusion is the finding that Ca^{2+} entry into neurons via NMDA glutamate receptors and voltage-sensitive Ca^{2+} channels increased delta-wave activity. Genetic deletion of these Ca^{2+} channels, or of a kinase closely linked to their function, decreased spontaneous sleep durations in mice and prevented increases in NREM and total sleep amounts after 8 h of sleep deprivation (Tatsuki et al., 2016; Wang et al., 2022). These results implicate regulation of Ca^{2+} flux across cell membranes in homeostatic responses to sleep loss.

Other findings linked sleep pressure to differences in chloride ion (Cl^-) flux through $GABA_A$ receptors that occur during waking and sleep. Sleep pressure led to more depolarization of the equilibrium potential for Cl^-, which increased synchrony among cortical neurons' On/Off rhythms. This increased synchrony resulted in increased signs of local sleep in the affected cortical region (Alfonsa et al., 2023).

There are, therefore, a wide variety of mechanisms operating at the levels of molecules, organelles, cells, and systems that function differently during waking and sleep. Processes linked to ion flux across cell membranes have been shown to promote generation of SWA in the cortex and to be involved in homeostatic responses. It remains to be determined which of these mechanisms are essential elements of the build-up of sleep need and of recovery from this need during SWA.

5.3.5 Summary

Acute sleep deprivation results in increases in the amount of sleep shown when sleep is again permitted, but there is not usually a 1:1 replacement of lost hours of sleep. This finding can be understood by recognizing that sleep duration is not itself the target of homeostatic regulation but is a mechanism that permits that regulation. The target is instead one or more changes in brain function that occur during waking and must be reversed; sleep is the mechanism that permits reversal of these changes.

One potential indication of what is being regulated is the finding that the depth of sleep, as indexed by the amount of either N3 sleep or SWA (during all sleep stages), increases preferentially during recovery sleep after deprivation. SWA increases more than sleep duration and comes close to making up for lost SWA. This observation suggests the possibility that the generation of slow EEG waves is the actual target of homeostatic regulation during sleep. Evidence that drugs such as benzodiazepines permit recuperative sleep, even though they suppress slow waves, indicates that this is probably not the case.

Instead, the amount of SWA appears to be a reliable marker of sleep homeostasis and to be closer than sleep duration to the regulated target process. This conclusion is strengthened by evidence that the total amount of SWA/SWS is preserved across a 24 h period. Thus, the amount of SWA/SWS generated during daytime naps is subtracted from the amount usually shown during sleep at night. Similarly, the amount of SWA/SWS decreases gradually over the course of the night, as the need to recover from waking is decreased by early-night SWA/SWS.

The process of gradually building up a need for SWA during waking and satisfying it during sleep has been summarized as the rise and fall of Process S. Modeling the dynamic changes in this hypothetical process produces robust predictions of how people and other mammals sleep. Despite the strength of these predictions, the identity and nature of the physiological process being indexed by SWA is uncertain, and there are questions as to which aspects of SWA are most closely related to the underlying recovery process.

Several molecular and cellular correlates of waking and of sleep have been identified in the brain. These include wake-related changes in DNA and mitochondria and patterns of transmembrane flux of several ions that affect neuronal activity. Mimicking extracellular ion patterns that are characteristic of sleep in local cortical regions can produce EEG patterns characteristic of SWS, suggesting that these changes are involved in increasing sleep after periods of waking. Other ion flux changes appear to be necessary in order to show typical homeostatic responses to short-term sleep loss. It remains to be determined which of these changes are essential to the build-up of sleep need and to the subsequent recovery process that together represent the essential elements of the hypothetical process S.

5.4 Alternatives to homeostatic regulation

5.4.1 Allostasis & chronic sleep loss

Most of the quantitative data used to model homeostatic regulation of SWA came from studies involving acute sleep deprivation in people and animals and from studies showing relatively precise homeostatic regulation of SWS amounts within a 24 h period (see **Figure 5.5**). Incomplete compensation for lost sleep after more extended sleep deprivation suggests that there are differences between the mechanisms that respond to brief and more extreme sleep loss. Animals may have evolved homeostatic mechanisms to respond to short-term sleep losses resulting from acute environmental stressors by immediate compensatory increases in sleep amounts and/or quality. But these mechanisms may not be adequate to respond to the experience of severe, longer-term deprivation.

In a few species, sustained reductions in sleep are part of a normal life program (e.g., related to seasonal breeding or migration; see Chapter 7) (Siegel, 2022), accompanied by other physiological adaptations. For most species, however, sustained reductions in sleep amounts over periods of days or weeks are probably rare outside of laboratory situations. These episodes of chronic sleep loss may not be addressed by the typical homeostatic responses seen in response to acute sleep loss and may evoke a different set of physiological adaptations.

Incomplete homeostasis in response to extreme physiological challenges has been linked to a process called allostasis. This concept refers to a pattern of regulatory changes in response to stressful, persistent physiological challenges that cannot be addressed by the usual homeostatic mechanisms. Allostasis has been interpreted as either an alternative way to preserve homeostasis or as a set of physiological adjustments that follow the failure of homeostasis (McEwen & Stellar, 1993; Skorucak et al., 2018; Sterling, 2012). The usefulness of the concept of allostasis has also been questioned (Day, 2005).

Allostatic adjustments are hypothesized to involve altered activity of the body's principal stress-response mechanisms (the hypothalamic-pituitary-adrenal (HPA) axis), other neural mechanisms, and the immune system. These adjustments may allow animals to better defend homeostatic set points or to shift defended set points temporarily to different values. While this may sound like a convenient way of circumventing homeostatic regulation of sleep/SWA or other fundamental needs, there is a cost involved in allostasis. Chronic allostatic adjustments are proposed to cause damage to physiological systems (referred to as allostatic load), which accumulates over time and increases the risk of developing a variety of stress-related diseases (McEwen, 2006).

Studies of chronic, partial sleep deprivation in rodents have produced varied results some of which indicated incomplete—and others complete—homeostatic responses. In some studies of chronic sleep loss, rats or mice were restricted over 3–5 consecutive days to 4–6 h sleep opportunities daily (versus their usual durations of 10–12 h or more). Daily sleep opportunities were either consolidated as a single block or spaced across the day as 1 h periods every 4 h, with the remaining time spent engaged in slow, forced walking to prevent sleep. Rats showed initial homeostatic increases in NREM sleep and/or SWA, but these increases were lost over days as restriction continued. As a result, only partial compensation had occurred by the end of the deprivation period (Deurveilher et al., 2012; Kim et al., 2012; Kim et al., 2007). Immediately after sleep restriction ended, rats showed large rebound increases in REM sleep, but rebound increases in NREM sleep and SWA either did not occur or were delayed until hours later (**Figure 5.6**). Overall, the rebound compensation that occurred did not make up for much of the lost NREM sleep or SWA, consistent with the idea of allostatic responses to chronic sleep loss.

Earlier studies used a disk-over-water (DOW) method to deprive rats of sleep (**Figure 5.7**). Two rats were housed separately with free access to food and water on a divided disk over a shallow pool of water; the disk was motorized and could be activated by a computer. When the computer detected sleep onset in the experimental rat's EEG (but not the control rat's EEG), the disk began to rotate so that both the experimental and control rats had to walk against the direction of rotation to avoid contacting the water.

After 4 days of continuous sleep deprivation for the experimental rats, there were large increases in REM sleep amounts as soon as recovery sleep was allowed, along with delayed and very modest increases in NREM sleep and even decreases in the rodent equivalent of N3 sleep (Rechtschaffen et al., 1999) (**Figure 5.8**). Sustained sleep loss in rats over even longer periods caused pathological changes that were life-threatening,

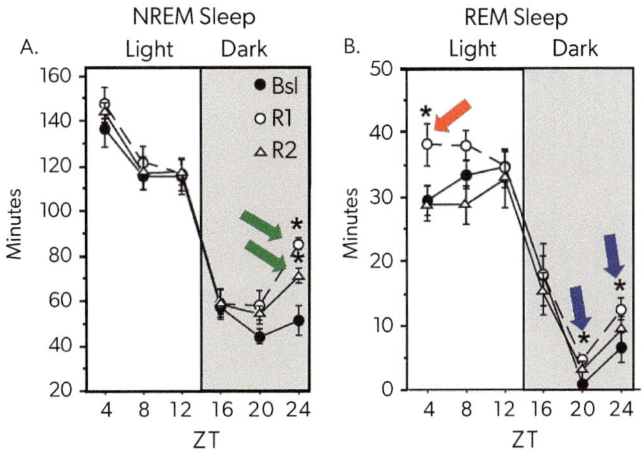

Figure 5.6 Rats were sleep-deprived for 3 h periods by walking on a motorized wheel, followed by 1 h sleep opportunities (3:1 protocol), continuously over 4 days. Daily patterns of NREM sleep (**A**) and REM sleep (**B**) amounts are shown for the baseline day before sleep restriction (Bsl, black circles), the first recovery day with free sleep after 4 days of the 3:1 sleep restriction protocol (R1, white circles), and during the second recovery day (R2, white triangles). Data are plotted against time of day (ZT: zeitgeber time). The white and gray regions represent the daily light and dark phases. NREM sleep showed no significant increase relative to baseline until the end of the first dark phase on R1 and showed a smaller significant increase on R2 (green arrows and * in **A**). **B.** However, there was an immediate, significant increase (*) in REM sleep at the beginning of the light phase on the first recovery day (red arrow) as soon as sleep restriction ended. REM sleep also showed a significant increase relative to baseline on R1 at two times during the dark phase (blue arrows and *). These results are consistent with chronically sleep-deprived rats showing a high priority for REM sleep during recovery sleep. They also indicate that some recovery of NREM sleep occurred, but it was delayed and strongly modulated by the light-dark cycle and/or by circadian phase. Adapted with permission of the American Physiological Society from Deurveilher, S. et al. (2012). Time-of-day modulation of homeostatic and allostatic sleep responses to chronic sleep restriction in rats. *Am J Physiol* 302:1411–1425. © American Physiological Society (2012). doi: 10.1152/ajpregu.00678.2011.

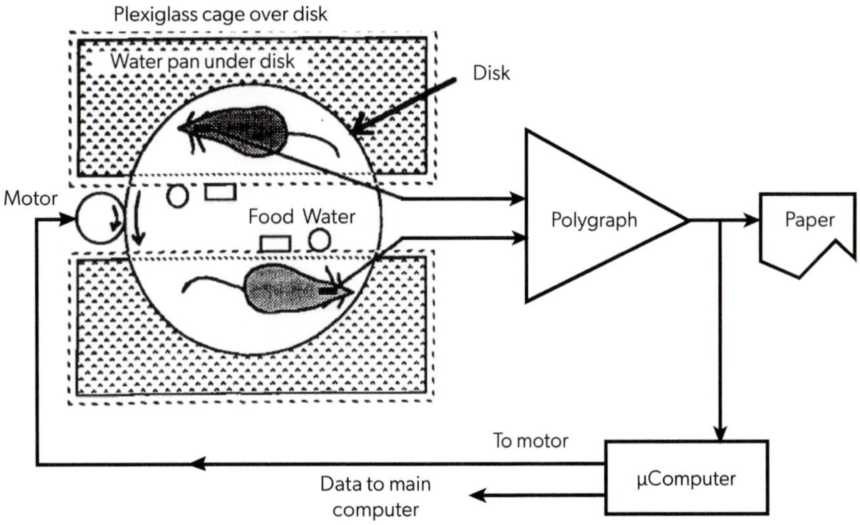

Figure 5.7 Disk-over-water (DOW) apparatus used to induce chronic sleep deprivation in rats over many days or weeks. Two rats were housed on the disk in separate compartments with free access to food and water; both were instrumented to record EEG. When the EEG indicated signs of sleep onset in the Experimental rat, a microcomputer recognized the pattern and turned on a motor to initiate rotation of a wheel, which in turn caused the disk to start rotating. If the rats did not start walking, they reached the edge of the disk and would contact the water in the pan under the disk. Thus, both rats had to walk whenever the Experimental rat started to show EEG signs of sleep to avoid contact with the water. Sleep onset in the Control rat, however, did not trigger rotation of the disk, so it was free to sleep at will, as long as the Experimental rat was awake (which was almost always). Control rats suffered a minor amount of sleep loss, but Experimental rats underwent severe sleep deprivation over the days of the experiment. Reprinted with permission of Oxford University Press and the Sleep Research Society from Bergmann, B. M. et al. (1989) Sleep deprivation in the rat: II. Methodology. *Sleep* 12(1): 5–12. © Sleep Research Society (1989). doi: 10.1093/sleep/12.1.5.

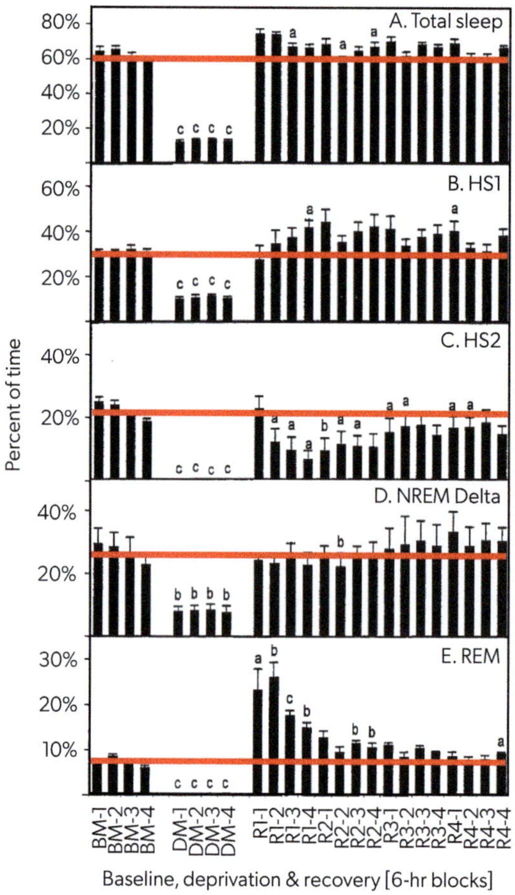

Figure 5.8 Responses of rats to four days of chronic sleep deprivation using the DOW method. Data are presented for four baseline days (BM-1 to BM-4) and four sleep deprivation days (DM-1 to DM-4). Data on each of 4 recovery days are presented in four 6 h segments during each day (R1-(1–4), R2-(1–4), etc.). Horizontal red lines are estimates of the mean values for each measure over the four baseline days to facilitate visualizing the changes from baseline during the recovery days. There was a very substantial decrease in the total percentage of the day spent asleep during deprivation days and a small rebound increase in total sleep time early in the recovery period (**A**). There was an immediate large increase in REM sleep at the start of R1, with increased amounts during part of the first 2 recovery days (**E**). There was a "negative rebound" (decrease) in HS2 sleep (**C**) (NREM sleep equivalent to N3 in people) and modest increases in HS1 (= N2 sleep) (**B**). Note that during sleep deprivation days, rats still expressed some lighter NREM sleep (HS1) and generated some NREM delta-band activity (**D**), but HS2 and REM sleep were essentially eliminated. Letters above the columns indicate statistically significant differences from baseline days: a = $p<0.05$, b = $p<0.01$, c = $p<0.001$. Adapted with permission of Oxford University Press and the Sleep Research Society from Rechtschaffen, A. et al. (1999) Effects of method, duration, and sleep stage on rebounds from sleep deprivation in the rat. *Sleep* 22:11–31. © Sleep Research Society (1999). doi: 10.1093/sleep/22.1.11.

which is consistent with the idea that extreme sleep loss imposes critical physiological costs (allostatic load); these findings are discussed in Chapter 14.

In contrast to the results in **Figure 5.6**, another study of long-term, partial sleep restriction in rats found robust preservation of SWA homeostasis, including complete recovery during two recovery days of the amount of slow-wave energy (SWA accumulated over time) lost during the restriction days in most cortical regions (Leemburg et al., 2010). This study differed in several ways from those discussed above: the strain of rats used, more complete scoring of sleep, recording from more cortical sites, and different methods of sleep restriction. Instead of continuous locomotion during deprivation periods, this study used the disk-over-water (DOW) method supplemented by continuous visual observation and interventions to distract rats and keep them awake as needed.

A study in mice, however, provided another line of evidence supporting the idea that chronic sleep loss changes homeostatic mechanisms and triggers allostatic adjustments (Clasadonte et al., 2014). Mice were sleep restricted over three days using continuous cycles of 4 h sleep deprivation (by forced walking on a treadmill) followed by 2 h sleep opportunities. At first, there were large increases in SWA during NREM sleep in the 2 h opportunities, but these decreased over the days of sleep restriction, despite accumulating sleep debt. Although there were also small increases in SWA (and theta-band activity) during the periods of forced waking, the total amount of SWA summed across wake and sleep episodes was chronically reduced over the days of sleep restriction and was still significantly decreased after a single recovery day (**Figure 5.9**). Without additional recovery days, it is not known whether there might have been more compensatory increases on later days.

In addition to finding incomplete homeostasis of SWA during chronic sleep loss in mice, this study also provided evidence for a mechanism that may be a component of allostatic responses. After two weeks of recovery from chronic sleep restriction, these mice (and controls with no previous sleep restriction) were acutely sleep-deprived for a single 6 h period using gentle handling (see Section 14.2 for a description of different sleep deprivation methods). After this acute sleep loss, mice that had previously experienced chronic restriction showed smaller rebound increases in NREM sleep amounts and in SWA during NREM sleep than naive control mice, and less increase in levels of the sleep-promoting neurochemical adenosine in one brain region (Clasadonte et al., 2014) (**Figure 5.10** (see Section 11.6 for a discussion of the role of adenosine).

These findings indicate that early homeostatic responses to sleep restriction in mice became inadequate as sleep loss

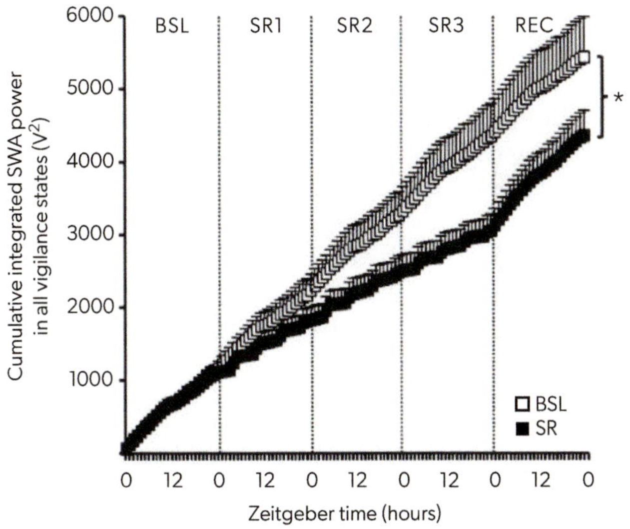

Figure 5.9 Integrated slow-wave activity (SWA) power across all vigilance states summed over 24 h periods in mice undergoing chronic sleep restriction. The white symbols (+ standard error of the mean) show the rate of accumulation of SWA on the baseline day (BSL), and these values are extrapolated across 3 days of sleep restriction (SR1-3) and the single recovery day (REC) (upper curve). During sleep restriction, mice were allowed 2 h sleep out of every 6 h for a total of 8 h of sleep daily. The rate of accumulation of SWA power across restriction and recovery days is shown by the black symbols (lower curve). SWA power was reduced on all restriction days and remained significantly decreased relative to predicted levels after the recovery day (*). * = p<.05. Reprinted with permission under a Creative Commons license (CC-BY-NC-SA) from Clasadonte, J. et al. (2014) Chronic sleep restriction disrupts sleep homeostasis and behavioral sensitivity to alcohol by reducing the extracellular accumulation of adenosine. *J Neurosci* 34:1879–1891. © The Authors (2014). doi: 10.1523/JNEUROSCI.2870-12.2014.

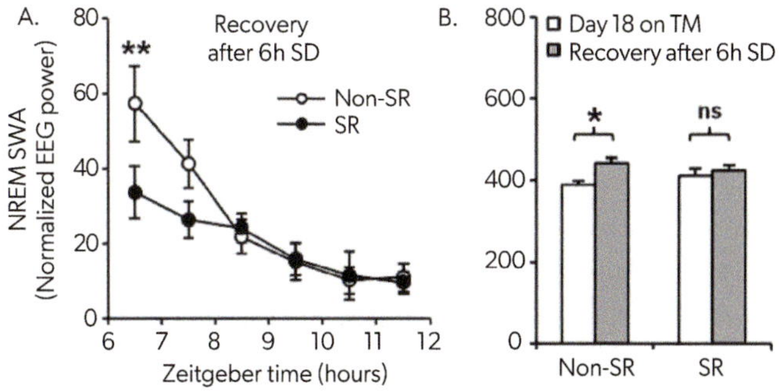

Figure 5.10 **A.** Power in the slow-wave activity (SWA) band during NREM sleep in mice after 6 h of sleep deprivation (Zeitgeber Time 0–6). Mice that had undergone three days of chronic sleep restriction (SR, filled symbols) two weeks earlier (see **Figure 5.9**) showed less rebound increase in SWA after acute sleep loss, compared to control mice that had not undergone sleep restriction (Non-SR, open symbols), which showed a robust homeostatic increase in SWA during the recovery period (Zeitgeber time 6–12). **B.** During 18 h on a recovery day after 6 h of sleep deprivation (gray column), control mice (Non-SR) showed a significant increase in NREM sleep duration compared to the same 18 h period during a baseline day before sleep deprivation (white column). Mice that had undergone three days of chronic sleep restriction 2 weeks earlier (SR) failed to show a homeostatic increase in NREM sleep duration after acute sleep deprivation. These altered homeostatic responses to acute sleep loss suggest that previous chronic sleep restriction triggered allostatic adjustments that altered later homeostatic responses to acute sleep loss. Reprinted with permission under a Creative Commons license (CC-BY-NC-SA) from Clasadonte, J. et al. (2014) Chronic sleep restriction disrupts sleep homeostasis and behavioral sensitivity to alcohol by reducing the extracellular accumulation of adenosine. *J Neurosci* 34:1879–1891.© The Authors (2014). doi: 10.1523/JNEUROSCI.2870-12.2014.

became chronic. In response, allostatic adjustments were triggered, including altered regulation of a critical sleep-promoting neurochemical, adenosine. This interpretation is supported by the observation that chronic sleep loss in rats altered expression of receptors for both adenosine and the wake-promoting neurotransmitter noradrenaline in several brain regions (Kim et al., 2012; Kim et al., 2015).

Studies aimed at similar issues have been conducted in rats. One study did not find that prior chronic sleep restriction for 4 days altered their homeostatic responses to acute sleep loss ~3 days later. This timing differed from the mouse study which assessed acute responses 2 weeks after the end of chronic sleep restriction. However, during a period of free sleep after chronic restriction and before the acute deprivation test, rats showed a decrease in their 24 h NREM delta power relative to their baseline values (Deurveilher et al., 2021). These results suggest that their typical, within-day (basal) homeostatic regulation of delta power had been altered by the experience of chronic sleep restriction, despite the lack of effect on responses to acute deprivation 3 days later.

Another study found that rats that were chronically sleep restricted for 5 days showed reduced levels of SWA during a free-sleep period after restriction ended (Guzeev et al., 2023), which resembled the reductions in NREM delta power during free sleep after chronic sleep loss in the rat studies discussed above (Deurveilher et al., 2012; Deurveilher et al., 2021). After a subsequent acute sleep loss, rats that had experienced chronic restriction showed rebound increases in SWA, but these levels were lower than those seen in control rats (Guzeev et al., 2023). Thus, there were both similarities and differences in results among the rat studies. The differences may be related to the age of the rats, the length of restriction, the methods of sleep deprivation, or the timing and nature of other tests that were used.

These results differed from those observed in mice, which showed substantial changes in homeostatic responses to acute sleep loss after chronic sleep restriction (Clasadonte et al., 2014). The differences between results in rat and mouse studies suggest that the way that SWS is homeostatically regulated differs between these species. Taken together, these studies provide evidence that chronic sleep loss altered basal, within-day homeostatic regulation in rats (Deurveilher et al., 2012; Deurveilher et al., 2021; Guzeev et al., 2023) and altered homeostatic responses to acute sleep loss in mice and, perhaps, less strongly in rats (Clasadonte et al., 2014; Guzeev et al., 2023).

Thus, some studies in rats provided evidence for reduced or altered SWS homeostatic responses after severe or prolonged sleep restriction and suggested that allostatic mechanisms were activated. The idea that acute and chronic sleep loss can elicit different responses is consistent with evidence that molecular, neurochemical, and behavioral effects of brief sleep deprivation in rats were modified when acute sleep loss was extended or repeated (Azogu et al., 2015; Junek et al., 2010), that chronic sleep restriction in mice altered later neurochemical and homeostatic responses to acute sleep loss (Clasadonte et al., 2014), and that chronic sleep loss in rats altered regulation of sleep-related neurotransmitter receptors (Kim et al., 2012; Kim et al., 2015).

An alternative interpretation of recovery from chronic sleep loss in rats invoked a settling-point model for homeostasis of sleep, and separated the concept of compensation for altered amounts of specific behavioral states (waking, NREM, and REM sleep) from the concept of compensation for EEG delta power. It concluded that chronic sleep loss in rats exceeded the capacity of a behavioral state homeostat to fully compensate for lost NREM sleep, while there was much less effect on the capacity for compensation of lost EEG delta power and REM sleep (Stephenson et al., 2015).

In contrast to some of these rodent studies, human studies showed that SWS/SWA are homeostatically regulated during chronic sleep restriction. SWS and delta power in people increased on each of 5 nights of restriction to a 4 h sleep opportunity (Åkerstedt et al., 2009a). Homeostasis of SWA was also preserved in people restricted to 6 h sleep nightly for a week. Recovery sleep after an acute 40 h sleep deprivation period was similar among those who had previously undergone a week of nightly sleep restriction and those who had experienced a week of extended (10 h) nightly sleep opportunities (Skorucak et al., 2018).

It is difficult to compare results in rodent studies of chronic sleep loss to those in people, in which sleep was restricted to 4–6 h over 5–7 days. In human studies, there was no evidence of a gradual attenuation of homeostatic responses (Skorucak et al., 2018; Åkerstedt et al., 2009a), as seen in several rodent studies. Adult humans typically have a consolidated 7–8 h sleep period nightly alternating with 16–17 h of waking, which may make them more capable of responding homeostatically to extended wake durations of 18–20 h daily. Small rodents, however, are polyphasic sleepers with many short sleep–wake bouts during both day and night, including up to 125 sleep–wake cycles/24 h (Le Bon et al., 2007; see, e.g., the bottom panel in **Figure 7.10**). This difference may contribute to different physiological responses in rodents and people to the sustained wake periods that are enforced during chronic sleep restriction cycles.

More research is needed to better understand the effects of acute vs. chronic sleep restriction in different species. This research would benefit from standardization of procedures across studies, including the method, pattern, and duration of chronic sleep restriction as well as the timing and method used for later acute sleep loss challenges.

5.4.2 Other ways of compensating for sleep loss

In interpreting these and other sleep deprivation studies, it is important to recognize that complete, long-term sleep deprivation in animal studies is virtually impossible. Short-term sleep deprivation in animal studies can be essentially complete if a human experimenter is continuously present and intervenes to prevent sleep. For longer-term studies, however, the inevitable delay between onset of a sleep episode and action to wake the animal results in at best a very large reduction in sleep amounts. Even a continuously walking rat can generate microsleeps.

Sleep deprivation can be achieved more completely in human studies in which the participant is motivated and willing to stay awake, unlike in animal studies in which the animal has the opposite motivation. Nevertheless, in long-term studies, the delays inherent in an experimenter responding to evidence of sleep will allow some sleep to occur. After long-term sleep loss, a person sitting with their eyes open may also generate microsleep episodes. In both animals and people, these brief sleep episodes are essentially all NREM sleep because REM sleep does not occur until after a substantial duration of NREM sleep. As a result, these studies can produce virtually total deprivation of REM sleep but not of NREM sleep (compare panels **B** and **E** in **Figure 5.8**).

Even if all sleep episodes could be prevented, both animals and people that are severely sleep-deprived also generate isolated slow EEG waves or show general EEG slowing while they are kept awake. In a mouse study of chronic sleep restriction that alternated 2 h sleep/4 h wake (treadmill walking) episodes, SWA increased during the sleep opportunities on the

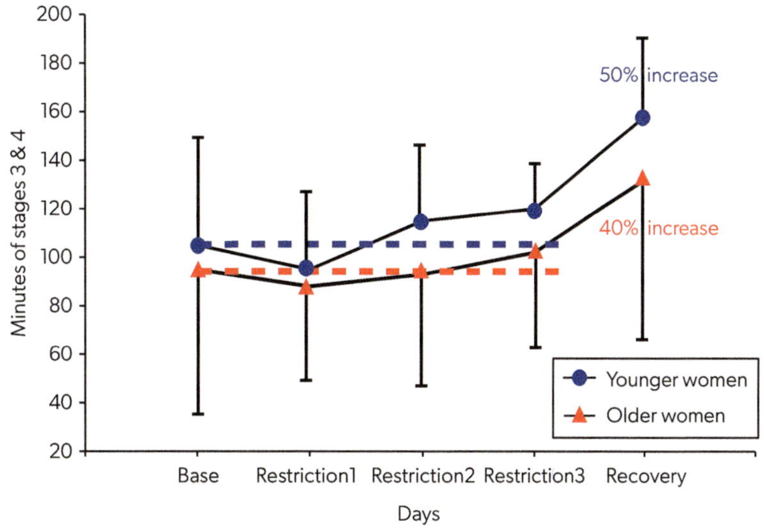

Figure 5.11 Younger women (20–30 years old, blue circles) and older women (55–65 years, red triangles) had sleep recorded at baseline (Base), then during three nights with sleep restricted to 4 h per night (01:00–05:00) (Restriction 1–3), and finally during a single recovery night (Recovery). The amount of N3 sleep (stages 3 and 4) was unaffected during the restriction nights, averaging about the same as on the baseline night (estimated as the dashed blue line for younger and red line for older women); means ± SD. Other sleep stages were reduced considerably. Nevertheless, there were increases of 40% (older) and 50% (younger) in N3 sleep during the recovery night relative to the baseline night. These results show that N3 sleep was preferentially preserved during restricted sleep opportunities. Nevertheless, it was also selectively increased during recovery sleep in response to the loss of either other sleep stages or total sleep amounts. Adapted with permission of Oxford University Press and the Sleep Research Society from Stenuit, P. & Kerkhofs, M. (2005) Age modulates the effects of sleep restriction in women. *Sleep* 28:1283–1288. © Sleep Research Society (2005). doi: 10.1093/sleep/28.10.1283.

first day of restriction but decreased from that peak on later days. However, while the mice walked on a treadmill during the wake periods, SWA *increased* over the days of restriction, indicating a growing, uncompensated need to produce SWA that was expressed even while walking (Clasadonte et al., 2014).

An increase in slower EEG activity has also been observed during REM sleep periods in people undergoing single episodes or repeated cycles of sleep restriction (Brunner et al., 1993; Brunner et al., 1990; Dijk, Brunner, et al., 1991), in rats undergoing chronic sleep restriction (Leemburg et al., 2010), and during brief entries into REM sleep in rats undergoing acute, selective REM sleep deprivation (Shea et al., 2008). These shifts toward producing slower EEG frequencies during waking or REM sleep may partially compensate for some of the SWA lost as a result of reduced NREM sleep. These findings demonstrate that the nervous system's drive to generate the slow EEG rhythms typical of deep NREM sleep is a physiological imperative that is not easily thwarted.

The physiological importance of slow EEG rhythms is also demonstrated by some surprising results in studies of chronic sleep restriction in people. Studies of men restricted nightly to 3 h of sleep (for 8 nights) or 4 h of sleep (for 2 nights) and of women restricted to 4 h of sleep (for 3 nights) found that SWS amounts were almost completely preserved during the 3 or 4 h sleep opportunities. In contrast, REM, N1, and N2 sleep amounts were strongly reduced (Brunner et al., 1990; Stenuit & Kerkhofs, 2005; Webb & Agnew, 1965).[5]

Despite the fact that SWS was largely or completely preserved during the restricted sleep nights, there were increases in SWS amounts relative to baseline levels during recovery nights. In the study involving women, these increases were dramatic: older women (55–65 years old) showed a 40% increase and younger women (20–30 years old) a 50% increase in SWS during recovery sleep, despite not losing any SWS during the restriction nights (Stenuit & Kerkhofs, 2005) (**Figure 5.11**). In a study involving men aged 46–55 years, SWS (Stages 3 and 4) was less completely preserved during 5 days of restriction to 4 h sleep nightly (66–89% of baseline duration). However, during a recovery night, SWS increased to the same extent as for older women in the previous study (41% greater than baseline). In a study involving 5 nights of 4 h time in bed (TIB), young men gradually concentrated their total nightly SWS amounts

[5] This is likely the case because people typically enter SWS as soon as they fall asleep, especially under restriction, and most SWS occurs in the first half of the sleep period, which is all that was available. REM and N2 sleep are more concentrated in the second half of a 7–8 h sleep period, which was never reached during 3 or 4 h sleep opportunities. There does not appear to be any homeostatic adjustment over days to attempt to replace the growing deficit in REM and N2 sleep by shifting these to earlier times in the short sleep opportunities.

into the first 3.8 h over the first few restriction nights but still showed a significantly increased amount of SWS during the first recovery night (Åkerstedt et al., 2009b).

During sleep restriction in these studies, participants lost large proportions of other sleep stages, were awake for longer than usual each day, but maintained most or all of their usual amounts of SWS. Yet they selectively increased SWS during a recovery night. These findings indicate that generating SWS is the preferred, perhaps most efficient, mechanism for recovering from the consequences of sleep loss (or of excess waking). This conclusion is consistent with the evidence that during chronic sleep restriction, or even during acute, selective REM sleep restriction, slow EEG activity starts to intrude into waking and REM sleep episodes.

5.4.3 Summary

Unlike the clear homeostatic increases in SWA after acute sleep loss in animals, chronic sleep restriction resulted in only transient or incomplete homeostatic increases in SWA over days of restriction in several studies. Another study, however, found robust compensation of SWA after chronic sleep loss in rats. The extent of homeostatic recovery of SWA observed in rodents may depend on which cortical regions are studied, on the deprivation methods and schedules used, as well as the species or strain being studied, all of which differed among these studies.

During recovery sleep after severe chronic sleep restriction, rodents tended to increase REM sleep immediately, but increases in SWS were delayed and weaker. In people, however, there were immediate increases in SWS after chronic, partial sleep loss. It is unclear whether this species difference depends on the relative effectiveness of the procedures used to prevent sleep, on the severity of sleep loss, or on differences in the usual sleep structure of people and rodents.

Allostatic responses to chronic sleep loss have been demonstrated in mice, resulting in altered homeostatic and neurochemical responses to later acute sleep loss. In rats, chronic sleep restriction altered within-day homeostatic processes, but it is unclear whether it affected later responses to acute sleep loss. These differences may reflect different degrees of tolerance of chronic sleep loss in mice and rats. Taken together, the results suggest that chronic sleep loss that exceeds the capacity for homeostatic regulation can trigger different adjustments in the operation of homeostatic regulatory mechanisms. Other ways in which animals and people adjust to extended sleep restriction, or even to selective REM sleep deprivation, include microsleeps and the intrusion of slow waves into either waking or REM sleep episodes.

An indication of the priority placed on SWS in people is the finding that the amount of SWS was selectively preserved during chronic sleep restriction, despite the reductions in other sleep stages. When free recovery sleep was later allowed, people showed large increases in SWS, even though this stage was uniquely preserved during restriction. These results suggest that SWS is especially important for recovering from the cumulative effects of both acute and chronic sleep loss in people.

5.5 Homeostatic regulation of REM sleep

5.5.1 Human studies

The evidence reviewed above supports the idea that SWS is homeostatically regulated in people and may serve as a preferred recovery state after any kind of sleep loss. But it does not clearly support homeostatic regulation of REM sleep. The amount of REM sleep generated is closely related to the circadian phase at which sleep occurs rather than to the length of time since REM sleep was last produced; see Section 2.5.1 and **Figures 2.10** and **5.4**.

Nevertheless, there is evidence that REM sleep is homeostatically regulated, but its regulation differs from that of either SWS or SWA. In people, homeostatic regulation of REM sleep after acute loss of all sleep may be obscured during recovery by the immediate increase in SWS that delays the first REM sleep episode (see **Figure 5.2**). Increases in REM sleep may not occur until later that night or during a second recovery night (Berger & Oswald, 1962; Bonnet & Rosa, 1987; Webb & Agnew, 1965). In one study, during a recovery night after 3 nights of restriction to 4 h sleep, REM sleep amounts increased over baseline values. These increases, however, were delayed and followed large SWS increases, even though REM sleep was reduced by half or more during restriction while SWS amounts were preserved intact throughout restriction (Stenuit & Kerkhofs, 2005). After 11 days awake, Randy Gardner showed 5-fold increases in Stage 4 sleep, which was concentrated early in his first recovery night, but he also showed 3-fold increases in REM sleep (Gulevich et al., 1966).

Studies of selective REM sleep deprivation in people also demonstrated its homeostatic regulation. These studies included selective REM sleep deprivation over a 5 h sleep period (Beersma et al., 1990) or over several nights (Agnew et al., 1967; Cartwright et al., 1967; Dement, 1960). Increases in REM sleep amounts were variable among participants during early recovery nights, but sometimes persisted over several nights (Cartwright et al., 1967; Dement, 1960). These findings show that deprivation of REM sleep leads to later increases, although not always immediately. The results also indicate that there is complexity in the response, depending in part on apparent competition with the pressure to produce SWS.

Another approach to studying homeostatic regulation of REM sleep in people is to assess the strength of the drive to produce REM sleep. One measure of this drive is the number of interventions required to selectively deprive people of REM sleep by waking them whenever they produce it. Several studies in people showed that repeatedly interrupting REM sleep expression as soon as it began increased the drive to enter REM sleep later in the night; that is, increasingly more interventions were needed later in the night to prevent REM sleep onset (Agnew et al., 1967; Cartwright et al., 1967; Endo et al., 1998).

A stronger drive to enter REM sleep late in the night could be explained by either the typical increase in circadian promotion of REM sleep during the second half of the night (see **Figures 2.9** and **2.10**), or by increased homeostatic pressure for REM sleep because of its loss earlier in the night. Studies that continued the deprivation procedure for several consecutive nights, however, provided evidence that cannot be explained by a circadian influence alone. At each time point during the third night of REM sleep interruptions, significantly more interventions were required than during the first night. The increased drive to enter REM sleep both early and late during the third night must reflect the cumulative homeostatic effects of reducing REM sleep during the first two nights (Endo et al., 1998) (**Figure 5.12**). Similarly, over 4 or 5 nights of "dreaming" deprivation, Dement reported a progressive increase over nights in the number of attempts to enter REM sleep, resulting in an average of nearly twice as many interventions to prevent REM sleep on the last night (19.3) as on the first (10.9) (Dement, 1960).

These several lines of evidence support the idea that REM sleep is homeostatically regulated, but also indicate that its expression after sleep loss is affected by other factors. Increased REM sleep after deprivation tends to be delayed and to occur gradually over multiple nights in humans. Delayed REM sleep recovery reflects the high priority for production of SWS immediately after sleep loss, whether recovery sleep starts at the beginning of the day or is delayed until the next night (Dijk, Brunner, et al., 1991), as well as the impact of the circadian promotion of REM sleep later in the night phase (**Figure 2.9**). These results differ from those observed in studies of rodents and cats, as discussed in the next section.

5.5.2 Animal studies

Total sleep deprivation[6] in rats over one or more days, or chronic partial deprivation, led to immediate increases in REM sleep at the start of the recovery period beginning in either the daily dark or light phase; increases in SWS were delayed (Borbély, 1982a; Deurveilher et al., 2012; Rechtschaffen et al., 1999; see **Figures 5.6**, and **5.8**). Either acute or chronic selective deprivation of REM sleep also increased later REM sleep amounts

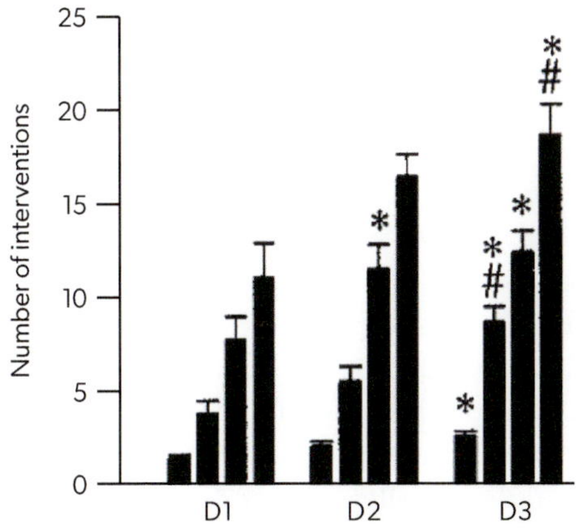

Figure 5.12 Participants underwent selective REM sleep deprivation by the experimenters waking them whenever they entered REM sleep. The figure shows the mean (+SEM) number of interventions required to interrupt REM sleep once it was initiated during each of four 2 h intervals over three successive nights (D1–3). There was a gradual increase in the number of interventions required during the course of each night. This finding might be related to an increasing circadian tendency to produce REM sleep later in the night and/or to an increased homeostatic drive for REM sleep because it was prevented early in the night. The significant increases in interventions required during the second, and especially the third, night, relative to the same time bins during the first night, are clear evidence of an increasing homeostatic pressure to produce REM sleep because of its selective deprivation during preceding nights. * Significantly different from the corresponding time bin on D1; # significantly different from the corresponding time bin on D2. Note that despite the increasing drive to produce REM sleep over the 3 nights, the circadian pattern of REM sleep probability was still expressed strongly during the third night. Reprinted with permission of the American Physiological Society from Endo, T. et al. (1998) Selective REM sleep deprivation in humans: effects on sleep and sleep EEG. *Am J Physiol* 274:R1186–R1194. © American Physiological Society (1998). doi: 10.1152/ajpregu.1998.274.4.R1186.

during recovery sleep opportunities (Morden et al., 1967; Shea et al., 2008), in some cases almost completely compensating for the lost REM sleep (McCarthy et al., 2016). In cats, hours of REM sleep deprivation by cold exposure was followed by robust recovery of REM sleep amounts within a 24 h period (Parmeggiani et al., 1980).

Other evidence supporting homeostatic regulation of REM sleep comes from studies of rats with suprachiasmatic nucleus lesions, which are discussed in Section 5.6. These results indicate very different priorities in people and rats for recovery of REM sleep vs. SWS after sleep loss.[7]

[6] This term refers to *attempts* to completely eliminate sleep, although all methods of deprivation allow brief periods during which sleep can occur (see **Figure 5.8**).

[7] Other species also respond differently to the loss of REM sleep. Neither starlings (*Sturnus vulgaris*) (van Hasselt et al., 2019) nor Australian magpies (*Cracticus tibicen tyrannica*) (Johnsson et al., 2021) showed homeostatic increases of REM sleep after its deprivation but did show NREM sleep homeostasis. However, this is not a universal trait among birds, since pigeons (*Columba livia*) showed homeostatic increases of REM sleep (but not SWA) after total sleep deprivation (Tobler & Borbély, 1988).

The effects of chronic, total sleep deprivation in rats for 1 or 4 days using the DOW method (Rechtschaffen et al., 1999) resulted in very large increases in the amount of REM sleep in rats as soon as sleep deprivation ended (see **Figure 5.8**). During recovery days, there were only small, delayed increases in NREM sleep, little change in delta activity during NREM sleep, and even decreases in high-amplitude NREM sleep (HS2, equivalent to human N3 sleep) (**Figure 5.8 C**).

If REM sleep is homeostatically regulated in both people and rats, why do these species show different immediate priorities when sleep is allowed after deprivation? One explanation relates to the fact that sleep-deprived rats are motivated to sleep whenever they possibly can, given the constraints of the deprivation procedure, for example, for the few seconds that they are carried backwards on a moving disk, wheel, or treadmill. In contrast, willing human volunteers cooperate in trying to stay awake during an experiment, rather than trying to sleep, so frank sleep episodes are unintentional, brief, and less common. As a result, rats, unlike people, regularly produce short episodes of NREM sleep during the deprivation period, which accumulate to significant amounts over days.

For lighter NREM sleep (HS1), these short episodes totaled about a third of baseline amounts (**Figure 5.8 B**). REM sleep, however, was completely prevented because it does not occur in rats without 5–10 min of preceding NREM sleep, a duration that was never produced during the deprivation procedure (**Figure 5.8 E**) (Benington & Heller, 1999; Deurveilher et al., 2012; Leemburg et al., 2010; Rechtschaffen et al., 1999). The longer rats underwent this sleep deprivation procedure, the more REM sleep they lost relative to the less severe loss of NREM sleep, leading to a stronger homeostatic drive to generate REM sleep.

A related interpretation derives from the hypothesis that the need for REM sleep arises as a response to prior NREM sleep (discussed in Sections 5.5.3 and 5.6) (Benington & Heller, 1994a; Benington & Heller, 1999; Moses et al., 1977). This hypothesis implies that the gradual accumulation of small amounts of NREM sleep during a lengthy sleep deprivation procedure would itself generate an increasing drive for REM sleep that cannot be even partially satisfied during the deprivation procedure.

Both the fact that there is a differential loss of NREM and REM sleep and the idea that the accumulation of small amounts of NREM sleep creates a specific need for REM sleep would predict a priority for rats to generate REM sleep as soon as sleep is allowed. In human sleep deprivation studies, it is unlikely that participants would accumulate significant durations of NREM sleep, so these arguments would not apply, and people would not develop a similar drive to immediately generate REM sleep during recovery.

Consistent with this interpretation, when rats were sleep-deprived using a gentle handling method (mostly distraction with novel objects and minimal or no actual contact; see Section 14.2), they could be virtually completely deprived of NREM sleep for a 6 h period at the beginning of the light phase. When allowed to sleep, they immediately showed large increases in NREM sleep and SWA, and only a small, delayed increase in REM sleep (Tobler & Borbély, 1990; Wang et al., 2023). However, this method was only applied for a single, acute sleep deprivation period, which may not have the same effect on regulatory systems as sustained, long-term deprivation.

A different approach to deprivation of REM sleep in rats is the use of antidepressant drugs that are known to reduce REM sleep amounts (McCarthy et al., 2016). Behavioral deprivation of REM sleep (by rotating a cylinder housing a rat whenever REM sleep was detected) resulted in full compensation for lost REM sleep within the next 1–2 days. Treatment with one class of antidepressants (selective serotonin reuptake inhibitors, SSRIs)[8] that reduced REM sleep to a similar extent did not result in later homeostatic increases. Treatment with a tricyclic antidepressant (which acts via multiple receptor types) also suppressed REM sleep, but most of the lost REM sleep was homeostatically compensated during recovery.

When rats were first behaviorally deprived of REM sleep and were then treated with an SSRI to extend the deprivation, they subsequently compensated for the amount of REM sleep lost by behavioral deprivation, but not for the amount attributable to the drug treatment (McCarthy et al., 2016). These results confirm that selective REM sleep deprivation activates homeostatic compensation for the loss but indicate that selectively enhancing serotonergic activity to reduce REM sleep evades this homeostatic mechanism.

5.5.3 Complexity of REM sleep regulation

Although there is clear evidence supporting homeostatic increases in REM sleep after selective or total sleep deprivation, there are also findings that are incompatible with homeostatic regulation. When people were asked to sleep on three successive nights for 8, 12, and 8 h, respectively, NREM sleep increased by ~32% during the night with the 12 h sleep opportunity. REM sleep, however, increased by ~90% because of the circadian phase during which the extra sleep occurred (07:00–11:00). This result is consistent with the high probability of producing REM sleep in the morning hours even after

[8] These drugs enhance serotonergic activity in the synapse by preventing the reuptake of released serotonin into the presynaptic terminal. High serotonergic activity is known to inhibit the expression of REM sleep; see Section 10.6.2.

a full night's sleep; see **Figure 2.10 A**. Despite the very large increase in total REM sleep during the morning hours, REM sleep during the following 8 h night was not reduced. It actually showed a small increase (~11%) relative to the amount shown on the first night (Feinberg et al., 1980).

Similarly, REM sleep accumulated during a daytime nap opportunity did not reduce the amount shown during the following night. In contrast, the amount of SWA or SWS during a nap reduced the amount shown during the next night, as would be expected for a homeostatically controlled system (Campbell et al., 2005; Werth et al., 1996).

Thus, deprivation of REM sleep (especially lengthy deprivation) leads to rebound increases, but increasing the amount of REM sleep does not lead to later decreases. This is an unusual, unidirectional form of homeostasis. A speculative interpretation is that organisms need a certain amount of REM sleep, perhaps to counter the effects of lengthy episodes of SWS (see Section 5.6). But there is presumably no harm in generating more REM sleep than is needed, so increases are not compensated by later reductions. A related view is that the normal expression of REM sleep includes both obligate (physiologically necessary) and facultative (optional) amounts (Parmeggiani et al., 1980). This interpretation implies that there is no harm in producing more REM sleep during ordinary NREM–REM cycles than is physiologically essential. In contrast, the generation of SWS may be important, but it may also have associated costs, so increases are compensated for by later decreases.

While changes in the duration of sleep stages have been the focus of many studies of SWS and REM sleep regulation, these measures give an incomplete picture of the brain's responses to lost sleep. It is possible, for example, that there is an intensity dimension to REM sleep as there is to SWS. For example, one report indicated that longer REM sleep deprivation in rats led to more intense muscular twitches during recovery REM sleep, a possible marker of more intense REM sleep expression (Morden et al., 1967).

In addition, there are "cross-over" effects between sleep stages, as described above (see Section 5.4.2). Sleep deprivation in people and rats led to intrusions of slow EEG activity into REM sleep and/or waking. Chronic reductions of other sleep stages while SWS amounts were preserved led to increases in SWS during recovery nights (Brunner et al., 1990; Stenuit & Kerkhofs, 2005; Webb & Agnew, 1965) (see **Figure 5.11**). Selective deprivation of REM sleep for one day in rats led to a large increase in REM sleep but also to a transient increase in the rat equivalent of SWS (Rechtschaffen et al., 1999). In people, 5 h of selective REM sleep deprivation was accompanied by a reduction in slow EEG frequencies in NREM sleep during the deprivation period (Beersma et al., 1990).

These effects demonstrate that the brain responds to selective loss of one sleep stage with more than just compensatory increases in the duration of the targeted stage. There are changes in neural activity during other vigilance states both concurrently and during recovery. In people, there is also preferential expression of SWA/SWS as part of the recovery process, regardless of which sleep stages were reduced.

5.5.4 Summary

Selective deprivation of REM sleep or reduced total sleep (including REM sleep) led to rebound increases in this stage during recovery opportunities in both people and rats. Although this finding is consistent with homeostatic regulation, the expression of rebound increases is affected by other factors in people. It is delayed by apparent competition with SWS and it is modulated by circadian regulation. SWS appears to be the preferred mechanism of recovery from the effects of chronic sleep loss in people, so that it is expressed preferentially during recovery sleep, even when SWS amounts have been preserved and REM sleep has been lost. Slow waves also intrude into both REM sleep and waking after extended sleep loss.

Restriction of either SWS or REM sleep results in rebound increases in the restricted stage, indicating that both stages are homeostatically regulated in people. After brief, total sleep deprivation (6 h), rats also show immediate increases in NREM sleep and SWA. After lengthy, sustained sleep loss, the expression of homeostatic need is different during recovery sleep in rats and people. Rats show immediate large increases in REM sleep after sustained sleep loss, but people show large, immediate increases in SWS.

One factor likely contributing to these differences is that incomplete loss of NREM sleep in rats during chronic sleep deprivation, along with complete loss of REM sleep, results in asymmetric drives for these stages during recovery sleep. The more complete loss of NREM sleep in people than rats during deprivation probably reflects the fact that cooperative human participants try to stay awake while rats try to sleep as much as possible during deprivation periods. There may also be differences in the usual regulation of sleep in species with single, lengthy sleep and wake phases (people) and polyphasic sleepers (rats). Other factors that contribute to different results include the relative effectiveness of achieving sleep loss over short and long periods of restriction, and the impact of circadian influences on sleep expression during recovery sleep.

Unlike the classical, bidirectional homeostatic regulation shown for SWS/SWA, expression of "excess" REM sleep during the day does not have the expected effect in reducing nighttime REM sleep. A speculative possibility is that there are different physiological consequences of these sleep stages that lead to this asymmetry. Excess REM sleep may be harmless, while excess SWS may have negative consequences, although it is uncertain what these are; see the discussion in Section 7.4.4.

5.6 Models of REM sleep regulation

There is no agreement on a single model for REM sleep regulation. The evidence for differences in how REM sleep is expressed after sleep deprivation in humans and rats, its unusual form of homeostatic regulation, its strong modulation by circadian phase, and its alternation with NREM sleep have resulted in the development of several different hypotheses.

BRAC: One early suggestion was that an underlying oscillator (a basic rest activity cycle, BRAC) regulates REM sleep timing in people by opening a limited REM sleep "window" with an ultradian periodicity (Kleitman, 1982), that is, one with a frequency greater than [*ultra*] one cycle per day [*dies*]. This model predicts that a long NREM sleep episode would be followed by a relatively short REM sleep episode (and vice versa), because the total cycle length is constrained to fit within the framework of one ultradian period (e.g., 90–110 min in people). This constraint would result in an overall *serial negative correlation* between the lengths of successive NREM and REM sleep episodes (**Figure 5.13 A**). As discussed below, that correlation has not been observed.

Circadian regulation: Studies using the forced desynchronization method (see Chapter 3) are especially useful for understanding the control of REM sleep in people because they permit assessment of the independent contributions of circadian and homeostatic mechanisms, which are not separable under usual 24 h living conditions. These studies (along with nap studies) demonstrated that the production of REM sleep in people is strongly related to circadian phase and less influenced by homeostasis (Carskadon & Dement, 1980; Czeisler, Zimmerman, et al., 1980; Endo et al., 1981).

Separate roles for circadian and homeostatic influences on REM sleep were also demonstrated by the effects of destruction of the suprachiasmatic nuclei (SCN), the principal mammalian circadian pacemaker (see Chapter 8). Destruction of the SCN in monkeys and rats resulted in a redistribution of sleep, wake, and water intake into short, irregular bouts that were not modulated by a circadian rhythm (see **Figure 8.11 B, C** and **8.12 B**). However, the total amount of REM sleep produced daily remained unchanged, indicating continued homeostatic regulation (Edgar et al., 1993; Ibuka & Kawamura, 1975). This interpretation was confirmed by the finding that sleep deprivation in rats with no circadian regulation of sleep after SCN

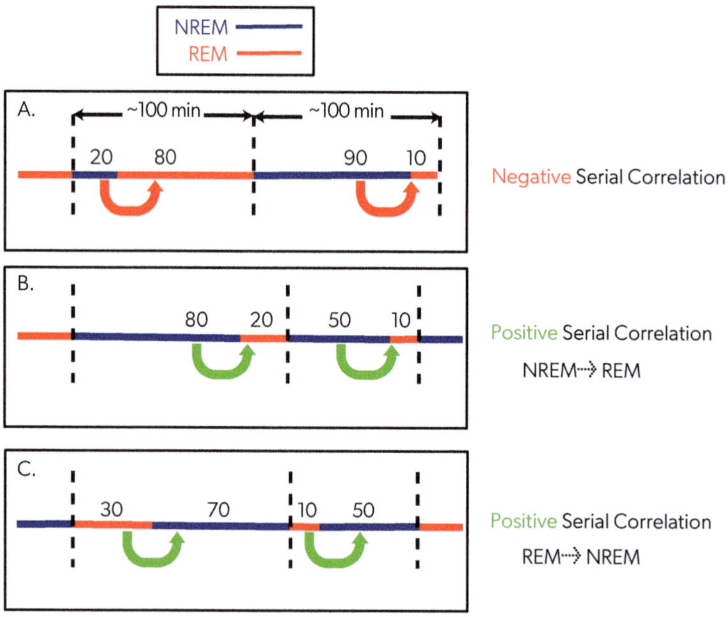

Figure 5.13 **A.** The Basic Rest-Activity Cycle (BRAC) hypothesis would predict that NREM–REM sleep cycles are constrained by an ultradian oscillator to show a combined period of 90–110 min (shown as ~100 min). Short NREM sleep episodes (e.g., 20 min; blue) would be followed by long REM sleep bouts (80 min; red); long NREM sleep bouts (90 min) would be followed by short REM sleep bouts (10 min) to add up to ~100 min. This would result in an overall negative serial correlation (red arrows) between adjacent NREM and REM sleep bouts. **B.** and **C.** These models are based on the assumption that NREM sleep creates a physiological need for REM sleep; thus, more NREM sleep should be linked to more REM sleep, resulting in a serial positive correlation. The **B** panel shows the most obvious prediction from this model: that longer NREM sleep bouts would be *followed* by longer REM sleep bouts (green arrows). The **C** panel shows that longer REM sleep bouts discharge the need for REM sleep, creating the opportunity for longer NREM sleep bouts before the need for REM sleep reaches threshold again. This also results in a positive serial correlation (green arrows) between NREM and REM sleep bout lengths, but in the opposite direction (i.e., *preceding* REM sleep bouts are correlated with the length of following NREM sleep bouts). The experimental evidence is consistent with model **C**.

ablation still resulted in increases in total sleep, NREM sleep, and REM sleep during recovery days (Mistlberger et al., 1983; Tobler et al., 1983).

Insight into how the circadian system influences REM sleep expression in rats was obtained from a study in which intact and SCN-ablated rats were selectively deprived of REM sleep, and attempts to initiate REM sleep were measured. SCN-ablated rats showed a reduced number of attempts to enter REM sleep relative to those shown by intact rats during their circadian rest phase. However, there was no difference in the number of attempts to enter REM sleep relative to intact rats during their active phases. Thus, an intact circadian system in rats promotes REM sleep expression during the circadian rest phase, but neither promotes nor inhibits REM sleep attempts during the active phase (Wurts & Edgar, 2000).

Taken together, these results show that the circadian and homeostatic systems regulate different aspects of REM sleep production. The circadian system determines the timing of REM sleep production within a day, but the amount of REM sleep produced is homeostatically regulated over the long term[9] even in the absence of circadian regulation.

REM sleep as a response to NREM sleep: Another hypothesis is that REM sleep is a response to the expression of NREM sleep: Cellular events that occur during NREM sleep create a neural state that must be reversed by generating REM sleep (Benington & Heller, 1994a; Benington & Heller, 1999; Moses et al., 1977). According to this hypothesis, the drive for SWS/SWA is a response to being awake, but the drive for REM sleep is a response to the amount of NREM sleep produced.

This hypothesis has the attractive feature of providing an explanation for the cycling between NREM and REM sleep throughout the human sleep phase: The neural consequences of generating NREM sleep create the need to enter REM sleep, and once that need is satisfied, NREM sleep can recur. As previously discussed, this hypothesis also offers an alternative explanation for the large REM sleep rebound seen after near-total, chronic sleep deprivation in rats (see **Figure 5.8**). Repeated brief NREM sleep episodes that inevitably occur during deprivation, but are never accompanied by REM sleep, will generate a gradual, selective increase in pressure to produce REM sleep, which cannot occur during the deprivation procedure. The result is the production of large amounts of REM sleep during recovery sleep.

The idea that REM sleep is a response to NREM sleep is also consistent with a hypothesis about the evolution of cortical desynchronization during REM sleep in most birds and mammals; see Section 7.4.4. This hypothesis proposes that early in the evolution of birds and mammals, all sleep was NREM. When brainstem REM sleep (atonia and REMs) first appeared, it was also accompanied by slow EEG activity in the cortex. Later in evolution, activation of the cortex was added to brainstem REM sleep, resulting in REM sleep as seen in most modern mammals and birds.

One hypothesis for why this occurred is that the growing capacity for learning and brain plasticity throughout the lifetime of advanced mammals and birds (Jarvis et al., 2005) resulted in structural or functional changes in the cortex or hyperstriatum (the avian equivalent) that were incompatible with sustaining NREM sleep, especially SWS, for long durations. Cortical activation was added to brainstem REM sleep to interrupt slow-wave production while still maintaining sleep. This idea and its relation to brain temperature and metabolic activity during sleep is discussed in Section 7.4.4.

A prediction of the hypothesis that REM sleep reverses brain changes that occur during NREM sleep is that the occurrence of REM sleep should depend on the accumulation of NREM sleep. This prediction was supported by evidence from a study of human sleep distributed in short naps across the day and night. It found that the occurrence of REM sleep onset was best predicted by the accumulation of minutes of NREM sleep, rather than by the passage of time (Johnson, 1980).

The most direct prediction from this hypothesis would be that longer NREM sleep episodes would cause the accumulation of more brain changes that would require longer REM sleep episodes to reverse. Statistically, this would result in a *serial positive correlation* between the length of NREM sleep episodes and the length of the following REM sleep episodes (**Figure 5.13 B**). This prediction was examined in studies of rats (Benington & Heller, 1994a; Benington & Heller, 1994b; Vivaldi et al., 1994), mice (Le Bon et al., 2007), and people (Barbato & Wehr, 1998). None of these studies found the negative serial correlations predicted by the BRAC hypothesis, but they also did not find positive serial correlations between the duration of NREM sleep and the following REM sleep episode. They did, however, find evidence for a serial positive correlation between the length of a NREM sleep episode and the length of the *preceding* (not following) REM sleep episode (**Figure 5.13 C**).

This result was interpreted in several related, but distinct, ways. Based on the hypothesis that REM sleep is the brain's response to NREM sleep, one interpretation is that longer REM sleep episodes deplete more of the drive for REM sleep that had accumulated as a result of earlier NREM sleep. This reduced drive for REM sleep then permits a longer NREM sleep episode to follow before the drive for REM sleep reaches threshold again and initiates another REM sleep bout (Benington & Heller, 1994b). This interpretation is logically consistent with the idea that REM sleep is a homeostatic response to the

[9] "Long-term" refers to the homeostatic regulation of REM sleep amounts over days (or longer) to distinguish it from "short-term" homeostasis, which is hypothesized to occur within a sleep period, as discussed later in this section.

occurrence of NREM sleep, although the observed results do not match the most intuitive prediction from the model: that the consequences of more NREM sleep should produce longer *following* periods of REM sleep.

Short-term homeostasis of REM sleep: Similar results were explained by a different model that proposes that REM sleep and NREM sleep are each regulated by independent homeostatic mechanisms within a sleep period. The interpretation of the finding that the length of a REM sleep episode was positively correlated with the length of the following NREM sleep episode focused on the concept of short-term homeostasis of REM sleep (Vivaldi et al., 1994).

In this model, a lengthy REM sleep episode exhausts the homeostatic drive for REM sleep, so there is time for a long NREM sleep episode before the independent drive for REM sleep again reaches threshold and initiates REM sleep. A short REM sleep episode does not fully exhaust the drive for REM sleep, so only a short NREM sleep episode can follow before the REM sleep initiation threshold is reached (Vivaldi et al., 1994). In this view, REM sleep is the target of homeostatic regulation and NREM sleep "fills in" the gaps between REM sleep episodes. A related model proposed that a period of REM sleep leads to a refractory period for initiating further REM sleep production, allowing for the expression of either NREM or waking until the refractory period ends (Le Bon, 2021).

These models (Le Bon, 2021; Vivaldi et al., 1994) do not depend on the idea that the production of NREM sleep generates the drive to produce REM sleep. Instead, they propose that each stage is regulated separately by its own long-term and short-term homeostatic mechanisms. The visual impression of linked NREM–REM cycles in plots of sleep stages is proposed to result from focusing on the small number of regular switches between these stages during the consolidated sleep of primates, including humans (e.g., 4–5 NREM–REM cycles per night). In contrast, polyphasic species like rats and mice show dozens or hundreds of short, alternating periods of wake, NREM, and REM sleep. REM sleep may be followed by waking or by NREM sleep. As a result, rodent sleep records do not give the same impression of rhythmic cycles alternating between NREM and REM sleep as seen in primate sleep records. The latter appear more compatible with models that propose a causal link between sleep stages, such as the idea that NREM sleep expression drives the production of REM sleep.

Ultradian/circadian influences: Other evidence for the complexity of REM sleep regulation comes from a unique study in which the REM sleep episodes of three people were recorded using PSG over 30 consecutive nights. The results suggested that multiple mechanisms, possibly including an ultradian oscillator, contributed to producing the observed patterns of REM sleep across the month of recordings (**Figure 5.14**).

Onset of the first REM sleep episode of the night was loosely tied to the timing of NREM sleep onset (although this is difficult to see in the single record illustrated), but later REM sleep episodes occurred at intervals unrelated to sleep onset. When plotted across 30 nights, later REM sleep episodes occurred in cycles of near-90 min length (different lengths in each individual) that scanned across the 24 h day (Schulz et al., 1975). A study in which people were given sleep opportunities for 7 min every 20 min over 24-36 h also concluded that the first REM sleep episode was linked to NREM sleep onset and later episodes recurred with a near-90 min rhythm (Lavie, 1987).

These results can be explained by assuming that the first REM sleep episode is gated by the onset of NREM sleep, while later episodes are controlled by an ultradian timer with a period of ~90 min that scans across the 24 h cycle, yielding a pattern like that shown in **Figure 5.14**.[10] While the nature of this hypothetical ultradian oscillator (BRAC?) is unknown, there is evidence that a different ultradian rhythm in mice is related to fluctuations in the level of the neurotransmitter dopamine in the striatum (Blum et al., 2014). Dopamine has also been linked to aspects of REM sleep regulation; see Section 10.4.2.

5.6.1 Summary

There are several models of how REM sleep is regulated. One model proposes that it represents the aroused phase of a basic rest–activity cycle (BRAC) that continues throughout the day and night. Another hypothesizes that REM sleep is a response to the expression of NREM sleep. REM sleep is also strongly regulated by the circadian system, and the expression of REM sleep in people can be delayed by the pressure to produce NREM sleep after sleep loss. REM and NREM sleep have also been proposed to be regulated homeostatically by two independent mechanisms. The timing of the first REM sleep episode of the night appears to be gated by the onset of NREM sleep, but the timing of later episodes appears instead to be influenced by an ultradian oscillator that is not tied to either clock time or sleep onset.

The predicted correlations between NREM and REM sleep durations based on the BRAC hypothesis and on one version of the hypothesis that REM sleep is a response to NREM sleep were not observed experimentally. But there were positive

[10] An alternative interpretation is that the three apparently nightly peaks of REM sleep in **Figure 5.14** are controlled by a single circadian oscillator that is not entrained, free-runs indefinitely with a period greater than 24 h, and promotes 3–4 REM sleep episodes nightly. This interpretation would require the existence of a non-entrainable circadian oscillator (or perhaps three or four such oscillators, each linked to a REM sleep episode), running independently of an entrainable circadian pacemaker. This interpretation seems physiologically less probable but cannot be ruled out based on the limited data available.

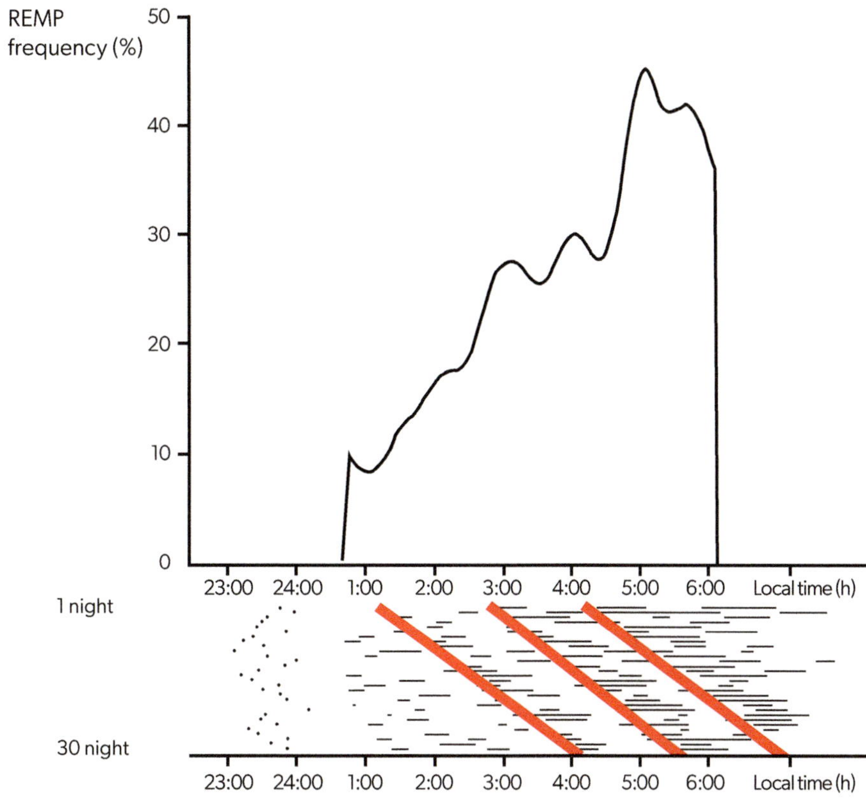

Figure 5.14 The timing of REM sleep shown by one human participant during 30 consecutive nights of PSG studies, plotted against time of day. **Top:** The probability of producing REM sleep during the night, averaged over the 30 nights of recording and showing the typical increasing probability of REM sleep over the course of the night. **Bottom:** For each of the 30 nights, the time of sleep onset is indicated by a dot (23:00–24:00) and REM sleep episodes are indicated by horizontal lines. The diagonal red lines indicate the apparent continuity in timing of REM sleep episodes scanning across the 30 recording nights. This pattern could reflect an ultradian oscillator with a period somewhat longer than 90 min (a rough estimate would be ~96 min), which would, as a result, scan across the 24 h time plot. An alternative (but unlikely) interpretation would be control by an un-entrained circadian mechanism. The timing of the first (brief) REM sleep episode of each night was reported to be weakly related to the onset of sleep, but later REM sleep episodes were not stably linked to either clock time or the time of sleep onset. Adapted with permission from Schulz, H. et al. (1975) Phase shift in the REM sleep rhythm. *Pflügers Arch* 358:203–212. © Springer: Nature (1975). doi: 10.1007/BF00587217.

correlations between the duration of REM sleep episodes and the duration of the following NREM episodes, which can be interpreted to support the hypothesis that REM sleep is a response to NREM sleep. An alternative interpretation is that both REM and NREM sleep are regulated exclusively by their own short-term, homeostatic regulators. In this view, the alternation between NREM and REM sleep in the consolidated sleep of people gives a visual impression of a causal interaction between these stages that is not supported by evidence from rodent species in which many rapid, irregular transitions among waking, NREM, and REM sleep occur throughout sleep periods.

REM sleep expression appears to be influenced by multiple mechanisms (circadian, ultradian, homeostatic, NREM-related). It may be difficult to observe the results predicted by any one model of REM sleep regulation because of the interactions among these several mechanisms. A more complete model of REM sleep regulation may need to incorporate the influence of, and interactions among, multiple mechanisms.

5.7 The two-process model of sleep regulation

5.7.1 Circadian clock regulation

A homeostatic model for the regulation of sleep (or any other motivated behavior) predicts that the drive to sleep will increase as the length of sleep deprivation (time awake) increases. The relationship between deprivation length and drive strength does not have to be linear (i.e., increase at the same rate over all possible lengths of deprivation), but it has to be monotonic (i.e., there are no reversals in the increasing trend). The strength of a drive at any point during deprivation must be equal to or greater than its strength at earlier time points.

We can conceptualize this requirement in relation to sleep regulation using the hypothetical Process S. We can think of S as a product (in the broadest sense) of wakefulness that accumulates in the brain as long as sleep has not occurred, and that is reduced only by sleep. As a result, the level of S (and therefore the drive to sleep) will increase as long as an individual does not sleep.

The behavior of the first participant studied by Patrick and Gilbert during nearly 4 days of sleep deprivation was, however, not consistent with the predictions of a pure homeostatic model. They noted that there was a marked daily rhythm of sleepiness, with a reduced level in the afternoon and evening, and increased sleepiness from midnight to noon, with the greatest amount around dawn (Patrick & Gilbert, 1896). In addition, during their recovery sleep, all three participants first woke in mid-morning, when they had clearly not made up for their lost sleep, and only then returned to sleep for a few more hours. Early reports by Kleitman and colleagues of the effects of sustained sleep deprivation also noted that sleepiness was intense during the night (e.g., 03:00–06:00) but was reduced during the daytime while sleep deprivation continued (Cooperman et al., 1934; Kleitman, 1923).

These descriptions fit the common experience of most people staying awake all night: they become increasingly sleepy during the early part of the night, reach a point of maximal sleepiness and lowest energy level late in the night ("about dawn" according to Patrick and Gilbert), and then gradually feel less sleepy as their habitual waking time approaches. As some workers experience after an overnight work shift, it may even be difficult to get to sleep at 8 or 9 in the morning after a night awake and to sustain a lengthy sleep phase once they do fall asleep. These observations are incompatible with a pure homeostatic model, which cannot explain why the drive for sleep would be stronger after 18 h than after 26 h of continuous waking. This reversal in the intensity of the sleep drive, despite continuing sleep deprivation and accumulating sleep debt, points to the involvement of a non-homeostatic mechanism, the circadian clock.

As described in Chapter 3, the circadian system operates in conjunction with homeostatic mechanisms to regulate virtually every aspect of physiology and behavior. A key difference between circadian and homeostatic regulatory systems is that the circadian system functions independently of direct feedback from the processes it regulates, while homeostasis depends critically on feedback (compare **Figures 5.1 C** and **5.15 B**). Circadian modulation of physiological processes occurs as a function of the passage of time, not as a response to physiological imbalances. It increases and decreases the probability of drives and their associated behaviors at certain daily phases, and its actions are independent of whether the evoked drives are satisfied or not (**Figure 5.15**). This lack of feedback regulation explains why sleepiness decreases and alertness increases during the usual waking phase of the circadian cycle in a person who has not slept overnight, even as homeostatic sleep debt continues to accumulate. Without sleep overnight, a feedback-based system would further increase sleepiness in the morning, rather than provoking alertness.

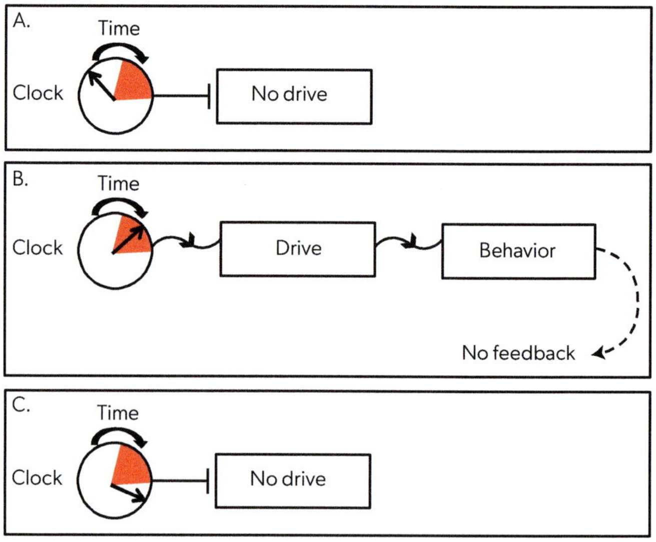

Figure 5.15 A model of how a circadian clock contributes to the expression of drives and motivated behaviors, drawn by analogy with the control-system model of homeostasis shown in **Figure 5.1**. The clock signals circadian phase to other systems as it expresses its internally generated rhythm. **A.** The curved black arrow represents the progress of the clock through time. At some times, when the clock's current phase (straight black arrow) points outside the red zone, it does not promote expression of the drive being modeled (e.g., hunger, thirst, sleepiness). **B.** When the clock's phase reaches circadian times within the red zone, it promotes expression of that drive. (The figure illustrates this change as all-or-none for simplicity. In fact, drive probability in most cases would increase and decrease gradually during part of the cycle, following a sinusoidal function, as represented by the curved line; see Process C in **Figure 5.16**.) **C.** Once the clock has passed out of the red zone, it no longer promotes that drive. Note that the oscillatory changes in the drive and in the behavior(s) it promotes depend only on the progress of the circadian clock through its phases. The consequences of the expression of the drive (eating, drinking, sleeping . . . or not doing so) do not generate a feedback signal (dashed arrow) that regulates whether the circadian clock continues to promote the drive, or not, in contrast to the critical role of feedback in a homeostatic system.

5.7.2 Combining homeostatic and circadian regulation

As discussed in Section 5.3, the roles of the homeostatic regulator for sleep and of the circadian clock were combined into a two-process model that is widely accepted as a description of how homeostatic and circadian systems interact to control sleep in people and other species (Achermann, 2004; Borbély, 2022; Borbély, 1982b; Daan et al., 1984). In a simple homeostatic model, the level of S rises during waking until it reaches an upper threshold value that triggers sleep onset. Sleep gradually reduces the level of S until it reaches a lower threshold value that triggers waking (**Figure 5.16 B**). The two-process model incorporates these elements but also adds a circadian clock that imposes a ~24 h rhythm on these threshold values (**Figure 5.16 A**), so that the probability of S reaching the sleep and wake thresholds is modified rhythmically (**Figure 5.16 C**).

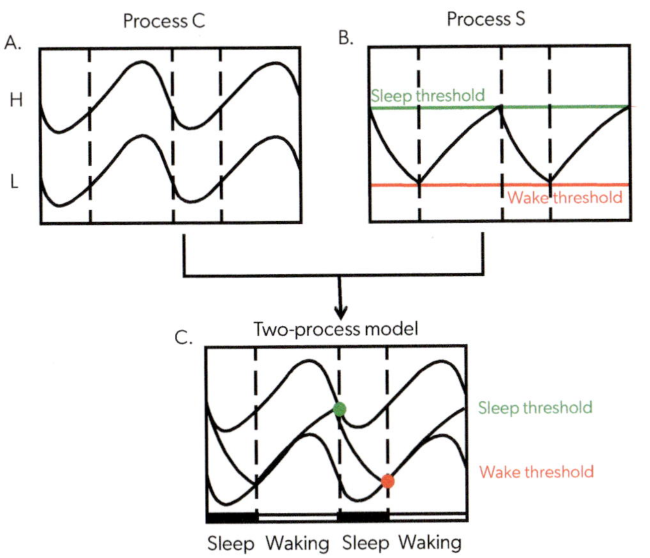

Figure 5.16 The two-process model of sleep regulation is illustrated through its component parts. **A.** Process C is a circadian mechanism that endogenously increases and decreases the probability that sleep will occur on a 24 h basis, continuously shifting the sleep (H) and wake (L) thresholds up and down in a sinusoidal fashion. **B.** Process S is a homeostatic mechanism that involves the accumulation of sleep need during wakefulness (ascending black line) until a sleep threshold value is reached (green line), which triggers sleep onset. During sleep, the expression of SWA results in (or is correlated with) a gradual decline in the level of S until it reaches a wake threshold (red line) when sleep ends. The need for sleep begins to accumulate again as soon as the individual wakes up. **C.** Combining these two elements produces a two-process model in which the homeostatic mechanism continues to operate (as in **B**), but the hypothetical straight-line thresholds are replaced by oscillating thresholds that continuously change the probability of sleeping or waking as a function of circadian time. The green and red circles indicate the intersections of the accumulation of Process S and the circadian thresholds for sleep onset and wake onset, respectively; the sleep period is the interval between those two points, shown by a black rectangle on the X axis. Adapted with permission of the Aerospace Medicine Association from Achermann, P. (2004) The two-process model of sleep regulation revisited. *Aviat Space Environ Med* 75(3, Suppl. 1):A37–A43. © Aerospace Medicine Association (2004). PMID:15018264.

The combined operation of these mechanisms is illustrated in **Figure 5.17**. If a person stays awake for a typical duration of ~16 h, the combination of rising S levels (ascending black curve) and the influence of the circadian clock will make it highly probable that he or she will fall asleep (**A**; downward blue arrow). While asleep (black rectangle), the level of S will fall (dashed black arrow) until it intersects with the wake threshold (which is also modulated by the circadian clock), and the person will wake up after ~8 h (upward blue arrow).

The impact of dual homeostatic/circadian regulation becomes clearer when someone does not fall asleep at their usual time because of shift work, partying, or other activities. The level of S will continue to rise during the extra hours awake (**Figure 5.17;** red curve) until the individual falls asleep at ~07:00 (**B**; downward green arrow) and the level of S starts to fall (dashed red arrow). The oscillation of the circadian clock continues regardless of the state of sleep or waking, so by that hour, it will have already passed through its daily phase of promoting sleep and be well into its phase of promoting waking (i.e., the rising arm of the circadian wake initiation threshold).

During the morning hours, hormonal, neural, and other mechanisms driven by the circadian clock increase the probability of waking and decrease the probability of staying asleep. Even if the high level of S overcomes the circadian influence and triggers sleep onset in the morning, the arousing impact of the circadian system at this phase will cause sleep to be both interrupted and prematurely ended (upward green arrow). When the level of S intersects the rising wake threshold (**Figure 5.17 C**), it will trigger waking even though the level of S has not fallen to its usual value at the time of waking. The residual amount of S will instead be retained and possibly contribute to an earlier onset of sleep during the next cycle.

Unlike the homeostatic system, which modulates drives depending on feedback from the processes it regulates (in engineering terms, it is a "closed-loop" system), the circadian system does not monitor the consequences of its output signals ("open-loop" system); see **Box 5.3**. After it signals that it is time to sleep, whether the individual sleeps or not, the clock keeps ticking toward its next daily phase of promoting waking. As early as 1896, long before the circadian structure of physiology was recognized, Patrick and Gilbert observed the consequences of this circadian influence in the daily rhythms of sleepiness and performance that characterized their sleep-deprived participants.

5.7.3 Other circadian-homeostatic interactions

Several experimental approaches have been used to tease apart the relative contributions of homeostatic and circadian mechanisms to the regulation of different aspects of sleep–wake

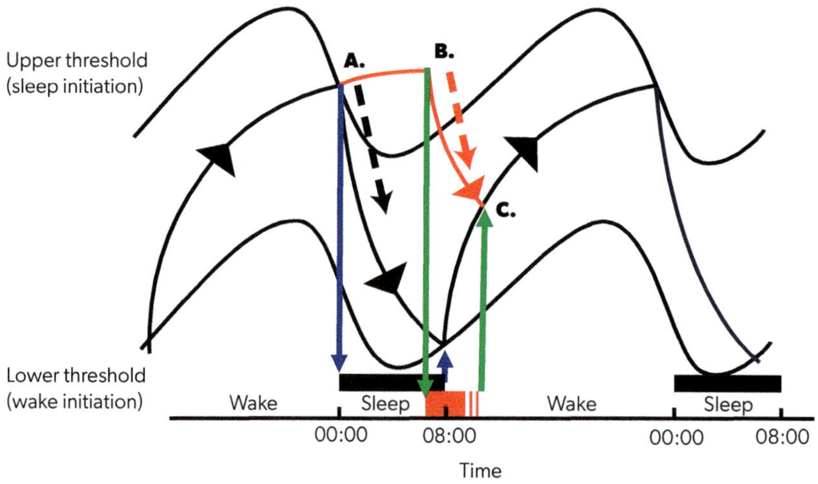

Figure 5.17 Implementation of the two-process model in one example. This illustration demonstrates how the two-process model predicts the impact of staying awake beyond the usual sleep-initiation threshold. During stable sleep–wake cycles, levels of S rise and fall (black curves with arrowheads), and wake and sleep (black rectangles) alternate regularly (**bottom**). The individual falls asleep daily around midnight (**A**; downward blue arrow) and sleeps until 8 AM (08:00; upward blue arrow), as illustrated by the black rectangle. The descending black curve and dashed black arrow indicate the decline in the value of S as the individual sleeps. When waking is extended beyond the usual bedtime; e.g., if an individual stays up overnight working an overnight shift without sleeping, levels of S (black curve) continue to increase from the point marked **A** (= midnight) to **B** (= 07:00) (ascending red line). When the individual falls asleep in the early morning (**B**: downward green arrow), levels of S decline as usual (descending red curve and dashed red arrow). However, the circadian clock has begun to promote arousal and reduce the probability of sleeping, independently of feedback from the lack of sleep. The result is that if the individual falls asleep at ~07:00, sleep (red box) will show disrupted continuity and will terminate early (upward green arrow) because of the arousing impact of the circadian clock. These processes promote waking while S is still highly elevated (**C**) relative to nights with normal sleep timing. As a result of not satisfying the sleep need represented by the level of S, the individual carries an increased sleep debt into the next day. Adapted with permission of the Aerospace Medicine Association from Achermann, P. (2004) The two-process model of sleep regulation revisited. *Aviat Space Environ Med* 75(3, Suppl.):A37–A43. © Aerospace Medicine Association (2004). PMID:15018264.

cycles. The results of these studies have contributed to mathematical simulations based on the two-process model that predict sleep parameters and alertness in a variety of situations (Achermann & Borbély, 2003; Dijk & Czeisler, 1995).

Studies of the relation between sleep–wake and body temperature rhythms in time-free environments showed how homeostatic and circadian mechanisms interact to regulate sleep timing and duration. In these studies, the circadian

BOX 5.3 Feedback and the Circadian Pacemaker

The circadian clock promotes functions like eating, sleeping, hormone release, or being active at various phases of its cycle. The consequences of performing these activities do not, however, exert classic, homeostatic feedback effects on the clock. By this we mean that the consequences of performing these functions do not determine whether the clock promotes increases or decreases of these functions.

Nevertheless, some clock-regulated outputs can affect the circadian clock in other important ways. For example, intense locomotor activity or the hormone estrogen, both of which are under circadian clock control, are among stimuli that can change the period of circadian rhythms (Morin et al., 1977; Mrosovsky, 1996; Rusak, 1981; Yamada et al., 1988). Stimulating acute increases in activity level can also phase shift the circadian system (Reebs & Mrosovsky, 1989) as can sleep deprivation (Antle & Mistlberger, 2000). The outputs of the SCN pacemaker control the circadian timing of sleep-wake states, but the firing rates of SCN neurons are also modified during REM and NREM sleep (Deboer et al., 2003).

These are a few examples of how the circadian system can be influenced by physiological processes whose timing it regulates; see **Figure 8.2** for an illustration of some of these relations. But this influence is different from the effects of feedback in a homeostatic system, in which the feedback consequences of expressing a drive, rather than the passage of time, determine when the drive begins and ends.

rhythm of body temperature is used as a reliable marker of the phase of the circadian clock. As described in Section 3.5.1, some people living in time-free environments (up to several months) showed a dissociation between body temperature rhythms and the timing of sleep and wake, which in normal environments cycle together. This dissociation resulted from people showing either very short or long sleep–wake cycles, while the period of the circadian temperature rhythm remained close to 24 h (Aschoff & Wever, 1976; Czeisler, Weitzman, et al., 1980).

In this condition of internal desynchronization, people fell asleep at a variety of circadian phases. When they fell asleep near the trough of their temperature rhythms, they showed short sleep phases, averaging ~7 h, but sometimes much shorter. When they fell asleep near their body temperature peak, however, they showed very long durations, averaging ~16 h at one phase. What these situations had in common was that participants woke up at similar circadian phases—when body temperatures had begun to increase, despite having slept for very different durations (Czeisler, Weitzman, et al., 1980) (**Figure 5.18**).

The state of internal desynchronization revealed the surprising fact that length of time awake (which determines how much of Process S has accumulated) had little impact on the length of the next sleep episode. Instead, the length of prior waking determined how much SWA would be produced during the next sleep episode. The duration of the sleep episode was instead indirectly determined by the circadian phase at which people fell asleep because they woke up at roughly the same circadian phase regardless of how long they had slept (Strogatz et al., 1986). Thus, Process S strongly affected the amount of SWA produced, while the length of sleep episodes was influenced by Process C.

The circadian system also interacts with the homeostatic drive for sleep to determine the timing of sleep onset and length of sleep under normal living conditions. A homeostatic model predicts that the longer someone is awake, the stronger will be their drive to sleep, so sleepiness should rise throughout the day and evening. Instead, young adults typically show a time of reduced probability of sleep onset during ~20:00–22:00 h, when their homeostatic sleep drive should be close to its daily maximum (Dantz et al., 1994; Dijk & Czeisler, 1994; Haimov &

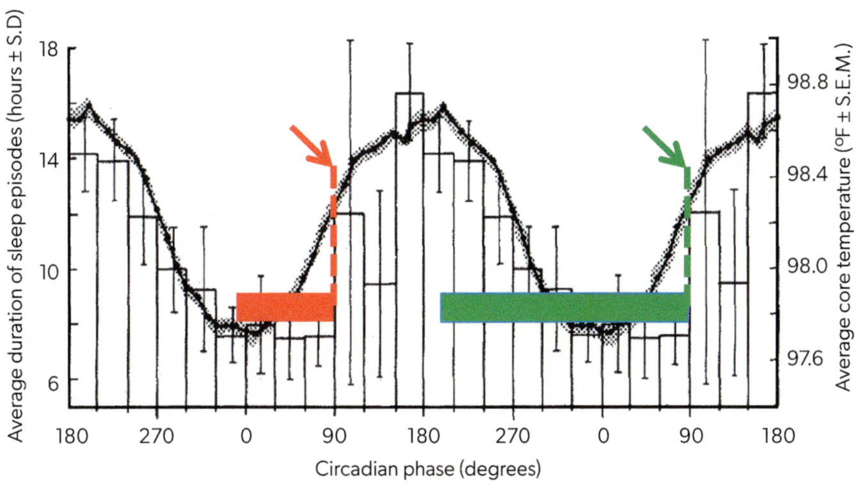

Figure 5.18 The white columns show the average duration of sleep (left Y axis) produced by human participants free-running in constant, time-free conditions when they fell asleep at each circadian phase (X axis). The average core body temperature waveform (black curve; right Y axis) is plotted against circadian phase (X axis, with the core temperature minimum set at 0 degrees). A single circadian cycle (360 degrees) is double-plotted to better illustrate the oscillations in sleep duration and body temperature. The plotted sleep durations are only those that occurred when the participants underwent spontaneous desynchronization (i.e., when their sleep–wake cycles ran with periods that differed significantly from the near-24 h rhythm of core body temperature) so they slept at all phases of the circadian temperature cycle. The shortest sleep durations (averaging ~7 h, but some were much shorter) were shown when sleep onset occurred near the body temperature minimum (0 degrees), while the longest durations (~16 h on average) occurred following sleep onset near the body temperature maximum (180 degrees). To illustrate these relations with specific examples, the red rectangle shows a rough estimate of where a 7 h sleep period, beginning near the body temperature minimum, would fall, and the green rectangle indicates where a sleep period of 16 h, beginning near the body temperature peak, would fall. In each case, average waking times (red and green arrows) occurred on the rising slope of the body temperature rhythm. (Note that the illustrated timing is only approximate because the X axis is plotted in circadian time of the participants, not in hours, while the rectangles used to illustrate sleep durations are plotted in standard hours.) Adapted with permission of Dr. Charles Czeisler and AAAS from Czeisler, C. A. et al. (1980) Human sleep: its duration and organization depend on its circadian phase. *Science* 210:1264–1267. © American Association for the Advancement of Science (1980). doi: 10.1126/science.7434029.

Lavie, 1997; Lavie, 1986; Strogatz et al., 1987). This "forbidden zone" for sleep onset is also called a wake maintenance zone.

Reduced sleepiness at this time of day is accompanied by other signs of increased arousal. Theta/alpha power in the EEG, which is a marker of the strength of the sleep drive (Cajochen et al., 1995), increases continuously during sustained waking but decreases specifically during this limited circadian phase (Aeschbach et al., 1997). During a forced desynchronization study, this was also a circadian phase of improved cognitive performance on vigilance and other performance tests (Wyatt et al., 1999). The wake maintenance zone is followed by the opening of a circadian sleep gate that increases the probability of falling asleep, and sleep onset typically follows within 1–2 h (Dijk et al., 1997). For a discussion of the physiological mechanisms involved, see Chapter 9, **Figures 9.8** and **9.9,** and Section 11.3.1.

Similarly, there is a relatively low probability of waking up late in the nightly sleep phase (the sleep maintenance zone), even though most of the accumulated homeostatic need for sleep would have been satisfied by that time (i.e., the level of S would be approaching its minimum). In each case, the circadian system helps to maintain the current state of waking or sleep late in each daily phase, in opposition to the influence of homeostasis. This role is important in maintaining the long, consolidated sleep and wake states seen in adult humans and other primates (Dijk & Czeisler, 1994; Dijk & Czeisler, 1995).

Many older people might object to this description of wake and sleep maintenance zones. They often find it quite easy to fall asleep in mid-evening and may also wake up much earlier than they typically did at a younger age and be unable to fall back asleep at 4 or 5 in the morning. Since the wake and sleep maintenance zones are produced by the circadian system acting against the influence of homeostasis, one explanation for these changes during aging is that there is a reduction in the strength of circadian signals during aging.

There is evidence from both animal and human research that the amplitude of the circadian pacemaker's oscillation decreases with age (Duffy et al., 1998; Nakamura et al., 2011); the related evidence is reviewed in detail in Chapter 8 (Sections 8.4.3 and 8.4.4). A weaker circadian signal in older people may be unable to counter the impact of homeostatic influences late in each daily phase, thereby contributing to the altered sleep patterns often reported by older people. Other mechanisms that might contribute to the shift in timing of sleep phases during aging are discussed in Sections 4.6.1 and 8.4.

5.7.4 Why have two regulatory mechanisms?

At first glance, it may seem counter-productive to regulate sleep—or any other motivated behavior—in part using a circadian timer that is not regulated by feedback about the current physiological state of an organism. What benefit would an organism get from ignoring information about its current sleep need and letting a relatively inflexible central timer influence sleep timing? The answer to this question lies in the predictive power of circadian timing. A system that combines the predictive power of a timer with the physiological responsiveness of a homeostatic regulator can be more effective than either mechanism acting alone.

The circadian clock sets the timing for sleep and other functions based on the patterns that have served a species well over evolutionary time. Thus, being active during the day and sleeping at night is adaptive for species that function best at high light intensities and are relatively helpless in the dark (humans, sparrows, and other diurnal species). The opposite is true for species with poor daytime vision, superb auditory abilities or night vision that permits functioning in low light or total darkness (bats, barn owls, and other nocturnal species). Adhering to the overall circadian program encoded in an animal's genome guarantees engagement with the environment when it is best able to obtain resources and is at lowest risk of predation or accident, as well as ensuring disengagement, rest, and sleep when the environment is most hostile to that species.

The daily temporal program set by the circadian system serves the needs of an individual well most of the time; the program is encoded in its genome precisely because it has succeeded for millennia. But it will fail in unusual circumstances that could not have been predicted by the genetic program. At those times, a deficit situation can arise (inadequate food, water, or sleep), and homeostatic regulators are activated in order to compensate for the current physiological need. That need reflects the gap between the target set by a homeostatic mechanism and what the circadian program has actually achieved. In this view, homeostatic drive mechanisms function as emergency backup systems that respond when an inherited, daily behavioral program fails to adequately meet an organism's needs.

This perspective differs from the traditional idea that homeostatic mechanisms are the primary regulators of motivated behaviors. The view that homeostatically regulated drives dominate the behavior of organisms was likely reinforced by the results of laboratory studies involving deprivation (e.g., of food or water) rather than by studies of organisms living in their natural environments. These laboratory studies showed that acute deprivation is highly effective in evoking drives and that these drives exert powerful control over the expression of behavior. One can condition a rat or a pigeon to perform impressive feats for water or food reward when they have been deprived of these resources.

Such laboratory studies, however, do not prove that deprivation-evoked drives are the usual regulators of daily

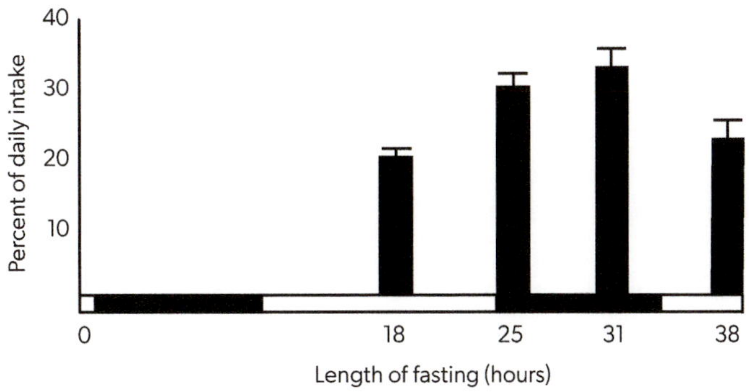

Figure 5.19 The impact of the time of day at which food is made available on the amount of food consumed by hungry rats. Rats in this study were deprived of food beginning at the same phase (0 on the X axis) and were then given a 2 h opportunity to eat after 18, 25, 31, or 38 h of deprivation. The average percentage of their normal total daily intake consumed in each 2 h period (+ standard error) (Y axis) is plotted against the time of day at which food was restored under a 14 h light–10 h dark cycle (illustrated on the X axis). Rats ate progressively more after 25 and 31 h than after 18 h of deprivation. However, after a longer duration (38 h), they ate only slightly more than after 18 h of fasting and less than after either 25 or 31 h. The fact that they were refed at a time of day when rats are programmed to eat very little (daytime) is likely responsible. There could also have been a minor effect of the presence of light. Adapted with permission of Elsevier, Ltd. from Bellinger, L. L. & Mendel, V. E. (1975) Effects of deprivation and time of refeeding on food intake. *Physiol Behav* 14(1):42–46. © (1975) Elsevier. doi: 10.1016/0031-9384(75)90139-0.

behavior in the natural environment. Outside the laboratory, organisms function primarily on the basis of daily (and seasonal) programs of behavior that are adequate to meet their needs under most circumstances. When these programs are effective, they *prevent* dangerous homeostatic imbalances from ever arising. This is a form of predictive homeostasis (Moore-Ede, 1986) that motivates behavior in order to avoid deficit situations, rather than to respond to deficits once they have occurred.[11] When these programs are inadequate, the homeostatic system responds by exerting control over behavior in order to correct the resulting deficit (reactive homeostasis).[12]

However, even under circumstances of deprivation and robust activation of homeostatic drive mechanisms, the internal circadian program continues to be expressed and to exert a strong influence on behavior. One illustration of this phenomenon is a laboratory study in which rats were deprived of food at different times for durations ranging from 18 h to 38 h and were then allowed to eat for 2 h. A homeostatic model would predict increasing hunger as the length of deprivation increased, resulting in increased intake of food when it became available. Instead, rats ate only slightly more after 38 h of deprivation than after 18 h, but considerably less than at the intervening 25 h and 31 h deprivation periods.

This surprising result reflects the fact that food was restored during the daily light phase after 18 and 38 h of deprivation and during the daily dark phase after 25 and 31 h of deprivation (Bellinger & Mendel, 1975) (**Figure 5.19**). Despite a strong homeostatic drive evoked by the longest period of food deprivation (38 h), the underlying rhythmic tendency for rats to eat more at night than during the day still strongly affected their behavior (Zucker, 1971).

A hybrid system involving both a homeostatic regulator sensitive to feedback and an internal timing system that predicts needs based on previous history is familiar to anyone who has used a programmable thermostat to control temperature in a home. The program anticipates the usual daily routine of a home's occupants, thereby increasing comfort and saving the cost of unnecessary heating or cooling. A typical pattern might involve a series of different temperature settings that are preferred for sleeping/getting up, when everyone is away at school or work, during the evening, and going to sleep again. A different program can accommodate the habitual (and therefore predictable) schedules of the family on weekends.

The programmed shifts in temperature set points (analogous to endogenous circadian cycles of shifting thresholds summarized in **Figure 5.17**) are designed to anticipate, rather than respond to, the most probable needs of the household based on their previous history. The program is not responsive to feedback from the house temperature, and it does not turn

[11] One illustration of this anticipatory role is that the mouse suprachiasmatic nucleus releases vasopressin to increase thirst and water intake late in its daily active phase (nighttime) in anticipation of physiological needs during the day. As a result, dehydration is prevented during the daytime without the mouse needing to leave the safety of a retreat to access water (Gizowski et al., 2016).

[12] The idea that rhythmically produced motivated behaviors, such as sleep, serve a preventive function was expressed clearly at a time when little was known about biological rhythms and their function. Von Economo wrote in 1930: "In this sense, the statement of Claparède that we sleep not because we are intoxicated [i.e., poisoned] by hypnotoxins but in order not to get intoxicated by them, is probably correct." This is likely a reference to Édouard Claparède, a Swiss neurologist (1873–1940) (von Economo, 1930, p. 257).

heating or cooling systems on or off. Instead, the program provides a series of changing thresholds at which a homeostatic mechanism can be activated that is sensitive to the current house temperature (i.e., responsive to feedback). When applied to physiology, this function has been named rheostasis, in contrast to homeostasis (from the Greek "rheo" meaning "flowing") (Mrosovsky, 1990).

Given the importance of circadian organization in the regulation of physiology and behavior, it is surprising to note the results of a 2011 survey about important concepts in physiology. The survey involved 81 postsecondary instructors in physiology and was aimed at identifying the top 5 out of 15 suggested core principles of physiology ("big ideas") that undergraduate physiology students need to learn about (Michael & McFarland, 2011). The concept of "homeostasis" was tied for the #1 ranking with "cell membrane". The concepts of circadian rhythmicity, and of the temporal structure of physiology in general, did not appear on the list of suggested core principles.

5.7.5 Summary

Regulation of sleep–wake timing has been modeled as consisting of a homeostatic process and a circadian process. The homeostatic buildup during waking of the need for sleep (S) and its discharge during sleep interact with continuously changing thresholds for triggering sleep and wake, which are set by a circadian clock (C). The interaction of these regulatory systems in people can account for a normal daily pattern of daytime waking and adequate sleep at night. It can also account for abnormally short and disrupted sleep when the dictates of these systems are ignored, and work or play replaces sleep during the circadian night phase.

The circadian contribution to the regulation of sleep also extends to reducing the probability of sleep onset late in the circadian day, despite a near-maximal buildup of S, and reducing the probability of early waking late in the circadian night, when S has reached a low level. This function reinforces the maintenance of lengthy, consolidated sleep and wake phases in primates, including humans. Reduced strength of circadian modulation during aging may contribute to altered timing of wake and sleep periods in older people.

The two-process model that was developed to account for the regulation of sleep through the interaction of S and C also serves as a useful model for the regulation of other motivated behaviors. Instead of a single, ideal set point reflecting the homeostatic wisdom of the body, the hybrid circadian/homeostatic system has a shifting set point that matches its regulatory activity to the organism's most likely needs at different times of day. The circadian timing system conserves energy by avoiding wasteful or dangerous expenditures at inappropriate daily phases, while allowing anticipation of needs that are highly likely to arise, and thereby preventing homeostatic deficits. The homeostatic system defends the series of regulated values set by the internal timer and provides a fail-safe mechanism to ensure that the organism can compensate for large, unanticipated deficits.

Literature cited

Achermann, P. (2004). The two-process model of sleep regulation revisited *Aviat Space Environ Med*, *75*(3, Supplement 1), A37–A43.

Achermann, P., & Borbély, A. A. (2003). Mathematical models of sleep regulation. *Front Biosci*, *8*(6), S683–S693. doi: 10.2741/1064

Achermann, P., Dijk, D. J., Brunner, D. P., & Borbély, A. A. (1993). A model of human sleep homeostasis based on EEG slow-wave activity: quantitative comparison of data and simulations. *Brain Res Bull*, *31*, 97–113.

Aeschbach, D., Matthews, J. R., Postolache, T. T., Jackson, M. A., Giesen, H. A., & Wehr, T. A. (1997). Dynamics of the human EEG during prolonged wakefulness: evidence for frequency-specific circadian and homeostatic influences. *Neurosci Lett*, *239*, 121–124.

Agnew, H. W., Webb, W. B., & Williams, R. L. (1967). Comparison of stage four and 1-REM sleep deprivation. *Percept Motor Skills*, *24*, 851–858.

Åkerstedt, T., Kecklund, G., Ingre, M., Lekander, M., & Axelsson, J. (2009a). Sleep homeostasis during repeated sleep restriction and recovery from EEG dynamics. *Sleep*, *32*(2), 217–222.

Åkerstedt, T., Kecklund, G., Ingre, M., Lekander, M., & Axelsson, J. (2009b). Sleep homeostasis during repeated sleep restriction and recovery: support from EEG dynamics. *Sleep*, *32*(2), 217–222.

Alfonsa, H., Burman, R. J., Brodersen, P. J. N., Newey, S. E., Mahfooz, K., Yamagata, T., ... Akerman, C. J. (2023). Intracellular chloride regulation mediates local sleep pressure in the cortex. *Nat Neurosci*, *26*(1), 64–78. doi: 10.1038/s41593-022-01214-2

Antle, M., & Mistlberger, R. (2000). Circadian clock resetting by sleep deprivation without exercise in the Syrian hamster. *J Neurosci*, *20*(24), 9326–9332.

Aschoff, J., & Wever, R. (1976). Human circadian rhythms: a multioscillatory system. *Fed Proc*, *35*, 2326–2332.

Azogu, I., de la Tremblaye, P. B., Dunbar, M., Lebreton, M., LeMarec, N., & Plamondon, H. (2015). Acute sleep deprivation enhances avoidance learning and spatial memory and induces delayed alterations in neurochemical expression of GR, TH, DRD1, pCREB and Ki67 in rats. *Behav Brain Res*, *279*, 177–190. doi: 10.1016/j.bbr.2014.11.015

Barbato, G., & Wehr, T. A. (1998). Homeostatic regulation of REM sleep in humans during extended sleep. *Sleep*, *21*(3), 267–276.

Beersma, D. G., & Daan, S. (2015). On the role of sleep intensity in a model of sleep regulation. *Sleep*, *38*(5), 661–662. doi: 10.5665/sleep.4646

Beersma, D. G., Dijk, D. J., Blok, C. G., & Everhardus, I. (1990). REM sleep deprivation during 5 hours leads to an immediate REM sleep rebound and to suppression of non-REM sleep intensity. *Electroencephalogr Clin Neurophysiol*, *76*(2), 114–122. doi: 10.1016/0013-4694(90)90209-3

Bellinger, L. L., & Mendel, V. E. (1975). Effects of deprivation and time of refeeding on food intake. *Physiol Behav*, *14*(1), 43–46.

Benington, J. H., & Heller, H. C. (1994a). Does the function of REM sleep concern non-REM sleep or waking? *Prog Neurobiol*, *44*, 433–449.

Benington, J. H., & Heller, H. C. (1994b). REM-sleep timing is controlled homeostatically by accumulation of REM-sleep propensity in non-REM sleep. *Am J Physiol*, *266*(6), R1992–R2000.

Benington, J. H., & Heller, H. C. (1999). Implications of sleep deprivation experiments for understanding of sleep homeostasis. *Sleep*, *22*(8), 1033–1037.

Berger, R. J., & Oswald, I. (1962). Effects of sleep deprivation on behaviour, subsequent sleep, and dreaming. *J Mental Sci*, *108*, 457–465.

Blum, I. D., Zhu, L., Moquin, L., Kokoeva, M. V., Gratton, A., Giros, B., & Storch, K. F. (2014). A highly tunable dopaminergic oscillator generates ultradian rhythms of behavioral arousal. *Elife*, *3*. doi: 10.7554/eLife.05105

Bonnet, M. H., & Rosa, R. R. (1987). Sleep and performance in young adults and older normals and insomniacs during acute sleep loss and recovery. *Biol Psychol, 25*, 153–172.

Borbély, A. (2022). The two-process model of sleep regulation: beginnings and outlook. *J Sleep Res, 31*(4), e13598. doi:10.1111/jsr.13598

Borbély, A. A. (1982a). Sleep regulation: circadian rhythm and homeostasis. In D. Ganten & D. W. Pfaff (Eds.), *Sleep. Clinical and Experimental Aspects* (pp. 83–103). Berlin: Springer-Verlag.

Borbély, A. A. (1982b). A two process model of sleep regulation. *Hum Neurobiol, 1*, 195–204.

Borbély, A. A., Åkerstedt, T., Benoit, O., Holsboer, F., & Oswald, I. (1991). Hypnotics and sleep physiology: a consensus report. *Eur Arch Psychiatry Clin Neurosci, 241*, 13–21.

Borbély, A. A., Baumann, F., Brandeis, D., Strauch, I., & Lehmann, D. (1981). Sleep deprivation: effect on sleep stages and EEG power density in man. *Electroencephalogr Clin Neurophysiol, 51*, 483–493.

Borbély, A. A., Daan, S., Wirz-Justice, A., & Deboer, T. (2016). The two-process model of sleep regulation: a reappraisal. *J Sleep Res, 25*(2), 131–143. doi: 10.1111/jsr.12371

Borbély, A. A., & Neuhaus, H. U. (1979). Sleep deprivation: effects on sleep and EEG in the rat. *J Comp Physiol, 133*, 71–87.

Brandt, J., & Leong, C. (2017). Benzodiazepines and Z-drugs: an updated review of major adverse outcomes reported on in epidemiologic research. *Drugs R D, 17*(4), 493–507. doi: 10.1007/s40268-017-0207-7

Brunner, D. P., Dijk, D. J., & Borbély, A. A. (1993). Repeated partial sleep deprivation progressively changes in EEG during sleep and wakefulness. *Sleep, 16*(2), 100–113.

Brunner, D. P., Dijk, D.-J., Münch, M., & Borbély, A. A. (1991). Effect of zolpidem on sleep and sleep EEG spectra in healthy young men. *Psychopharmacology, 104*, 1–5.

Brunner, D. P., Dijk, D. J., Tobler, I., & Borbély, A. A. (1990). Effect of partial sleep deprivation on sleep stages and EEG power spectra: evidence for non-REM and REM sleep homeostasis. *Electroencephalogr Clin Neurophysiol, 75*, 492–499.

Cajochen, C., Brunner, D. P., Kräuchi, K., Graw, P., & Wirz-Justice, A. (1995). Power density in theta/alpha frequencies of the waking EEG progressively increases during sustained wakefulness. *Sleep, 18*(10), 890–894.

Campbell, S. S., Murphy, P. J., & Stauble, T. N. (2005). Effects of a nap on nighttime sleep and waking function in older subjects. *J Am Geriatr Soc, 53*(1), 48–53.

Cannon, W. B. (1929). Organization for physiological homeostasis. *Physiol Rev, 9*(3), 399–431.

Carskadon, M. A., & Dement, W. C. (1980). Distribution of REM sleep on a 90 minute sleep-wake schedule. *Sleep, 2*(3), 309–317.

Carskadon, M. A., & Dement, W. C. (2011). Normal human sleep: an overview. In M. H. Kryger, T. Roth & W. C. Dement (Eds.), *Principles and Practice of Sleep Medicine* (5th ed., pp. 16–26). St. Louis: Elsevier.

Cartwright, R. D., Monroe, L. J., & Palmer, C. (1967). Individual differences in response to REM deprivation. *Arch Gen Psychiatr, 16*, 297–303.

Christ, G., de Koninck, J., Hébert, M., Carrier, J., Lamarche, C., & Dufour, S. (1996). Body temperature and the return of slow wave activity in extended sleep. *Electroencephalogr Clin Neurophysiol, 98*, 42–50.

Clasadonte, J., McIver, S. R., Schmitt, L. I., Halassa, M. M., & Haydon, P. G. (2014). Chronic sleep restriction disrupts sleep homeostasis and behavioral sensitivity to alcohol by reducing the extracellular accumulation of adenosine. *J Neurosci, 34*(5), 1879–1891. doi: 10.1523/JNEUROSCI.2870-12.2014

Cooperman, N. R., Mullin, F. J., & Kleitman, N. (1934). Studies on the physiology of sleep. XI. Further observations on the effects of prolonged sleeplessness. *Am J Physiol, 107*(3), 589–593.

Czeisler, C. A., Weitzman, E. D., Moore-Ede, M. C., Zimmerman, J. C., & Knauer, R. S. (1980). Human sleep: its duration and organization depend on its circadian phase. *Science, 210*(4475), 1264–1267.

Czeisler, C. A., Zimmerman, J. C., Ronda, J. M., Moore-Ede, M. C., & Weitzman, E. D. (1980). Timing of REM sleep is coupled to the circadian rhythm of body temperature in man. *Sleep, 2*, 329–346.

Daan, S., Barnes, B. M., & Strijkstra, A. M. (1991). Warming up for sleep? Ground squirrels sleep during arousals from hibernation. *Neurosci Lett, 128*(2), 265–268.

Daan, S., Beersma, D. G. M., & Borbély, A. A. (1984). Timing of human sleep: recovery process gated by a circadian pacemaker. *Am J Physiol, 246*, R161–R178.

Dantz, B., Edgar, D. M., & Dement, W. C. (1994). Circadian rhythms in narcolepsy: Studies on a 90 minute day. *Electroencephalogr Clin Neurophysiol, 90*, 24–35.

Day, T. A. (2005). Defining stress as a prelude to mapping its neurocircuitry: no help from allostasis. *Prog Neuropsychopharmacol Biol Psychiatry, 29*(8), 1195–1200. doi: 10.1016/j.pnpbp.2005.08.005

Deboer, T., & Tobler, I. (2000). Slow waves in the sleep electroencephalogram after daily torpor are homeostatically regulated. *NeuroReport, 11*(4), 881–885.

Deboer, T., Vansteensel, M. J., Détári, L., & Meijer, J. H. (2003). Sleep states alter activity of suprachiasmatic nucleus neurons. *Nat Neurosci, 6*(10), 1086–1090. doi: 10.1038/nn1122

Dement, W. C. (1960). The effect of dream deprivation. *Science, 131*(3415), 1705–1707.

Deurveilher, S., Rusak, B., & Semba, K. (2012). Time-of-day modulation of homeostatic and allostatic sleep responses to chronic sleep restriction in rats. *Am J Physiol Regul Integr Comp Physiol, 302*(12), R1411–1425. doi: 10.1152/ajpregu.00678.2011

Deurveilher, S., Shewchuk, S. M., & Semba, K. (2021). Homeostatic sleep and body temperature responses to acute sleep deprivation are preserved following chronic sleep restriction in rats. *J Sleep Res, 30*(5), 1–14. doi: 10.1111/jsr.13348

Dijk, D.-J. (2009). Regulation and functional correlates of slow wave sleep *J Clin Sleep Med, 5*(2), S6–S15.

Dijk, D.-J., Brunner, D. P., & Borbély, A. A. (1991). EEG power density during recovery sleep in the morning. *Electroencephalogr Clin Neurophysiol, 78*(3), 203–214.

Dijk, D.-J., Cajochen, C., Tobler, I., & Borbély, A. A. (1991). Sleep extension in humans: sleep stages, EEG power spectra and body temperature. *Sleep, 14*(4), 294–306.

Dijk, D. J., & Czeisler, C. A. (1994). Paradoxical timing of the circadian rhythm of sleep propensity serves to consolidate sleep and wakefulness in humans. *Neurosci Lett, 166*, 63–68.

Dijk, D. J., & Czeisler, C. A. (1995). Contribution of the circadian pacemaker and the sleep homeostat to sleep propensity, sleep structure, electroencephalographic slow waves, and sleep spindle activity in humans. *J Neurosci, 15*, 3526–3538.

Dijk, D. -J., Shanahan, T. L., Duffy, J., Ronda, J., & Czeisler, C. (1997). Variation of electroencephalographic activity during non-rapid eye movement and rapid eye movement sleep with phase of circadian melatonin rhythm in humans. *J Physiol, 505*(3), 851–858.

Ding, F., O'Donnell, J., Xu, Q., Kang, N., Goldman, N., & Nedergaard, M. (2016). Changes in the composition of brain interstitial ions control the sleep-wake cycle. *Science, 352*(6285), 550–555. doi: 10.1126/science.aad4821

Duffy, J., Dijk, D.-J., Klerman, E., & Czeisler, C. (1998). Later endogenous circadian temperature nadir relative to an earlier wake time in older people. *Am J Physiol, 275*, R1478–R1487.

Edgar, D. M., Dement, W. C., & Fuller, C. A. (1993). Effect of SCN lesions on sleep in squirrel monkeys: evidence for opponent processes in sleep-wake regulation. *J Neurosci, 13*, 1065–1079.

Endo, S., Kobayashi, T., Yamamoto, T., Fukuda, H., Sasaki, M., & Ohta, T. (1981). Persistence of the circadian rhythm of REM sleep: a variety of experimental manipulations of the sleep-wake cycle. *Sleep, 4*(3), 319–328.

Endo, T., Roth, C., Landolt, H.-P., Werth, E., Aeschbach, D., Achermann, P., & Borbély, A. A. (1998). Selective REM sleep deprivation in humans: effects on sleep and sleep EEG. *AJP: Regul Integr Comp Physiol, 274*, R1186–R1194.

Feinberg, I., Fein, G., & Floyd, T. C. (1980). EEG patterns during and following extended sleep in young adults. *Electroencephalogr Clin Neurophysiol, 50*, 467–476.

Feinberg, I., Fein, G., Walker, J. M., Price, L. J., Floyd, T. C., & March, J. D. (1977). Flurazepam effects on slow-wave sleep: stage 4 suppressed but number of delta waves constant. *Science, 198*(4319), 847–848.

Feinberg, I., Maloney, T., & March, J. D. (1992). Precise conservation of NREM period 1 (NREMP1) delta across naps and nocturnal sleep: implications for REM latency and NREM/REM alternation. *Sleep, 15*(5), 400–403.

Fothergill, E., Guo, J., Howard, L., Kerns, J. C., Knuth, N. D., Brychta, R., … Hall, K. D. (2016). Persistent metabolic adaptation 6 years after "The Biggest Loser" competition. *Obesity (Silver Spring), 24*(8), 1612–1619. doi: 10.1002/oby.21538

Frank, M. G. (2021). Challenging sleep homeostasis. *Neurobiol Sleep Circ Rhythms, 10*, 100060. doi:10.1016/j.nbscr.2021.100060

Franken, P., Tobler, I., & Borbély, A. A. (1991). Sleep homeostasis in the rat: simulation of the time course of EEG slow-wave activity. *Neurosci Lett, 130*, 141–144.

Gizowski, C., Zaelzer, C., & Bourque, C. W. (2016). Clock-driven vasopressin neurotransmission mediates anticipatory thirst prior to sleep. *Nature, 537*(7622), 685–688. doi: 10.1038/nature19756

Gross, C. G. (1998). Claude Bernard and the constancy of the internal environment. *Neuroscientist, 4*, 380–385.

Gulevich, G., Dement, W. C., & Johnson, L. (1966). Psychiatric and EEG observations on a case of prolonged (264 hours) wakefulness. *Arch Gen Psychiatr, 15*, 29–35.

Guzeev, M. A., Kurmazov, N. S., & Ekimova, I. V. (2023). [Chronic sleep restriction in rats leads to a weakening of compensatory reactions in response to acute sleep deprivation]. *Zh Nevrol Psikhiatr Im S S Korsakova, 123*(5. Vyp. 2), 35–42. doi: 10.17116/jnevro202312305235

Haimov, I., & Lavie, P. (1997). Circadian characteristics of sleep propensity function in healthy elderly: a comparison with young adults *Sleep, 20*(4), 294–300.

Herculano-Houzel, S. (2012). The remarkable, yet not extraordinary, human brain as a scaled-up primate brain and its associated cost. *Proc Natl Acad Sci U S A, 109*(Suppl 1), 10661–10668. doi: 10.1073/pnas.1201895109

Hubbard, J., Gent, T. C., Hoekstra, M. M. B., Emmenegger, Y., Mongrain, V., Landolt, H. P., … Franken, P. (2020). Rapid fast-delta decay following prolonged wakefulness marks a phase of wake-inertia in NREM sleep. *Nat Commun, 11*(1), 1–16. doi: 10.1038/s41467-020-16915-0

Ibuka, N., & Kawamura, H. (1975). Loss of circadian rhythm in sleep-wakefulness cycle in the rat by suprachiasmatic nucleus lesions. *Brain Res, 96*, 76–81.

Jarvis, E. D., Güntürkün, O., Bruce, L., Csillag, A., Karten, H., Kuenzel, W., … Consortium, A. B. N. (2005). Avian brains and a new understanding of vertebrate brain evolution. *Nat Rev Neurosci, 6*(2), 151–159. doi: 10.1038/nrn1606

Johnson, L. C. (1980). The REM cycle is a sleep-dependent rhythm. *Sleep, 2*(3), 299–307.

Johnsson, R. D., Connelly, F., Vyssotski, A. L., Roth II, T. C., & Lesku, J. A. (2021). Homeostatic regulation of NREM sleep, but not REM sleep, in Australian magpies. *Sleep, 45*(2), zsab218. doi:10.1093/sleep/zsab218

Ju, Y. S., Ooms, S. J., Sutphen, C., Macauley, S. L., Zangrilli, M. A., Jerome, G., … Holtzman, D. M. (2017). Slow wave sleep disruption increases cerebrospinal fluid amyloid-beta levels. *Brain, 140*(8), 2104–2111. doi: 10.1093/brain/awx148

Junek, A., Rusak, B., & Semba, K. (2010). Short-term sleep deprivation may alter the dynamics of hippocampal cell proliferation in adult rats. *Neuroscience, 170*(4), 1140–1152. doi: 10.1016/j.neuroscience.2010.08.018

Kang, J. E., Lim, M. M., Bateman, R. J., Lee, J. J., Smyth, L. P., Cirrito, J. R., … Holtzman, D. M. (2009). Amyloid-β dynamics are regulated by orexin and the sleep-wake cycle. *Science, 326*(5955), 1005–1007. doi: 10.1126/science.1180962

Kilduff, T. S., Sharp, F. R., & Heller, H. C. (1982). [14 C]2-deoxyglucose uptake in ground squirrel brain during hibernation. *J Neurosci, 2*, 143–157.

Kim, Y., Bolortuya, Y., Chen, L., Basheer, R., McCarley, R. W., & Strecker, R. E. (2012). Decoupling of sleepiness from sleep time and intensity during chronic sleep restriction: evidence for a role of the adenosine system. *Sleep, 35*(6), 861–869. doi: 10.5665/sleep.1890

Kim, Y., Elmenhorst, D., Weisshaupt, A., Wedekind, F., Kroll, T., McCarley, R. W., … Bauer, A. (2015). Chronic sleep restriction induces long-lasting changes in adenosine and noradrenaline receptor density in the rat brain. *J Sleep Res, 24*(5), 549–558. doi: 10.1111/jsr.12300

Kim, Y., Laposky, A., Bergmann, B., & Turek, F. (2007). Repeated sleep restriction in rats leads to homeostatic and allostatic responses during recovery sleep. *Proc Natl Acad Sci USA, 104*(25), 10697–10702. doi: 10.1073/pnas.0610351104

Kleitman, N. (1923). Studies on the physiology of sleep. I. The effects of prolonged sleeplessness on man. *Am J Physiol, 66*, 67–92.

Kleitman, N. (1982). Basic rest-activity cycle - 22 years later. *Sleep, 5*(4), 311–317.

Klerman, E. B., Boulos, Z., Edgar, D. M., Mistlberger, R. E., & Moore-Ede, M. C. (1999). Circadian and homeostatic influences on sleep in the squirrel monkey: sleep after sleep deprivation. *Sleep, 22*(1), 45–59.

Larkin, J., & Heller, H. (1999). Sleep after arousal from hibernation is not homeostatically regulated. *Am J Physiol, 276*, R522–R529.

Lavie, P. (1986). Ultrashort sleep-waking schedule. III. "Gates" and "forbidden zones" for sleep. *Electroencephalogr Clin Neurophysiol, 63*(5), 414–425.

Lavie, P. (1987). Ultrashort sleep-wake cycle: timing of REM sleep. Evidence for sleep-dependent and sleep-independent components of the REM cycle. *Sleep, 10*(1), 62–68.

Le Bon, O. (2021). An asymmetrical hypothesis for the NREM-REM sleep alternation-what is the NREM-REM cycle? *Front Neurosci, 15*, 627193. doi:10.3389/fnins.2021.627193

Le Bon, O., Popa, D., Streel, E., Alexandre, C., Lena, C., Linkowski, P., & Adrien, J. (2007). Ultradian cycles in mice: definitions and links with REMS and NREMS. *J Comp Physiol A, 193*(10), 1021–1032. doi: 10.1007/s00359-007-0253-7

Leemburg, S., Vyazovskiy, V. V., Olcese, J., Bassetti, C. L., Tononi, G., & Cirelli, C. (2010). Sleep homeostasis in the rat is preserved during chronic sleep restriction. *Proc Natl Acad Sci USA, 107*(36), 15939–15944.

McCarthy, A., Wafford, K., Shanks, E., Ligocki, M., Edgar, D. M., & Dijk, D. J. (2016). REM sleep homeostasis in the absence of REM sleep: effects of antidepressants. *Neuropharmacology, 108*, 415–425. doi: 10.1016/j.neuropharm.2016.04.047

McEwen, B. S. (2006). Sleep deprivation as a neurobiologic and physiologic stressor: allostasis and allostatic load. *Metabolism Clin Exp, 55*(Supplement 2), S20–S23. doi: 0.1016/j.metabol.2006.07.008

McEwen, B. S., & Stellar, E. (1993). Stress and the individual. Mechanisms leading to disease. *Arch Intern Med, 153*, 2093–2101.

Michael, J., & McFarland, J. (2011). The core principles ("big ideas") of physiology: results of faculty surveys. *Adv Physiol Educ, 35*(4), 336–341. doi: 10.1152/advan.00004.2011

Mistlberger, R. E., Bergmann, B. M., Waldenar, W., & Rechtschaffen, A. (1983). Recovery sleep following sleep deprivation in intact and suprachiasmatic nuclei-lesioned rats. *Sleep, 6*, 217–233.

Moore-Ede, M. C. (1986). Physiology of the circadian timing system: predictive versus reactive homeostasis. *Am J Physiol, 250*, R735–R752.

Morden, B., Mitchell, G., & Dement, W. C. (1967). Selective REM sleep deprivation and compensation phenomena in the rat. *Brain Res, 5*, 339–349.

Morin, L. P., Fitzgerald, K. M., & Zucker, I. (1977). Estradiol shortens the period of hamster circadian rhythms. *Science, 196*, 305–307.

Moses, J., Lubin, A., Johnson, L. C., & Naitoh, P. (1977). The rapid eye movement cycle is a sleep-dependent rhythm. *Nature, 265*, 360–361.

Mrosovsky, N. (1990). *Rheostasis: The Physiology of Change*. New York: Oxford University Press.

Mrosovsky, N. (1996). Locomotor activity and non-photic influences on circadian clocks. *Biol Rev, 71*, 343–372.

Nakamura, T. J., Nakamura, W., Yamazaki, S., Kudo, T., Cutler, T., Colwell, C. S., & Block, G. D. (2011). Age-related decline in circadian output. *J Neurosci, 31*(28), 10201–10205. doi: 10.1523/jneurosci.0451-11.2011

Ooms, S., Overeem, S., Besse, K., Rikkert, M. O., Verbeek, M., & Claassen, J. A. (2014). Effect of 1 night of total sleep deprivation on cerebrospinal fluid β-amyloid 42 in healthy middle-aged men: a randomized clinical trial. *JAMA Neurol, 71*(8), 971–977. doi: 10.1001/jamaneurol.2014.1173

Parmeggiani, P. L., Cianci, T., Calasso, M., Zamboni, G., & Perez, E. (1980). Quantitative analysis of short term deprivation and recovery of desynchronized sleep in cats. *Electroencephalogr Clin Neurophysiol, 50*, 293–302.

Patrick, G. T. W., & Gilbert, J. A. (1896). On the effects of loss of sleep. *Psych Rev, 3*(5), 469–483.

Popov, V. I., & Bocharova, L. S. (1992). Hibernation-induced structural changes in synaptic contacts between mossy fibres and hippocampal pyramidal neurons. *Neuroscience, 48*(1), 53–62.

Prabhakar, N. R., & Semenza, G. L. (2015). Oxygen sensing and homeostasis. *Physiology (Bethesda), 30*(5), 340–348. doi: 10.1152/physiol.00022.2015

Rechtschaffen, A., Bergmann, B. M., Gilliland, M. A., & Bauer, K. (1999). Effects of method, duration, and sleep stage on rebounds from sleep deprivation in the rat. *Sleep, 22*(1), 11–31.

Reebs, S. G., & Mrosovsky, N. (1989). Large phase-shifts of circadian rhythms caused by induced running in a re-entrainment paradigm: The role of pulse duration and light. *J Comp Physiol A, 165*, 819–825.

Ross, J. J. (1965). Neurological findings after prolonged sleep deprivation. *Arch Neurol, 12*, 399–403.

Rusak, B. (1981). Vertebrate behavioral rhythms. In J. Aschoff (Ed.), *Biological Rhythms* (pp. 183–205). New York: Plenum Press.

Schifano, F., Chiappini, S., Corkery, J. M., & Guirguis, A. (2019). An insight into Z-drug abuse and dependence: an examination of reports to the European Medicines Agency Database of Suspected Adverse Drug Reactions. *Int J Neuropsychopharmacol, 22*(4), 270–277. doi: 10.1093/ijnp/pyz007

Schulz, H., Dirlich, G., & Zulley, J. (1975). Phase shift in the REM sleep rhythm. *Pflügers Archiv, 358*, 203–212.

Shea, J., Mochizuki, T., Sagvaag, V., Aspevik, T., Bjorkum, A., & Datta, S. (2008). Rapid eye movement (REM) sleep homeostatic regulatory processes in the rat: changes in the sleep–wake stages and electroencephalographic power spectra. *Brain Res, 1213*, 48–56. doi: 10.1016/j.brainres.2008.03.062

Siegel, J. M. (2022). Sleep function: an evolutionary perspective. *Lancet Neurol, 21*(10), 937–946. doi: 10.1016/s1474-4422(22)00210-1

Skorucak, J., Arbon, E. L., Dijk, D. J., & Achermann, P. (2018). Response to chronic sleep restriction, extension, and subsequent total sleep deprivation in humans: adaptation or preserved sleep homeostasis? *Sleep, 41*(7), 1–17. doi:10.1093/sleep/zsy078

Speakman, J. R., Levitsky, D. A., Allison, D. B., Bray, M. S., de Castro, J. M., Clegg, D. J., … Westerterp-Plantenga, M. S. (2011). Set points, settling points and some alternative models: theoretical options to understand how genes and environments combine to regulate body adiposity. *Dis Model Mech, 4*(6), 733–745. doi: 10.1242/dmm.008698

Stenuit, P., & Kerkhofs, M. (2005). Age modulates the effects of sleep restriction in women. *Sleep, 28*(10), 1283–1286.

Stephenson, R., Caron, A. M., & Famina, S. (2015). Behavioral sleep-wake homeostasis and EEG delta power are decoupled by chronic sleep restriction in the rat. *Sleep, 38*(5), 685–697. doi: 10.5665/sleep.4656

Sterling, P. (2012). Allostasis: a model of predictive regulation. *Physiol Behav, 106*(1), 5–15. doi: 10.1016/j.physbeh.2011.06.004

Strijkstra, A., & Daan, S. (1998). Dissimilarity of slow-wave activity enhancement by torpor and sleep deprivation in a hibernator. *Am J Physiol, 275*, R1110–R1117.

Strogatz, S. H., Kronauer, R. E., & Czeisler, C. A. (1986). Circadian regulation dominates homeostatic control of sleep length and prior wake length in humans. *Sleep, 9*, 353–364.

Strogatz, S. H., Kronauer, R. E., & Czeisler, C. A. (1987). Circadian pacemaker interferes with sleep onset at specific times each day: role of insomnia. *Am J Physiol, 253*, R172–R178.

Tatsuki, F., Sunagawa, G. A., Shi, S., Susaki, E. A., Yukinaga, H., Perrin, D., ... Ueda, H. R. (2016). Involvement of Ca^{2+}-dependent hyperpolarization in sleep duration in mammals. *Neuron, 90*(1), 70–85. doi: 10.1016/j.neuron.2016.02.032

Thomas, D. W., Dorais, M., & Bergeron, J., -M. (1990). Winter energy budgets and costs of arousal for hibernating little brown bats, *Myotis lucifugus*. *J Mammal, 71*(3), 475–479.

Tobler, I., & Borbély, A. A. (1988). Sleep and EEG spectra in the pigeon (*Columba livia*) under baseline conditions and after sleep deprivation. *J Comp Physiol A, 163*(6), 729–738.

Tobler, I., & Borbély, A. A. (1990). The effect of 3-h and 6-h sleep deprivation on sleep and EEG spectra of the rat. *Behav Brain Res, 36*, 73–78.

Tobler, I., Borbély, A. A., & Groos, G. (1983). The effect of sleep deprivation on sleep in rats with suprachiasmatic lesions. *Neurosci Lett, 42*, 49–54.

van Hasselt, S. J., Rusche, M., Vyssotski, A. L., Verhulst, S., Rattenborg, N. C., & Meerlo, P. (2019). The European starling (Sturnus vulgaris) shows signs of NREM sleep homeostasis but has very little REM sleep and no REM sleep homeostasis. *Sleep, 43*(6), zsz311. doi: 10.1093/sleep/zsz311

Varga, A. W., Wohlleber, M. E., Giménez, S., Romero, S., Alonso, J. F., Ducca, E. L., ... Osorio, R. S. (2016). Reduced slow-wave sleep is associated with high cerebrospinal fluid Aβ42 levels in cognitively normal elderly. *Sleep, 39*(11), 2041–2048. doi: 0.5665/sleep.6240

Vivaldi, E. A., Ocampo, A., Wyneken, U., Roncagliolo, M., & Zapata, A. M. (1994). Short term homeostasis of active sleep and the architecture of sleep in the rat. *J Neurophysiol, 72*(4), 1745–1755.

von Economo, C. (1930). Sleep as a problem of localization. *J Nerv Ment Dis, 71*(3), 249–259.

Wang, L., & Aton, S. J. (2022). Ultrastructural analyses reflect the effects of sleep and sleep loss on neuronal cell biology. *Sleep, 45*(5), zsac047. doi:10.1093/sleep/zsac047

Wang, L. C. H. (1979). Time patterns and metabolic rates of natural torpor in the Richardson's ground squirrel. *Can J Zool, 57*, 149–155.

Wang, Y., Melgers, M., Meijer, J. H., & Deboer, T. (2023). Comparison of sleep deprivation and a low dose of ketamine on sleep and the electroencephalogram in Brown Norway rats. *J Sleep Res, 32*(5), e13863. doi:10.1111/jsr.13863

Wang, Y., Minami, Y., Ode, K. L., & Ueda, H. R. (2022). The role of calcium and CaMKII in sleep. *Front Syst Neurosci, 16*, 1–15. doi: 10.3389/fnsys.2022.1059421

Webb, W. B., & Agnew, H. W. (1965). Sleep: effects of a restricted regime. *Science, 150*(3704), 1745–1747.

Werth, E., Dijk, D.-J., Achermann, P., & Borbély, A. A. (1996). Dynamics of the sleep EEG after an early evening nap: experimental data and simulations. *Am J Physiol, 271*, R501–R510.

Wirtshafter, D., & Davis, J. D. (1977). Set points, settling points, and the control of body weight. *Physiol Behav, 19*, 75–78.

Wurts, S. W., & Edgar, D. M. (2000). Circadian and homeostatic control of rapid eye movement (REM) sleep: promotion of REM tendency by the suprachiasmatic nucleus. *J Neurosci, 20*(11), 4300–4310.

Wyatt, J. K., Ritz-De Cecco, A., Czeisler, C. A., & Dijk, D.-J. (1999). Circadian temperature and melatonin rhythms, sleep, and neurobehavioral function in humans living on a 20-h day. *Am J Physiol, 277*, R1152–R1163.

Xie, L., Kang, H., Xu, Q., Chen, M. J., Liao, Y., Thiyagarajan, M., ... Nedergaard, M. (2013). Sleep drives metabolite clearance from the adult brain. *Science, 342*(6156), 373–377. doi: 10.1126/science.1241224

Yamada, N., Shimoda, K., Ohi, K., Takahashi, S., & Takahashi, K. (1988). Free-access to a running wheel shortens the period of free-running rhythm in blinded rats. *Physiol Behav, 42*, 87–91.

Zada, D., Sela, Y., Matosevich, N., Monsonego, A., Lerer-Goldshtein, T., Nir, Y., & Appelbaum, L. (2021). Parp1 promotes sleep, which enhances DNA repair in neurons. *Mol Cell, 81*(24), 4979–4993.e4977. doi: 10.1016/j.molcel.2021.10.026

Zucker, I. (1971). Light-dark rhythms in rat eating and drinking behavior. *Physiol Behav, 6*, 115–126.

CHAPTER 6

Cultural and Environmental Effects on Sleep

6.1 OVERVIEW

This chapter reviews how culture and the linked factors of geography and technology affect the regulation of sleep. It describes national differences in sleep patterns; the role of socioeconomic and ethnic factors within large, diverse nations; and the impact of environmental, social, and technological influences. It discusses the evidence related to whether access to electric lighting has changed historical sleep patterns and durations. A final topic related to sleep and cultural differences is the controversy centered on the risks and benefits of infants sharing a sleeping space with their parents or sleeping in a separate room.

6.2 Cultural, social, and geographic influences on sleep

Most of the descriptions of normal human sleep in the preceding chapters emerged from studies conducted in laboratories that were established in the 20th century or later. The sleep environments in these laboratories were designed to mimic many of the conditions in the homes of people in contemporary "industrial" societies.[1] One important exception, however, is that in most laboratory studies the participant sleeps alone, which is important for research and clinical studies to avoid any impact of bed partners on sleep patterns or quality. Sleeping alone, however, is not the norm for many adults in these societies.

Sleep laboratory conditions include the following features:

- individual sleeping spaces that are physically isolated from adjacent functional spaces, which in peoples' homes would be areas used for cooking, eating, entertainment, or socializing;
- a heavily padded sleep surface with a variety of covers and pillows;
- complete darkness or very low light intensity;
- physical barriers that reduce or eliminate environmental noise;
- regulatory systems that maintain stable room temperatures;
- a single, continuous, nocturnal sleep opportunity (except for MSLT and similar studies; see Section 2.7).

These were not, however, typical sleep conditions for most people in industrial societies until the recent past; nor are they typical of conditions in some current societies. These were also not the conditions under which people slept in the more distant past when the resources and devices needed to produce these environmental features were not available.

The single nightly sleep opportunity that is standard in laboratory studies is also not a universal pattern among adults in current societies. Midday naps (siestas) among adults, for example, are common in some traditional societies, where heat or water stress threaten human and animal health at that time of day. They are also common and considered normative in some African, Asian, and Mediterranean cultures, and those in the western hemisphere influenced by them; but they are uncommon in other Asian countries, northern Europe, and parts of North America. The typical afternoon timing of siestas may be related to an increased tendency for sleepiness (post-lunch dip) that can be observed in adults who do not usually nap at that time as well as in other primates (Carskadon & Dement, 1992); see **Figures 2.11** and **8.11 C**.

An example of sleep patterns in a society in which siestas are common was summarized in a study of Greek

[1] This term is used as a shorthand for the increasingly urbanized societies in much of the world today that function on the basis of large-scale agricultural, industrial, and post-industrial economies. These societies are contrasted to 'traditional' or preindustrial societies that rely primarily on hunting, gathering, herding, and small-scale agriculture.

adolescents (14–18 years old). It found that nearly half the group reported regular siestas and an equal proportion reported occasional siestas, with a median duration of 2 h (range: 0.5–4.5 h). Although some of these adolescents reported problems with daytime sleepiness (as do many in non-siesta societies), it is not surprising that those having regular siestas were less likely to express such complaints (Paraskakis et al., 2008).

Sleeping during the day might be expected to contribute to increased difficulty in falling asleep at night. However, a survey of >500,000 people in China found that the 20% reporting daytime napping had a significantly lower risk of reporting insomnia symptoms than those who did not nap (Chen et al., 2018), suggesting a complex interaction between daytime napping and perceived nightly sleep quality.

The attitudes toward napping may be changing in some historically "non-siesta" societies (e.g., Japan). Some businesses have begun to permit and even encourage short afternoon naps among their employees. Nap facilities available for rent are found in business districts and airports in cities in several countries (**Figure 6.1**).

Daytime sleep is virtually universal in young children, but it follows different developmental paths depending on culturally determined practices. Parents of young children (up to 3 years old) in 17 countries, including 12 predominantly Asian countries (including India, Japan, China, Thailand, Philippines, and others) and five predominantly Caucasian "Western" nations (United Kingdom, United States, Canada, Australia, New Zealand), reported that their children took similar length naps. Those in Asian countries, however, had later bedtimes at night, resulting in somewhat shorter total daily sleep durations (e.g., 11.6 h in Japan vs. 13.3 h in New Zealand) (Mindell et al., 2010). In a similar internet-based survey asking about sleep in older children (3–6 years old) in 13 countries, parents in Asian countries still reported later bedtimes, but also more common daytime naps than in Western countries, resulting in daily sleep totals that were quite similar across countries. By 5 years of age, however, 60.7% of children in Asian countries, but only 6.8% of children in Western countries, still took naps (Mindell et al., 2013).

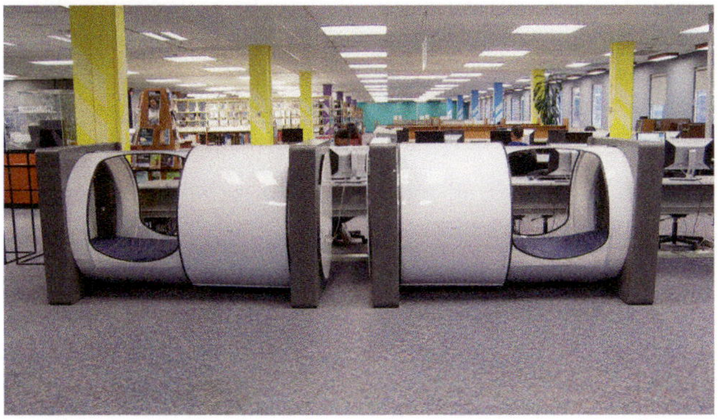

Figure 6.1 Sleep pods were installed to allow students to take naps in a library at the British Columbia Institute of Technology. Dillon Hodgin/CBC Licensing.

The consolidated daily wake phase that emerges during development and is maintained in some societies during adulthood often changes again with advancing age. Whether aging itself or the relaxation of work and family demands after retirement age is responsible, a bimodal pattern that includes an afternoon nap, or even a polyphasic pattern with more than one daily nap, may reappear in older people.

Other cultural practices also have an impact on sleep timing. One example is found among adult Muslims who observe Ramadan annually by not eating or drinking during daylight hours for a full lunar month. This practice shifts food intake and other behaviors to different times of day than is typical during the rest of the year. Studies have shown delayed sleep onset and reduced total sleep times during Ramadan as well as an increased tendency to sleep during the day (Roky et al., 2003; Roky et al., 2001).

Less formally prescribed, but nevertheless prevalent, cultural practices can affect sleep timing. There are, for example, significant cultural differences in the timing of major daily meals that interact with sleep and work schedules. During a visit to Barcelona, Spain in the 1990s, I was surprised to find that I could not get an evening meal served in a restaurant as early as 20:00. In fact, native Barcelonans were hardly beginning to gather for predinner drinks at that hour, with dinner following at 22:00 or later. The groups settling in for dinner at that time included families with very young children.[2]

A typical daily schedule in Spain involved eating the major meal of the day in the early afternoon, followed by a siesta period, then work hours extending into the evening, followed by a lighter late-night meal. Thus, meal timing, sleep schedules, and work schedules were linked together into a pattern that differed from that typically observed in North America and other non-siesta regions. For a description of the origin of this daily pattern and how economic pressures and changing lifestyles have more recently put it at risk, see https://tinyurl.com/y38w4tvq.

Formal surveys of sleep timing in other countries have described various patterns. Questions asked of >35,000 respondents across 10 countries resulted in reports of quite different sleep characteristics, self-reported sleep quality, and daytime sleepiness. Average reported sleep duration was ~7.5

[2] When questioned about this habit, one Barcelonan asserted that residents of Madrid were more extreme and often did not start their late-night meal before midnight; I did not have a chance to verify this claim.

h across these countries, but national means ranged from 6.9 h in Japan to 13.4 h in Portugal. Regular napping was reported by 12% of Japanese and 42.4% of Brazilian respondents. There were also large differences in self-reported poor sleep, symptoms of insomnia, or feeling very or dangerously sleepy during the day, with the proportion reporting daytime sleepiness ranging from 6.2% in China to 24.5% in South Africa (Soldatos et al., 2005). Even among adolescents in more similar, English-speaking countries (Australia and the United States), there were some differences in sleep patterns: Australian adolescents had later school start times, had bedtimes set more frequently by parents, and slept ~47 min longer on school nights than their American counterparts (Short et al., 2013).

These surveys necessarily drew samples from only a few locations in large, diverse countries (e.g., China, United States, India). Multiethnic nations, especially those with a history of diverse immigration sources, include significant cultural and demographic differences within their borders. Samples drawn from different groups and regions within these countries also have sleep characteristics that differ from their national averages.

In studies involving relatively ethnically homogeneous samples within single nations, environmental and personal factors were linked to sleep characteristics. In population samples drawn from African Americans, higher levels of psychosocial stress, neighborhood violence, and other problems were associated with more reports of poor quality and short sleep, objectively more disrupted sleep, and increased sympathetic arousal during sleep. Perceived high levels of social cohesion were, however, associated with better sleep quality. The effects on sleep of neighborhood problems were mediated in part by depressive symptoms and psychological distress (Johnson, Lisabeth, Hickson, et al., 2016; Johnson, Lisabeth, Lewis, et al., 2016; Kim et al., 2022; Mellman et al., 2018).

A longitudinal study involving a sample of mostly (95%) White children in the United Kingdom found that reported sleep problems increased as a function of reduced family income, lower maternal education achievement, and maternal anxiety and depression (Barazzetta & Ghislandi, 2017). More reported insomnia symptoms in an adult sample from China were also associated with lower socioeconomic status, living alone, or a history of health problems (Chen et al., 2018).

An Australian study examined the relations between social factors and sleep patterns from birth to age 6 or 7 years. Infants who began as short sleepers and continued in that pattern had poorer physical, emotional, and social health than typical sleepers. Both personal attributes of the children (irritability, nocturnal coughing, restless sleep) and family characteristics, such as household size and financial hardship, predicted persistent poor sleep quality, and later negative health outcomes (Magee et al., 2014).

A study of middle-aged women compared native-born, White women to immigrants to the United States from non-English-speaking countries (China, Japan, and several Hispanic countries). It found that sleep complaints were less common among the immigrant women than among native-born White women. The recent immigrants also reported fewer sleep complaints than those from their own ethnic background who had been born in the United States (Hale et al., 2014).

Among more established immigrants, those who were most strongly acculturated to English language usage showed the largest increase in sleep complaints. This tendency may be related to adoption of more typical American lifestyles and health behaviors by those who became more integrated into their new environment. Alternatively, since these results were based on self-reports, the impact of the degree of acculturation may have been related to adopting more typical American attitudes, terminology, and expectations in relation to sleep quality (Hale et al., 2014).

6.2.1 Summary

Despite the limitations of self-reports in most studies, the evidence indicates that there are broad differences in sleep patterns among nations, particularly in sleep durations and timing during the day, and in parental regulation of children's sleep. Local cultural practices influence the way people sleep, especially in relation to the presence or absence of daytime siestas beyond the typical age of starting school in some societies. These practices appear to be changing over time, but in both directions, with increasing and decreasing frequencies of daytime sleep in different countries. Traditional sleep patterns in each society reflect differences in the way daily schedules integrate the timing of sleep, work, school attendance, and meals.

Within countries, sleep patterns and perceived sleep quality are also modified by income, education, and ethnic/racial composition. Local environmental factors, including exposure to noise or violence, and family socioeconomic status are related to reported quality of sleep, and these may act in part through effects on psychological health. Cultural factors, such as perceived social cohesion in a stressful environment or the degree of integration of immigrants into their new environments, also influence self-reports of sleep quality.

6.3 Cultural anthropology of sleep

Few cultural anthropologists or historians have shown much academic interest in sleep until recently. Anthropologists studying traditional societies reported incidentally on some aspects of how sleep was organized because sleeping arrangements are related to other features of social organization. For example, where people with different social roles sleep was reported in relation to patterns of mother–infant contact, housing structures, and the social impacts of puberty. According to one author, most historians studying documents, such as diaries and reports of travelers from the past, paid little attention to references to sleep because their focus was on more active and dramatic aspects of life (Ekirch, 2001).

Two anthropologists published an extensive review of what was known about sleep in preindustrial societies from the perspective of cultural anthropology (Worthman & Melby, 2002). At the time of their review, they reported that there were virtually no studies available that focused specifically on sleep in cultures other than industrial societies (but see Section 6.6 for more recent empirical studies). Thus, they relied on a combination of participant self-reports and observations by anthropologists of a handful of traditional societies to reach some tentative generalizations, which are summarized here.

One lesson from Worthman and Melby's review of studies related to these societies is that features of current sleep practices, whether in the sleep laboratory or in industrial societies in general, are not inevitable. They reflect culturally determined choices related to the social and physical environments in which we sleep. Current sleep practices in industrial societies reflect their technological ecology, which provides access to resources permitting a high degree of physical and social isolation, physical comfort, and environmental control. These resources include building materials, bedding technology, and systems to control light, temperature, and noise levels. Worthman and Melby also pointed out that the blankets, bedding, and covers typical of industrial societies would not be welcome in many places because they would attract bedbugs and fleas, and require frequent washing and maintenance to control these parasites.

People in traditional human societies have more limited access to materials and resources to construct sleep environments, and resources vary greatly depending on where they live (rain forests, river valleys, open plains, mountains, the Arctic, deserts, etc.). As a result, their ability to control temperature, noise, and light are limited, as is their ability to protect themselves from the hazards that might be associated with sleeping at night.

The lifestyles, belief systems, and social structures that developed in these different environments influence sleep just as they influence daytime behaviors. The features of sleep that vary among cultures include where individuals sleep, what structures they sleep in (if any), who sleeps together or separately, and how sleep patterns change with age, social status, or current events.

Environmental and cultural factors result in a variety of sleeping arrangements in traditional societies, but rarely, if ever, in a single individual sleeping alone and in physical isolation from others. Individuals might share a type of bed with one or more family members or visitors, or they could sleep "alone" (i.e., on their own sleeping surface), but even then, typically in a shared family or communal sleeping space. In these situations, sleepers might have physical contact with at least some members of the group. They would also be exposed to auditory, visual, and olfactory stimuli from others nearby, related to snoring, sexual behavior, or digestion (Smit et al., 2019; Worthman & Melby, 2002).

Important factors that influence sleeping arrangements in traditional societies include those that affect most aspects of life (wealth, social status, gender, age) as well as those that are specifically related to sleeping at night. The latter factors depend on the local ecology but typically include fears related to a variety of potential hazards: low temperatures at night; nocturnal predators (e.g., large canids or felids); parasites (fleas, bedbugs); nocturnal agents that spread diseases (e.g., mosquitoes); attacks from other groups; or attacks from witches and nocturnal spirits (Musharbash, 2013).

A study of the Warlpiri Aboriginal community at Yuendumu, Northern Australia reported that single men or families formed defensive "sleeping rows" for the night. Those on the outside edges of the rows were considered "socially senior," which meant that they were most capable of detecting danger and responding effectively to it (Musharbash, 2013).

People in traditional societies often sleep not only with other people nearby but also with other species (as do some pet owners in industrial societies). Thus, in different cultures people share their indoor domestic sleeping spaces with dogs, goats, sheep, fowl, camels, and others. A subset of individuals (usually adolescent boys and young men) might be required to sleep in open areas with the group's herds, often some distance away from a tribal center, to protect the herds against both human and animal predation.

Communal or family fires are used for cooking and warmth, but they are also a defense against many nocturnal dangers because they frighten potential predators and increase the visibility of other threats. Smoke from fires is useful in repelling insects, but it also impairs air quality, especially indoors. Fires are also noisy and bright and carry substantial risk of causing burns to nearby sleepers or of spreading dangerously. They require attention from people who might need to be awake periodically during the night to ensure that they are both maintained and contained.

In societies without scheduled work hours, sleep times are more flexibly distributed across the 24 h cycle than in those with rigid work schedules. In societies that rely on gathering and foraging, individuals work and rest periodically in a relatively unstructured way. The timing of sleep can change depending on social and environmental conditions and events, and parents may not set sleeping hours for even very young members of the group (Worthman & Melby, 2002). The Ugandan poet, Okot p'Bitek, described how children in a village sleep and wake when they feel the need, without parents setting specific schedules (p'Bitek, 1989), while the American historian Lewis Mumford emphasized that in industrial societies organic functions like eating and sleeping are scheduled to occur in relation to clock time, not on the basis of how people feel (Mumford, 1934).

Daytime naps or drowsy states are common in some societies, and their frequency may increase after extended waking during preceding nights, a time sometimes spent socializing, dancing, story-telling, and engaging in rituals. In some societies, sleep loss at night is used as a way of promoting dissociated cognitive states (e.g., encouraging visions), and as a test of endurance that may be the topic of boasting to others, particularly among men. (Boasting of how little one has slept is also not uncommon in industrial societies.) In some cultures, individuals stressed or bored during a social interaction engage in what has been called "check-out sleep," in which they simply fall asleep during the interaction (Worthman & Melby, 2002).

6.3.1 Summary

This brief summary of the limited information available indicates that sleep timing in traditional societies is often less rigid than is typical in industrial societies. The distinctions that laboratory studies make between wake and sleep states may also not apply as clearly to people who engage periodically in intermediate states, like drowsiness or light dozing, at any time of day or night. In the absence of EEG recordings from people in those societies, however, it is difficult to make direct comparisons.

Some common features of sleep in traditional societies are that few people sleep completely alone; they are typically in close contact with other people, and often animals, while they sleep. They also sleep in situations in which they are much less protected than in industrial societies from aspects of their environment, including temperature/humidity changes, noise, potential predators, and disease vectors.

Fires are of central importance for most cultures because they are used for cooking and provide warmth as well as some degree of protection from nocturnal predators and insects. However, fires also require attention periodically during the night and carry their own risks related to smoke inhalation, burns, and uncontrolled spread.

6.4 Control of lighting

6.4.1 History of nocturnal illumination

The most salient difference between night and day is the level of environmental illumination; most adult humans sleep in the darkness of night and are active primarily during the day. The human visual system allows us to interact most effectively with the environment during daylight and leaves us relatively helpless, and potentially vulnerable, in darkness. Light at night from the moon and stars is irregularly available, depending on cloud cover and lunar phase. Even at its brightest, natural illumination at night is too dim to permit most kinds of productive activities and to allow easy detection of, and defense against, nocturnal dangers.

Our strongly day-adapted visual system and diurnal activity preference have shaped the organization of our sleep–wake cycles. They have also generated a wealth of mythology, art, and folklore that evoke the dangers of darkness and the night. For example, the Protestant *Book of Common Prayer* (1928) includes: "Lighten our darkness, we beseech thee, O Lord, and by thy great mercy defend us from all perils and dangers of this night."

Humans have had some influence over illumination in their environment for millennia because of their unique ability to control fire. Wood, coal, oil, and similar materials that feed fires may, however, require considerable effort or cost to obtain, and they are not readily available in some places where people live. When burned, they also provide more heat than useful illumination, and the resulting fires are difficult to control and to transport to where they are needed. Technological advances gave people better control of illumination and more flexibility because they could use candles and torches or burn oil or kerosene in lamps. Although these sources were more portable and easier to control than open fires, they were expensive for most people and still provided only limited illumination, along with considerable heat and a high risk of causing fires.[3] These features reduced their usefulness as a practical replacement for daylight, except for the very wealthiest.

In the late 19th century, however, the harnessing of electric power and the invention of the commercially viable electric light bulb changed the cost/benefit ratio dramatically. With the subsequent development of urban (and later, rural) grids for electrical power distribution,[4] along with light bulbs that

---

[3] Virtually every major (and minor) city has experienced one or more historical "great fires" that destroyed some or all of the city, caused the deaths of dozens or hundreds of residents, and left many more homeless. See https://en.wikipedia.org/wiki/List_of_fires for one list.

[4] See http://tinyurl.com/lj33nph for an interesting description of the early struggles among Edison, Tesla, and Westinghouse to develop and control the electrification of New York City.

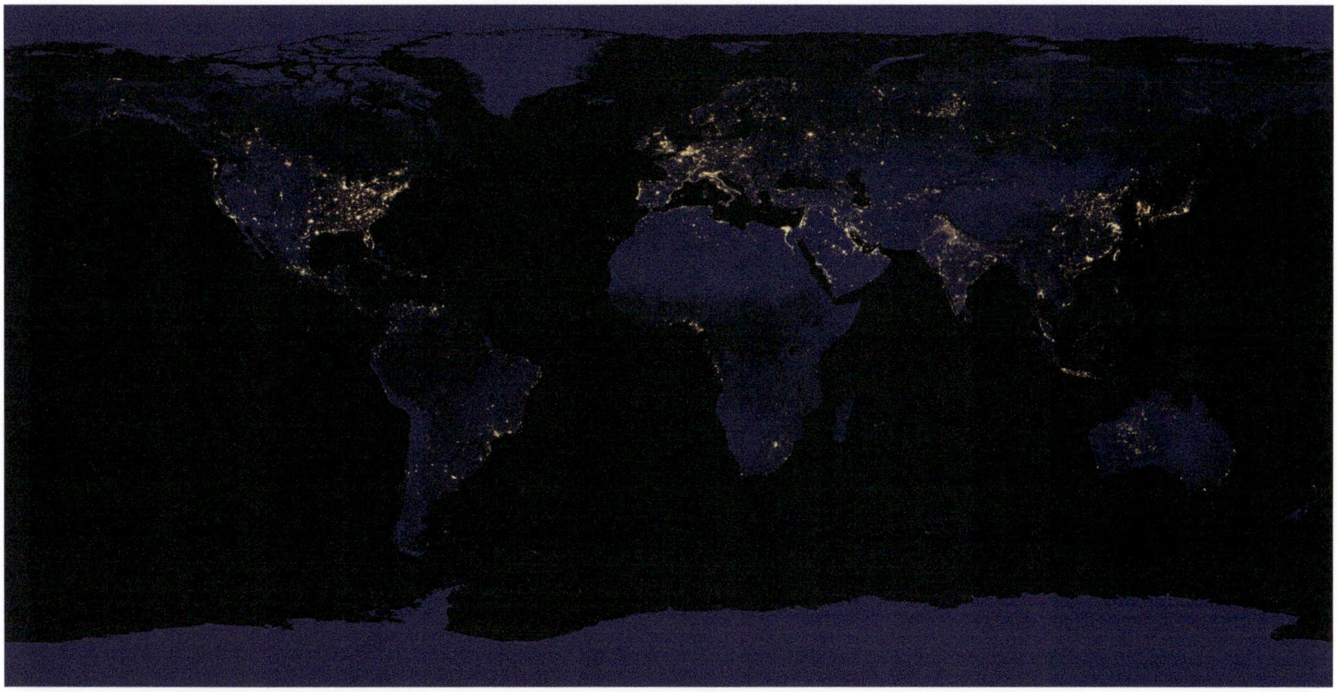

Figure 6.2 A 2012 composite photograph showing the earth as it would look if it were simultaneously night everywhere (which it never is). The brightness of electrical illumination at night is an indicator of the density of population in regions with electricity, including regions that contrast with their surroundings, for example, the banks and delta of the River Nile in North Africa, the US eastern seaboard, northern Germany, and the east coasts of Japan and China, among others. Reprinted from NASA: https://eoimages.gsfc.nasa.gov/images/imagerecords/79000/79765/dnb_land_ocean_ice.2012.13500x6750.jpg.

produced relatively bright light with minimal heat, the general population could for the first time extend the length of the personal "day" during which work could be done effectively and safely. Soon factories could be lit 24 h a day at reasonable cost with a light intensity that permitted productive work, and electrically powered engines could replace the less effective steam engines that powered industry before that time.

As a result, the expensive machinery in factories could repay investment costs more rapidly by being run continuously. People were then called on to work during night hours to keep these productive activities going. Illumination of public spaces during the night added to the safety of the environment by reducing the "perils and dangers" of the night and thereby encouraged the growth of a variety of other social and entertainment activities at night. These, in turn, brought people out of their homes in larger numbers and created new commercial opportunities. These were addressed increasingly by businesses providing a variety of late-night services, including entertainment venues, restaurants, gas stations, and others, especially in growing urban centers.

The impacts of the initial technological revolution that depended on electricity was further amplified by the invention of the telegraph and telephone in the 19th century and then of entertainment media that were also based on electricity. There was a rapid growth of leisure-time and work tools: phonographs (and their descendants, tape players, compact disks, DVDs), cinema, radio, television, computers, portable phones, smartphones, tablets, the internet, and streaming services. These electrically powered tools extended opportunities for work, education, and entertainment activities to any time of day or night for much of the population, rather than affecting only industrial workers.[5]

6.4.2 Lighting and sleep

The availability of cheap nocturnal illumination not only changed peoples' habits and ability to perform work, but also affected the illumination of the sleep environment and the quality of sleep. There is a strong correlation between the satellite-measured, local light intensity in a location and reported sleep problems among its inhabitants. Higher environmental light intensities are associated with shorter sleep, delayed sleep onsets, earlier awakening, and more dissatisfaction with sleep quality. Although high light levels at night are also strongly correlated with high population densities that could contribute to these problems (**Figure 6.2**), controlling for population

[5] Many kinds of work and educational activities were conducted remotely via the internet during the peak of the COVID-19 pandemic in 2020–22, and increased participation in remote work and education has since continued for a substantial number of people.

density did not eliminate the link between bright nights and delayed/problematic sleep (Ohayon & Milesi, 2016). In a group of older participants, poorer objective and subjective sleep quality were also associated with higher measured light levels in the bedroom at night (Obayashi et al., 2014).

Artificial illumination also affects the behavior of other species. Male birds that lived closer to artificial light sources showed earlier singing in the morning and had more mating success. Seasonal patterns regulated by day length were also affected, so that female birds living in those areas laid eggs earlier than did those in similar habitats without artificial illumination (Kempenaers et al., 2010).[6]

Studying how our control of lighting has altered sleep was prompted in one case by an interest in whether seasonally changing night lengths affect human physiology. Thomas Wehr and colleagues at the US National Institutes of Health studied several aspects of how seasonal changes in the ratio of light to dark alter human behavior and physiology, including sleep. To assess whether people show photoperiodic responses (i.e., seasonal physiological and behavioral changes related to changing day/night ratios; see Section 9.2), they compared the effects of spending 8 h vs. 14 h in darkness each night in a laboratory during a 4-week period. During weeks with long nights, most participants extended their sleep time (in one study from 7.6 to 10.6 h) and divided their sleep into two or more bouts, with intervening periods spent lying awake quietly in the dark (**Figure 6.3**). People also showed reduced fatigue, higher energy levels, and better moods in the long-night condition (Wehr, 1991; Wehr, 1999; Wehr et al., 1993).

Based on a historical review of diaries and other documents going back centuries, Roger Ekirch concluded that this kind of segmented sleep was a normal pattern in northern Europe (and elsewhere) before the 19th century, especially during the long nights of winter. These documents referred to "first sleep," which lasted from sometime after sunset until about midnight, followed by waking for a short period, and then "second sleep," leading to dawn. The period of waking around midnight was reportedly occupied by quiet rest, contemplation, prayer, social interactions, or sexual activity (Ekirch, 2001; Ekirch, 2016). This pattern resembled some of the sleep patterns observed by Wehr and colleagues during 14 h nights in a laboratory (**Figure 6.3**).

In laboratory studies, several physiological measures in addition to sleep changed during 14 h nights. The duration of

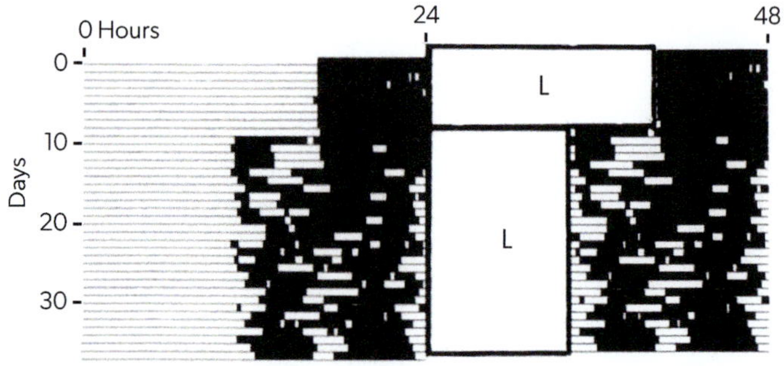

Figure 6.3 A man who showed changes in the organization of his sleep phase when he was studied first during a long-day (=short-night) condition (16 h light and 8 h dark) and then two weeks later in a short-day condition (10 h light and 14 h dark). The light phases are shown as white areas labeled L and sleep is shown as black areas. This individual showed a single, well-consolidated sleep phase in the short-night condition shown at the top. When sleeping in the long-night condition, however, he showed irregular lengthy interruptions of sleep, lengthened sleep-onset latencies, and, eventually, a strikingly bimodal sleep pattern, with distinct early and late sleep phases during the long night. Hours are shown across the top of the figure and days from top to bottom; the 24 h sleep–wake records are double-plotted on a 48 h scale. Reprinted with permission of Oxford University Press from Wehr, T. A. (1991) The durations of human melatonin secretion and sleep respond to changes in daylength (photoperiod). *J Clin Endocrinol Metab* 73:1276–1280. © The Endocrine Society (1991). doi: 10.1210/jcem-73-6-1276.

active secretion of melatonin[7] lengthened in one study from 10.3 to 11.9 h, and there were similar changes in the length of secretion of the pituitary hormone prolactin. In 8 h nights, prolactin levels rose shortly after sleep onset, which is consistent with other observations that prolactin secretion occurred during the peak of N3 sleep early in the night (Sassin et al., 1973; Spiegel et al., 1995). In 14 h nights, however, prolactin levels rose early in the dark phase while participants were still lying quietly awake, and long before the peak of N3 sleep occurred (Wehr et al., 1993).

The independence of prolactin secretion from sleep was confirmed in a later study, which found that levels rose during the subjective night even in people who were kept awake continuously for >24 h (Waldstreicher et al., 1996). Thus, the secretion patterns of melatonin and prolactin are linked to darkness and circadian phase, not to sleep, and presumably would have changed seasonally when people living in non-equatorial regions, without easy access to artificial lighting, were exposed to long nights.

[6] Effects of artificial illumination have also been observed on species ranging from the microbial population in drainage ditches to migrating birds and foraging bats. See https://tinyurl.com/ybpo2qv4 for a description of these changes and references to the related literature, and Sanders et al., 2021 for a meta-analysis of the diverse behavioral, endocrine, and reproductive effects of artificial nocturnal illumination on a range of species.

[7] See Chapter 9 for a discussion of the control of melatonin production and its role in sleep regulation. In relation to studies discussed here, it is important to know that significant amounts of melatonin are secreted by the pineal gland only at night and that light exposure rapidly reduces melatonin levels.

These experimental and historical observations imply that our improved control of lighting and the availability of cheap electrical power could have changed the duration and pattern of sleep, and its linked physiological functions, as traditional societies evolved into industrial societies with control of electricity. It is, however, difficult to find empirical evidence demonstrating that these changes occurred during the last 150 years, spanning the transition from a pre-electric world to today. Observational studies of sleep (e.g., using actigraphy) and survey studies, which are now commonly conducted in various populations, did not exist until recent decades. To try to address this question, researchers have turned to other approaches (see Section 6.5).

6.4.3 Summary

Control of fire undoubtedly played a critical role in human evolution by providing protection and warmth as well as facilitating food preparation, but its benefits were partially offset by some associated costs and risks. Control of electricity over the last century and a half dramatically reshaped human societies, providing cheap, bright illumination at night that altered many people's work schedules and eventually allowed development of opportunities for 24 h access to work, information, and entertainment. Whether it also dramatically modified human sleep patterns is less clear.

There is experimental evidence that some people develop bimodal sleep patterns under conditions of long nights in a laboratory setting. The idea that this segmented sleep pattern occurred more broadly in the pre-electric era is supported by historical writings describing bimodal nocturnal sleep patterns in northern European winters and perhaps also in other places and seasons.

6.5 Observational and experimental studies of sleep in preindustrial societies

Since we cannot study sleep in our pre-electric era ancestors, we must rely on other methods to develop inferences about their likely sleep patterns. As previously discussed, other approaches to understanding sleep patterns in the absence of electricity include examining written records that have survived from the recent past (Ekirch, 2001), studying anthropological reports that include incidental observations related to sleep in traditional societies (Worthman & Melby, 2002), or extrapolating from the results of laboratory studies that mimic the long, dark nights that some ancestral humans would have experienced in winter (Wehr et al., 1993).

More recently, there have been empirical studies of sleep in people who choose to live without electricity for a period of time and in members of surviving traditional societies that do not have access to electricity. These studies were aimed at collecting direct observational (and some experimental) data on how people sleep without access to electric lighting as ancestral human groups must have done.

In one study, a very small group of adults and children in Germany spent 8 weeks (during August–September, a time of year when nights would be relatively short in southern Germany) with no electricity, running water, or other modern amenities and were allowed only a campfire. There was an increase in the adults' average sleep duration relative to their baseline sleep (from 5.7 to 7.2 h), resulting from earlier bedtimes and longer times in bed (TIB). It is unlikely that this was a rebound increase in response to their habitual short sleep because the long sleep durations emerged only gradually and persisted over several weeks (Piosczyk et al., 2014). It is possible, however, that these results reflect differences, other than access to electricity, between 21st century life in urban Germany and in a camping environment.

A different approach was taken by researchers who studied people currently living in traditional societies without access to electricity. These studies took place in relatively remote regions of Haiti, Tanzania, Madagascar, Bolivia, and the Kalahari desert in southern Africa. Most studies used actigraphy to track the sleep–wake patterns of participants, but some also used questionnaires or portable PSGs for a few participants. Some researchers also had the opportunity to study related groups that lived in close proximity to each other with only one group having access to electric lighting. These groups were studied in Argentina, Brazil, and Vanuatu (an island nation in the South Pacific). These very challenging field studies generally involved relatively small numbers of participants.

The results of these studies provide a mixed picture of how adults without access to electricity sleep in these diverse traditional societies. Some studies reported evidence of segmented sleep patterns at least some of the time—in one case, primarily among nursing mothers (Knutson, 2014; Samson, Manus, et al., 2017; Smit et al., 2019)—while others did not (de la Iglesia et al., 2015; Samson, Crittenden, et al., 2017; Yetish et al., 2015). Some studies did not report daytime naps, while others reported frequent naps (Samson, Crittenden, et al., 2017; Samson, Manus, et al., 2017; Smit et al., 2019) or occasional naps (Yetish et al., 2015). Sleep durations reported in these studies were similar to, or shorter than, those in most studies conducted in industrial societies (~5.7–7.9 h), and most studies found fairly high levels of wake after sleep onset (WASO), reflecting relatively long TIBs (Knutson, 2014; Samson, Crittenden, et al., 2017; Samson, Manus, et al., 2017).

The absence of segmented sleep in three equatorial groups in one study led to the interpretation that this was not a pattern typical of traditional societies without access to electricity but was more likely an adaptation to the long winter

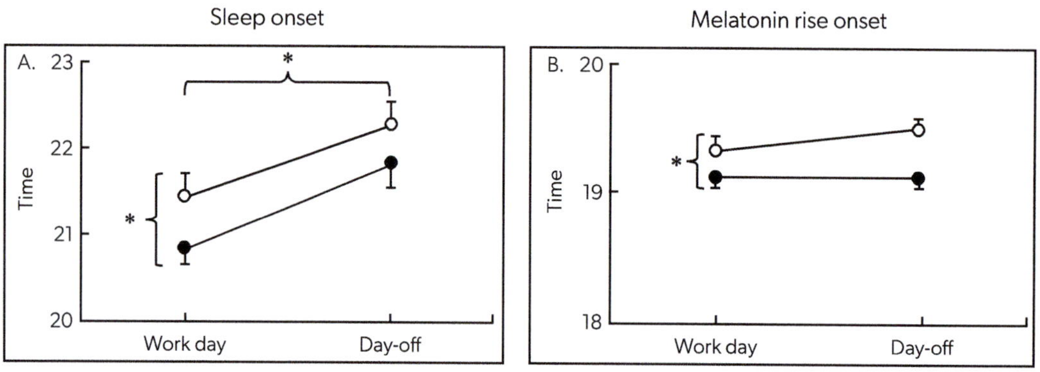

Figure 6.4 **A.** Brazilian rubber tappers' average sleep onset time (Y axis), showing that those with access to electric light (white symbols) had significantly later sleep onsets on workdays than those without access to electricity (black symbols). Sleep onset was further delayed in all participants on days off relative to workdays. **B.** For the same participants, the timing of melatonin secretion onset was delayed in those with access to electricity relative to those without access. There was no significant change from workdays to days off work. * indicates a statistically significant difference. Reprinted with permission from Moreno, C. R. C. et al. (2015) Sleep patterns in Amazon rubber tappers with and without electric light at home. *Sci Rep* 5:14074. Licensed under a Creative Commons Attribution 4.0 International License (http://creativecommons.org/licenses/by/4.0/). doi: 10.1038/srep14074.

nights experienced in northern Europe (Yetish et al., 2015). In response, Ekirch noted that historical documents included references to segmented sleep in both winter and summer in Europe, and in many other locations, including some more southerly regions (Ekirch, 2016).

The impact of light exposure on sleep was inconsistent among studies. In one study, TIB was closely tied to sunrise and sunset (Samson, Manus, et al., 2017), but another reported that participants typically woke before dawn (although timing varied with season) and did not go to sleep until hours after sunset (Yetish et al., 2015). When some participants who lacked electricity were given access to battery-operated field lights, there was little change in sleep pattern (Samson, Manus, et al., 2017).

These studies also noted that factors other than light exposure had important effects on sleep patterns. Thus, high humidity levels were associated with increased WASO (Samson, Crittenden, et al., 2017) as were high levels of noise at night (Samson, Manus, et al., 2017). High temperatures increased sleep durations in one study (Samson, Manus, et al., 2017), while another reported that high temperatures early in the night inhibited sleep, resulting in more sleep occurring during the cooler second half of the night (Yetish et al., 2015).

In studies involving comparisons between related groups living near each other, one found that those with electricity in Argentina slept 0.75–1.0 h less (depending on season) than those who relied on natural lighting, primarily because of later bedtimes. These results support the idea that access to electric lighting delayed sleep onset and reduced its duration (de la Iglesia et al., 2015).

Traditional horticulturists on Tanna island in Vanuatu, who had access to electricity, had delayed sleep onsets and slightly shorter nighttime sleep relative to those without electric lighting (although almost all had access to small, portable, solar-powered LED lights). But when daytime naps were included, total sleep time did not differ between the groups. The authors noted that the benign climate, lack of predators, and easy access to food may have contributed to the relatively longer total sleep times (7.5–7.9 h) in this environment than among other traditional groups that had been studied (Smit et al., 2019).

A combination of questionnaires and actigraphy were used to study the sleep of two groups of Brazilians who were not traditional hunter–gatherers. They were rubber plantation workers who were transported from their villages to work during the week. One group had access to electricity and went to sleep later throughout the week and woke up earlier on days off than those exposed only to natural lighting, sleeping ~0.5 h less according to questionnaires. The evening rise of melatonin in those with electricity was delayed by ~0.33 h. These results indicated a small effect of artificial lighting on the onset of melatonin secretion and the timing and duration of sleep, even though the light intensity available was very dim (Moreno et al., 2015) (**Figure 6.4**).

6.5.1 Summary

Since these studies on small numbers of participants with different ethnic backgrounds were conducted in different seasons and in varied regions, it is not surprising that results were not consistent; the principal findings are summarized in **Table 6.1**. There was support for an impact of electric lighting in delaying the timing of both sleep and melatonin secretion. A frequent effect of easy access to electric light was a small delay in timing

Table 6.1 Field Studies of Electricity Use and Sleep Patterns

Publication	Population	Comparison	Method	Sleep Duration	WASO	Segmentation?	Naps	Effects of Light Condition	Other Factors	Comments
Piosczyk et al., 2014	German "reality" TV show participants	Electricity; then no-electricity while camping	Actigraphy	Increased: 5.7→7.2 h	?	No		Earlier sleep onset while camping		Unlikely to be rebound sleep
Knutson, 2014	Haiti	No electricity	Actigraphy	7.0 h	2.3 h	Some				
Samson et al., 2017A	Tanzania: hunter/ gatherers	No electricity	Actigraphy	6.5 h	High	No	Yes: 50%		Humidity/ temperature	High humidity disrupted sleep, increased WASO
Samson et al., 2017B	Madagascar	No electricity	Actigraphy/ PSG	6.5 h	High	Frequent, especially males	Yes	Field lanterns only: no effect on sleep	Noise increased WASO	Some PSG studies; similar results
Yetish et al., 2015	Tanzania, Kalahari, Bolivia	No electricity	Actigraphy	5.7-7.1 h	Some	No; probably only in northern Europe winter	Summer, yes (22%)	Awake before dawn	Temperature is important	Slept in cooler 2nd half of night
de la Iglesia et al., 2015	Argentina: hunter/ gatherers	Compared two groups, with & without electricity	Actigraphy	Elec: Summer: 6.27 h Winter: 7.53 h No Elec: Summer: 6.98 h Winter: 8.47 h	?	No		With electricity: shorter sleep, especially in winter		Timing of sleep onset determined length of sleep periods
Moreno et al., 2015	Brazil: rubber tappers	Compared two groups, with & without electricity	Questionnaire, actigraphy, melatonin assays	Elec: Work: 7.5 h Days off: 8.4 h No elec: Work days: 8.0 h Days off: 8.8 h	?	?		Delayed melatonin onset with electricity		30 min delay in melatonin onset, but less by actigraphy
Smit et al., 2019	Melanesia: horticulturists	Compared two groups, with & without electricity, (except for solar torches)	Actigraphy & interviews	Electricity: 7.4 h + naps No electricity: 7.9 h	Some	Yes, especially nursing mothers, but not regularly timed	Yes, frequent	Delayed sleep onset with electricity; both groups used solar torches	Large effects of light at night among breast-feeding mothers	Electricity affected timing of onset, but not total 24 h sleep
Ekirch, 2016	Commented that segmented sleep occurred in all seasons and was not only a Northern European or winter phenomenon.									

of sleep onset and a corresponding reduction in nocturnal sleep duration, but the groups without electricity did not show dramatically different sleep durations from those typically found in industrial societies.

Sleep segmentation and daytime naps were virtually absent in some groups but appeared variably in others. Thus, neither segmented sleep nor daytime naps in adults appear to be universal characteristics of sleep in current, traditional societies. The results also demonstrated that factors other than light, such as environmental noise, humidity, temperature at night, and the general ease or difficulty of living conditions have significant effects on the timing and duration of sleep. The generality of these conclusions is limited by the fact that most studies were conducted in regions less than 20° from the equator, and therefore did not include groups living in more extreme northern or southern latitudes where seasonal changes in day length would be more pronounced.

These studies provided valuable information about how human societies adapt their sleep patterns under different environmental, technological, and cultural conditions and about a number of factors that modify sleep patterns. Their findings did not, however, converge on a single form of "natural" human sleep that is expressed in the absence of electric lighting. The available evidence suggests that there was probably never a single human way of sleeping, even in pre-electric times. Rather, there were many specific adaptations to local environmental conditions that varied across groups, geography, and time.[8]

6.6 Sleep patterns over recent decades

6.6.1 Have sleep durations decreased?

There are claims that developing control over lighting during the last 150 years has produced a decline in average sleep durations, resulting in the world's population being united by chronic sleep deprivation in comparison to our preindustrial ancestors. Others have argued that there is no convincing evidence of systematic changes in sleep durations over this period, in part because estimates of sleep durations in previous centuries are largely anecdotal. The studies reviewed in the preceding section do not make a convincing case for either side, although small duration differences were observed in comparisons between related groups with and without access to electricity (de la Iglesia et al., 2015; Moreno et al., 2015). A question that is somewhat easier to address is what the effects on sleep have been of more recent technological developments, namely, computers and smartphones that connect users to entertainment, information, and work via the pervasive, never-sleeping internet.

A study that summarized reported sleep patterns in 15 countries from the 1960s to the 2000s found that sleep durations increased in some countries and decreased in others, as did the prevalence of very short and long sleep durations, but with no universal trend across countries (Bin et al., 2012). Surveys of American adults from 1985 to 2012 found a weak trend toward shorter sleep and an increasing percentage of people reporting <6 h sleep nightly until 2004. It was around 2007 that smartphones began to be introduced, and the years since then have seen smartphones and access to the internet become almost universal, yet there was no evidence of a subsequent trend toward shorter sleep among adults up to 2012 (Ford et al., 2015).

Studies using different methods reported minimal changes over recent decades up to 2013. A review of mostly laboratory PSG studies and a smaller number of actigraphy studies for the period 1960–2013 found no systematic decline in average sleep durations (Youngstedt et al., 2016). Laboratory studies would not provide useful information about people's habits in their usual daily lives, but actigraphy studies also did not indicate significant changes.

A more recent survey of adult Americans confirmed that there was no increase in reported short sleep in the 2004–12 period, but identified a significant trend toward more reports of short sleep from 2013–17. This change was most pronounced among Hispanic respondents and even more so among non-Hispanic Black populations, groups that already had shorter sleep durations than non-Hispanic Whites at the starting point (Sheehan et al., 2019).

Time-use studies[9] in Canada for the period 1985–2010 found small increases in reported sleep durations and decreases in short sleep among respondents 15 years and older, despite increases in reported screen time (Leech, 2017). A large time-use study among people over 10 years old in South Korea for the years 2004–19 also found a recent trend toward longer sleep times. These increases were almost entirely attributable to delayed waking on weekends, especially Saturdays, with little change during the work week (Jang et al., 2023). A large-scale, time-use study of people >15 years old in the United States

[8] A similar conclusion was reached about other aspects of human life by the historian and author Yuval Harari in his book *Sapiens*, in which he wrote that across historical time humans have not exhibited a single, natural way of life, but only many variations shaped by different cultural choices (Harari, 2014).

[9] Rather than simply self-reporting length of sleep, or bedtime and wake time, participants in these studies track and record the timing of all of their activities each day.

also reported a recent trend toward small increases in sleep durations in at least some subgroups. This increase was mostly attributable to earlier bedtimes (Basner & Dinges, 2018), in contrast to the later wake times in the Korean survey data.

These results were interpreted as possibly reflecting the partial success of recent advertising campaigns warning of the risks of inadequate sleep and promoting better sleep habits among Americans (Basner & Dinges, 2018). It is, however, difficult to verify the impact of such public health campaigns in the context of other changing social and environmental conditions. This interpretation was questioned based on the results mentioned earlier that sleep durations declined from 2013 to 2017, especially in minority racial/ethnic groups (Sheehan et al., 2019), although an interview-based study reported that American sleep durations increased again in the 2017–20 period, particularly influenced by longer sleep on "free" (non-work) days (Di et al., 2022).

Ideal studies to assess societal trends over time would involve a substantial number of people whose sleep is monitored while they engage in their usual patterns of activity, with these studies repeated over decades for the same age group. Such studies do not yet exist, and in their absence, the available data related to recent changes in sleep duration among adults in general are mixed. Studies are clearer in pointing to further reductions in sleep durations among ethnic/racial groups that were already at higher risk of short sleep. In addition, when there are recent trends toward longer sleep, these changes are often attributable to more makeup sleep on free days. There are inconsistent findings about the benefits of such makeup sleep on human health (see Section 14.6) because the extra sleep comes at the expense of increasing instability in circadian sleep–wake schedules and social jetlag (see Section 4.4.4).

Whether or not there has been a recent trend toward shorter sleep does not address the question of whether adults currently get enough sleep, a question that depends on agreement about how much sleep people need (Horne, 2011; Watson et al., 2015) (see discussion in Section 14.1). The consensus among most experts, including the US Centers for Disease Control is that insufficient sleep is currently a significant public health problem.[10] Regardless of whether there is a continuing trend toward shorter sleep among adults, the conclusion that many people in industrial societies do not get enough sleep raises concerns about the impacts on health and human performance of chronic inadequate sleep, as discussed in Chapters 13–15.

Despite recent reports of both small increases and decreases in sleep durations among adults, there are more consistent results for children and young adolescents, with some variation among countries (Matricciani et al., 2011). It appears that access to new technologies has affected the sleep of these groups over recent decades and has had consequences for their daily functioning (for a recent review, see Matricciani et al., 2017). For example, a study of Finnish adolescents from 1984 to 2011 reported increasing insomnia symptoms and tiredness as well as poorer academic performance up to 2008, after which these trends flattened out (Kronholm et al., 2015). Spanish children (aged 2–14) showed decreasing sleep durations (including siestas) from 1987 to 2011, with the prevalence of short sleep increasing from 30% to 45% of this age group (de Ruiter et al., 2016).

A meta-analysis of publications related to children and adolescents found a strong association between the use of media devices near bedtime and shorter sleep, poorer sleep quality, and increased daytime sleepiness (Carter et al., 2016). A summary of time-use and survey studies of American adolescents also reported an increase from 2009 to 2015 in reports of short sleep durations (<7 h), which was associated with increased use of new media (Twenge et al., 2017).

Using electronic devices late in the day after presumed bedtimes will delay actual sleep onset. In addition, light from device screens (especially in the blue part of the visible spectrum) can further delay sleep by causing circadian phase delays, increasing arousal, and suppressing the circadian-regulated melatonin signal that helps facilitate sleep onset (Chang et al., 2015; Green et al., 2017); see Section 9.2.2 and **Figure 9.3**. These effects depend on the duration, intensity, and wavelength of the light exposure. Whether computer screens used for 2 h before bedtime emitted short-wavelength light was more important than the intensity of the light exposure in a study of young adults. Blue light exposure disrupted melatonin onset and temperature decline at bedtime, disrupted sleep continuity, decreased N3 sleep and total sleep time, and increased daytime sleepiness (Green et al., 2017).

Although interacting through social media may be arousing and delay sleep onset, a study involving 30 min of social media use on smartphones while wearing glasses that selectively blocked blue wavelengths found no effect on subjective arousal levels, and only small reductions in total sleep duration and N2 sleep (Combertaldi et al., 2021). Blocking blue light exposure, use of smartphones with smaller screens, and a short exposure period may have contributed to reducing effects on sleep compared to the study using blue-light emitting computer screens for a 2 h period (Green et al., 2017).

Together, these findings indicate that social media use around bedtime caused a small decrease in sleep amounts, independent of illumination effects. However, adding exposure to significant amounts of short-wavelength light from electronic devices and having longer periods of exposure produced important effect on sleep parameters and daytime functioning.

---

[10] See https://tinyurl.com/2cxsv8f7 for a summary of the frequency of insufficient sleep in the United States generally and in different states during 2013–2022.

The type of activity involving electronic devices and the nature of the device are also important. A study that obtained self-reports from teenagers about device use before bedtime and in bed found that delays in sleep onset were related to the type of activity involved and the device being used. Activities that were more interactive and open-ended (e.g., using phones, laptops, watching social media videos, playing on gaming consoles) tended to cause larger delays in sleep onset than passively watching television (Pillion et al., 2022).

Watching television was, in fact, the most common media-related activity in the hour before sleep in a survey of a broad age range of people. However, this was not the case for younger people, who used cell phones more often than older groups, had more difficulty falling asleep, and had less refreshing sleep (Gradisar et al., 2013). Thus, for young people, shortened sleep as a result of using electronic media around bedtime can be attributed to a combination of postponement of sleep onset to engage in these activities and delaying effects of illumination on melatonin secretion and the circadian system, especially when the use involves open-ended, interactive activities.

Despite the lack of clarity as to how adult sleep has trended over recent decades, the results for children and adolescents are much more consistent in showing shorter sleep durations that are linked to increased electronic media use near bedtime.

6.6.2 Cultural impacts on children's sleep

Evidence of recently increasing sleep problems among children and adolescents (see Section 4.4 for a discussion of the effects of school schedules on sleep in adolescents) should be considered in a historical context. The current concerns about children's sleep are not unique to this era; similar themes were expressed decades ago in relation to other important cultural and technological changes at that time, according to two reviews (Matricciani et al., 2012; Stearns et al., 1996). Information about children's sleep during the period from the middle of the 19th to the early 20th century was obtained from a variety of sources, including articles in magazines and opinion pieces as well as more traditional research reports.

According to these reviews, magazines included little discussion of sleep itself during the 19th century, although there was some advice provided about warm coverings and baby's body position. An 1863 article described allowing a baby to sleep on its back (supine position) as dangerous and likely to damage the developing skull. This idea contrasts sharply to the current advice related to preventing infant crib death (sudden infant death syndrome, or SIDS), which recommends that babies up to a year of age sleep on their backs, as reflected in "back to sleep" campaigns (now called "safe to sleep") (https://safetosleep.nichd.nih.gov/).

By the early 20th century, articles began to discuss children's sleep as a problem that needed attention. This shift in focus was related to other societal changes occurring at that time:

- a growing, urban middle class with increasing wealth that permitted ownership of larger houses;
- reductions in family sizes and infant mortality rates, leading to a more intense focus on the health of individual children;
- a reduction in the number of live-in maids who were responsible for childcare;
- the growth of the disciplines of medicine and behavioral psychology and the associated use of popular media for practitioners to provide advice about health issues.

Among other changes that occurred at that time were the replacement of traditional cradles (usually kept near a parent or sibling to permit rocking) with stationary cribs.[11] In addition, smaller families and larger houses resulted in fewer children needing to sleep together, which facilitated placing an infant's crib in a separate room. This trend was linked to changes in the lifestyles of the urban middle class, including increasing popularity of entertaining guests at home in the evening; the perceived need to isolate sleeping children from noisy new home appliances, such as vacuum cleaners and washing machines; and a reported increased interest in parental recreational activities, including sex, that were seen to require separation from children (Stearns et al., 1996).

Articles providing advice about children's sleep became a standard element of magazines aimed at women in the 1920s and 30s, with a focus on the problem of inadequate sleep in children. The idea that children were not getting enough sleep and risked developing "chronic fatigue" was linked to the "frenzied pace" of modern life in this era and the impact of recent inventions on children's sleep. These included electric lighting, radio, movie theaters as well as automobiles and appliances that contributed to environmental noise. Some magazine articles were critical of the impact on sleep of the time demands associated with both schoolwork and entertainment. Listening to radio late at night (mostly by boys) and reading (mostly by girls) were cited in one article as two examples of entertainment forms that deprived children of sleep (Matricciani et al., 2012; Stearns et al., 1996).

[11] Research in both mice and people has recently shown that slow, automated rocking during a sleep period reduced sleep onset latency, increased total sleep time and the amount of deep NREM sleep and, for humans, increased sleep spindles and slow oscillations, and improved memory consolidation (Kompotis et al., 2019; Perrault et al., 2019); see Section 18.12.

Thus, the current concern about how much sleep children and adolescents get is not a new phenomenon. Social and technological changes that influenced the behaviors of children have prompted concerns in the past. It is also clear that a range of cultural factors can influence what durations of sleep are considered by parents and health experts to be appropriate for different age groups. There is now, however, also empirical evidence about how social structures, such as school schedules, and access to screen-based technologies, can shorten and disrupt sleep, especially in adolescents (see Chapter 4). There is also considerable evidence documenting the impact of chronic short and disrupted sleep on cognitive functions and mental and physical health (see Chapters 13–15).

6.6.3 Summary

Current concerns about how the time demands of people's busy lives affect sleep patterns are not new; this topic was raised in relation to social and technological developments early in the 20th century. The accelerating pace of technological change in the 21st century (home computers, smartphones/tablets, and the internet), however, has prompted studies investigating whether sleep durations have fallen further over recent decades.

Survey studies among adults provided mixed evidence related to changes over recent decades in sleep durations (which were likely inadequate to start with) as well as evidence for further decreases in sleep amounts in some minority groups. Similar studies of children and adolescents in recent years, however, reported shorter sleep durations and more sleep problems that are linked to several aspects of the use of electronic media near bedtime. Both the time spent on media use and the effects on the circadian system of screens that emit short-wavelength light have significant negative effects on sleep quality and duration in this age group.

6.7 The co-sleeping controversy

6.7.1 Co-sleeping and SIDS

Another cultural issue that affects the sleep of children, especially infants, is the appropriateness of co-sleeping. Co-sleeping (or bed-sharing) refers to the practice of a newborn or young infant sharing a sleeping surface with their mother (and often another parent). This practice is usually, but not always, distinguished from room-sharing, in which the infant is in a separate bed, but in the same room as the parent(s). A systematic review noted that key terms in the literature such as "bed-sharing" and "breastfeeding" are used inconsistently across publications, making comparisons difficult (Baddock et al., 2019).

The debates around the potential risks and benefits of co-sleeping are among the most heated in the field of sleep medicine, with strongly held views and published evidence supporting both sides of the issue. A 2006 review of 40 parenting books that addressed this issue and were available in the United States at that time found that 41% were negative about co-sleeping and 28% were positive (although the strength of these views varied), while the remainder did not explicitly endorse either view (Ramos & Youngclarke, 2006).

A critical review of this topic summarized the findings of nearly 600 publications, including scientific reports, reviews, and opinion pieces and discussed the weaknesses of the available empirical evidence (Mileva-Seitz et al., 2017). The authors' summary indicated that Western medical advice is predicated on two concerns: that bed-sharing increases the risk to infants of smothering and that it may slow the development of independence and self-regulation, often referred to as "self-soothing." Those favoring the practice instead start from the idea that co-sleeping is a natural, ancient practice that is consistent with primate and human biology but has been demonized by Western medicine (McKenna et al., 2007). Given the different starting points of these discussions, it is not surprising that they lead to very different conclusions about the balance of risks and benefits.

These different opinions are echoed in the stark differences in prevalence of co-sleeping across nations. In some countries, it is a virtually universal practice (e.g., several African countries and Mongolia), while surveys in other countries found that only ~6% of respondents indicated that they practiced co-sleeping (Italy, Israel, Ukraine) (Mileva-Seitz et al., 2017). These national estimates obscure the fact that within some countries the prevalence of the practice also varies with socioeconomic status and cultural background, especially in large, multicultural nations (Luijk et al., 2013; McKenna et al., 2007).

One reason for the strong division of opinion is that the issue of co-sleeping is entangled with several related child-rearing controversies. One issue is the unresolved question of the cause(s) of SIDS (sudden infant death syndrome: unexplained death of an otherwise healthy infant, typically in the first few months of life).[12] It is suspected by some to be related to respiratory failure, which typically leaves no detectable signs and is difficult to trace to a specific cause.

---

[12] This term is used in different ways. Some use it to refer to any unexplained death in early infancy, while others reserve its use for situations in which no plausible risk factors can be identified. They note that, at a population level, cases of sudden death that occur in what are clearly high-risk co-sleeping situations are likely the result of smothering, in which case "unexplained" is not an appropriate characterization. On the other hand, it is often impossible to identify a direct cause in individual cases, so "SIDS" is frequently used as a diagnosis by exclusion that does not imply a specific cause.

The risk of SIDS drives arguments on both sides. One view is endorsed by the American Academy of Pediatrics (AAP) (TFOSIDS, 2016). It states that there is an increased risk of SIDS or of smothering young infants if they co-sleep with an adult on soft surfaces (e.g., couches, armchairs) or on parental beds with pillows and blankets. This risk is further increased if the parents are overly sleepy because of consumption of medications, alcohol, or street drugs (Carpenter et al., 2013). The risk of SIDS is also strongly increased by exposure of the infant to parental smoking.[13] The AAP recommended that infants up to 12 months of age sleep on their backs in the same room as parents, but in a separate side bed with an appropriate firm surface and lack of soft bedding or other hazardous materials (TFOSIDS, 2016).[14]

Co-sleeping advocates, however, argue that having immediate contact with an infant may reduce the risk of SIDS by facilitating rapid responses to evidence of respiratory or other distress and by synchronizing maternal–infant breathing patterns (Mileva-Seitz et al., 2017). The evidence of increased risk of SIDS is interpreted as being related primarily to the high-risk conditions and behaviors previously mentioned rather than to the fact of co-sleeping itself. Advocates argue that the statistical association of co-sleeping with SIDS does not establish that co-sleeping itself is a risk factor for SIDS in the absence of these high-risk conditions (Marinelli et al., 2019). This view is also reflected in guidelines from the UK's National Institute for Health and Care Excellence (NICE, 2014).

6.7.2 Breastfeeding, crying, sleep, and development

Other issues that are linked to where an infant sleeps include how best to support breastfeeding and how to respond to an infant crying during the night (Blunden et al., 2011; Marinelli et al., 2019; St James-Roberts, 2007). Having infants in a separate room (or even in a separate bed) during the night creates the requirement for active decisions about when to retrieve and feed them and when to intervene and comfort them if they are crying. In contrast, distressed or hungry infants in the parental bed could have immediate access to their mothers.

In studies related to breastfeeding and co-sleeping, it is difficult to determine the direction of causality. Facilitating breastfeeding is often cited as an argument in favor of co-sleeping because there are numerous studies showing that bed-sharing infants continue to breastfeed for more weeks than those who do not bed-share (Baddock et al., 2019; Ball, 2003). However, either of two causal interpretations is plausible. Mothers who are committed to breastfeeding could bring babies to the parental bed for convenience (i.e., a decision to breastfeed leads to more co-sleeping). Alternatively, choosing to co-sleep could promote more frequent and persistent breastfeeding (i.e., co-sleeping leads to more breastfeeding).

A related issue is the impact of co-sleeping on infant crying and soothing. One review examined the impact of close infant contact (including increased, but not exclusive, bed-sharing) on reducing infant crying. It noted that the evidence supports an overall reduction in the total amount of crying relative to infants being cared for in a "Western" model (i.e., mostly sleeping in a separate room). However, there were no differences in two other measures that likely contribute more to parental distress and sleep loss than the overall amount of crying, namely, the amount of inconsolable crying and fussing/crying for >3 h daily. This review also noted that increases in sleep amounts do not necessarily reduce infant crying; structured behavioral treatments are very effective in reducing sleep problems that have become established in children, but despite sleep improvements, they may not reduce infant crying (St James-Roberts, 2007).

Sleeping arrangements and decisions about breastfeeding could also affect the sleep of both mothers and infants. One study found that mothers who room-shared showed objectively poorer sleep quality than those who did not (Volkovich et al., 2018). Interpreting this result is not straightforward. It is possible that fussy infants with poor self-soothing skills were more likely to be brought into the parental bedroom and to subsequently disrupt maternal sleep. Alternatively, having an infant share the parental bedroom for other reasons could have given mothers more opportunity to wake up and respond to normal sounds from an infant who was not particularly fussy. As in most studies reviewed here, however, it is difficult to discuss causality, in part because the motivations for co-sleeping or room-sharing and its frequency and duration were not documented.

A rare experimental study that used PSG to record maternal sleep involved two groups of mothers: those who regularly slept separately from their infants and those who were regular bed-sharers. During the study, each mother slept under both conditions with their infants. The sleep of mothers in the bed-sharing condition showed a small percentage decrease in NREM stages 3 and 4 and an increase in stages 1 and 2 sleep

[13] There is a four-fold increased risk of future SIDS in siblings of infants who died of SIDS, but these findings are ambiguous. They may indicate either common environmental factors or shared genetic vulnerability, for example, to cardiovascular, respiratory, or immune system abnormalities (Glinge et al., 2023).

[14] The idea that co-sleeping could be risky to infants is not new. There is a well-known bible story (1 Kings 3:16–28, King James Version) in which King Solomon used a clever, but cruel, trick to determine which of two women was the mother of a living infant and which the mother of one who died during the night because she "lay on him."

as well as more frequent but shorter arousals, regardless of the mothers' usual sleeping arrangements (Mosko et al., 1997).

A meta-analysis involving seven studies of the effects on maternal sleep of breastfeeding found that breastfeeding mothers slept an average of about 14 min longer than non-breastfeeding mothers (Srimoragot et al., 2023). The studies that were summarized did not all report on sleeping arrangements, and those that did indicated a mixture of co-sleeping in a bed, room-sharing, and not co-sleeping. Because co-sleeping and breastfeeding may be correlated, it is not clear whether sleeping arrangements influenced the small sleep duration differences found in relation to breastfeeding.

Potential links between co-sleeping and the sleep of infants have also been examined. Some studies, but not others, found a positive association between co-sleeping and infant sleep problems or increased number of arousals, but the results depended on how infant sleep was assessed. Maternal reports indicated shorter sleep in co-sleeping infants, but overnight monitoring studies reported no consistent differences. Infant arousals were also seen as problematic in some studies but not in others, suggesting that the attitudes of individual mothers were important determinants of how they interpreted the sleep of their infants in relation to co-sleeping (Baddock et al., 2019).

As with breastfeeding, the causal relations between co-sleeping and mothers' or infants' sleep quality are uncertain. Do fussy babies get brought to the parental bed more often to reduce parental sleep disruption ("reactive co-sleeping") or does "intentional co-sleeping" disrupt infant sleep by exposing infants to stimuli from the parents? The same concerns apply to studies showing differences in other outcomes between infants who do and do not co-sleep: physiological measures, child health conditions, and achievement of independence. In addition to reporting conflicting results, these studies cannot determine causal relations because they are primarily cross-sectional and correlational. In addition, they do not typically report the factors that led to decisions to co-sleep, which could help clarify the causal links (Baddock et al., 2019; Cook et al., 2023; Mileva-Seitz et al., 2017).

The few longitudinal studies available provide little evidence for long-lasting effects of sleeping arrangements on development. A study of infants over the period of 3–18 months of age sleeping in the same room as parents or in a separate room found little difference in their sleep quality (Volkovich et al., 2018). Children who did or did not co-sleep as infants also showed no significant psychological or functional differences by 18 years of age (Okami et al., 2002).

6.7.3 Cultural and societal contexts

Because most research on this topic depends on parental reports, cross-cultural studies can be influenced by differences in the way terminology is used by different groups. Parents and researchers in different regions may interpret phrases like "co-sleeping," "sleep problems," and even "infant crying" differently (Cook et al., 2023; Sadeh et al., 2011). Waking or crying at night, for example, may be defined as problems in some cultural contexts but not in others.

Describing motivations for co-sleeping is also problematic. The difference between "reactive" and "intentional" co-sleeping may be well-defined theoretically, but this can be a difficult distinction for parents to make in practice. Parental decisions about infant sleep may be fluid and subject to change with the parents' experience of a particular infant and their evolving goals for the infant. Parents may be influenced by the infant's temperament, age, and tolerance of the current sleeping arrangement, among other factors, to change their sleeping arrangements, and it may happen more than once during early infancy.

Defining co-sleeping in real-world situations can also be a challenge. Infants sleeping in a separate room, for example, may be brought into the parental bed to breastfeed and then remain there for some or all of the night (Ball, 2003). As a result, the choice to describe an infant as a co-sleeper or not and the distinction between reactive and intentional co-sleeping may both be ambiguous. There is a need for larger-scale, experimental, and longitudinal studies to begin to sort out the impacts of the many factors involved in parental choices related to sleeping arrangements. There is also a need for better understanding of how to interpret the terminology used to describe sleeping arrangements and the choices parents make (Cook et al., 2023; Mileva-Seitz et al., 2017).

The debate about co-sleeping practices highlights several issues related to sleep in infants and in people in general. One issue is whether there is a natural ("biological") form and social structure for human, and especially infant, sleep that has been transformed by cultural influences and inventions to the potential detriment of health. A second issue is the basis for the large differences in the frequency with which co-sleeping occurs in different countries and, within some countries, in different ethnocultural and socioeconomic groups. A third issue is the need for better evidence related to the impact of different sleeping arrangements on infants' sleep, and their ability to develop self-soothing during the night, as well as on parental sleep patterns and quality.

Finally, there are different views about what the best strategy is for encouraging healthy outcomes for infants. One option is to continue the argument for and against co-sleeping, but with better data and more information about outcomes for parents and infants. Another option is to acknowledge that co-sleeping occurs to varying extents (among countries, cultural groups, and within individual families over time) and to focus instead on encouraging a reduction in the well-known

BOX 6.1 Fertility and Mortality Rates

Both female fertility rates and infant mortality rates have fallen dramatically across the world. From 1950 to 2021, the total fertility rate (live births per woman) fell from 2.84 to 1.52 in more developed regions and from 5.94 to 2.44 in less developed regions (**Figure 6.5A**). Infant mortality rates/1,000 live births dropped from 60.4 to 4.0 in more developed regions and from 165.2 to 30.3 in less developed regions (**Figure 6.5B**). Data were downloaded from a 2022 United Nations Population data site with different groupings than are currently used. Comparable data can be viewed for different time periods at: https://population.un.org/dataportal/home.

Both fertility and infant mortality rates were undoubtedly much higher before 1950, and the trends seen since then are likely continuing. Over a more recent, shorter interval (2000-2017), worldwide mortality in children under 5 years old fell by nearly 50%, despite a world population increase of 1 billion people and continuing large national and regional differences in wealth (September 17, 2019 edition of the *New York Times*; https://tinyurl.com/yxuxb2ag).

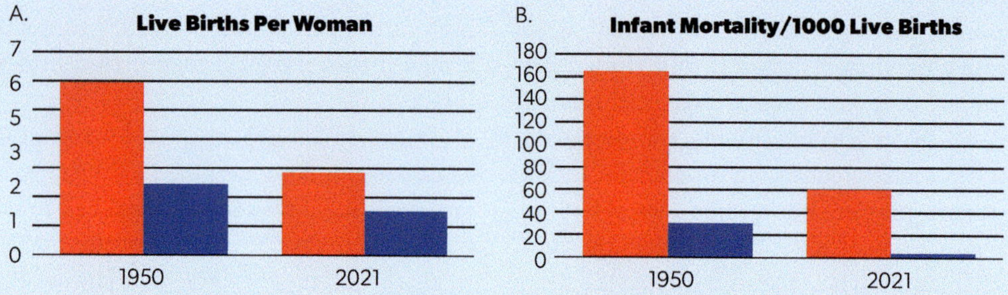

Figure 6.5 **A.** Live births per woman in 1950 and 2021 in the world's less developed regions (red) and more developed regions (blue). **B.** Similar statistics for the rates of infant mortality/1000 live births.

health risks associated with specific parental behaviors and with features of the sleep environment (Marinelli et al., 2019).

These arguments can also be placed in the broader context of long-term changes in demographic and health conditions affecting infants. Preindustrial societies had high infant mortality rates, which were reduced by improvements in sanitation, disease control, and nutrition in wealthy industrial societies. Associated with high infant mortality rates were high female fertility rates, which also fell with industrialization, growing wealth, and increasing female educational attainment. Thus, high fertility rates and high infant mortality rates can both be considered "natural" aspects of preindustrial human ecology that have been altered by public health measures, scientific developments, education, and growing wealth. See **Box 6.1** for a summary of recent changes in fertility and infant mortality rates.

If co-sleeping posed a small risk to infants in traditional societies with their high rates of both fertility and infant mortality, it was likely a very minor factor relative to other risks (e.g., infectious diseases, malnutrition) and not one likely to impede population growth on its own. The same small risk would loom much larger in wealthy, industrial societies that generally protect infants against much greater threats and where family sizes typically average one to two children. It is in this cultural context that the AAP recommended that very young infants should sleep on safe surfaces immediately adjacent to their parents.

6.7.4 Summary

The question of whether human infants should sleep in immediate proximity to their mothers, as other primate infants do, remains contentious. Some arguments focus on the potential hazards of co-sleeping in the form of bed-sharing (e.g., risk of smothering or SIDS). This concern relates especially to high-risk situations such as parental smoking, the presence of bed coverings and soft pillows, and mothers/parents who may have diminished awareness because of substance use, medication, or other factors.

Others argue that the safety concerns of Western medical experts are exaggerated because humans (and other primates) have co-slept with their infants for millennia, and our species has survived and thrived, perhaps too successfully. In addition, they cite the potential benefits of co-sleeping for both infants and mothers, including more breastfeeding and easier access to infants to detect respiratory or other health problems.

These debates are further complicated because discussions of co-sleeping intersect with other contentious issues, such as dealing with infant crying, encouraging breastfeeding, and helping infants achieve self-regulation. Most studies related to co-sleeping are correlational and cross-sectional, making it difficult to reach conclusions about causality. Studies of co-sleeping may also not distinguish clearly between intentional and reactive co-sleeping. While this distinction is important for interpreting the results of studies, it can also be difficult to apply to real-world situations in which parents may be flexible or inconsistent in their use of co-sleeping. There is a need for more longitudinal studies of the use and consequences of co-sleeping for infant sleep and development as well as for parental sleep.

The potential risks of direct co-sleeping (bed-sharing) in wealthier societies needs to be evaluated in relation to the very low rates of both infant mortality and female fertility in these societies. Given this context, the AAP recommendation that very young infants should sleep on a side bed near their parents without potentially dangerous bedding seems like a reasonable compromise. More cross-cultural research is needed to evaluate the risks and advantages of co-sleeping in different countries and ethnocultural contexts.

Literature cited

Baddock, S. A., Purnell, M. T., Blair, P. S., Pease, A. S., Elder, D. E., & Galland, B. C. (2019). The influence of bed-sharing on infant physiology, breastfeeding and behaviour: a systematic review. *Sleep Med Rev, 43*, 106–117. doi: 10.1016/j.smrv.2018.10.007

Ball, H. L. (2003). Breastfeeding, bed-sharing, and infant sleep. *Birth, 30*(3), 181–188.

Barazzetta, M., & Ghislandi, S. (2017). Family income and material deprivation: do they matter for sleep quality and quantity in early life? Evidence from a longitudinal study. *Sleep, 40*(3), 1–9. doi: 10.1093/sleep/zsw066

Basner, M., & Dinges, D. F. (2018). Sleep duration in the United States 2003-2016: first signs of success in the fight against sleep deficiency? *Sleep, 41*(4), zsy012. doi:10.1093/sleep/zsy012

Bin, Y. S., Marshall, N. S., & Glozier, N. (2012). Secular trends in adult sleep duration: a systematic review. *Sleep Med Rev, 16*(3), 223–230. doi: 10.1016/j.smrv.2011.07.003

Blunden, S. L., Thompson, K. R., & Dawson, D. (2011). Behavioural sleep treatments and night time crying in infants: challenging the status quo. *Sleep Med Rev, 15*(5), 327–334. doi: 10.1016/j.smrv.2010.11.002

Carpenter, R., McGarvey, C., Mitchell, E. A., Tappin, D. M., Vennemann, M. M., Smuk, M., & Carpenter, J. R. (2013). Bed sharing when parents do not smoke: is there a risk of SIDS? An individual level analysis of five major case-control studies. *BMJ Open, 3*, e002299. doi: 10.1136/bmjopen-2012-002299

Carskadon, M. A., & Dement, W. C. (1992). Multiple sleep latency tests during the constant routine. *Sleep, 15*, 396–399.

Carter, B., Rees, P., Hale, L., Bhattacharjee, D., & Paradkar, M. S. (2016). Association between portable screen-based media device access or use and sleep outcomes: a systematic review and meta-analysis. *JAMA Pediatr, 170*(12), 1202–1208. doi: 10.1001/jamapediatrics.2016.2341

Chang, A. M., Aeschbach, D., Duffy, J. F., & Czeisler, C. A. (2015). Evening use of light-emitting eReaders negatively affects sleep, circadian timing, and next-morning alertness. *Proc Natl Acad Sci U S A, 112*(4), 1232–1237. doi: 10.1073/pnas.1418490112

Chen, Y., Kartsonaki, C., Clarke, R., Guo, Y., Yu, C., Bian, Z., … China Kadoorie Biobank, S. (2018). Characteristics and correlates of sleep duration, daytime napping, snoring and insomnia symptoms among 0.5 million Chinese men and women. *Sleep Med, 44*, 67–75. doi: 10.1016/j.sleep.2017.11.1131

Combertaldi, S. L., Ort, A., Cordi, M., Fahr, A., & Rasch, B. (2021). Pre-sleep social media use does not strongly disturb sleep: a sleep laboratory study in healthy young participants. *Sleep Med, 87*, 191–202. doi: 10.1016/j.sleep.2021.09.009

Cook, G., Carter, B., Wiggs, L., & Southam, S. (2023). Parental sleep-related practices and sleep in children aged 1–3 years: a systematic review. *J Sleep Res, 22*, e14120. doi:10.1111/jsr.14120

de la Iglesia, H. O., Fernandez-Duque, E., Golombek, D. A., Lanza, N., Duffy, J. F., Czeisler, C. A., & Valeggia, C. R. (2015). Access to electric light is associated with shorter sleep duration in a traditionally hunter-gatherer community. *J Biol Rhythms, 30*(4), 342–350. doi: 10.1177/0748730415590702

de Ruiter, I., Olmedo-Requena, R., Sanchez-Cruz, J. J., & Jimenez-Moleon, J. J. (2016). Changes in sleep duration in Spanish children aged 2-14 years from 1987 to 2011. *Sleep Med, 21*, 145–150. doi: 10.1016/j.sleep.2015.12.021

Di, H., Guo, Y., Daghlas, I., Wang, L., Liu, G., Pan, A., … Shan, Z. (2022). Evaluation of sleep habits and disturbances among US adults, 2017-2020. *JAMA Netw Open, 5*(11), e2240788. doi:10.1001/jamanetworkopen.2022.40788

Ekirch, A. R. (2001). Sleep we have lost: pre-industrial slumber in the British Isles. *Am Histor Rev, 106*(2), 343–386.

Ekirch, A. R. (2016). Segmented sleep in preindustrial societies. *Sleep, 39*(3), 715–716. doi: 10.5665/sleep.5558

Ford, E. S., Cunningham, T. J., & Croft, J. B. (2015). Trends in self-reported sleep duration among US adults from 1985 to 2012. *Sleep, 38*(5), 829–832. doi: 10.5665/sleep.4684

Glinge, C., Rossetti, S., Oestergaard, L. B., Stampe, N. K., Lynge, T. H., Skals, R., … Tfelt-Hansen, J. (2023). Risk of sudden infant death syndrome among siblings of children who died of sudden infant death syndrome in Denmark. *JAMA Netw Open, 6*(1), e2252724. doi: 10.1001/jamanetworkopen.2022.52724

Gradisar, M., Wolfson, A. R., Harvey, A. G., Hale, L., Rosenberg, R., & Czeisler, C. A. (2013). The sleep and technology use of Americans: findings from the National Sleep Foundation's 2011 Sleep in America poll. *J Clin Sleep Med, 9*(12), 1291–1299. doi: 10.5664/jcsm.3272

Green, A., Cohen-Zion, M., Haim, A., & Dagan, Y. (2017). Evening light exposure to computer screens disrupts human sleep, biological rhythms, and attention abilities. *Chronobiol Int, 34*(7), 855–865. doi: 10.1080/07420528.2017.1324878

Hale, L., Troxel, W. M., Kravitz, H. M., Hall, M. H., & Matthews, K. A. (2014). Acculturation and sleep among a multiethnic sample of women: the Study of Women's Health Across the Nation (SWAN). *Sleep, 37*(2), 309–317. doi: 10.5665/sleep.3404

Harari, Y. N. (2014). *Sapiens: A Brief History of Mankind.* Toronto: McLelland & Stewart.

Horne, J. (2011). The end of sleep: "sleep debt" versus biological adaptation of human sleep to waking needs. *Biol Psychol, 87*(1), 1–14. doi: 10.1016/j.biopsycho.2010.10.004

Jang, Y., Jun, J. S., & Jung, K.-Y. (2023). Trends in sleep duration in Korea: the Korean time use survey. *Sleep Med, 103*, 24–28. doi: 10.1016/j.sleep.2023.01.025

Johnson, D. A., Lisabeth, L., Hickson, D., Johnson-Lawrence, V., Samdarshi, T., Taylor, H., & Diez Roux, A. V. (2016). The social patterning of sleep in African Americans: associations of socioeconomic position and neighborhood characteristics with sleep in the Jackson Heart Study. *Sleep, 39*(9), 1749–1759. doi: 10.5665/sleep.6106

Johnson, D. A., Lisabeth, L., Lewis, T. T., Sims, M., Hickson, D. A., Samdarshi, T., Taylor, H., & Diez Roux, A. V. (2016). The contribution of psychosocial stressors to sleep among African Americans in the Jackson Heart Study. *Sleep, 39*(7), 1411–1419. doi: 10.5665/sleep.5974

Kempenaers, B., Borgstrom, P., Loes, P., Schlicht, E., & Valcu, M. (2010). Artificial night lighting affects dawn song, extra-pair siring success, and lay date in songbirds. *Curr Biol, 20*(19), 1735–1739. doi: 10.1016/j.cub.2010.08.028

Kim, B., Troxel, W. M., Dubowitz, T., Hunter, G. P., Ghosh-Dastidar, B., Chaix, B., … Duncan, D. T. (2022). Mediating role of psychological distress in the associations between neighborhood social environments and sleep health. *Sleep, 45*(8), zsac087. doi:10.1093/sleep/zsac087

Knutson, K. L. (2014). Sleep duration, quality, and timing and their associations with age in a community without electricity in Haiti. *Am J Hum Biol, 26*(1), 80–86. doi: 10.1002/ajhb.22481

Kompotis, K., Hubbard, J., Emmenegger, Y., Perrault, A., Muhlethaler, M., Schwartz, S., … Franken, P. (2019). Rocking promotes sleep in mice through rhythmic stimulation of the vestibular system. *Curr Biol, 29*(3), 392–401. doi: 10.1016/j.cub.2018.12.007

Kronholm, E., Puusniekka, R., Jokela, J., Villberg, J., Urrila, A. S., Paunio, T., … Tynjala, J. (2015). Trends in self-reported sleep problems, tiredness and related school performance among Finnish adolescents from 1984 to 2011. *J Sleep Res, 24*(1), 3–10. doi: 10.1111/jsr.12258

Leech, J. A. (2017). Changes in sleep duration and recreational screen time among Canadians, 1998–2010. *J Sleep Res, 26*(2), 202–209. doi: 10.1111/jsr.12479

Luijk, M. P., Mileva-Seitz, V. R., Jansen, P. W., van IJzendoorn, M. H., Jaddoe, V. W., Raat, H., … Tiemeier, H. (2013). Ethnic differences in prevalence and determinants of mother-child bed-sharing in early childhood. *Sleep Med, 14*(11), 1092–1099. doi: 10.1016/j.sleep.2013.04.019

Magee, C. A., Gordon, R., & Caputi, P. (2014). Distinct developmental trends in sleep duration during early childhood. *Pediatrics, 133*(6), e1561–e1567. doi: 10.1542/peds.2013-3806

Marinelli, K. A., Ball, H. L., McKenna, J. J., & Blair, P. S. (2019). An integrated analysis of maternal-infant sleep, breastfeeding, and sudden infant death syndrome research supporting a balanced discourse. *J Hum Lact, 35*(3), 510–520.

Matricciani, L., Bin, Y. S., Lallukka, T., Kronholm, E., Dumuid, D., Paquet, C., & Olds, T. (2017). Past, present, and future: trends in sleep duration and implications for public health. *Sleep Health, 3*(5), 317–323. doi: 10.1016/j.sleh.2017.07.006

Matricciani, L., Olds, T., & Petkov, J. (2011). In search of lost sleep: secular trends in the sleep time of school-aged children and adolescents. *Sleep Med Rev, 16*(3), 203–211. doi: 10.1016/j.smrv.2011.03.005

Matricciani, L. A., Olds, T. S., Blunden, S., Rigney, G., & Williams, M. T. (2012). Never enough sleep: a brief history of sleep recommendations for children. *Pediatrics, 129*(3), 548–556. doi: 10.1542/peds.2011-2039

McKenna, J. J., Ball, H. L., & Gettler, L. T. (2007). Mother-infant cosleeping, breastfeeding and sudden infant death syndrome: what biological anthropology has discovered about normal infant sleep and pediatric sleep medicine. *Am J Phys Anthropol, Suppl 45*, 133–161. doi: 10.1002/ajpa.20736

Mellman, T. A., Bell, K. A., Abu-Bader, S. H., & Kobayashi, I. (2018). Neighborhood stress and autonomic nervous system activity during sleep. *Sleep, 41*(6), zsy059. doi: 10.1093/sleep/zsy059

Mileva-Seitz, V. R., Bakermans-Kranenburg, M. J., Battaini, C., & Luijk, M. P. (2017). Parent-child bed-sharing: the good, the bad, and the burden of evidence. *Sleep Med Rev, 32*, 4–27. doi: 10.1016/j.smrv.2016.03.003

Mindell, J. A., Sadeh, A., Kwon, R., & Goh, D. Y. (2013). Cross-cultural differences in the sleep of preschool children. *Sleep Med, 14*(12), 1283–1289. doi: 10.1016/j.sleep.2013.09.002

Mindell, J. A., Sadeh, A., Wiegand, B., How, T. H., & Goh, D. Y. (2010). Cross-cultural differences in infant and toddler sleep. *Sleep Med, 11*(3), 274–280. doi: 10.1016/j.sleep.2009.04.012

Moreno, C. R., Vasconcelos, S., Marqueze, E. C., Lowden, A., Middleton, B., Fischer, F. M., Louzada, F. M., & Skene, D. J. (2015). Sleep patterns in Amazon rubber tappers with and without electric light at home. *Sci Rep, 5*, 14074. doi: 10.1038/srep14074

Mosko, S., Richard, C., & McKenna, J. (1997). Maternal sleep and arousal during bedsharing with infants. *Sleep, 20*(2), 142–150.

Mumford, L. (1934). *Technics and Civilization.* Chicago: The University of Chicago Press.

Musharbash, Y. (2013). Night, sight, and feeling safe: an exploration of aspects of Warlpiri and western sleep. *Aust J Anthropol, 24*, 48–63. doi: 10.1111/taja.12021

NICE. (2014). Addendum to Clinical Guideline 37, Postnatal Care: routine postnatal care of women and their babies. Retrieved January 12, 2020, from https://www.nice.org.uk/guidance/cg37/evidence/fullguideline-addendum-485782238

Obayashi, K., Saeki, K., & Kurumatani, N. (2014). Association between light exposure at night and insomnia in the general elderly population: the HEIJO-KYO cohort. *Chronobiol Int, 31*(9), 976–982. doi: 10.3109/07420528.2014.937491

Ohayon, M. M., & Milesi, C. (2016). Artificial outdoor nighttime lights associate with altered sleep behavior in the American general population. *Sleep, 39*(6), 1311–1320. doi: 10.5665/sleep.5860

Okami, P., Weisner, T., & Olmstead, R. (2002). Outcome correlates of parent-child bedsharing: an eighteen-year longitudinal study. *Dev Behav Pediatr, 23*(4), 244–253.

p'Bitek, O. (1989). *Song of Lawino.* Nairobi, Kenya: East African Educational Publishers Ltd.

Paraskakis, E., Ntouros, T., Ntokos, M., Siavana, O., Bitsori, M., & Galanakis, E. (2008). Siesta and sleep patterns in a sample of adolescents in Greece. *Pediatr Int, 50*(5), 690–693. doi: 10.1111/j.1442-200X.2008.02632.x

Perrault, A. A., Khani, A., Quairiaux, C., Kompotis, K., Franken, P., Muhlethaler, M., Schwartz, S., & Bayer, L. (2019). Whole-night continuous rocking entrains spontaneous neural oscillations with benefits for sleep and memory. *Curr Biol, 29*(3), 402–411. doi: 10.1016/j.cub.2018.12.028

Pillion, M., Gradisar, M., Bartel, K., Whittall, H., & Kahn, M. (2022). What's "app"-ning to adolescent sleep? Links between device, app use, and sleep outcomes. *Sleep Med, 100*, 174–182. doi: 10.1016/j.sleep.2022.08.004

Piosczyk, H., Landmann, N., Holz, J., Feige, B., Riemann, D., Nissen, C., & Voderholzer, U. (2014). Prolonged sleep under Stone Age conditions. *J Clin Sleep Med, 10*(7), 719–722. doi: 10.5664/jcsm.3854

Ramos, K. D., & Youngclarke, D. M. (2006). Parenting advice books about child sleep: cosleeping and crying it out. *Sleep, 29*(12), 1616–1623.

Roky, R., Chapotot, F., Benchekroun, M. T., Benaji, B., Hakkou, F., Elkhalifi, H., & Buguet, A. (2003). Daytime sleepiness during Ramadan intermittent fasting: polysomnographic and quantitative waking EEG study. *J Sleep Res, 12*(2), 95–101.

Roky, R., Chapotot, F., Hakkou, F., Benchekroun, M. T., & Buguet, A. (2001). Sleep during Ramadan intermittent fasting. *J Sleep Res, 10*(4), 319–327.

Sadeh, A., Mindell, J., & Rivera, L. (2011). "My child has a sleep problem": a cross-cultural comparison of parental definitions. *Sleep Med, 12*(5), 478–482. doi: 10.1016/j.sleep.2010.10.008

Samson, D. R., Crittenden, A. N., Mabulla, I. A., Mabulla, A. Z., & Nunn, C. L. (2017). Hadza sleep biology: evidence for flexible sleep-wake patterns in hunter-gatherers. *Am J Phys Anthropol, 162*(3), 573–582. doi: 10.1002/ajpa.23160

Samson, D. R., Manus, M. B., Krystal, A. D., Fakir, E., Yu, J. J., & Nunn, C. L. (2017). Segmented sleep in a nonelectric, small-scale agricultural society in Madagascar. *Am J Hum Biol, 29*(4). doi: 10.1002/ajhb.22979

Sanders, D., Frago, E., Kehoe, R., Patterson, C., & Gaston, K. J. (2021). A meta-analysis of biological impacts of artificial light at night. *Nat Ecol Evol, 5*(1), 74–81. doi: doi: 10.1038/s41559-020-01322-x

Sassin, J. F., Frantz, A. G., Kapen, S., & Weitzman, E. D. (1973). The nocturnal rise of human prolactin is dependent on sleep. *J Clin Endocr Metab, 37*, 436–440.

Sheehan, C. M., Frochen, S. E., Walsemann, K. M., & Ailshire, J. A. (2019). Are U.S. adults reporting less sleep?: findings from sleep duration trends in the National Health Interview Survey, 2004–2017. *Sleep, 42*(2), zsy221. doi:10.1093/sleep/zsy221

Short, M. A., Gradisar, M., Lack, L. C., Wright, H. R., Dewald, J. F., Wolfson, A. R., & Carskadon, M. A. (2013). A cross-cultural comparison of sleep duration between US And Australian adolescents: the effect of school start time, parent-set bedtimes, and extracurricular load. *Health Educ Behav, 40*(3), 323–330. doi: 10.1177/1090198112451266

Smit, A. N., Broesch, T., Siegel, J. M., & Mistlberger, R. E. (2019). Sleep timing and duration in indigenous villages with and without electric lighting on Tanna Island, Vanuatu. *Sci Rep, 9*(1), 17278. doi:10.1038/s41598-019-53635-y

Soldatos, C. R., Allaert, F. A., Ohta, T., & Dikeos, D. G. (2005). How do individuals sleep around the world? Results from a single-day survey in ten countries. *Sleep Med, 6*(1), 5–13. doi: 10.1016/j.sleep.2004.10.006

Spiegel, K., Luthringer, R., Follenius, M., Schaltenbrand, N., Macher, J. P., Muzet, A., & Brandenberger, G. (1995). Temporal relationship between prolactin secretion and slow-wave electroencephalic activity during sleep. *Sleep, 18*(7), 543–548.

Srimoragot, M., Hershberger, P. E., Park, C., Hernandez, T. L., & Izci Balserak, B. (2023). Infant feeding type and maternal sleep during the postpartum period: a systematic review and meta-analysis. *J Sleep Res, 32*(2), e13625. doi:10.1111/jsr.13625

St James-Roberts, I. (2007). Helping parents to manage infant crying and sleeping: a review of the evidence and its implications for services. *Child Abuse Rev, 16*(1), 47–69. doi: 10.1002/car.968

Stearns, P. N., Rowland, P., & Giarnella, L. (1996). Children's sleep: sketching historical change. *J Soc Hist, 30*(2), 345–366.

TFOSIDS. (2016). SIDS and other sleep-related infant deaths: updated 2016 recommendations for a safe infant sleeping environment. *Pediatrics, 138*(5), 1–12. doi: 10.1542/peds.2016-2938

Twenge, J. M., Krizan, Z., & Hisler, G. (2017). Decreases in self-reported sleep duration among U.S. adolescents 2009-2015 and association with new media screen time. *Sleep Med, 39*, 47–53. doi: 10.1016/j.sleep.2017.08.013

Volkovich, E., Bar-Kalifa, E., Meiri, G., & Tikotzky, L. (2018). Mother-infant sleep patterns and parental functioning of room-sharing and solitary sleeping families: a longitudinal study from 3 to 18 months. *Sleep, 41*(2), zsx207. doi: 10.1093/sleep/zsx207

Waldstreicher, J., Duffy, J. F., Brown, E. N., Rogacz, S., Allan, J. S., & Czeisler, C. A. (1996). Gender differences in the temporal organization of prolactin (PRL)

secretion: evidence for a sleep-independent circadian rhythm of PRL levels–a clinical research center study. *J Clin Endocr Metab, 81*, 1483–1487.

Watson, N. F., Badr, M. S., Belenky, G., Bliwise, D. L., Buxton, O. M., Buysse, D., Dinges, D. F., Gangwisch, J., ... Tasali, E. (2015). Joint consensus statement of the American Academy of Sleep Medicine and Sleep Research Society on the recommended amount of sleep for a healthy adult: methodology and discussion. *Sleep, 38*(8), 1161–1183. doi: 10.5665/sleep.4886

Wehr, T. A. (1991). The durations of human melatonin secretion and sleep respond to changes in daylength (photoperiod). *J Clin Endocr Metab, 73*, 1276–1280.

Wehr, T. A. (1999). The impact of changes in nightlength (scotoperiod) on human sleep. In F. W. Turek & P. C. Zee (Eds.), *Regulation of Sleep and Circadian Rhythms* (pp. 263–285). Boca Raton: CRC Press.

Wehr, T. A., Moul, D. E., Barbato, G., Giesen, H. A., Seidel, J. A., Barker, C., & Bender, C. (1993). Conservation of photoperiod-responsive mechanisms in humans. *Am J Physiol, 265*(4 Pt 2), R846–R857.

Worthman, C. M., & Melby, M. K. (2002). Toward a comparative developmental ecology of human sleep. In M. A. Carskadon (Ed.), *Adolescent Sleep Patterns: Biological, Social, and Psychological Influences* (pp. 69–117). New York: Cambridge University Press.

Yetish, G., Kaplan, H., Gurven, M., Wood, B., Pontzer, H., Manger, P. R., Wilson, C., McGregor, R., & Siegel, J. M. (2015). Natural sleep and its seasonal variations in three pre-industrial societies. *Curr Biol, 25*(21), 2862–2868. doi: 10.1016/j.cub.2015.09.046

Youngstedt, S. D., Goff, E. E., Reynolds, A. M., Kripke, D. F., Irwin, M. R., Bootzin, R. R., Khan, N., & Jean-Louis, G. (2016). Has adult sleep duration declined over the last 50+ years? *Sleep Med Rev, 28*, 69–85. doi: 10.1016/j.smrv.2015.08.004

CHAPTER 7

Sleep in Other Species

7.1 OVERVIEW

Animal models have been, and continue to be, of critical importance for our understanding of both the mechanisms and functions of sleep. This chapter describes limitations on the use of electrophysiological measures to study sleep across species and discusses how behavioral criteria can be applied to identify sleep in species for which electrophysiological criteria cannot be used. It discusses the large differences in sleep patterns that have been described among mammalian species and the characteristics that have been correlated with the amounts of sleep and of sleep stages.

This chapter also discusses the existence, mechanisms, and possible functions of a sleep pattern in birds and marine mammals that differs dramatically from that seen in terrestrial mammals, including humans; namely, sleep that occurs in one cerebral hemisphere at a time (unihemispheric sleep). It reviews evidence for dramatic changes in sleep patterns associated with adaptations to seasonal environmental changes, including during migration in some bird species.

The evidence for diverse sleep patterns among species, and within species at different life stages, is discussed in relation to understanding both the regulation of sleep and its flexibility in accommodating other needs and functions.

7.2 Measuring sleep across species

7.2.1 Measuring sleep using EEG features

In order to develop and test hypotheses about the functions of sleep, we need to be able to account for how sleep varies during development in people (Chapter 4), in different cultural and physical environments (Chapter 6), and among a variety of species (Aulsebrook et al., 2016). The first step toward species comparisons, however, is to decide which species sleep and how we can measure their sleep accurately.

It is not hard to guess without the benefit of EEG recordings when the family dog, hamster, or canary has fallen asleep. They show characteristic features that we also see in other (human) family members. They stop moving and interacting with the environment, close their eyes, and become noticeably unresponsive to external events. In addition, each animal adopts a species-characteristic sleep posture: a dog may curl up in a bed like a horizontal snail (**Figure 7.1**); a cat adopts a "sphinx" posture; a hamster rolls into a ball in its nest; and

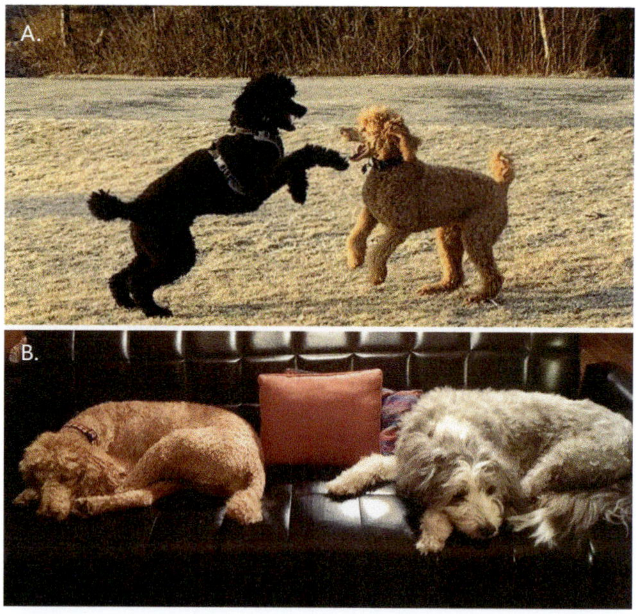

Figure 7.1 We are likely to be able to judge with good reliability whether familiar mammals are asleep or awake based strictly on behavioral criteria, without recording EEG activity. The dogs in **A** (Nellie on the right and her kid brother Gus) are standing, apparently in motion, and interacting with each other; we would readily judge them to be awake. The two dogs in **B** (Nellie and her friend Marcus) have very different postures, with eyes closed, and are apparently not interacting with each other or the environment; they seem likely to be asleep. (Personal photographs)

a canary clamps its feet tightly to a perch and tucks its beak under a wing.

But would you be equally confident in deciding whether a pet goldfish that is hanging motionless in the water, or a turtle with its head withdrawn into its shell is awake or asleep? What about a fruit fly sitting motionless on the kitchen counter? Is it asleep? In fact, does it sleep (**Figure 7.2**)?

EEG criteria that are generally similar to those used for humans can be applied to identify sleep and its stages in other mammals and in birds. The signals that are recorded from the human scalp are generated by electrical activity occurring in the large neocortex (a part of the cerebrum) that overlies the rest of the brain in all mammals (see Section 2.2.1). The size and complexity of the neocortex vary among mammals, but its fundamental six-layered structure is common to mammalian species, so sleep recordings from different mammals look relatively similar. The cerebral structures of other vertebrate classes, however, do not include a six-layered neocortex.

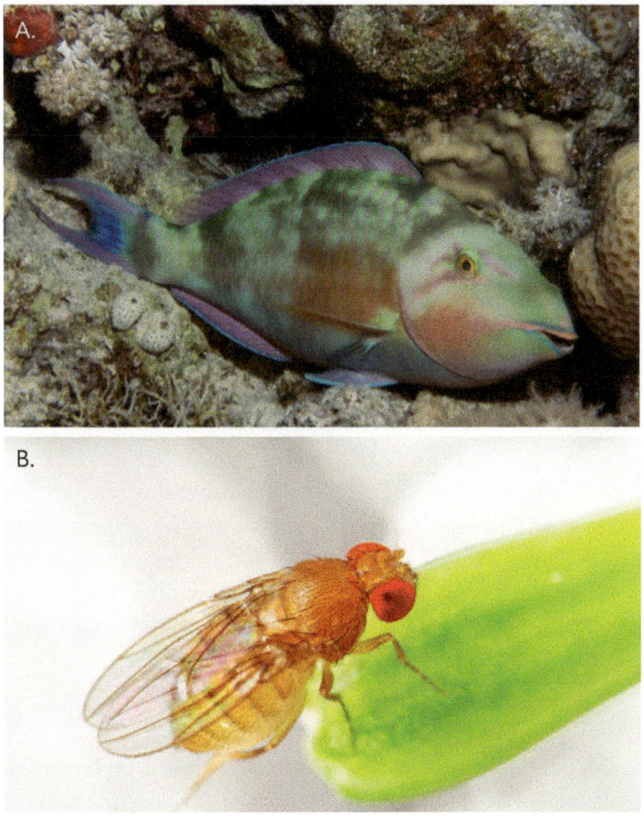

Figure 7.2 Although applying casual behavioral criteria may be effective in deciding whether a familiar mammal is awake or asleep (as in **Figure 7.1**), it is much more challenging when studying other vertebrates or invertebrates. **A.** The Pacific longnose parrotfish (*Hipposcarus longiceps*) illustrated here was described in a caption as sleeping at night. But based on its posture, and in the absence of eyelids, we might judge it to be resting, lying in wait for prey, or sleeping. Paul Vinten/Shutterstock.com. **B.** In the case of an invertebrate like the fruit fly (*Drosophila* sp.), its apparent immobility is ambiguous, and its eyes again provide no obvious clue about its state. Alexky/Shutterstock.com.

Birds are most similar to mammals because both groups have an elaborate cerebral structure that arises from the embryonic dorsal telencephalon (forebrain) and overlies subcortical structures, such as the basal ganglia, diencephalon, and brainstem. These structures are called the cortex or neocortex in mammals and the pallium in birds (until recently called the hyperstriatum) (Jarvis et al., 2005). The avian pallium, however, is not layered; it is organized in a nuclear fashion, more like mammalian subcortical structures. Despite their organizational differences, these cerebral structures perform many similar functions in organizing behavior in both groups (Jarvis et al., 2005).

The combination of similar functions but different structures in the cortex and pallium raises the question of how the components of these structures are related to each other. A partial answer is that some cellular components of the pallium and cortex have similar molecular markers and input/output connections. There is also evidence that the cells forming the mammalian cortex and the avian (and reptilian) dorsal ventricular ridge (part of the pallium) have common developmental origins (Karten, 1997). Thus, many of the basic cellular elements that make up the mammalian cortex appear to be homologous to those found in birds (i.e., they have an ancient, common evolutionary origin). Modifications that occurred later in the separate evolutionary histories of birds and mammals resulted in stacking of cells in tissue layers in the cortex and packing of homologous elements into nuclei in the pallium (Dugas-Ford & Ragsdale, 2015; Jarvis et al., 2005; Karten, 1991).

Given these significant structural differences between mammals and birds, it is somewhat surprising that EEG recordings obtained from the brains of birds show electrical patterns that resemble those from mammals (Low et al., 2008). EEG patterns in birds include low-amplitude activity during waking and REM sleep and high-amplitude, slower oscillations during NREM sleep. One difference is that avian REM sleep episodes are typically very brief (<10 s), relative to those in mammals, and occupy very little of the sleep phase (van Hasselt et al., 2019). Despite these EEG similarities, there is no evidence that birds generate other EEG features characteristic of mammalian sleep, including cortical sleep spindles and hippocampal sharp-wave ripples (Rattenborg et al., 2011; van der Meij et al., 2019).

Other vertebrate classes (reptiles, amphibians, fish) have not been studied as often as mammals and birds, but most researchers agree that they do sleep. Some have concluded that these species show sleep that is homologous to the sleep of birds and mammals, based on evidence of brain electrical patterns, changes in response thresholds, and homeostatic regulation of their sleep state; for a review, see Tobler, 2005). Others, however, have questioned whether the available evidence convincingly demonstrates that the rest states of other vertebrates are physiologically or functionally equivalent to the sleep states of mammals (Siegel, 2008).

There is evidence, however, that a forebrain structure in reptiles may be developmentally homologous to the cortex of mammals (Karten, 1991; Karten, 1997) and that the "cortices" of reptiles, birds, and mammals could have evolved from a three-layered structure in a common ancestor of all three groups (Laurent et al., 2016). Despite these suggestions of homology, the different cerebral anatomy in nonmammalian/avian vertebrates makes brain electrical recordings difficult to interpret and to compare to those from mammals or birds.

The electrophysiological features recorded from cerebral structures of sleeping reptiles are not identical to those seen during either NREM or REM sleep in birds and mammals, which leaves room for argument about which state reptilian sleep resembles more closely (Flanigan et al., 1974; Rattenborg, 2006b; Siegel, 2008; Vorster & Born, 2015). Studies in a variety of reptiles identified electrophysiological features in their sleep that resembled features of mammalian REM sleep, NREM sleep, or both. These different conclusions could be related to the different neural targets of the recordings (Albeck et al., 2022) or the species studied (for references, see Albeck et al., 2022; Rattenborg, 2006b; Siegel, 2008).

A report of bursts of eye movements alternating with periods without eye movements during sleep in a lizard (the Australian dragon, *Pogona vitticeps*) (Shein-Idelson et al., 2016) suggested the existence of a very high-frequency alternation (~80 s period) between NREM-like and REM-like sleep in a reptile.[1] A subsequent study of a different diurnal lizard (*Laudakia vulgaris*) found a similar high-frequency cycle of changing probabilities of slower and faster EEG activity, eye movements, and muscle twitches during sleep (Albeck et al., 2022).

Despite these suggestions of REM sleep-like activity in reptiles, most researchers concluded that sleep in reptiles is more similar to mammalian NREM sleep than to REM sleep. For example, the large, sharp EEG waves observed during sleep or anesthesia in reptiles have been proposed to represent analogs or precursors of sharp waves originating in the hippocampus, or of cortical slow waves, both of which occur during mammalian NREM sleep (Aulsebrook et al., 2016; Flanigan et al., 1974; Rattenborg, 2006b; Tisdale et al., 2018; Zepelin et al., 2005). If sleep in current reptiles is similar to mammalian and avian NREM sleep, it would be likely that a form of NREM sleep characterized the early vertebrates that were common ancestors of these groups. This assumption leads to the conclusion that REM sleep evolved more recently in both birds and mammals (see Section 7.4.4). It remains to be seen how recent evidence supporting the existence of two sleep states in reptiles will be integrated into this view of the evolution of REM sleep.

[1] A later article raised questions about whether these reported eye movements actually occurred during sleep (Aulsebrook et al., 2016).

7.2.2 Behavioral criteria for sleep

When we turn to invertebrate species, the fundamental organization of the nervous system is so different that it is unlikely that they would generate EEG signals similar to those recorded from mammalian brains. If EEG criteria cannot be applied to decide whether and how invertebrates (and many vertebrates) sleep, an alternative approach is to apply behavioral criteria, as we do informally for our nonhuman housemates. Given the very large differences in physiology and behavior in species ranging from invertebrates to mammals, it is important to agree on a set of objective behavioral criteria that discriminate sleep from other behavioral states across these taxonomic groups.

An early proposal was that four criteria can be used to identify behavioral sleep and to distinguish it from other states (similar to those attributed to Piéron, 1913 in Meisel et al., 2011), as applied to the caiman (*Caiman sclerops*, a small crocodilian reptile; see Flanigan Jr. et al., 1973). A fifth criterion related to homeostatic regulation of sleep was added later (Campbell & Tobler, 1984), resulting in the following formal behavioral criteria for identifying sleep in any species:

1. During preparation for sleep, the animal orients toward a specific sleeping site and adopts a species-characteristic posture (which varies greatly among species; see **Figure 7.3**).
2. The animal becomes immobile (i.e., stops voluntary activity and shows reduced mobility).
3. The animal shows an elevated threshold for reacting or awakening in response to external stimuli.
4. Moderately intense stimuli lead to more or less rapid reversal of state to full waking.
5. Deprivation of the opportunity to sleep leads subsequently to increased pressure to sleep (i.e., an increased probability of falling asleep) and to a rebound increase in sleep duration (i.e., lost sleep is, at least partially, compensated for during a recovery opportunity). In other words, sleep is homeostatically regulated (see Chapter 5).

Note that these criteria are intended to distinguish sleep not only from the usual waking behaviors of organisms, which is relatively easy to do, but also from the state of rest while fully

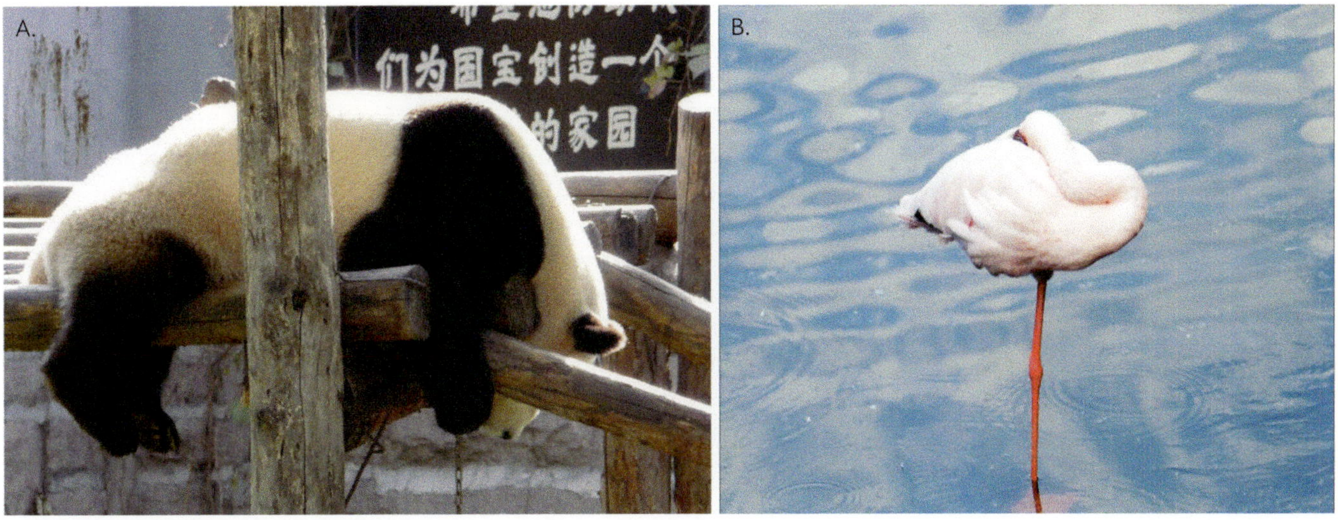

Figure 7.3 **A.** The spontaneously adopted sleep posture of a giant panda (*Ailuropoda melanoleuca*) living in an outdoor enclosure at the Beijing zoo (Personal photograph). **B.** The typical sleep posture of a flamingo (likely *Phoenicopterus sp.*), standing on one leg, in water, with head firmly tucked under one wing. Galina Skornyakova/Shutterstock.com.

awake, which is more challenging.[2] These criteria also distinguish sleep from less common states which sleep can resemble, at least superficially. These include stupor (unresponsiveness as a result of brain injury, toxic drugs, or a psychiatric condition), torpor (as in hibernation), or coma (sometimes irreversible loss of consciousness, usually as a result of brain trauma).

An organism that is fully awake, but resting quietly with eyes closed may meet the first two criteria (immobility and a species-characteristic posture) but can respond immediately to external stimuli (typically sounds; with eyes closed, it will not respond to most visual stimuli). Therefore, it does not show an elevated response threshold and fails to meet criterion 3. An organism during a metabolic-, injury- or drug-induced stupor, during hibernation, or while in a coma will meet criteria 1–3 but will not show rapid waking in response to moderately intense stimuli (criterion 4), and may not respond at all to external stimuli. If aroused from a stupor by an intense intervention, however, the organism will not later increase the time spent in that state (criterion 5). The organism has no physiological need to be in a state of stupor for a specific duration; thus, "deprivation" of that state does not result in a compensatory increase.

The final criterion—rebound increases after deprivation—is critical for distinguishing sleep from other inactive states because it incorporates the view that sleep is the expression of a drive similar to other powerful, instinctual drives (e.g., hunger, thirst) that are homeostatically regulated. Organisms that cannot satisfy these drives show: 1) increasing motivation to do so; and 2) a rebound increase in the amount or intensity of the related behavior (eating, drinking, sleeping) when deprivation ends. These features reflect the pressure to satisfy an important need (see Chapter 5). Thus, these five criteria together identify a unique behavioral state, different from wakefulness as well as from other states of inactivity, which represents the expression of an important instinctual drive.

Adding these behavioral criteria to the electrophysiological and regulatory features described in Chapters 2 and 5, we can generate a definition of sleep that is broadly applicable across species: Sleep consists of one or more neurobehavioral states that are rapidly reversible to waking by moderate-intensity sensory stimulation. It is characterized by unique patterns of neural activity and regulated by both homeostatic and circadian mechanisms. During sleep, animals adopt a species-typical posture/location, show reduced activity, and diminished, but not absent, responsiveness to environmental stimuli.

7.2.3 Summary

Recordings from the neocortex or pallium in mammals and birds, respectively, show EEG features during both NREM and REM sleep that are relatively similar. It is less clear whether other vertebrate species show similar EEG patterns. There are different views as to whether the EEG patterns of reptiles resemble either REM or NREM sleep of mammals, but most researchers view reptilian sleep as more similar to NREM sleep. Recent research suggests the possibility, however, that reptiles produce two rapidly alternating sleep states with characteristics that resemble those of NREM and REM sleep. The results of recordings in reptiles may depend on which brain structure is targeted.

---

[2] Many people have attempted to simulate sleep at some point for the benefit of a parent or partner by mimicking criteria 1–4, with varying degrees of success.

The large differences in neural organization between vertebrate and invertebrate species make it unlikely that the electrophysiological correlates of human/mammalian sleep will be identified in invertebrates. There are also situations in which EEG recordings are not available in mammals and other vertebrates, so behavioral criteria must be applied to study their sleep. A set of five behavioral criteria have been developed that are used to determine whether sleep is present in any species. These distinguish sleep from waking and from other states that involve reductions in activity and environmental responsiveness. These criteria define a unique neurobehavioral state that is the expression of an important instinctual drive.

7.3 Sleep in invertebrates

The five behavioral criteria originally established for vertebrates have also been applied to determine whether invertebrate species sleep. Most of this research has involved fruit flies (*Drosophila melanogaster*) and honeybees (*Apis mellifera*), but there are also studies of cockroaches, scorpions, spiders, cuttlefish, octopus, and nematode worms.

The first two criteria (immobility and a characteristic posture) can be readily demonstrated in several invertebrate species and are typically shown only at some circadian phases, which is also characteristic of sleep in many mammals.[3] However, these features could also occur during rest while awake. A change in responsiveness to the environment is one of the defining characteristics of sleep, but not of quiet rest. Elevated thresholds to respond to external stimuli have been demonstrated in immobile fruit flies and honeybees (Hendricks et al., 2000; Huber et al., 2004; Kaiser, 1988), which encourages interpretation of this state as being at least "sleep-like." In support of this interpretation, there is also behavioral and electrophysiological evidence for lighter and deeper sleep stages in fruit flies, characterized by differences in the degree of reduction in environmental responsiveness (van Alphen et al., 2013).

The final test for whether one interprets inactive, quiet periods in an invertebrate as functionally similar to mammalian sleep is whether there is a rebound increase in the duration of this state after a period of deprivation. Studies in fruit flies and cockroaches, for example, have shown that there are later increases in a sleep-like state of immobility after its deprivation (Hendricks et al., 2000; Huber et al., 2004; Tobler, 1983). A neural mechanism has also been identified that mediates the effects of sleep deprivation on later sleep in fruit flies (Liu et al., 2016). Some deprivation effects were time of day-dependent, which can also be seen in mammals, and there were sex differences under some conditions (Huber et al., 2004). Biological sex and sex hormone profiles have also been shown to affect homeostatic responses to sleep loss in mammals (Armitage et al., 2001; Carrier et al., 2017; Deurveilher et al., 2011; Dib et al., 2021).

Despite some observed differences from mammals, several reviews have concluded that the behavioral criteria for sleep (Campbell & Tobler, 1984) have been satisfied for fruit flies as well as for other invertebrates (Hendricks et al., 2000; Meisel et al., 2011; Raizen et al., 2008; Sauer et al., 2004; Shaw et al., 2000; Zimmerman et al., 2008).[4] There is even evidence that a central nervous system is not required for an organism to meet the behavioral criteria for sleep. Nighttime rest was documented in a species of jellyfish (a Cnidarian which has a distributed nerve net rather than a central nervous system) (Seymour et al., 2004). The criteria for reduced responsiveness during this state and for compensatory increases when deprived of nightly rest were later shown in a different jellyfish species (Nath et al., 2017).

One issue with sleep deprivation studies, whether in mammals, insects, or other species, is the need to distinguish the effects of sleep loss on later behavior from the effects of what experimenters do to deprive animals of sleep (see discussion in Section 13.1). Fruit flies are usually prevented from sleeping or resting by disturbing them enough to make them active. This sleep deprivation method forces flies to show higher levels of activity (and therefore energy expenditure) than they would otherwise show spontaneously at that time. A later increase in a sleep-like state could reflect homeostatic regulation of energy balance, rather than of sleep. In this interpretation, flies that are forced to expend more energy compensate with a later decrease in energy expenditure (i.e., increase their inactivity). Arguing against this interpretation is evidence that the length of sleep after disturbances is not correlated with the amount of activity that was provoked in either fruit flies (Hendricks et al., 2000; Shaw et al., 2000) or honeybees (Sauer et al., 2004), as might be expected if the target of homeostasis were energy balance.

Some sleep deprivation methods applied to rodents also force them to increase activity (e.g., by walking on a motorized treadmill or wheel) in order to prevent sleep, which will also increase their energy expenditure. However, in studies during which rodents showed large increases in voluntary

[3] In the case of the nematode worm *C. elegans*, the phases of immobility occur at specific life stage transitions during its very brief (~2 week) lifespan (Raizen et al., 2008).

[4] Whether there are also distinct sleep stages in species other than mammals and birds is less clear. In addition to reports of REM-like sleep features in reptiles (see Section 7.2.1), there are reports of regular cycles of active (REM-like) and inactive sleep in cuttlefish (*Sepia officinalis*) (Iglesias et al., 2019) and octopus (*Octopus insularis*) (Medeiros et al., 2021), and of periodic retinal and leg movements during their sleep phase in jumping spiders (*Evarcha arcuata*) (Rossler et al., 2022).

activity, they did not show later increases in sleep durations (Hanagasioglu & Borbély, 1982). Sleep deprivation in people requires little or no change in activity (especially during a constant routine procedure), but it still increases the need for sleep. This evidence supports the interpretation that rebound sleep increases are not simply a product of energy homeostasis. However, one complication demonstrated in people is that being awake itself consumes more energy than sleeping, even during a constant routine (Jung et al., 2011). As a result, even in the absence of increased activity, keeping a person awake will necessarily increase their energy expenditure.

While it is generally accepted that an increased sleep drive after sleep loss in both vertebrates and invertebrates reflects sleep homeostasis and is not primarily a response to increased energy expenditure, energy balance may still be relevant to sleep regulation. Some theories of the function of sleep are specifically related to its role in the regulation of energy balance and the allocation of energy resources (see Benington & Heller, 1995; Schmidt, 2014).

Another approach to the question of whether invertebrate and mammalian sleep states are similar is to ask whether they serve similar functions. As discussed in Chapters 17 and 18, there is a large body of evidence showing that sleep after learning strengthens some types of memory consolidation in mammals. Studies addressing this issue in both fruit flies and honeybees also found evidence that sleeping after learning facilitated later retrieval of learned information (Beyaert et al., 2012; Donlea et al., 2017; Donlea et al., 2011; Ganguly-Fitzgerald et al., 2006; Zwaka et al., 2015).

Although some interpretational issues remain, sleep or a similar, sleep-like state is clearly seen in several invertebrate species and in at least one group that does not have a central nervous system. Comparative studies of sleep in fruit flies have been especially valuable because of the wealth of genetic information and tools available for this species. Studies in this speccies have provided insights into the effects of several genes and biochemical pathways that are linked to arousal regulation and sleep in both insects and mammals (Allebrandt et al., 2013; Koh et al., 2008; Seugnet et al., 2006; Shaw et al., 2000; Xu et al., 2005). Some sleep-related genes, however, appear to serve different functions in different species (Xu et al., 2005); for reviews, see (Crocker & Sehgal, 2010; Joiner, 2016; Zimmerman et al., 2008).

7.3.1 Summary

There is probably no definitive answer to the question of whether the "same" brain state (sleep, as defined originally in relation to the mammalian brain) is expressed in organisms like invertebrates with very differently organized nervous systems. Nevertheless, many nonhuman vertebrates and invertebrates have clearly met the five behavioral criteria used to identify sleep and to distinguish it from other inactive states.

There are clear similarities in sleep across species but also some differences that are probably inevitable when comparing behavior and physiology among phylogenetically distant groups. The best conclusion one can reach for now on the basis of behavioral criteria, similarity of function, and overlap in physiological regulation, is that sleep as observed in mammals, or a very similar sleep-like state, occurs in many, and perhaps all, animal species.

7.4 Differences in sleep patterns among mammals

7.4.1 Background

If we restrict the discussion to mammals, the basic electrophysiological characteristics of the sleeping brain are similar across species, yet there are striking species differences in the patterns of sleep. Total sleep duration, as well as amounts of different sleep stages (expressed either as absolute durations or as proportions of total sleep time), vary widely among those species that have been studied. These differences have been attributed to physiological/anatomical features (e.g., metabolic rates, brain, or body sizes), ecological niches (e.g., diet or habitat), and phylogeny (species relatedness). Researchers have correlated differences in these physiological/ecological variables with differences in how species sleep to try to develop a coherent explanation for the observed variations.

We can illustrate the general goal of this approach with some obviously untrue examples. If ground-dwelling primates showed REM sleep but tree-dwelling primates did not, it would suggest that this sleep stage is linked to a particular ecological adaptation in some primates. Alternatively, if all primates showed REM sleep and no other mammalian order did, that might indicate that the phylogenetic history of one mammalian order determined the presence of REM sleep. Unfortunately, none of the actual correlations that have been observed are as specific or as absolute as these fanciful examples.

It is also important to note that by the early 21st century, sleep had been recorded electrophysiologically in only ~3% of mammalian species (Zepelin et al., 2005), and complete assessments of sleep had been performed in only 50 of 80,000 vertebrate species (~0.06%) (Siegel, 2008). Thus, generalizations about mammals (and, even more so, about vertebrates) based on these limited samples should be considered tentative.

Among mammalian species that have been studied, total daily sleep duration ranged from short (~2 h in elephants; ~3 h in horses; and ~4.5 h in giraffes) to very long (17–19 h) in armadillos, opossums, and bats. Both the absolute duration of REM

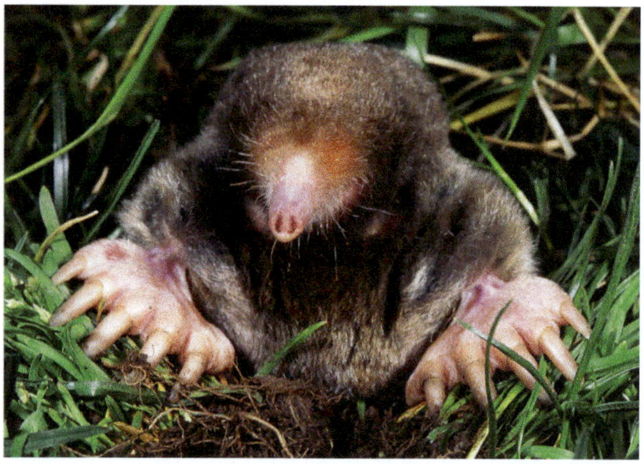

Figure 7.4 Moles (e.g., the common mole, *Scalopus aquaticus*, shown here) and humans have roughly the same average sleep durations and proportions of REM sleep amounts, yet these species share virtually nothing else in relation to habitat, diet, behavior, phylogeny, or reliance on sensory systems. Reprinted with permission, courtesy of © Dr. Kenneth C. Catania, Vanderbilt University.

sleep per 24 h and the percentage of total sleep time occupied by REM sleep also ranged widely, from 0.5 h (~17%) in horses to 7 h (~50%) in opossums. For references, see (Gravett et al., 2017; Siegel, 2005; Zepelin et al., 2005).

Adult humans are unremarkably middle-of-the-road among mammals, showing a total sleep duration of ~8 h daily, of which 2 h (25%) is REM sleep. Identifying species with a relatively similar sleep pattern gives little indication that these sleep features can be explained by factors like similar ecological niches, trophic levels (what they eat), or phylogenetic relatedness. For example, common eastern moles (*Scalopus aquaticus*) show quite similar sleep durations (~8.4 h daily, with ~25% REM sleep)[5] (Allison & Van Twyver, 1970) but have little else in common with us physiologically, ecologically, or phylogenetically. They live in underground burrows, rarely come aboveground, eat mostly earthworms and insects, have degenerate eyes with limited vision, and rely heavily on tactile and olfactory sensory systems (**Figure 7.4**).

7.4.2 Ecological/circadian correlates of sleep timing

Ecological/circadian models have been proposed as one approach to making sense of the available data on sleep amounts (Meddis, 1975; Siegel, 2009). These models attribute differences in sleep patterns to the pressures resulting from species occupying a particular temporal niche (e.g., nocturnality vs. diurnality) in combination with other ecological factors (e.g., diet, availability of shelter, predator–prey relations). Because of the dramatic environmental differences between day and night, specializations that adapt species to function very effectively during one part of the day–night cycle may also make them uncompetitive at other times. Diurnally active birds and primates have acute daytime vision, but relatively poor night vision; nocturnally active bats have exquisite abilities to navigate and hunt by echolocation in darkness or low light at night, but have relatively poor daytime vision (**Figure 7.5**). Each species is adapted to function best, and therefore to be most active, at particular times of day.

The best strategy for a species is to avoid engaging in activity at the "wrong" time of day (which is energy-costly, unlikely to be effective, and likely to generate high risk) by

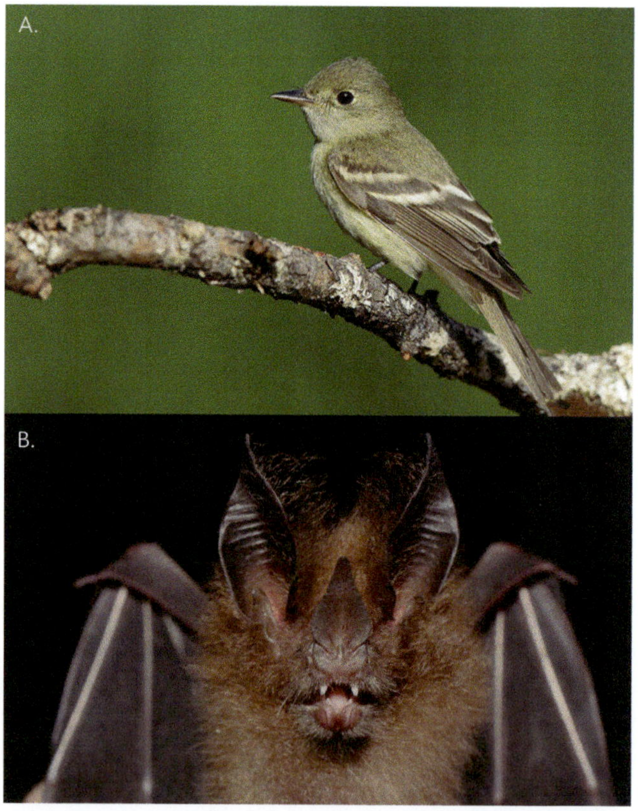

Figure 7.5 **A.** A diurnally adapted bird, the Acadian flycatcher (*Empidonax virescens*; Agami photoagency/Shutterstock.com), and **B.** a nocturnally adapted little, big-eared bat (*Micronycteris megalotis*; Mendesbio/Shutterstock.com). Note the different relative sizes of eyes (not easily visible in the bat, beside the prominent "nose-leaf") and ears (not visible in the flycatcher) in these two flying predators that are both adapted to catching and eating insects. The flycatcher relies primarily on vision during the day for hunting, and the bat relies primarily on sound echolocation during the night. The nose-leaf in the bat is apparently an adaptation that is used to focus its echolocation calls.

[5] One difference from adult humans, however, is that these moles sleep in multiple short bouts throughout the day and night, which may be related to their underground lifestyle.

retreating to a relatively safe shelter (e.g., nest, underground burrow, treetop, cave) and sleeping. Avoiding potential risks and ineffective energy expenditure at one time of day (their rest/sleep phase) also ensures that they have more energy resources to devote to activity when it will do the most good with the least risk.

Preindustrial humans with diurnally adapted visual systems, for example, would have been poorly equipped to hunt, forage, or farm at night and would have been at high risk of encountering nocturnal predators that are better adapted to darkness. Nights would have been better spent in shelter and at rest. Ecological-circadian models thus relate species differences in sleep timing to the ecological pressures under which a species evolved rather than to species differences in physiological functions (for more discussion, see Chapter 16).

The impact of temporal niches may determine the daily phase at which each species sleeps, but other explanations are needed for features such as total sleep duration, bout timing, and proportions of different sleep stages. An example of an ecological interpretation of sleep amounts and timing relates to the fact that many ungulates (hoofed species, like horses, zebras, antelopes, etc.) are vulnerable prey animals, some of which live in relatively open habitats with little shelter. They typically sleep in brief bouts and have short total daily sleep durations (~3–5 h). This sleep structure can serve an antipredator function by avoiding lengthy periods of unconsciousness in animals that are protected mainly by their ability to detect and outrun potential predators. In addition, their relatively energy-poor plant diets require that they graze for many hours daily, limiting the time available for sleep. On the other hand, carnivores like felids (cats, both large and small), wolves, and ferrets, which are less vulnerable to predation and eat energy-rich, but infrequent meals, can afford to sleep (and conserve their energy) for many hours daily (~12.5–14.5 h daily for cats).

This explanation for why herbivorous ungulates and carnivores sleep differently is based on ideas about the functions of these sleep patterns in relation to predation risk and energy requirements. Functional explanations, however, are very difficult to test experimentally. Selected examples like these can sound plausible for some species, but there are also counter-examples. Adult elephants, which are herbivores, but which most predators avoid (except for large prides of lions), show extremely short sleep durations (see next section). Small, relatively defenseless prey species, like rats and hamsters, sleep for as long as predators like cats. Predation risk and diet are plausible contributors to shaping the sleep patterns of ungulates and carnivores, but they alone do not readily account for mammalian sleep patterns in general. Other variables have also been considered.

7.4.3 Physiological correlates of sleep and NREM–REM cycle durations

Among these variables are several physiological/anatomical characteristics that have been correlated with species differences in the length of sleep and of the NREM–REM cycle. Total sleep time correlates negatively with both brain weight and body weight (correlation coefficient of about −0.55), so that large mammals sleep less than small mammals (Siegel, 2005; Zepelin & Rechtschaffen, 1974). Consistent with this correlation are the findings from actigraphic studies in the wild of sleep in two adult female African elephants (*Loxodonta africana*), the largest living land mammals. They showed the shortest daily sleep length of any mammal that has been studied (~2 h) and occasionally went for days with no apparent sleep (Gravett et al., 2017).

This correlation has been attributed to the impact of body size on metabolism and energy balance in endotherms (animals that maintain an elevated body temperature using physiological mechanisms; largely, birds and mammals).[6] Endothermy requires high levels of energy expenditure (i.e., a high metabolic rate) to maintain body temperature above that of the environment. Large mammals have lower metabolic rates because they have a small ratio of external surface area to body mass (and, in some cases, insulating layers of fur, skin, and fat), so they lose heat to the environment very slowly. Small mammals have proportionately larger surface areas in relation to their body mass, so they lose heat rapidly to the external environment, driving up their energy requirements. Since metabolic rates are reduced during sleep, smaller mammals can use longer sleep durations to reduce their overall energy costs, while large mammals, which retain heat more effectively, would have less need to sleep in order to conserve metabolic energy.

However, if one divides mammals up in relation to their ecological trophic level (i.e., type and quality of food consumed), the robust negative correlation between body size and sleep duration does not apply uniformly. There was a very strong negative correlation between sleep duration and body mass among herbivores (−0.8) (**Figure 7.6**), but there was no similar correlation with body mass among the carnivores and omnivores that have been studied (Siegel, 2005). It is unclear why this should be the case, but it indicates that body mass

[6] A few other groups have also evolved a form of endothermy, including some sharks, tunas, and their relatives as well as some insects (Block & Finnerty, 1994). Most other vertebrates are ectothermic (i.e., they use external resources to regulate body temperature). A lizard can bask in the sunshine to raise its temperature, and a snake can go underground to cool off, but they do not rely on internal mechanisms of heat production and cooling as mammals and birds do.

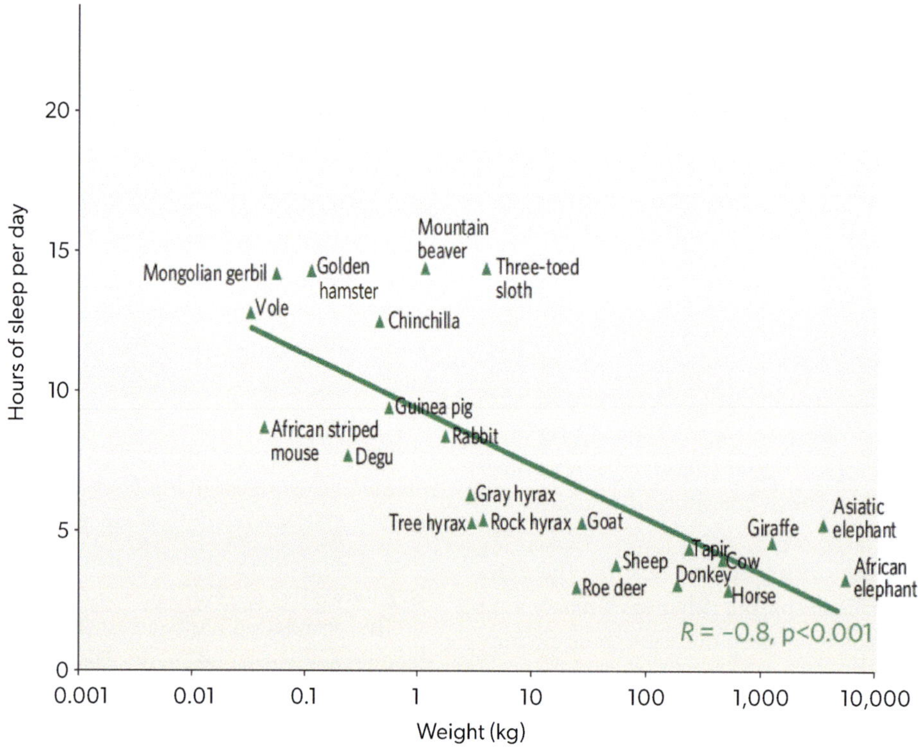

Figure 7.6 There is a robust negative correlation (regression line indicating R = −0.8) between the body size of herbivores and the average hours of sleep they show daily. Despite the strength of this correlation among these species, there is no significant correlation between these variables in carnivores or omnivores that have been studied. Note that the actigraphically recorded sleep duration of the African elephant was later found to be ~2 h daily or less (Gravett et al., 2017), bringing it even closer to the regression line than illustrated here. Reprinted with permission from Siegel, J. (2005) Clues to the functions of mammalian sleep. *Nature* 437:1264–1271. © Springer:Nature (2005). doi: 10.1038/nature04285.

(and metabolic rate) alone cannot account for sleep duration differences among mammals in general.

Even more robust correlations exist between the length of the NREM–REM sleep cycle and both metabolic rate (−0.82) and brain weight (+0.89). Thus, small mammals with high metabolic rates and small brains have shorter NREM–REM sleep cycles than large mammals with low metabolic rates and large brains (Zepelin et al., 2005). A similar relationship exists within a human lifespan. Babies have shorter NREM–REM sleep cycles than adults, which is consistent with their smaller bodies, smaller brains, and higher metabolic rates. These results imply that the length of the NREM–REM cycle is closely tied to a mammal's metabolic rate (which is linked to body size) and its degree of encephalization. This measure refers to the extent to which a species has a large brain, particularly one larger than can be explained by its relative body size.

7.4.4 Monotremes and the evolution of REM sleep

Studies have also assessed how the relative proportion and absolute amount of REM sleep are related to ecological and taxonomic relationships. As discussed above, many (but not all) researchers have concluded that reptiles, unlike birds and mammals, do not generate REM sleep (Eiland et al., 2001; Zepelin et al., 2005); but see Section 7.2.1). This interpretation raises the possibility that the presence of REM sleep is related to endothermy, which is broadly present only in birds and mammals among vertebrates.

The mammalian subclass Prototheria (better known as monotremes) presents an interesting test case for the hypothesis that endothermy is closely tied to REM sleep production. These few existing species (the echidnas and the platypus) have the unique feature among mammals of laying eggs rather than bearing live young. They are all endothermic, but they also maintain a lower core temperature (~32 °C) than is typical of other mammals.

The observation that birds and other mammals show both endothermy and REM sleep predicts the presence of REM sleep in endothermic monotremes. Yet, one echidna species (the short-beaked echidna, *Tachyglossus aculeatus*) appears not to show REM sleep, while another (*Zaglossus* sp.) does (Zepelin et al., 2005). In addition, the platypus (*Ornithorhynchus anatinus*) is among mammalian REM sleep champions, generating 6–8 h daily (Siegel et al., 1998; Siegel et al., 1999). The variability in REM sleep among monotremes is puzzling and seems to contradict the idea that there is an obligatory link between REM sleep and endothermy.

Monotremes, however, may be a special case, one that also raises an intriguing suggestion about how REM sleep evolved. Their REM sleep (defined by rapid eye movements and atonia during sleep) is accompanied by cortical slow waves, not an activated cortical pattern, as shown by other mammals (Siegel et al., 1998; Siegel et al., 1999). Monotremes may represent the persistence of an early stage in the evolution of REM sleep in which rapid eye movements and atonia ("brainstem REM sleep") occur along with cortical slow waves rather than cortical activation ("forebrain REM sleep") (Lesku et al., 2011; Siegel et al., 1998); see Chapter 10. The few monotremes that exist today may be descended from animals that developed early forms of both endothermy and REM sleep to different extents.

Ostriches (*Struthio camelus*), which are part of a lineage of relatively primitive birds (ratites), also show mixed REM sleep features. They show brainstem REM sleep features (eye closure, rapid eye movements, reduced tone in neck muscles, leading to drooping of the head and neck) that are accompanied variably by either forebrain slow waves (as in monotremes) or an activated EEG (as in other birds and mammals). Adult ostriches also differ from most other birds that have been studied in showing very large amounts of REM sleep (~6 h daily) (Lesku et al., 2011).

However, the mixed features of REM sleep are apparently not universal among ratites. Another member of this group, the elegant crested tinamou (*Eudromia elegans*), shows brainstem REM sleep features accompanied only by forebrain EEG activation, as in most other bird species (Tisdale et al., 2017). With so few species studied from this group, it is unclear whether mixed or standard REM sleep features are more common among ratites.

One interpretation of the unusual REM sleep features of monotremes and ostriches is that species that were distant ancestors of mammals and birds might have produced only slow waves during sleep, as modern reptiles are usually assumed to do. Some groups later evolved brainstem REM sleep features that were expressed periodically during part of the slow-wave sleep phase, leading to the mixed pattern still seen in some monotremes and variably in ostriches. The groups that evolved into most modern mammals and birds added exclusive forebrain EEG activation during REM sleep, leading to the characteristic features of NREM–REM sleep cycles now seen in their descendants (Siegel et al., 1998).

7.4.5 Why is mammalian REM sleep needed?

If this evolutionary narrative is correct, it raises two questions. Why did brainstem REM sleep evolve in the first place? And why was cortical activation added subsequently? One potential response to the second question is the hypothesis that REM sleep is a response to the physiological consequences of the lengthy production of slow waves during NREM sleep (see Section 5.6) (Benington & Heller, 1994; Benington & Heller, 1999; Moses et al., 1977). The suggestion is that the potential for damage to a complex brain, especially the cortex, as a result of long-sustained, slow-wave activity (SWA) is counteracted by the cortical activation occurring during REM sleep, while the global benefits of sleep are preserved.

REM sleep has been proposed to reverse unidentified cellular or network changes that occur during NREM sleep, perhaps related to burst-firing patterns, EEG synchronization, or lowered metabolic rates. One possibility is that the changes in transmembrane ion flux that occur in neurons during NREM sleep and are associated with producing SWA (see Section 5.3.4), or other synaptic or cellular changes during SWA, may not be physiologically sustainable over long periods.

This formulation fits well with the evidence that the total daily amount of SWA is defended in modern mammals with appropriate increases and decreases. SWS produced during a daytime nap is compensated by reduced amounts at night, and deprivation of SWS leads to rebound increases. This symmetrical form of homeostatic regulation suggests that the benefits of sufficient SWA are offset by the potential harms of excess SWA. Deprivation of REM sleep also produces later compensatory increases, but there does not appear to be compensation for excess REM sleep, which presumably lacks a similar potential to cause neural harm (see Section 5.5.3).

During SWS cortical neurons show bursts of firing during each Up phase, and there are complex patterns of information exchange among the cortex, thalamus, and hippocampus. These activities may be critical to stabilizing memory and facilitating brain plasticity in general; see Chapters 17 and 18. But there is also evidence that REM sleep plays a role in some forms of memory consolidation, and the sequence of NREM followed by REM sleep facilitates plasticity in the brain (see Sections 17.4, 17.8, and 18.10). Thus, the alternating pattern of sleep stages may also be functionally important for complex, highly plastic brains.

Another idea relates to the effects of sustained, low brain/body temperature during NREM sleep. Hypothermia during NREM sleep is beneficial because it conserves energy, and the nocturnal "dipping" pattern of body temperature in people is protective against development of vascular diseases (see Section 14.8). Despite the rapid firing of cortical neurons during bursts of activity in each On phase of slow waves, the overall level of metabolic activity in the brain during NREM sleep (indexed by glucose metabolism) is reduced by nearly a third relative to waking. During REM sleep, metabolism rises to approach the levels of the waking brain (Buchsbaum et al., 1989). There are general physiological benefits associated with the low temperatures and low metabolic activity characteristic of NREM sleep. But sustained low brain temperatures and metabolic activity over long periods of sleep may challenge the integrity of neural functional connectivity (see **Box 5.2** in Section 5.3.4).

In addition to rewarming and reactivating the cortex to address the consequences of reduced metabolism and brain temperature, REM sleep may also help prepare the brain for

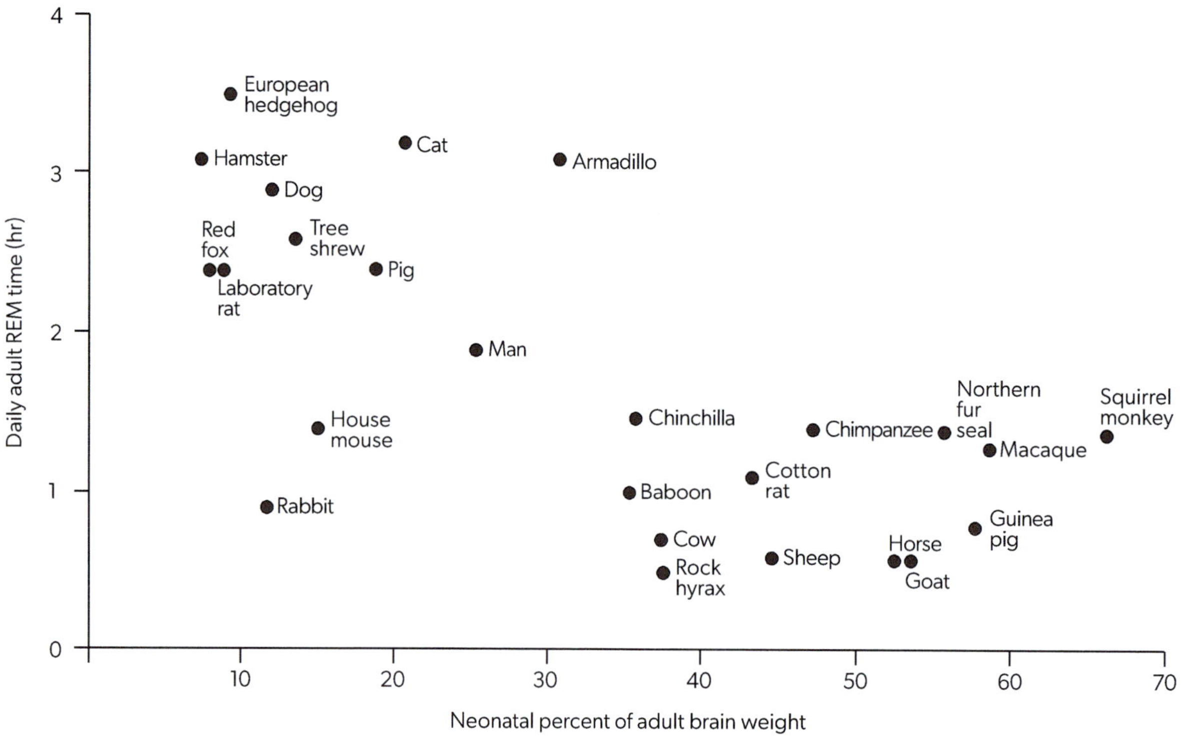

Figure 7.7 Daily adult REM sleep duration (Y axis) is plotted against a measure of maturity at birth (X axis) for several mammalian species, illustrating the negative relation between the amount of adult REM sleep and maturity of the young at birth. The measure of maturity at birth (precocity) is the brain weight of newborn young expressed as a percentage of the brain weight achieved in mature adults. The brains of very precocial guinea pig pups at birth weigh nearly 60% of adult brain weight and those of squirrel monkey neonates weigh ~66% of adult brains, while the brains of very altricial hamsters at birth weigh less than 10% of adult brains. Humans ("Man") fall near the middle of both distributions, with about 2 h of REM sleep as adults and an intermediate percentage of adult brain weight at birth, consistent with mixed precocial and altricial features. Reprinted with permission of Elsevier, Ltd. from Zepelin, H. (1989) Mammalian sleep. In M. H. Kryger, et al. (Eds.), *Principles and Practice of Sleep Medicine* (1st edition, pp. 30–49). © Elsevier, 1989.

waking activities (Siegel, 2022; Wehr, 1992). REM sleep episodes are often followed by very brief wake episodes (see, e.g., Figure 10.10). In people, REM sleep amounts increase progressively during the second half of the night and, if allowed to sleep freely, people usually wake spontaneously out of REM sleep. Waking out of REM sleep allows for a rapid transition to full alertness, while waking out of SWS results in periods of sleep inertia that may impede normal waking functions (see Section 2.3.3).

7.4.6 Endothermy and REM sleep

A factor that has been correlated with the amount of REM sleep shown by a species is how mature (precocial) or immature (altricial) the young are at birth (see Figure 4.3, Section 4.2.2). There is a strong positive correlation between how altricial neonates are (linked to how short gestation is) and the amount of REM sleep shown in infancy (**Figure 7.7**) (Jouvet-Mounier et al., 1969; Zepelin et al., 2005).

Cats and rats are born at an early developmental stage and show a great deal of REM sleep at birth (~90% of their total sleep), while REM sleep makes up only 15% of total sleep in precocial guinea pigs at birth (Jouvet-Mounier et al., 1969). Similarly, premature human infants show higher REM sleep amounts than full-term infants (see Georgoulas et al., 2021; **Figure 4.2**). Despite steep reductions in REM sleep amounts during early development (**Figure 7.8**), mammals that are altricial at birth (including humans) still wind up showing higher percentages of REM sleep than precocial species as adults (**Figures 7.7 and 7.8**). The platypus, which is born in an extremely altricial state, shows a record duration of up to 8 h of REM sleep daily as an adult (Siegel et al., 1998; Siegel et al., 1999).[7]

Altricial and precocial mammals differ at birth in several ways, in addition to the physical features illustrated in **Figure 4.3**. Altricial neonates show relatively immature regulation of heart rate, breathing, and thermoregulation, functioning

[7] To add to the unusual sleep characteristics of ostriches discussed above, ostrich chicks do not show large amounts of REM sleep, as do mammalian young, but express less REM sleep and shorter REM-sleep bout lengths as newly hatched chicks than as adults. A developmental *increase* in REM sleep amounts has not been documented in any other species (Lyamin et al., 2021).

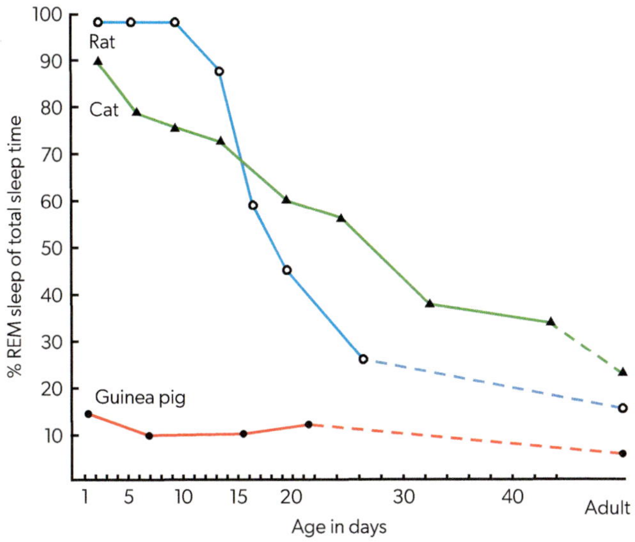

Figure 7.8 Examples of amounts of REM (or active) sleep as a percentage of total sleep time (Y axis) in infancy and in adulthood among both altricial species (rat and cat) and a very precocial species, guinea pig. Note that the altricial species have much higher REM sleep percentages at birth (consistent with the prevalence of REM sleep earlier *in utero* for precocial species), but that these levels fall throughout their lives. Despite this decline, these species still have higher REM sleep percentages as adults than adult guinea pigs. Adapted with permission of John Wiley & Sons from Jouvet-Mounier et al. (1969) Ontogenesis of the states of sleep in rat, cat, and guinea pig during the first postnatal month. *Dev Psychobiol* 2(4):216-239, 1969. © John Wiley and Sons (1969) doi: 10.1002/dev.420020407.

basically as ectotherms (Zepelin et al., 2005). Maturation of the nervous system during development results in improved physiological homeostasis, including the development of endothermy, along with reductions in REM sleep durations (**Figure 7.8**). However, even as adults, mammals lose normal homeostatic regulation of body temperature and metabolism during REM sleep, unlike during NREM sleep. This was demonstrated by evidence that cooling the hypothalamic mechanism that normally responds to cooling by increasing metabolic rates to restore a higher temperature, does not trigger increased metabolism during REM sleep (Glotzbach & Heller, 1976).

One interpretation is that ectothermy in young, altricial mammals and birds during their long periods of REM sleep allows them to channel the energy they acquire during early development to rapid growth, rather than to maintenance of elevated body temperatures. The energetic costs of temperature regulation and growth in the young are shared by the care-giving parents through the nutrition and body heat they provide. This resource is not available to nonmammalian/avian vertebrates, which are precocial at hatching and do not receive parental care. This altricial developmental strategy is considered to be typical of mammals, while having precocial young at birth is a secondary adaptation acquired by a subset of mammals (Zepelin et al., 2005).

Thus, the links between endothermy, maturity at birth, and amounts of REM sleep are complex. Across taxonomic groups, those that show endothermy as adults (birds and mammals) generate REM sleep, while ectotherms (e.g., reptiles) appear not to do so (but see the discussion in Section 7.2.1), suggesting a strong linkage between REM sleep and endothermy. However, altricial mammals, which are essentially ectothermic at birth, show very large amounts of REM sleep, and levels of REM sleep decline steeply as they mature and become endothermic (**Figure 7.8**). Nevertheless, during REM sleep as adults, they again become ectothermic.

Thus, REM sleep and endothermy seem to be linked in opposite ways phylogenetically (REM sleep is characteristic of endotherms) and developmentally (becoming endothermic during development is associated with reducing amounts of REM sleep). Nevertheless, it remains the case that ectothermy is characteristic of REM sleep throughout development. One caution, however, is that there is uncertainty whether "REM/active sleep" very early in development is the same physiological state as REM sleep in mature animals (see Section 4.2.2).

There remain unanswered questions about how REM sleep amounts relate to endothermy. Altricial mammals during infancy show large amounts of REM sleep, including its characteristic ectothermy. Assuming that this is an energy-conserving/growth promoting strategy in neonates that can rely on parental nutrition and warmth, it is unclear why they continue to show larger amounts of REM sleep than precocial species once they are fully mature, adult homeotherms (**Figures 7.7** and **7.8**). The several links among mammalian/avian REM sleep, thermoregulation, and developmental maturity suggest that these features are related, but it remains speculative what these relations imply about the functions of REM sleep and the mechanisms that drove its evolution. Fitting the (so-far) unique features of REM sleep in ostriches into this puzzle will be an additional challenge (Lyamin et al., 2021).

7.4.7 Phylogeny and sleep

Species that are closely phylogenetically related (i.e., share a relatively recent common ancestor), may show similarities in their sleep patterns (e.g., the brief sleep bout lengths and short total sleep amounts seen in many ungulates). However, some closely related species also share physical characteristics and fill similar ecological niches, making it difficult to disentangle the roles of common ancestry and shared ecology/trophic levels. There is some evidence suggesting that phylogenetic relatedness is important. Indian and African elephants, the two extant elephant species, share many obvious physical characteristics and behaviors, but their closest living relatives, manatees (*Trichechus inunguis*) and the more distantly related rock hyrax (*Procavia capensis*), share few of these features. Yet, the hyrax, manatee, and African elephants all have remarkably short durations of REM sleep, which may be a result of their common ancestry (Gravett et al., 2012; Gravett et al., 2017; Mukhametov et al., 1992).

Humans and many other primates generally show a single consolidated daily sleep episode (as adults), but also share a tendency toward midday napping (the post-lunch dip). This tendency is reflected in afternoon decreases in alertness in some human societies and in regular afternoon sleep periods (siestas) in others (see Section 4.3). In a study of squirrel monkeys in constant light conditions, this afternoon dip was also reflected in reduced wakefulness in the middle of an otherwise consolidated wake period, suggesting that this feature may be a common primate characteristic (see **Figure 8.11 C**).

The tendency for related species to show similar sleep characteristics has raised questions about the interpretation of some correlations that were reported between physiological parameters and sleep. Some of the species contributing data to these correlations are closely related phylogenetically, so shared phylogeny might contribute to correlations that were originally attributed to shared physiological features (Lesku et al., 2008). A reanalysis of these correlations, taking phylogenetic relatedness into account, concluded that although some previously reported correlations were potentially confounded by common phylogeny, the following remained reliable:

- The duration of SWS is negatively correlated with body mass, brain mass, basal metabolic rate, and duration of gestation (i.e., animals with smaller bodies and brains, lower basal metabolic rates, and shorter gestation periods have more SWS).
- The amount of REM sleep in adults is negatively correlated with the length of gestation and the degree of precociality at birth; that is, animals with short gestation periods and less mature young at birth show more REM sleep, even as adults (**Figure 7.8**).
- The proportion of total sleep occupied by REM sleep is positively correlated with a higher degree of encephalization; that is, proportionately more REM sleep is associated with a larger brain size relative to body mass (Lesku et al., 2008).

7.4.8 Issues in comparing sleep patterns among species

Researchers have studied the anatomical/physiological correlates of different sleep features in the hope that strong correlations would suggest the likely functions served by different sleep patterns. One caution with respect to these correlations is that they may be sensitive to the methods used to assess sleep. EEG recordings are typically collected in a laboratory, but there is evidence that laboratory living conditions can result in different patterns of sleep and activity than are shown in the natural habitat (see **Figure 3.7**) (Vanin et al., 2012). For example, sloths were reported to sleep ~16 h daily in the laboratory, but a telemetry-based study of a small number of free-living sloths found that they slept <10 h daily (Rattenborg et al., 2008). The use of actigraphy in the natural habitat can also produce results that differ from those obtained using only observational methods with either captive or free-living animals, as was reported for elephants (Gravett et al., 2017).

Another issue is identifying the appropriate physiological variable to correlate with sleep features. The assumption that sleep is related to brain function suggests that measures related to the brain should be used. Measures used previously included total brain mass, mass of the cerebrum, and the ratio of brain mass to body mass. The best measure to use would presumably be one that is most closely related to the functions served by sleep, but that remains the subject of continuing debate (see Chapter 16).

Measures of brain mass similar to those that have been correlated with sleep features have also been correlated with other functions, including cognitive abilities. But recent analyses indicated that cognitive differences between species were not well correlated with total brain mass nor with the mass of the cerebrum. Instead, the most robust correlations were with the total number of cortical neurons (Herculano-Houzel, 2012; Herculano-Houzel et al., 2014).

While measures like total neuronal numbers and brain mass may sound closely related, they can be dissociated. Total cerebral mass could be higher in one species than another for different reasons: increased numbers of either neurons or glia (or both), increased sizes of individual neurons or glia, or both. For example, the elephant cerebral cortex has twice the mass of the human cortex but includes only about 1/3 as many neurons (Herculano-Houzel et al., 2014). Identifying brain-related measures that are closely related to the functions of sleep may help clarify the basis for the diversity of sleep amounts and patterns observed among species.

7.4.9 Summary

Although some strong correlations have been reported between sleep parameters and physiological measures, they leave many unanswered questions. Among herbivores, total sleep amounts increase as body mass decreases, but that relationship is not seen among omnivores and carnivores. It is unclear whether this difference represents an interaction between the effects of trophic level (type of food consumed) and body mass or some other factor. Phylogenetic relatedness may also contribute to some similarities in sleep among closely related species, and it can complicate analyses of other correlates of sleep features.

The expression of REM sleep has been linked to the evolution of endothermy in birds and mammals in contrast to most other vertebrates. However, REM sleep amounts are very high in most young mammals while they are essentially ectothermic, and the amount of REM sleep decreases as they mature and become endothermic. Thus, endothermy and REM sleep appear to be linked in opposite ways during phylogeny and ontogeny.

Species that are altricial at birth initially show more REM-like sleep than precocial species, which is consistent with evidence that mammals at earlier developmental stages show more REM sleep. Because maintaining homeothermy is energetically costly, the large amounts of REM sleep may reduce energy costs because it involves suspension of homeothermy. The energy saved can be devoted to rapid growth, while the young rely on the energy resources provided by parental birds and mammals to stay warm. However, why altricial species continue to show more REM sleep than precocial species once both have reached full maturity as adult endotherms is unknown.

The appearance in some species of unusual REM sleep patterns that combine slow EEG waves with brainstem REM features (e.g., atonia, REMs) suggests that the modern version of REM sleep seen in people, most mammals, and birds may have evolved in stages, but the forces contributing to these evolutionary changes are unknown. It is possible that highly complex brains that rely to a large extent on plasticity benefit from forebrain REM sleep for several reasons. These include reversing potentially harmful effects on neural function or connectivity that may occur during long-sustained NREM sleep; rewarming the brain to avoid the consequences of hypothermia during NREM sleep; and facilitating consolidation of plastic changes that occur during waking, either alone or in combination with NREM sleep.

The hope that comparative analyses would provide insights into the functions served by different durations of sleep and of sleep stages has been only partially fulfilled. Metabolic rate, brain size, and altriciality are correlated with some sleep parameters, but these correlations are neither simple nor universal. A better understanding of how these physiological features relate to sleep characteristics in different species is needed. Evaluating some less-studied measures related to brain structure and function may help clarify the functional significance of species differences in sleep features and amounts.

7.5 Unihemispheric sleep

7.5.1 Cetaceans

A remarkable feature of sleep in some species is the capacity to show electrophysiologically defined sleep in one cerebral hemisphere while the other hemisphere remains awake. Cetaceans (whales, dolphins, and porpoises) nearly always sleep one hemisphere at a time (unihemispheric sleep). While one hemisphere shows the EEG signs of sleep, the whale or dolphin continues to breathe (which requires rising to the surface) and frequently to swim, presumably with its motor system controlled by the waking hemisphere (Lyamin, Manger, et al., 2008).

While one hemisphere sleeps, the contralateral eye (connected to the sleeping hemisphere) is typically closed, and the eye connected to the waking hemisphere remains fully or partially open. The optic chiasm in cetaceans is almost fully decussated (crossed); that is, retinal projections from one eye cross almost entirely to the opposite hemisphere. As a result, during unihemispheric sleep, the waking hemisphere gets its usual visual input, while the sleeping hemisphere gets very little, if any. Some small dolphins swim continuously throughout their lives, including during sleep episodes, presumably aided by visual input from their open eye. Others remain relatively motionless near the surface (or on the bottom of a tank in captivity) for periods of time while sleeping unihemispherically.

In the best-studied cetacean, the bottlenose dolphin (*Tursiops truncatus*), each cerebral hemisphere sleeps a total of about 4 h daily, but not at the same time as the opposite hemisphere. Sleep occurs primarily at night, with periods of sleep alternating between hemispheres at approximately 1 h intervals (**Figure 7.9**). Similar alternation of sleep between the hemispheres has been observed in beluga whales (*Delphinapterus leucas*). These patterns contrast to the usual pattern in terrestrial species; e.g., the laboratory rat, of simultaneous sleep–wake cycling in the two hemispheres (**Figure 7.10**) (Siegel, 2005).

Cetaceans are also remarkable because their sleep includes only high- or medium-voltage EEG patterns, typical of NREM sleep in terrestrial mammals. REM sleep, characterized by a low-voltage EEG pattern and motor paralysis, is either completely absent or at least undetectable by the EEG criteria usually applied to other mammals (Lyamin, Manger, et al., 2008).

The independence of both sleep production and sleep need in the two hemispheres was illustrated by the results of sleep-deprivation studies in dolphins (Oleksenko et al., 1992). To deprive only one hemisphere of SWS (0.5–3 Hz) sleep, a dolphin was stimulated to wakefulness whenever that hemisphere showed sleep with substantial SWA, but the dolphin was not disturbed while the contralateral hemisphere slept. The first indication of the independence of sleep regulation in each hemisphere was that the hemisphere that was allowed to sleep freely showed no increase in sleep duration while the other hemisphere was being sleep-deprived.

A second important finding was that during a later recovery period when both hemispheres were free to sleep, there were large increases in delta-wave sleep primarily in the previously sleep-deprived hemisphere. The non-deprived hemisphere showed variable responses: sometimes lower or (rarely)

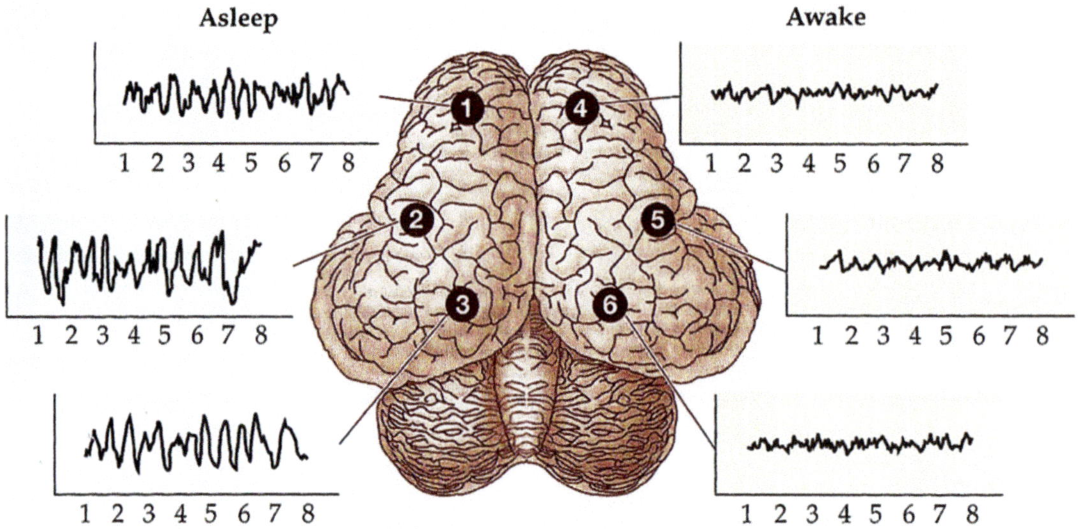

Figure 7.9 Illustration of electrophysiological recordings made simultaneously from the two hemispheres of a bottlenose dolphin (*Tursiops truncatus*), showing high-voltage slow activity from three cortical sites on the left along with low-voltage, fast activity in three parallel sites on the right. Adapted with permission of Oxford University Press from Purves et al. (2001) *Neuroscience*, 5th Edition © Oxford University Press, and with permission of Elsevier, Ltd. from Mukhametov, L. M. et al. (1977) Interhemispheric asymmetry of the electroencephalographic sleep patterns in dolphins. *Brain Res* 134:581–584. © Elsevier (1977).

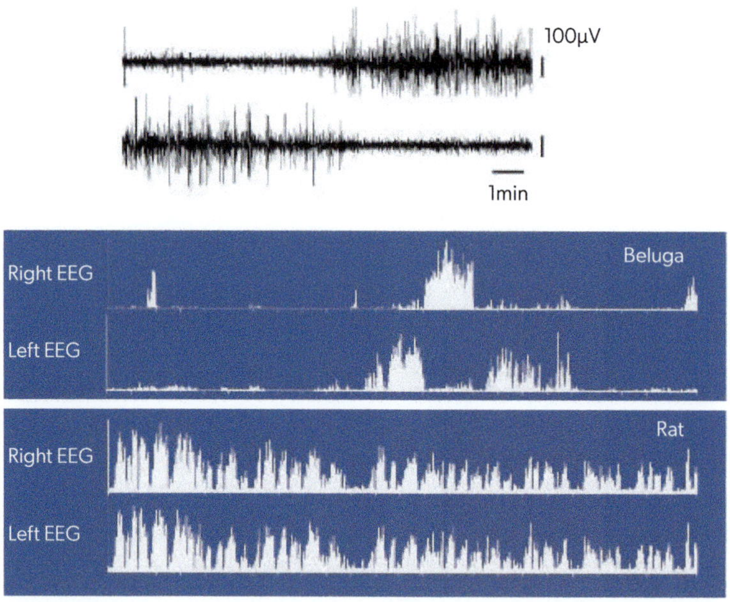

Figure 7.10 The top panel shows the EEG patterns of waking (low voltage) and sleep (high voltage) alternating between the two hemispheres of a beluga whale. The lower panel shows the distribution of 1–3 Hz activity during 12 h of EEG recordings from both left and right cortices of a beluga whale (above) and a rat (below). The beluga showed slow EEG activity consistent with sleep only during a limited time window, and in one cortex or the other, but never in both at the same time. The rat showed a typical polyphasic sleep pattern with many bouts of slow EEG alternating rapidly with periods lacking slow EEG activity, but this pattern appeared synchronously in the two hemispheres. Reprinted with permission from Siegel, J. (2005) Clues to the functions of mammalian sleep. *Nature* 437:1264–1271 © Springer: Nature (2005). doi: 10.1038/nature04285.

somewhat higher than baseline levels of sleep during recovery sleep. Rebound increases in SWS were less consistent than in terrestrial mammals (see Chapter 5), and they were not strictly proportional to the length of prior deprivation. Rebound increases in SWS were similarly inconsistent during recovery from either uni- or bihemispheric sleep deprivation.

Another effect of either uni- or bihemispheric sleep deprivation was an increase in the rate at which sleep alternated between hemispheres during the recovery period. This observation may be explained by competition between the hemispheres for the opportunity to sleep. Sleep deprivation of either both or only one hemisphere would result in increased pressure for a deprived hemisphere (or both) to fall asleep after a shorter wake duration, causing the other hemisphere to wake earlier than usual. This change would, in turn, result in increased sleep pressure in the contralateral, awakened hemisphere (especially if it had also been sleep-deprived), which would also tend to fall asleep earlier. As a result, there would be a more rapid alternation of sleep episodes between hemispheres (Oleksenko et al., 1992).

7.5.2 Unihemispheric sleep in other mammals

Unihemispheric sleep has never been observed in terrestrial mammals, but it occurs to varying degrees in other aquatic and semi-aquatic mammals. Thus, the aquatic manatee (*Trichechus inunguis*) shows partially asynchronous SWA patterns in the two hemispheres (Mukhametov et al., 1992). In addition, a number of seal species have been studied, including both "true seals" (members of the family Phocidae) and "fur (or eared) seals" and sea lions (family Otariidae). Species in both groups are amphibious, spending part of their lives at sea and part on land. To the limited extent that they have been studied, phocids appear to show only bilateral sleep. Phocids are able to remain submerged for very long periods of time without breathing, during which they may be able to show sustained bihemispheric sleep, and awaken only when they need to rise to the surface to breathe (see discussion in Section 7.5.5) (Lyamin, Kosenko, et al., 2008).

The Northern elephant seal (*Mirounga angustirostris*) is another phocid species, which showed repeated deep dives in the Pacific Ocean during which it often slept. In this species, however, sleep at sea was relatively brief, averaging <2 h/day. However, in contrast to other phocids, a very large percentage of this limited sleep time at sea was REM sleep (29%). In contrast, they averaged ~11 h of sleep daily on land, and a similar, or slightly larger percentage of that time was spent in REM sleep (Kendall-Bar et al., 2023).

Fur seals (otariids), on the other hand, have a much more limited capacity to hold their breath under water, and they showed mostly unihemispheric sleep in the water. Their sleep in water included very little REM sleep (~1%), similarly to other amphibious seals and walruses, which showed REM sleep amounts of 1–11% (Kendall-Bar et al., 2023). Fur seals in captivity often slept one hemisphere at a time, paddling idly on their sides on the water surface, using the flipper that is contralateral to the waking hemisphere and keeping the eye on that side open. The waking hemisphere presumably kept them swimming while the other hemisphere slept (Lyamin et al., 2017).

But when otariids are on land, and the need to breathe at the water's surface is not an issue, they show bihemispheric sleep, including ~5% REM sleep and a curled-up body posture. If they were deprived selectively of bihemispheric, high-voltage EEG sleep while on land, but were permitted unihemispheric sleep, they showed more unihemispheric sleep, but also showed increasingly frequent attempts to enter bihemispheric sleep. These findings suggest that, despite their lack of bihemispheric sleep while in the water, otariids have a specific drive and preference for this type of sleep when they are on land (Lyamin, Kosenko, et al., 2008; Lyamin et al., 2017).

7.5.3 Avian unihemispheric sleep and mammalian asymmetries

Among mammals, only fully aquatic or amphibious species are known to regularly show unihemispheric sleep, but the phenomenon has been reported in several bird species. Birds have been shown to produce both bihemispheric sleep, accompanied by bilateral eye closure, and unihemispheric NREM sleep, accompanied by contralateral eye closure (Libourel et al., 2023; Low et al., 2008; Ookawa & Gotoh, 1965; Rattenborg et al., 1999) (**Figure 7.11**). REM sleep (which is very brief in most birds) does not occur unihemispherically and has been observed only during bihemispheric sleep (Rattenborg et al., 2000).

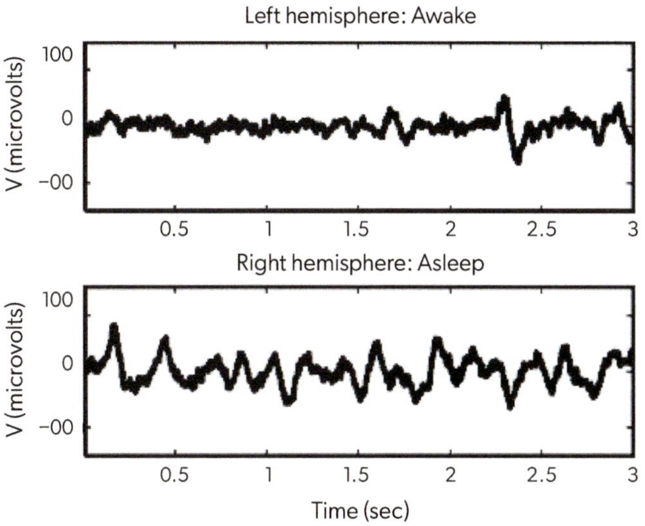

Figure 7.11 Typical EEG recordings taken simultaneously from the two hemispheres of a zebra finch (*Taeniopygia guttata*), showing low-voltage activity typical of waking in the left hemisphere (top) while the right hemisphere showed high-voltage activity typical of sleep (bottom). Reprinted with permission from Low, P.S. et al. (2008) Mammalian-like features of sleep structure in zebra finches. *PNAS* 105:9081–9086. © National Academy of Sciences, USA (2008). doi: 10.1073/pnas.0703452105.

Evidence from a study of mallard ducks (*Anas platyrhynchos*) suggests the likely functional significance of the choice between uni- and bihemispheric sleep. Four ducks were housed singly in a linear arrangement of transparent boxes. They showed different sleep patterns depending on their positions in the row. The two central birds that were surrounded by conspecifics on either side tended to show primarily bilateral sleep and bilateral eye closure. The two "edge" birds showed >150% increase in unilateral sleep and unilateral eye closure relative to the central birds. Most striking was the observation that in the great majority of sleep episodes, the two edge birds had a strong tendency to sleep with their open eyes facing away from the group and toward the periphery (**Figure 7.12**).

This was not the case for the central birds during their less frequent episodes of unihemispheric sleep. Edge birds also tended to show more SWS in the hemisphere connected to the closed eye. Evidence that presentation of threatening visual stimuli to the open eye led to rapid awakening supported the interpretation that the occurrence and orientation of unihemispheric sleep serves an antipredator function (Rattenborg et al., 1999). The tendency to sleep with one eye open, as well as increasing amounts of such "monocular" sleep in the presence of potential threats, have also been reported in some reptiles, including a species of crocodile (Kelly et al., 2015).

Another species, the great frigate bird (*Fregata minor*), engages in extended, non-stop flights of up to 10 days over regions of open ocean. During these flights, they show dramatically reduced total sleep times and increased asymmetry in sleep between the hemispheres (**Figure 7.13**). This pattern presumably allows the bird to continue flying under the control of a waking hemisphere, while still obtaining the benefits of some amount of sleep (Rattenborg et al., 2016).

The ability of some birds to implement unihemispheric or asymmetric sleep as needed is consistent with, and probably facilitated by, several features: a strong visual decussation in the chiasm; few interhemispheric connections; and very strongly lateralized eye positions. This arrangement also makes them able to engage in two different visual behaviors simultaneously (Rattenborg et al., 1999).

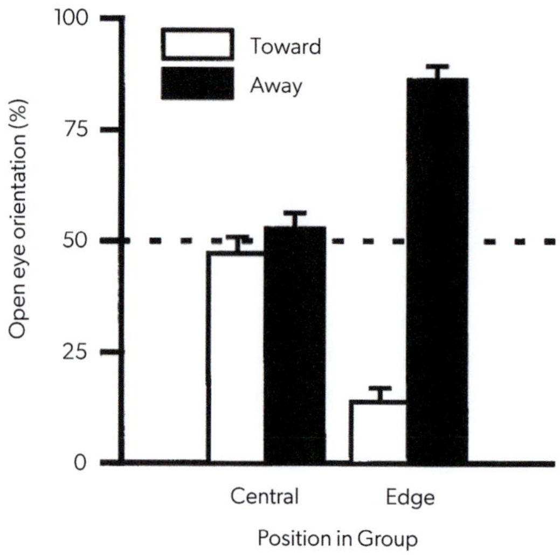

Figure 7.12 Four ducks were housed in a linear array in transparent boxes that allowed recording of eye closures and EEG. When one eye was open, the contralateral hemisphere showed a low voltage EEG characteristic of waking; when it was closed, the contralateral hemisphere showed an EEG pattern typical of sleep. Ducks showing unilateral eye closure while housed on the Edge of the array (right columns) were much more likely to keep open the eye that faced away from the group (black) than the eye facing toward the group (white). Ducks in a Central position (left columns) had either eye open about equally often when they showed unilateral eye opening. These findings are consistent with birds adjusting their unihemispheric vigilance patterns as an anti-predator mechanism, depending on where they were located within a "flock." Reprinted with permission of Elsevier, Ltd. from Rattenborg, N.C. et al. (1999) Facultative control of avian unihemispheric sleep under the risk of predation. *Behav Brain Res* 105:163–172. © Elsevier (1999). doi: 10.1016/s0166-4328(99)00070-4.

Fully terrestrial mammals do not show unihemispheric sleep, but the left and right cortices may show modest degrees of asymmetry under some conditions. For example, there is a shift in people toward more errors in localizing sound

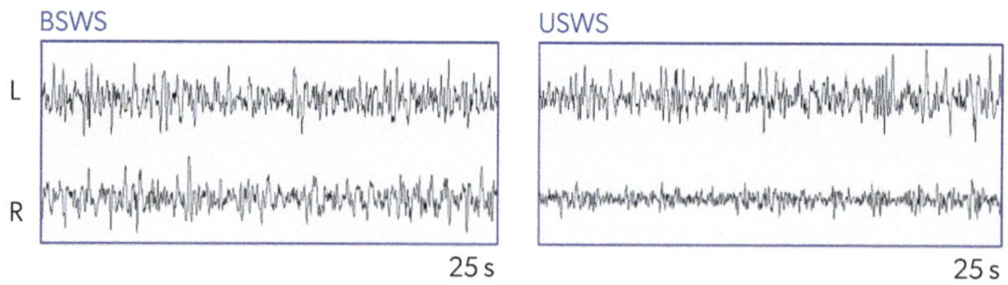

Figure 7.13 Examples of EEG patterns from the left (L) and right (R) sides of the brain of a great frigate bird (*Fregata minor*) during flight. The left side shows an example of bihemispheric SWS (BSWS) and the right side an example of unihemispheric SWS (USWS). High-voltage activity in each panel indicates sleep, while the low-voltage pattern in the right panel is consistent with waking. Reprinted with permission of Springer:Nature from Rattenborg N.C. et al. (2016) Evidence that birds sleep in mid-flight. *Nat Commun* 7:10.1038/ncomms12468. © The Authors (2016). Licensed under a Creative Commons Attribution 4.0 International License. (http://creativecommons.org/licenses/by/4.0/). doi: 10.1038/ncomms12468.

stimuli presented on the left side as drowsiness increases. These results suggest that alertness in the right hemisphere is more strongly suppressed early during the transition to sleep (Bareham et al., 2014).

A study of people experiencing a "first-night effect" (or novel-environment effect) while sleeping (for up to 90 min during a daytime nap) in an unfamiliar laboratory found increased vigilance and reduced NREM sleep depth only in the left hemisphere, as indexed by the amount of SWA (see Section 2.6.2). In particular, there was reduced SWA in a set of cortical structures that are grouped as the default mode network (DMN),[8] suggesting that this cortical system on the left side was engaged with passively monitoring the environment during sleep (Tamaki et al., 2016).

During N3 sleep, each hemisphere of participants was presented separately with a series of identical noises that were interrupted by single "oddball" stimuli with different features. Oddball stimuli presented to the left hemisphere triggered EEG and behavioral responses with higher probability and shorter latency than those presented to the right hemisphere, suggesting a more alert state in the left hemisphere. These lateral asymmetries disappeared when participants were tested during their second or third nap in the laboratory, when the novel-environment effect would have dissipated (Tamaki et al., 2016).

There have also been reports of some left–right asymmetries in the strengths of EEG frequency bands during different sleep stages in people (Roth et al., 1999). Some EEG asymmetries during sleep could be the product of functional specialization of the hemispheres (e.g., language, motor, or other functions). Other asymmetries may be the product of selectively increased activity of parts of one hemisphere during waking tasks. Increased activity of a cortical region during waking results in increased amounts of SWA in those regions during later sleep; see Section 12.6.2 for a discussion of these "use-dependent effects" on sleep EEG characteristics.

This capacity for expressing minor, localized EEG differences during sleep in terrestrial mammals could have been the basis for the evolution of partially asymmetric and, ultimately, fully unihemispheric sleep in amphibious and aquatic mammals, all of which evolved from originally terrestrial forms.

[8] The DMN includes several brain regions, primarily the medial prefrontal, inferior parietal, and posterior parietal cortices. They show highly correlated activity when people are awake and alert but are not actively engaged in any specific cognitive activity (Mason et al., 2007; Raichle, 2009; Raichle et al., 2001). Components of the DMN, especially frontal regions, tend to become uncoupled from the rest of the DMN during SWS (Horovitz et al., 2009). Reduced SWA in the DMN on one side suggests that it remained more correlated with other components and more activated, which could reflect alert, unfocused attention to the environment.

7.5.4 Physiology and anatomy of unihemispheric sleep

An analysis of acetylcholine (ACh) content in the hemispheres of sleeping northern fur seals (*Callorhinus ursinus*, an otariid species) demonstrated the degree to which sleep regulatory mechanisms can function independently in each cerebral hemisphere. In other mammals, cortical ACh levels are elevated bilaterally during both waking and REM sleep but are strongly reduced during NREM sleep.[9] In fur seals, both hemispheres showed decreased ACh levels during bihemispheric NREM sleep, as expected. But only the sleeping hemisphere showed low ACh levels during unihemispheric sleep, while the waking hemisphere continued to show high ACh levels (**Figure 7.14**) (Lapierre et al., 2007).

There is little information about how either EEG activity or ACh levels are controlled independently in the two cortices of aquatic mammals. One feature that may be involved is that cetaceans have a smaller corpus callosum (the principal commissure connecting the two cortices) relative to terrestrial mammals. This reduced size presumably reflects fewer direct connections between the two cortices and, therefore, less coordination of neural activity between them. In the same species, however, the posterior commissure (a brainstem pathway connecting subcortical regions) is very enlarged. These differences from typical mammalian anatomical features are not seen, however, in either phocid or otariid seals. Thus, these anatomical features do not appear to be essential to producing unihemispheric sleep in otariid seals, but they may facilitate it in obligate unihemispheric sleepers like cetaceans (Lyamin, Manger, et al., 2008).

One way of trying to better understand the role of a reduced corpus callosum is to examine the impact of its absence in people. The corpus callosum is sometimes surgically cut in people to prevent the bilateral spread of epileptic seizures ("split-brain" preparation), but there is little information about the sleep physiology of these patients. A study of two women who underwent this surgery indicated a reduction in the interhemispheric propagation of slow oscillations during sleep, but no unusual asymmetries in sleep EEG in general (Avvenuti et al., 2020).

Studies of a small number of people who lack a corpus callosum because of a rare condition in which it does not develop prenatally (callosal agenesis) found few differences in sleep patterns relative to controls. There were hints of reduced EEG coherence between the hemispheres (referring to second-to-second differences in the phases of EEG waves), but no evidence of actual dissociations of sleep–wake states between the two hemispheres

[9] ACh is critically involved in activating the cortex during both waking and REM sleep. For a discussion of the role of ACh, see Chapters 10 and 11.

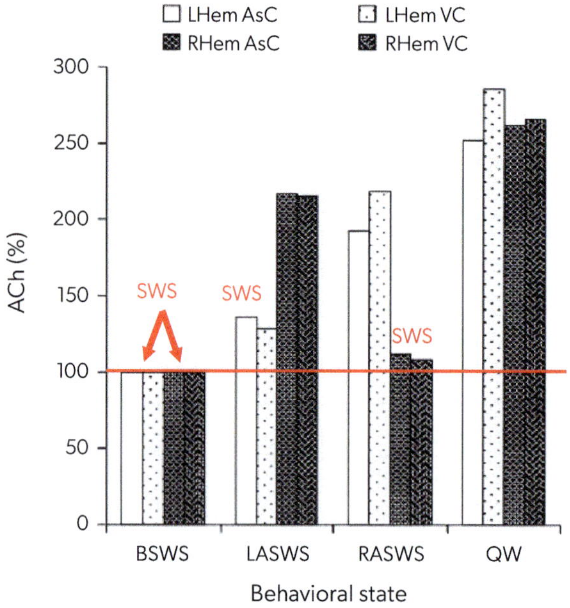

Figure 7.14 Northern fur seals (*Callorhinus ursinus*) show both bilateral and unilateral cortical sleep patterns. Acetylcholine (ACh) levels were measured in association cortex (AsC) and visual cortex (VC) in both the left and right hemispheres (LHem, RHem) while the animals were in bilateral sleep, were awake, or were showing slow-wave sleep (SWS) only in the left or right hemisphere. Values are expressed as a percentage of ACh levels when in bilateral sleep (=100%; red line), during which ACh levels in other species that show only bilateral sleep would be very low (red arrows). When the fur seals were in quiet wake (QW), both regions in both hemispheres showed much higher ACh levels than when they were in bilateral slow-wave sleep (BSWS). When only the left hemisphere was asleep (LASWS), ACh levels were highly elevated in the right hemisphere (dark bars) but only slightly in the left hemisphere (light bars). When only the right hemisphere was asleep (RASWS), ACh levels were elevated only in the left hemisphere (light bars). These results demonstrate the robust independence of ACh levels in the two hemispheres during unihemispheric sleep. Adapted with permission of Dr. Jerome Siegel and SfN from Lapierre, J.L. et al. (2007) Cortical acetylcholine release is lateralized during asymmetrical slow-wave sleep in northern fur seals. *J Neurosci* 27:11999–12006. © Society for Neuroscience (2007). doi: 10.1523/JNEUROSCI.2968-07.2007.

(Nielsen et al., 1992). Thus, complete absence of the corpus callosum developmentally or following surgery in people does not on its own reproduce the strongly asymmetric sleep patterns of aquatic mammals and birds.

7.5.5 Functions of unihemispheric sleep in marine mammals

There are several hypotheses for why unihemispheric sleep arose through convergent evolution in cetaceans and some seals. Like other mammals, these species cannot extract oxygen from water as fish do and must breathe air, so they hold their breath underwater and come to the surface to breathe. Phocids, which have not been shown to generate unihemispheric sleep, are capable of holding their breath underwater for long periods of time, with dives lasting from many minutes up to 2 h. This ability would allow them to sleep bilaterally for extended periods underwater without having to swim to the surface to breathe (Kendall-Bar et al., 2023; Lyamin, Manger, et al., 2008). Otariids, however, typically dive for only a few minutes at a time, so they would be able to sleep bilaterally for only very short periods before needing to surface. As a result, they would have very fragmented sleep if they generated only bilateral sleep in the water.

These observations suggest that unihemispheric sleep in otariids (and cetaceans) may in part be an adaptation permitting sustained sleep periods alternately in each hemisphere, while still allowing the motor behaviors (swimming and surfacing) needed to permit breathing to continue, under the control of the contralateral hemisphere.

A second class of functions served by this adaptation is allowing maintenance of close contact with conspecifics, and continuous assessment of predation risks, as suggested above for birds. Cetaceans range widely in size, but even very large whales are subject to predation when they are young (and in some cases even as adults), primarily by killer whales and large sharks, which also prey on smaller cetaceans and seals of any age. Thus, constant vigilance and close contact with other vigilant pod members are needed to reduce predation risk. In the open ocean environment, there is no secure refuge, so cetaceans and seafaring seals must balance the need for sleep with the need for constant antipredator vigilance, like ungulates living on wide-open prairies. Maintaining alertness in one hemisphere while the other sleeps may serve this antipredator function.

This hypothesis is supported by some observational results. A pod of four Pacific white-sided dolphins (*Lagenorhyncus obliquidens*), that were studied in captivity, swam in tight formations during their nightly sleep phase. The dolphins typically alternated having one eye open and the other closed (presumably reflecting alternating unihemispheric sleep), with the position of the closed eye linked to their lateral position in the pod. In contrast to ducks housed in a row (Rattenborg et al., 1999), the dolphins typically kept open the eye that faced *toward*, not away from, other members of the pod. These observations suggest that the highest priority while swimming through dark waters at night was to maintain visual contact and close proximity to the rest of the pod (Goley, 1999).

A final set of pressures that may have influenced the evolution of this sleep pattern relates to thermal balance. Water is much more efficient than air at transferring heat; estimates suggest that heat loss from a body in cold ocean water may be 90-fold faster than in dry air (Manger, 2006).[10]

Mammals expend a very large part of their energy intake to maintain a high, homeostatically defended body temperature (up to 80% of calories consumed, by some estimates), so they face a serious energy-balance challenge in aquatic environments where they can lose heat rapidly to the cold water. This challenge is met by several adaptations to reduce heat loss, including insulating layers of heavy blubber and countercurrent heat exchange mechanisms in the circulatory system. But on the production side of the heat equation, mammals rely on the activity of large muscle groups as a major source of metabolic heat.

In terrestrial mammals, large muscle activity is much reduced during SWS and essentially absent during the atonia of REM sleep (during which, thermoregulation is also suspended). Thus, another driver of the evolution of unihemispheric sleep in aquatic mammals may have been the cost of lost heat production if they were to become immobile during sleep, and especially if they expressed REM sleep atonia. The lack of bihemispheric SWS in the water among cetaceans and otariids, and the virtual absence of REM sleep while in the water may both be adaptations that permit continued swimming, allowing sustained high heat production and counteracting the risks of heat loss.

In addition, glial cells in the brain are known to generate metabolic heat, particularly in response to the neurotransmitter norepinephrine, levels of which are high during waking but low in both SWS and REM sleep (see Chapter 11). Cetaceans have unusually high densities of glia in their cortices. Maintenance of high levels of glial heat production alternately in each waking hemisphere could help preserve normal brain temperature and function (Lyamin, Manger, et al., 2008; Manger, 2006). One hypothesis about the function of REM sleep in terrestrial species is to help protect neural tissue from the effects of low temperatures during long NREM sleep episodes (Siegel, 2022; Wehr, 1992). The combination of continuous heat production from large-muscle activity and sustained glial heat production during unihemispheric sleep may explain why these species can forego the need for REM sleep.

[10] The same principle applies to heat transfer in the opposite direction. That is why a person can put a hand into the dry, hot air of a 200° C (392° F) oven for a few seconds with no harm done (without touching metal, which is also a good heat conductor), while putting a hand into 100° C (212° F) water for the same duration would cause major tissue damage.

7.5.6 Revisiting behavioral criteria for sleep

Many of the features of unihemispheric sleep are inconsistent with the behavioral criteria discussed earlier for identifying sleep in animals (Section 7.2.2). In violation of these criteria, some cetaceans or seals may not adopt a unique posture for sleep, and they may not reduce or stop gross motor activity. Another behavioral criterion for sleep is a reduction in responsiveness to external stimuli, but in cetaceans (and birds) there may be little or no reduction in vigilance by the organism as a whole, despite the closure of one eye during unihemispheric sleep.

A final criterion, normally applied to the whole animal, is that sleep deprivation should lead to later rebound increases in sleep duration/intensity. The limited information available indicates weak homeostatic regulation of SWS that is expressed only in the selectively deprived hemisphere (Lyamin, Manger, et al., 2008). Thus, these species do not meet the behavioral criteria for sleep at the whole-organism level (Siegel, 2008), but they appear to satisfy the criteria of reduced motor activity, reduced environmental responsiveness, state reversibility, and homeostatic regulation at the level of each hemisphere.

One interpretation of these sleep features in aquatic mammals is that sleep as manifest in terrestrial mammals is not essential to animals in general. Alternatively, one might conclude that sleep is of such physiological importance that animals have evolved innovative solutions to preserve its essential features in environments that would not appear compatible with sleep. A better understanding of the sleep adaptations of aquatic mammals and their implications for understanding the functions of sleep will depend on future studies of these remarkable species. These studies are, however, difficult to conduct because of the very large size and inaccessibility of some species, and the challenging aquatic environments in which they live.

7.5.7 Summary

The sleep of seagoing mammals differs from that of terrestrial mammals in several ways. Cetaceans (always) and most otariid seals (while they are in the water) sleep one hemisphere at a time and show little or no REM sleep. Elephant seals appear to be an exception in that they show substantial REM sleep both on land and during deep ocean dives. Seals, however, show bihemispheric sleep while on land, including small, variable amounts of REM sleep. Depriving one hemisphere of sleep in dolphins caused substantial, but inconsistent, rebound sleep increases in that hemisphere, but did not increase sleep in the other hemisphere during either sleep loss or recovery sleep. In fur seals while on land, selective deprivation of bihemispheric sleep led to increasing pressure to produce it.

Many birds also show unihemispheric or strongly asymmetric sleep, which may serve an antipredator function as well as facilitating uninterrupted, long-distance flights over periods of days (see Section 7.6).

The anatomical characteristics of cetaceans that may be associated with unihemispheric sleep include strongly decussated optic projections, a small corpus callosum, and increased size of the posterior commissure. These anatomical features do not, however, appear to be necessary in otariid seals to allow unihemispheric sleep and its associated independent regulation of ACh levels in the two hemispheres.

The evolution of unihemispheric sleep and reduced or absent REM sleep in mammals in the ocean may have been driven by several factors:

- the need to continue large muscle activity and norepinephrine-dependent glial thermogenesis to maintain brain and body temperature in the cold ocean;
- the need to continue swimming and surfacing to permit breathing;
- the need to maintain awareness of and visual contact with conspecifics; and
- the risk of predation in the absence of any form of shelter in the open ocean.

The differences in sleep between birds/aquatic mammals and terrestrial mammals raise questions about how to apply behavioral criteria to measure sleep and about the neural level at which sleep is regulated and sleep need is satisfied. This issue is discussed further in Chapter 12.

7.6 Seasonal changes in sleep

People who live a significant distance away from the equator are familiar with the changes in our environment that occur through the seasons. As the northern hemisphere gradually tilts toward and away from the sun over the course of the earth's annual wobbly orbit, the photoperiod (daylength) gradually increases and decreases, while the southern hemisphere experiences the opposite shifts. These changes range up to the extremes of continuous darkness during mid-winter and continuous daylight during mid-summer in arctic and antarctic regions. Even in more temperate zones, these photoperiod changes result in large seasonal variations in the amount of solar energy reaching the earth's surface, with dramatic effects on temperature and precipitation. A host of secondary changes in ground cover, food availability, and the presence of plant and animal populations produce radically different ecological conditions in winter and summer.

People in many human societies today use technology to control light and temperature in their environments, which reduces seasonal effects on their physiology, behavior, and sleep patterns. As mentioned in Chapter 6, in pretechnological societies, human sleep may once have been more responsive to the seasons. Even today, some people in temperate zones undergo seasonal changes in activity and sleep patterns, showing, for example, longer sleep and more food intake during the winter compared to the summer (Hardin et al., 1991). Some of these changes may reflect behavioral choices made in response to low temperatures and challenging weather conditions in winter. But there is also evidence that endocrine systems in some people remain responsive to photoperiod changes (Wehr, 1991).

In many animal species, seasonal changes are far more dramatic and strongly tied to endocrine signals that track photoperiod. The physiological mechanisms in mammals that are involved in measuring and responding to changing photoperiods are discussed in more detail in Chapter 9. Briefly, the principal mediator of these seasonal changes in many species is the secretion pattern of the hormone melatonin by the pineal gland (Goldman, 2001).

Under the control of photoperiodic and other signals, animals respond to seasonal environmental changes with a variety of strategies. These include ceasing reproduction during some annual phases and concentrating it in others; migrating seasonally to and from more temperate regions; or hibernating in their usual home territories. Species that neither migrate nor hibernate may still undergo quite dramatic seasonal changes in behavior, reproductive function, endocrine and immune system function, diet, coloration, and coat quality.

Seasonal changes include altered daily patterns of activity that imply changes in the organization of sleep, such as switching among predominantly diurnal, nocturnal, and crepuscular (around dawn and/or dusk) activity patterns across the seasons (Nyholm, 1965; Reebs, 2002; Rusak, 1981). For example, oryx antelopes living in the Arabian desert slept during both day and night in the winter, but slept less in the summer and primarily during extreme midday heat (up to 40° C) (Davimes et al., 2018). Even species that sleep at the same time of day in different seasons may change their sleep amounts significantly.

Among bird species that migrate southward in the fall and northward in the spring, some that are day-active in other seasons fly primarily at night during migration, presumably to reduce predation by diurnal predators such as hawks. Those that breed in far northern regions during continuous summer daylight show a variety of activity patterns, including entrained 24 h rhythms (perhaps in response to small changes in light intensity or temperature), free-running rhythms, or arrhythmic activity patterns (Steiger et al., 2013). Although sleep was not measured directly in most studies, these altered activity patterns imply substantial changes in the timing and amounts of sleep.

When sleep was recorded directly from male pectoral sandpipers (*Calidris melanotos*) during their short breeding season in the Arctic, many showed reduced sleep amounts when they were competing for mating opportunities. Those that showed the largest reductions in sleep (i.e., showed longest periods of waking and activity) were most successful in mating and in siring offspring, demonstrating a trade-off between sleep duration and reproductive success under these conditions (Lesku et al., 2012).

Another species, chinstrap penguins (*Pygoscelis antarcticus*), studied while nesting on an Antarctic island in December (when daylength is very long), showed both bihemispheric and unihemispheric NREM sleep. This sleep occurred in extremely short bouts (averaging ~4 sec durations), but the birds still accumulated 11.5–12.0 h of sleep per hemisphere daily (Libourel et al., 2023). Given that they were nesting in a very crowded colony situation with a high risk of predation, this sleep pattern may be an adaptation to permit vigilance during nesting while obtaining substantial amounts of sleep.

When small, migratory songbirds are caged and exposed to seasonal changes in photoperiod, they develop physiological and behavioral characteristics in the spring and fall that are typical of birds during actual migrations. In their cages, these diurnally active birds show altered activity and sleep patterns, including the nighttime expression of intense "zugunruhe" (migratory restlessness; **Figure 7.15**), which is oriented in the compass direction to which free-living birds would migrate in that season (Kramer, 1950). During expression of zugunruhe, brain regions involved in processing information relevant to migratory orientation reverse the timing of their spontaneous activation from day to night. This observation indicates that there is a broad reorganization of brain functions related to sleep and other behaviors to permit migration (Rastogi et al., 2011).

White-crowned sparrows (*Zonotrichia leucophrys gambelii*) engage in remarkable seasonal migrations. Those that breed in Alaska, for example, migrate in the fall to southern California and back again in the spring (~4,300 km [2,700 mi] each way). When they were housed in cages and exposed to annual photoperiod changes, they shortened and reorganized sleep during the fall and spring seasons when they would normally migrate (Jones et al., 2010). EEG recordings from caged sparrows in migratory and nonmigratory states showed that the migratory state involved reducing sleep durations from ~8 h to ~3 h nightly, including a reduction in SWA. In addition, REM sleep was both reduced in amount and concentrated early in the night, rather than at the end of the night, as during the nonmigratory phase (Rattenborg et al., 2004) (**Figure 7.16**).

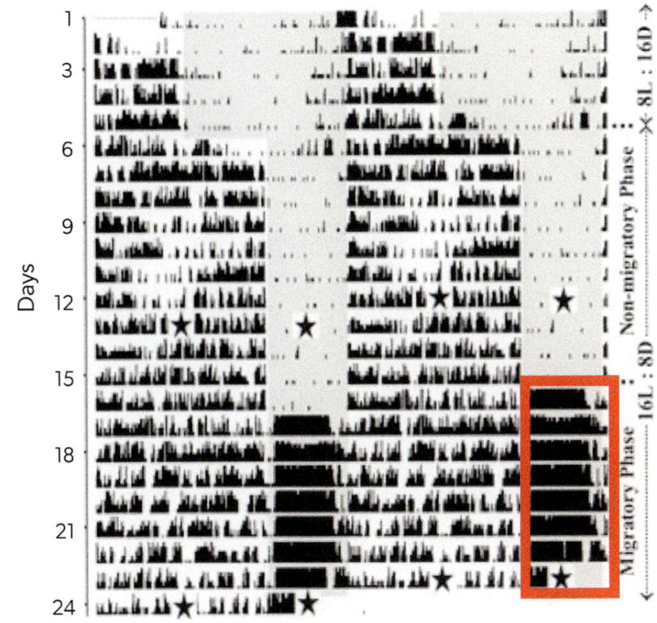

Figure 7.15 Activity record (black markings; double-plotted to show 48 h periods) of a caged black-headed bunting (*Emberiza melanocephala*) housed initially in a short-day photoperiod for 5 days (8 h of light daily, shown as white areas) and after transfer (on Day 6) to a long-day photoperiod (16 h of light daily), during which it was initially in nonmigratory condition. In this condition, the bunting was active almost exclusively during the daily light phase. After 12 days in the long photoperiod, it entered a migratory condition and started to show intense nocturnal activity (zugunruhe) (red box) along with continued activity during the day. Stars represent times during which other birds were removed to study patterns of gene expression in the brain. Reprinted with permission of John Wiley & Sons Ltd. from Rastogi, A. et al. (2011) Phase inversion of neural activity in the olfactory and visual systems of a night-migratory bird during migration. *Eur J Neurosci* 34:99–109. © The Authors (2011). Journal compilation © Federation of European Neuroscience Societies and Blackwell Publishing. doi: 10.1111/j.1460-9568.2011.07737.x.

Blackpoll warblers (*Setophaga striata*) migrate in the fall from eastern North America to the Caribbean or the northern part of South America. Their southward migration is almost entirely over open ocean, where they cannot land and sleep. These tiny birds (~12 g body weight) were equipped with geolocators (0.5 g) that permitted estimation of their locations. During their fall migration, some birds flew over the Atlantic Ocean for several days, covering an average of ~2,500 km (1,550 mi) without the possibility of stopping (DeLuca et al., 2015) (**Figure 7.17**). A later study of this same species showed even longer flights over the Atlantic which averaged 60 h (range = 48–96 h), during which they could not have landed in order to sleep (DeLuca et al., 2019).

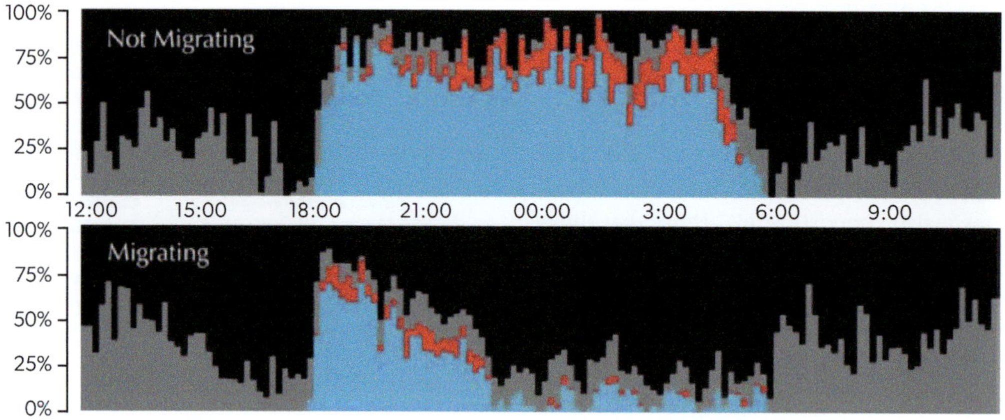

Figure 7.16 Sleep EEG was recorded in a laboratory from white-crowned sparrows (*Zonotrichia leucophrys gambelii*) that were in their nonmigratory phase (top panel) and migratory phase (bottom panel). Recordings were made in lighting cycles with 12 h of light daily (light phase: 06:00–18:00) to eliminate any immediate impact of lighting condition. The percentage of each state (Y axis) is shown across a 24 h period (X axis) with different colors. Black = waking, gray = drowsiness, blue = slow-wave sleep, and red = REM sleep. During the migratory phase, birds showed increased nocturnal wakefulness (especially beginning around 23:00 h), reduced slow-wave sleep, and reduced REM sleep. REM sleep was also concentrated at the beginning of the night (~18:00) rather than being most intense late in the night (~03:00–05:00) as in nonmigratory birds. Reprinted with permission from Rattenborg N.C. et al. (2004) Migratory sleeplessness in the white-crowned sparrow (*Zonotrichia leucophrys gambelii*). *PLoS Biol* 2:924–936. © 2004 Rattenborg et al. Creative Commons Attribution License (CC-BY). doi: 10.1371/journal.pbio.0020212.

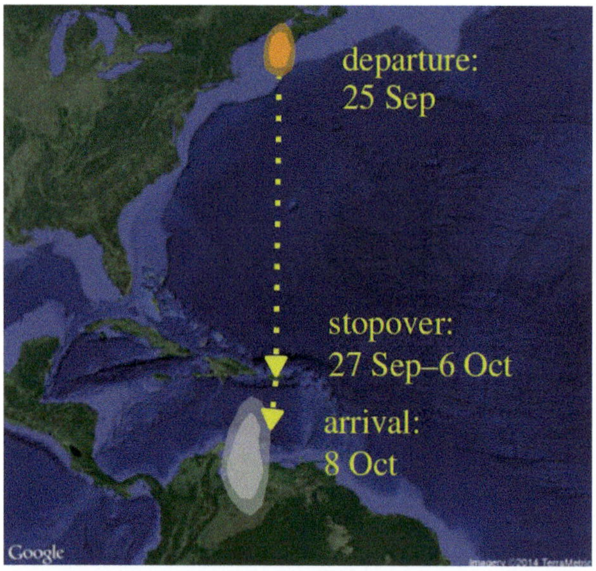
departure:
25 Sep
stopover:
27 Sep–6 Oct
arrival:
8 Oct
Google

Figure 7.17 The inferred flight path of a male blackpoll warbler (*Setophaga striata*) over the ocean from Nova Scotia to the eastern Caribbean, derived from a recovered geolocator device that had been attached to the bird during its migration. The orange region represents the area in which the bird was active before departure and the white region represents the area where the bird was active after its migratory flight. Note that the bird flew over open ocean for ~2–3 days between stopovers (triangles) during each of the two legs of its migration. Reprinted with permission of The Royal Society (UK) from DeLuca, W.V. et al. (2015) Transoceanic migration by a 12 g songbird. *Biol Lett* 11:20141045. © The Authors (2015); published by the Royal Society. Permission conveyed through Copyright Clearance Center, Inc. doi: 10.1098/rsbl.2014.1045. Imagery © TerraMetrics, LLC (2015)- www.terrametrics.com.

It is not yet feasible to record the sleep of such small birds while in flight. But in the much larger great frigate bird (*Fregata minor*), EEG recordings were obtained while they flew continuously for periods of up to 10 days over the Pacific Ocean near the Galapagos Islands. Their total NREM sleep was drastically reduced relative to when they were on land, and there was an increase in sleep asymmetry between the hemispheres, extending to unihemispheric sleep while in flight (Rattenborg et al., 2016); see **Figure 7.13**. Whether smaller migratory species show partial or complete unihemispheric sleep during sustained flights of up to 4 days (DeLuca et al., 2019) has not been determined, but this might be a mechanism for preserving at least some sleep during continuous multiday flights (Rattenborg, 2006a).

These findings indicate that sleep-regulatory mechanisms in long-distance migrants and in species exposed to extreme seasonal changes, such as continuous light, are flexibly adapted to these conditions. They show dramatic changes in both the duration and the temporal distribution of sleep in these circumstances, to the extent that sleep may even be suspended for periods of time. Large reductions in sleep have also been reported shortly after birth in killer whale and dolphin mothers and their newborns (Lyamin et al., 2005), although the extent of these reductions has been questioned (Gnone et al., 2006; Sekiguchi et al., 2006). The idea of flexibility in sleep regulatory systems is reinforced by evidence from other species in which circadian rest–activity rhythms can be suppressed under some circumstances (Bloch et al., 2013), implying large changes in the amounts and/or temporal distribution of sleep.

7.6.1 Summary

Seasonal changes in photoperiod trigger a broad array of ecological changes that affect species in temperate zones. Humans may show some physiological changes related to photoperiod, and other changes in habits and activities may occur because of the constraints imposed by extreme temperatures. Animals address seasonal challenges by combinations of physiological changes, hibernation, and migration.

Some birds that breed at extreme latitudes during long or continuous daily illumination may show strong reductions in sleep amounts related to competition for mating opportunities. At least one species, however, showed many, extremely short uni- and bihemispheric sleep episodes while nesting and still accumulated large amounts of daily sleep.

Birds that are diurnally active in the nonmigratory season show dramatic changes in sleep patterns during migrations, including large increases in nocturnal activity, reduced NREM and REM sleep amounts, and redistribution of REM sleep during the sleep period. Some birds may take advantage of partial unihemispheric sleep to get some sleep during lengthy migration bouts or multiday flights that are incompatible with landing and engaging in bihemispheric sleep.

Different sleep amounts and patterns among species with different life histories indicate that sleep has been strongly modified by ecological factors over the course of evolutionary time. The results related to migration and seasonal change demonstrate that sleep can also be regulated flexibly within the lifetimes of individual animals. The extent of this flexibility varies among species, but these findings indicate that for some species the functions served by sleep (see Chapters 16 and 19) can be temporarily altered, postponed, or satisfied in different ways in response to other critical needs.

Literature cited

Albeck, N., Udi, D. I., Eyal, R., Shvartsman, A., & Shein-Idelson, M. (2022). Temperature-robust rapid eye movement and slow wave sleep in the lizard Laudakia vulgaris. *Commun Biol*, *5*(1), 1310. doi: 10.1038/s42003-022-04261-4

Allebrandt, K. V., Amin, N., Muller-Myhsok, B., Esko, T., Teder-Laving, M., Azevedo, R. V., ... Roenneberg, T. (2013). A K(ATP) channel gene effect on sleep duration: from genome-wide association studies to function in Drosophila. *Mol Psychiatry*, *18*(1), 122–132. doi: 10.1038/mp.2011.142

Allison, T., & Van Twyver, H. (1970). Sleep in the moles, *Scalopus aquaticus* and *Condylura cristata*. *Exp Neurol*, *27*, 564–578.

Armitage, R., Smith, C., Thompson, S., & Hoffmann, R. (2001). Sex differences in slow-wave activity in response to sleep deprivation. *Sleep Res Online*, *4*(1), 33–41.

Aulsebrook, A. E., Jones, T. M., Rattenborg, N. C., Roth, T. C., 2nd, & Lesku, J. A. (2016). Sleep ecophysiology: integrating neuroscience and ecology. *Trends Ecol Evol*, *31*(8), 590–599. doi: 10.1016/j.tree.2016.05.004

Avvenuti, G., Handjaras, G., Betta, M., Cataldi, J., Imperatori, L. S., Lattanzi, S., ... Bernardi, G. (2020). Integrity of corpus callosum is essential for the cross-hemispheric propagation of sleep slow waves: a high-density EEG study in split-brain patients. *J Neurosci*, *40*(29), 5589–5603. doi: 10.1523/JNEUROSCI.2571-19.2020

Bareham, C. A., Manly, T., Pustovaya, O. V., Scott, S. K., & Bekinschtein, T. A. (2014). Losing the left side of the world: rightward shift in human spatial attention with sleep onset. *Sci Rep*, *4*, 5092. doi: 10.1038/srep05092

Benington, J. H., & Heller, H. C. (1994). Does the function of REM sleep concern non-REM sleep or waking? *Prog Neurobiol*, *44*, 433–449.

Benington, J. H., & Heller, H. C. (1995). Restoration of brain energy metabolism as the function of sleep. *Prog Neurobiol*, *45*, 347–360.

Benington, J. H., & Heller, H. C. (1999). Implications of sleep deprivation experiments for understanding of sleep homeostasis. *Sleep*, *22*(8), 1033–1037.

Beyaert, L., Greggers, U., & Menzel, R. (2012). Honeybees consolidate navigation memory during sleep. *J Exp Biol*, *215*(Pt 22), 3981–3988. doi: 10.1242/jeb.075499

Bloch, G., Barnes, B. M., Gerkema, M. P., & Helm, B. (2013). Animal activity around the clock with no overt circadian rhythms: patterns, mechanisms and adaptive value. *Proc Roy Soc Lon B*, *280*(1765), 20130019. doi: 10.1098/rspb.2013.0019

Block, B. A., & Finnerty, J. R. (1994). Endothermy in fishes: a phylogenetic analysis of constraints, predispositions, and selection pressure. *Environ Biol Fish*, *40*(283–302).

Buchsbaum, M. S., Gillin, J. C., Wu, J., Hazlett, E., Sicotte, N., Dupont, R. M., & Bunney Jr., W. E. (1989). Regional cerebral glucose metabolic rate in human sleep assessed by positron emission tomography. *Life Sci*, *45*(15), 1349–1356.

Campbell, S. S., & Tobler, I. (1984). Animal sleep: A review of sleep duration across phylogeny. *Neurosci Biobehav Rev*, *8*, 269–300.

Carrier, J., Semba, K., Deurveilher, S., Drogos, L., Cyr-Cronier, J., Lord, C., & Sekerovick, Z. (2017). Sex differences in age-related changes in the sleep-wake cycle. *Front Neuroendocrinol*, *47*, 66–85. doi: 10.1016/j.yfrne.2017.07.004

Crocker, A., & Sehgal, A. (2010). Genetic analysis of sleep. *Gene Dev*, *24*(12), 1220–1235. doi: 10.1101/gad.1913110

Davimes, J. G., Alagaili, A. N., Bhagwandin, A., Bertelsen, M. F., Mohammed, O. B., Bennett, N. C., ... Gravett, N. (2018). Seasonal variations in sleep of free-ranging Arabian oryx (Oryx leucoryx) under natural hyperarid conditions. *Sleep*, *41*(5), zsy038. doi: 10.1093/sleep/zsy038

DeLuca, W. V., Woodworth, B. K., Mackenzie, S. A., Newman, A. E. M., Cooke, H. A., Phillips, L. M., ... Norris, D. R. (2019). A boreal songbird's 20,000 km migration across North America and the Atlantic Ocean. *Ecology*, *100*(5), e02651. doi:10.1002/ecy.2651

DeLuca, W. V., Woodworth, B. K., Rimmer, C. C., Marra, P. P., Taylor, P. D., McFarland, K. P., ... Norris, D. R. (2015). Transoceanic migration by a 12 g songbird. *Biol Lett*, *11*(4), 20141045. doi: 10.1098/rsbl.2014.1045

Deurveilher, S., Rusak, B., & Semba, K. (2011). Female reproductive hormones alter sleep architecture in ovariectomized rats. *Sleep*, *34*(4), 519–530.

Dib, R., Gervais, N. J., & Mongrain, V. (2021). A review of the current state of knowledge on sex differences in sleep and circadian phenotypes in rodents. *Neurobiol Sleep Circad Rhythms*, *11*, 1–11. doi: 10.1016/j.nbscr.2021.100068

Donlea, J. M., Alam, M. N., & Szymusiak, R. (2017). Neuronal substrates of sleep homeostasis; lessons from flies, rats and mice. *Curr Opin Neurobiol*, *44*, 228–235. doi: 10.1016/j.conb.2017.05.003

Donlea, J. M., Thimgan, M. S., Suzuki, Y., Gottschalk, L., & Shaw, P. J. (2011). Inducing sleep by remote control facilitates memory consolidation in Drosophila. *Science*, *332*(6037), 1571–1576. doi: 10.1126/science.1202249

Dugas-Ford, J., & Ragsdale, C. W. (2015). Levels of homology and the problem of neocortex. *Annu Rev Neurosci*, *38*, 351–368. doi: 10.1146/annurev-neuro-071714-033911

Eiland, M. M., Lyamin, O. I., & Siegel, J. M. (2001). State-related discharge of neurons in the brainstem of freely moving box turtles, *Terrapene carolina major*. *Arch Ital Biol*, *139*, 23–36.

Flanigan Jr., W. F., Wilcox, R. H., & Rechtschaffen, A. (1973). The EEG and behavioral continuum of the crocodilian, *Caiman sclerops*. *Electroencephalogr Clin Neurophysiol*, *34*, 521–538.

Flanigan, W. F., Jr., Knight, C. P., Hartse, K. M., & Rechtschaffen, A. (1974). Sleep and wakefulness in chelonian reptiles. I. The box turtle, *Terrapene carolina*. *Arch Ital Biol*, *112*, 227–252.

Ganguly-Fitzgerald, I., Donlea, J., & Shaw, P. J. (2006). Waking experience affects sleep need in *Drosophila*. *Science*, *313*(5794), 1775–1781.

Georgoulas, A., Jones, L., Laudiano-Dray, M. P., Meek, J., Fabrizi, L., & Whitehead, K. (2021). Sleep-wake regulation in preterm and term infants. *Sleep*, *44*(1), zsaa148. doi:10.1093/sleep/zsaa148

Glotzbach, S. F., & Heller, H. (1976). Central nervous regulation of body temperature during sleep. *Science*, *194*(4264), 537–539.

Gnone, G., Moriconi, T., & Gambini, G. (2006). Sleep behaviour: activity and sleep in dolphins. *Nature, 441*(7096), E10–E11. doi: 10.1038/nature04899

Goldman, B. (2001). Mammalian photoperiodic system: formal properties and neuroendocrine mechanisms of photoperiodic time measurement. *J Biol Rhythms, 16*(4), 283–301.

Goley, P. D. (1999). Behavioral aspects of sleep in Pacific white-sided dophins (*Lagenorhynchus obliquidens*, Gill 1865). *Mar Mamm Sci, 15*(4), 1054–1064.

Gravett, N., Bhagwandin, A., Lyamin, O. I., Siegel, J. M., & Manger, P. R. (2012). Sleep in the rock hyrax, Procavia capensis. *Brain Behav Evol, 79*(3), 155–169. doi: 10.1159/000335342

Gravett, N., Bhagwandin, A., Sutcliffe, R., Landen, K., Chase, M. J., Lyamin, O. I., ... Manger, P. R. (2017). Inactivity/sleep in two wild free-roaming African elephant matriarchs – Does large body size make elephants the shortest mammalian sleepers? *PLoS One, 12*(3), e0171903. doi: 10.1371/journal.pone.0171903

Hanagasioglu, M., & Borbély, A. A. (1982). Effects of voluntary locomotor activity on sleep in the rat. *Behav Brain Res, 4*, 359–368.

Hardin, T. A., Wehr, T. A., Brewerton, T., Kasper, S., Berrettini, W., Rabkin, J., & Rosenthal, N. E. (1991). Evaluation of seasonality in six clinical populations and two normal populations. *J Psychiatr Res, 25*(3), 75–87.

Hendricks, J. C., Finn, S. M., Panckeri, K. A., Chavkin, J., Williams, J. A., Sehgal, A., & Pack, A. I. (2000). Rest in drosophila is a sleep-like state. *Neuron, 25*(1), 129–138.

Herculano-Houzel, S. (2012). The remarkable, yet not extraordinary, human brain as a scaled-up primate brain and its associated cost. *Proc Natl Acad Sci U S A, 109 Suppl 1*, 10661–10668. doi: 10.1073/pnas.1201895109

Herculano-Houzel, S., Avelino-de-Souza, K., Neves, K., Porfirio, J., Messeder, D., Mattos Feijo, L., ... Manger, P. R. (2014). The elephant brain in numbers. *Front Neuroanat, 8*, 46. doi: 10.3389/fnana.2014.00046

Horovitz, S. G., Braun, A., Carr, W., Picchioni, D., Balkin, T., Fukunaga, M., & Duyn, J. H. (2009). Decoupling of the brain's default mode network during deep sleep. *Proc Natl Acad Sci USA, 106*(27), 11376–11381.

Huber, R., Hill, S. L., Holladay, C., Biesiadecki, M., Tononi, G., & Cirelli, C. (2004). Sleep homeostasis in *Drosophila melanogaster*. *Sleep, 27*(4), 628–639.

Iglesias, T. L., Boal, J. G., Frank, M. G., Zeil, J., & Hanlon, R. T. (2019). Cyclic nature of the REM sleep-like state in the cuttlefish *Sepia officinalis*. *J Exp Biol, 222 (Pt 1)*, jeb174862. doi:10.1242/jeb.174862

Jarvis, E. D., Güntürkün, O., Bruce, L., Csillag, A., Karten, H., Kuenzel, W., ... Consortium, A. B. N. (2005). Avian brains and a new understanding of vertebrate brain evolution. *Nat Rev Neurosci, 6*(2), 151–159. doi: 10.1038/nrn1606

Joiner, W. J. (2016). Unraveling the evolutionary determinants of sleep. *Curr Biol, 26*(20), R1073–R1087. doi: 10.1016/j.cub.2016.08.068

Jones, S. G., Paletz, E. M., Obermeyer, W. H., Hannan, C. T., & Benca, R. M. (2010). Seasonal influences on sleep and executive function in the migratory White-crowned Sparrow (Zonotrichia leucophrys gambelii). *BMC Neurosci, 11*(1), 87. doi: 10.1186/1471-2202-11-87

Jouvet-Mounier, D., Astic, L., & Lacote, D. (1969). Ontogenesis of the states of sleep in rat, cat, and guinea pig during the first postnatal month. *Dev Psychobiol, 2*(4), 216–239.

Jung, C. M., Melanson, E. L., Frydendall, E. J., Perreault, L., Eckel, R. H., & Wright, K. P. (2011). Energy expenditure during sleep, sleep deprivation and sleep following sleep deprivation in adult humans. *J Physiol, 589*(1), 235–244. doi: 10.1113/jphysiol.2010.197517

Kaiser, W. (1988). Busy bees need rest, too. *J Comp Physiol A, 163*, 565–584.

Karten, H. J. (1991). Homology and evolutionary origin of the 'neocortex'. *Brain Behav Evol, 38*, 264–272.

Karten, H. J. (1997). Evolutionary developmental biology meets the brain: the origins of mammalian cortex. *Proc Natl Acad Sci USA, 94*, 2800–2804.

Kelly, M. L., Peters, R. A., Tisdale, R. K., & Lesku, J. A. (2015). Unihemispheric sleep in crocodilians? *J Exp Biol, 218*(Pt 20), 3175–3178. doi: 10.1242/jeb.127605

Kendall-Bar, J. M., Williams, T. M., Mukherji, R., Lozano, D. A., Pitman, J. K., Holser, R. R., ... Costa, D. P. (2023). Brain activity of diving seals reveals short sleep cycles at depth. *Science, 380*, 260–265.

Koh, K., Joiner, W. J., Wu, M. N., Yue, Z., Smith, C., J., & Sehgal, A. (2008). Identification of SLEEPLESS, a sleep-promoting factor. *Science, 321*(5887), 372–376. doi: 10.1126/science.1155942

Kramer, G. (1950). Orientierte Zugaktivität gekäfigter Singvögel. *Naturwissenschaften, 37*(8), 188.

Lapierre, J. L., Kosenko, P. O., Lyamin, O. I., Kodama, T., Mukhametov, L. M., & Siegel, J. M. (2007). Cortical acetylcholine release is lateralized during asymmetrical slow-wave sleep in northern fur seals. *J Neurosci, 27*(44), 11999–12006. doi: 10.1523/jneurosci.2968-07.2007

Laurent, G., Fournier, J., Hemberger, M., Müller, C., Naumann, R., Ondracek, J. M., ... Yamawaki, T. (2016). Cortical evolution: introduction to the reptilian cortex. In G. Buzsáki & Y. Christen (Eds.), *Micro-, Meso- and Macro-Dynamics of the Brain* (pp. 23–33). Cham: Springer International Publishing.

Lesku, J., Roth, T., Rattenborg, N., Amlaner, C., & Lima, S. (2008). Phylogenetics and the correlates of mammalian sleep: a reappraisal. *Sleep Med Rev, 12*(3), 229–244. doi: 10.1016/j.smrv.2007.10.003

Lesku, J. A., Meyer, L. C. R., Fuller, A., Maloney, S. K., Dell'Omo, G., Vyssotski, A. L., & Rattenborg, N. C. (2011). Ostriches sleep like platypuses. *PLoS ONE, 6*(8), e23203. doi: 10.1371/journal.pone.0023203.g001

Lesku, J. A., Rattenborg, N. C., Valcu, M., Vyssotski, A. L., Kuhn, S., Kuemmeth, F., ... Kempenaers, B. (2012). Adaptive sleep loss in polygynous pectoral sandpipers. *Science, 337*, 1654–1658.

Libourel, P. A., Lee, W. Y., Achin, I., Chung, H., Kim, J., Massot, B., & Rattenborg, N. C. (2023). Nesting chinstrap penguins accrue large quantities of sleep through seconds-long microsleeps. *Science, 382*(6674), 1026–1031. doi: 10.1126/science.adh0771

Liu, S., Liu, Q., Tabuchi, M., & Wu, M. N. (2016). Sleep drive is encoded by neural plastic changes in a dedicated circuit. *Cell, 165*, 1347–1360. doi: 0.1016/j.cell.2016.04.013

Low, P. S., Shank, S. S., Sejnowski, T. J., & Margoliash, D. (2008). Mammalian-like features of sleep structure in zebra finches. *Proc Natl Acad Sci U S A, 105*(26), 9081–9086. doi: 10.1073/pnas.0703452105

Lyamin, O., Pryaslova, J., Lance, V., & Siegel, J. (2005). Animal behaviour: continuous activity in cetaceans after birth. *Nature, 435*(7046), 1177. doi: 10.1038/4351177a

Lyamin, O. I., Kibalnikov, A. S., & Siegel, J. M. (2021). Sleep in ostrich chicks (Struthio camelus). *Sleep, 44*(5), zsaa259. doi:10.1093/sleep/zsaa259

Lyamin, O. I., Kosenko, P. O., Lapierre, J. L., Mukhametov, L. M., & Siegel, J. M. (2008). Fur seals display a strong drive for bilateral slow-wave sleep while on land. *J Neurosci, 28*(48), 12614–12621. doi: 10.1523/jneurosci.2306-08.2008

Lyamin, O. I., Manger, P. R., Ridgway, S. H., Mukhametov, L. M., & Siegel, J. M. (2008). Cetacean sleep: an unusual form of mammalian sleep. *Neurosci Biobehav Rev, 32*(8), 1451–1484. doi: 10.1016/j.neubiorev.2008.05.023

Lyamin, O. I., Mukhametov, L. M., & Siegel, J. M. (2017). Sleep in the northern fur seal. *Curr Opin Neurobiol, 44*, 144–151. doi: 10.1016/j.conb.2017.04.009

Manger, P. R. (2006). An examination of cetacean brain structure with a novel hypothesis correlating thermogenesis to the evolution of a big brain. *Biol Rev, 81*(02), 293. doi: 10.1017/s1464793106007019

Mason, M. F., Norton, M. I., Van Horn, J. D., Wegner, D. M., Grafton, S. T., & Macrae, C. N. (2007). Wandering minds: the default mode network and stimulus-independent thought. *Science, 315*(5810), 393–395.

Meddis, R. (1975). On the function of sleep. *Anim Behav, 23*, 676–691.

Medeiros, S. L. S., Paiva, M. M. M., Lopes, P. H., Blanco, W., Lima, F. D., Oliveira, J. B. C., ... Ribeiro, S. (2021). Cyclic alternation of quiet and active sleep states in the octopus. *iScience, 24*(4), 102223. doi: 10.1016/j.isci.2021.102223

Meisel, D. V., Byrne, R. A., Mather, J. A., & Kuba, M. (2011). Behavioral sleep in *Octopus vulgaris*. *Vie Milieu, 61*(4), 185–190.

Moses, J., Lubin, A., Johnson, L. C., & Naitoh, P. (1977). The rapid eye movement cycle is a sleep-dependent rhythm. *Nature, 265*, 360–361.

Mukhametov, L. M., Lyamin, O. I., Cetyrbok, I. S., Vassilyev, A. A., & Diaz, R. P. (1992). Sleep in an Amazonian manatee, *Trichechus inunguis*. *Experientia, 48*, 417–419.

Nath, R. D., Bedbrook, C. N., Abrams, M. J., Basinger, T., Bois, J. S., Prober, D. A., ... Goentoro, L. (2017). The jellyfish *Cassiopea* exhibits a sleep-like state. *Curr Biol, 27*(19), 2984–2990. doi: 10.1016/j.cub.2017.08.014

Nielsen, T., Montplaisir, J., & Lassonde, M. (1992). Sleep architecture in agenesis of the corpus callosum: laboratory assessment of four cases. *J Sleep Res, 1*, 197–200.

Nyholm, E. S. (1965). Zur O'kologie von Myotis mystacinus (Leisl.) und M. daubentoni (Leisl.) (Chiroptera). *Annales Zoologici Fennici, 2*(2), 77–123.

Oleksenko, A., Mukhametov, L., Polyakova, I., Supin, A., & Kovalzon, V. (1992). Unihemispheric sleep deprivation in bottlenose dolphins. *J Sleep Res, 1*, 40–44.

Ookawa, T., & Gotoh, J. (1965). Electroencephalogram of the chicken recorded from the skull under various conditions. *J Comp Neurol, 124*, 1–14.

Raichle, M. E. (2009). A paradigm shift in functional brain imaging. *J Neurosci, 29*(41), 12729–12734. doi: 10.1523/jneurosci.4366-09.2009

Raichle, M. E., MacLeod, A. M., Snyder, A. Z., Powers, W. J., Gusnard, D. A., & Shulman, G. L. (2001). A default mode of brain function. *Proc Natl Acad Sci USA, 98*(2), 676–682.

Raizen, D. M., Zimmerman, J. E., Maycock, M. H., Ta, U. D., You, Y. J., Sundaram, M. V., & Pack, A. I. (2008). Lethargus is a *Caenorhabditis elegans* sleep-like state. *Nature, 451*(7178), 569–572. doi: 10.1038/nature06535

Rastogi, A., Kumari, Y., Rani, S., & Kumar, V. (2011). Phase inversion of neural activity in the olfactory and visual systems of a night-migratory bird during migration. *Eur J Neurosci, 34*(1), 99–109. doi: 10.1111/j.1460-9568.2011.07737.x

Rattenborg, N. C. (2006a). Do birds sleep in flight? *Naturwissenschaften, 93*(9), 413–425. doi: 10.1007/s00114-006-0120-3

Rattenborg, N. C. (2006b). Evolution of slow-wave sleep and palliopallial connectivity in mammals and birds: a hypothesis. *Brain Res Bull, 69*(1), 20–29. doi: 10.1016/j.brainresbull.2005.11.002

Rattenborg, N. C., Amlaner, C. J., & Lima, S. L. (2000). Behavioral, neurophysiological and evolutionary perspectives on unihemispheric sleep. *Neurosci Biobehav Rev, 24*, 817–842.

Rattenborg, N. C., Lima, S. L., & Amlaner, C. J. (1999). Facultative control of avian unihemispheric sleep under the risk of predation. *Behav Brain Res, 105*(2), 163–172.

Rattenborg, N. C., Mandt, B. H., Obermeyer, W. H., Winsauer, P. J., Huber, R., Wikelski, M., & Benca, R. M. (2004). Migratory sleeplessness in the white-crowned sparrow (*Zonotrichia leucophrys gambelii*). *PLoS Biol, 2*(7), 924–936. doi: 10.1371/journal.pbio.0020212.g001

Rattenborg, N. C., Martinez-Gonzalez, D., Roth, T. C., 2nd, & Pravosudov, V. V. (2011). Hippocampal memory consolidation during sleep: a comparison of mammals and birds. *Biol Rev Camb Philos Soc, 86*(3), 658–691. doi: 10.1111/j.1469-185X.2010.00165.x

Rattenborg, N. C., Voirin, B., Cruz, S. M., Tisdale, R., Dell'Omo, G., Lipp, H. P., … Vyssotski, A. L. (2016). Evidence that birds sleep in mid-flight. *Nat Commun, 7*, 12468. doi: 10.1038/ncomms12468

Rattenborg, N. C., Voirin, B., Vyssotski, A. L., Kays, R. W., Spoelstra, K., Kuemmeth, F., … Wikelski, M. (2008). Sleeping outside the box: electroencephalographic measures of sleep in sloths inhabiting a rainforest. *Biol Lett, 4*, 402–405. doi: 0.1098/rsbl.2008.0203

Reebs, S. G. (2002). Plasticity of diel and circadian activity rhythms in fishes. *Rev Fish Biol Fisheries, 12*(4), 349–371.

Rossler, D. C., Kim, K., De Agro, M., Jordan, A., Galizia, C. G., & Shamble, P. S. (2022). Regularly occurring bouts of retinal movements suggest an REM sleep-like state in jumping spiders. *Proc Natl Acad Sci U S A, 119*(33), e2204754119. doi: 10.1073/pnas.2204754119

Roth, C., Achermann, P., & Borbély, A. (1999). Frequency and state specific hemispheric asymmetries in the human sleep EEG. *Neurosci Lett, 271*, 139–142.

Rusak, B. (1981). Vertebrate behavioral rhythms. In J. Aschoff (Ed.), *Biological Rhythms*. (pp. 183–205). New York: Plenum Press.

Sauer, S., Herrmann, E., & Kaiser, W. (2004). Sleep deprivation in honey bees. *J Sleep Res, 13*, 145–152.

Schmidt, M. H. (2014). The energy allocation function of sleep: a unifying theory of sleep, torpor, and continuous wakefulness. *Neurosci Biobehav Rev, 47*, 122–153. doi: 0.1016/j.neubiorev.2014.08.001

Sekiguchi, Y., Arai, K., & Kohshima, S. (2006). Sleep behaviour: sleep in continuously active dolphins. *Nature, 441*(7096), E9-E10. doi: 10.1038/nature04898

Seugnet, L., Boero, J., Gottschalk, L., Duntley, S. P., & Shaw, P. J. (2006). Identification of a biomarker for sleep drive in flies and humans. *Proc Natl Acad Sci USA, 103*(52), 19913–19918. doi: 10.1073/pnas.0609463104

Seymour, J. E., Carrette, T. J., & Sutherland, P. A. (2004). Do box jellyfish sleep at night? *Med J Aust, 181*(11-12), 707. doi: 10.5694/j.1326-5377.2004.tb06529.x

Shaw, P. J., Cirelli, C., Greenspan, R. J., & Tononi, G. (2000). Correlates of sleep and waking in *Drosophila melanogaster*. *Science, 287*(5459), 1834–1837. doi: 10.1126/science.287.5459.1834

Shein-Idelson, M., Ondracek, J. M., Liaw, H.-P., Reiter, S., & Laurent, G. (2016). Slow waves, sharp waves, ripples and REM in sleeping dragons. *Science, 352*(6285), 590–595.

Siegel, J. M. (2005). Clues to the functions of mammalian sleep. *Nature, 437*(7063), 1264–1271. doi: 10.1038/nature04285

Siegel, J. M. (2008). Do all animals sleep? *Trends Neurosci, 31*(4), 208–213. doi: 10.1016/j.tins.2008.02.001

Siegel, J. M. (2009). Sleep viewed as a state of adaptive inactivity. *Nat Rev Neurosci, 10*, 747–753. doi: 0.1038/nrn2697

Siegel, J. M. (2022). Sleep function: an evolutionary perspective. *Lancet Neurol, 21*(10), 937–946. doi: 10.1016/s1474-4422(22)00210-1

Siegel, J. M., Manger, P. R., Nienhuis, R., Fahringer, H. M., & Pettigrew, J. D. (1998). Monotremes and the evolution of rapid eye movement sleep. *Phil Trans R Soc Lond B, 353*, 1147–1157.

Siegel, J. M., Manger, P. R., Nienhuis, R., Fahringer, H. M., Shalita, T., & Pettigrew, J. D. (1999). Sleep in the platypus. *Neuroscience, 91*(1), 391–400.

Steiger, S. S., Valcu, M., Spoelstra, K., Helm, B., Wikelski, M., & Kempenaers, B. (2013). When the sun never sets: diverse activity rhythms under continuous daylight in free-living arctic-breeding birds. *Proc Biol Sci, 280*(1764), 20131016. doi: 10.1098/rspb.2013.1016

Tamaki, M., Bang, J. W., Watanabe, T., & Sasaki, Y. (2016). Night watch in one brain hemisphere during sleep associated with the first-night effect in humans. *Curr Biol, 26*(9), 1190–1194. doi: 10.1016/j.cub.2016.02.063

Tisdale, R. K., Lesku, J. A., Beckers, G. J. L., & Rattenborg, N. C. (2018). Bird-like propagating brain activity in anesthetized Nile crocodiles. *Sleep, 41*(8), zsy105. doi: 10.1093/sleep/zsy105

Tisdale, R. K., Vyssotski, A. L., Lesku, J. A., & Rattenborg, N. C. (2017). Sleep-related electrophysiology and behavior of tinamous (*Eudromia elegans*): tinamous do not sleep like ostriches. *Brain Behav Evol, 89*(4), 249–261. doi: 10.1159/000475590

Tobler, I. (1983). Effect of forced locomotion on the rest–activity cycle of the cockroach. *Behav Brain Res, 8*, 351–360.

Tobler, I. (2005). Phylogeny of sleep regulation. In M. H. Kryger, T. Roth & W. C. Dement (Eds.), *Principles and Practice of Sleep Medicine* (5th ed., pp. 112–125). St. Louis: Elsevier (Saunders).

van Alphen, B., Yap, M. H., Kirszenblat, L., Kottler, B., & van Swinderen, B. (2013). A dynamic deep sleep stage in Drosophila. *J Neurosci, 33*(16), 6917–6927. doi: 10.1523/JNEUROSCI.0061-13.2013

van der Meij, J., Martinez-Gonzalez, D., Beckers, G. J. L., & Rattenborg, N. C. (2019). Intra-'cortical' activity during avian non-REM and REM sleep: variant and invariant traits between birds and mammals. *Sleep, 42*(2), 1–13. doi: 10.1093/sleep/zsy230

van Hasselt, S. J., Rusche, M., Vyssotski, A. L., Verhulst, S., Rattenborg, N. C., & Meerlo, P. (2019). The European starling (Sturnus vulgaris) shows signs of NREM sleep homeostasis but has very little REM sleep and no REM sleep homeostasis. *Sleep, 43*(6), zsz311. doi: 10.1093/sleep/zsz311

Vanin, S., Bhutani, S., Montelli, S., Menegazzi, P., Green, E. W., Pegoraro, M., … Kyriacou, C. P. (2012). Unexpected features of Drosophila circadian behavioural rhythms under natural conditions. *Nature, 484*, 371–375. doi: 10.1038/nature10991

Vorster, A. P., & Born, J. (2015). Sleep and memory in mammals, birds and invertebrates. *Neurosci Biobehav Rev, 50*, 103–119. doi: 10.1016/j.neubiorev.2014.09.020

Wehr, T. A. (1991). The durations of human melatonin secretion and sleep respond to changes in daylength (photoperiod). *J Clin Endocr Metab, 73*, 1276–1280.

Wehr, T. A. (1992). A brain-warming function for REM sleep. *Neurosci Biochem Rev, 16*, 379–397.

Xu, Y., Padiath, Q. S., Shapiro, R. E., Jones, C. R., Wu, S. C., Saigoh, N., . . . Fu, Y.-H. (2005). Functional consequences of a CKIδ mutation causing familial advanced sleep phase syndrome. *Nature, 434*, 640–644.

Zepelin, H., & Rechtschaffen, A. (1974). Mammalian sleep, longevity, and energy metabolism. *Brain Behav Evol, 10*, 425–470.

Zepelin, H., Siegel, J. M., & Tobler, I. (2005). Mammalian sleep. In M. H. Kryger, T. Roth & W. C. Dement (Eds.), *Principles and Practice of Sleep Medicine* (4th ed., pp. 91–100). St. Louis: Elsevier.

Zimmerman, J. E., Naidoo, N., Raizen, D. M., & Pack, A. I. (2008). Conservation of sleep: insights from non-mammalian model systems. *Trends Neurosci, 31*(7), 371–376. doi: 10.1016/j.tins.2008.05.001

Zwaka, H., Bartels, R., Gora, J., Franck, V., Culo, A., Gotsch, M., & Menzel, R. (2015). Context odor presentation during sleep enhances memory in honeybees. *Curr Biol, 25*(21), 2869–2874. doi: 10.1016/j.cub.2015.09.069

C.

Physiological Mechanisms

CHAPTER 8

Suprachiasmatic Nuclei, Sleep, and Aging

8.1 OVERVIEW

This chapter reviews the role of the principal circadian pacemaker in mammals, the suprachiasmatic nuclei (SCN), in regulating circadian rhythms and sleep. It reviews evidence that the SCN is an autonomous oscillator and a system pacemaker. It also reviews the mechanisms by which the SCN is entrained by lighting cycles and the routes by which its output affects sleep. It discusses the effects of SCN ablations on the temporal distribution of sleep, sleep homeostasis, and the total amount of sleep within a day.

This chapter then reviews the hypothesis that degenerative changes in the SCN and reductions in its rhythm amplitude contribute to changes in sleep patterns during aging. Finally, it reviews evidence related to the surprising finding that older people are less affected by sleep loss than younger people. Factors that may be involved are discussed, including the impact of the circadian phase of testing, aging effects on the amplitude of circadian rhythms, and the design of studies comparing younger and older participants.

8.2 Physiological mechanisms generating daily rhythms

8.2.1 Introduction

Imagine living in a perpetual twilight state, a condition in which you cannot sustain full wakefulness and are rarely fully asleep and at rest. Rather, your state fluctuates irregularly moment-to-moment between brief wakefulness and fitful, unsatisfying sleep. This condition is difficult for most of us to imagine, but it appeared to be the state of a woman with damage to a critical part of her hypothalamus that controls daily rhythms (Cohen & Albers, 1991) and of animals that had undergone experimental destruction of the same brain region. As discussed in Section 8.3.1, these findings hint at one of the important functions served by circadian modulation of sleep and wake states in people.

8.2.2 Suprachiasmatic nuclei as a rhythm generator

Almost all aspects of our normal physiology and behavior, responsiveness to drugs, and many clinical conditions show daily rhythms, a few of which are illustrated in **Figure 8.1**. So, it might seem improbable that a single brain structure would be responsible for organizing the many systems that control these diverse functions.

Yet, early experimental work pointed to the idea that the mammalian circadian system is controlled by a single central clock, which serves as its pacemaker (i.e., the endogenous timer that controls its overall periodicity). The search for this pacemaker was guided by the fact that light is the principal zeitgeber for circadian rhythms (see Chapter 3), so the pacemaker must have access to information about daily lighting cycles. It must also be able to regulate many different downstream effector systems (i.e., neural, endocrine, and other mechanisms that directly control behavior and physiology).

The model in **Figure 8.2** illustrates the essential components of a circadian system that can perform these functions. These include a central, independently rhythmic pacemaker; an entrainment pathway by which light can affect the pacemaker; and output pathways that allow the pacemaker to influence an array of effector systems that control physiological and behavioral processes, including those that regulate sleep.

Since the work of Curt Richter in the early part of the 20th century (Chapter 3), it was clear that light could affect the central pacemaker in mammals only via a retinal route (see, e.g., Richter, 1971).[1] Knowledge of the essential role

[1] This statement is not true of other species, including other vertebrates, whose circadian clock mechanisms are often directly light sensitive as well as receiving light input indirectly via other structures including the retina.

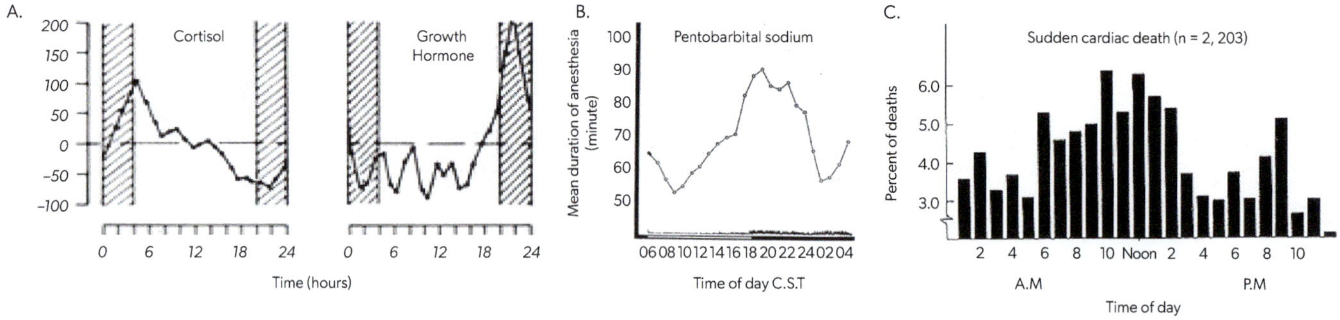

Figure 8.1 **A.** Two examples of daily hormone rhythms in people, showing the amplitude of each expressed as percent deviations from its 24 h mean (= 0). The hatched areas represent sleep phases, and white areas are waking time. Note the difference in timing of peak and trough levels between cortisol and growth hormone. Reprinted with permission from Aschoff, J. (1978) Circadiane Rhythmen im endocrinen System. *Klin Wochenschr* 56:425–435. © Springer:Nature (1978). doi: 10.1007/BF01477056. **B.** The duration of anesthesia induced in rats that were given a fixed dose of an anesthetic (pentobarbital sodium) at different times of day. Data are plotted as 3 h moving averages. Average sleeping times ranged from as little as 53 min to as much as 90 min depending on daily phase. A recording of the colony activity level is shown at the bottom of the record, above the white and black bars, indicating the colony's light-dark cycle. Reprinted with permission of John Wiley & Sons from Scheving, L.E. et al. (1968) A circadian susceptibility rhythm in rats to pentobarbital sodium. *Anat Rec* 160: 741–749. © John Wiley and Sons (1968). Permission conveyed through Copyright Clearance Center, Inc. doi: 10.1002/ar.1091600409. **C.** Daily population rhythms of the number of sudden cardiac deaths plotted against the time of day at which they occurred. Fatal heart attacks peaked in frequency during the morning and early afternoon, with a relatively protected phase during the night. Reprinted with permission from Muller, J.E. et al. (1987) Circadian variation in the frequency of sudden cardiac death. *Circulation* 75:131–138, 1987, © Wolters Kluwer Health (P&E) Limited (1987), American Heart Association. Reprinted with permission of the Licensor through PLSclear. doi: 10.1161/01.cir.75.1.131.

played by retinal photoreception guided the hunt for the circadian pacemaker in mammals, which involved tracing retinal projections into the brain and assessing the involvement of their known targets in circadian regulation. Destruction of several retinal projections or their termination zones in the brains of rodents did not eliminate circadian rhythm entrainment, although it did modify aspects of the entrained pattern (Moore & Eichler, 1972; Rusak, 1977a; Stephan & Zucker, 1972b). Anatomical studies in rats, however, identified a previously controversial retinal projection that terminated in the hypothalamus, called the retinohypothalamic tract (RHT) (Hendrickson et al., 1972; Moore & Lenn, 1972). The RHT innervates a tiny structure that lies directly above the optic chiasm, the suprachiasmatic nuclei (SCN) (**Figures 8.3**). The presence of the RHT projection has since been confirmed in many species, including in humans using a postmortem, tract-tracing method (Dai et al., 1998).

Ablation of the SCN in rats and hamsters caused the loss of normal nocturnality under a lighting cycle, confirming its role as a target of light information needed to entrain the circadian system. But its destruction also eliminated circadian rhythms, resulting in arrhythmic patterns of behavior and physiology, consistent with the loss of a circadian pacemaker (Moore & Eichler, 1972; Rusak, 1977b; Stephan & Zucker, 1972a; Witte et al., 1998) (**Figure 8.4**).

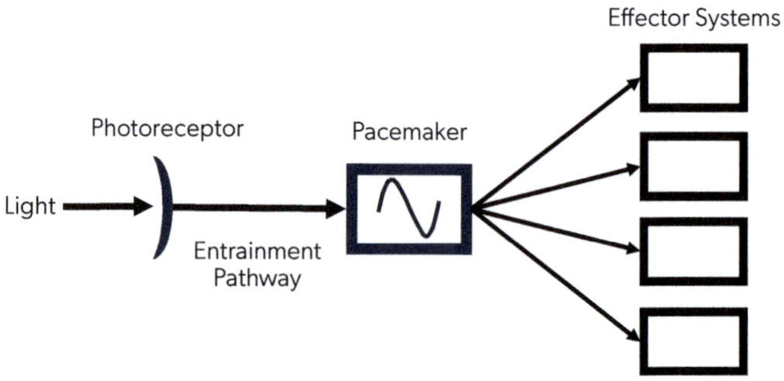

Figure 8.2 This simplified model illustrates the essential elements of a circadian system in mammals. There is a central pacemaker that is intrinsically rhythmic (indicated by the sine wave); a photoreceptor system in the retina that responds to daily light-dark signals; an entrainment pathway that conveys this photic information to the pacemaker; and various outputs from the pacemaker that influence the function of many effector systems. These effectors produce changes in the physiology and behavior of the organism. They include other parts of the nervous system (and the motor, sensory, and other functions they regulate), the endocrine system, and components of the immune system.

Research over the following decades developed a comprehensive picture of the anatomy, physiology, and function of the SCN as a pacemaker for the mammalian circadian system (Meijer & Rietveld, 1989; Rusak & Zucker, 1979). This tiny, paired nucleus, comprising only ~16,000–20,000 neurons in

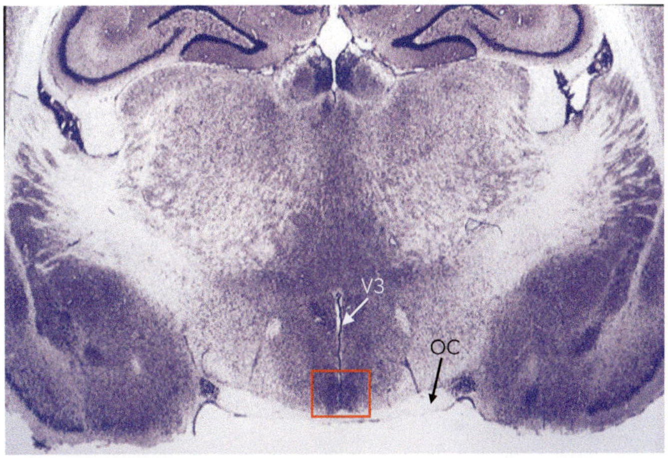

Figure 8.3 A coronal section at the level of the caudal optic chiasm (OC) of the brain of a golden hamster (*Mesocricetus auratus*), stained with cresyl violet to show cell bodies. The optic chiasm appears at the bottom of the section as a thick white horizontal band, beginning to form the optic tracts. Embedded in the chiasm at the midline are the darkly staining suprachiasmatic nuclei (red box) surrounding the base of the third ventricle (V3). Adapted with permission from Rusak, B. (1977) The role of the suprachiasmatic nuclei in the generation of circadian rhythms in the golden hamster, *Mesocricetus auratus*. *J Comp Physiol A* 118: 145–164. © Springer:Nature (1977). doi: 10.1007/BF00611819.

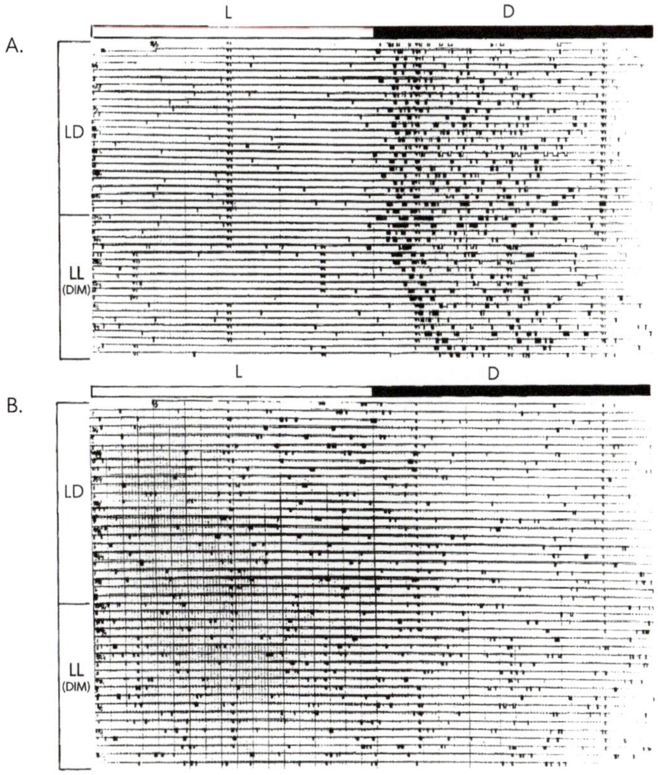

Figure 8.4 Records of contacts with a drinking tube (probably representing both drinking and activities like chewing) in two golden hamsters (*Mesocricetus auratus*). **A.** The behavior of an intact hamster in a light (L)–dark (D) cycle and in constant very dim light (LL Dim), as indicated on the left of the record. Behavior was strongly nocturnal in a LD cycle and free-ran with a period slightly longer than 24 h in constant dim light. **B.** A similar record for a hamster with a lesion of the suprachiasmatic nuclei, showing a lack of normal nocturnality in an LD cycle, and the absence of a free-running rhythm in constant conditions. (The appearance of vertical lines in the charts is an artefact of channel numbers on the paper used in the electromechanical recorders that generated these records in the days before laboratory computers.) Adapted with permission from Rusak, B. (1977) The role of the suprachiasmatic nuclei in the generation of circadian rhythms in the golden hamster, *Mesocricetus auratus*. *J Comp Physiol A* 118: 145–164. © Springer:Nature (1977). doi: 10.1007/BF00611819.

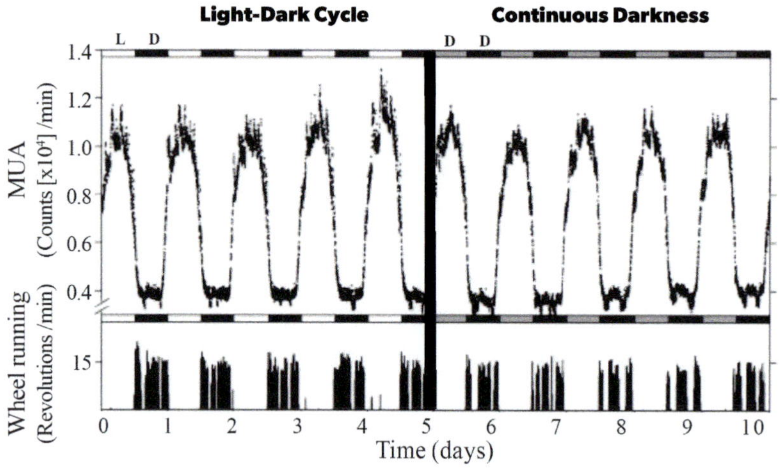

Figure 8.5 Daily suprachiasmatic nucleus (SCN) neuronal firing rhythms (top) and activity rhythms (bottom) recorded simultaneously from mice. The firing-rate rhythm was acquired using an electrode implanted into the SCN, which recorded from an unknown number of neurons simultaneously [a multiple-unit activity (MUA) recording]. under a light–dark cycle (LD; left side) for 5 days and in continuous darkness (DD; right side) for 5 days, as indicated at the top. The nocturnal wheel-running rhythm under the LD cycle continued with a period near 24 h in DD. The SCN firing-rate rhythm peaked during the daily L phase (white) in LD and in the corresponding subjective day phase (light gray) under DD. It persisted in constant conditions with a robust rhythm that was only slightly reduced in amplitude relative to the LD condition. Adapted with permission of Dr. Takahiro Nakamura et al. and the Society for Neuroscience from Nakamura, T.J. et al., (2011) Age-related decline in circadian output. *J Neurosci* 31:10201–05. © The Authors (2011). doi: 10.1523/JNEUROSCI.0451-11.2011.

rodents (Moore et al., 2002; van den Pol, 1980), plays the three distinct roles required of a pacemaker: It generates an intrinsic circadian rhythm, it is entrained by environmental lighting cycles, and it imposes its periodicity on other physiological systems; see **Figure 8.2**.

Molecular mechanisms in the cells of the SCN (See **Box 8.1** and **Figure 8.8**) generate a circadian rhythm that is approximately 24 h in length. The resulting cellular rhythmicity is detectable in intact animals in vivo as a daily rhythm of neuronal firing rates in both light–dark cycles and continuous darkness (Inouye & Kawamura, 1979; Nakamura et al., 2011) (**Figure 8.5**). But this finding does not prove that the rhythmicity is generated by the SCN; many structures in the brain show daily rhythms in an intact animal. These rhythms could be intrinsic to these structures or could be imposed on them by clocks elsewhere in the animal.

The critical evidence that the SCN functions as an intrinsically rhythmic oscillator is that it continues to generate persistent circadian rhythms of neural firing (and rhythms of neuropeptide secretion) even when cultured in vitro, in the absence of any rhythmic external signals, and without contact with other tissues (Bos & Mirmiran, 1990; Gillette, 1987; Green & Gillette, 1982; Groos & Hendriks, 1982; Prosser & Gillette, 1989; Yamazaki et al., 2000) (**Figure 8.6**).

Within the SCN, the capacity to express sustained circadian rhythmicity is the product of an intracellular mechanism rather than being an emergent property of a network of neurons. Individual neurons in explanted SCN tissues in vitro can express independent circadian firing-rate rhythms with different periods, which therefore run out of phase with each other (Welsh et al., 1995) (**Figure 8.7**). The rhythm-generating mechanism within single SCN cells involves a set of clock genes that interact to generate a ~24 h molecular rhythm that is self-sustaining. See **Box 8.1** and **Figure 8.8** for a summary of the molecular mechanisms that have been shown to underlie circadian rhythm generation in the mammalian SCN.

Although the timekeeping machinery is intracellular, network interactions among cells are important for coordinating and stabilizing the expression of a common circadian period across the population of SCN neurons. They are synchronized in vivo through direct electrical interactions as well as through the release of neurotransmitters and neuropeptides that are critical to the production of coherent circadian rhythms from the entire nucleus (Aton & Herzog, 2005; Colwell, 2000; Long et al., 2004; Piggins & Cutler, 2003; Yamaguchi et al., 2003).

A surprising feature of network connections among SCN cells emerged following a genetic ablation that prevented individual neurons from generating circadian rhythms in vitro. Despite the lack of rhythmicity in isolated neurons, when coupling among cells was allowed, noisy circadian rhythms emerged in the output of the neuronal population (Ko et al., 2010). Thus, network interactions in an intact SCN not only synchronize the independent cycles of individual neurons into a common periodicity but also promote oscillation at the population level, even when individual neurons cannot generate their own independent rhythms.

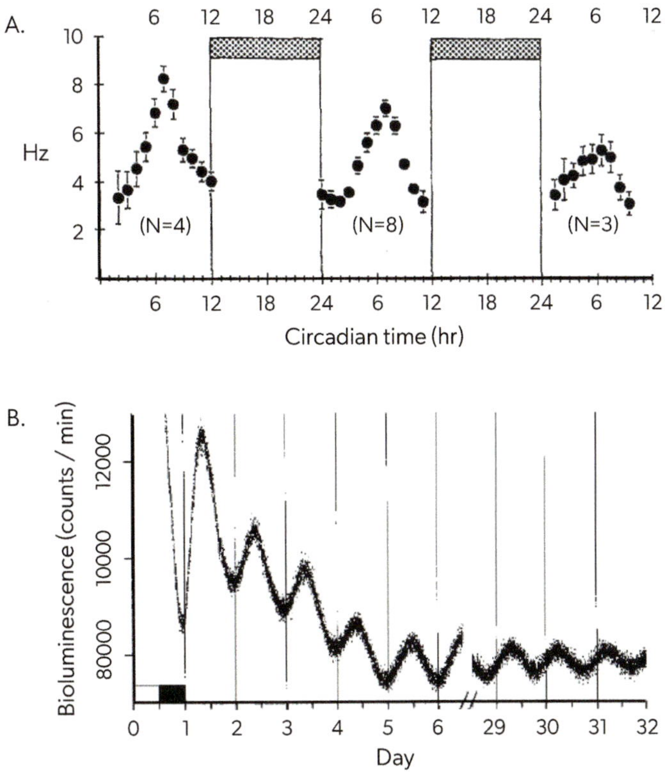

Figure 8.6 **A.** Average multiple-unit neuronal firing rates (spikes/sec or Hz; Y axis) recorded from a rat suprachiasmatic nucleus (SCN) in an in vitro brain slice preparation. The SCN tissue was bathed in artificial cerebrospinal fluid that kept it alive in vitro for several days. Recordings were made only during the time corresponding to the light phase of the light-dark cycle (dark phases shown as hatched bars at the top) to which the rat had been exposed before it was killed and the SCN explant was prepared. The typical firing-rate peak seen in vivo during the daily light phase or subjective day (see **Figure 8.5**) was preserved for several days in the isolated SCN slice preparation in the absence of any external cycle. Reprinted with permission of the Society for Neuroscience from Prosser, R.A. & Gillette, M.U. (1989) The mammalian circadian clock in the suprachiasmatic nuclei is reset in vitro by cyclic adenosine monophosphate (cAMP). *J Neurosci* 9:1073–1081, 1989. © Society for Neuroscience (1989). doi: 10.1523/JNEUROSCI.09-03-01073.1989. **B.** Activity of a cultured rat SCN explant in vitro measured by the bioluminescence generated using a reporter gene (luciferase) linked to the promoter of a circadian clock gene (*Per1*). Despite the gradual reduction in rhythm amplitude over the early days of the study, the circadian cycle persisted for at least 32 days, when the study ended. (Note the gap in the record between day 6 and day 29 of the study.) The inset at the bottom of the first column shows the light-dark cycle to which the rat had been exposed before it was killed and the explant was prepared. Reprinted with permission of the AAAS from Yamazaki, S. et al. (2000) Resetting central and peripheral circadian oscillators in transgenic rats. *Science* 288:682–685. © American Association for the Advancement of Science (2000); permission conveyed through Copyright Clearance Center, Inc. doi: 10.1126/science.288.5466.682.

8.2.3 SCN pacemaker function

The intrinsic, independent rhythmicity of the SCN shows that it is a self-sustaining circadian oscillator. To demonstrate that it is the oscillator serving as the pacemaker for circadian rhythms in physiology and behavior, however, requires evidence that it controls the periodicity of these overt rhythms. The elimination of most circadian rhythms by destruction of the SCN showed that these rhythms cannot be expressed without the SCN. But loss of a central pacemaker is only one potential interpretation of those findings.

A study that supported a pacemaker interpretation used knife cuts around the SCN to form an island of hypothalamic tissue that was separated from the rest of the brain. It allowed neuronal firing-rate rhythms to persist in the SCN and its surrounding island, but brain regions outside the knife cuts lost their circadian firing-rate rhythms (Inouye & Kawamura, 1979). These effects of lesions and knife cuts strengthened the interpretation of a pacemaker function for the SCN, but other lines of evidence were needed to confirm its role.[2]

[2] This is generally true of ablation studies. When an experimenter ablates a brain structure and observes the behavior or physiology of an animal, it is only possible to describe the deficits that occur or capacities that remain in the absence of that structure. We cannot infer directly what the normal function of the ablated structure is. Ablation studies allow us to generate testable hypotheses about the structure's role, but studies using other methods are necessary to demonstrate its normal function.

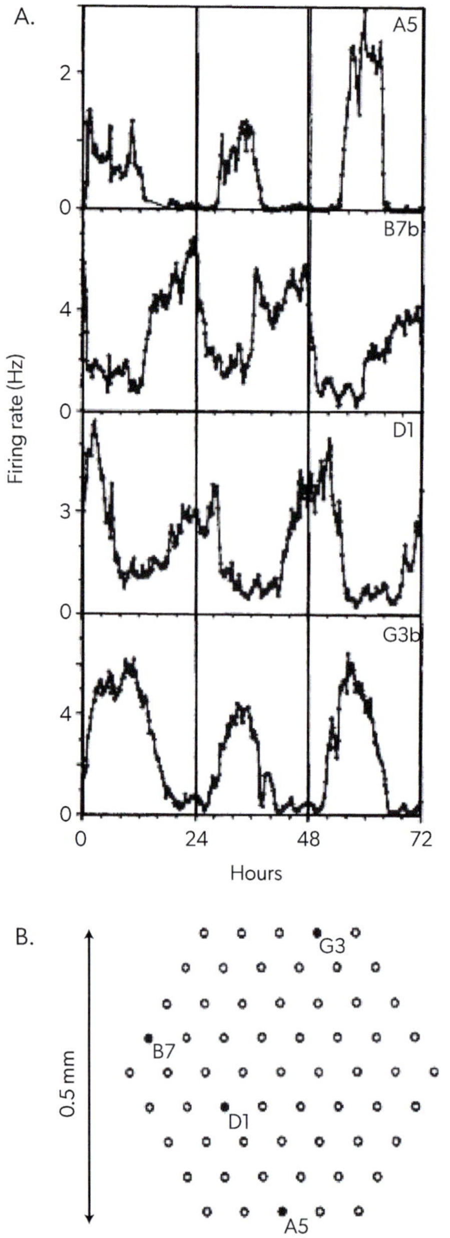

Figure 8.7 **A.** The firing-rates (Y axis) of four individual neurons in the rat suprachiasmatic nucleus (SCN) that were recorded from an isolated in vitro culture preparation. The SCN was explanted onto a surface consisting of an array of 61 miniature electrode contacts, shown in **B**, with the location of each neuron that was recorded successfully over a 72 h period (X axis) identified with its number (A5, B7, D1 & G3). The cultured SCN tissue grew in contact with the surface electrodes, which were sampled to identify individual neurons that were sufficiently close to the electrodes to generate good electrical signals. Each of the illustrated neurons showed a robust circadian, firing-rate rhythm, but the periods and phases of the expressed rhythms differed among neurons. Reprinted with permission of Elsevier, Ltd. from Welsh, D.K. et al. Individual neurons dissociated from rat suprachiasmatic nucleus express independently phased circadian firing rhythms. *Neuron* 14:697–706; © Elsevier (1995). doi: 10.1016/0896-6273(95)90214-7.

Evidence supporting a pacemaker function for the SCN came from a series of studies involving transplantation of SCN tissue. Early SCN transplantation studies demonstrated a striking example of functional recovery following neural transplantation. An SCN derived from a fetal brain was implanted into the brain of an adult rodent that was arrhythmic after an SCN lesion; the transplant restored behavioral circadian rhythms (Sawaki et al., 1984; Silver et al., 1996). This finding further strengthened the case for the SCN as the pacemaker, but it was still subject to other interpretations. For example, the transplanted SCN might restore a missing chemical that is necessary for another structure to generate circadian rhythmicity. Other evidence was needed to show that the transplanted SCN was itself the pacemaker driving the restored rhythm.

The most convincing evidence for the SCN functioning as a pacemaker came from a study involving cross-transplantation of SCN tissue between genetic mutant and wild-type hamsters. Wild-type hamsters express circadian rhythms with a period that is very close to 24 h. Those with a mutation in the *tau* gene have abnormally short circadian rhythms: ~20 h in the homozygote (i.e., the mutation occurs in both paired alleles of the *tau* gene), and ~22 h in the heterozygote (one mutated and one wild-type allele) (Ralph & Menaker, 1988).

When the SCN was ablated in hamsters with either 20 h or 24 h rhythms, both sets of animals lost their ability to generate circadian activity rhythms. However, when a heterozygous *tau* mutant (~22 h) hamster without an SCN received an SCN from a wild-type hamster, the circadian rhythm that emerged showed a period near the wild-type value of 24 h. Conversely, when an SCN-ablated, wild-type hamster received an SCN from a homozygous *tau* mutant (~20 h) hamster, it developed a short-period circadian rhythm (Ralph et al., 1990) (**Figure 8.9**). Even though the rest of the cells in the recipient animal's brain and body were genetically different, it was the genotype of the transplanted SCN that controlled the circadian periodicity of the animal's behavior. The capacity to transfer period, the defining characteristic of a circadian oscillator, by transplanting only the SCN is a convincing demonstration of its role as a pacemaker for the circadian system.

Transplantation of a fetal SCN into the brain of an SCN-ablated hamster restored circadian rhythmicity but not the ability to entrain to lighting cycles. The lack of entrainment likely reflects the inability of retinal ganglion cells to form normal, functional connections with the transplanted SCN. In animals with an intact SCN, cutting the optic nerves innervating it allowed the transected retinal ganglion cell axons to grow back into the native SCN, but they did not form appropriate synaptic connections and could not support entrainment by light (Johnson et al., 1988). It is likely that if any transplanted fetal SCNs were innervated by native retinal ganglion cells, they would similarly fail to form functional connections.

BOX 8.1 Clock Genes Involved in Circadian Rhythm Generation

The molecular mechanisms responsible for circadian rhythm generation in the mammalian SCN involve a set of core genes that participate in nested positive and negative feedback loops of mRNA expression (transcription from DNA to mRNA in the nucleus), protein synthesis (translation by mRNA on ribosomes in the cytoplasm), and transport and metabolism of the proteins. The key elements in mammals are a pair of genes (*clock* and *bmal1*, or related genes), whose protein products promote the expression of another pair of genes (members of the *period* (*per*) and *cryptochrome (cry)* gene families) (**Figure 8.8 A**).

The protein products of *per* and *cry* genes (PER/CRY) gradually accumulate to high levels in the cytoplasm, dimerize (link together), and then enter the nucleus where they inhibit the further promotion of *per/cry* transcription by *clock* and *bmal1*. As a result, PER/CRY protein levels gradually decline until they reach a level low enough to release the positive transcription promoters (*clock/bmal1*) from their inhibition, allowing the cycle to begin again.

This transcription/translation feedback loop (TTFL) constitutes one of three interacting regulatory loops that together form the key elements of the intracellular mammalian circadian clock (**Figure 8.8 B**). Because of the time constants involved in the expression, accumulation, and degradation of these gene products, and the indirect, negative feedback relations among them, this molecular machinery generates a continuous, self-sustaining intracellular cycle with a ~24 h period (Zhang & Kay, 2010).

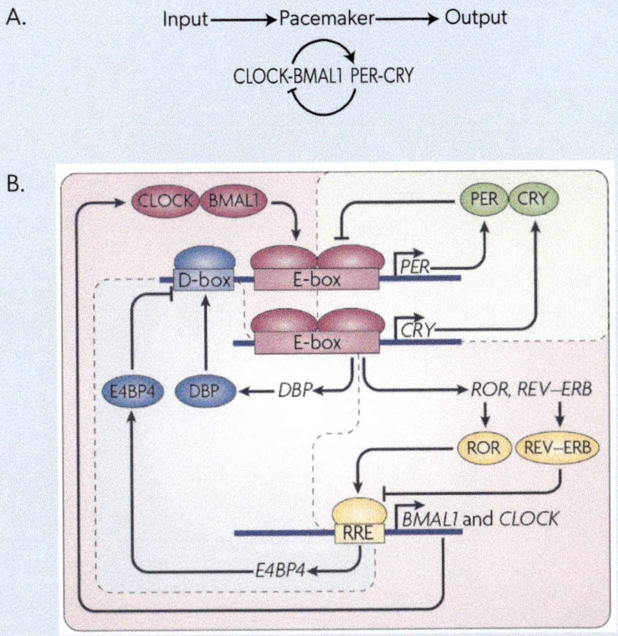

Figure 8.8 **A.** A simple model of the core loop of a molecular circadian clock in a mammalian cell that receives environmental inputs and serves as a pacemaker for a variety of rhythms through its outputs. The core pacemaker consists of a positive limb (→) including two genes coding for proteins (CLOCK-BMAL1) that promote transcription of mRNAs coding for two other proteins (PER and CRY). The negative limb of this cycle (--|) involves the proteins PER-CRY, which act to inhibit the transcription of CLOCK/BMAL1. **B.** A more detailed molecular model of the mechanism responsible for generating circadian rhythms in SCN neurons and other mammalian cells. The mechanism consists of three interlocking loops of gene expression and feedback. The core loop (summarized in **A**) consists of the transcription of mRNAs from the genes *bmal1* and *clock* (bottom) which produce the corresponding proteins BMAL1 and CLOCK (top, purple). These proteins bind to an E-box element in the promoters of the genes *per* and *cry*, which activates the production of their protein products (PER and CRY, green). These proteins accumulate in the cytoplasm until they enter the nucleus where they inhibit the further activation of their own genes by CLOCK and BMAL1, thereby reducing further production of PER and CRY. The gradual fall in levels of PER and CRY disinhibits the promotion of their transcription by CLOCK and BMAL1 and permits the cycle to restart. In conjunction with the other interlocking feedback loops illustrated; i.e., the DBP loop (blue) and the REV-ERB loop (yellow), this feedback process generates a self-sustaining cycle of gene transcription and RNA translation that oscillates with a near-24 h period. Reprinted with permission from Zhang, E.E. & Kay, S.A. (2010) Clocks not winding down: unravelling circadian networks. *Nat Rev Mol Cell Biol* 11:764–776. © Springer:Nature (2010). doi: 10.1038/nrm2995.

BOX 8.1 Continued

Although these genes are the canonical components (i.e., those recognized as standard) of the intracellular clock, there is also evidence that different members of gene families can substitute for each other to varying degrees. Thus, loss of any one molecular component may not abolish rhythmicity, with the exception that *bmal1* may be an essential clock component (McDearmon et al., 2006). The cyclicity of the core clock genes has also been shown to be modulated by an increasingly complex network of other molecular mechanisms as well as by post-translational changes in some of the proteins involved (Buhr & Takahashi, 2013; Zhang & Kay, 2010).

While the core genes in this system are usually referred to as "clock genes" because of their central roles in circadian rhythm generation, they likely have other regulatory effects on cell physiology. Thus, manipulations of these genes or their products could alter aspects of physiology either because of their roles as core components of the circadian clock machinery or because some are also involved in promoting gene transcription related to non-circadian mechanisms (von Schantz, 2008).

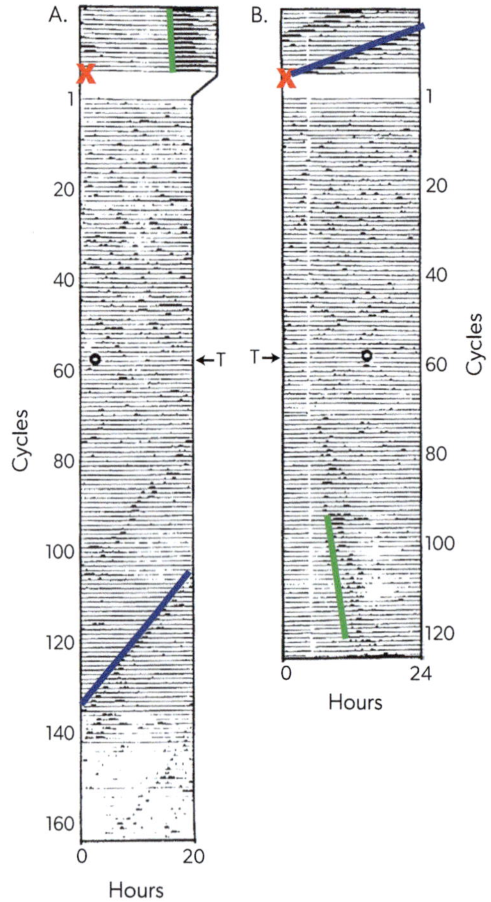

Figure 8.9 Effects of transplantation of fetal suprachiasmatic nucleus (SCN) tissue in hamsters that had SCN ablations. The top of each column shows 24 h periods of activity recording of individual golden hamsters with successive days plotted from top to bottom. **A.** The running-wheel activity record of a wild-type hamster in constant darkness showed a robust circadian rhythm with a period slightly longer than 24 h (green line). The hamster underwent surgery to ablate its SCN (SCNx; red X) and was returned to its running-wheel cage after recovery. From day 1 until just before day 60 it showed the typical disruption of circadian rhythmicity that follows SCN destruction. At that time, it underwent a second surgery to transplant fetal SCN tissue into its brain (T, black circle). The fetal tissue was derived from a homozygous mutant hamster (*tau-/-*) that would express a ~20 h rhythm if it were tested as an adult. After about one week, the recipient hamster began to express a free-running circadian rhythm with a period of ~19.5 h (note that the time base of the display changed from 24 to 20 h on day 1 to make it easier to see the near-20 h rhythm; blue line). **B.** The reciprocal study was conducted with a heterozygous mutant hamster (*tau+/-*) that showed a robust ~21.7 h rhythm (blue line) when it was intact, became arrhythmic after SCN ablation (red X), and then received a fetal SCN transplant from a wild-type hamster (T, black circle). After ~10 days, a free-running circadian rhythm emerged, but in this case the *tau*-mutant hamster expressed a wild-type period of 24.2 h (green line) after receiving the wild-type SCN. Adapted with permission of Dr. Martin Ralph and AAAS from Ralph, M.R. et al. (1990) Transplanted suprachiasmatic nucleus determines circadian period. *Science* 523:117–120. © American Association for the Advancement of Science (1990); permission conveyed through Copyright Clearance Center, Inc. doi: 10.1126/science.2305266.

8.2.4 Mechanisms of entrainment

The identification of the RHT projection to the SCN (Hendrickson et al., 1972; Moore & Lenn, 1972) led to the initial ablation studies that demonstrated the role of the SCN in the expression of circadian rhythms. In rodents, the RHT consists of fibers rising from the optic chiasm directly into the overlying SCN, so it is difficult to selectively lesion the RHT without also destroying much of the SCN and therefore disrupting circadian rhythmicity. The resulting loss of normally entrained rhythms is ambiguous with respect to the entrainment role of the RHT because, without an SCN, there is no surviving rhythm to be entrained.

In one study, however, horizontal knife cuts were used successfully in hamsters to transect the RHT while preserving much of the SCN intact. As a result, circadian rhythms were preserved but, as indicated above, the hamsters could not entrain to lighting cycles. They generated free-running rhythms in light–dark cycles, as if their SCNs were effectively in constant darkness because of the loss of RHT input. These results confirmed that the RHT plays an essential role in photic entrainment of the circadian pacemaker (Johnson et al., 1988).

It was reasonable to assume that the retinal ganglion cells forming the RHT receive light information from the classical rod and cone photoreceptors in the retina that serve all known visual functions in mammals. However, this assumption was challenged by evidence that mice with genetic defects that result in a gradual loss of most or all photoreceptors were still able to entrain to light–dark cycles, in some cases without even an increase in the threshold intensity needed for entrainment (Foster et al., 1991).

The solution to the puzzle of how mammals lacking rod and cone photoreceptors in their retinas could still entrain to retinal illumination involved the identification of a novel photopigment in the mammalian retina, melanopsin (also called Opn4) (Provencio et al., 2000). There are several other opsins found in the retinas of mammals and other vertebrates, all of which are most sensitive to short wavelength light in the blue and violet parts of the spectrum. They serve functions related to detecting light intensity, as opposed to the familiar visual functions related to detecting form, color, and movement, served by rods and cones (Guido et al., 2022; Hannibal, 2021).

Unlike classical photopigments, melanopsin is not found in photoreceptors in the outer nuclear layer of the retina, but in a specialized class of retinal ganglion cells that were not previously known to be directly photoreceptive. Like all retinal ganglion cells, the axons of these photosensitive cells project into the brain through the optic nerves, but they project selectively to a few targets, including reaching the SCN via the RHT (Hannibal et al., 2002; Hattar et al., 2002) (**Figure 8.10**). These ganglion cells are very large and have broad receptive fields, which would not be useful for performing ordinary visual functions. They are appropriate, however, for gathering information about the general level of illumination, which is highly relevant for circadian rhythm entrainment. Intrinsically photoreceptive, melanopsin-containing retinal ganglion cells could therefore provide entrainment-related light information to the SCN even in the absence of classical rod and cone photoreceptors.

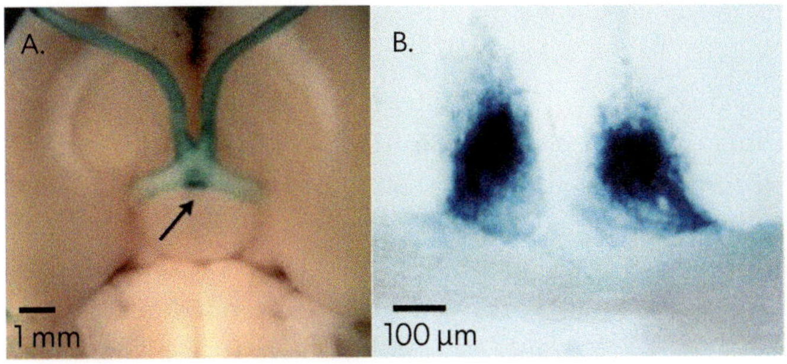

Figure 8.10 Melanopsin-containing retinal ganglion cells project to the suprachiasmatic nuclei (SCN) in the mouse. By genetically linking a reporter gene to the melanopsin gene, melanopsin-containing cells and their projections were visualized and are shown stained blue in these images. **A.** A view of the ventral surface of a mouse brain showing the blue-stained optic nerves meeting in the optic chiasm and the dark blue color of the SCN seen through the caudal edge of the chiasm (arrow). **B.** A cross-section of the mouse hypothalamus at the caudal edge of the chiasm showing the dark blue staining of the SCN because of its strong innervation by melanopsin-containing retinal ganglion cells. Adapted with permission of of Dr. Samer Hattar and AAAS from Hattar, S. et al. (2002) Melanopsin-containing retinal ganglion cells: architecture, projections, and intrinsic photosensitivity. *Science* 295:1065–1070. © American Association for the Advancement of Science (2002); permission conveyed through Copyright Clearance Center, Inc. doi: 10.1126/science.1069609.

Eliminating melanopsin production by knocking out the melanopsin gene, however, did not completely eliminate circadian rhythm responses to light (Ruby et al., 2002). This finding was explained by the fact that, like other retinal ganglion cells, melanopsin-containing cells also receive input from rod and cone photoreceptors (Belenky et al., 2003). While these ganglion cells were no longer directly photoreceptive in the absence of melanopsin, they still received light information from rod and cone photoreceptors, which they conveyed via the RHT. When melanopsin was eliminated in mice that also lacked classical photoreceptors, however, entrainment was eliminated (Hattar et al., 2003; Panda et al., 2003).

Thus, entrainment in mammals depends on the convergence of light information from rod/cone photoreception and from melanopsin-mediated photoreception onto specialized ganglion cells that form the RHT projection to the SCN. This system is present in both sighted mammals and in subterranean mammals that are functionally blind with respect to ordinary vision. In these species, melanopsin-containing ganglion cells form almost all of the optic nerve, while in sighted species they represent only ~1% of the optic nerve; for a review, see Hannibal, 2021.

Melanopsin-containing ganglion cells convey light information for circadian entrainment and for other functions related to global illumination. These are considered "photic" functions that are separate from classical visual functions. Because melanopsin is most sensitive to the short-wavelength (blue) part of the spectrum (Berson et al., 2002; Lucas et al., 2014), light in this wavelength range is most effective in shifting circadian rhythms and suppressing melatonin production, while longer wavelength light is less effective (Lockley et al., 2003).

Photic functions include pupillary constriction in response to increasing light levels, which is mediated by projections from melanopsin-containing ganglion cells to brain regions other than the SCN (Hattar et al., 2003). The joint role of melanopsin-containing cells in both photic reflexes and circadian rhythm entrainment is reinforced by evidence that the strength of pupillary constriction in response to light is correlated with a function related to the circadian system, namely, the timing of sleep onset. Young adults with the strongest pupillary constriction responses to light have the most delayed sleep timing (van der Meijden et al., 2016). These results imply that individuals with a more light-sensitive melanopsin system generate both stronger pupillary reflexes and more robust circadian delays in response to light exposure in the evening (the delay zone of the phase response curve; see **Figures 3.3** and **3.4**).

Melanopsin is also involved in mediating photic effects on sleepiness. When a nocturnal rodent (e.g., a mouse) is exposed to bright light, it typically responds by falling asleep, regardless of time of day, while darkness at night tends to promote waking. These responses are mediated by melanopsin-containing ganglion cells (Altimus et al., 2008; Lupi et al., 2008) but with involvement of classical photoreceptors; for a review, see Muindi et al., 2014.

In people, nighttime light exposure has the opposite effect: it increases arousal (Campbell et al., 1993; Chang et al., 2013). Evening light exposure would promote this arousing effect as well as generating phase delays of the circadian system, thereby contributing to delaying the time of sleep onset. The dual effects of enhanced delay shifts and arousal mediated by the same mechanism can account for why people with a more light-sensitive melanopsin system also tend to have later sleep onsets (van der Meijden et al., 2016).

8.2.5 Circadian mechanisms in other tissues

Rhythms of clock gene expression (versus metabolic or physiological rhythms) have been recorded from many tissues in the brain and body. Some rhythms persist for many cycles when tissues are cultured in vitro, while others fade in amplitude over several cycles but may be restored by manipulations of the culture medium. Fading rhythmicity in some cases may reflect loss of synchrony among component cellular oscillators (Abe et al., 2002; Balsalobre et al., 1998; Davidson et al., 2005; Gibbs et al., 2008; Granados-Fuentes, Saxena, et al., 2004; Guilding et al., 2010; Sakhi et al., 2014; Yamazaki et al., 2000; Young, 2006).

Some of these molecular rhythms depend on input from the SCN pacemaker in order to translate into overt rhythms in physiology or metabolism (Allen et al., 2001). Daily rhythms of clock genes in several different peripheral tissues were abolished by SCN lesions in hamsters; some of these rhythms, but not others, were restored by SCN transplants. Critically, the genotype of the transplanted SCN determined the timing of the peripheral tissue rhythms (Guo et al., 2006).

Other neural tissues, including the retina, olfactory bulbs, and lateral habenula, show circadian rhythms of physiological activity that persist for at least a few cycles when they are cultured in vitro or are studied in vivo in the absence of the SCN (Granados-Fuentes, Saxena, et al., 2004; Sakhi et al., 2014; Terman et al., 1993; Tosini & Menaker, 1996; Zhao & Rusak, 2005). Olfactory bulbs, which sustained robust circadian rhythms in vitro, were entrained by the SCN in intact organisms (Granados-Fuentes, Prolo, et al., 2004).

These results indicate that the capacity for at least damped circadian oscillation at the level of gene expression is inherent in many, or most, cell types throughout the body, and that some extra-SCN tissues are capable of generating circadian rhythms independently of the SCN. The SCN functions as a pacemaker for most of these rhythms but may interact differently with other tissues depending on the extent to which they are intrinsically rhythmic.

The capacity for circadian rhythm generation in many extra-SCN tissues is consistent with evidence that behavioral rhythms can be expressed after SCN lesions under special conditions in rats and other species. For example, robust rhythms with circadian characteristics appeared when rats were exposed to cycles of timed daily feeding or during continuous treatment with methamphetamine. The existence of these rhythms must depend on extra-SCN oscillators in the brain and/or in peripheral tissues; for reviews, see (Honma & Honma, 2009; Mistlberger, 1994).

There has been increasing interest in how peripheral circadian mechanisms interact with the central pacemaker to regulate physiological functions. Most body tissues show rhythms of gene expression, including those of the core circadian clock genes, but many other mRNAs are also expressed rhythmically. Nearly half of all mouse mRNAs studied in 12 organs showed daily rhythms; these included

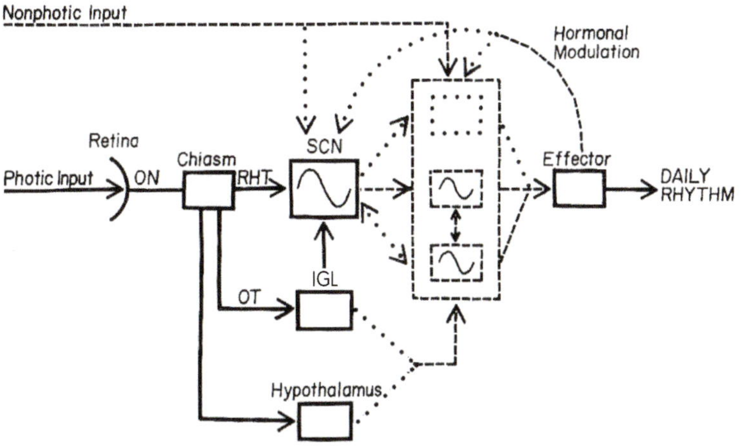

Figure 8.11 A more complex conceptual model of the the mammalian circadian system incorporating multiple components that influence overt rhythm production (as of 1982). An endogenously self-sustained oscillator is represented by a sine wave. Solid lines represent projection pathways that were known at that time; dashed lines represent pathways known to exist based on functional evidence but were unidentified; and dotted lines represent possible interactions for which there was no compelling functional evidence. The figure shows an entrainment pathway originating in the retina, entering the brain via the optic nerve (ON), and reaching the suprachiasmatic nuclei (SCN) via the retinohypothalamic tract (RHT); see text for more details. Another part of the photic pathway involves a projection reaching the intergeniculate leaflet (IGL) in the thalamus, which projects to the SCN. Other retinal fibers terminate in hypothalamic regions adjacent to the SCN. The SCN projects via direct neural pathways and secretory mechanisms to other systems, some of which are also endogenously rhythmic and some of which are not. Whether photic input reaching the IGL and/or hypothalamic regions near the SCN also influences these other systems directly is unknown. Some extra-SCN rhythmic systems may reciprocally influence the SCN or interact with each other and their various outputs influence the expression of overt daily rhythms in physiology and behavior. The resulting rhythmic outputs (e.g., gonadal or adrenal hormones) may, in turn, influence either or both the SCN and extra-SCN oscillator systems and modulate their rhythmicity. In addition to photic information, nonphotic input can clearly affect daily rhythms by acting outside the SCN, but in some species may potentially affect the SCN pacemaker itself. Adapted with permission from Rusak, B. (1982) Physiological models of the rodent circadian system; pp. 62–74. In: Aschoff, J. et al. (Eds.) *Vertebrate Circadian Systems*. © Springer-Verlag, Berlin, 1982.

not only mRNAs that code for proteins, but also non-coding RNAs, which may serve regulatory functions (Zhang et al., 2014). A study of gene expression in 46 different tissues from postmortem human tissues found that many mRNAs were rhythmic, that some rhythm patterns differed between male and female tissues, and that many showed decreases in rhythm amplitude in tissues from older people (Talamanca et al., 2023).

Circadian oscillations in peripheral tissues have been shown to be important for the normal function of organs like the heart, kidney, and lungs (e.g., Gibbs et al., 2014; Martino et al., 2008; Young, 2006). Some organ oscillations are regulated directly by the daily rhythm of adrenal corticosteroid secretion (Balsalobre et al., 2000; Gibbs et al., 2014; Leliavski et al., 2015), which is in turn controlled by the SCN pacemaker (Moore & Eichler, 1972). Others are influenced by SCN regulation of components of the autonomic nervous system (Bartness et al., 2001; Buijs et al., 2003) and by light information reaching hypothalamic targets adjacent to the SCN, which receive limited retinal inputs (Husse et al., 2015).

These findings require that a model of the mammalian circadian system must include components in addition to those core elements shown in **Figure 8.2**. At the time **Figure 8.11** was made (1982), some of these components had been identified while the existence of others could be inferred from the available evidence. These components included: modulation of photic effects by other parts of the visual system (Harrington, 1997; Harrington & Rusak, 1986; Rusak, 1977a); factors other than light that influence the overt expression of circadian rhythms (see Sections 3.4 and 3.6) (Mrosovsky, 1996); the influence on the pacemaker of outputs from some processes and organs that it regulates (see **Box 5.3**); and complex interactions between the pacemaker and other circadian oscillators in the brain and in other parts of the body (Honma & Honma, 2009; Mistlberger, 1994; Stephan, 1986).

8.2.6 Nocturnal and diurnal species

Although most studies of retinal input to the SCN have been conducted with nocturnal species, a few have involved diurnally active species. The overall temporal patterns of SCN firing rates and of spontaneous clock gene expression are similar in nocturnal and diurnal rodents (Inouye & Kawamura, 1979; Mrosovsky et al., 2001; Sato & Kawamura, 1984; Yan et al., 1999). This evidence indicates that a species' usual activity type is determined outside the SCN. This might occur as a result of SCN signals being translated differently by target tissues that control overt activity, but there is also evidence implicating the involvement of the retina in determining activity type (Doyle et al., 2008).

Despite the similarity of rhythm generation in the SCN among species, responsiveness of SCN neurons to retinal illumination and to electrical activation of the RHT differ between nocturnal and diurnal species that have been studied. Approximately 80% of photically responsive SCN neurons in nocturnal rats and hamsters are activated by retinal illumination, consistent with a critical role for the excitatory amino acid glutamate in entrainment of the SCN in these species (De Vries et al., 1994; Ebling, 1996; Meijer et al., 1986). In species that are typically day-active, a smaller proportion of photically responsive cells are activated by retinal illumination, and the majority are inhibited (Jiao et al., 1999; Meijer et al., 1989).

In one diurnal species (*Rhabodmys pumilio*), stimulation of the optic chiasm in an in vitro SCN slice preparation resulted in about equal proportions of excited and inhibited SCN neurons, in contrast to the mouse SCN where ~88% of responses to chiasm stimulation were excitatory. The inhibitory inputs to the SCN reflected direct RHT projections rather than the presence of an intervening inhibitory synapse (Schoonderwoerd, de Torres Gutierrez, et al., 2022). Models of the effects of retinal input to the SCN that are based on predominant activation of SCN neurons by retinal illumination may not apply fully to the influence of light on diurnal species.

Some studies in humans have used functional magnetic resonance imaging (fMRI) to examine the effects of retinal illumination on neural activity in the hypothalamus and have reported net activation in response to light (McGlashan et al., 2018; Vimal et al., 2009). Because of the limited resolution of the imaging methods used, these analyses targeted a larger hypothalamic region than the SCN alone. A recent study that used a higher strength magnet to focus on a smaller region centered on the SCN found instead that retinal illumination had a net suppressive effect on activity in this region (Schoonderwoerd, de Rover, et al., 2022). This observation is consistent with the dominant inhibitory responses observed using single-cell recordings in a few other diurnal species (Jiao et al., 1999; Meijer et al., 1989; Schoonderwoerd, de Torres Gutierrez, et al., 2022).

These findings suggest that a complete model of photic regulation of SCN activity will require understanding the effects of inhibitory retinal input on SCN function in people and other diurnal species as well as in nocturnal species, in which inhibitory responses also occur but are less common.

8.2.7 Summary

The mammalian circadian system includes a central pacemaker in the SCN of the hypothalamus. The SCN is a self-sustaining oscillator that generates circadian rhythms based on intracellular cycles of gene transcription, translation, and protein modification in individual neurons. These individual cellular rhythms are in turn synchronized among SCN neurons, resulting in circa-24 h rhythms of SCN neuronal firing rates that persist in vitro.

The role of the SCN as a pacemaker for the circadian system was confirmed by several lines of evidence: SCN neural and secretory rhythms persist indefinitely while the structure is isolated from all rhythmic inputs in vitro; most measurable physiological and behavioral rhythms are lost after destruction of the SCN; transplantation of the SCN into an animal that is arrhythmic after SCN lesions restores rhythmicity; and, critically, the period of the restored rhythm is determined by the genotype of the transplanted SCN, not that of the host organism.

The SCN interacts with a complex hierarchy of other oscillatory systems with varying degrees of self-sustaining capacity both within the brain and in other organs and tissues. The integration of these rhythms into a single circadian framework depends on the integrity of the SCN.

A subset of retinal ganglion cells form the RHT, which terminates in the SCN and is principally responsible for its photic entrainment and, as a result, for the synchronization of the physiology and behavior of mammals to the day–night cycle. The RHT includes axons from retinal ganglion cells that contain melanopsin, a photopigment with peak sensitivity in the blue/violet part of the visual spectrum. These cells are intrinsically photoreceptive as well as receiving input from classical rod and cone photoreceptors. These ganglion cells form a photic system that provides information about levels of general illumination that regulates functions like pupillary constriction in response to increased illumination. This photic system is especially suited to responding to the global illumination changes that occur during day–night cycles and entrain circadian rhythms.

While most light-responsive SCN neurons in nocturnal species are activated by retinal illumination, a minority are suppressed. In the few diurnal species that have been studied, the majority of photically responsive SCN neurons are inhibited by retinal illumination, while evidence from humans is mixed because of technical limitations in imaging this tiny nucleus. The best current evidence, however, indicates that the SCN of humans is more suppressed than activated by retinal illumination, consistent with other diurnally active species. Physiological models of photic entrainment need to incorporate the minority of inhibitory responses to light found in nocturnal species and the dominance of inhibitory responses in diurnal species, likely including humans.

8.3 Role of the SCN in sleep regulation

8.3.1 SCN ablation effects on sleep

The involvement of the SCN pacemaker in the circadian regulation of sleep was demonstrated by studies showing that circadian sleep rhythms were lost after SCN ablations in rats and squirrel monkeys (*Saimiri sciureus*). Unlike in intact animals (**Figures 8.12 A** and **8.13 A**), after SCN ablations sleep and activity were distributed in short, ultradian (high-frequency) bouts throughout 24 h periods (Eastman et al., 1984; Edgar et al., 1993; Ibuka & Kawamura, 1975; Mistlberger et al., 1987) (**Figures 8.12 B, C,** and **8.13 B**). In intact rats, ultradian sleep–wake cycles are present throughout both the day and night, but circadian modulation strongly biases rats to sleep mostly in the day and be active mostly at night (**Figure 8.13 A**). After loss of the SCN, these ultradian sleep–wake cycles persisted and were very robust but were no longer modulated by circadian phase (**Figure 8.13 B**).

Despite disruption of the normal circadian organization of sleep–wake cycles, the homeostatic regulation of sleep remained intact. SCN-ablated rats and mice showed rebound increases in sleep amounts after sleep deprivation (Easton et al., 2004; Mistlberger, 2005; Mistlberger et al., 1983; Tobler et al., 1983). These results support the conclusion that separate physiological mechanisms are responsible for the circadian and homeostatic aspects of sleep–wake regulation, as discussed in Chapter 5.

The rapid, irregular alternation of short sleep and wake bouts observed in squirrel monkeys and rats after SCN ablation may be related to the activity of an ultradian (<24 h) oscillator. Alternatively, it may result from short-term homeostatic regulation in the absence of circadian modulation of sleep and wake. An animal that is awake for a short period (at any time) would acquire some sleep debt (i.e., an increased level of substance S; see Chapter 5). As time awake lengthened, homeostasis would increasingly promote sleep onset to reverse the accumulated sleep debt. After SCN ablation, this tendency would not be opposed by the wake-promoting action of the circadian pacemaker. As a result, the animal would fall asleep, and after only a brief sleep period, it would have repaid this small sleep debt (i.e., reduced substance S levels) and would wake up. Once awake, it would again start to accumulate sleep debt, and the short, irregular cycles of sleep and wake would continue as illustrated in **Figure 8.13 B**.

In intact adult monkeys (and people), the circadian wake-promoting function of the SCN during the day allows accumulation of a very large (usually day-long) sleep debt

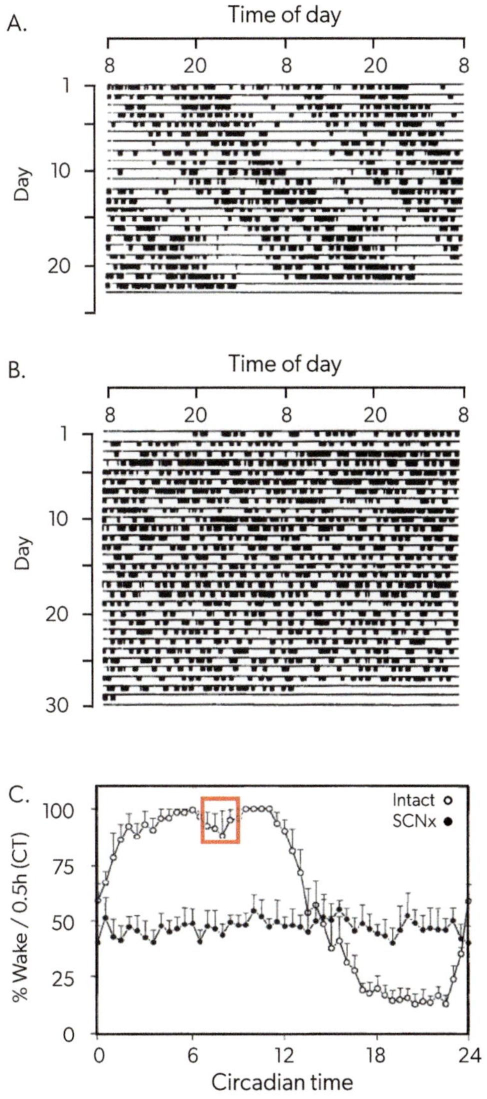

Figure 8.12 The effects of SCN ablations on circadian rhythms in squirrel monkeys (*Saimiri sciureus*). **A.** A free-running drinking rhythm (contacts with a drinking spout) with a period >24 h generated by an intact squirrel monkey housed in constant light, double-plotted on a 48 h time base. **B.** The lack of circadian organization of drinking in a monkey after complete SCN ablation. **C:** The circadian rhythm of waking (Y axis) in intact (white symbols) and SCN-ablated (black symbols) monkeys is shown as a plot of the percentage of each 0.5 of a circadian hour (=1/48 of a circadian cycle) during which the monkeys were awake, plotted against circadian time (X axis). The robust circadian rhythm of wake probability in intact monkeys is abolished by SCN ablations. The red box outlines a period of reduced waking during the middle of the circadian wake phase in intact monkeys, which may be analogous to the human "post-lunch dip." Adapted with permission of the authors and Society for Neuroscience from Edgar, D.M. et al. (1993) Effect of SCN lesions on sleep in squirrel monkeys: evidence for opponent processes in sleep–wake regulation. *J Neurosci* 13:1065–1079. © Society for Neuroscience (1993). doi: 10.1523/JNEUROSCI.13-03-01065.1993.

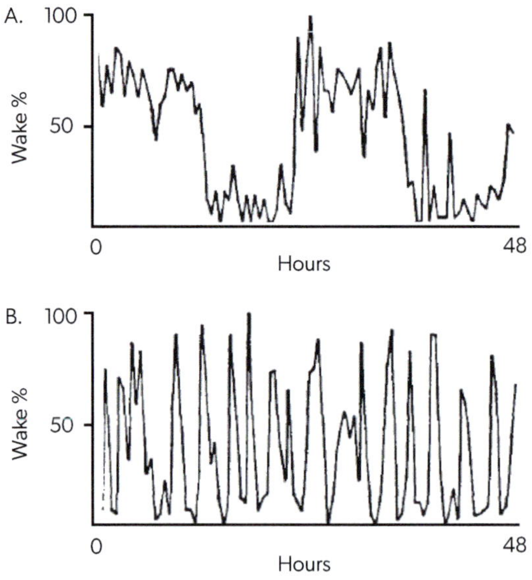

Figure 8.13 **A.** Percentage of a 48 h period spent awake (Y axis) by an intact rat (*Rattus norvegicus*) free-running in constant dim light, showing a robust circadian rhythm of wake along with a superimposed higher frequency (ultradian) rhythm of wake and sleep during two successive, subjective active and rest phases. **B.** A similar 48 h record of percentage time awake in a rat with a complete SCN ablation, showing the loss of circadian rhythmicity but preservation of robust ultradian cyclicity of wake and sleep. Adapted with permission of Oxford University Press from Mistlberger, R.E. et al. (1987) Relationships among wake episode lengths, contiguous sleep episode lengths, and electroencephalographic delta waves in rats with suprachiasmatic nuclei lesions. *Sleep* 10:12–24. © Sleep Research Society (1987); permission conveyed through Copyright Clearance Center, Inc. doi: 10.1093/sleep/10.1.12.

that is discharged at night during a lengthy, sustained sleep phase. The combination of this large sleep debt and the sleep-promoting function of the SCN at night can together sustain sleep for hours at night. Without the SCN's promotion of sustained periods of wake and sleep, only short-term, homeostatic regulation affects the arousal state of monkeys, producing a rapid, irregular alternation of sleep and wake indefinitely and a 50% probability of being awake or asleep at any time (**Figure 8.12 C**).

This interpretation implies that one function of an intact circadian system in primates is to permit consolidation of lengthy, sustained waking during the day and sleep at night. The circadian system acts to maintain state stability by opposing the effects of either highly elevated or strongly depleted homeostatic sleep pressure late in the waking and sleep phases, respectively, as discussed in Section 5.7.3. One exception to the delay imposed by the circadian system in responding to cumulative sleep need is the increase in sleepiness among adult humans in early or mid-afternoon (Haimov & Lavie, 1997; Strogatz et al., 1987b) (see Section 6.2). This tendency is also reflected in the reduced wakefulness of squirrel monkeys after midday that is highlighted by the red box in **Figure 8.12** C, representing what appears to be the squirrel monkey equivalent of the human post-lunch dip/siesta hour (see Figure 2.11).

Although rats with SCN lesions showed severe disruption of their sleep–wake cycles, they showed no change in overall amounts of sleep, consistent with their preserved homeostatic regulation of sleep (Eastman et al., 1984; Ibuka & Kawamura, 1975; Mistlberger et al., 1983; Tobler et al., 1983; Trachsel et al., 1992). In contrast to this finding, SCN ablation in squirrel monkeys resulted in a large increase (~3–4 h) in the total amount of sleep, consisting mostly of increased N1 sleep (drowsiness or very light sleep) at the expense of waking (Edgar et al., 1993).

These contrasting results could be related to the role of the circadian system in generating the different daily patterns of sleep in these species. Primates have strong circadian wake- and sleep-promoting influences during the day and night, respectively. Rats are polycyclic sleepers, so they sleep at all circadian phases but with a tendency to be awake more often at night and less often during the day (see **Figure 8.13 A**). SCN lesions in monkeys eliminate the strong circadian influences that inhibit daytime sleep, so more light sleep can emerge. Loss of the weaker circadian modulation of sleep–wake in rats may have less effect, so total sleep amounts are not changed. This interpretation, however, does not explain the ~2 h increase in total sleep time in SCN-ablated mice, which are also polycyclic sleepers (Easton et al., 2004). It is possible that the SCN promotes sleep during the rest phase and waking during the active phase to different extents in different species, regardless of overall sleep–wake pattern.

In people, the impact of not having the wake-promoting influence of the circadian system during the day can be inferred from a clinical case report of the woman we described at the beginning of this chapter. During surgery to remove a hypothalamic tumor, she sustained damage that likely included the SCN. She showed frequent, irregular bouts of drowsiness alternating with activity and agitation, disrupted continuity of both sleep and wake, and unstable body temperature rhythms (**Figure 8.14 A**).

This patient gave no indication of consistent deficits during cognitive testing, but during repeated testing over several days, she unpredictably showed either normal or very poor performance on the same tests. The deficits emerged as she switched rapidly from fully alert to drowsy and unresponsive within a short test session, resulting in difficulty sustaining attention and performance (Cohen & Albers, 1991) (**Figure 8.14 B**). Without a sustained circadian arousal signal from the SCN during the day, she could not maintain daytime alertness; similarly, her sleep at night was frequently disrupted in the absence of a circadian sleep signal.

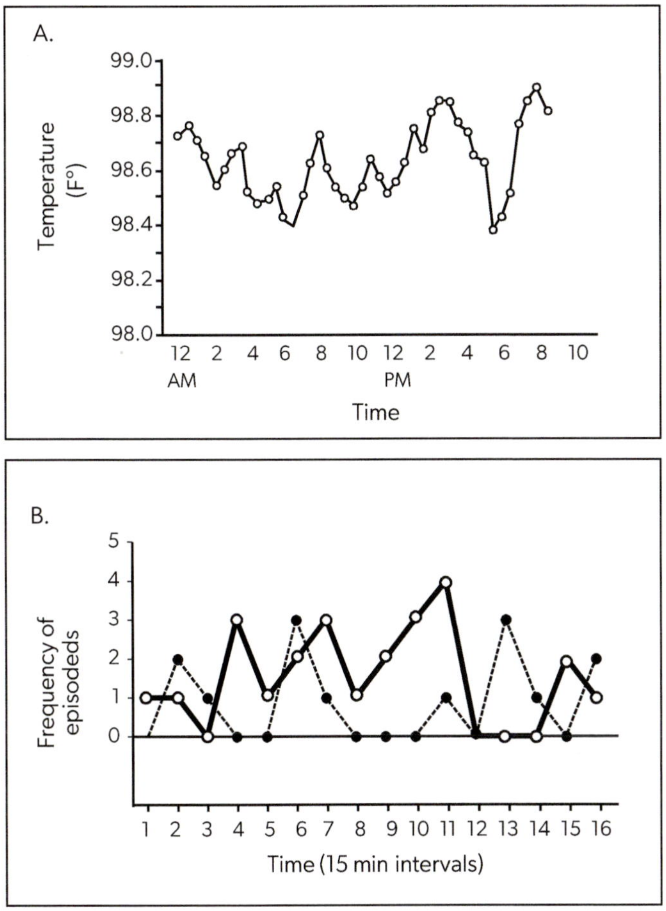

Figure 8.14 **A.** Body temperature averaged over 3 days (Y axis), plotted against time of day (X axis), from a patient who had undergone neurosurgery to remove a hypothalamic tumor. She showed a highly irregular 24 h pattern of body temperature as well as disrupted sleep–wake rhythms. The surgery involved removal of a portion of her hypothalamus that apparently included the suprachiasmatic nuclei (SCN). **B.** The same patient was observed for a 4 h daytime period during which she underwent cognitive testing. The number of episodes she showed of lethargy or actual sleep onset (dotted line), and of agitation, restlessness, or excessive activity (solid black line) are plotted for every 15 min segment. The individual showed irregular, unpredictable fluctuations in levels of consciousness and activation during the test period. Adapted with permission of Wolters Kluwer Lippincott from Cohen, R.A. & Albers, E. (1991) Disruption of human circadian and cognitive regulation following a discrete hypothalamic lesion: a case study. *Neurology* 41:726–729. © American Academy of Neurology (1991). doi: 10.1212/wnl.41.5.726.

Although a role for SCN damage in producing these symptoms seems likely, neither a tumor, nor surgery to remove it, would produce damage limited to a single small structure. Thus, damage to nearby hypothalamic nuclei that are known to be involved in regulating body temperature, sleep, and arousal (see Chapter 11) could also have contributed to some of these symptoms.

8.3.2 How SCN outputs affect sleep

There are several routes by which the SCN can modulate sleep probability on a circadian basis. The loss of firing-rate rhythms in some brain regions after they were separated by knife cuts from the SCN (Inouye & Kawamura, 1979) imply that these structures and the systems they regulate depend for their rhythmicity on direct input from the SCN.

There are direct anatomical projections from the SCN to several brain regions that influence sleep (Canteras et al., 2011; Swanson & Cowan, 1975; Zhang et al., 2009). These include the ventrolateral preoptic nucleus (VLPO) (Deurveilher et al., 2002; Sun et al., 2001), which plays an important role in the regulation of NREM sleep (see Chapter 11). There are indirect projections from the SCN to the locus coeruleus (Aston-Jones et al., 2001), the source of brain norepinephrine, which is involved in the regulation of both waking/arousal and REM sleep timing (see Chapter 10).

There are also indirect projections from the SCN to the paraventricular hypothalamic nucleus (PVN). The PVN is involved in regulation of pineal melatonin secretion (Klein et al., 1983), which helps facilitate sleep onset as well as playing a role in regulating seasonal phenomena in many species (see Chapter 9). The PVN and the dorsomedial hypothalamic nucleus (DMH) are also important relay points for circadian input from the SCN that reaches sympathetic and parasympathetic divisions of the autonomic nervous system (Bartness et al., 2001; Buijs et al., 2003). These links provide a mechanism for the SCN to regulate global changes in autonomic balance that are characteristic of different circadian phases as well as of sleep and wake states.

The SCN projects directly to the lateral and posterior hypothalamus which contain neurons that are the source of the peptides hypocretin and melanin concentrating hormone (MCH) (Abrahamson et al., 2001). These neurons project widely in the brain, including throughout the cortex, and play an important role in the regulation of sleep and waking (see Chapter 11). The SCN also projects to several other brain regions, including the septum, paraventricular thalamic nucleus, lateral habenula, and bed nucleus of the stria terminalis (Canteras et al., 2011; Swanson & Cowan, 1975; Zhang et al., 2009).

SCN efferent projections to different targets are selectively involved in the expression of different rhythms. Dorsal projections from the SCN terminate directly in the subparaventricular zone (SPZ) and the DMH, which serve as relays that convey circadian information to other neural targets, including those involved in regulating sleep and waking (Deurveilher & Semba, 2005; Saper et al., 2005). Ablation of these structures have differential effects on daily rhythms. Damage to the DMH in rats greatly reduced the amplitude of circadian rhythms of sleep, waking, and cortisol, among other rhythms, but did not affect rhythms of melatonin production (Chou et al., 2003), which are regulated through the PVN (Klein et al., 1983). Ablation of one part of the SPZ reduced the amplitude of sleep–wake and locomotor activity rhythms, but damage to an adjacent region had a larger effect on body temperature rhythms (Lu et al., 2001).

In addition to these direct and indirect neural projections from the SCN, there is also evidence that diffusible neurochemicals secreted by SCN cells can convey, or influence, rhythmicity. In one study, fetal SCNs enclosed in a semipermeable membrane were implanted into the brain of SCN-ablated hamsters. The membrane had pore sizes that permitted chemicals to move between the transplants and the host brain but that were too small for the formation of synaptic connections between them. Nevertheless, circadian activity rhythms were restored, demonstrating that a chemical circadian signal reached the brain by diffusion from the transplanted SCN (Silver et al., 1996).

A candidate chemical promoter of sleep that is produced by SCN projection neurons is a peptide[3] called prokineticin 2 (PK2). Its mRNA is co-localized in SCN neurons that contain other peptides, including vasopressin (VP), vasoactive intestinal peptide (VIP), and gastrin-releasing peptide (GRP) (Masumoto et al., 2006). Expression of the mRNA coding for PK2 is high during the daytime (the rest phase for mice and rats) and low at night (their active phase). Both the SCN and many structures to which it projects express high levels of a specific PK2 receptor. Microinjection of PK2 into the lateral ventricle of rats during the night phase to mimic high daytime levels strongly suppressed activity (Cheng et al., 2002; Zhang et al., 2009). The effects of these treatments may be mediated in part by PK2 acting within the SCN itself as well as on other neural targets.

The widespread projections from the SCN that contain PK2 suggest that it plays a role in signaling circadian time to several neural systems regulating sleep, activity, and other functions (Zhang et al., 2009). Knockout of the gene coding for the PK2 receptor in mice resulted in altered activity rhythms in both lighting cycles and constant conditions but generally preserved rhythmicity (Prosser et al., 2007). However, knockout of the gene for PK2 itself reduced both spontaneous sleep amounts (especially NREM sleep) and homeostatic increases after sleep deprivation (Hu et al., 2007). An analysis of patterns of cellular transcription in the SCN indicated that PK2 and its receptors are involved in rhythm production and affect the period and amplitude of the ensemble circadian oscillation in the SCN (Morris et al., 2021). Thus, PK2 plays an important role in the regulation of both circadian rhythms and sleep homeostasis.

[3] Peptides are short chains of linked amino acids; proteins are longer chains.

Other SCN peptides that co-localize with PK2 mRNA have important roles in rhythm regulation and in maintenance of internal rhythmicity within the SCN. VP is a peptide that is produced by a subset of SCN efferent neurons and is secreted with a circadian rhythm in vitro (Gillette, 1987). VP-immunoreactive (ir) neurons project from the SCN to several of its target regions (Abrahamson & Moore, 2001). These neurons are involved in aspects of circadian rhythm regulation, including contributing to integrating activity among SCN neurons (Mieda, 2019).

VP levels in the cerebrospinal fluid (CSF) of rats show a daily rhythm, with levels normally higher during the daily light phase when rats are least active (Kruisbrink et al., 1987). Ablation of the SCN eliminates the VP rhythm in the CSF and reduces its level to the detection limit of assays (Schwartz & Reppert, 1985). In addition to VP projections to other brain regions, VP-ergic SCN neurons send both axons and dendrites into and through the walls of the immediately adjacent third ventricle in mice. This feature provides a route by which the SCN can affect VP levels in the CSF, which can influence all of the brain through the ventricular system (Taub et al., 2021).

Neurons in the SCN that contain the peptide neuromedin S (NMS) also play an important role in maintaining SCN rhythm integrity and driving the period of the SCN rhythm (Lee et al., 2015) as well as providing important efferent information to systems involved in seasonal changes in physiology (Porcu et al., 2022).

Some SCN neurons within the retinorecipient portion of the nucleus contain the peptide VIP. VIP and its receptor VPAC2, which is found in ~35% of SCN neurons, are critically involved in mediating photic effects on the SCN as well as being essential to generating SCN population firing-rate rhythms and normal circadian behavioral rhythms (Hamnett et al., 2021; Piggins & Cutler, 2003). VIP is co-localized in SCN neurons with other peptides (peptide histidine isoleucine [PHI] and GRP). Injection of VIP, GRP, or PHI into the SCN of hamsters caused circadian rhythm phase shifts that mimicked those produced by retinal illumination (Piggins et al., 1995).

8.3.3 Summary

As for other circadian rhythms, daily sleep–wake rhythms are eliminated by destruction of the SCN, resulting in a pattern of short, alternating bouts of sleep and waking throughout the day–night cycle in both rodents and primates. Despite the loss of circadian organization, homeostatic regulation of sleep in response to deprivation remains intact. Total amounts of sleep are preserved in rats after SCN ablation, but in squirrel monkeys and mice, there is an increase in the amount of primarily light sleep. These results may be related to differences in how strongly the intact SCN modulates sleep and wake probability at different circadian phases or to other species differences.

Projections directly from the SCN, or from relay nuclei to which it projects, reach many brain regions known to be involved in sleep–wake regulation as well as autonomic control systems that contribute to the regulation of arousal levels in different sleep–wake states. Circadian modulation of the probability of sleep may depend on both neural modulation of the SCN's targets by the changing firing rates of SCN efferents and by secretion of SCN peptides.

Peptides produced in the SCN act within the nucleus to enhance the integrity of circadian oscillations and mediate photic responses as well as affecting neural targets to which the SCN projects. The peptide PK2 acts within the SCN and elsewhere to affect circadian rhythms, inhibit activity, and promote sleep, especially NREM sleep. It is co-localized in the SCN with VP which is secreted into the CSF and can thereby affect all of the brain.

Thus, the SCN influences sleep via direct and indirect projections to brain regions known to be involved in sleep–wake regulation. It also contains several peptides that act within the SCN to regulate the integrity of rhythm generation, affect photic responsiveness of SCN neurons, and influence sleep–wake rhythms and homeostatic regulation of sleep amounts.

8.4 Role of the circadian system in aging effects on sleep

8.4.1 Changes in sleep timing

Changes in sleep features during aging (see Chapter 4) have prompted studies of how the circadian system may be involved. These have focused on how aging alters SCN anatomy and physiology as well as overall circadian organization. A related issue is whether aging- and/or disease-related changes in the circadian system contribute to the extreme disruption of sleep and circadian rhythmicity that characterizes many older people who develop dementia (Vitiello & Prinz, 1989; Witting et al., 1990).

One change that is typical of human aging is an advance in the timing of sleep and waking to earlier phases of the day–night cycle (see Chapter 4). Circadian entrainment models suggest that an advance of sleep–wake timing could be the result of a shortening of the circadian rhythm period with aging. A shorter clock period predicts a more advanced phase of entrainment relative to the external cycle (see **Figure 3.5**).

Some studies in animal models reported shorter circadian periods in older animals, for example, in golden hamsters (*Mesocricetus auratus*) (Pittendrigh & Daan, 1974). But a later study of hamsters that were kept in constant dim light from a young age throughout their natural lifespans (1–2 years) found no evidence for a systematic shortening of circadian periods with age (Duffy, Viswanathan, et al., 1999). There have been mixed results in studies of other species, which does not encourage a simple interpretation of advanced human sleep timing in older people as the result of shorter circadian periods.

In human studies, core body temperature was used as one marker of the pacemaker's circadian phase in studies conducted using constant routines and forced desynchronization. There was no evidence of substantially shorter circadian periods in older relative to younger people (Czeisler et al., 1999; Duffy et al., 1998). These studies found that temperature fell less and rose earlier during the night in older people on their usual schedules, which was associated with a reduced ability to maintain sleep in the second half of the sleep period. As a result, waking in older people occurred at an earlier phase of their circadian rhythms than in younger people. The resulting earlier wake time could also expose older people to more phase-advancing effects of morning light, which would predict a shift to earlier timing of the next sleep onset (Duffy et al., 1998; Duffy, Dijk, et al., 1999). Other studies that used different methods did not confirm a shift in phase relation between sleep and circadian phase markers in older people (Carrier et al., 2009; Kim et al., 2014) or found that some rhythms (e.g., the phase of waking) were shifted but not others (Yoon et al., 2003).

Although these differences remain to be resolved, it appears that several factors, other than a shorter circadian period, could contribute to earlier timing of sleep and wake in older people. These include shifts in the timing of sleep–wake rhythms relative to individuals' circadian cycles and altered shape and timing of the body temperature rhythm (Czeisler et al., 1999; Duffy et al., 1998).

Another likely contributor to earlier sleep onset in older people is a reduction in the robustness of the circadian-regulated wake maintenance zone late in the daily wake phase and the sleep-maintenance zone late in the night; see Section 11.3.1 (Deboer et al., 2004; Strogatz et al., 1987a; Zeitzer et al., 2003; Zhang et al., 2004). A multiple nap study (75 min nap opportunities, every 225 min) compared sleep propensity rhythms of 20–31 year-olds to those of 57–74 year-olds. There were shorter sleep-onset latencies and longer sleep episodes in the older group during the nap opportunity scheduled at 22:00 h, which falls during the usual wake maintenance zone of the younger group, indicating reduced strength of the circadian wake-maintenance function (Münch et al., 2005).

8.4.2 Changes in light exposure and sensitivity

Daily light exposure is critical to entraining circadian rhythms and affecting their amplitude. People living in industrial societies in temperate zones get relatively little exposure to the bright light intensities that are most effective in entraining rhythms, especially outside the summer months (Espiritu et al., 1994; Hébert et al., 1998). There is also evidence that older people get less daily exposure to entraining light intensities than younger people, especially older women (Campbell et al., 1988; Mishima et al., 2001).

Older people housed in care environments get even less light exposure; those with dementia living in a care home received only about a quarter of the light exposure of those with comparable levels of dementia living at home (Olsen et al., 2016). Among patients with severe dementia who were institutionalized, those who were exposed to higher levels of light intensity were more alert, had better quality of life, and went to sleep later than those with lower levels of light exposure (Münch et al., 2017). Thus, the intensity of daily light exposure appears to be one factor that affects the timing of sleep onset among older people, including those institutionalized with dementia.

However, one study reported that very physically and psychologically healthy older people (average age 66), who had no sleep complaints, took no medications, and had volunteered for a research project, actually had more daily light exposure than a comparison group of younger people (average age 23) (Scheuermaier et al., 2010). It is probably critical that the older participants were mostly retired, and the younger people were mostly employed or students. Retirees who were healthy and fit enough could presumably take advantage of their increased free time to engage in more sustained outdoor activities. Many older people, however, have chronic health conditions, including excess weight, vascular disease, arthritis, and other joint conditions that could limit mobility and restrict outdoor activities, so this finding may not be applicable to the general population of older people.

Even exposure to comparable light intensities could have different effects on circadian rhythms of older people than younger people. Healthy older people with no medical complaints showed reduced circadian rhythm phase-shifts compared to younger people in response to moderate light intensities (Duffy et al., 2007). One factor that could contribute to reduced photic responsiveness in older people is the development of cataracts that reduce light transmission to the retina. In addition, progressive yellowing of the lens during aging specifically reduces transmission in the blue region of the spectrum that is most effective in stimulating melanopsin-containing retinal ganglion cells (Berson et al., 2002; Brøndsted et al., 2013; Lucas et al., 2014; Turner et al., 2010); see Section 8.2.4.

In older golden hamsters (which undergo similar changes in their lenses), there was a large reduction relative to young animals in the effectiveness of light in shifting circadian rhythms and regulating gene expression in the SCN (Zhang et al., 1996). However, the observed maximum 50% reduction in light transmission through the lens during aging in hamsters was too small to explain the large reduction in light-induced phase shifts, indicating that other mechanisms were involved (Zhang et al., 1998). In addition, older hamsters showed greatly reduced phase shifts in response to non-photic,[4] as well as photic, phase-shifting stimuli (van Reeth et al., 1992), implying a more general change in the sensitivity of the circadian system to phase-shifting stimuli.

A human study found that the lenses of 76-year-olds transmitted 33–45% of short wavelength (blue) light when compared to the lenses of 18-year-olds (Brøndsted et al., 2013), which is similar to the reduction in old hamsters (Zhang et al., 1998). Unlike in hamsters, however, there were no significant differences in phase-shifting responses to bright light (2 or 3 h of 2000–8000 lux) between younger and older people (Kim et al., 2014; Kripke et al., 2007). The absence of age differences in response to sustained, bright light does not rule out differences in sensitivity to the lower light intensities typically experienced in indoor environments (e.g., hundreds of lux). People in temperate zones may be exposed to intensities >1,000 lux only briefly in winter months but for longer in summer (Espiritu et al., 1994; Hébert et al., 1998).

Some older people who develop severe cataracts receive artificial lens implants.[5] Studies of sleep in patients who had this surgery found that there were no consistent effects on the timing of sleep or circadian rhythms, or on sleep quality (Brøndsted et al., 2017; Yan & Wang, 2016). One review concluded that subjective sleep quality was transiently better in those receiving lenses that preserved blue-light transmission compared to those that did not, but that this small difference was lost over time (Lee et al., 2021). A comparison of patients who received clear vs. blue-light blocking lenses after cataract removal noted a slower rise of melatonin levels to a lower nighttime peak in those who received the blue-light blocking lens, both compared to their preoperative baseline and to controls receiving clear lenses. These results indicate that reduced

[4] The category of "non-photic" stimuli includes a variety of stimuli other than light. In animal studies the stimuli used are dark pulses (against a light background) or one of several drug treatments that provoke increased activity levels in nocturnal rodents and cause circadian rhythm phase shifts (Mrosovsky, 1996).

[5] Implanted lenses usually filter ultraviolet (UV) light to reduce the risk of damage to the retina from sunlight, but some lenses are also blue-light filtered, which would reduce input to the melanopsin-based photic system.

melanopsin signaling affected the amplitude of the melatonin rhythm, but there were no clear effects on sleep (Brøndsted et al., 2017).

Although altered visual system function in older people can affect some circadian features, this does not appear to be a major contributor to altered sleep timing. An alternative interpretation is that a reduction in light-induced phase shifts in laboratory studies may reflect a more general change in the organization and responsiveness of the circadian system, rather than a change in photic entrainment mechanisms. This interpretation is consistent with the evidence cited above that there is a reduction in older hamsters of phase-shift amplitude in response to both photic and non-photic stimuli (van Reeth et al., 1992).

8.4.3 Changes in sleep quality and circadian rhythm amplitude

Changes in the organization of sleep in older people include reduced continuity of sleep, resulting in an increase in the duration of wake after sleep onset (WASO) (see **Figure 4.5**), more daytime naps, more N1 sleep and—at least in older men—less N3 sleep. One potential explanation for the less consolidated sleep of older adults is that they have a reduced amplitude of circadian modulation of sleep and waking compared to younger people. As summarized below, aging reduces the amplitude of several daily rhythms. These results suggest that what is reduced during aging is the amplitude of circadian pacemaker signals that drive these rhythms. This interpretation is supported by evidence that the amplitude of oscillation of the SCN pacemaker itself is reduced during aging (see Section 8.4.4).

The SCN pacemaker in adult humans confines sleep largely to the rest phase of the circadian cycle and waking to the active phase. Ablation of the SCN causes a loss of circadian regulation of sleep in animals (and apparently in people), resulting in alternating short bouts of waking and sleep (or sleepiness) at all times of day and night. The less extreme changes in sleep seen in older people (i.e., intermittent waking during the night and more napping during the day) could in theory result from a reduction in the strength of signals produced by the SCN, in contrast to their complete absence after SCN ablation.

Because it is not possible to measure the strength of SCN rhythmicity directly in people, an alternative is to measure rhythmicity in more accessible functions that are tightly regulated by the SCN. One of these is the pineal gland's secretion of its principal hormonal product, melatonin. Under the control of the SCN (Klein et al., 1983), melatonin levels increase early in the night, peak during the night, and fall toward the end of the night. The rise of melatonin plays an important role in regulating sleep timing in people; see Chapter 9 for a discussion of its role.

The amplitude of daily rhythms of melatonin secretion, body temperature, and several hormones (e.g., growth hormone) were reported to be markedly reduced during aging, consistent with the idea that there is a reduction in the amplitude of many or all SCN-regulated rhythms (Magri et al., 2004; Mahlberg et al., 2006; Pérez-Medina-Carballo et al., 2022; van Coevorden et al., 1991; Weitzman et al., 1982; Zhao et al., 2002). The lifetime course of changes in melatonin rhythms has not been fully mapped, but melatonin peak levels at night have been reported to start to decline as early as the third decade of life (Kennaway et al., 1999). There is also evidence that older people (average age 69 years) who habitually napped (at least twice a week for at least 30 min) had lower amplitude melatonin rhythms than those who were not habitual nappers (Deantoni et al., 2024).

A related issue is that the degree of sleep disturbance in adults with primary insomnia is correlated with the extent of pineal calcification[6] (Mahlberg et al., 2009). Calcification of the pineal gland increases with age and reduces melatonin production; see Section 9.6.3 for further discussion. Taken together with the evidence related to napping patterns, these results suggest that less robust melatonin rhythmicity (presumably a reflection of the amplitude of the pacemaker signal) is associated with less sequestering of sleep to the night phase and waking to the day phase.

One study that used a 30 h constant routine (with no sleep and restricted mobility; see Section 3.5.2), however, did not observe a group difference in melatonin rhythm amplitude between younger (18–30 years) and older (64–81 years) participants. The design and results of the study raise some important issues. Participants were carefully screened to ensure that they were very healthy, took no medications, and had no sleep complaints (Zeitzer et al., 1999). The hypothesis we are considering is that lower-amplitude circadian rhythms (including that of melatonin production) contribute to sleep complaints, so this last criterion may have unintentionally excluded older participants with lower-amplitude daily rhythms.

Despite the lack of an overall group difference in melatonin secretion, there was evidence of reduced rhythm amplitudes even among these highly selected, healthy older participants. The 15% of the older age group with the lowest amplitude rhythms had much lower peak melatonin levels than the 15% of the younger group with lowest amplitude rhythms. The melatonin rhythms of the 15% in each age group with the highest amplitude rhythms did not differ (Zeitzer et al., 1999) (**Figure 8.15**).

[6] This is the process of deposition of calcium in the pineal tissue, which reduces its capacity to secrete melatonin. It occurs variably among people, and the specific factors influencing the process are unknown.

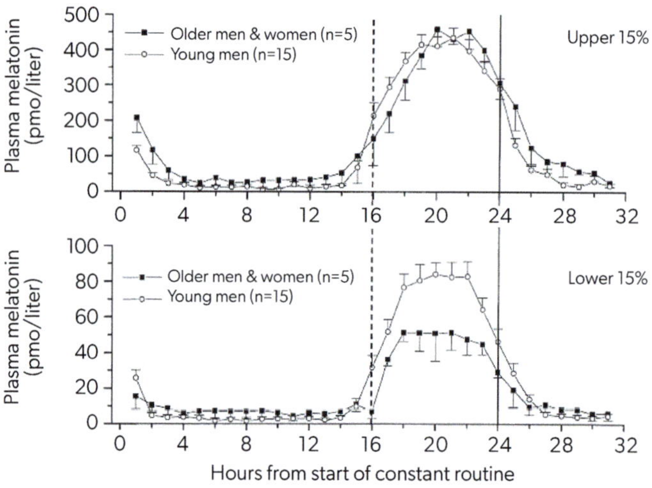

Figure 8.15 Comparison of the plasma melatonin rhythms of younger and older participants during constant routine studies lasting ~30 h. There were no statistically significant differences between the groups as a whole. The data shown, however, are from the top and bottom 15th percentiles of rhythm amplitudes generated in each age group. Those with the highest amplitude rhythms (top panel) showed similar patterns in both age groups. The subsets of participants in each group with the lowest amplitude rhythms (bottom panel: note the different ranges on the upper and lower Y axes) showed large differences, with the older participants (black symbols) showing lower amplitude rhythms than the younger participants (white symbols). The dashed and solid vertical lines indicate the approximate start and end of bedtime, respectively, before the beginning of the constant routine. Reprinted with permission of Elsevier, Ltd. from Zeitzer J.M. et al. (1999) Do plasma melatonin concentrations decline with age? *Am J Med* 107:432–436. © Elsevier (1999). doi: 10.1016/s0002-9343(99)00266-1.

These results raise several issues related to measurement and comparison of melatonin rhythms as markers of the circadian system. One issue is that there are large individual differences in nocturnal melatonin levels, regardless of age (Mahlberg et al., 2006), which can make it difficult to detect group differences in melatonin rhythms. These results also emphasize the difficulties inherent in designing cross-sectional studies to compare physiological measures in younger and older populations, as discussed in Section 4.7. For example, older people willing and able to participate in a 30 h constant routine (Zeitzer et al., 1999) or in a challenging protocol involving 60 h of alternating, very short sleep and wake periods, as described below (Buysse et al., 2005), represent a highly selected subset of that age group. Generalizability from these participants to the broader population of less healthy older people may be limited.

Screening to ensure a lack of sleep complaints, excellent health, and absence of drug treatments has both advantages and disadvantages. An advantage is that drugs that are more commonly used by older than younger people, such as non-steroidal anti-inflammatories (e.g., ibuprofen, aspirin, often prescribed to treat joint pain/arthritis symptoms) (Cardinali & Ritta, 1983; Surrall et al., 1987), and β-adrenergic antagonists (e.g., atenolol, propranolol, prescribed to control high blood pressure) (Murphy et al., 1996; Stoschitzky et al., 1999) suppress melatonin production and can disturb sleep. Thus, exclusion of people with these conditions who take these drugs is necessary in order to assess whether there are direct effects of aging on sleep.

A disadvantage, however, is that the inclusion/exclusion criteria may further contribute to studying older people who are "physiologically young" relative to their chronological age and atypical of their age group. Chronological age has been proposed to be less important than the overall rate of physiological aging in determining how melatonin rhythms change over the lifespan (Muehlroth & Werkle-Bergner, 2020).

Age differences in the amplitudes of other circadian rhythms have been documented. Sleep propensity rhythms were compared between younger (19–26 years) and older (65–78 years) participants when they were given 7 min sleep opportunities every 20 min across the day and night. The older group showed greatly reduced sleep amounts during the nighttime opportunities, reflecting a reduced intensity of sleep drive during that phase (Haimov & Lavie, 1997).

A similar study compared sleep propensity and body temperature rhythms between older and younger participants (average ages: 76 vs. 23 years) when they experienced 30 min sleep opportunities (lights out and lying down) alternating with 60 min wake periods (lights on and out of bed) continuously for 60 h. There was a reduced amplitude in the rhythm of sleep propensity in the older group, as reflected in multiple measures of sleep, but there was no apparent reduction in the amplitude of the daily body temperature rhythm (Buysse et al., 2005). Masking effects on body temperature resulting from changes in posture, activity, and light exposure during the sleep and wake periods may have obscured differences in temperature rhythmicity, as suggested by the results of the study described below that was designed to eliminate masking effects.

This study used a forced desynchronization protocol (see Section 3.5.2) during which sleep opportunities of 9 h 20 min length were scheduled every 28 h for 18–23 cycles. This allowed assessment of body temperature rhythms independently of potential masking effects of light, activity, or posture. Unmasked circadian temperature rhythms of older (average age 68) and younger (average age 23) participants were studied with minimal contrast in illumination during the wake and sleep phases to reduce the possibility of photic masking effects on temperature. Under these conditions, the amplitudes of the unmasked circadian body temperature rhythms of older people were smaller than those of younger people, and temperatures were lower overall (Duffy et al., 1998) (**Figure 8.16**). These results are consistent with the conclusion that the unmasked amplitude of several SCN-driven rhythms is reduced in older people.

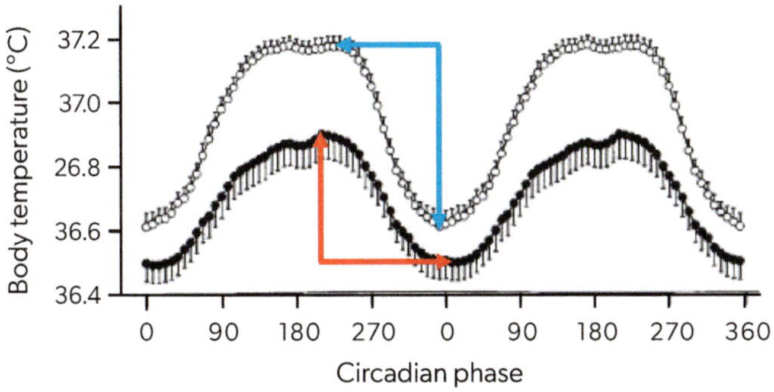

Figure 8.16 The mean (±SEM) body temperature rhythms in groups of participants who were younger (white symbols) and older (black symbols), plotted against circadian phase, with circadian phase 0 corresponding to the low point of the body temperature rhythm. Data are shown as mean values/30 min intervals +/- SEM and are double-plotted (= 2 circadian cycles) to facilitate visualization of the patterns. Participants were studied in a forced desynchronization protocol involving 28 h "days" to unmask the endogenous circadian rhythm of body temperature. Average body temperature was consistently lower in the older participants. The peak-to-trough amplitude of the temperature rhythm in the younger group (blue arrows) was ~0.58° C, and that of the older group (red arrows) was ~0.40° C, representing a ~31% reduction in the unmasked circadian rhythm amplitude in older people. Adapted with permission of the American Physiological Society from Duffy J.F. et al. (1998) Later endogenous circadian temperature nadir relative to an earlier wake time in older people. *Am J Physiol* 275:R1478–R1487. © American Physiological Society (1998); permission conveyed through Copyright Clearance Center, Inc. doi: 10.1152/ajpregu.1998.275.5.r1478.

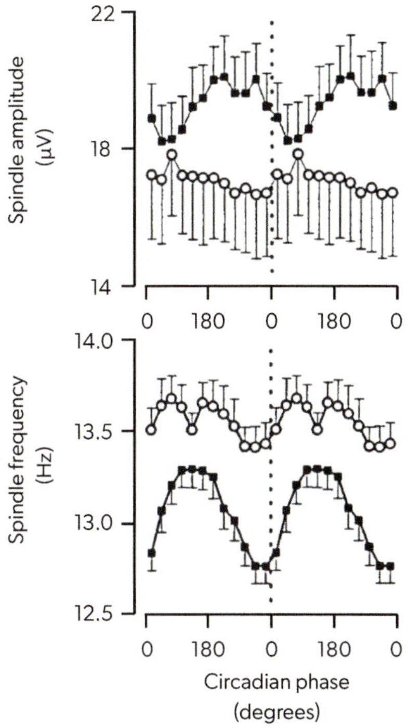

Figure 8.17 Reduction of the circadian variation in sleep spindle amplitudes (top) and in the dominant frequency of spindles (bottom) in older people (white symbols) compared to young people (black symbols) during a forced desynchronization protocol. Data are double-plotted to show two circadian cycles against circadian phase (X axis) shown in degrees of a cycle with 0 degrees representing the lowest average body temperature. Note that the average dominant frequency and the average amplitude of spindles differed between groups, and that the unmasked circadian variation in each measure was much smaller in the older group. Adapted with permission of Elsevier, Ltd. from Wei, H.G. et al. Attenuated amplitude of circadian and sleep-dependent modulation of electroencephalographic sleep spindle characteristics in elderly human subjects. *Neurosci Lett* 260:29–32. © Elsevier (1999). doi: 10.1016/s0304-3940(98)00851-9.

In addition to rhythms of sleep propensity, rest-activity, melatonin production, and body temperature, other rhythms have also been reported to show reduced amplitudes in older people (Dijk et al., 2000). These include rhythms of urinary output (Duffy et al., 2016); the dominant frequency of sleep spindles (**Figure 8.17**) (Wei et al., 1999); other features of sleep under free-running and entrained conditions (Weitzman et al., 1982); cortisol and several other hormones (van Coevorden et al., 1991); gene expression rhythms (Talamanca et al., 2023); and human performance (Duffy et al., 1998).

8.4.4 Aging effects on rhythmicity of the SCN

A different approach to studying aging effects on circadian rhythm amplitude is to measure the rhythmicity of the SCN itself, which can be done most directly in animal models, although there is also relevant human data. There have been reports in rodent studies of reduced amplitude during aging of physiological rhythms controlled by the SCN, including sleep, and of the rhythmicity of the SCN itself (Cai & Wise, 1996; Li & Satinoff, 1995; Rosenberg et al., 1979; Satinoff et al., 1993). The amplitude of SCN firing-rate rhythms recorded from intact mice in vivo, for example, was reduced as early as middle age (Nakamura et al., 2011) (**Figure 8.18**).

A study of dissociated SCN neurons in culture also found lower amplitude and more irregular firing-rate rhythms in individual SCN neurons taken from middle-aged vs. young mice (Aujard et al., 2001). In another mouse study conducted in vivo, disrupted sleep–wake rhythms in older mice were associated with reduced amplitudes of firing-rate rhythms, dissociated rhythms among SCN neurons, and abnormal electrophysiological features that could disrupt communication among neurons (Farajnia et al., 2012).

Another approach to evaluating how aging affects pacemaker rhythmicity is to study daily rhythms of peptide levels in the SCN. Postmortem immunocytochemical studies in both rats and humans demonstrated reductions with

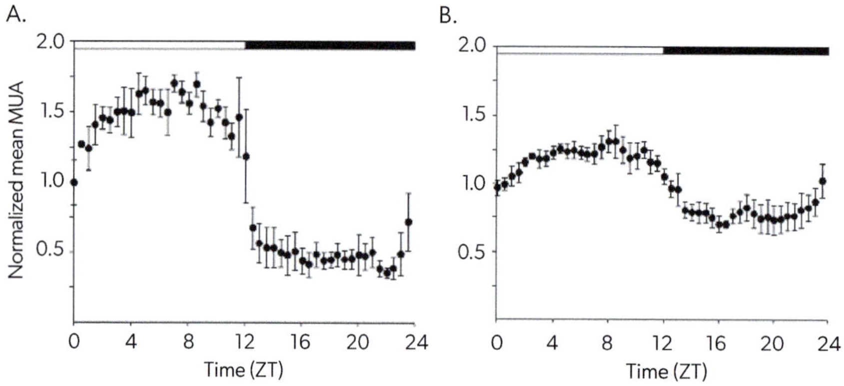

Figure 8.18 Multiple unit activity (MUA) (Y axis) recorded from neurons in the SCN of (**A**) young (~4 months old) and (**B**) middle-aged (~15 months old) mice averaged over 5 days in light-dark conditions (indicated at the top), plotted against time of day (X axis). There was a large reduction in the amplitude of the MUA rhythm in the older mice, implying a reduced output signal from the SCN to its efferent targets. Reprinted with permission of the Society for Neuroscience from Nakamura, T.J. et al. (2011) Age-related decline in circadian output. *J Neurosci* 31:10201–10205. © The Authors (2011). doi: 10.1523/JNEUROSCI.0451-11.2011.

aging in several measures related to SCN peptides. These included reduced numbers of VP-immunoreactive (VP-ir) neurons; reduced amplitude of the daily rhythm of VP-ir in the SCN (**Figure 8.19**); reduced number of VIP-ir cells; reduced levels and lost rhythmicity of VIP mRNA; and reduced rhythmicity of mRNA for a VIP receptor (Chee et al., 1988; Hofman & Swaab, 1994; Kalló et al., 2004; Kalsbeek et al., 2010; Swaab et al., 1985).

Reductions in the number of VP neurons in the SCN or their content of VP could have several different effects on circadian rhythms. VP acts within the SCN to maintain rhythm integrity, and VP-ir neurons form some of the principal projections from the SCN to other brain regions. Genetic deletion of one class of VP receptors in mice resulted in disruption of activity rhythms in constant darkness (Li et al., 2009). Loss of this receptor can also affect behavior indirectly by reducing the expression of the gene that codes for PK2, an efferent signal from the SCN that affects activity rhythms (see Section 8.3.2) (Li et al., 2009). VP helps sustain robust circadian rhythms that resist rapid resetting by external signals, so knockout of VP receptors in mice resulted in more rapid shifts of behavioral and molecular rhythms (Yamaguchi et al., 2013).

The importance of VP signaling for the integrity of behavioral rhythms is supported by evidence that the amount of VP-ir staining in their SCNs of common voles (*Microtus arvalis*) was correlated with spontaneous differences in the strength of their circadian activity rhythms (Gerkema et al., 1994). The critical factor determining whether voles showed circadian behavioral rhythms appeared to be the rhythmic release of VP from SCN neurons onto target systems. Voles that showed daily rhythms of VP-ir in the SCN also generated daily activity rhythms. Behaviorally arrhythmic voles instead

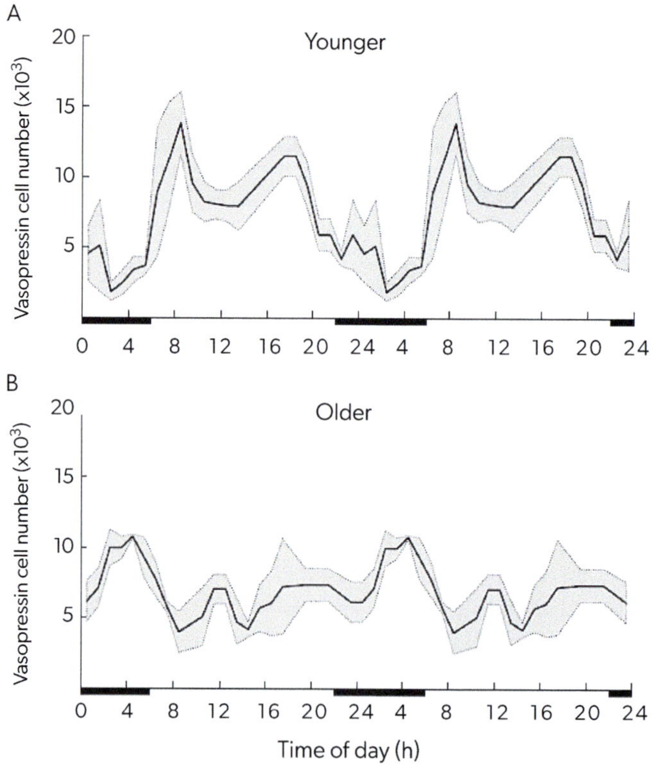

Figure 8.19 A smoothed, double-plot (48 h) of the average number (±SEM) of vasopressin-immunoreactive neurons (Y axis) in postmortem preparations of the suprachiasmatic nuclei from people who were younger (6–46 years) (Top) and older (50–91 years) (Bottom). Data are plotted against the reported clock time of death (X axis). Individuals had died because of various acute and chronic diseases or accidents. Reprinted with permission of Elsevier, Ltd. from Hofman, M.A. & Swaab, D.F. (1994) Alterations in circadian rhythmicity of the vasopressin-producing neurons of the human suprachiasmatic nucleus (SCN) with aging. *Brain Res* 651:134–142. © Elsevier (1994). doi: 10.1016/0006-8993(94)90689-0.

had continuously high levels of VP-ir in the SCN, probably because of reductions in its rhythmic release from the SCN, onto its efferent targets (Jansen et al., 2007).

In addition to a reduction in the amplitude of the daily rhythm of SCN VP-ir among older people (see **Figure 8.19**) (Hofman & Swaab, 1994; Swaab et al., 1985), there is a profound reduction in the amount of SCN VP-ir in dementia patients who died with Alzheimer's disease (AD) (Harper et al., 2008; Swaab et al., 1985; Wu et al., 2007). Patients with AD often show earlier and more severe disruptions of sleep–wake cycles and circadian organization than healthy controls (see Section 15.5). Increased fragmentation of activity in dementia patients, as recorded months before death, was associated with lower numbers of VP-ir neurons in the SCN in postmortem studies (Harper et al., 2008).

VIP-ir neurons in the ventral SCN are the target of retinal projections containing glutamate, the peptide PACAP, and melanopsin, which convey light information that entrains circadian rhythms (Hannibal et al., 2002; van den Pol & Tsujimoto, 1985). In aged rats, the density of both VIP and PACAP receptors in the SCN were decreased (Kalló et al., 2004), which could reduce the impact of the lighting cycle on daily rhythms and alter their entrainment. Loss of either VIP or of its receptors also disrupted the firing-rate rhythms of SCN neurons as well as behavioral rhythms expressed under constant conditions (Aton et al., 2005; Aton & Herzog, 2005; Piggins & Cutler, 2003).

Thus, VIP neurons play an important role in maintaining the synchrony of SCN oscillators and the integrity and amplitude of circadian signaling from the SCN to other brain regions. Reduced VIP signaling during aging could therefore contribute to reduced amplitude of sleep and other daily rhythms. One postmortem study of the SCN involved people who had died with or without AD (at about age 90) and had been studied with actigraphy within the preceding 18 months. There was a robust positive correlation between the number of VIP-ir neurons in the SCN and greater amplitude of the daily activity rhythm (Wang et al., 2015). This study did not find significant correlations of VP-ir neuron numbers with the amplitude of behavioral rhythms, nor any difference in activity rhythm parameters between those with and without AD, except for a large delay in activity onset in those with AD. The differences from other studies with respect to SCN VP-ir and rhythmicity may be related to differences in the methods used to estimate VP-ir cell numbers.

These lines of evidence suggest that both aging and the brain damage that occurs in AD can disrupt the circadian organization of sleep–wake and other rhythms. Contributors to the observed changes include reduced amplitude of circadian pacemaker oscillation (as seen in VP-ir levels and in reduced and disrupted electrophysiological rhythms) combined with loss of VIP cells and reduced photic signaling to the circadian system (Hofman & Swaab, 2006). The interpretation that reduced photic signaling during aging has a negative effect on expression of daily rhythms is supported by evidence that increased daytime light exposure helped consolidate sleep and rest-activity rhythms in some older patients with dementia, including those with AD (Ancoli-Israel et al., 2003; Van Someren et al., 1997).

Decreases in VP-ir and VIP-ir could reflect either reduced VP/VIP cell numbers or a loss of peptide production from unchanged cell numbers. Some studies of aging rats and monkeys indicated that there was little cell loss in the SCN, suggesting that reduced VP production accounts for the decrease in immunoreactivity observed in other studies (Madeira et al., 1995). The brains of people who died with dementia, however, provided anatomical evidence consistent with actual cell loss in the SCN (Harper et al., 2008).

Other studies reached contradictory conclusions about whether the loss of VP occurs in aging without dementia as well as in AD patients, or only in AD patients (Lim et al., 2014; Wu & Swaab, 2007). A study that reported a correlation between reduced VP neuron numbers and disrupted activity rhythms did not detect an association with the amplitude of rhythms. Amplitudes of both body temperature and activity rhythms were instead correlated with reduced numbers of neurons containing neurotensin (Harper et al., 2008), a peptide that is also found in the human dorsal SCN (Mai et al., 1991). Different conclusions among these studies are likely related to the use of different methods to estimate the loss of neurons and peptides.

Regardless of whether VP and VIP are lost from the SCN because of cell death or because of reduced peptide production or release from surviving cells, the net effect would be to have less peptide release both within the SCN and at its efferent targets. Extrapolating from the results of animal studies in which SCN VP and VIP systems were experimentally disrupted, aging would be expected to produce a combination of impaired rhythmicity in individual SCN neurons, reduced synchrony of the SCN neuronal population, and a reduced amplitude of synchronizing signals from the SCN to target tissues (Aton et al., 2005; Aton & Herzog, 2005; Jansen et al., 2007; Piggins & Cutler, 2003).

These predictions are supported by electrophysiological recordings in vivo and in vitro from the SCN. These studies found an age-related reduction in the amplitude of SCN firing-rate rhythms in mice (Leise et al., 2013; Nakamura et al., 2011) (see **Figure 8.18**) that was attributable to reduced synchrony of circadian rhythms among individual SCN neurons (Ramkisoensing & Meijer, 2015). In vitro studies also found lower amplitude free-running rhythms of expression of the circadian clock gene *period2* in SCN tissue from old mice compared to young mice (Nakamura et al., 2015). The low-amplitude, disrupted rhythm of VP content of the SCN detected postmortem in older people (Hofman & Swaab, 1994) (see **Figure 8.19**) is consistent with the evidence from animal studies of a reduction in the amplitude of SCN pacemaker rhythmicity and outputs.

Lower amplitude signals from the SCN pacemaker likely contribute to the expression of less robust behavioral and physiological rhythms during aging, at least in some older people (Ramkisoensing & Meijer, 2015). It is also possible that circadian oscillations in other tissues decline in amplitude or in responsiveness to SCN input during aging, which would also contribute to reductions in the amplitude of measurable rhythms (see Monk, 2005; Yamazaki et al., 2002). A reduction in the strength of SCN signals reaching target structures could also contribute to weaker sleep and wake maintenance zones, which are a product of the circadian system (Deboer et al., 2004; Strogatz et al., 1987a; Zeitzer et al., 2003; Zhang et al., 2004). The predicted result of this weakening would be a shift toward earlier timing of both sleep onset and morning waking in older people.

8.4.5 Summary

One consistently observed feature of sleep in older people is an advance in the timing of both sleep onset and waking. Among the factors potentially contributing to these changes are altered waveforms of circadian rhythms (e.g., body temperature); a shift in timing of sleep relative to the circadian pacemaker; reduced phase-shifting effects of light and other stimuli; increased morning light exposure because of earlier awakening; and reductions in the strength of circadian inputs that generate the sleep and wake maintenance zones.

Aging results in reduced photic input to the retina because of cataract formation and yellowing of the lens, which could contribute to reduced entraining effects of light and altered phases of sleep timing. Although reduced phase-shifting effects of light have been reported in older people and animals, changes in phase-shifting and in sleep timing do not appear to be related primarily to altered light input. Phase-shifts in response to non-photic stimuli were also reduced in older animals, suggesting that the effects of aging are more related to changes in the pacemaker than to altered photic input.

Comparisons between age groups of behavioral and physiological rhythms in people show mixed results across studies. Most studies reported reduced amplitudes in several physiological and behavioral rhythms in older people, including rhythms of melatonin production and body temperature that are closely tied to the circadian pacemaker.

Discrepancies among studies may reflect individual differences in the effects of aging on the circadian system and the impact of the inclusion and exclusion criteria used in these studies. Cross-sectional comparisons of people of different ages are challenging in part because of the exclusion criteria that must be applied to participants in demanding experimental protocols, which affect different age groups to varying extents. Nevertheless, studies using constant routines and forced desynchronization protocols, which control for a number of these potential confounding factors, generally found lower amplitude physiological rhythms in older people.

Several changes in SCN function have been reported to occur during aging in both people and animals, which are likely to weaken circadian modulation of sleep and waking. These changes include reduced amplitude and integrity of SCN neuronal firing-rate rhythms in animal models; reduced VP amounts or release; reduced prokineticin 2 signaling; lower VIP and neurotensin levels; reduced mRNA levels for VIP and its receptors; reduced number of detectable VP-ir and VIP-ir neurons; and reduced light input reaching the SCN from the retina.

Less robust circadian signals from the SCN would be less effective in consolidating sleep and waking and restricting them to separate circadian phases. As a result, older people would be predicted to show reduced activation and an increased tendency to nap during the day as well as less-consolidated sleep at night. In AD patients, who often develop severe sleep–wake disruptions as the disease progresses, there is evidence of reductions of VP-ir in the SCN beyond those attributable to age.

Changes to the organization and circadian patterning of sleep and waking are linked to the degree of integrity of the SCN pacemaker system in different situations. The reduced amplitude of signaling from the SCN during healthy aging reduces the amplitude of sleep–wake and other rhythms. Damage to the SCN as a result of neural degeneration in patients with advanced AD results in severely disrupted sleep–wake rhythms. Total ablation of the SCN in experimental animals produces a complete loss of circadian regulation of sleep and waking.

8.5 Are older people less affected by sleep loss?

The evidence summarized in the preceding sections can help clarify interpretation of other findings related to sleep and aging. One surprising finding is that older research participants often show less impact of sleep loss on alertness and cognitive performance than do younger participants. The evidence supporting this conclusion comes from two kinds of studies: 1) After acute sleep restriction, older people show less impairment of daytime performance and less daytime sleepiness than younger people. 2) When kept awake for a full 24 h, older people show fewer performance deficits during the night and are less likely to fall asleep unintentionally. The following sections review some of the related evidence and its interpretation.

8.5.1 Daytime sleepiness after sleep loss

Population-based surveys indicate that older people take more daytime naps than younger people (Ohayon & Zulley, 1999). One possible explanation is that older people have more disrupted sleep and produce less N3 or REM sleep overnight, especially among older men, which does not satisfy their homeostatic sleep needs. Daytime naps could then serve as a compensatory response to inadequate nighttime sleep. This idea was tested in a study involving healthy people who were younger (20–30 years), middle-aged (40–55 years), or older (66–83 years).

As expected, during a baseline night, older participants slept less at night, had less N3, more awakenings and more wake after sleep onset (WASO). Daytime sleepiness was then assessed during the next day with Multiple Sleep Latency Tests (MSLTs; see Section 2.7). In contrast to the prediction that older participants with objectively lower quality sleep during the preceding night would fall asleep faster during the day, they had significantly longer sleep onset latencies during five daytime nap opportunities than young and middle-aged participants (Dijk et al., 2010) (**Figure 8.20**).

A potential explanation is that older people have a weaker homeostatic drive for sleep, accounting for both less N3 and total sleep at night and longer latencies to fall asleep during the day. To test their homeostatic drive, the same participants also had their N3 sleep deliberately disrupted for 2 nights. Participants in all groups responded with similar decreases in their MSLT latencies the next day, indicating that the older participants did not have a deficit in homeostatic responses to reduced N3 sleep (Dijk et al., 2010). Another study measured daytime sleep latencies using MSLTs on younger (~24 years) and older participants (~83 years) before and after a night of total sleep deprivation. The older participants shortened their daytime sleep latencies after sleep loss by at least as much as the younger participants, consistent with an intact homeostatic response (Reynolds et al., 1991).

The sleepiness of older people was also assessed using the Maintenance of Wakefulness Test (MWT) (Sullivan & Kushida, 2008), in which participants are given instructions to *not* fall asleep while they sit comfortably in bed during daytime tests of up to 40 min each, typically in very dim light. Younger and older women were studied using the MWT twice daily during 3 consecutive days after being restricted to 4 h sleep during each preceding night. No one fell asleep during MWTs on a baseline day, but young women fell asleep frequently during tests on days following sleep restriction, while older women rarely did. Older women also showed little change in self-reported sleepiness and no systematic change in tests of vigilance. Younger women, however, reported progressively increased sleepiness and decreased vigilance, especially following the third restriction night (Stenuit & Kerkhofs, 2005). Thus, older women showed reduced daytime sleepiness and vigilance impairment compared to younger women after repeated sleep restriction.

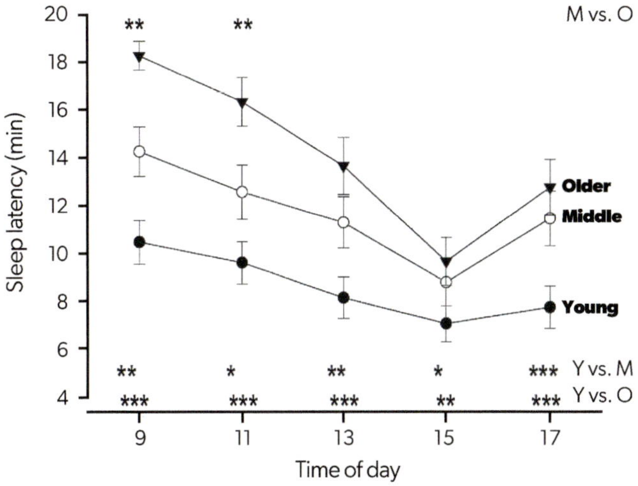

Figure 8.20 Results of Multiple Sleep Latency Tests that were given at the times indicated on the X axis for participants who were Young (Y: mean ~25 years; black circles), Middle-Aged (M: mean ~48 years; white circles) and Older (O: mean ~71 years; black triangles). Statistically significant differences in the comparisons indicated are shown by *, **, ***, indicating p values of <.05, <.01 and <.001, respectively. Latencies to fall asleep during these daytime tests were significantly longer in older participants at all times tested, especially for the Young vs. Older comparisons (Y vs. O), which were significant at all times tested, despite older participants having objectively poorer sleep quality during the preceding night. Reprinted with permission of Oxford University Press from Dijk D.-J. et al. (2010) Age-related reduction in daytime sleep propensity and nocturnal slow wave sleep. *Sleep* 33:211–223. © Sleep Research Society (2010); permission conveyed through Copyright Clearance Center, Inc. doi: 10.1093/sleep/33.2.211.

Findings from these studies that older people show less objective and subjective evidence of sleepiness during the day than younger participants seem inconsistent with self-reports (Reynolds et al., 1991) and population-based survey studies (Foley et al., 1995; Ohayon & Zulley, 1999), indicating frequent daytime napping by older participants. One potential contributor to this finding is that older participants in laboratory studies constitute an unusually healthy sample drawn from the population they represent.

For example, inclusion in one study required that older participants not take medications that might affect sleep, have no major illnesses or sleep complaints, and have a regular bedtime between 22:00 and midnight (Dijk et al., 2010). In contrast, in the general population, people in this age group (66-83 years) often have a variety of chronic illnesses, take multiple medications, have frequent sleep complaints, and have earlier habitual bedtimes (Foley et al., 1995). Although some older participants in one of these studies took a variety of medications, they were also reported to be vigorous, physically active, and socially engaged (Reynolds et al., 1991).

Older women have better preserved sleep quality than older men (Rediehs et al., 1990); see Section 4.6. It is, therefore, possible that inclusion of a larger number of older women in studies could bias results toward showing less daytime sleepiness than suggested by population-based studies. In one study reviewed above, the older and younger groups were 81% and 52% female, respectively (Dijk et al., 2010). In another, there was a somewhat higher proportion of women in the older group (55%) than in the younger group (38%) (Reynolds et al., 1991), and a third study included only women in both groups (Stenuit & Kerkhofs, 2005). Regardless of differences in the proportions of women in the older groups, all three studies reported that older participants had less subjective and objective daytime sleepiness after sleep loss than younger participants.

An alternative interpretation might be that the latency to fall asleep is simply not a good measure of actual sleepiness, despite the fact that MSLT latencies are reliably related to cumulative sleep loss that is produced in different ways (Carskadon & Dement, 1981; Carskadon & Dement, 1987); see Section 13.2.2. The lengthened sleep latencies of older participants could, instead, reflect an impaired ability to initiate and maintain sleep, despite being subjectively very "sleepy." This interpretation, however, cannot explain other findings; namely, that older people self-report less daytime sleepiness than young people after overnight sleep loss and, as discussed in the next section, show fewer deficits in vigilance and performance tests.

8.5.2 Performance during and after sleep loss

Another set of surprising age-related differences relate to how cognitive performance is affected by sleep loss. Studies have included both nighttime tests during sustained waking and daytime tests after overnight sleep restriction. Older women showed a small decrement in performance on vigilance tests[7] after one night of restriction to 4 h sleep, but their performance remained stable after 2 and 3 nights of similar sleep restriction. Young women, however, showed progressively worse performance over the 3 days of restriction (Stenuit & Kerkhofs, 2005). Similarly, young men (~23 years) were compared to older men (~67 years) on a test of simulated driving performance during mid-afternoon after one night with 5 h sleep. Compared to the older group, the younger men reported more subjective sleepiness, had more driving errors, and showed a larger increase in alpha and theta frequencies in their EEGs (consistent with increased sleepiness) (Filtness et al., 2012).

In contrast to these results, a study comparing women in their 20s to those in their 60s found no difference in the decline in PVT lapses during hours 24–40 of continuous sleep loss. However, younger women showed large increases in "false starts" (anticipatory responses), while older women showed no increases, suggesting differences in motivation or strategy related to task performance during sleep loss. After an 8 h recovery sleep, younger women were also sleepier than the older women and continued to show more false starts (Urrila et al., 2007).

Thus, older people in many studies show less impact of sleep loss on daytime performance than younger people, just as they show less increase in apparent sleepiness (assessed by self-report, MWTs, and MSLTs). These results could suggest that older people need less sleep to function optimally, so their performance is less affected by sleep loss; however, there are alternative interpretations.

In evaluating daytime studies of alertness and performance, it is important to consider the times at which participants were tested. When men were given frequent, very short sleep opportunities throughout a 24 h day, older men showed a weaker tendency to fall asleep than younger men in early morning hours but a stronger tendency to fall asleep in the evening hours (Haimov & Lavie, 1997). Consistent with this age-related difference in sleepiness at different times of day, young women reported more sleepiness than older women in the morning after 3 nights of sleep restricted to 5 h. They also showed slower reaction times than older women on a test of sustained attention in the morning, but the size of these differences in performance and self-reported sleepiness decreased during tests later in the afternoon (Stenuit & Kerkhofs, 2005).

These results reflect the fact that morning tests occurred at a preferred phase for older people, who are typically early risers and tend to have morning chronotypes, but at the least preferred phase for younger people, who typically have more delayed chronotypes (May et al., 1993; Roenneberg et al., 2004) (see Chapter 4). None of these studies included late evening tests, which would likely have favored younger participants. Therefore, some of the apparently reduced impact of sleep loss on older participants may be attributable to testing them at their more preferred circadian phase, in contrast to the younger participants. In one study showing no effect of age on PVT lapses during sleep loss, tests were given every 2 h over 38 h of waking, so they would have overlapped all circadian

[7] The test used in this and many other studies was the Psychomotor Vigilance Test. It is described and discussed in detail in Section 13.3.1.

phases of both groups (Urrila et al., 2007). This procedure may have contributed to less apparent benefit for performance of older participants than in studies involving only morning tests.

Tests of simulated driving after sleep restriction, however, which showed better performance in older participants, were conducted in mid-afternoon (Filtness et al., 2012), which could be considered a relatively neutral time with respect to circadian phase preferences. Thus, there is consistent evidence that daytime alertness and performance in older people are less affected by prior sleep loss than younger people. However, the apparent extent of these age-related differences may be influenced by the time of day of testing, given the characteristic differences in chronotype of different age groups.

A second method that has been used frequently to study the impact of sleep loss is to keep participants awake continuously for a 24 h period or longer and to evaluate performance at different times during the sleep deprivation period. One study that used this approach compared vigilance performance between participants who were younger (18–29 years) and older (65–76 years) while they stayed awake for 26 h. During hours 16–24 of continuous waking (approximately their usual sleep period), the older group showed less impaired performance than the younger group, were less likely to fall asleep unintentionally, and reported less subjective sleepiness. These results were surprising because sleep recordings during a baseline night before sleep deprivation showed that the older group had poorer sleep quality than the younger group. A night of worse sleep would be expected to make people more sensitive to the impact of further sleep loss, yet the older group showed less subjective and objective sleepiness during the next day (**Figure 8.21**) (Duffy et al., 2009).

In a similar study, older men (~66 years) showed less impairment in vigilance performance than younger men (~25 years) during a 40 h sleep deprivation procedure (Adam et al., 2006). In this study and others (e.g., Bonnet & Rosa, 1987), older people showed fewer performance deficits when they were kept awake and tested at night and were less likely to fall asleep. These results are consistent with findings from daytime studies that the vigilance performance of older people is less affected by sleep loss. However, interpreting these results depends on distinguishing the impacts of circadian phase and of sleep loss on performance and sleepiness, as discussed in the following section.

8.5.3 Sleep-circadian confounds

Studies of performance during sustained sleep loss suggest that losing sleep causes fewer deficits in vigilance and less subjective sleepiness in older than younger people. The results of a study of performance during 40 h of waking (**Figure 8.22**) (Adam et al., 2006), however, point to a different interpretation. During the first ~15 h of testing, both groups showed a similar number of lapses (failures to respond to a stimulus within the allowed time window), but young participants responded significantly more quickly to the stimuli than the older group.

Starting at ~16 h of waking (beginning of the usual sleep phase), there was a steep decline in the performance of the younger group, which involved both increased lapses (solid red arrow, bottom panel, **Figure 8.22**) and slower average responses to the stimuli (solid red arrow, top panel, **Figure 8.22**) than in the older group. This trend continued until they had been awake for about 25 h, at the beginning of the next subjective day. The older participants showed much less decline in performance during the interval of 16–25 h of waking (green arrows, **Figure 8.22**). This difference in the rate of decline during the subjective night resulted in older participants performing better than younger participants during this phase. Self-reported sleepiness followed a similar pattern with older men reporting significantly less sleepiness during hours 21–31 of waking.

If sleep loss caused the decline in performance in young men, their performance should have continued to deteriorate throughout the 25–40 h interval, during which sleep loss continued to accumulate. Instead, their performance gradually improved during the later hours of sustained waking (subjective day phase; dashed red arrows, **Figure 8.22**), until it did not differ significantly from that of the older participants after 40 h of sleep deprivation. Among older participants, after a shallow decline during the subjective night, performance remained essentially stable during the following subjective day (Adam et al., 2006).

These results indicate that performance differences between groups were not a result of differences in response to sleep loss alone but also reflected differences between the groups in the circadian modulation of vigilance performance and subjective sleepiness. The cause of the steep decline in performance in young people after 16 h of waking is ambiguous. It could be the result of being kept awake for longer than 16 h or the result of the impact of a circadian mechanism that promotes sleep during the subjective night phase, or both. The steady improvement in performance in young participants beginning at about 08:00 (i.e., after 25 h awake), despite continued and accumulating sleep loss, is unambiguous. If sleep loss were the critical factor, their performance should have continued to deteriorate, but instead it improved steadily up to the end of the study at hour 40.

This initial deterioration and later improvement in performance reflect the impact of robust circadian modulation of alertness as young participants passed through their subjective night and day phases. This observation is consistent with what Patrick and Gilbert had reported in 1896 about their young participants: that during sustained wakefulness, sleepiness reached a peak near dawn, but alertness increased as the day

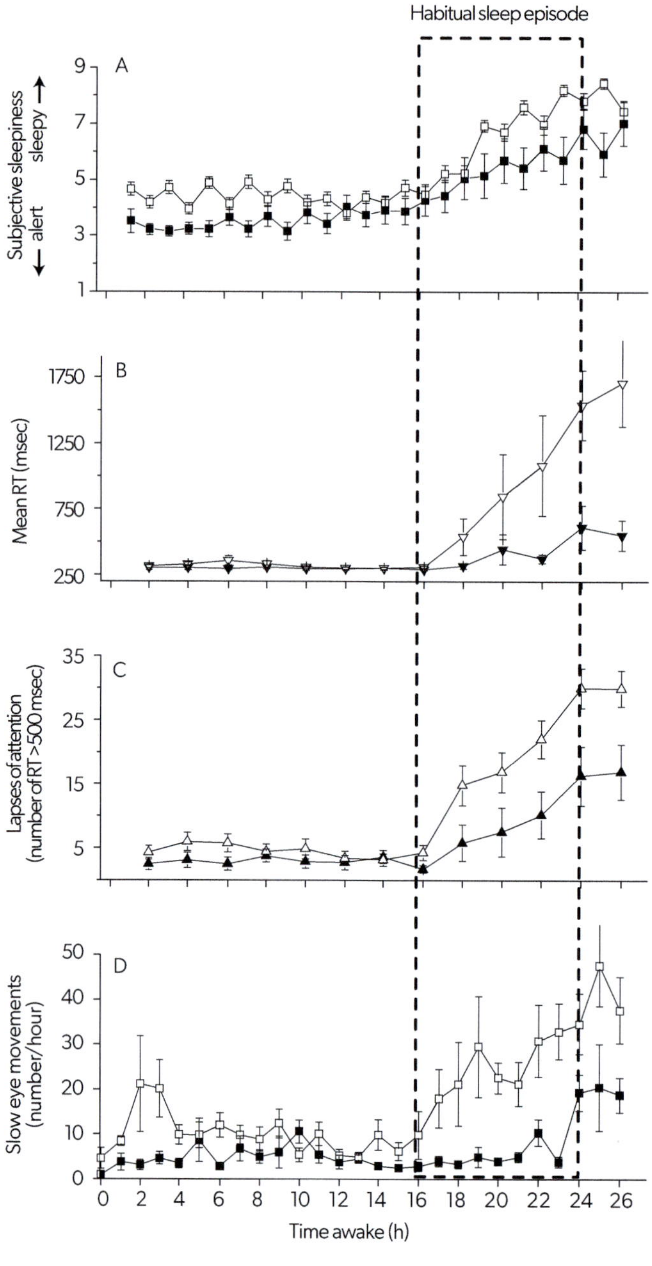

Figure 8.21 Young participants (18–29 years; white symbols) and older participants (65–76 years; black symbols) were kept awake for 26 h and tested for their vigilance performance and sleepiness; the area outlined with dashes indicates the habitual sleep period. **A.** Self-reported sleepiness was higher in the young participants, especially at night. **B.** Average response latencies in the vigilance task rose throughout the night in young people but showed only a slight change in older people. **C.** Lapses of attention during the vigilance task similarly rose steeply during the night in young people and less so in the older group. **D.** Slow, rolling eye movements while awake at night (a marker of sleepiness) increased more in the younger than in the older participants. The test of sustained attention used in this study was the Psychomotor Vigilance Test; see the text in Section 13.3.1 for a description of the test and of the measures represented in panels B and C. Reprinted with permission of John Wiley and Sons from Duffy, J.F. et al. (2009) Healthy older adults better tolerate sleep deprivation than young adults. *J Am Geriatr Soc* 57:1245–1251. © The Authors; Journal compilation © The American Geriatrics Society (2009); permission conveyed through Copyright Clearance Center, Inc. doi: 10.1111/j.1532-5415.2009.02303.x.

progressed, despite continuing sleep deprivation (see Chapter 6). This interpretation is also supported by evidence from a number of studies involving cognitive performance in young participants that are reviewed in Section 13.5.

The older participants did not show a similarly steep decline in performance at the beginning of the subjective night; nor did they show similar, gradual improvement during the next subjective day. These results support the interpretation that

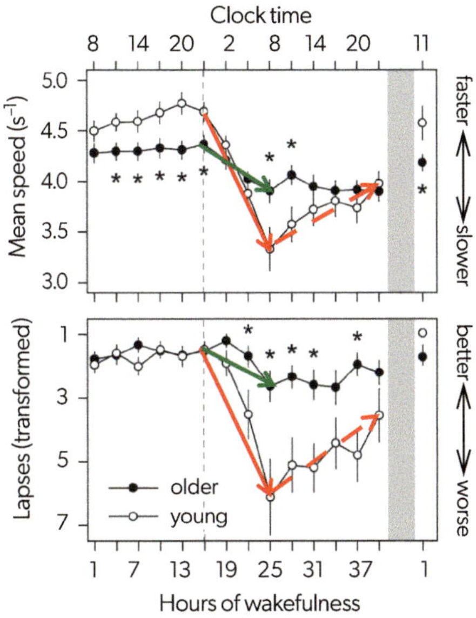

Figure 8.22 Speed of responses (top panel) and number of lapses (bottom panel) shown by young men (mean age 25; white symbols) and older men (mean age 66; black symbols) on Psychomotor Vigilance Tests during 40 h of continuous waking. Asterisks mark significant group differences. Note that the data for lapses are plotted inversely so that worse performance is shown by changes in the same direction (downward) for both speed of responses and lapses of attention. Young men showed steep declines in performance (solid red arrows) over hours 15–25 of waking, followed by a a shallower rise during hours 25–40 (dashed red arrows). Older men showed a a much less severe decline in performance (green arrows) and relatively stable performance during hours 25–40. Young men showed faster responses than older men when tested during daytime (up to hour 16: vertical line) but performed more poorly when kept awake during the subjective night. Their performance recovered during the second subjective day (after hour 25) to be equivalent to that of older men by the end of the study (hour 40). The gray bar indicates a 10.5 h opportunity for recovery sleep, and the symbols to the right of the bar represent performance recovery to normal daytime levels the next morning, 1 h after waking from their recovery sleep opportunity. Adapted with permission of Oxford University Press from Adam, M. et al. (2006) Age-related changes in the time course of vigilant attention during 40 hours without sleep in men. *Sleep* 29:55–57. © Sleep Research Society (2006); permission conveyed through Copyright Clearance Center, Inc. doi: 10.1093/sleep/29.1.55.

the differences between the two age groups resulted primarily from weak circadian modulation of both sleepiness and alertness in older participants and strong circadian modulation in younger participants.

Similar evidence was not available in the study involving 26 h of sleep deprivation (Duffy et al., 2009) (see **Figure 8.21**) because it did not extend substantially into a second subjective day. The independent influences of sleep loss and of circadian phase on performance during the night are completely confounded in studies extending over only about 24 h (see the discussion of this issue in Groeger et al., 2008). As a result, the reason for worse deterioration of performance in young people than in older people cannot be determined in ~24 h studies. But the results available in the 40 h study (**Figure 8.22**; see also Section 13.5) show clearly that older people perform better than young people when kept awake and tested at night because they are less affected by circadian phase, not because they are more resistant to the effects of sleep loss.

This interpretation is consistent with evidence that the amplitude of the circadian pacemaker's oscillation and of many measurable rhythms declines with age (see **Figures 8.15 to 8.19**). As a result, older people experience reduced promotion of arousal during the day and reduced promotion of sleep at night. Young people show a steep decline in performance when tested during their subjective night because their circadian system strongly promotes sleep during that phase, contributing to poor performance on tasks requiring attention and alertness. Older people show less performance impairment during that phase because their low-amplitude circadian rhythms produce a weaker sleep-promoting effect, not because they are less sensitive to the effects of sleep loss. Similarly, younger people experience a stronger circadian arousal signal during the day, which contributes to their better performance relative to older participants during daytime tests (see **Figure 8.22, top panel**).

The idea that the physiology of younger people is more affected by circadian phase is supported by the results of the forced desynchronization study discussed earlier (Section 8.4.3) (Duffy et al., 1998). Younger and older participants living with scheduled sleep opportunities at 28 h intervals to unmask effects of circadian rhythms were studied for their rates of calculation performance. Based on a figure in that publication showing the rates of calculation performance in both groups, one can estimate the peak-to-trough range of performance quality across a circadian cycle, calculated as standard deviations (Z scores) from their average performance during the wake phase.

For young people, the full peak-to-trough range of performance was ~1.25 standard deviations; for older participants, the range was only ~0.8 standard deviations. Thus, the amplitude of the performance rhythm in seniors, driven by an unmasked circadian mechanism, was only about 64% of that in young people. This value is remarkably similar to the estimated ratio of body-temperature rhythm amplitudes in these participants, shown in **Figure 8.16**. The young participants showed a total body temperature range of ~0.6°C across a circadian cycle, while the older group showed a range of ~0.4°C, which is 67% of the amplitude shown by the young group (Duffy et al., 1998).

A study of younger (~26 years) and older (~55 years) postmenopausal women undergoing alternating cycles of short (1 h each) wake and sleep opportunities for 48 h found a similar reduction in the amplitude of several rhythms in the older women. These included rhythms of melatonin levels, several sleep parameters, and post-nap alertness. Using the amplitude of the rhythm of sleep-onset latencies across nap opportunities as a measure of circadian variation in sleep promotion, the older women showed a rhythm amplitude that was 62% of that shown by younger women (Pérez-Medina-Carballo et al., 2022).[8]

Despite a general recognition that the circadian system is one of the two principal mechanisms influencing sleep propensity, its importance is not always considered in studying the effects of sleep loss on performance over 24 h periods. How performance changes during 24 h of sleep deprivation does not reflect the effects of sleep loss alone. The circadian impact on performance and alertness is critically involved, and its modification during aging accounts for much of the age-related difference in performance quality and sleepiness observed in these studies during sustained waking. Whether we can determine how much sleep loss (or excess waking) contributes to the observed deficits during extended waking and how much results from circadian modulation is discussed in **Box 8.2**.

8.5.4 Factors affecting sleep in aging

While the hypothesis of circadian amplitude decline in older people can account for many results in studies of sleepiness and performance during sleep loss, it cannot explain the longer latencies and reduced probability of sleep onset during daytime tests in seniors. Reduced promotion of arousal during the day in older people as a result of lower-amplitude input from the pacemaker would predict the opposite result—an increased probability of sleep onset. These findings may relate instead to changes in sleep-regulatory systems.

There is evidence, for example, that there are age-related changes in the capacity to generate sleep. One study explored this possibility by keeping older and younger participants in bed during 12 h overnight and during 4 h in the afternoon for a week in order to try to "saturate" sleep capacity (i.e., to achieve

[8] One study of healthy older and younger men also found a ~35% reduction in the amplitude of body temperature rhythms in older men under normal living conditions but, contrary to most results cited, this difference was lost under constant routine conditions. However, the study also reported large declines in performance and alertness in the younger men relative to the older men in the subjective night during the constant routine (Monk, 1991).

BOX 8.2 Estimating Effects of Sleep Loss Alone

Despite the confounding influence of circadian effects, it seems likely that extended sleep loss (or accumulated effects of waking) also affects alertness and performance. Can we estimate the degree to which sleep loss contributes to performance deficits independently of circadian phase? If the *only* factor affecting performance were circadian modulation, the prediction would be that performance at equivalent circadian times would be similar during two successive days spent awake. In other words, in a study conducted over 40 h of waking, performance should be similar at 24:00 on both days (e.g., hours 16 and 40 of waking) (Adam et al., 2006).

In fact, performance in that study was considerably worse at hour 40 than hour 16 using measures of lapses and response latencies in the younger group, and it was slightly worse in the older group (**Figure 8.22**). The difference in performance at equivalent circadian phases could be considered a rough measure of the impact of sleep loss itself, independent of the alerting or sleep-promoting effects of the circadian system.

Although this rough estimate suggests that younger participants were more impaired by sleep loss itself than older participants (in addition to the effects of circadian phase), it depends on the doubtful proposition that the effects of sleep loss and circadian phase are additive and act independently of each other. The evidence, however, indicates that is not the case.

For example, sleep loss in people appears to reduce the amplitude of circadian rhythms, so the circadian impact on performance would be smaller during sleep loss, and peak performance levels would be reduced. The evidence supporting this idea comes from studies of circadian rhythms of gene expression measured in blood samples obtained from people after chronic sleep restriction. Many gene products that oscillated during normal sleep conditions showed reduced oscillation amplitudes after sleep loss (Archer et al., 2014; Arnardottir et al., 2014; Möller-Levet et al., 2013).

Animal studies also provide several lines of evidence supporting the idea of cross-talk between circadian and sleep-regulatory systems:

- Adenosine is a critical regular of sleep homeostasis (see Section 11.5.1). Applications of adenosine to the SCN also affect the physiology of SCN neurons and alter circadian behavioral rhythms (Antle et al., 2001; Chen & van den Pol, 1997).

BOX 8.2 Continued

- The firing rates of individual SCN neurons recorded from intact rats changed systematically as they alternated between sleep and waking states across ultradian cycles (Deboer et al., 2003).
- A mutation in the *Clock* gene involved in generating circadian rhythms also affected sleep homeostasis (Naylor et al., 2000).
- Knock-outs of several clock genes altered homeostatic regulation of sleep, and sleep deprivation affected brain expression of core circadian clock genes (Franken, 2013).
- Acute sleep deprivation caused phase shifts of rodent circadian rhythms (Antle & Mistlberger, 2000).

Where these sleep-circadian interactions occur is not clear. Changes in SCN firing-rates during different sleep stages may reflect direct effects on the pacemaking system, but it is unknown which correlates of sleep states mediate these effects (e.g., body temperature, activity level). Other influences on regulation of core clock genes (e.g., *per* expression) occur in "peripheral" targets (which in this sense includes the cortex, for example) but not in the SCN (Abe et al., 2001; Wakamatsu et al., 2001).

Regardless of the targets affected and the mediators involved, the net result of these examples of overlapping physiological regulation is that they can influence behavioral measures. So it is not surprising that a study in humans concluded that sleep loss and circadian phase interact nonlinearly in their effects on performance (Van Dongen & Dinges, 2003). These crossover effects and nonlinear interactions indicate that we cannot assume that the behavioral effects of sleep loss and circadian phase are independent and additive, making it very difficult to accurately estimate the impact of sleep loss itself on performance during lengthy periods of sleep deprivation.

the maximum amount of sleep that can be generated in 24 h). The initial sleep durations were very long, probably reflecting homeostatic responses to chronic insufficient sleep before the study, but durations reached a stable value by the fifth day of the study.

Older participants slept less than younger participants from the beginning and never achieved similar total sleep durations throughout the week. Stable total sleep amounts at the end of the study were ~9 h daily in the younger group and ~7.5 h in the older group (Klerman & Dijk, 2008) (**Figure 8.23**). Thus, a reduced capacity to generate sleep may contribute to the longer sleep onset latencies of older participants during the day as well as to their shorter sleep durations at night. If the values achieved at steady-state by the end of the week of sleep extension represent the actual sleep needs (rather than only sleep capacity) of these groups, this may also contribute to differences in performance during sleep restriction. Being restricted to 4 h of sleep nightly, for example, would result in effectively less nightly sleep loss, relative to need, for older people (7.5 – 4 = 3.5 h loss) than for younger people (9 – 4 = 5 h loss).

A related hypothesis is that being awake does not create as strong a sleep need for the brains of older people, so that equal lengths of time awake do not generate as much sleep drive as for younger people. A globally reduced sleep drive could contribute to longer sleep onset latencies during daytime, reduced production of N3 sleep at night, and a reduced impact of sleep loss on cognitive performance overnight (Dijk et al., 2010).

One challenge to the circadian-amplitude explanation for differences in effects of sleep loss across ages is that not all rhythms are reported to have a reduced amplitude in older people, and there is little consensus about which rhythms are affected. Studies discussed above reported reduced amplitude of the following rhythms in older people: body temperature; features of sleep spindle production; sleep propensity; rest-activity; melatonin production; cortisol and several other hormones; and vigilance performance But some studies did not find reduced amplitudes of melatonin rhythms or sleep-propensity rhythms in older people (Dijk et al., 2000) (see Section 8.4.2), nor in the amplitude of body temperature rhythms (Buysse et al., 2005).

Several factors likely contributed to these inconsistencies. Experimental procedures that eliminate potential effects of masking or homeostatic processes may be critical to demonstrating changes in rhythm amplitude. In addition, the criteria used to recruit participants, especially older participants, may influence whether aging effects on rhythm amplitude are detected (see Sections 4.6 and 8.4.3).

Despite evidence from animal studies that the rhythmicity of the SCN pacemaker itself is reduced, it is also possible that only a subset of overt rhythms show decreased amplitude. Some body tissues and systems may be less dependent than others on signals from the SCN because they have the capacity to generate their own circadian rhythms either transiently or indefinitely (see Section 8.2.5). In addition, there are multiple neural and neuroendocrine routes by which information from the SCN can reach different systems, and these mechanisms may be altered to different extents during aging.

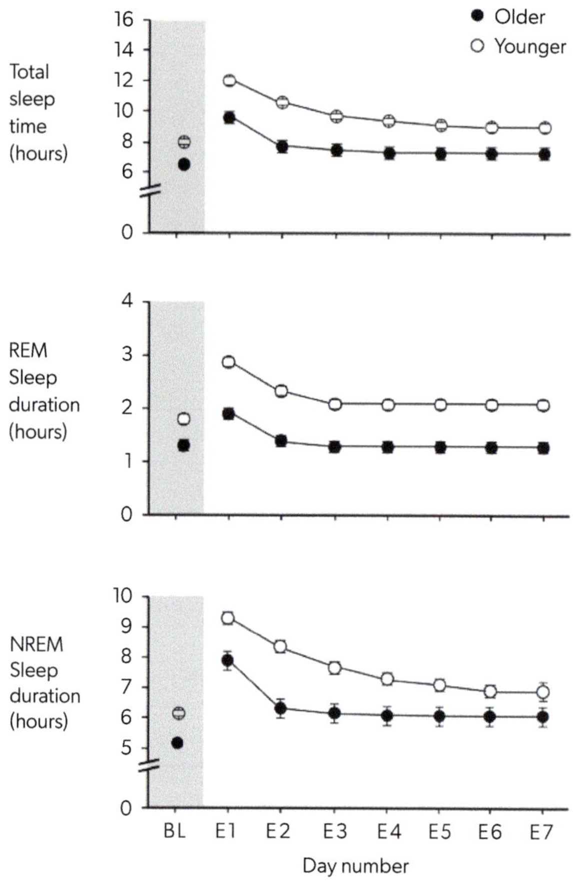

Figure 8.23 Individuals who were younger (white symbols) and older (black symbols) participated in PSG sleep studies for one night, with timing that matched their habitual sleep timing at home (BL, shaded area). They were then given both a 12 h sleep opportunity at night and a 4 h sleep opportunity during the afternoon daily for 7 days (E1–E7). Both groups showed an initial increase in amounts of total sleep (top), REM sleep (middle), and NREM sleep (bottom) when allowed a total of 16 h time in bed daily, suggesting a chronic sleep debt relative to sleep need. These values decreased to stable but still increased amounts during later days of the study (except for REM sleep in the older group, which returned to baseline durations). The durations of total sleep, REM sleep, and NREM sleep during each 24 h period were greater in the younger participants throughout the study, indicating a reduced need and/or capacity for older participants to increase sleep durations. Reprinted with permission of Elsevier, Ltd. from Klerman, E.B. & Dijk, D.-J. (2008) Age-related reduction in the maximal capacity for sleep--implications for insomnia. *Curr Biol* 18:1118–1123. © Elsevier (2008). doi: 10.1016/j.cub.2008.06.047.

8.5.5 Summary

Older people in population-based, observational studies tend to report more daytime naps and more disrupted nocturnal sleep than young people. But the interpretation of these findings is unclear because in experimental situations they also show longer latencies to fall asleep during the day, even when sleep deprived. These apparent inconsistencies probably reflect the fact that these studies are asking different questions.

Some laboratory studies are aimed at determining the extent to which sleep and circadian regulatory mechanisms change as a function of aging itself. They select exceptionally fit older participants for these very challenging studies, thereby excluding many of the variables that affect sleep in the general population, which would make it impossible to address the impact of aging alone. These include increases in primary sleep disorders, health conditions that affect sleep, and the use of medications to treat these conditions, some of which can affect sleep.

Longer latencies to fall asleep during daytime nap opportunities among older people could reflect either a slower buildup of sleep need while awake or a reduced physiological capacity to generate sleep, as suggested by their more limited ability to increase total daily sleep durations.

Better vigilance performance and reduced sleepiness in older people when kept awake at night are probably not the result of a reduced impact of sleep loss on their physiology. Instead, these differences appear to reflect reductions during aging in the amplitude of circadian rhythms that promote nighttime sleep and daytime alertness. Studies that extend waking beyond 24 h show that declining alertness and performance in young participants reverses direction during the following subjective day, despite accumulating sleep loss. Older people, with few exceptions, show a shallower decline in performance during the night and little if any recovery of performance during the following daytime tests. These results indicate that better performance during sleep loss at night among older people is not primarily caused by differences in the effects of sleep loss but rather to differences in the strength of the circadian drive promoting sleep at night.

The high amplitude circadian modulation of alertness/sleepiness in young people promotes better consolidation of sleep at night and more alertness during the day, but at the cost of larger negative effects on performance and alertness when they stay awake at night. Reduced circadian amplitude in older people impairs consolidation of sleep at night and reduces peak alertness during the day but also allows better preservation of performance and alertness when kept awake overnight.

When given 16 h sleep opportunities daily, young people showed maximal daily sleep amounts that were ~1.5 h longer than those of older people. These results suggest that their sleep need may be greater, so restriction to the same nightly sleep amount (e.g., 4 h) may represent a larger effective reduction relative to sleep need for young people.

There is evidence in both people and animals that the amplitude of several circadian rhythms, including that of the SCN pacemaker, are reduced during aging. The evidence from measures closely tied to the pacemaker, such as core temperature

Table 8.1 Studying Sleep and the Effects of Sleep Loss During Aging: Factors Affecting Outcomes

Types of Studies
• Population-based observational studies (usually involving self-reports)
• Laboratory studies conducted at one or more times of day after sleep loss
• Tests conducted around the clock during continuous sleep loss in a constant routine or during ultradian sleep–wake cycles
• Tests conducted using forced desynchronization
• Tests conducted during brief awakenings from sleep
Participant Selection (see Chapter 4 **for more discussion)**
• Survivor effects
• Participants' representativeness of the general population in different age ranges
• Differential impacts of the application of the same exclusion criteria to different age groups
Types of Measures Taken
• Self-reported sleep patterns
• Self-reported sleepiness
• Unintentional sleep onsets
• Multiple Sleep Latency Tests
• Maintenance of Wakefulness Tests
• Performance on tests of vigilance (e.g., Psychomotor Vigilance Tests)
• Performance on other cognitive tests
• Homeostatic responses to sleep loss
• EEG measures (e.g., waking theta as a measure of sleepiness)
Interpreting Results
• Sleep need versus sleep production capacity: effects on responses to sleep loss
• Impact of circadian phase of testing on comparisons among age groups
• Influence of circadian rhythm amplitude vs. sleep loss during the night
• Different indices of circadian amplitude: body temperature, melatonin, cortisol, sleep features, gene expression rhythms

and melatonin secretion, indicate that their amplitudes are decreased by ~25–33% in older people compared to younger people (e.g., **Figure 8.16**; see Section 8.5.3). Other oscillations, including those of SCN VP-ir levels in human postmortem tissue, firing rates of SCN neurons in mice, and sleep spindle frequencies in people show even larger age-related reductions in amplitude (**Figures 8.17 to 18.19**). This circadian amplitude reduction may occur because of reduced coherence among component oscillators in the circadian system, both within the SCN and between the SCN and other oscillators.

Both technical differences in the way studies are run and the selection criteria applied to older participants may influence whether particular circadian rhythms are found to show reduced amplitude in experiments involving older people. Amplitude reductions observed for some physiological and behavioral rhythms may not appear in other rhythms, perhaps because of a greater capacity for independent rhythm generation in some regulatory systems.

Designing studies comparing participants from two different age groups appears superficially simple. However, there are many factors related to the design of studies involving older participants that make these studies difficult to interpret. Some of the factors that can affect the results of studies on this topic are summarized in **Table 8.1**.

Literature cited

Abe, H., Honma, S., Namihira, M., Masubuchi, S., & Honma, K. (2001). Behavioural rhythm splitting in the CS mouse is related to clock gene expression outside the suprachiasmatic nucleus. *Eur J Neurosci*, *14*(7), 1121–1128. doi: 10.1046/j.0953-816x.2001.01732.x

Abe, M., Herzog, E. D., Yamazaki, S., Straume, M., Tei, H., Sakaki, Y., … Block, G. D. (2002). Circadian rhythms in isolated brain regions. *J Neurosci*, *22*(1), 350–356.

Abrahamson, E. E., Leak, R. K., & Moore, R. Y. (2001). The suprachiasmatic nucleus projects to posterior hypothalamic arousal systems. *NeuroReport*, *12*(2), 435–440.

Abrahamson, E. E., & Moore, R. Y. (2001). Suprachiasmatic nucleus in the mouse: retinal innervation, intrinsic organization and efferent projections. *Brain Res*, *916*, 172–191.

Adam, M., Rétey, J., Khatami, R., & Landolt, H.-P. (2006). Age-related changes in the time course of vigilant attention during 40 hours without sleep in men. *Sleep*, *29*(1), 55–57.

Allen, G., Rappe, J., Earnest, D., & Cassone, V. (2001). Oscillating on borrowed time: Diffusible signals from immortalized suprachiasmatic nucleus cells regulate circadian rhythmicity in cultured fibroblasts. *J Neurosci*, *21*(20), 7937–7943.

Altimus, C. M., Guler, A. D., Villa, K. L., McNeill, D. S., LeGates, T. A., & Hattar, S. (2008). Rods-cones and melanopsin detect light and dark to modulate sleep independent of image formation. *Proc Natl Acad Sci USA*, *105*(50), 19998–20003. doi: 10.1073/pnas.0808312105

Ancoli-Israel, S., Gehrman, P., Martin, J. L., Shochat, T., Marler, M., Corey-Bloom, J., & Levi, L. (2003). Increased light exposure consolidates sleep and strengthens circadian rhythms in severe Alzheimer's disease patients. *Behav Sleep Med, 1*(1), 22–36.

Antle, M., & Mistlberger, R. (2000). Circadian clock resetting by sleep deprivation without exercise in the Syrian hamster. *J Neurosci, 20*(24), 9326–9332.

Antle, M., Steen, N., & Mistlberger, R. (2001). Adenosine and caffeine modulate circadian rhythms in the Syrian hamster. *NeuroReport, 12*(13), 2901–2905.

Archer, S. N., Laing, E. E., Moller-Levet, C. S., van der Veen, D. R., Bucca, G., Lazar, A. S., … Dijk, D. J. (2014). Mistimed sleep disrupts circadian regulation of the human transcriptome. *Proc Natl Acad Sci U S A, 111*(6), E682–E691. doi: 10.1073/pnas.1316335111

Arnardottir, E. S., Nikonova, E. V., Shockley, K. R., Podtelezhnikov, A. A., Anafi, R. C., Tanis, K. Q., … Pack, A. I. (2014). Blood-gene expression reveals reduced circadian rhythmicity in individuals resistant to sleep deprivation. *Sleep, 37*(10), 1589–1600. doi: 10.5665/sleep.4064

Aston-Jones, G., Chen, S., Zhu, Y., & Oshinsky, M. (2001). A neural circuit for circadian regulation of arousal. *Nat Neurosci, 4*(7), 732–738.

Aton, S. J., Colwell, C. S., Harmar, A. J., Waschek, J., & Herzog, E. D. (2005). Vasoactive intestinal polypeptide mediates circadian rhythmicity and synchrony in mammalian clock neurons. *Nat Neurosci, 8*(4), 476–483.

Aton, S. J., & Herzog, E. D. (2005). Come together, right … now: synchronization of rhythms in a mammalian circadian clock. *Neuron, 48*(4), 531–534. doi: 10.1016/j.neuron.2005.11.001

Aujard, F., Herzog, E., & Block, G. (2001). Circadian rhythms in firing rate of individual suprachiasmatic nucleus neurons from adult and middle-aged mice. *Neuroscience, 106*(2), 255–261.

Balsalobre, A., Brown, S., Marcacci, L., Tronche, F., Kellendonk, C., Reichardt, H., … Schibler, U. (2000). Resetting of circadian time in peripheral tissues by glucocorticoid signaling. *Science, 289*, 2344–2347.

Balsalobre, A., Damiola, F., & Schibler, U. (1998). A serum shock induces circadian gene expression in mammalian tissue culture cells. *Cell, 93*, 929–937.

Bartness, T. J., Song, C. K., & Demas, G. E. (2001). SCN efferents to peripheral tissues: implications for biological rhythms. *J Biol Rhythms, 16*(2), 196–204.

Belenky, M. A., Smeraski, C. A., Provencio, I., Sollars, P. J., & Pickard, G. E. (2003). Melanopsin retinal ganglion cells receive bipolar and amacrine cell synapses. *J Comp Neurol, 460*(3), 380–393. doi: 10.1002/cne.10652

Berson, D., Dunn, F. A., & Takao, M. (2002). Phototransduction by retinal ganglion cells that set the circadian clock. *Science, 295*(5557), 1070–1073. doi: 10.1126/science.1067262

Bonnet, M. H., & Rosa, R. R. (1987). Sleep and performance in young adults and older normals and insomniacs during acute sleep loss and recovery. *Biol Psychol, 25*, 153–172.

Bos, N. P. A., & Mirmiran, M. (1990). Circadian rhythms in spontaneous neuronal discharges of the cultured suprachiasmatic nucleus. *Brain Res, 511*, 158–162.

Brøndsted, A. E., Haargaard, B., Sander, B., Lund-Andersen, H., Jennum, P., & Kessel, L. (2017). The effect of blue-blocking and neutral intraocular lenses on circadian photoentrainment and sleep one year after cataract surgery. *Acta Ophthalmol, 95*(4), 344–351. doi: 10.1111/aos.13323

Brøndsted, A. E., Lundeman, J. H., & Kessel, L. (2013). Short wavelength light filtering by the natural human lens and IOLs -- implications for entrainment of circadian rhythm. *Acta Ophthalmol, 91*(1), 52–57. doi: 10.1111/j.1755-3768.2011.02291.x

Buhr, E., & Takahashi, J. (2013). Molecular components of the mammalian circadian clock. *Handb Exp Pharmacol, 217*, 3–27.

Buijs, R. M., la Fleur, S. E., Wortel, J., van Heyningen, C., Zuiddam, L., Mettenleiter, T. C., … Niijima, A. (2003). The suprachiasmatic nucleus balances sympathetic and parasympathetic output to peripheral organs through separate preautonomic neurons. *J Comp Neurol, 464*(1), 36–48. doi: 10.1002/cne.10765

Buysse, D., Monk, T., Carrier, J., & Begley, A. (2005). Circadian patterns of sleep, sleepiness and performance in older and younger adults. *Sleep, 28*(11), 1365–1376.

Cai, A., & Wise, P. M. (1996). Age-related changes in the diurnal rhythm of CRH gene expression in the paraventricular nuclei. *AJP: Physiol Endocrinol Metab, 270*, E238–E243.

Campbell, S. S., Dawson, D., & Anderson, M. W. (1993). Alleviation of sleep maintenance insomnia with timed exposure to bright light. *J Am Geriatr Soc, 41* (8), 829–836.

Campbell, S. S., Kripke, D. F., Gillin, J. C., & Hrubovcak, J. C. (1988). Exposure to light in healthy elderly subjects and Alzheimer's patients. *Physiol Behav, 42*, 141–144.

Canteras, N. S., Ribeiro-Barbosa, É. R., Goto, M., Cipolla-Neto, J., & Swanson, L. W. (2011). The retinohypothalamic tract: comparison of axonal projection patterns from four major targets. *Brain Res Rev, 65*(2), 150–183. doi: 10.1016/j.brainresrev.2010.09.006

Cardinali, D. P., & Ritta, M. N. (1983). The role of prostaglandins in neuroendocrine junctions: studies in the pineal gland and the hypothalamus. *Neuroendocrinology, 36*(2), 152–160. doi: 10.1159/000123452

Carrier, J., Monk, T. H., Reynolds, C. F., Buysse, D. J., & Kupfer, D. J. (2009). Are age differences in sleep due to phase differences in the output of the circadian timing system? *Chronobiol Int, 16*(1), 79–91. doi: 10.3109/07420529908998714

Carskadon, M. A., & Dement, W. C. (1981). Cumulative effects of sleep restriction on daytime sleepiness. *Psychophysiology, 18*(2), 107–113.

Carskadon, M. A., & Dement, W. C. (1987). Daytime sleepiness: quantification of a behavioral state. *Neurosci Biobehav Rev, 11*, 307–317.

Chang, A. M., Scheer, F. A., Czeisler, C. A., & Aeschbach, D. (2013). Direct effects of light on alertness, vigilance, and the waking electroencephalogram in humans depend on prior light history. *Sleep, 36*(8), 1239–1246. doi: 10.5665/sleep.2894

Chee, C. A., Roozendaal, B., Swaab, D. F., Goudsmit, E., & Mirmiran, M. (1988). Vasoactive intestinal polypeptide neuron changes in the senile rat suprachiasmatic nucleus. *Neurobiol Aging, 9*, 307–312.

Chen, G., & van den Pol, A. (1997). Adenosine modulation of calcium currents and presynaptic inhibition of GABA release in suprachiasmatic and arcuate nucleus neurons. *J Neurophysiol, 77*, 3035–3047.

Cheng, M., Bullock, C., Li, C., Lee, A., Bermak, J., Belluzzi, J., Weaver, D., Leslie, F., & Zhou, Q.-Y. (2002). Prokineticin 2 transmits the behavioural circadian rhythm of the suprachiasmatic nucleus. *Nature, 417*, 405–410.

Chou, T. C., Scammell, T. E., Gooley, J. J., Gaus, S. E., Saper, C. B., & Lu, J. (2003). Critical role of dorsomedial hypothalamic nucleus in a wide range of behavioral circadian rhythms. *J Neurosci, 23*(33), 10691–10702.

Cohen, R. A., & Albers, H. E. (1991). Disruption of human circadian and cognitive regulation following a discrete hypothalamic lesion: a case study. *Neurology, 41*, 726–729.

Colwell, C. S. (2000). Rhythmic coupling among cells in the suprachiasmatic nucleus. *J Neurobiol, 43*(4), 379–388.

Czeisler, C., Duffy, J. F., Shanahan, T. L., Brown, E. N., Mitchell, J., Rimmer, D., … Kronauer, R. E. (1999). Stability, precision, and near-24-hour period of the human circadian pacemaker. *Science, 284*, 2177–2181.

Dai, J., Van Der Vliet, J., Swaab, D., & Buijs, R. M. (1998). Human retinohypothalamic tract as revealed by in vitro postmortem tracing. *J Comp Neurol, 397*, 757–770.

Davidson, A. J., London, B., Block, G. D., & Menaker, M. (2005). Cardiovascular tissues contain independent circadian clocks. *Clin Exp Hypertens, 27*(2/3), 307–311.

Deantoni, M., Reyt, M., Baillet, M., Dourte, M., De Haan, S., Lesoinne, A., … Schmidt, C. (2024). Napping and circadian sleep-wake regulation during healthy aging. *Sleep, 47*(5), zsad287. doi:10.1093/sleep/zsad287

Deboer, T., Overeem, S., Visser, N. A., Duindam, H., Frolich, M., Lammers, G. J., & Meijer, J. H. (2004). Convergence of circadian and sleep regulatory mechanisms on hypocretin-1. *Neuroscience, 129*(3), 727–732. doi: 10.1016/j.neuroscience.2004.07.049

Deboer, T., Vansteensel, M. J., Détári, L., & Meijer, J. H. (2003). Sleep states alter activity of suprachiasmatic nucleus neurons. *Nat Neurosci, 6*(10), 1086–1090. doi: 10.1038/nn1122

Deurveilher, S., Burns, J., & Semba, K. (2002). Indirect projections from the suprachiasmatic nucleus to the ventrolateral preoptic nucleus: a dual tract-tracing study in rat. *Eur J Neurosci, 16*(7), 1195–1213. doi: 10.1046/j.1460-9568.2002.02196.x

Deurveilher, S., & Semba, K. (2005). Indirect projections from the suprachiasmatic nucleus to major arousal-promoting cell groups in rat: implications for the circadian control of behavioural state. *Neuroscience, 130*(1), 165–183. doi: 10.1016/j.neuroscience.2004.08.030

De Vries, M. J., Treep, J. A., De Pauw, E. S. D., & Meijer, J. H. (1994). The effects of electrical stimulation of the optic nerves and anterior optic chiasm on the circadian activity rhythm of the Syrian hamster: Involvement of excitatory amino acids. *Brain Res, 642*, 206–212.

Dijk, D.-J., Duffy, J. F., & Czeisler, C. A. (2000). Contribution of circadian physiology and sleep homeostasis to age-related changes in human sleep. *Chronobiol Int, 17*(3), 285–311. doi: 10.1081/cbi-100101049

Dijk, D.-J., Groeger, J., Stanley, N., & Deacon, S. (2010). Age-related reduction in daytime sleep propensity and nocturnal slow wave sleep. *Sleep, 33*(2), 211–223.

Doyle, S. E., Yoshikawa, T., Hillson, H., & Menaker, M. (2008). Retinal pathways influence temporal niche. *Proc Natl Acad Sci USA, 105*(35), 13133–13138. doi: 10.1073/pnas.0801728105

Duffy, J., Dijk, D.-J., Klerman, E., & Czeisler, C. (1998). Later endogenous circadian temperature nadir relative to an earlier wake time in older people. *Am J Physiol, 275*, R1478–R1487.

Duffy, J., Scheuermaier, K., & Loughlin, K. (2016). Age-related sleep disruption and reduction in the circadian rhythm of urine output: contribution to nocturia? *Curr Aging Sci, 9*, 34–43.

Duffy, J., Viswanathan, N., & Davis, F. C. (1999). Free-running circadian period does not shorten with age in female Syrian hamsters. *Neurosci Lett, 271*, 77–80.

Duffy, J. F., Dijk, D.-J., Hall, E. F., & Czeisler, C. A. (1999). Relationship of endogenous circadian melatonin and temperature rhythms to self-reported preference for morning or evening activity in young and older people. *J Investig Med, 47*(3), 141–150.

Duffy, J. F., Willson, H. J., Wang, W., & Czeisler, C. A. (2009). Healthy older adults better tolerate sleep deprivation than young adults. *J Am Geriatr Soc, 57*(7), 1245–1251. doi: 10.1111/j.1532-5415.2009.02303.x

Duffy, J. F., Zeitzer, J. M., & Czeisler, C. A. (2007). Decreased sensitivity to phase-delaying effects of moderate intensity light in older subjects. *Neurobiol Aging, 28*(5), 799–807.

Eastman, C. I., Mistlberger, R. E., & Rechtschaffen, A. (1984). Suprachiasmatic nuclei lesions eliminate circadian temperature and sleep rhythms in the rat. *Physiol Behav, 32*, 357–368.

Easton, A., Meerlo, P., Bergmann, B., & Turek, F. W. (2004). The suprachiasmatic nucleus regulates sleep timing and amount in mice. *Sleep, 27*(7), 1307–1318.

Ebling, F. J. P. (1996). The role of glutamate in the photic regulation of the suprachiasmatic nucleus. *Prog Neurobiol, 50*(2/3), 109–132.

Edgar, D. M., Dement, W. C., & Fuller, C. A. (1993). Effect of SCN lesions on sleep in squirrel monkeys: evidence for opponent processes in sleep-wake regulation. *J Neurosci, 13*, 1065–1079.

Espiritu, R. C., Kripke, D. F., Ancoli-Israel, S., Mowen, M. A., Mason, W. J., Fell, R. L., … Kaplan, O. J. (1994). Low illumination experienced by San Diego adults: association with atypical depressive symptoms. *Biol Psychiatry, 35*, 403–407.

Farajnia, S., Michel, S., Deboer, T., vanderLeest, H. T., Houben, T., Rohling, J. H., … Meijer, J. H. (2012). Evidence for neuronal desynchrony in the aged suprachiasmatic nucleus clock. *J Neurosci, 32*(17), 5891–5899. doi: 10.1523/JNEUROSCI.0469-12.2012

Filtness, A. J., Reyner, L. A., & Horne, J. A. (2012). Driver sleepiness-comparisons between young and older men during a monotonous afternoon simulated drive. *Biol Psychol, 89*(3), 580–583. doi: 10.1016/j.biopsycho.2012.01.002

Foley, D. J., Monjan, A. A., Brown, S. L., Simonsick, E. M., Wallace, R. B., & Blazer, D. G. (1995). Sleep complaints among elderly persons: An epidemiologic study of three communities. *Sleep, 18*, 425–432.

Foster, R. G., Provencio, I., Hudson, D., Fiske, S., De Grip, W., & Menaker, M. (1991). Circadian photoreception in the retinally degenerate mouse (rd/rd). *J Comp Physiol [A], 169*, 39–50.

Franken, P. (2013). A role for clock genes in sleep homeostasis. *Curr Opin Neurobiol, 23*(5), 864–872. doi: 10.1016/j.conb.2013.05.002

Gerkema, M. P., van der Zee, E. A., & Feitsma, L. E. (1994). Expression of circadian rhythmicity correlates with the number of arginine-vasopressin-immunoreactive cells in the suprachiasmatic nucleus of common voles, *Microtus arvalis*. *Brain Res, 639*, 93–101.

Gibbs, J., Ince, L., Matthews, L., Mei, J., Bell, T., Yang, N., … Loudon, A. (2014). An epithelial circadian clock controls pulmonary inflammation and glucocorticoid action. *Nat Med, 20*(8), 919–926. doi: 10.1038/nm.3599

Gibbs, J. E., Beesley, S., Plumb, J., Singh, D., Farrow, S., Ray, D. W., & Loudon, A. S. I. (2008). Circadian timing in the lung; a specific role for bronchiolar epithelial cells. *Endocrinology, 150*(1), 268–276. doi: 10.1210/en.2008-0638

Gillette, M. U. (1987). The hypothalamic suprachiasmatic nuclei: circadian patterns of vasopressin secretion and neuronal activity in vitro *Brain Res Bull, 19*, 135–139.

Granados-Fuentes, D., Prolo, L., Abraham, U., & Herzog, E. D. (2004). The suprachiasmatic nucleus entrains, but does not sustain, circadian rhythmicity in the olfactory bulb. *J Neurosci, 24*(3), 615–619. doi: 10.1523/JNEUROSCI.4002-03.2004

Granados-Fuentes, D., Saxena, M. T., Prolo, L. M., Aton, S. J., & Herzog, E. D. (2004). Olfactory bulb neurons express functional, entrainable circadian rhythms. *Eur J Neurosci, 19*(4), 898–906.

Green, D. J., & Gillette, R. (1982). Circadian rhythm of firing rate recorded from single cells in the rat suprachiasmatic brain slice. *Brain Res, 245*, 198–200.

Groeger, J., Viola, A., Lo, J., von Schantz, M., Archer, S., & Dijk, D.-J. (2008). Early morning executive functioning during sleep deprivation is compromised by a *PERIOD3* polymorphism. *Sleep, 31*(8), 1159–1167.

Groos, G., & Hendriks, J. (1982). Circadian rhythms in electrical discharge of rat suprachiasmatic neurones recorded in vitro. *Neurosci Lett, 34*, 283–288.

Guido, M. E., Marchese, N. A., Rios, M. N., Morera, L. P., Diaz, N. M., Garbarino-Pico, E., & Contin, M. A. (2022). Non-visual opsins and novel photo-detectors in the vertebrate inner retina mediate light responses within the blue spectrum region. *Cell Mol Neurobiol, 42*(1), 59–83. doi: 10.1007/s10571-020-00997-x

Guilding, C., Hughes, A. T., & Piggins, H. D. (2010). Circadian oscillators in the epithalamus. *Neuroscience, 169*(4), 1630–1639. doi: 10.1016/j.neuroscience.2010.06.015

Guo, H., Brewer, J. M., Lehman, M. N., & Bittman, E. L. (2006). Suprachiasmatic regulation of circadian rhythms of gene expression in hamster peripheral organs: effects of transplanting the pacemaker. *J Neurosci, 26*(24), 6406–6412. doi: 10.1523/JNEUROSCI.4676-05.2006

Haimov, I., & Lavie, P. (1997). Circadian characteristics of sleep propensity function in healthy elderly: a comparison with young adults *Sleep, 20*(4), 294–300.

Hamnett, R., Chesham, J. E., Maywood, E. S., & Hastings, M. H. (2021). The cell-autonomous clock of VIP receptor VPAC2 cells regulates period and coherence of circadian behaviour. *J Neurosci, 41*(3), 502–512. doi: 10.1523/JNEUROSCI.2015-20.2020

Hannibal, J. (2021). Comparative neurology of circadian photoreception: the retinohypothalamic tract (RHT) in sighted and naturally blind mammals. *Front Neurosci, 15*, 1–15. doi:10.3389/fnins.2021.640113

Hannibal, J., Hindersson, P., Knudsen, S. M., Georg, B., & Fahrenkrug, J. (2002). The photopigment melanopsin is exclusively present in pituitary adenylate cyclase-activating polypeptide-containing retinal ganglion cells of the retinohypothalamic tract. *J Neurosci, 22*(1), RC191.

Harper, D. G., Stopa, E. G., Kuo-Leblanc, V., McKee, A. C., Asayama, K., Volicer, L., … Satlin, A. (2008). Dorsomedial SCN neuronal subpopulations subserve different functions in human dementia. *Brain, 131*, 1609–1617. doi: 10.1093/brain/awn049

Harrington, M. E. (1997). The ventral lateral geniculate nucleus and the intergeniculate leaflet: interrelated structures in the visual and circadian systems. *Neurosci Biobehav Rev, 21*(5), 705–727.

Harrington, M. E., & Rusak, B. (1986). Lesions of the thalamic intergeniculate leaflet alter hamster circadian rhythms. *J Biol Rhythms, 1*, 309–325.

Hattar, S., Liao, H. W., Takao, M., Berson, D. M., & Yau, K. W. (2002). Melanopsin-containing retinal ganglion cells: architecture, projections, and intrinsic photosensitivity. *Science, 295*(5557), 1065–1070. doi: 10.1126/science.1069609

Hattar, S., Lucas, R. J., Mrosovsky, N., Thompson, S., Douglas, R. H., Hankins, M. W., … Yau, K. W. (2003). Melanopsin and rod–cone photoreceptive systems account for all major accessory visual functions in mice. *Nature, 424*(6944), 75–81. doi: 10.1038/nature01761

Hébert, M., Dumont, M., & Paquet, J. (1998). Seasonal and diurnal patterns of human illumination under natural conditions. *Chronobiol Int, 15*(1), 59–70. doi: 10.3109/07420529808998670

Hendrickson, A. E., Wagoner, N., & Cowan, W. M. (1972). An autoradiographic and electron microscopic study of retino-hypothalamic connections. *Z Zellforsch Mikrok Anat, 135*(1), 1–26. doi: 10.1007/BF00307084

Hofman, M., & Swaab, D. (2006). Living by the clock: the circadian pacemaker in older people. *Aging Res Rev, 5*(1), 33–51. doi: 10.1016/j.arr.2005.07.001

Hofman, M. A., & Swaab, D. F. (1994). Alterations in circadian rhythmicity of the vasopressin-producing neurons of the human suprachiasmatic nucleus (SCN) with aging. *Brain Res, 651*, 134–142.

Honma, K., & Honma, S. (2009). The SCN-independent clocks, methamphetamine and food restriction. *Eur J Neurosci, 30*(9), 1707–1717. doi: 10.1111/j.1460-9568.2009.06976.x

Hu, W.-P., Li, J.-D., Zhang, C., Boehmer, L., Siegel, J., & Zhou, Q.-Y. (2007). Altered circadian and homeostatic sleep regulation in prokineticin 2-deficient mice. *Sleep, 30*(3), 247–256.

Husse, J., Eichele, G., & Oster, H. (2015). Synchronization of the mammalian circadian timing system: Light can control peripheral clocks independently of the SCN clock: alternate routes of entrainment optimize the alignment of the body's circadian clock network with external time. *Bioessays, 37*(10), 1119–1128. doi: 10.1002/bies.201500026

Ibuka, N., & Kawamura, H. (1975). Loss of circadian rhythm in sleep-wakefulness cycle in the rat by suprachiasmatic nucleus lesions. *Brain Res, 96*, 76–81.

Inouye, S. I. T., & Kawamura, H. (1979). Persistence of circadian rhythmicity in a mammalian hypothalamic "island" containing the suprachiasmatic nucleus. *Proc Natl Acad Sci USA, 76*, 5962–5966.

Jansen, K., Van der Zee, E. A., & Gerkema, M. P. (2007). Vasopressin immunoreactivity, but not vasoactive intestinal polypeptide, correlates with expression of circadian rhythmicity in the suprachiasmatic nucleus of voles. *Neuropeptides, 41*(4), 207–216. doi: 10.1016/j.npep.2007.04.003

Jiao, Y. Y., Lee, T. M., & Rusak, B. (1999). Photic responses of suprachiasmatic area neurons in diurnal degus (*Octodon degus*) and nocturnal rats (*Rattus norvegicus*). *Brain Res, 817*(1-2), 93–103. doi: 10.1016/s0006-8993(98)01218-9

Johnson, R. F., Moore, R. Y., & Morin, L. P. (1988). Loss of entrainment and anatomical plasticity after lesions of the hamster retinohypothalamic tract. *Brain Res, 460*, 297–313.

Kalló, I., Kalamatianos, T., Piggins, H. D., & Coen, C. W. (2004). Ageing and the diurnal expression of mRNAs for vasoactive intestinal peptide and for the VPAC2 and PAC1 receptors in the suprachiasmatic nucleus of male rats. *J Neuroendocrinol, 16*(9), 758–766. doi: 10.1111/j.1365-2826.2004.01232.x

Kalsbeek, A., Fliers, E., Hofman, M. A., Swaab, D. F., & Buijs, R. M. (2010). Vasopressin and the output of the hypothalamic biological clock. *J Neuroendocrinol, 22*(5), 362–372. doi: 10.1111/j.1365-2826.2010.01956.x

Kennaway, D., Lushington, K., Dawson, D., Lack, L., van den Heuvel, C., & Rogers, N. (1999). Urinary 6-sulfatoxymelatonin excretion and aging: new results and a critical review of the literature. *J Pineal Res, 27*, 210–220.

Kim, S., Benloucif, S., Reid, K., Weintraub, S., Kennedy, N., Wolfe, L., & Zee, P. (2014). Phase-shifting response to light in older adults. *J Physiol, 592*(1), 189–202. doi: 0.1113/jphysiol.2013.262899

Klein, D. C., Smoot, R., Weller, J. L., Higa, S., Markley, S. P., Creed, G. J., & Jacobowitz, D. M. (1983). Lesions of the paraventricular nucleus area of the hypothalamus disrupt the suprachiasmatic→ spinal cord circuit in the melatonin rhythm generating system. *Brain Res Bull, 10*(5), 647–652. doi: 10.1016/0361-9230(83)90033-3

Klerman, E. B., & Dijk, D. J. (2008). Age-related reduction in the maximal capacity for sleep-implications for insomnia. *Curr Biol, 18*(15), 1118–1123. doi: 10.1016/j.cub.2008.06.047

Ko, C. H., Yamada, Y. R., Welsh, D. K., Buhr, E. D., Liu, A. C., Zhang, E. E., ... Takahashi, J. S. (2010). Emergence of noise-induced oscillations in the central circadian pacemaker. *PLoS Biol, 8*(10), e1000513. doi: 10.1371/journal.pbio.1000513

Kripke, D. F., Elliott, J. A., Youngstedt, S. D., & Rex, K. M. (2007). Circadian phase response curves to light in older and young women and men. *J Circad Rhythms, 5*, 4. doi: 10.1186/1740-3391-5-4

Kruisbrink, J., Mirmiran, M., van der Woude, T. P., & Boer, G. J. (1987). Effects of enhanced cerebrospinal fluid levels of vasopressin, vasopressin antagonist or vasoactive intestinal polypeptide on circadian sleep-wake rhythm in the rat. *Brain Res, 419*, 76–86.

Lee, I. T., Chang, A. S., Manandhar, M., Shan, Y., Fan, J., Izumo, M., ... Yanagisawa, M. (2015). Neuromedin s-producing neurons act as essential pacemakers in the suprachiasmatic nucleus to couple clock neurons and dictate circadian rhythms. *Neuron, 85*(5), 1086–1102. doi: 10.1016/j.neuron.2015.02.006

Lee, T. M., Loh, E. W., Kuo, T. C., Tam, K. W., Lee, H. C., & Wu, D. (2021). Effects of ultraviolet and blue-light filtering on sleep: a meta-analysis of controlled trials and studies on cataract patients. *Eye (Lond), 35*(6), 1629–1636. doi: 10.1038/s41433-020-01132-2

Leise, T., Harrington, M., Molyneux, P., Song, I., Queenan, H., Zimmerman, E., ... Biello, S. (2013). Voluntary exercise can strengthen the circadian system in aged mice. *Age, 35*, 2137–2152. doi: 10.1007/s11357-012-9502-y)

Leliavski, A., Dumbell, R., Ott, V., & Oster, H. (2015). Adrenal clocks and the role of adrenal hormones in the regulation of circadian physiology. *J Biol Rhythms, 30*(1), 20–34. doi: 10.1177/0748730414553971

Li, H., & Satinoff, E. (1995). Changes in circadian rhythms of body temperature and sleep in old rats. *Am J Physiol Regul Integr Comp Physiol, 269*, R208–R214.

Li, J. D., Burton, K. J., Zhang, C., Hu, S. B., & Zhou, Q. Y. (2009). Vasopressin receptor V1a regulates circadian rhythms of locomotor activity and expression of clock-controlled genes in the suprachiasmatic nuclei. *Am J Physiol Regul Integr Comp Physiol, 296*(3), R824–830. doi: 10.1152/ajpregu.90463.2008

Lim, A. S., Ellison, B. A., Wang, J. L., Yu, L., Schneider, J. A., Buchman, A. S., Bennett, D. A., & Saper, C. B. (2014). Sleep is related to neuron numbers in the ventrolateral preoptic/intermediate nucleus in older adults with and without Alzheimer's disease. *Brain, 137*(Pt 10), 2847–2861. doi: 10.1093/brain/awu222

Lockley, S. W., Brainard, G. C., & Czeisler, C. A. (2003). High sensitivity of the human circadian melatonin rhythm to resetting by short wavelength light. *J Clin Endocrinol Metab, 88*(9), 4502–4505. doi: 10.1210/jc.2003-030570

Long, M. A., Jutras, M. J., Connors, B. W., & Burwell, R. D. (2004). Electrical synapses coordinate activity in the suprachiasmatic nucleus. *Nat Neurosci, 8*(1), 61–66. doi: 10.1038/nn1361

Lu, J., Zhang, Y.-H., Chou, T. C., Gaus, S. E., Elmquist, J. K., Shiromani, P. J., & Saper, C. B. (2001). Contrasting effects of ibotenate lesions of the paraventricular nucleus and subparaventricular zone on sleep-wake cycle and temperature regulation. *J Neurosci, 21*(13), 4864–4874.

Lucas, R. J., Peirson, S. N., Berson, D. M., Brown, T. M., Cooper, H. M., Czeisler, C. A., ... Brainard, G. C. (2014). Measuring and using light in the melanopsin age. *Trends Neurosci, 37*(1), 1–9. doi: 10.1016/j.tins.2013.10.004

Lupi, D., Oster, H., Thompson, S., & Foster, R. G. (2008). The acute light-induction of sleep is mediated by OPN4-based photoreception. *Nat Neurosci, 11*(9), 1068–1073. doi: 10.1038/nn.2179

Madeira, M. D., Sousa, N., Santer, R. M., Paula-Barbosa, M. M., & Gundersen, H. J. G. (1995). Age and sex do not affect the volume, cell numbers, or cell size of the suprachiasmatic nucleus of the rat: an unbiased stereological study. *J Comp Neurol, 361*, 585–601.

Magri, F., Sarra, S., Cinchetti, W., Guazzoni, V., Floravanti, M., Cravello, L., & Ferrari, E. (2004). Qualitative and quantitative changes in melatonin levels in physiological and pathological aging and in centenarians. *J Pineal Res, 36*(4), 256–261. doi: 10.1111/j.1600-079X.2004.00125.x

Mahlberg, R., Kienast, T., Hadel, S., Heidenreich, J. O., Schmitz, S., & Kunz, D. (2009). Degree of pineal calcification (DOC) is associated with polysomnographic sleep measures in primary insomnia patients. *Sleep Med, 10*(4), 439–445. doi: 10.1016/j.sleep.2008.05.003

Mahlberg, R., Tilmann, A., Salewski, L., & Kunz, D. (2006). Normative data on the daily profile of urinary 6-sulfatoxymelatonin in healthy subjects between the ages of 20 and 84. *Psychoneuroendocrinology, 31*(5), 634–641. doi: 10.1016/j.psyneuen.2006.01.009

Mai, J. K., Kedziora, O., Teckhaus, L., & Sofroniew, M. V. (1991). Evidence for subdivisions in the human suprachiasmatic nucleus. *J Comp Neurol, 305*, 508–525.

Martino, T. A., Oudit, G. Y., Herzenberg, A. M., Tata, N., Koletar, M. M., Kabir, G. M., ... Sole, M. J. (2008). Circadian rhythm disorganization produces profound cardiovascular and renal disease in hamsters. *Am J Physiol Regul Integr Comp Physiol, 294*(5), R1675–R1683. doi: 10.1152/ajpregu.00829.2007

Masumoto, K.-h., Nagano, M., Takashima, N., Hayasaka, N., Hiyama, H., Matsumoto, S.-i., ... Shigeyoshi, Y. (2006). Distinct localization of prokineticin 2 and prokineticin receptor 2 mRNAs in the rat suprachiasmatic nucleus. *Eur J Neurosci, 23*(11), 2959–2970. doi: 10.1111/j.1460-9568.2006.04834.x

May, C. P., Hasher, L., & Stoltzfus, E. R. (1993). Optimal time of day and the magnitude of age differences in memory. *Psychol Sci, 4*(3), 326–330.

McDearmon, E. L., Patel, K. N., Ko, C. H., Walisser, J. A., Schook, A. C., Chong, J. L., ... Takahashi, J. S. (2006). Dissecting the functions of the mammalian clock protein BMAL1 by tissue-specific rescue in mice. *Science, 314*(5803), 1304–1308. doi: 10.1126/science.1132430

McGlashan, E. M., Poudel, G. R., Vidafar, P., Drummond, S. P. A., & Cain, S. W. (2018). Imaging individual differences in the response of the human suprachiasmatic area to light. *Front Neurol, 9*, 1022. doi: 10.3389/fneur.2018.01022

Meijer, J. H., Groos, G. A., & Rusak, B. (1986). Luminance coding in a circadian pacemaker: The suprachiasmatic nucleus of the rat and the hamster. *Brain Res, 382*, 109–118.

Meijer, J. H., & Rietveld, W. J. (1989). Neurophysiology of the suprachiasmatic circadian pacemaker in rodents. *Physiol Rev, 69*, 671–707.

Meijer, J. H., Rusak, B., & Harrington, M. E. (1989). Photically responsive neurons in the hypothalamus of a diurnal ground squirrel. *Brain Res, 501*, 315–323.

Mieda, M. (2019). The network mechanism of the central circadian pacemaker of the SCN: do AVP neurons play a more critical role than expected? *Front Neurosci, 13*, 139. doi:10.3389/fnins.2019.00139

Mishima, K., Okawa, M., Shimizu, T., & Hishikawa, Y. (2001). Diminished melatonin secretion in the elderly caused by insufficient environmental illumination. *J Clin Endocrinol Metab, 86*(1), 129–134.

Mistlberger, R. (2005). Circadian regulation of sleep in mammals: role of the suprachiasmatic nucleus. *Brain Res Rev, 49*(3), 429–454. doi: 10.1016/j.brainresrev.2005.01.005

Mistlberger, R. E. (1994). Circadian food-anticipatory activity: formal models and physiological mechanisms. *Neurosci Biobehav Rev, 18*, 171–195.

Mistlberger, R. E., Bergmann, B. M., & Rechtschaffen, A. (1987). Relationships among wake episode lengths, contiguous sleep episode lengths, and electroencephalographic delta waves in rats with suprachiasmatic nuclei lesions. *Sleep, 10*, 12–24.

Mistlberger, R. E., Bergmann, B. M., Waldenar, W., & Rechtschaffen, A. (1983). Recovery sleep following sleep deprivation in intact and suprachiasmatic nuclei-lesioned rats. *Sleep, 6*, 217–233.

Möller-Levet, C. S., Archer, S. N., Bucca, G., Laing, E. E., Slak, A., Kabiljo, R., ... Dijk, D. J. (2013). Effects of insufficient sleep on circadian rhythmicity and expression amplitude of the human blood transcriptome. *Proc Natl Acad Sci U S A, 110*(12), E1132–E1141. doi: 10.1073/pnas.1217154110

Monk, T. H. (1991). Sleep and circadian rhythms. *Exp Gerontol, 26*, 233–234.

Monk, T. H. (2005). Aging human circadian rhythms: conventional wisdom may not always be right. *J Biol Rhythms, 20*(4), 366–374. doi: 10.1177/0748730405277378

Moore, R. Y., & Eichler, V. B. (1972). Loss of circadian adrenal corticosterone rhythm following suprachiasmatic lesions in the rat. *Brain Res, 42*, 201–206.

Moore, R. Y., & Lenn, N. J. (1972). A retinohypothalamic projection in the rat. *J Comp Neurol, 146*, 1–14.

Moore, R. Y., Speh, J. C., & Leak, R. K. (2002). Suprachiasmatic nucleus organization. *Cell Tissue Res, 309*(1), 89–98. doi: 10.1007/s00441-002-0575-2

Morris, E. L., Patton, A. P., Chesham, J. E., Crisp, A., Adamson, A., & Hastings, M. H. (2021). Single-cell transcriptomics of suprachiasmatic nuclei reveal a Prokineticin-driven circadian network. *EMBO J, 40*(20), e108614. doi:10.15252/embj.2021108614

Mrosovsky, N. (1996). Locomotor activity and non-photic influences on circadian clocks. *Biol Rev, 71*, 343–372.

Mrosovsky, N., Edelstein, K., Hastings, M. H., & Maywood, E. S. (2001). Cycle of period gene expression in a diurnal mammal (Spermophilus tridecemlineatus): implications for nonphotic phase shifting. *J Biol Rhythms, 16*(5), 471–478. doi: 10.1177/074873001129002141

Muehlroth, B. E., & Werkle-Bergner, M. (2020). Understanding the interplay of sleep and aging: methodological challenges. *Psychophysiology, 57*(3), e13523. doi: 10.1111/psyp.13523

Muindi, F., Zeitzer, J. M., & Heller, H. C. (2014). Retino-hypothalamic regulation of light-induced murine sleep. *Front Syst Neurosci, 8*, 135. doi: 10.3389/fnsys.2014.00135

Murphy, P. J., Myers, B. L., & Badia, P. (1996). Nonsteroidal anti-inflammatory drugs alter body temperature and suppress melatonin in humans. *Physiol Behav, 59*, 133–139.

Münch, M., Knoblauch, V., Blatter, K., Schröder, C., Schnitzler, C., Kräuchi, K., Wirz-Justice, A., & Cajochen, C. (2005). Age-related attenuation of the evening circadian arousal signal in humans. *Neurobiol Aging, 26*(9), 1307–1319. doi: 10.1016/j.neurobiolaging.2005.03.004

Münch, M., Schmieder, M., Bieler, K., Goldbach, R., Fuhrmann, T., Zumstein, N., ... Cajochen, C. (2017). Bright light delights: effects of daily light exposure on emotions, rest-activity cycles, sleep and melatonin secretion in severely demented patients. *Curr Alzheimer Res, 14*(10), 1063–1075. doi: 10.2174/1567205014666170523092858

Nakamura, T. J., Nakamura, W., Tokuda, I. T., Ishikawa, T., Kudo, T., Colwell, C. S., & Block, G. D. (2015). Age-related changes in the circadian system unmasked by constant conditions. *eNeuro, 2*(4). doi: 10.1523/ENEURO.0064-15.2015

Nakamura, T. J., Nakamura, W., Yamazaki, S., Kudo, T., Cutler, T., Colwell, C. S., & Block, G. D. (2011). Age-related decline in circadian output. *J Neurosci, 31*(28), 10201–10205. doi: 10.1523/jneurosci.0451-11.2011

Naylor, E., Bergmann, B., Krauski, K., Zee, P., Takahashi, J., Vitaterna, M., & Turek, F. (2000). The circadian *Clock* gene mutation alters sleep homeostasis in the mouse. *J Neurosci, 20*(21), 8138–8143.

Ohayon, M. M., & Zulley, J. (1999). Prevalence of naps in the general population. *Sleep Hypnos, 1*, 88–97.

Olsen, C., Pedersen, I., Bergland, A., Enders-Slegers, M. J., Jøranson, N., Calogiuri, G., & Ihlebaek, C. (2016). Differences in quality of life in home-dwelling persons and nursing home residents with dementia - a cross-sectional study. *BMC Geriatr, 16*, 1–11. doi:10.1186/s12877-016-0312-4

Panda, S., Provencio, I., Tu, D., Pires, S., Rollag, M., Castrucci, A., ... Hogenesch, J. (2003). Melanopsin in required for non-image-forming photic responses in blind mice. *Science, 301*(5632), 526–527.

Pérez-Medina-Carballo, R., Kosmadopoulos, A., Boudreau, P., Robert, M., Walker, C. D., & Boivin, D. B. (2022). The circadian variation of sleep and alertness of postmenopausal women. *Sleep, 46*(2), zsac272. doi:10.1093/sleep/zsac272

Piggins, H. D., Antle, M., & Rusak, B. (1995). Neuropeptides phase shift the mammalian circadian pacemaker. *J Neurosci, 15*, 5612–5622.

Piggins, H. D., & Cutler, D. J. (2003). The roles of vasoactive intestinal polypeptide in the mammalian circadian clock. *J Endocrinol, 177*(1), 7–15.

Pittendrigh, C. S., & Daan, S. (1974). Circadian oscillations in rodents: a systematic increase of their frequency with age. *Science, 186*, 548–550.

Porcu, A., Nilsson, A., Booreddy, S., Barnes, S. A., Welsh, D. K., & Dulcis, D. (2022). Seasonal changes in day length induce multisynaptic neurotransmitter switching to regulate hypothalamuc network activity and behavior. *Sci Adv, 8*, 1–18.

Prosser, H. M., Bradley, A., Chesham, J. E., Ebling, F. J. P., Hastings, M. H., & Maywood, E. S. (2007). Prokineticin receptor 2 (Prokr2) is essential for the regulation of circadian behavior by the suprachiasmatic nuclei. *Proc Natl Acad Sci USA, 104*(2), 648–653. doi: 10.1073/pnas.0606884104

Prosser, R. A., & Gillette, M. U. (1989). The mammalian circadian clock in the suprachiasmatic nuclei is reset *in vitro* by cAMP. *J Neurosci, 9*, 1073–1081.

Provencio, I., Rodriguez, I., Jiang, G., Hayes, W., Moreira, E., & Rollag, M. (2000). A novel human opsin in the inner retina. *J Neurosci, 20*(2), 600–605.

Ralph, M. R., Foster, R. G., Davis, F. C., & Menaker, M. (1990). Transplanted suprachiasmatic nucleus determines circadian period. *Science, 247*, 975–978.

Ralph, M. R., & Menaker, M. (1988). A mutation of the circadian system in golden hamsters. *Science, 241*, 1225–1227.

Ramkisoensing, A., & Meijer, J. H. (2015). Synchronization of biological clock neurons by light and peripheral feedback systems promotes circadian rhythms and health. *Front Neurol, 6*, 128. doi: 10.3389/fneur.2015.00128

Rediehs, M. H., Reis, J. S., & Creason, N. S. (1990). Sleep in old age: focus on gender differences. *Sleep, 13*(5), 410–424.

Reynolds, C. F., III, Jennings, J. R., Hoch, C. C., Monk, T., Berman, S., Hall, F., ... Kupfer, D. (1991). Daytime sleepiness in the healthy "old old": a comparison to young adults. *J Am Geriatr Soc, 39*, 957–962.

Richter, C. P. (1971). Inborn nature of the rat's 24-hour clock. *J Comp Physiol Psych, 75*(1), 1–4.

Roenneberg, T., Kuehnle, T., Pramstaller, P. P., Ricken, J., Havel, M., Guth, A., & Merrow, M. (2004). A marker for the end of adolescence. *Curr Biol, 14*(24), R1038–R1039. doi: 10.1016/j.cub.2004.11.039

Rosenberg, R. S., Zepelin, H., & Rechtschaffen, A. (1979). Sleep in young and old rats. *J Gerontol, 34*(4), 525–532.

Ruby, N., Brennan, T., Xie, X., Vinh, C., Franken, P., Heller, H., & O'Hara, B. (2002). Role of melanopsin in circadian responses to light. *Science, 298*(5601), 2211–2213.

Rusak, B. (1977a). Involvement of the primary optic tracts in mediation of light effects on hamster circadian rhythms. *J Comp Physiol A, 118*, 165–172.

Rusak, B. (1977b). The role of the suprachiasmatic nuclei in the generation of circadian rhythms in the golden hamster, *Mesocricetus auratus J Comp Physiol A, 118*, 145–164.

Rusak, B., & Zucker, I. (1979). Neural regulation of circadian rhythms. *Physiol Rev, 59*(3), 449–526. doi: 10.1152/physrev.1979.59.3.449

Sakhi, K., Wegner, S., Belle, M. D., Howarth, M., Delagrange, P., Brown, T. M., & Piggins, H. D. (2014). Intrinsic and extrinsic cues regulate the daily profile of mouse lateral habenula neuronal activity. *J Physiol, 592*(22), 5025–5045. doi: 10.1113/jphysiol.2014.280065

Saper, C. B., Scammell, T. E., & Lu, J. (2005). Hypothalamic regulation of sleep and circadian rhythms. *Nature, 437*(7063), 1257–1263. doi: 10.1038/nature04284

Satinoff, E., Li, H., Tcheng, T. K., Liu, C., McArthur, A., Medanic, M., & Gillette, M. U. (1993). Do the suprachiasmatic nuclei oscillate in old rats as they do in young ones? *Am J Physiol, 265*, R1216–R1222.

Sato, T., & Kawamura, H. (1984). Circadian rhythms in multiple unit activity inside and outside the suprachiasmatic nucleus in the diurnal chipmunk (*Eutamias sibiricus*). *Neurosci Res, 1*, 45–52. doi: 10.1016/0168-0102(84)90029-4

Sawaki, Y., Nihonmatsu, I., & Kawamura, H. (1984). Transplantation of the neonatal suprachiasmatic nuclei into rats with complete bilateral suprachiasmatic lesions. *Neurosci Res, 1*, 67–72.

Scheuermaier, K., Laffan, A. M., & Duffy, J. F. (2010). Light exposure patterns in healthy older and young adults. *J Biol Rhythms, 25*(2), 113–122. doi: 10.1177/0748730410361916

Schoonderwoerd, R. A., de Rover, M., Janse, J. A. M., Hirschler, L., Willemse, C. R., Scholten, L., ... Meijer, J. H. (2022). The photobiology of the human circadian clock. *Proc Natl Acad Sci U S A, 119*(13), e2118803119. doi: 10.1073/pnas.2118803119

Schoonderwoerd, R. A., de Torres Gutierrez, P., Blommers, R., van Beurden, A. W., Coenen, T. C. J. J., Klett, N. J., ... Meijer, J. H. (2022). Inhibitory responses to retinohypothalamic tract stimulation in the circadian clock of the diurnal rodent *Rhabdomys pumilio*. *FASEB J, 36*(8), e22415. doi: 10.1096/fj.202200477R

Schwartz, W. J., & Reppert, S. M. (1985). Neural regulation of the circadian vasopressin rhythm in cerebrospinal fluid: a pre-eminent role for the suprachiasmatic nuclei. *J Neurosci, 5*(10), 2771–2778.

Silver, R., LeSauter, J., Tresco, P. A., & Lehman, M. N. (1996). A diffusible coupling signal from the transplanted suprachiasmatic nucleus controlling circadian locomotor rhythms. *Nature, 382*, 810–813.

Stenuit, P., & Kerkhofs, M. (2005). Age modulates the effects of sleep restriction in women. *Sleep, 28*(10), 1283–1286.

Stephan, F. K. (1986). Coupling between feeding- and light-entrainable circadian pacemakers in the rat. *Physiol Behav, 38*, 537–544.

Stephan, F. K., & Zucker, I. (1972a). Circadian rhythms in drinking behavior and locomotor activity of rats are eliminated by hypothalamic lesions. *Proc Natl Acad Sci USA, 69*, 1583–1586.

Stephan, F. K., & Zucker, I. (1972b). Rat drinking rhythms: central visual pathways and endocrine factors mediating responsiveness to environmental illumination. *Physiol Behav, 8*, 315–326.

Stoschitzky, K., Sakotnik, A., Lercher, P., Zweiker, R., Maier, R., Liebmann, P., & Lindner, W. (1999). Influence of betablockers on melatonin release. *Eur J Clin Pharmacol, 55*, 111–115.

Strogatz, S. H., Kronauer, R. E., & Czeisler, C. A. (1987a). Circadian pacemaker interferes with sleep onset at specific times each day: role in insomnia. *Am J Physiol, 253*, R172–R178.

Strogatz, S. H., Kronauer, R. E., & Czeisler, C. A. (1987b). Circadian pacemaker interferes with sleep onset at specific times each day: role of insomnia. *Am J Physiol, 253*, R172–R178.

Sullivan, S. S., & Kushida, C. A. (2008). Multiple Sleep Latency Test and Maintenance of Wakefulness Test. *Chest, 134*(4), 854–861. doi: 10.1378/chest.08-0822

Sun, X., Whitefield, S., Rusak, B., & Semba, K. (2001). Electrophysiological analysis of suprachiasmatic nucleus projections to the ventrolateral preoptic area in the rat. *Eur J Neurosci, 14*, 1257–1274.

Surrall, K., Smith, J. A., Okala, B., Othman, H., & Patrick, D. J. (1987). Effect of ibuprofen and indomethacin on human plasma melatonin. *J Pharm Pharmacol, 39*(10), 840–843.

Swaab, D. F., Fliers, E., & Partiman, T. S. (1985). The suprachiasmatic nucleus of the human brain in relation to sex, age and senile dementia. *Brain Res, 342*, 37–44.

Swanson, L. W., & Cowan, W. M. (1975). The efferent connections of the suprachiasmatic nucleus of the hypothalamus. *J Comp Neurol, 160*, 1–12.

Talamanca, L., Gobet, C., & Naef, F. (2023). Sex-dimorphic and age-dependent organization of 24-hour gene expression rhythms in humans. *Science, 379*, 478–483.

Taub, A., Carbajal, Y., Rimu, K., Holt, R., Yao, Y., Hernandez, A. L., LeSauter, J., & Silver, R. (2021). Arginine vasopressin-containing neurons of the suprachiasmatic nucleus project to CSF. *eNeuro, 8*(2). doi:10.1523/ENEURO.0363-20.2021

Terman, J. S., Remé, C. E., & Terman, M. (1993). Rod outer segment disk shedding in rats with lesions of the suprachiasmatic nucleus. *Brain Res, 605*, 256–264.

Tobler, I., Borbély, A. A., & Groos, G. (1983). The effect of sleep deprivation on sleep in rats with suprachiasmatic lesions. *Neurosci Lett, 42*, 49–54.

Tosini, G., & Menaker, M. (1996). Circadian rhythms in cultured mammalian retina. *Science, 272*, 419–421.

Trachsel, L., Edgar, D., WF, S., Heller, H., & Dement, W. (1992). Sleep homeostasis in suprachiasmatic-lesions rats: effects of sleep deprivation and triazolam administration. *Brain Res, 589*, 253–261.

Turner, P. L., Van Someren, E. J., & Mainster, M. A. (2010). The role of environmental light in sleep and health: effects of ocular aging and cataract surgery. *Sleep Med Rev, 14*(4), 269–280. doi: 10.1016/j.smrv.2009.11.002

Urrila, A. S., Stenuit, P., Huhdankoski, O., Kerkhofs, M., & Porkka-Heiskanen, T. (2007). Psychomotor vigilance task performance during total sleep deprivation in young and postmenopausal women. *Behav Brain Res, 180*(1), 42–47. doi: 10.1016/j.bbr.2007.02.019

van Coevorden, A., Mockel, J., Laurent, E., Kerkhofs, M., L'Hermite-Baléreaux, M., Decoster, C., ...Van Cauter, E. (1991). Neuroendocrine rhythms and sleep in aging men. *Am J Physiol, 260*(4 Part 1), E651–E661.

van den Pol, A. N. (1980). The hypothalamic suprachiasmatic nucleus of rat: intrinsic anatomy. *J Comp Neurol, 191*, 661–702.

van den Pol, A. N., & Tsujimoto, K. L. (1985). Neurotransmitters of the hypothalamic suprachiasmatic nucleus: immunocytochemical analysis of 25 neuronal antigens. *Neuroscience, 15*, 1049–1086.

van der Meijden, W. P., Van Someren, J. L., Te Lindert, B. H., Bruijel, J., van Oosterhout, F., Coppens, J. E., ... Van Someren, E. J. (2016). Individual differences in sleep timing relate to melanopsin-based phototransduction in healthy adolescents and young adults. *Sleep, 39*(6), 1305–1310. doi: 10.5665/sleep.5858

Van Dongen, H., & Dinges, D. (2003). Investigating the interaction between the homeostatic and circadian processes of sleep–wake regulation for the prediction of waking neurobehavioural performance. *J Sleep Res, 12*(181-187).

van Reeth, O., Zhang, Y., Zee, P. C., & Turek, F. W. (1992). Aging alters feedback effects of the activity-rest cycle on the circadian clock. *Am J Physiol Regul Integr Comp Physiol, 263*, R981–R986.

Van Someren, E. J. W., Kessler, A., Mirmiran, M., & Swaab, D. F. (1997). Indirect bright light improves circadian rest-activity rhythm disturbances in demented patients. *Biol Psychiatry, 41*, 955–963.

Vimal, R. L. P., Pandey-Vimal, M.-U. C., Vimal, L.-S. P., Frederick, B. B., Stopa, E. G., Renshaw, P. F., ... Harper, D. G. (2009). Activation of suprachiasmatic nuclei and primary visual cortex depends upon time of day. *Eur J Neurosci, 29*(2), 399–410. doi: 10.1111/j.1460-9568.2008.06582.x

Vitiello, M., & Prinz, P. N. (1989). Alzheimer's disease: sleep and sleep/wake patterns. *Clin Geriatr Med, 5*(2), 289–299.

von Schantz, M. (2008). Phenotypic effects of genetic variability in human clock genes on circadian and sleep parameters. *J Genet, 87*, 513–519.

Wakamatsu, H., Yoshinobu, Y., Aida, R., Moriya, T., Akiyama, M., & Shibata, S. (2001). Restricted-feeding-induced anticipatory activity rhythm is associated with a phase-shift of the expression of mPerl and mPer2 mRNA in the cerebral cortex and hippocampus but not in the suprachiasmatic nucleus of mice. *Eur J Neurosci, 13*(6), 1190–1196. doi: 10.1046/j.0953-816x.2001.01483.x

Wang, J. L., Lim, A. S., Chiang, W. Y., Hsieh, W. H., Lo, M. T., Schneider, J. A., ... Saper, C. B. (2015). Suprachiasmatic neuron numbers and rest-activity circadian rhythms in older humans. *Ann Neurol, 78*(2), 317–322. doi: 10.1002/ana.24432

Wei, H. G., Riel, E., Czeisler, C. A., & Dijk, D.-J. (1999). Attenuated amplitude of circadian and sleep-dependent modulation of electroencephalographic sleep spindle characteristics in elderly human subjects. *Neurosci Lett, 260*, 29–32.

Weitzman, E. D., Moline, M. L., Czeisler, C. A., & Zimmerman, J. C. (1982). Chronobiology of aging: temperature, sleep-wake rhythms and entrainment. *Neurobiol Aging, 3*, 299–309.

Welsh, D. K., Logothetis, D. E., Meister, M., & Reppert, S. M. (1995). Individual neurons dissociated from rat suprachiasmatic nucleus express independently phased circadian firing rhythms. *Neuron, 14*, 697–706.

Witte, K., Schnecko, A., Buijs, R. M., van der Vliet, J., Scalbert, E., Delagrange, P., ... Lemmer, B. (1998). Effects of SCN lesions on circadian blood pressure rhythm in normotensive and transgenic hypertensive rats. *Chronobiol Int, 15*(2), 135–145. doi: 10.3109/07420529808998678

Witting, W., Kwa, I., Eikelenboom, P., Mirmiran, M., & Swaab, D. (1990). Alterations in the circadian rest-activity rhythm in aging and Alzheimer's disease. *Biol Psychiatry, 27*, 563–572.

Wu, Y.-H., & Swaab, D. F. (2007). Disturbance and strategies for reactivation of the circadian rhythm system in aging and Alzheimer's disease. *Sleep Med, 8*(6), 623–636. doi: 10.1016/j.sleep.2006.11.010

Wu, Y.-H., Zhou, J.-N., Van Heerikhuize, J., Jockers, R., & Swaab, D. (2007). Decreased MT1 melatonin receptor expression in the suprachiasmatic nucleus in aging and Alzheimer's disease. *Neurobiol Aging, 28*, 1239–1247. doi: 0.1016/j.neurobiolaging.2006.06.002

Yamaguchi, S., Isejima, H., Matsuo, T., Okura, R., Yagita, K., Kobayashi, M., & Okamura, H. (2003). Synchronization of cellular clocks in the suprachiasmatic nucleus. *Science, 302*, 1408–1412.

Yamaguchi, Y., Suzuki, T., Mizoro, Y., Kori, H., Okada, K., Chen, Y., ... Okamura, H. (2013). Mice genetically deficient in vasopressin V1a and V1b receptors are resistant to jet lag. *Science, 342*(6154), 85–90.

Yamazaki, S., Numan, R., Abe, M., Hida, A., Takahashi, R.-I., Ueda, M., ... Tei, H. (2000). Resetting central and peripheral circadian oscillators in transgenic rats. *Science, 288*(5466), 682–685. doi: 10.1126/science.288.5466.682

Yamazaki, S., Straume, M., Tei, H., Sakaki, Y., Menaker, M., & Block, G. D. (2002). Effects of aging on central and peripheral mammalian clocks. *Proc Natl Acad Sci U S A, 99*(16), 10801–10806. doi: 10.1073/pnas.152318499

Yan, L., Takekida, S., Shigeyoshi, Y., & Okamura, H. (1999). *PER*1 and *PER*2 gene expression in the suprachiasmatic nucleus: circadian profile and the compartment-specific response to light. *Neuroscience, 94*(1), 141–150.

Yan, S. S., & Wang, W. (2016). The effect of lens aging and cataract surgery on circadian rhythm. *Int J Ophthalmol, 9*(7), 1066–1074. doi: 10.18240/ijo.2016.07.21

Yoon, I. Y., Kripke, D. F., Elliott, J. A., Youngstedt, S. D., Rex, K. M., & Hauger, R. L. (2003). Age-related changes of circadian rhythms and sleep-wake cycles. *J Am Geriatr Soc, 51*(8), 1085–1091.

Young, M. E. (2006). The circadian clock within the heart: potential influence on myocardial gene expression, metabolism, and function. *Am J Physiol Heart Circ Physiol, 290*(1), H1–H16. doi: 10.1152/ajpheart.00582.2005

Zeitzer, J. M., Buckmaster, C. L., Parker, K. J., Hauck, C. M., Lyons, D. M., & Mignot, E. (2003). Circadian and homeostatic regulation of hypocretin in a primate model: implications for the consolidation of wakefulness. *J Neurosci, 23*(8), 3555–3560.

Zeitzer, J. M., Daniels, J. E., Duffy, J. F., Klerman, E. B., Shanahan, T. L., Dijk, D.-J., & Czeisler, C. A. (1999). Do plasma melatonin concentrations decline with age? *Am J Med, 107*, 432–436.

Zhang, C., Truong, K. K., & Zhou, Q. Y. (2009). Efferent projections of prokineticin 2 expressing neurons in the mouse suprachiasmatic nucleus. *PLoS One, 4*(9), e7151. doi: 10.1371/journal.pone.0007151

Zhang, E. E., & Kay, S. A. (2010). Clocks not winding down: unravelling circadian networks. *Nat Rev Mol Cell Biol, 11*(11), 764–776. doi: 10.1038/nrm2995

Zhang, R., Lahens, N. F., Ballance, H. I., Hughes, M. E., & Hogenesch, J. B. (2014). A circadian gene expression atlas in mammals: implications for biology and medicine. *Proc Natl Acad Sci U S A, 111*(45), 16219–16224. doi: 10.1073/pnas.1408886111

Zhang, S., Zeitzer, J., Yoshida, Y., Wisor, J., Nishino, S., Edgar, D., & Mignot, E. (2004). Lesions of the suprachiasmatic nucleus eliminate the daily rhythm of hypocretin-1 release. *Sleep, 27*(4), 619–627.

Zhang, Y., Brainard, G., Zee, P., Pinto, L., Takahashi, J., & Turek, F. (1998). Effects of aging on lens transmittance and retinal input to the suprachiasmatic nucleus in golden hamsters. *Neurosci Lett, 258*, 167–170.

Zhang, Y., Kornhauser, J. M., Zee, P. C., Mayo, K. E., Takahashi, J. S., & Turek, F. W. (1996). Effects of aging on light-induced phase-shifting of circadian behavioral rhythms, Fos expression and CREB phosphorylation in the hamster suprachiasmatic nucleus. *Neuroscience, 70*, 951–961.

Zhao, H., & Rusak, B. (2005). Circadian firing-rate rhythms and light responses of rat habenular nucleus neurons *in vivo* and *in vitro*. *Neuroscience, 132*(2), 519–528. doi: 10.1016/j.neuroscience.2005.01.012

Zhao, Z.-Y., Xie, Y., Fu, Y.-R., Bogdan, A., & Touitou, Y. (2002). Aging and the circadian rhythm of melatonin: a cross-sectional study of Chinese subjects 30-110 yr of age. *Chronobiol Int, 19*(6), 1171–1182. doi: 0.1081/CBI-120015958

CHAPTER 9

Pineal Gland and Melatonin

9.1 OVERVIEW

The pineal gland is an important component of the vertebrate circadian system that is closely linked to the function of the suprachiasmatic nuclei (SCN). This chapter reviews the mechanisms by which secretion of the hormone melatonin by the mammalian pineal is regulated by the SCN and by retinal illumination reaching the SCN. As context for a discussion of the role of pineal melatonin in regulating sleep, the chapter summarizes background information about how melatonin acts in regulating seasonal phenomena and how it shifts circadian rhythms. It then discusses several ways that melatonin influences sleep by acting on the SCN as well as on mechanisms regulating body temperature. This chapter also reviews evidence related to the use of melatonin treatments for sleep problems in different populations and reasons for caution in its use.

9.2 The pineal gland and the circadian system

9.2.1 Background

An important component of the circadian system in most vertebrate species is the pineal gland, a name derived from the same root as "pine," presumably because its shape resembles that of a pine nut (Lokhorst, 2021; Shoja et al., 2016). The pineal is a unique, globular structure that in mammals is located in the brain near the junction of the cerebrum and cerebellum, connected to the habenular complex (part of the epithalamus) via the pineal stalk. The fact that the pineal gland is not a lateralized structure, but centrally positioned near the convergence point of several veins and sinuses (the principal drainage routes from the brain), led to the generation of many hypotheses about its functions in the prescientific era. One famous example is presented in **Box 9.1**.

The principal hormonal product of the pineal gland, melatonin, is derived via two enzymatic steps from the neurotransmitter serotonin (Axelrod & Wurtman, 1966; Klein & Moore, 1979). It is produced by many tissues in the body, where it has local effects, including influencing cellular metabolism (Acuña-Castroviejo et al., 2014). Melatonin produced by the pineal gland, however, appears to be unique in its systemic effect on expression of daily rhythms. Pineal melatonin is secreted rhythmically into the cerebrospinal fluid (CSF) that bathes the central nervous system, where it affects many targets via high-affinity melatonin receptors (Vanecek et al., 1987; Weaver et al., 1989; Weaver et al., 1993). Melatonin and its metabolites that can be detected in the CSF, blood, and saliva are largely or entirely a product of the pineal gland (Lewy, Tetsuo, et al., 1980).

Experimental evidence that accumulated beginning in the 20th century suggested a less exalted role for the pineal than Descartes had proposed, but one that is nevertheless important in the regulation of sleep and circadian rhythms. The SCN and pineal have been linked closely throughout vertebrate phylogeny; for example, they jointly regulate circadian rhythms in birds (Takahashi & Menaker, 1982a). In intact birds, the avian pineal is entrained by light–dark cycles so that it secretes high levels of melatonin in the dark phase and little or none during the light phase. Like the mammalian SCN (see Chapter 8), the avian pineal is also a competent, autonomous circadian oscillator. It generates at least several circadian cycles of melatonin production in vitro under constant environmental conditions, but with decreasing amplitude. Even in vitro, the avian pineal can still be entrained by lighting cycles because it is directly light sensitive, unlike the mammalian SCN (Takahashi et al., 1980).

The pineal is not only a light-entrainable, self-sustained oscillator in birds; it is also part of the pacemaker system that sets the phase of overt rhythms, including daily activity rhythms. The study leading to this conclusion involved transplanting a pineal from a "donor" house sparrow (*Passer domesticus*) housed in one lighting cycle into a recipient sparrow that had been housed in a different lighting cycle. The recipient sparrow was arrhythmic in constant conditions after its pineal had

BOX 9.1 The Pineal: Seat of the Soul?

(based on Lokhorst, 2021; Lokhorst & Kaitaro, 2001; http://tinyurl.com/l3adaeb)

The pineal is well known in popular culture in part because René Descartes, the 17th century French philosopher, described it as the "seat of the soul." This conclusion was based on its unique, central position in the brain, its presumed mobility, and the belief that it floated in the sinuses, which were said to be filled with "animal spirits." Animal spirits were believed to flow from the brain down hollow tubes to muscles, which they could inflate, thereby being responsible for muscle contractions and the resulting limb movements and behaviors that the brain controls.

Descartes was a dualist who believed that humans, unlike animals, possessed an immortal, immaterial soul as well as a material body. Voluntary human activity was seen as the product of a decision made by the soul to produce a particular action. Implementing that decision, however, required that the immaterial soul must somehow interact with the mechanisms of the material body.

Descartes considered the midline position of the pineal at the confluence of the sinuses and its undivided structure to be important for two reasons. First, he concluded that sensory perceptions (presumed to be a function of the soul) are experienced as unitary events, even if they originate, for example, from two separate eyes or ears. Although two ears receive sound information independently, the person perceives only a single sound. Somehow these separate inputs must reach a unitary mechanism that interprets them as a single experience. Similarly, he concluded that a person could produce only one thought at a time, despite the fact that the brain structures that presumably give rise to thoughts are all bilaterally duplicated.

Descartes' inference (note that he was a philosopher who operated by deduction, not an experimentalist) was that only a unitary structure could serve as the mechanism that gives rise to a person's experience of unitary perceptions and could ensure that a bilaterally symmetrical brain generates only one thought at a time. The pineal was his candidate for this role.

In relation to behavior, Descartes believed that because of the pineal's location, its minute movements could direct the flow of animal spirits through pores and into the many "channels" that lead from the brain to the body. A decision (by the soul) to generate an action would cause a subtle movement of the pineal that directed animal spirits to the appropriate muscles to produce the desired behavior. Therefore, Descartes deduced that the pineal had the role of mediating perceptual, cognitive, and motor interactions between the immaterial soul and the material body.

been surgically removed (pinealectomy). Implanting a pineal restored free-running activity rhythms beginning from a phase predicted by the lighting cycle to which the donor had been exposed, not that of the recipient bird. Thus, the pineal conveyed both rhythmicity and the phase of its own rhythm to the recipient bird, reflecting its role as a critical component of the circadian pacemaking system (Zimmerman & Menaker, 1979).

9.2.2 Mammalian SCN-pineal interactions

In mammals, unlike birds, the pineal is not a circadian pacemaker. The mammalian pineal lacks the capacity to oscillate independently in vitro or to respond directly to external lighting cues. Nevertheless, it generates a very robust daily rhythm in vivo, with melatonin production restricted to the night (**Figure 9.1**).

This daily rhythm in mammals is controlled by a surprisingly indirect pathway originating in the SCN. The SCN projects dorsally to the hypothalamic paraventricular nucleus (PVN). Neurons in the PVN project monosynaptically onto neurons in the spinal cord, which send projections outside the central nervous system to the superior cervical ganglion (SCG) of the sympathetic nervous system. The SCG projects via the nervi conarii (i.e., pineal nerves) to the pineal gland, where their release of the neurotransmitter norepinephrine (NE) stimulates the production and secretion of melatonin (Moore, 1996; Moore & Klein, 1974) (**Figure 9.2**). Because the external light–dark cycle entrains the circadian firing-rate rhythm of the SCN (see Chapter 8), and therefore its output signals to the PVN, lighting cycles indirectly control the timing of the rhythm of melatonin release from the pineal gland.

The steps by which the SCN controls pineal activity were identified in studies of nocturnal rodents, principally rats (Moore, 1996; Moore & Klein, 1974). SCN neurons spontaneously generate a circadian firing-rate rhythm in constant darkness or when cultured in vitro, with low activity during the subjective night and high activity during the subjective day (see Chapter 8). Under a lighting cycle, light input reaching the SCN via the retinohypothalamic tract further increases the firing rates of most SCN cells in nocturnal animals (Meijer et al., 1986). As a result, SCN neural activity, which is high during the subjective day in constant darkness, is raised even higher in vivo during the light phase of a light–dark cycle. This cycle of high SCN activity during the day and low activity at

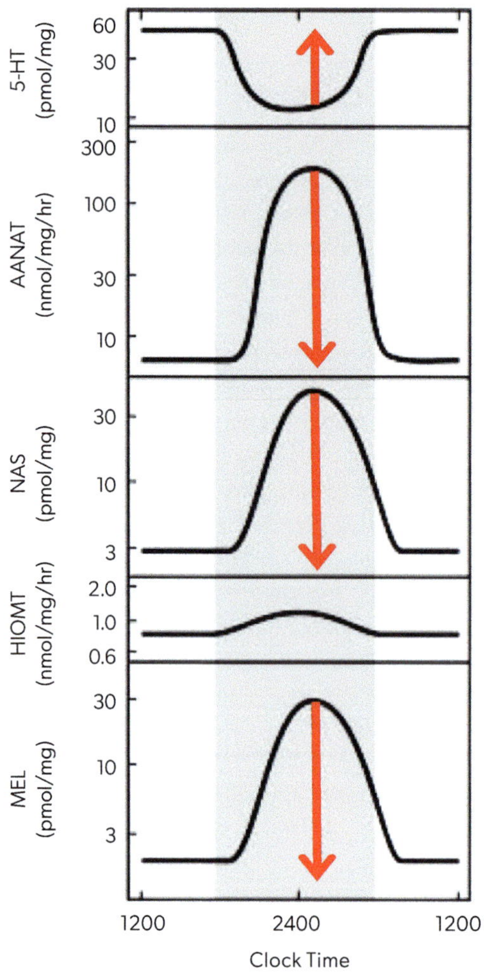

Figure 9.1 Daily rhythms of pineal serotonin (5-HT), N-acetyl serotonin (NAS), melatonin (MEL), and the enzymes that regulate the conversion steps from 5-HT to melatonin (AANAT and HIOMT). Enzymatic activity of AANAT increases at the beginning of the night (shaded area) and it catalyzes the conversion of serotonin to N-acetyl-serotonin (NAS), which is catalyzed by HIOMT to melatonin. Because of its conversion to NAS, levels of serotonin in the pineal decline in parallel to the nighttime increases in NAS and melatonin. The red arrows show the direction of the effects that would result from light exposure at night, which reduces AANAT activity and therefore reduces production of both NAS and melatonin from serotonin, resulting in increased serotonin levels. Adapted with permission from Klein, D.C. (2004) The 2004 Aschoff/Pittendrigh Lecture: Theory of the origin of the pineal gland—a tale of conflict and resolution. *J Biol Rhythms* 19:264–279. © Sage Publications (2004). doi: 10.1177/0748730404267340.

night ultimately ensures that pineal melatonin is released only at night.

This impact of SCN rhythmicity results from the fact that SCN input to the PVN is primarily inhibitory, mediated by the release of GABA, the principal SCN neurotransmitter (Moore & Speh, 1993). The PVN is key to regulation of the pineal gland because its neural activity triggers the spinal cord-SCG network to cause release of NE and initiate the conversion of serotonin to melatonin in the pineal (**Figure 9.2**) (Klein et al., 1983; Moore, 1996). Melatonin production is also facilitated by the activity in the pineal of a prostaglandin (PGE2), a lipid molecule that has hormone-like effects (Cardinali & Ritta, 1983). Since the pineal does not store melatonin, it is produced and secreted simultaneously.

The high daytime firing rate of SCN GABAergic neurons inhibits PVN neurons, which prevents activation of this circuit and production of melatonin during the day (**Figure 9.2 A**). SCN activity starts to decrease in the evening hours because of its intrinsic neural firing-rate rhythm (see Figures 8.5 and 8.6) and because of the loss of activation by light when darkness falls. Decreasing SCN activity at night reduces inhibition of the PVN, which permits the disinhibited (i.e., activated) PVN to trigger the pineal gland to start producing melatonin. As a result, melatonin levels start to rise late in the evening (**Figure 9.2 B**).

The SCN also contains melatonin receptors; when melatonin acts on these receptors, it inhibits the activity of most SCN neurons (Mason & Brooks, 1988; Shibata et al., 1989; Stehle et al., 1989; Ying et al., 1996). The potent inhibition of SCN firing rates by physiological doses of melatonin are mediated by the MT_1 melatonin receptor subtype (Liu et al., 1997). Once SCN firing rates start to fall spontaneously at night and melatonin levels start to rise, the circulating melatonin further inhibits SCN neural activity (**Figure 9.2 B** and **C**). Inhibition of the SCN further disinhibits the PVN-pineal circuit, causing an accelerating increase in melatonin production and release.

In addition, a small number of neurons in the rat SCN release the excitatory neurotransmitter glutamate in the PVN and at other targets (Cui et al., 2001; Hermes et al., 1996; Sun et al., 2001). This projection to the PVN also contributes to melatonin production at night by directly activating PVN neurons (Perreau-Lenz et al., 2003; Perreau-Lenz et al., 2004).

Melatonin levels remain high through much of the night (unless it is interrupted by artificial illumination) until the spontaneous increase in SCN neural activity as morning approaches begins to shut down melatonin production (**Figure 9.2 A;** see **Figure 9.7**). As a result, in mammals, as in other vertebrates, the pineal secretes melatonin only at night and only in darkness, consistent with its designation as the "hormone of darkness" (Utiger, 1992). As reviewed in Section 9.5, the rise of melatonin levels in the evening is a physiological signal that promotes behavior appropriate to the night phase, including sleep onset in people.

In nocturnal rodents, retinal illumination increases the firing rates of a large majority of light-responsive SCN neurons, which would contribute to inhibition of the PVN-pineal circuit and a rapid fall in melatonin levels (red arrows in **Figure 9.1**).

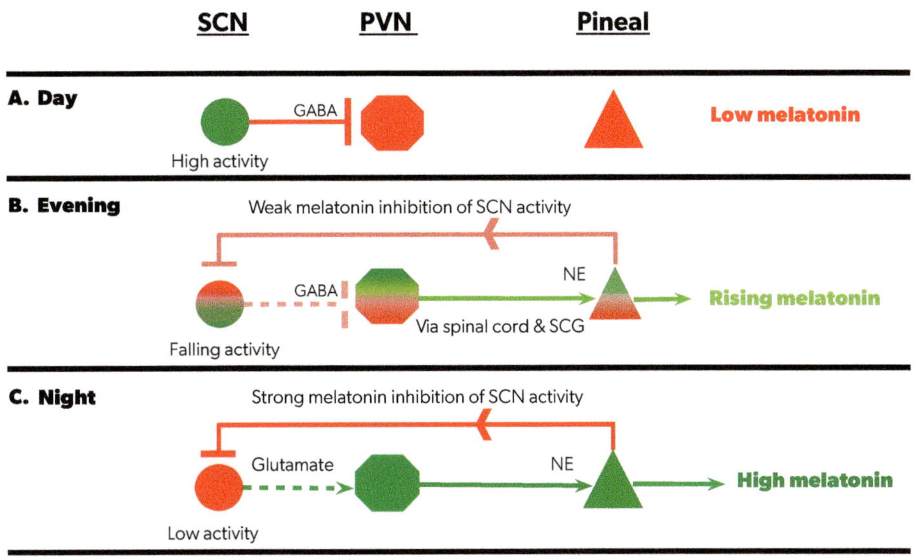

Figure 9.2 A model of the interactions between the suprachiasmatic nuclei (SCN) and pineal gland that trigger the release of melatonin in nocturnal rodents. Red lines indicate inhibition, green arrows represent activation. Green symbols indicate high activity, and red symbols indicate suppressed activity. **A. Day**: The SCN generates a spontaneous daily firing-rate rhythm with high activity during the subjective day that is further increased by light exposure during the day, because light activates most SCN neurons in nocturnal rodents. Since most SCN neurons release the inhibitory neurotransmitter GABA, this high rate of firing causes release of GABA (solid red line) onto cells in the hypothalamic paraventricular nucleus (PVN), which inhibits their activity. As a result, PVN neurons do not activate the circuit that causes the pineal gland to release melatonin. **B. Evening:** In the early evening, the firing rate of SCN neurons declines spontaneously and is further reduced by decreasing light intensity, thereby reducing the amount of GABA inhibition reaching the PVN (dashed pink line). When released from inhibition, PVN neurons increase their activity. They project to the spinal cord where they activate cells that project to the superior cervical ganglion (SCG) of the sympathetic nervous system. Sympathetic neurons from the SCG project via the nervi conarii to the pineal gland where they release norepinephrine (NE), which triggers the production of melatonin from serotonin and its release into the cerebrospinal fluid. Melatonin that is released binds to receptors on neurons in the SCN, which inhibits SCN neurons (solid pink line) and further reduces their already decreasing firing rates. **C. Night:** Low firing rates of SCN GABA neurons allows the PVN to strongly drive the circuit that releases NE, which activates the pineal gland's production and release of melatonin. High levels of melatonin further inhibit the SCN (solid red line)**.** A small subset of SCN neurons also use glutamate to activate PVN neurons (dashed green arrow), thereby further reinforcing the production of melatonin at night. Late in the subjective night (not illustrated), spontaneous increases in firing of SCN neurons start to inhibit the PVN, reducing both melatonin production and its inhibition of the SCN, and eventually restoring the daytime condition shown in **A**.

In the few diurnal rodents that have been studied, however, more cells are inhibited than activated by retinal illumination or optic nerve stimulation (Jiao et al., 1999; Meijer et al., 1989; Schoonderwoerd, de Torres Gutierrez, et al., 2022). Similarly, the most recent evidence, based on high-resolution fMRI studies, shows that the overall human SCN response to illumination is a reduction in neural activity (Schoonderwoerd, de Rover, et al., 2022); see Section 8.2.6.

Despite these species differences in the responses of subsets of SCN neurons to retinal illumination, light at night reduces melatonin levels in people (Lewy, Wehr, et al., 1980) as it does in nocturnal rodents. We do not know how light-suppressed and light-activated neurons in the SCN of people or other diurnal species influence the activity of SCN projections to different targets. Whatever mechanism is involved, SCN neuronal responses to light input must ultimately produce a reduction in activity in the PVN-pineal pathway and its production of melatonin.

In people, illumination as dim as ordinary room light in the evening can delay the onset of the melatonin rise and shorten the overall length of melatonin secretion at night (Gooley et al., 2011; Phillips et al., 2019). Even exposure to light from computer screens or electronic books during the evening can reduce melatonin secretion and thereby modify sleep (Lockley et al., 2003). The effects of evening illumination in people combined with the arousing effects of many computer-linked activities, results in increased levels of arousal at bedtime, delays in melatonin secretion onset, delays in sleep onset, reduced sleep quality, and impaired morning alertness (Cajochen et al., 2011; Carter et al., 2016; Chang et al., 2015; Green et al., 2017) (**Figure 9.3**).

The effects of artificial illumination at night have been proposed to contribute to both delayed and shorter sleep in the general population, as compared to people without access to electric lighting. The evidence related to this idea is discussed in Sections 6.5 and 6.6. In addition, the sensitivity of the circadian/pineal system to light exposure in the evening has special implications for adolescents who already have a delayed phase preference, including those with a diagnosis of delayed sleep

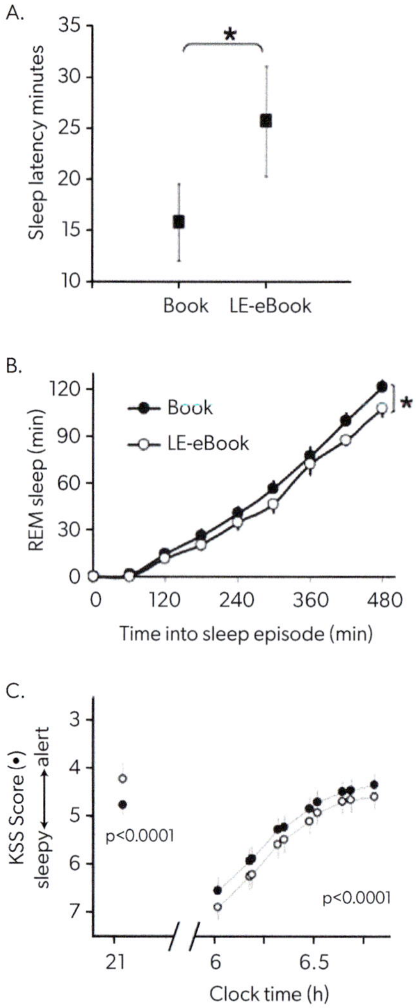

Figure 9.3 Participants in this study read the same text either from a traditional paper book or a light-emitting ebook (LE-ebook) during several hours in the evening. Their sleep and sleepiness were assessed after several days of the same experience. **A.** ebook readers showed a significantly longer latency to fall asleep. **B.** ebook readers (white symbols) accumulated significantly less REM sleep (Y axis) by the end of the sleep period (X axis) than paper book readers (black symbols). **C.** Subjective sleepiness was measured using the Karolinska Sleepiness Scale (KSS) (Y axis). At 9 PM (21 h), those using e-books (white symbol) were significantly less sleepy and more alert than those reading a paper book (black symbol). Beginning after waking at 6 AM, those who used ebooks were consistently sleepier during the morning hours than those who read a paper book, presumably because of reduced sleep quality/duration during the night. Clock time is shown on the X axis. Reprinted with permission from Chang A-M et al. (2015) Evening use of light-emitting eReaders negatively affects sleep, circadian timing, and next-morning alertness. *Proc Natl Acad Sci USA* 112:1232–1237. doi: 10.1073/pnas.1418490112.

phase syndrome (DSPS) (see Sections 4.4.4 and 4.4.5). Those with DSPS are even more sensitive than healthy controls to both the phase-delaying and melatonin-suppressing effects of evening illumination (Aoki et al., 2009; Watson et al., 2018). They are also very likely to be awake and exposed to room lighting and computer screens after sunset.

9.2.3 Summary

The pineal gland is an ancient structure that is closely tied to the circadian system in vertebrates. In birds, it is a directly light-entrainable component of the circadian pacemaker system. Its principal product is the hormone melatonin, which is released only at night and in darkness. The mammalian pineal is activated to produce melatonin through a pathway beginning in the hypothalamic PVN. Activation of the PVN-pineal system results in the release of the neurotransmitter NE onto the pineal, which causes synthesis and release of melatonin.

In mammals, the pineal production of melatonin has fallen under the control of the retina-SCN system that generates circadian rhythms and entrains them to day–night cycles. High firing rates of SCN neurons inhibit the PVN-pineal pathway during the daytime. The spontaneous decline of SCN neural activity to low nighttime levels, along with a decrease in illumination, disinhibits the PVN-pineal pathway, resulting in stimulation of the pineal gland to produce and release melatonin. Melatonin acts on receptors in the SCN at night to further inhibit its neural activity and thereby accelerate melatonin production. The onset of melatonin production marks the transition into the circadian night phase.

Late in the night phase, the spontaneous rise in SCN neural activity inhibits the PVN and eventually terminates melatonin production, so it is low or absent during the day. Even moderate light exposure in the evening, e.g., from electronic readers and computer screens, can delay onset of melatonin secretion, shorten sleep, and impair morning alertness. Sufficiently bright light exposure at any time during the night also suppresses melatonin production.

This background information on the regulation of melatonin secretion leads to the question of what role melatonin plays in the regulation of sleep. To provide a context for this topic, it is useful to first review two other known functions of melatonin: its involvement in regulating seasonal changes in behavior and physiology and its ability to shift and entrain circadian rhythms. The next two sections review these topics.

9.3 Seasonal physiological regulation: a model for melatonin's function

The involvement of melatonin in regulation of seasonal changes in physiology is one of its best-studied and least controversial functions. Although this may sound like an odd topic to discuss in the context of this chapter, it provides important lessons for understanding how melatonin functions in regulating sleep.

During the earth's annual circuit around the sun, it gradually tilts its polar regions toward and away from the sun. As a result, the day and night phases on the earth's surface steadily lengthen and shorten across the year, except near the equator where they are always ~12 h long. In many (but not all) species living in regions away from the equator, this gradual change in day and night length is the critical signal that triggers physiological and behavioral changes that adapt them to seasonal changes in their environments. Another term for daylength is "photoperiod" (and for night length, the less commonly used "scotoperiod"), so these changes are described as photoperiodic phenomena. These include the onset of a limited breeding season at one time of year, followed by gonadal regression and stopping reproduction during another season. Among other seasonal adaptations shown by various species are hibernation, migration, fat deposition, altered social/aggressive behavior, changes in coat color and quality, and altered immune system function (Nelson et al., 1990; Nelson et al., 1995).

The effects of the changing light:dark ratio within the 24 h day are mediated physiologically in many species by changes in the duration of melatonin secretion, which reflect the length of the night phase (Bartness et al., 1993; Hastings et al., 1985). As summarized above, pineal release of melatonin starts as night falls and stops as dawn approaches. As a result, the lengthening nights in the fall increase the duration of melatonin secretion, while the shortening nights as summer approaches decrease melatonin production. The changing duration of melatonin secretion across the year is a critical signal that initiates physiological and behavioral adaptations in anticipation of the challenges and opportunities that characterize each season (Goldman, 2001).

Changes in night length are thus encoded physiologically as changes in the duration of melatonin secretion, which are controlled by the SCN-PVN-pineal circuit. As a result, destruction of the SCN prevents these photoperiodic responses (Rusak & Morin, 1976). Interpreting the daylength information encoded in the length of the melatonin signal also requires a mechanism that can measure it, but organisms other than humans do not have access to external timers. Instead, the melatonin signal is decoded by several brain regions in the hypothalamus and nearby structures. Melatonin binds to these structures via high-affinity receptors (Vanecek et al., 1987; Weaver et al., 1989; Weaver et al., 1993) to trigger a broad array of seasonal changes. While in some mammals the SCN is itself a critical target on which melatonin acts to signal photoperiod changes (Bartness et al., 1991), in others the anterior hypothalamus, pars tuberalis of the pituitary complex, and nearby regions are involved instead (Bartness et al., 1991; Bartness et al., 1993; Leitner & Bartness, 2010).

Small rodents like golden hamsters (*Mesocricetus auratus*) or Siberian hamsters (*Phodopus sungorus*) have short gestation periods (2–3 weeks), so they are sexually active in the spring to ensure birth and development of their young in that season. They stop reproduction in the autumn once nights start to lengthen and melatonin durations increase. Infusing animals with long durations of melatonin artificially also triggers a switch to the nonbreeding state. This evidence might suggest that long durations of melatonin secretion suppress reproduction (i.e., that melatonin is antigonadal). Comparisons among species show that this is not the case. Large mammals, including sheep, deer, and their relatives, have long gestation periods (e.g., 5–7 months), so they must be sexually active in the autumn in order to ensure that their young are also born in the spring.

Thus, lengthening nights and increasing melatonin durations in the autumn signal the *onset* of reproductive development and sexual activity in short-day breeders with long gestation periods (deer, sheep), but they signal the *end* of reproductive activity in long-day breeders with short gestation periods (small rodents). Lengthening nights and increasing melatonin durations neither promote nor inhibit reproduction directly. Rather, seasonal changes in melatonin durations provide information about how the length of the night is changing, and therefore about the time of year. The same night-length signal is then interpreted physiologically in different, species-characteristic ways in order to have the appropriate effects on the reproductive (and other) systems of species that have very different seasonal strategies.

9.3.1 Summary

For many species living in non-equatorial regions, dramatic environmental changes across the annual cycle have critical implications for their survival and reproductive success. To prepare for these seasonal transformations, many species use changes in the length of the night as signals to trigger a host of physiological and behavioral adaptations. The retina-SCN-pineal circuit functions as a transducer that converts information about changing night-length into changes in the duration of melatonin secretion. This signal is interpreted by the brain as information about the time of year, so the circadian system functions as "a clock for all seasons" (Pittendrigh & Daan, 1976b).

An important lesson about melatonin that emerges from research on photoperiodism is that the duration of melatonin does not determine the current physiological state of animals, including their reproductive condition. In other words, melatonin is neither directly pro- nor antigonadal. Instead, the changing pattern of melatonin secretion provides information about time—in this case, the time of year—which has different, often opposite, physiological consequences for different species. We will return to this lesson in discussing the role of melatonin in sleep regulation.

9.4 Melatonin as a chronobiotic

A separate line of research related to melatonin adds another complication related to interactions between the SCN and the pineal. When taken orally by people or injected into other species, melatonin can phase shift the circadian system (Lewy et al., 1992; Underwood, 1986). Treatments that phase shift a rhythm can also entrain that rhythm if they are given periodically (within a limited range of periods).[1] Consistent with melatonin's phase-shifting effects, daily melatonin treatments every 24 h in rats or people entrain their circadian rhythms to the treatment schedule (Arendt et al., 1997; Cassone et al., 1986b; Redman et al., 1983; Sack et al., 1991) (**Figure 9.4**), although effects are not equally robust for all rhythms (Arendt et al., 1997).

The entraining effects of melatonin occur via its action on the SCN. This conclusion comes from evidence that melatonin phase-shifts and entrains circadian rhythms in intact rats but not in rats that have undergone SCN ablations (Cassone et al., 1986a; Redman et al., 1983). In addition, melatonin applied directly to the SCN in brain slice preparations shifts the SCN's in vitro circadian firing-rate rhythm (McArthur et al., 1991). Thus, with respect to sleep–wake and other rhythms, melatonin acts as a chronobiotic, a drug that can affect circadian timekeeping, in this case by acting on the SCN (Arendt & Skene, 2005). These phase-shifting effects are mediated by MT_2 receptors, but with a contribution from MT_1 receptors, at least in mice, and possibly in people (Dubocovich et al., 2005; Liu et al., 1997).

In human studies, circadian phase is often referenced to the timing of the spontaneous rise in melatonin levels above a minimal threshold, studied in darkness or under very dim illumination in order not to suppress or delay the endogenous rise. This phase is defined as the dim-light melatonin onset (DLMO) (Lewy & Sack, 1989). In people, this phase typically occurs in the evening near the peak of the circadian body-temperature rhythm (~21:00). The timing of the DLMO varies among individuals, depending on their habitual entrained phase, and it is influenced by age and gender; see Section 4.4.2.

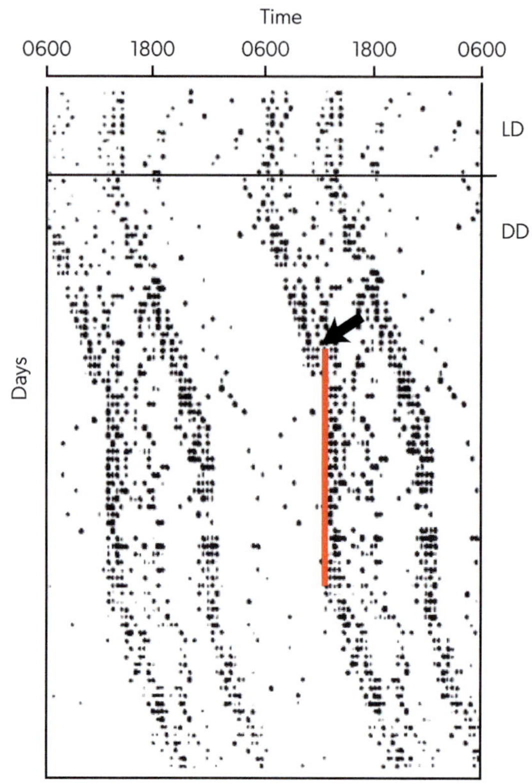

Figure 9.4 A. Wheel-running activity record of a rat entrained initially to a light–dark cycle (LD) with 14 h of light daily (16:00-06:00); the 24 h record is double-plotted (48 h) to improve visualization of the activity pattern. Activity was confined largely to the daily dark phase in the LD cycle. On the day indicated by the horizontal black line, the rat was transferred to continuous darkness (DD) for the remainder of the record. It showed a free-running rhythm with a period greater than 24 h. Daily melatonin injections began at the time indicated by the black arrow and were continued daily at the times indicated by the vertical red line. The activity rhythm became entrained so activity began shortly after the daily injection phase, adopting a 24 h rhythm. When injections stopped, the rat resumed a free-running rhythm with a period longer than 24 h. Saline injections did not entrain activity rhythms, nor could rats with suprachiasmatic nuclei ablations be entrained by daily melatonin injections. Adapted with permission of Dr. Vincent Cassone and Sage Publications from Cassone, V.M. et al. (1986) Dose-dependent entrainment of rat circadian rhythms by daily injection of melatonin. *J Biol Rhythms* 1:219–229. © Sage Publications (1986). doi: 10.1177/074873048600100304.

The DLMO in adults generally precedes habitual sleep onset by ~1–2 h (Shochat et al., 1997).

Treatment with melatonin in the late afternoon, ~5–6 h before the DLMO in most people (= 6–7 h before anticipated sleep onset), causes the largest phase advances of the circadian system (as indexed, e.g., by the timing of the endogenous DLMO). Taking melatonin in the early morning soon after waking instead produces maximal phase delays, which are typically smaller than advance shifts resulting from afternoon/

[1] Entrainment can be modeled as a daily phase shift that compensates for the difference in period between an external cycle (e.g., melatonin given every 24 h) and an internally generated, non-24 h circadian rhythm; see Chapter 3. For circadian clocks, entrainment is generally possible only within a limited range of periods near 24 h.

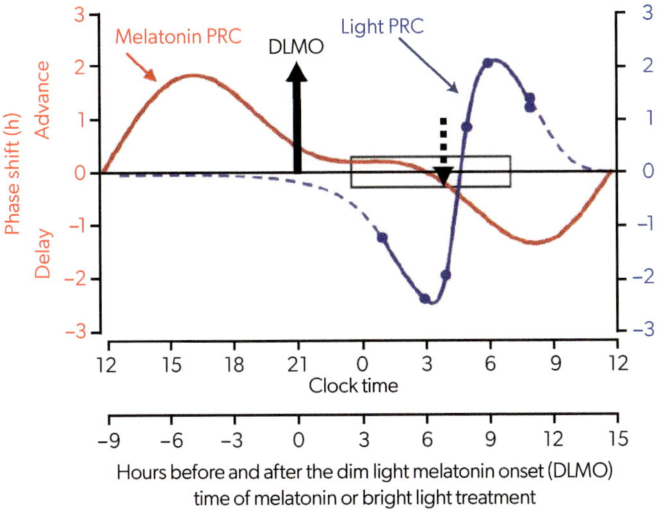

Figure 9.5 Phase response curves (PRCs) for light (2 h at 3500 lux; blue) and melatonin (3 mg; red) in people. Y axis: The curves show the size of delay shifts (– values) and advance shifts (+ values) of the circadian system caused by melatonin or light treatments at different circadian phases**.** The bottom X axis shows the number of hours before or after the time of onset of melatonin secretion in the evening under dim lighting conditions (DLMO = time 0, indicated by the solid black arrow) at which the melatonin treatments or light pulses were given. The upper X axis shows the estimated equivalent clock times under normal living conditions (DLMO = 21:00 clock time). The rectangle represents a typical 7.5 h sleep phase, and the dashed black arrow indicates the approximate trough of the circadian body temperature rhythm. Data points to which the Light PRC curve was fitted are shown as blue symbols; the dashed parts of the light PRC indicate estimates based on other studies for data points that were not collected in this study. Adapted with permission of Elsevier, Ltd. from Eastman, C.I. & Burgess, H.J. (2009) How to travel the world without jet lag. *Sleep Med Clin* 4:241-255. © Elsevier (2009). doi: 10.1016/j.jsmc.2009.02.006.

evening treatments (Burgess et al., 2010) (**Figure 9.5**). The timing of the switch from advance to delay shifts depends on the melatonin dose but typically occurs several hours after the DLMO, near the trough of the body temperature rhythm (dashed arrow, **Figure 9.5**) (Breslow et al., 2013; Eastman & Burgess, 2009).

Based on its chronobiotic properties, melatonin has been used to entrain circadian rhythms in people who express unentrained (free-running) rhythms in the presence of normal day–night cycles; see **Box 9.2**.

Melatonin rhythms play a critical role in regulating sleep timing and maintaining synchrony to the external day–night cycle. Daily melatonin treatments can generate phase shifts large enough to synchronize the free-running rhythms of many people with an unentrained circadian system, whether they are blind or sighted (Lewy et al., 2002; McArthur et al., 1996; Sack et al., 2000; Sack et al., 1991) (**Figure 9.7**). Participants who

BOX 9.2 Unentrained Rhythms in People

Most people who cannot entrain their daily rhythms to day–night cycles are blind, but some sighted people may also fail to entrain (Hayakawa et al., 2005; Klein et al., 1993; Lockley et al., 1997; McArthur et al., 1996; Miles et al., 1977). Legal "blindness" usually refers to severely impaired conscious light and form perception. The visual tracts responsible for conscious visual functions are separate from the RHT that brings photic information to the SCN (see Section 8.2.4). As a result, a person with damage to the visual cortex or lateral geniculate nuclei, for example, could be functionally and legally blind but still have an intact RHT projecting to the SCN, which can mediate normal entrainment. Severe retinal damage or loss of the eyes, however, will result in no light information reaching either the SCN or other brain structures.[a] Many people with no photic input to the SCN, and a small number of sighted people (see below), cannot entrain to 24 h day–night cycles (Czeisler et al., 1995). Instead, they may show disrupted daily sleep–wake patterns or clear free-running circadian rhythms (e.g., of their melatonin production) under normal day–night living conditions. Approximately 30% of blind people show unentrained circadian rhythms (Dr. Steven Lockley, personal communication, 2023).

Failure to entrain to 24 h cycles can result in serious disruption of peoples' sleep patterns and their lives, as was documented by one individual (J. X.) who kept careful records of his sleep–wake cycles over many months (Miles et al., 1977). His records showed that he expressed a near-25 h free-running rhythm in sleep tendencies, which would sometimes coincide with the external night, but would gradually slip out of phase, delaying by ~1 h daily. Attempts to synchronize him to 24 h cycles with rigid scheduling of bedtimes, wake times, and meal patterns were ineffective, and he continued to be sleepy in line with his 25 h internally generated rhythms.

Despite his sleep complaints, J. X. did not have an intrinsic sleep disorder. His sleep disruption resulted from a periodic mismatch between the dictates of his internal 25 h clock and the requirements of a 24 h world to which he could not entrain stably. His sleep was consolidated and normal in length only when his circadian sleep phase coincided with the external night. But his symptoms reemerged spontaneously at regular intervals and persisted until his free-running internal clock cycled back into phase with the external world (Miles et al., 1977).

A similar effect was documented in several completely blind people living in a 24 h world, along with evidence that the periodic disruption of sleep was closely related to the timing of melatonin production (i.e., the timing of their subjective

BOX 9.2 Continued

nights). When the nocturnal sleep phase coincided with the phase of an unentrained melatonin production rhythm, their sleep was lengthy and consolidated. When the melatonin rhythm peaked during the daytime, they were sleepy or napped during the day, and had short, disrupted sleep at night (St. Hilaire & Lockley, 2015); **Figure 9.6**.

[a]A subset of people with visual system damage affecting the RHT may still entrain to daily cycles, probably in response to non-photic cues (Czeisler et al., 1995).

entrained to daily melatonin treatments showed improvements in their sleep at night, including spending less time awake after sleep onset (Sack et al., 2000; Sack & Lewy, 1997). Note, however, that melatonin can only synchronize people's sleep–wake cycles to a 24.0 h schedule if their unentrained rhythms run with a period relatively close to 24 h, as in **Figure 9.7**.

The phase-shifting function of melatonin has also been adapted to help accelerate re-entrainment during simulated jet lag and to help workers adjust to shifting work schedules (Eastman & Burgess, 2009; Sack & Lewy, 1997; Smith & Eastman, 2012), thus reducing the negative impacts of jet lag or shift work on sleep and other daily rhythms (see Section 13.8). The sleep benefits of using melatonin to treat symptoms caused by jet lag or shift work are the indirect result of helping to shift the circadian clock toward a desired phase, rather than being a direct effect of melatonin on sleep processes.

These effects require treatments to be timed appropriately, according to the melatonin sensitivity curve, in order to produce the needed phase shift (**Figure 9.5**). If the state of a person's circadian system has been disrupted by jet lag or shift work, an independent marker of circadian phase is needed

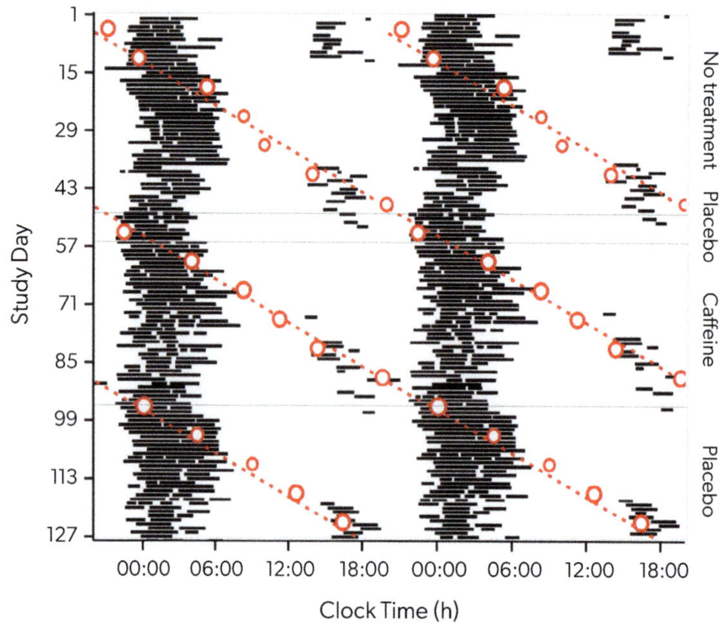

Figure 9.6 A double-plotted record (48 h) of the self-reported nocturnal sleep and nap episodes (black bars) of a totally blind person living normally at home on a 24 h schedule over ~18 weeks (left Y axis). Superimposed on the sleep record are red circles representing the calculated peak times of producing the principal urinary metabolite of melatonin, aMT6s (6-sulfatoxymelatonin), as an indicator of the phasing of the non-entrained circadian pacemaker. The size of each symbol is related to the reliability of the fitted circadian phase marker, with smaller symbols representing a larger error in the fits. The individual was studied under several conditions, separated by the gray horizontal lines and labeled on the right Y axis. The first condition involved no treatment, followed by a daily placebo treatment. The next condition involved a daily dose of caffeine at 10:00, followed by another placebo treatment. The periods estimated for the different conditions are shown as a dotted red line. Estimates did not differ significantly among conditions: 24.51 h with no treatment and 24.59 h for both the placebo and caffeine conditions. Sleep and waking showed an oscillatory pattern over weeks as the non-24 h pacemaker cycled in and out of phase with the 24.0 h societal schedule, resulting in weeks of good sleep alternating with weeks of bad sleep. When peak melatonin production fell in or near the nocturnal phase (~00:00–08:00 h), the sleep episodes tended to be long and sustained, and there was no napping recorded (see ~Days 10–20, 55–70). When melatonin production peaked during the daytime, there were naps in the afternoon (near the time of peak melatonin production), and nocturnal sleep (which occurred during the individual's subjective day phase) tended to be short and more irregular (see ~Days 40–50, 75–90). The morning caffeine treatment had an immediate alerting effect but had no apparent influence on the circadian regulation of sleep-wake or melatonin production. Reprinted with permission from St. Hilaire, M.A. & Lockley, S.W. (2015) Caffeine does not entrain the circadian clock but improves daytime alertness in blind patients with non-24-hour rhythms. *Sleep Med* 16(6): 800–804. © The Authors (2015). Published by Elsevier B.V. This is an open access article under the CC BY license (http://creativecommons.org/licenses/by/4.0/).

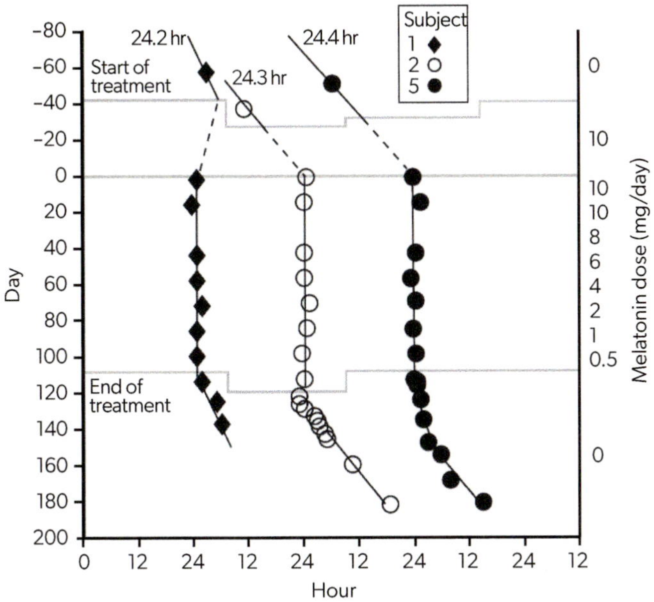

Figure 9.7 The effects of melatonin treatment on endogenous circadian rhythms of melatonin production in totally blind humans. Three participants who entrained to daily melatonin treatments were later retested with a range of melatonin doses. They had free-running periods of 24.2, 24.3, and 24.4 h at baseline, as indicated at the top of the figure. The right-hand Y axis shows the daily doses of melatonin (in mg) used during each segment of the study, starting with 10 mg nightly. Daily melatonin treatments entrained the endogenous circadian rhythm of melatonin production to 24.0 h at doses down to 0.5 mg/day. The endogenous rise of melatonin levels was assessed periodically after a 1–2 day washout with no treatment. After melatonin capsules were replaced with placebo capsules without the participants' knowledge (End of treatment), rhythms began to free-run again with periods longer than 24 h. The record for participant #5 (black circles) shows an example of a persistent after-effect of entrainment. After treatment ended, the free-running period stayed very close to 24 h for ~3 weeks (days 110–135) before it lengthened toward the baseline 24.4 h rhythm. Participants #1 & #2 (white circles and black diamonds) showed more limited persistence of a near-24 h rhythm for about 10 days before the >24 h free-run began. See Section 9.7.2 for a discussion of circadian after-effects. Reprinted with permission of the Massachusetts Medical Society from Sack, R.L. et al. (2000) Entrainment of free-running circadian rhythms by melatonin in blind people. *N Engl J Med* 343:1070–1077. © Massachusetts Medical Society (2000). doi: 10.1056/NEJM200010123431503.

in order to time treatments correctly. Treating someone with melatonin at an unknown circadian phase could fail to produce phase shifts or could cause shifts in the opposite direction of what is needed.

9.4.1 Summary

Acute treatments with melatonin can shift the phase of the SCN pacemaker, resulting in substantial phase advances and smaller phase delays at different circadian phases. Treatments in the late afternoon ~6–7 h before projected sleep onset cause the largest phase advances, and treatments in the early morning hours cause the largest phase delays. Because of this ability to shift the circadian pacemaker, repeated daily melatonin treatments can also entrain the rhythms of people and animals with unentrained free-running rhythms, including totally blind people who cannot be entrained by lighting cycles. This phase-shifting function of melatonin adds additional complexity to understanding how and when melatonin can affect sleep, as discussed in the next section.

9.5 Melatonin and sleep

9.5.1 Endogenous melatonin and sleep

There have been many proposed benefits of using melatonin. The mid-1990s saw the publication of scientific papers, popular books, and magazine articles that heralded (in the words of one enthusiastic title) "the melatonin miracle." The benefits attributed to using melatonin covered a broad range, including improving sleep, treating jet lag and other circadian rhythm disorders, reducing cancer risk, increasing sexual potency, limiting cell death following brain injury, reversing aging, and extending lifespan.

Some of these claims relate to the well-documented function of melatonin as a scavenger of free oxygen radicals, which can damage cellular DNA and are linked to many medical conditions (Galano et al., 2018; Reiter et al., 1995). Findings in model systems have suggested the potential for using melatonin to treat these conditions, but for most of them there is a lack of definitive, clinical evidence demonstrating benefits in people.

The most extensive and convincing evidence of benefits from melatonin treatments in people relates to its role in treating circadian rhythm disorders and regulating sleep timing. The starting point for discussing the role of melatonin in regulating sleep is the physiological evidence reviewed earlier that melatonin secretion in mammals is controlled by signals from the SCN. In people, as in other species, melatonin levels are very low during the day until the circadian system triggers a steep increase late in the evening. Within 1–2 h after the spontaneous rise in melatonin levels, people typically become sleepy and normally go to sleep at that time.

Several studies examined the relation between spontaneous melatonin levels and sleepiness. In one study, young men were moderately sleep restricted (one night with a 5 h sleep opportunity). They were then assessed for their ability to fall asleep during 7 min opportunities every 20 min during a total of 29 h while melatonin levels were measured. Sleepiness

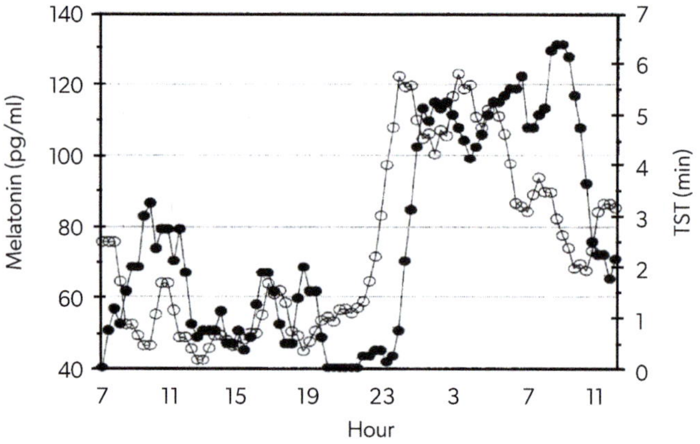

Figure 9.8 Average levels of sleepiness and melatonin production in 5 young men who were allowed 5 h of sleep the night before the study. Sleepiness was measured by giving them 7 min sleep opportunities in total darkness every 20 min continuously for 29 h. The measure of sleepiness was the total amount of sleep produced during each 7 min opportunity (TST) (black symbols, right Y axis). Melatonin levels (left Y axis, white symbols) were also measured throughout the 29 h of the study. Data were time-locked to the onset of melatonin secretion to allow data from participants to be combined. Melatonin levels and sleepiness were both low during the day. Sleepiness started to increase steeply about 1.5–2 h after melatonin levels started to rise (~22 h). Similarly, the decrease in melatonin levels in the morning preceded the steep decline in sleepiness. Reprinted with permission of the American Physiological Society from Shochat, T. et al. (1997) Nocturnal melatonin onset is phase locked to the primary sleep gate. *Am J Physiol* 273:R364–R370. © American Physiological Society (1997); permission conveyed through Copyright Clearance Center, Inc. doi: 10.1152/ajpregu.1997.273.1.R364.

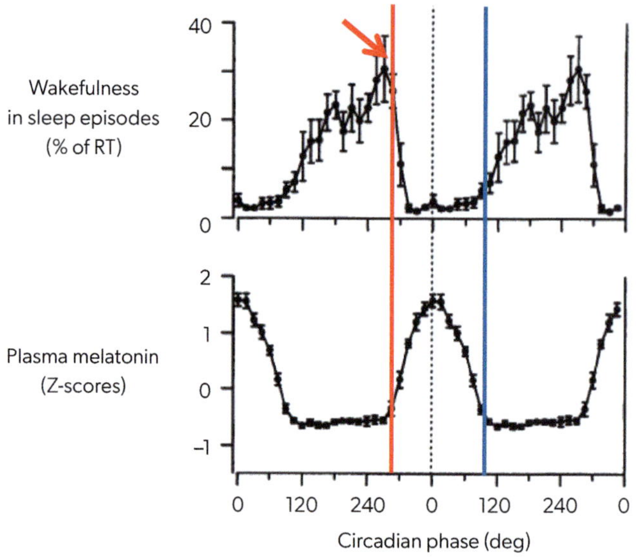

Figure 9.9 A forced desynchronization protocol (28 h cycles with sleep permitted for 9.33 h during each cycle) in temporal isolation permits analysis of the effects of endogenous melatonin secretion on sleep characteristics, since sleep is scheduled to occur in all possible phase relations to the free-running circadian melatonin rhythm. All data are double-plotted to show two full circadian cycles. The top panel shows the average percentage of recording time during which the participants were awake for all scheduled 9.33 h sleep opportunities, which reflects high physiological arousal and difficulty sleeping. Average melatonin levels (bottom panel) are plotted on the X axis in degrees of a circle, relative to the timing of the peak melatonin levels, set at 0 degrees. This phase would be equivalent to ~04:00 during typical entrainment to a 24 h cycle. Wakefulness during scheduled sleep opportunities was high when melatonin levels were low, peaking (red arrow) just before melatonin levels started to rise (red line; at ~300°). The abrupt drop in wakefulness at this phase corresponded to the onset of melatonin secretion and was maintained for as long as melatonin levels were elevated. Wakefulness began to increase again only when melatonin levels had fallen to low values (by ~95°; blue line). Adapted with permission of John Wiley & Sons from Dijk D.-J. et al. (1997) Variation of electroencephalographic activity during non-rapid eye movement and rapid eye movement sleep with phase of circadian melatonin rhythm in humans. *J Physiol* 505.3:851–858. © The Physiological Society (1997); permission conveyed via Copyright Clearance Center doi: 10.1111/j.1469-7793.1997.851ba.x.

was quantified as the minutes of sleep produced during each 7 min sleep opportunity. Sleepiness increased 1.5–2 h after melatonin levels started to rise and fell after melatonin levels started to decline in the morning (Shochat et al., 1997) (**Figure 9.8**).

Another study involved a forced desynchronization protocol (see Section 3.5.2) in constant dim light, during which participants were allowed 9.33 h of sleep every 28 h. Because their circadian clocks could not entrain to the imposed 28 h sleep/wake schedule, their rhythms free-ran with a circadian period. As a result, the scheduled sleep opportunities coincided with all possible phases of participants' circadian rhythms over the course of several weeks. The length of time spent awake during each scheduled sleep period reflected how difficult it was for participants to sleep at each circadian phase (i.e., how wakeful they were).

The highest level of wakefulness was found during sleep opportunities that were scheduled late in the subjective day phase (red arrow, top panel, **Figure 9.9**) (Dijk et al., 1997). This phase corresponds in normal environments to the wake-maintenance zone (also called "sleep forbidden zone") during the evening, when the circadian system promotes waking in opposition to the rising homeostatic drive to sleep after many hours of being awake (Dijk & Czeisler, 1994; Shochat et al., 1997) (see Section 5.7.3).

Immediately after this peak in alertness, circulating melatonin levels started to rise (**Figure 9.9, bottom panel**), and there was an abrupt decrease in wakefulness, which was maintained as long as melatonin levels were elevated (i.e., between the red and blue lines in **Figure 9.9**). The phase at which melatonin started to rise (circadian phase ~300°) can be considered the beginning of the subjective night, while the end of melatonin secretion (blue line) marked subjective dawn (Wehr et al., 2001). Thus, rising melatonin levels mark the end of the wake-maintenance zone and the transition to the circadian night phase, which for people includes the principal sleep period (Vandenheuvel et al., 2005).

There are robust correlations between the onset of melatonin secretion and increases in sleep propensity as well as between the end of melatonin secretion and waking. But a correlation does not establish that high melatonin levels are the cause of the onset of sleepiness. Melatonin and sleepiness rhythms could coincide, for example, because both are controlled in parallel by the SCN pacemaker. Establishing a causal relation requires experimental studies that manipulate melatonin levels, as discussed in the next section.

9.5.2 Effects of exogenous melatonin

Studies involving administration of exogenous melatonin have provided several insights into its physiological role. These studies have used a wide array of doses, producing blood levels ranging from those typically produced at night physiologically to values a thousandfold higher. The effects of supraphysiological doses may not reflect melatonin's normal physiological function. The results have been somewhat inconsistent across studies that used different doses, administered them at different times of day or night under different circumstances, and involved people who differed in age, gender, and health status.

Nevertheless, there is a consensus across most studies that melatonin treatments promote drowsiness and more rapid onset of sleep than a placebo treatment when given to healthy people during the day or in the evening before endogenous melatonin has started to rise. In most studies, there were also increases in the duration of sleep, although this depended on the study design (Arendt et al., 1997; Dollins et al., 1994; Lavie, 1997; Tzischinsky & Lavie, 1994; Zhdanova, 2005).

It is important to distinguish the sleep-*promoting* effects of melatonin from hypnotic (sleep-*inducing*) effects of other drugs used as sleep aids. Drugs such as barbiturates (e.g., phenobarbital, secobarbital) and opioid narcotics (e.g., codeine, morphine, oxycodone, fentanyl) have dramatically dose-dependent effects. Low doses of codeine (found in some pain and cough-suppressant medications) may cause drowsiness in some people. At progressively higher doses, opioids (especially more potent forms) cause sustained sleepiness, induced sleep, profound anesthesia, and ultimately suppression of breathing and death.

Repeated low doses of opioids that increase sleepiness eventually produce tolerance (needing increased doses) and may lead to addiction. Stopping intake of opioids after lengthy treatments can produce withdrawal symptoms, which can include rebound insomnia, severe cravings, gastrointestinal symptoms, and others. In addition, the physiological characteristics of opioid- or barbiturate-induced sleep differ from those of normal sleep, including suppressed N3 and/or REM sleep.[2] Similar statements can be made about the effects of benzodiazepines and related drugs that act on γ-aminobutyric acid-A ($GABA_A$) receptors to inhibit neural activity, although most are less potent and have a greater margin of safety than opioids or barbiturates.

None of these statements is true with respect to the effects of melatonin. Melatonin can induce drowsiness and promote earlier sleep onset at low physiological doses (only at certain times of day), but higher doses do not force sleep onset and usually do not further increase the level of drowsiness. Even massively higher than physiological doses do not cause anesthesia or death (Lerner & Nordlund, 1978). There is no evidence of developing tolerance to its effects, and melatonin also does not reduce amounts of REM sleep, N3, or slow-wave activity (Arbon et al., 2015; Scheer et al., 2012).

Either endogenous or exogenous melatonin is typically effective in promoting sleep when a person is in environmental circumstances that permit and encourage sleep onset and is willing to sleep. When motivated to stay awake, people may choose to do so for hours after the spontaneous rise of melatonin in the evening. Over a wide range of doses, melatonin does not induce sleep against an individual's will, nor in the presence of strong wake-promoting factors. In contrast to the effects of melatonin, high enough doses of barbiturate, opioid, or benzodiazepine hypnotics will cause loss of consciousness regardless of environmental circumstances, time of day, or the individual's motivation to stay awake.[3]

These differences probably relate to the physiological level at which each class of drugs act. Hypnotic drugs act on neural mechanisms that normally generate sleep as well as on separate neural mechanisms that affect levels of consciousness and basic physiological functions, such as breathing (Franks, 2008). Melatonin, in contrast, appears to act at an earlier stage of the process that leads to sleep onset, perhaps by depressing wake-promoting systems (Lavie, 1997) or affecting body temperature (Hughes & Badia, 1997); see Section 9.5.4. Metaphorically, this has been described as "opening the sleep

---

[2] The first commercially available barbiturate, Veronal, produced by Bayer, was widely used. One account of its effects in a diary described "heavier" sleep that was also more broken up, resulting in little increase in total duration (Flower, 1932).

[3] One benzodiazepine, triazolam, increased sleep in rats during the day (when they had an accumulated sleep need) but did not do so in rats without a sleep need. SCN-ablated rats, who have only high-frequency sleep–wake cycles and therefore do not spontaneously accumulate a strong sleep need, did not respond to the same doses with increased sleep (Edgar et al., 1991; Trachsel et al., 1992). These results imply that triazolam, at least at the doses used, only increased sleepiness in animals with an existing sleep need.

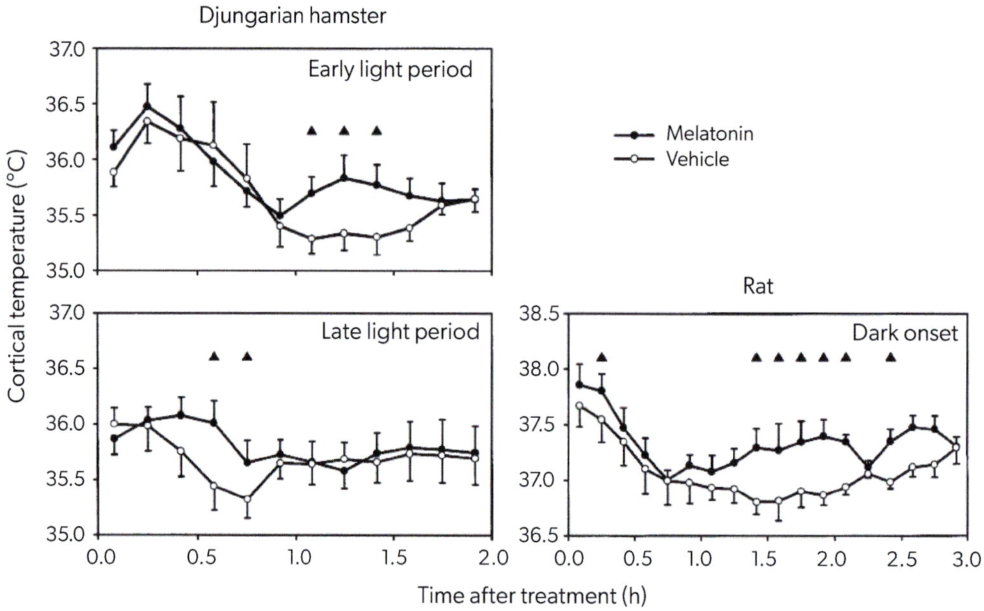

Figure 9.10 Cortical temperatures (Y axis) recorded from two nocturnal rodent species: Djungarian hamsters (*Phodopus sungorus*, Left panel) and rats (*Rattus norvegicus*, Right panel). Animals were injected with melatonin (black symbols) or control vehicle (white symbols) at different phases of a light-dark cycle (early or late light period for hamsters and at dark onset for rats). Time since injections is shown on the X axis. Melatonin caused statistically significant increases in brain temperature (time points marked with black triangles) in both species, which were accompanied by small increases in waking and decreases in sleep amounts. Melatonin treatment in these nocturnal species increased brain temperature and disrupted sleep, in contrast to its effects in people. Reprinted with permission of Elsevier, Ltd. from Huber, R. et al. (1998) Effect of melatonin on sleep and brain temperature in the Djungarian hamster and the rat. *Physiol Behav* 65:77-82. © Elsevier (1998). doi: 10.1016/s0031-9384(98)00125-5.

gate" (Shochat et al., 1997), or transitioning to the circadian night phase. As a result, melatonin *facilitates* the transition to sleep, but the actual production of sleep involves the same neural mechanisms that normally initiate and maintain sleep, so the sleep produced is also physiologically normal.

Another important characteristic of hypnotic drugs is that their sleep-inducing effects occur in both nocturnal and diurnal species; either a mouse or a person can be anesthetized with a barbiturate. Endogenous melatonin, however, is secreted at night, regardless of the activity type of the species, so physiological levels of melatonin cannot normally promote sleep in nocturnally active species. This evidence implies that melatonin treatments should have different effects in diurnal and nocturnal species, by transitioning each species to their respective night phases.

Body temperature cycles in mammals are closely linked to activity types, with high temperatures during circadian active phases and lower temperatures during rest phases. As discussed in more detail in Section 9.5.3, melatonin given to people lowers their core temperatures, but that is not the case for nocturnal species. A study of two nocturnal rodent species, Djungarian hamsters (*Phodopus sungorus*) and rats, found that large doses of melatonin given at some daily phases *increased* brain temperature and reduced or disrupted sleep (Huber et al., 1998) (**Figure 9.10**). Melatonin treatments also increased core body temperature in nocturnal golden hamsters (*Mesocricetus auratus*) (Rusak et al., 2001). These pharmacological effects are consistent with nocturnal rodents being most active at night when endogenous melatonin levels are high.

Consistent with these results, when rats housed in either constant darkness or constant light were injected daily with melatonin, they entrained their activity rhythms to the treatments so that the onset of activity followed immediately after injections, when melatonin levels were highest (Armstrong et al., 1986; Cassone et al., 1986b) (see **Figure 9.4**). These results show that increased melatonin levels act as a physiological timing signal for the beginning of the subjective night; the resulting changes in physiology and behavior depend on the activity type of the species being studied.[4] This interpretation is analogous to the role of seasonal changes in melatonin duration in

[4] Activation of melatonin receptors may also have minor pharmacological effects on sleep. Rats treated with a synthetic drug that is a partial agonist, primarily at one subtype of melatonin receptor (MT_2), showed increased NREM sleep during the daily light phase but not during the dark phase (Ochoa-Sanchez et al., 2011). These effects were mediated by MT_2 receptors in the thalamic reticular nucleus, which helps regulate cortical EEG oscillations (see Chapter 12). The doses used to demonstrate these effects in nocturnal rodents were very high (equivalent to 3–7 g in an adult human) (Hardeland, 2010), and the effects only occurred at a time of day when melatonin is normally not produced.

animals acting as a signal for the time of year, and the consequent physiological changes in physiology and behavior being dependent on the specific reproductive/seasonal strategies of each species (see Section 9.3).

9.5.3 Effects of dose and timing of melatonin

Consistent with the evidence for sleepiness in people increasing shortly after the rise of melatonin in the evening, melatonin treatments aimed at facilitating earlier sleep onsets should be taken ~1–2 h before intended bedtime (see **Figure 9.8**), a phase when it has minimal phase-shifting effect (see **Figure 9.5**). This timing is very different from that required to maximally phase advance the circadian clock (late afternoon/early evening) or delay it (early morning) in order to shift daily rhythms (e.g., as a treatment for jet lag).

The oral dose of melatonin required to phase shift the circadian system or promote sleepiness during the day in people can be as low as 0.1–0.3 mg, which produces blood levels that are close to physiological values at night (~150–200 pg/mL or lower, depending on age). These levels apparently saturate available melatonin receptors, so higher doses produce similar immediate effects (Breslow et al., 2013; Burgess et al., 2010; Dollins et al., 1994; Gooneratne et al., 2012).

Because melatonin has a very short half-life (~30–60 min), a 2 mg dose given to people in an immediate-release formulation produces elevations above baseline for only 3–4 h (Aldhous et al., 1985). Many commercially available melatonin products are sold as 3–10 mg doses, which will produce supraphysiological levels. These may not be any more effective than lower doses in promoting earlier sleep onset, but higher doses (or a sustained-release formulation) can have longer-lasting effects by maintaining elevated blood levels for longer (Aldhous et al., 1985). In a group of older people (average age 75) tested with a combined immediate- and sustained-release melatonin formulation, blood levels remained elevated for up to 10 h (Gooneratne et al., 2012). It is unclear, however, whether a sustained elevation in melatonin levels later in the night actually improves overall sleep quality any more than short-acting doses that promote early sleep onset and are rapidly metabolized (Hardeland, 2013).

Sustaining high blood levels over many hours can also have undesirable effects. High levels extending into the wake phase may increase the risk of morning drowsiness or have other unintended effects. In a study of a blind man with a long free-running circadian period (approaching 25 h), daily low doses of melatonin (0.5 mg) produced phase advances that entrained him to a 24 h rhythm, but high doses (10–20 mg) shortened his period somewhat without producing entrainment (Lewy et al., 2002). This finding may reflect the fact that high doses sustained elevated melatonin levels for longer and therefore affected both the targeted advance portion of the melatonin phase response curve and the delay portion several hours later, resulting in less net phase advance than the low dose treatment (see **Figure 9.5**), and therefore failing to entrain him.

Someone with a habitually late timing of sleep might take a dose of melatonin about 1 h before desired sleep onset (e.g., at 22:00) to try to get to sleep earlier. This timing may increase sleepiness about an hour later, but it will affect only a shallow part of the phase advance zone of the PRC, which peaked hours earlier. Supraphysiological doses at that time may instead affect more of the phase delay portion of the curve starting ~4–5 h later. Producing phase delays of the circadian clock that controls the timing of sleep onset would be counterproductive when trying to shift to an earlier bedtime.

Although there is no consensus about how melatonin facilitates the transition to sleep in people, effects of melatonin on SCN neural activity and on body temperature regulation (see Section 9.5.4) are likely involved. Melatonin probably acts in part by inhibiting the SCN's wake-promoting function in the evening when high levels of SCN neural activity sustain waking in the face of elevated homeostatic sleep drive (see **Figure 9.9**). This idea is consistent with melatonin's inhibitory effect on most SCN neurons (Liu et al., 1997; Mason & Brooks, 1988; Stehle et al., 1989; Ying et al., 1996). Inhibiting SCN neural activity late in the day would free sleep-regulatory systems from the effects of the circadian wake-maintenance zone and allow them to trigger sleep onset in response to the accumulated homeostatic sleep drive. This proposed mechanism is consistent with the idea that melatonin does not induce sleep but is permissive for the transition to sleep when other sleep-promoting conditions are in place.

One finding suggests that this gating function of melatonin may be quantitatively different in men and women. Young adults of both genders were studied in constant routines. Both groups fell asleep at the same time, but women showed an earlier onset and end of endogenous melatonin secretion and a higher amplitude melatonin rhythm than men. As a result, compared to men, sleep onset in women was delayed relative to the onset of their melatonin production (Cain et al., 2010).

9.5.4 Role of body temperature in sleep regulation

Melatonin's effects on human sleep may also be mediated in part by its influence on body temperature regulation. Preparing for sleep by relaxing, lying down, and turning off lights causes immediate peripheral vasodilation (opening of surface blood vessels in hands and feet). That results in warming of the skin surface and increased heat loss from the extremities, causing a gradual fall in core body temperature. The timing of these temperature changes predicts the timing of sleep onset (**Figure 9.11**),

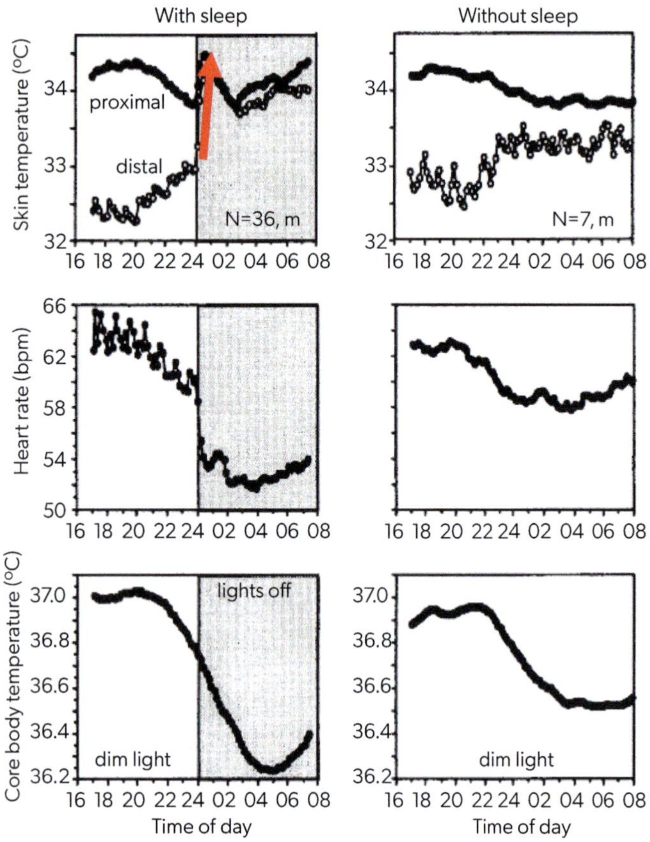

Figure 9.11 The left panels show the impact of turning off lights and giving participants permission to sleep (With sleep, left panels) or having them remain awake in dim constant light (Without sleep, right panels) on skin temperature (top), heart rate (middle) and core body temperature (bottom). Skin temperature was measured at both proximal (trunk) and distal (hand or foot) sites. Darkness (shaded area) and preparation for sleep caused declines in heart rate and core temperature, but sharp increases in skin temperature, especially at the distal extremities. All of these changes were either absent or much smaller if participants remained in dim light and were not permitted to sleep (right column). The red arrow illustrates the sharp increase in skin temperature at the distal skin sites. These changes presumably reflect strong distal vasodilation, followed by a drop in core body temperature, which appear to be important signals for sleep onset. Adapted with permission of Springer:Nature from Kräuchi, K. & Wirz-Justice, A. (2001) Circadian clues to sleep onset mechanisms. *Neuropsychopharmacology* 25:S92–S96. © American College of Neuropsychopharmacology (2001). doi: 10.1016/S0893-133X(01)00315-3.

suggesting that peripheral heat loss may serve as an important signal for the transition to sleep (Kräuchi et al., 2000; Ortiz-Tudela et al., 2014).

Treatment with exogenous melatonin also reduces core body temperature by promoting heat loss from the body surface (Cagnacci et al., 1992; Dollins et al., 1994; Hughes & Badia, 1997). The effects of melatonin on sleep onset may be mediated in part by the resulting fall in core temperature. These effects of melatonin on body temperature are also linked to its effects on the circadian system. There is a strong positive correlation between how much body temperature falls in response to different doses of melatonin given in the evening and how much phase advance of the circadian system they produce (Deacon & Arendt, 1995).

The role of core temperature change as a mediator of melatonin's sleep-promoting effects was further supported by evidence that spontaneous changes in core temperature during sleep onset depended on the rising level of melatonin at that time. Suppressing melatonin production by giving a β-adrenergic antagonist ("beta-blocker"), which prevents NE from affecting the pineal gland, reduced the amplitude of the body temperature rhythm in people by 40% (Cagnacci et al., 1992). Bright light exposure at night, which suppressed melatonin production, prevented the fall in core body temperature until lights were turned off (**Figure 9.12**). Replacing the missing melatonin with two doses of exogenous melatonin (1.0 mg + 0.75 mg) restored the typical body temperature decline, despite continuing bright light exposure (Cagnacci et al., 1993) (**Figure 9.12**).

These findings demonstrate that the endogenous release of melatonin at night is necessary to lower core body temperature, which, in turn, facilitates sleep onset. The opposite effect of melatonin on brain temperature in nocturnal rodents (Huber et al., 1998) (see **Figure 9.10**) emphasizes the fact that increases in melatonin levels at night trigger different physiological responses depending on the activity-type of a species.

A role for temperature changes in regulating sleep is supported by evidence that subtle increases in skin temperature, with little effect on core body temperature, can influence sleep continuity and quality. Artificially inducing a very small increase in skin temperature in the trunk region and upper limbs resulted in increased amounts of slow-wave sleep (SWS) and better sleep continuity, especially in older participants (Raymann et al., 2008). The increase in SWS amounts was striking because it reached levels not usually observed in healthy older people sleeping under typical laboratory conditions.

An exception to the effects of melatonin in reducing body temperature is in women during the luteal (post-ovulatory) phase of natural menstrual cycles. During the luteal phase, women showed elevated body temperatures throughout the day and a blunted decrease at night, resulting in an overall higher average temperature and lower-amplitude rhythm. The onset of melatonin secretion at night was also delayed during the luteal phase relative to the follicular phase, but the overall patterns of melatonin rhythms were similar across menstrual cycle phases. Supraphysiological doses of melatonin given during the day strongly reduced temperature during the follicular phase, but had no effect on the elevated temperatures shown during the luteal phase (Cagnacci et al., 1996).

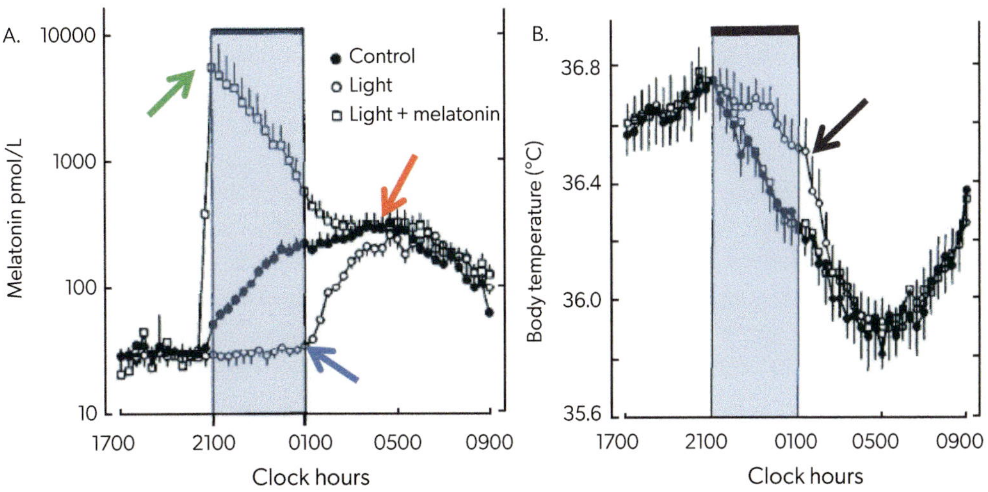

Figure 9.12 **A.** Melatonin levels of women who stayed awake until 01:15 and remained in near-darkness (<10 lux, black circles) or were exposed to bright light (3000 lux, white circles) from 21:00 until 01:00 (blue rectangle), or to both bright light and oral melatonin (1.0 mg at 20:30 and 0.75 mg at 23:00) (white squares). In darkness during preparation for sleep, melatonin levels rose starting at 21:00 to peak near 04:00 (red arrow). Light exposure completely suppressed the melatonin rise until lights were turned off at 01:00 (blue arrow). Exogenous melatonin produced a very high level of melatonin for several hours despite bright light exposure (green arrow; note the log scale on the Y axis). **B.** Body temperature patterns of these women during the same procedures. Body temperature fell continuously from peak values (~21:00) to trough values (~05:00) in both women kept in darkness and in those who were exposed to bright light but were treated with melatonin during the light exposure period. The values overlap so closely that the symbols for those treated with melatonin and those producing it endogenously are difficult to distinguish. Those exposed to bright light alone from 21:00 to 01:00 (white circles) showed elevations of body temperature during light exposure, and a steep fall after lights were turned off (01:00; black arrow). Taken together, these results show that the typical fall in body temperature at night depends on the endogenous rise of melatonin levels and that this effect on body temperature can be mimicked very closely by exogenous melatonin. Melatonin levels after treatment with this amount of exogenous melatonin during bright light exposure were more than 10-fold higher than the levels of endogenous melatonin secreted in darkness, but they had identical effects on the rate of fall of body temperature. Adapted with permission from Cagnacci, A. et al. (1993) The effect of light on core body temperature is mediated by melatonin in women. *J Clin Endocrinol Metab* 76(4):1036–1038. © Oxford University Press (1993); permission conveyed through Copyright Clearance Center, Inc. doi: 10.1210/jcem.76.4.8473378.

One possibility is that the effects of melatonin that are seen in men and in women in the follicular phase are blocked by the thermogenic effects of increased progesterone levels during the luteal phase. This idea is supported by evidence obtained from two women who no longer had menstrual cycles—an older, postmenopausal woman and a young woman who had been surgically ovariectomized as a medical treatment. Progesterone treatments in these women replicated the features of spontaneous body temperature rhythms seen during the luteal phase, including both overall increased temperatures and reduced rhythm amplitude (less decrease at night) (Cagnacci et al., 1996).

Control of body temperature is linked to regulation of sleep in several other ways. As discussed in Section 7.4.5, birds and mammals differ from most vertebrates in being homeothermic (as adults) and showing REM sleep. In addition, sleep onset and end are both closely tied to the daily rhythm of body temperature in people. In entrained conditions, people fall asleep on the descending slope of body temperature a few hours after their evening temperature peak and after the onset of melatonin secretion. They wake up spontaneously on the ascending temperature slope, a few hours after the nocturnal temperature trough, when melatonin levels have fallen.

Under forced desynchronization conditions, the circadian temperature rhythm becomes dissociated from the scheduled sleep–wake cycles. People show abnormally short or long sleep durations because they wake up spontaneously during rising temperature phases that are no longer appropriately timed with respect to the timing of sleep episodes (Czeisler et al., 1980) (see Section 5.7.3 and **Figure 5.18**).

Another link between regulation of body temperature and sleep relates to the physiological mechanisms involved. The preoptic area, which plays a critical role in the regulation of sleep (see Section 11.3), also houses the core regulatory systems involved in body temperature control. Neurons in the preoptic/anterior hypothalamic area respond to changes in the temperature of this region by altering firing rates. These neurons are involved in maintaining temperature within a homeostatically defended range as well as in inducing fever when needed (Boulant, 2000).

Artificially heating the preoptic region (which mimics a rise in core temperature) causes increased firing of warm-sensitive preoptic neurons and promotes heat loss from the skin surface as a homeostatic response to the apparent increase in core temperature. The same treatment also increases sleep propensity. Similarly, the daily peak of core body temperature occurs in mid-evening and is followed by increasing melatonin levels, peripheral heat loss, falling core temperatures, and an increased likelihood of falling asleep in the next 2 h. In addition, warm-sensitive neurons increase their firing rates during naturally occurring NREM sleep, which would also activate heat-loss mechanisms (Alam et al., 1995a; Szymusiak & McGinty, 2008). Thus, the same brain region and probably some of the same neurons that are involved in homeostatic regulation of body temperature by promoting heat loss also play a role in increasing sleep propensity (Gilbert et al., 2004).

Firing-rate changes in response to local preoptic area heating are shown during both waking and NREM sleep. However, these responses are lost during REM sleep, which is characterized by a general absence of homeostatic regulation of body temperature (Alam et al., 1995b; Glotzbach & Heller, 1976), resulting in elevated or decreased brain temperatures, depending on species (Csernai et al., 2019; Kawamura & Sawyer, 1965; Parmeggiani, 2007).

Amounts, timing, and continuity of REM and NREM sleep are also affected by environmental temperature. Both people and rats sleeping at different ambient temperatures show different proportions of REM and NREM sleep. Men who slept with no covers and wearing only shorts showed the highest amounts of SWS and REM sleep at 29° C, and lower amounts in either colder or warmer environments (Haskell et al., 1981). Male rats also showed the largest amounts of REM sleep at one ambient temperature and less at higher and lower temperatures, but the temperature giving peak levels varied depending on their prior adaptation to different temperature environments (Schmidek et al., 1972).

9.5.5 Summary

The role of melatonin in sleep regulation can be viewed through the lens of its role in regulating photoperiodic responses in mammals. In photoperiodic species, melatonin amounts do not directly control reproductive, immune, and other functions that change seasonally. Instead, increasing and decreasing night lengths determine the duration of melatonin secretion, which provides a physiological signal indicating the season of the year. Systems downstream from the melatonin signal determine the physiological profiles appropriate for that season, which can be entirely opposite in species that have different breeding seasons.

Similarly, the principal effects of melatonin on mammalian sleep do not involve direct regulation of sleep mechanisms. The spontaneous decline of SCN neural activity in the evening starts a mutually reinforcing interaction with the pineal gland. The result of that interaction is a steep rise in melatonin levels that signals the transition into the circadian night phase. Downstream systems receive that signal and initiate the physiological changes in each species that are appropriate to that circadian phase. In people, the appropriate physiological state for the night phase includes sleep.

Despite the strong evidence that endogenous melatonin facilitates the transition to the circadian night phase, the effects on sleep of pharmacological treatments with melatonin are more complicated. The first issue is that the goal of the treatment must determine its timing. If the goal is to facilitate earlier sleep onset, melatonin can be taken ~1–2 h before desired bedtime. Melatonin can increase drowsiness and facilitate a more rapid transition to sleep in people at this phase under appropriate, sleep-conducive, environmental conditions. At this phase, however, it has only a small phase-shifting effect.

If the goal, instead, is to phase shift the circadian system (and therefore sleep timing) to treat conditions such as jet lag or delayed sleep phase syndrome (see Chapter 4), the timing would be very different. The effects of melatonin vary from causing advances in the evening hours, before spontaneous onset of melatonin secretion, to causing delays in the late night/early morning. Dosing is also important. Small physiological doses shortly before bedtime have relatively brief effects that can promote earlier sleep onset. But very large doses taken at that time may remain physiologically available into the morning, causing either drowsiness or unintended rhythm delays. The phase-shifting effects of melatonin are sufficient to produce entrainment to a 24 h schedule of melatonin treatments in both rats and people who are expressing near-24 h, free-running rhythms.

The timing of spontaneous sleep onset is closely tied to increased heat loss from the periphery and a resulting fall in core body temperature. The evidence that these temperature changes are caused by the increase in melatonin levels at night includes the fact that bright light or blocking β-adrenergic activity, both of which prevent melatonin production, also prevent the fall in body temperature. Maintenance of elevated body temperature by light at night is not a direct effect of light exposure on temperature regulation; exogenous melatonin can restore the temperature fall despite continued bright light exposure. It is an effect that is mediated by blocking production of endogenous melatonin. These effects of melatonin are shown in men and in women during the follicular phase of the menstrual cycle. They are absent in women during the luteal phase, probably because of the thermogenic effect of high progesterone levels.

There are other close links between regulation of body temperature and sleep: both are regulated in part by neurons in the preoptic area; only homeothermic vertebrates (birds and mammals) generate REM sleep; homeostatic temperature regulation in adults of these species is absent only during REM sleep; and ambient temperatures influence the amounts of REM and NREM sleep produced. Thus, both regulation of sleep timing and the composition of sleep are related to temperature regulatory mechanisms. Melatonin plays a key role in the timing of sleep onset in people in part because of its action in lowering core body temperature.

9.6 Clinical uses of melatonin

9.6.1 Melatonin treatment of sleep problems

Melatonin is widely available as an over-the-counter (OTC) treatment that is promoted for sleep problems, disrupted rhythms, and jet lag. Children with various developmental and psychiatric disorders who had sleep difficulties often received prescription medicines, but among nonprescription treatments, melatonin was the second most commonly recommended by American psychiatrists (after antihistamines) (Owens et al., 2010).

Most early studies of melatonin's effectiveness as a sleep treatment had combinations of design features that would not allow strong conclusions: small numbers of participants; a wide variety of clinical conditions; open-label (i.e., not blinded) study designs; use of only subjective (parental) ratings; relatively brief durations of treatment; and a lack of placebo controls. More recent studies, however, have used more rigorous, blinded, placebo-controlled designs.

Melatonin treatment was reported to be more effective in children with disrupted or irregular sleep–wake schedules than in other groups. Its effectiveness was demonstrated in studies with children who were blind and/or had neurodevelopmental disorders (e.g., attention deficit hyperactivity disorder, autism, or one of several genetic developmental disorders), which are often associated with serious sleep problems (Kamara & Beauchaine, 2020). Studies in these groups and others using both uncontrolled and placebo-controlled designs generally found that nightly melatonin treatments decreased sleep onset latencies, improved consolidation of sleep and waking periods, and sometimes increased total sleep durations (Braam et al., 2008; Dodge & Wilson, 2001; Garfinkel et al., 2011; Gringras et al., 2012; Gringras et al., 2017; Jan & O'Donnell, 1996; Miano & Ferri, 2010; Schroder et al., 2019; Schwichtenberg & Malow, 2015; van Geijlswijk, Korzilius, et al., 2010; van Geijlswijk, van der Heijden, et al., 2010; Wirojanan et al., 2009).

Melatonin was also reported to significantly advance sleep onset in children (and in some adults) with delayed sleep phase disorder or sleep-onset insomnia (see the definition of insomnia in **Box 4.3**) (Carr et al., 2007; van Geijlswijk, Korzilius, et al., 2010; van Maanen et al., 2017; Wasdell et al., 2008). Depending on the timing of treatments, these effects could reflect melatonin either increasing drowsiness or phase-advancing the circadian system (see **Figure 9.5**).

The effectiveness of melatonin for treating sleep problems in both children and adults has, however, been disputed. Meta-analyses of the effectiveness of melatonin for treating sleep disorders reported little evidence for effectiveness, except for producing small advances in sleep onsets (Buscemi et al., 2005; Buscemi et al., 2006). These analyses were criticized for not evaluating effectiveness in selected groups for which there is consistent evidence (e.g., children with developmental disorders), and for including research that had not ensured the appropriate timing of treatments relative to circadian phase (Ahuja et al., 2006). Since the effects of melatonin are strongly circadian-phase dependent, including studies with inappropriate timing (or dosing; see Section 9.5.3) would dilute and obscure potential treatment effects.

More recent meta-analyses and reviews included better-controlled studies and, in some cases, addressed the critical issues of drug timing and effects on different subgroups. Reported effects in some groups appeared robust, but there were smaller benefits in others. The conclusions of these reviews are generally consistent: appropriately timed melatonin improves sleep and its timing in children with intellectual disabilities and sleep problems (Braam et al., 2009), in children with autism spectrum disorder (Rolling et al., 2022; Schroder et al., 2019), and in children and adolescents with sleep-onset insomnia (Wei et al., 2020) or delayed sleep phase disorder (van Geijlswijk, Korzilius, et al., 2010). In adults, there is also weak or moderate support for the use of melatonin to treat jet lag and promote earlier sleep onset (including in military personnel), but not for treatment of shift-work disorders (Costello et al., 2014).

Despite the recent availability of better-quality studies, there remains a need for larger, long-term, well-controlled trials in well-characterized clinical populations (Bruni et al., 2015; Wei et al., 2020). These studies need to pay particular attention to timing and dosing of melatonin in order to reach more robust conclusions about its effectiveness for sleep problems in different groups.

Since melatonin is a natural hormone and is not patentable, there is little incentive for pharmaceutical companies to fund expensive, large-scale studies of melatonin. Some companies have instead developed patented, sustained-release melatonin formulations and novel melatonin analogs that act as agonists on melatonin receptors. These drugs have also been the subject of numerous studies; for a review, see Atkin et al., 2018. A sustained-release formulation of melatonin (Circadin™)

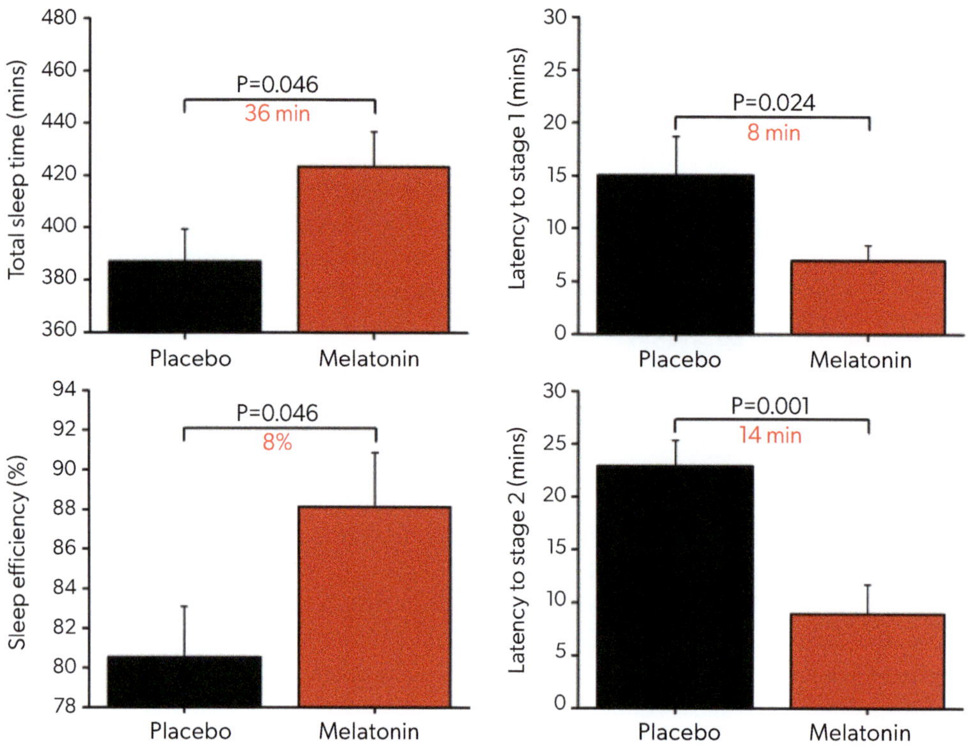

Figure 9.13 Nightly melatonin treatment (red columns; 2.5 mg, ~1 h before bedtime for about 3 weeks) improved sleep features relative to blinded placebo treatments (black columns) in hypertensive patients taking a variety of beta-adrenergic antagonists to control blood pressure. Significant differences between placebo and melatonin treatments are shown above the data. These include a 36 min increase in sleep time, an 8% increase in sleep efficiency, an 8 min decrease in latency to Stage 1 sleep, and a 14 min decrease in latency to Stage 2 sleep (red labels). Reprinted with permission of Oxford University Press from Scheer, F.A.J.L. et al. (2012) Repeated melatonin supplementation improves sleep in hypertensive patients treated with beta-blockers: a randomized controlled trial. *Sleep* 35:1295–1402. © Sleep Research Society (2012). doi: 10.5665/sleep.2122.

was shown to be effective in improving sleep in several populations (e.g., Roth et al., 2015; Wade et al., 2010). A melatonin analog (Ramelteon^{TM}), was approved by the US Food and Drug Administration for treatment of sleep-onset insomnia (Reynoldson et al., 2008), and another (Tasimelteon^{TM}) was approved for treatment of non-24 h sleep–wake disorder (Lockley et al., 2015). Melatonin analogs have also been approved, or submitted for regulatory approval, in other countries for treating insomnia and/or circadian entrainment disorders.

Another melatonin analog, agomelatine (Valdoxan^{TM}), was approved in some jurisdictions for the treatment of depression.[5] The antidepressant effects of agomelatine were attributed to its action as an antagonist at serotonin $(5\text{-HT})_{2C}$ receptors, which are hypothesized to be involved in mood regulation. Its function as an agonist at melatonin receptors is presumably responsible for its sleep-promoting effects, which may also indirectly improve depressive symptoms (Guardiola-Lemaitre et al., 2014; Yang et al., 2016). A role for better sleep in improving symptoms of depression is supported by evidence that psychological treatments aimed specifically at poor sleep quality can improve outcomes in patients undergoing standard treatments for depression and other psychiatric conditions (Cunningham & Shapiro, 2018; Wagley et al., 2013; Watanabe et al., 2011); see Section 15.3.2.

9.6.2 Impaired melatonin production

Patients with impaired melatonin production provide another opportunity to assess its role in sleep regulation. Single-case studies of individuals (e.g., a 14-year old boy) with tumors that reduced melatonin production reported disrupted sleep–wake cycles that were normalized by nightly melatonin treatments (Etzioni et al., 1996). People who were being treated with β-blockers to control hypertension or improve cardiovascular function by reducing NE activity had suppressed melatonin secretion at night. In these patients, melatonin given 1 h before bedtime increased sleep duration and efficiency, reduced the latency to initiate N1 and N2 sleep, and increased sleep durations (Scheer et al., 2012) (**Figure 9.13**).

[5] Disclosure: I previously conducted basic neurophysiological research on agomelatine and related drugs as a paid consultant for the company (Servier) that developed agomelatine.

A rare genetic defect interferes with the production of 5-hydroxytryptophan, which is the precursor of serotonin (5-hydroxytryptamine). As a result, this abnormality also prevents the production of melatonin, which is produced by enzymatic modification of serotonin. Patients with this condition did not show a nocturnal rise in melatonin and experienced severe sleep disruption, including daytime sleepiness, multiple naps, and irregular, but extended, nocturnal sleep periods. In one patient, treatment with 5-hydroxytryptophan restored more normal melatonin secretion and sleep–wake rhythms (Leu-Semenescu et al., 2010) (**Figure 9.14**). Sleep improvement may have been related to changes in both serotonin and melatonin production. Melatonin could have helped promote more regular sleep at night, while serotonin may have helped to maintain daytime alertness and to reduce napping. The nature of the involvement of serotonin in sleep and wake regulation is, however, a matter of continuing debate (see Section 10.5).

An example of a moderate reduction of melatonin production is seen in women diagnosed with premenstrual dysphoric disorder (PDD), as compared to healthy controls. Patients with PDD had delayed onset and lower amplitude melatonin rhythms, along with increased amounts of SWS, but reduced N2 sleep, throughout their menstrual cycles (Parry et al., 1997; Shechter et al., 2012). Taking 2 mg of a slow-release melatonin formulation nightly only during the luteal phase reduced negative mood ratings, especially during premenstrual days (the last days of the luteal phase). Although it was restricted to the luteal phase, nightly melatonin treatments reduced SWS and increased N2 sleep (i.e., reversed baseline sleep features) throughout the menstrual cycle (Moderie et al., 2021).

Another approach to evaluating the role of melatonin is to study the effects of surgically removing the pineal (pinealectomy). In rats, pinealectomy caused no significant changes in sleep patterns or parameters, except for reducing power in the theta frequency band during REM sleep (Fisher & Sugden, 2010). Pinealectomy did cause a small, but significant, reduction in core body temperature during the night, which is consistent with evidence that melatonin increases brain temperature in nocturnal rodents (Huber et al., 1998). Pinealectomy also resulted in a (nonsignificant) reduction in wake time during the daily dark phase, when melatonin levels and activity levels are normally highest in nocturnal rodents (Fisher & Sugden, 2010).

A very small fraction of brain tumors in people involve the pineal gland and require pinealectomy; there have been a few studies of sleep in these patients before and after surgery. One study reported that people with normal nocturnal increases in melatonin before surgery showed no significant changes in sleep parameters or rest–activity cycles after pinealectomy (Slawik et al., 2016). The lack of effects on sleep of surgical

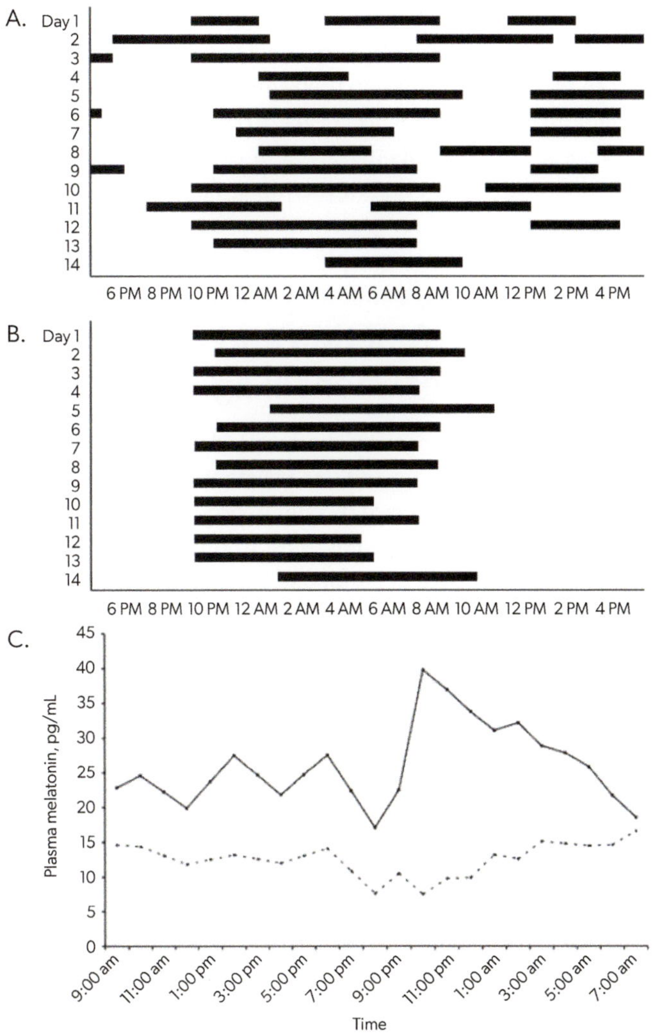

Figure 9.14 **A.** Episodes of sleep (black bars) across 24 h periods (X axis) for 2 weeks (Y axis), according to daily sleep logs. These were recorded by an individual with a genetic defect (sepiapterin reductase deficiency) that ultimately interferes with the production of serotonin and melatonin (as well as dopamine, but that was being treated with replacement therapy). **B.** A similar sleep log after 8 months of daily treatment with the serotonin precursor 5-hydroxytryptophan. Before treatment, the man showed excessive sleep durations, 1–3 daily sleep periods with irregular timing, and daytime sleepiness. After treatment, sleep durations were reduced to normal lengths, and sleep was generally consolidated and restricted to the nighttime. **C.** 24 h melatonin profiles in this man before (dotted line) and after (solid line) 5-hydroxytryptophan treatment. Before treatment, he had low melatonin levels and no nocturnal peak; a low-amplitude melatonin peak appeared after treatment, with typical nocturnal phasing. Adapted with permission from Leu-Semenescu, S. et al. (2010) Sleep and rhythm consequences of a genetically induced loss of serotonin. *Sleep* 33:307–314. © Sleep Research Society and Oxford University Press (2010). doi: 10.1093/sleep/33.3.307.

removal of the pineal is not what would be predicted based on evidence that people with pharmacologically suppressed melatonin production had sleep problems that were improved by melatonin treatments (Scheer et al., 2012) (see **Figure 9.13**), nor with some of the results discussed in the next section. More studies are needed to determine which factors contribute to disturbed or normal sleep patterns in the absence of pineal melatonin production in people.

9.6.3 Pineal function and melatonin treatment in aging

Older people, and especially those with dementia, often have disrupted sleep patterns and low melatonin levels, leading to the suggestion that reduced melatonin production might contribute to their sleep symptoms. Most studies have found highest levels of melatonin in childhood and a decline throughout life, resulting in very low levels in older people and in older people with dementia (Kennaway et al., 1999; Kim et al., 2014; Magri et al., 2004; Mahlberg et al., 2006; Sack et al., 1986; Zhao et al., 2002) (**Figure 9.15**). The elevation of melatonin levels during the day and the lack of a nocturnal peak in elderly, demented patients (Magri et al., 2004) is consistent with other evidence for disruption of circadian rhythms and loss of SCN neurons in dementia patients (see Sections 8.4.4 and 15.5).

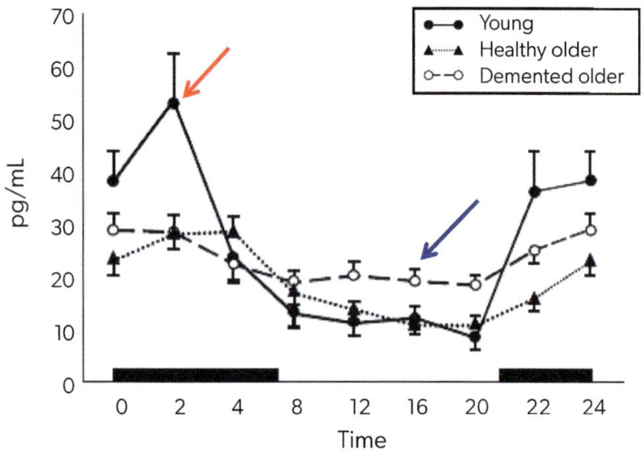

Figure 9.15 Levels of plasma melatonin (pg/mL; Y axis) plotted against time of day (X axis) in adults who were young (black circles; mean age = ~37 y), older (black triangles; mean age = ~82 y), or older and demented (white circles; mean age = ~81 y). The lighting cycle is illustrated on the X axis, with darkness during 21:00–07:00. Melatonin levels in young people started to rise in the early night and peaked in the middle of the dark phase (red arrow), and this increase differed significantly from both other groups at that phase. The older group showed a very attenuated rise in levels at night. The demented older group (both Alzheimer's disease and vascular dementia patients) had especially low amplitude melatonin rhythms with significantly higher levels than the other groups during the daytime (blue arrow). Adapted with permission of John Wiley & Sons from Magri, F. et al. (2004) Qualitative and quantitative changes in melatonin levels in physiological and pathological aging and in centenarians. *J Pineal Res* 36:256–261. © Blackwell Munksgaard (2004). doi: 10.1111/j.1600-079X.2004.00125.x.

There is, however, inconsistent evidence about the extent and timing of decreases in melatonin rhythm amplitude across the lifespan (see discussion in Section 8.4.3). Several factors probably contribute to different findings. One is that people of the same age can have quite different melatonin levels, varying as much as 20-fold. This high variability within age groups makes it difficult to compare levels across age groups (Mahlberg et al., 2006). In one study that compared younger and older people, the amplitudes of plasma melatonin rhythms among those with the most robust rhythms in each group were identical. However, among those with the lowest amplitude rhythms in each group, the older group had much lower amplitudes (Zeitzer et al., 1999); see discussion in Section 8.4.3 and **Figure 8.15**. Other factors include methodological differences among studies (e.g., people studied under usual living conditions vs. in a constant routine), the selection criteria for inclusion in a study, and variable effects of progressive calcification of the pineal during aging.

There are robust positive correlations between the volume of uncalcified (therefore presumably still secretory) pineal tissue in older people and the amount of nightly melatonin produced (Mahlberg et al., 2009; Sigurdardottir et al., 2016). Increased pineal calcification has been associated with reductions in total sleep time, sleep efficiency, and REM sleep amounts in patients with insomnia (Mahlberg et al., 2009). The implication that reduced melatonin production during aging is linked to worse sleep quality is supported by the results of a large, population-based study of men >65 years old. Among those not taking β-blockers (which would reduce melatonin levels), low melatonin production was associated with reduced total sleep time and reduced sleep efficiency (Saksvik-Lehouillier et al., 2015). The reduction in REM sleep amounts seen in those with more pineal calcification is also consistent with the finding that treatment with melatonin receptor agonists increases REM sleep amounts (Cajochen et al., 1997), and that evening light exposure both delays the rise of melatonin and reduces overnight accumulation of REM sleep (Chang et al., 2015); see **Figure 9.3 B.**

If disruption of sleep in aging and dementia is related in part to a loss of robust melatonin rhythmicity, nightly treatment with melatonin might be expected to help restore sleep–wake organization. A well-controlled study of elderly patients with Alzheimer's disease (AD) and disrupted sleep–wake patterns, however, found ambiguous results after 2 months of treatment with melatonin. There were no significant improvements in sleep parameters assessed by actigraphy, except for a nonsignificant trend toward better sleep quality, and there were also reports from caregivers that patients showed improved sleep (Singer et al., 2003). A study of older people with insomnia reported significant improvements in self-reported sleep quality during 6 months of treatment with a prolonged-release form of melatonin (Wade et al., 2010). A meta-analysis of studies of the effects of melatonin treatments on patients with AD reported an increase in sleep duration of <30 min and marginal benefits for sleep efficiency (Xu et al., 2015).

Several factors could have contributed to these variable outcomes, in addition to the use of different measures (self-reports, caregiver reports, and actigraphy). There is a decline in the number of SCN neurons that show immunoreactivity for the melatonin 1 (MT1) receptor during aging and an even more profound reduction among those in late stages of AD. In one postmortem study, the number of neurons that were immunoreactive for MT1 receptors in the central SCN of young people averaged 225.8. In older people and those with early AD, averages were 129 and 132.5, respectively, and in those in late AD, 26.1 (Wu et al., 2007). A similar reduction during aging in mice could account for the loss of a biochemical effect of melatonin on the SCN in older mice (von Gall & Weaver, 2008). If melatonin acts via the circadian system to influence sleep/wake organization, the reduction in SCN neurons with melatonin receptors could weaken responses to treatment in some patients.

The melatonin treatment dosage is also important. Low receptor numbers may suggest the possibility that higher doses would be more effective. However, giving high melatonin doses to older people could be counterproductive if they result in residual elevation of melatonin levels during the day or late in the sleep phase, when melatonin can promote circadian system delays, and therefore delayed sleep onsets. These issues are of special concern in older people because rates of drug metabolism are usually reduced in this population.

There is also evidence that the length of treatment is important. A naturalistic study of older people in group-living homes, some of whom had AD, reported modest benefits of nightly melatonin treatments for sleep duration and sleep latency. Some of these benefits, however, emerged only gradually over treatment periods lasting up to 18 months (Riemersma-van der Lek et al., 2008). Similarly, melatonin treatments resulted in earlier sleep onset among older insomnia patients within a few weeks of starting treatments, but other improvements, such as better overall sleep quality and increased morning alertness, were only evident after 6 months of treatment (Wade et al., 2010). A meta-analysis also concluded that melatonin was more effective in improving sleep in patients with AD when treatments were continued for more than 4 weeks (Xu et al., 2015). The implications of these results for interpreting how melatonin improves sleep in older people are discussed in Section 9.7.

9.6.4 Summary

There is substantial evidence that melatonin treatments are effective in promoting earlier sleep onset, synchronizing daily rhythmicity, and improving sleep in some populations. These include children with developmental disorders, blind people, and those with drug-induced reductions in melatonin levels. Its effectiveness in other populations is less certain, except for producing small advances in sleep onset. Sustained-release formulations of melatonin and melatonin receptor agonists have been developed and approved for treatment of specific sleep- or rhythm-related disorders in several jurisdictions.

Several conditions that are accompanied by reduced melatonin levels are associated with sleep problems that can be improved by treatments to increase melatonin levels. These include patients taking β-blockers, women with premenstrual dysphoric disorder, and those with a rare genetic abnormality that prevents production of serotonin and melatonin.

Declining melatonin production during aging can contribute to sleep problems in older people, but the evidence for effectiveness of melatonin treatments is mixed. Failure to improve sleep may be related to an aging-related decline in the number of melatonin receptors, which has been documented in the SCN of older people, especially those with AD. There is evidence, however, that longer durations of treatment can produce more improvement in sleep in older people and in those with dementia. These findings suggest that melatonin might improve sleep in this population indirectly by its effect on circadian rhythms, as discussed in the next section.

9.7 Melatonin and circadian amplitude

9.7.1 Melatonin influences on SCN rhythmicity

The finding that better sleep quality emerged only gradually during daily melatonin treatments in some older patients suggests that melatonin has actions beyond its immediate phase-shifting or sleep-promoting effects. Several lines of evidence suggest that these actions involve reversing aging-related declines in circadian rhythm amplitude. These decreases in amplitude have been shown in several daily rhythms, including those of melatonin production, body temperature, REM sleep distribution, cortisol secretion, sleep propensity, and others; see Section 8.4.3, and **Figures 8.15**, **8.16**, and **8.17**. One likely contributor to reduced rhythmicity in some functions is reduced rhythm amplitude of the SCN pacemaker itself; see Section 8.4.4 and **Figures 8.18** and **8.19**.

The mechanisms responsible for the reductions observed in physiological and behavioral rhythms are generally not known, but some findings hint at a role for rhythms of melatonin interactions with the SCN. Knockout mice that lacked MT_1 receptors showed flattened daily rhythms of REM sleep and of serum corticosterone levels (Comai et al., 2015; Comai et al., 2013). Reduced melatonin receptor numbers and blunted melatonin rhythms during aging could impair the feedback relations between the SCN and pineal (involving MT_1 receptors; see Liu et al., 1997), which reinforce the daily rhythmicity of SCN activity (see Section 9.2.2 and **Figure 9.2**. In addition, attenuated adrenal corticosteroid rhythms that depend on the SCN (Moore & Eichler, 1972) normally convey daily rhythmicity to a number of target organs (Balsalobre et al., 2000; Bering et al., 2023; Gibbs et al., 2014; Leliavski et al., 2015). Loss of amplitude of SCN rhythms could therefore result directly in reduced rhythmicity of the pineal and adrenal glands as well as a cascade of diminished rhythmicity in other systems controlled indirectly by output from the SCN.

Based on evidence of how the SCN generates circadian rhythms (see Section 8.2.2), the age-related reduction in SCN firing-rate rhythms probably reflects loss of rhythm amplitude in individual oscillating neurons and/or reduced synchrony among these pacemaker components (see **Figure 8.7**). Nightly melatonin treatments over periods of weeks or months could boost the amplitude of oscillation in individual neurons and induce phase shifts that increase the synchrony among the oscillators comprising the pacemaker. The resulting higher amplitude SCN rhythm would strengthen its circadian output signals and ultimately increase the amplitude of overt daily rhythms, including sleep–wake rhythms.

Effects consistent with this interpretation were reported in rats whose activity rhythms were severely disrupted by housing them in bright constant light. Daily melatonin injections restored a better organized rhythm in some rats, with activity concentrated in the hours immediately after injections (defining the subjective night) (Armstrong et al., 1986; Chesworth et al., 1987). The entraining effects of melatonin depend on its action on the SCN; after SCN ablations, melatonin could not entrain activity rhythms in rats (Armstrong et al., 1986; Cassone et al., 1986a). The idea that the SCN is the critical target on which exogenous melatonin acts is consistent with its high density of melatonin receptors in younger people and animals (Reppert et al., 1988; Vanecek et al., 1987), which decreases with age (Wu et al., 2007).

The proposed role for melatonin in boosting the rhythmicity of the mammalian SCN is supported by other lines of evidence. Rats housed in constant bright light lengthen their free-running circadian periods and many gradually lose the integrity of their activity rhythms over days. If rats were first pinealectomized, however, their activity rhythms became disrupted almost immediately in constant light, suggesting that their SCN had less robust rhythms that were more susceptible to further disruption by constant light (Cassone, 1992). Evidence from in vitro slice preparations of the golden hamster SCN is consistent with this idea. The SCNs from hamsters that had previously undergone pinealectomy had reduced amplitude circadian firing-rate rhythms relative to those from intact controls (Rusak & Yu, 1993).

The idea that melatonin acts to increase SCN oscillation amplitude is further supported by evidence that a single, systemic injection of melatonin or of a melatonin receptor agonist increased the amplitude of rhythms controlled by the SCN; namely, the rhythms of endogenous melatonin release and of body temperature (Castanho et al., 2014). Injecting melatonin directly into the SCN had a similar effect in enhancing the amplitude of subsequently assessed endogenous melatonin rhythms (Bothorel et al., 2002).

The loss of a reinforcing effect of melatonin rhythms on SCN rhythmicity may contribute to the decreased amplitude of SCN firing-rate rhythms when the SCN is transferred from an intact animal to an in vitro preparation, but there are obviously many other differences between these two conditions. Although an SCN firing-rate rhythm persists in vitro, the amplitude of the rhythm declines over several cycles when it is first isolated. This observation contrasts to the sustained, high-amplitude oscillation shown by the SCN in intact organisms housed in constant darkness (compare **Figures 8.5** and **8.6**).

Melatonin could also affect other systems in the brain or in other body tissues, some of which are weakly or robustly rhythmic on their own; see Section 8.2.5. Many organs and tissues have melatonin receptors on which it can act (Morgan et al., 1994), while others may be synchronized indirectly, for example, by responding to body temperature cycles, which are modulated by nightly increases in melatonin (see Section 9.5.4), or in response to adrenal corticosteroid rhythms. In summary, melatonin treatments may strengthen the rhythm amplitude of SCN neurons, increase synchrony among these neurons, and increase synchrony among multiple organs including the SCN; for a review, see Hardeland, 2013. These systemic changes in circadian organization, which would emerge over time during melatonin treatments, could result ultimately in more robust sleep–wake cycles.

The available evidence strongly supports the idea that the pineal and SCN of mammals form a mutually reinforcing rhythmic system, even though the mammalian pineal is not intrinsically rhythmic (Cassone et al., 1993). In that respect, their relations partially resemble those in other vertebrates such as birds, in which the pineal is intrinsically rhythmic and forms a compound pacemaker system together with the SCN (Takahashi & Menaker, 1982a; Takahashi & Menaker, 1982b).

The proposed effects of exogenous melatonin would likely take substantial time to strengthen circadian amplitude and ultimately to affect sleep consolidation in older people, in part because of the age-related reduction in melatonin receptors in the SCN and, perhaps, other tissues (von Gall & Weaver, 2008) and especially in those with AD or other forms of brain damage (Wu et al., 2007).

9.7.2 Persistence of melatonin effects

Another feature of melatonin treatments is the persistence of some of its circadian effects for days or weeks after treatments end, despite its very short half-life (30–60 min at a physiological dose in people). As previously described, a single injection of melatonin can have effects on the amplitude of the SCN-controlled endogenous melatonin rhythm for at least 2 days (Bothorel et al., 2002; Castanho et al., 2014). Similarly, some rats housed in constant light whose disrupted rhythms were organized by daily melatonin injections showed persistence of circadian rhythmicity for several days after injections ended (Armstrong et al., 1986).

Among patients who were being treated with β-blockers that reduce melatonin production, nightly melatonin treatments for 3 weeks increased total sleep amounts, improved sleep efficiency, and reduced latency to N2 sleep onset. The latency effect persisted for at least one follow-up night after drug treatment had ended (Scheer et al., 2012).

These findings cannot be explained by the immediate, pharmacological effects of melatonin on sleep propensity, activity, or other rhythms but imply instead that it has long-lasting, indirect effects. The observed effects can be attributed to melatonin acting on the circadian system by increasing the synchrony and amplitude of the SCN's oscillation (and perhaps the synchrony among other organs). The resulting increased amplitude of daily rhythms promotes improved sleep (Scheer et al., 2012; Scheer et al., 2004) and is preserved over several cycles. Presumably the loss of reinforcing rhythmic input after melatonin treatments are discontinued allows the circadian rhythm amplitude to gradually decline again.

Related effects on circadian period were found in the study illustrated in **Figure 9.7**. One of the blind participants, whose endogenous melatonin rhythm initially free-ran with a 24.4 h rhythm (#5, black circles), entrained stably with a 24.0 h rhythm while receiving nightly melatonin treatments for several months. She then continued to show a near-24 h rhythm for ~25 days after treatment ended, before starting to show a gradually lengthening period. Participant #2 (open circles) showed a similar persistence of a near-24 h rhythm until ~10 days after treatment ended, when a longer period gradually reemerged (Sack et al., 2000).

These results indicate that nightly melatonin treatments imposed a 24.0 h periodicity on the SCN pacemaker that controls endogenous melatonin secretion. These changes to the SCN were preserved in the form of after-effects of entrainment that persisted for days or weeks after treatments ended. Based on a model of entrainment (see discussion in **Box 9.3**), these effects imply that daily melatonin treatments imposed a reorganization of component oscillators in the circadian system. The organization of the oscillator population determines the period of the system as well as influencing the amplitude of oscillation.

Analogous effects on the persistent robustness of rhythms have been demonstrated using another agent, bright daytime illumination. In the diurnally active four-striped mouse (*Rhabdomys pumilio*), bright light during the day increased the amplitude of daily activity rhythms relative to dim daytime lighting. When released to free-running conditions in constant darkness for 4 days, mice coming from brighter lighting cycles continued to express higher amplitude circadian activity rhythms and showed different free-running periods than those transferred from dim lighting cycles. In addition, when hypothalamic slices were prepared from these mice and studied in vitro, firing-rate rhythms of the SCN had higher amplitudes in brain slices from mice that had been exposed to bright, as compared to dim, daytime lighting. Recordings from the slice preparations indicated that these effects were related to increased excitability of individual SCN neurons (Bano-Otalora et al., 2021).

In Syrian hamsters (*Mesocricetus auratus*), brighter light during the day increased activity levels at night in middle-aged and (less robustly) in old animals (Labyak et al., 1998). In rats, bright daytime illumination amplified rhythms of activity and sleep–wake (Witting et al., 1993). In people, increased daytime illumination produced larger amplitude melatonin rhythms (i.e., higher peaks at night) (Takasu et al., 2006). These examples probably all represent effects of the amplitude of the entraining cycle on the amplitude of the SCN's rhythm that drives the overt rhythms of activity, sleep–wake, and melatonin production.

These findings indicate that higher amplitude rhythms of either lighting cycles or melatonin reaching the SCN increase the amplitude of overt daily rhythms in both nocturnal and diurnal species. When the persistence of these changes was examined after withdrawal of the light or melatonin signal, effects on circadian amplitude often continued for a period of time. These findings are consistent with the interpretation that increasing circadian amplitude depends on reorganizing the circadian oscillator system and/or altering the excitability of pacemaker neurons, and that the changes induced can persist for days or weeks after the treatments end.

BOX 9.3 Oscillators, Coupling, and After-Effects

A circadian pacemaker expresses its native period when free-running in constant conditions (typically in continuous darkness). When entrained to a zeitgeber cycle, it expresses a different period (that of the zeitgeber cycle). When it is then released to constant conditions again, it often expresses a free-running period that differs from its initial period for days or weeks, despite identical conditions during the second test (Pittendrigh, 1974). Similar after-effects can be observed after single delay or advance phase-shifts of a circadian clock, which, respectively, lengthen or shorten the subsequent free-running circadian period for one or more cycles. These phenomena are related to the fact that the circadian pacemaker is a complex system including multiple oscillators.

The core concepts explaining after-effects were originally developed based on a model of the circadian pacemaker as being composed of two coupled (mutually entrained) oscillators, but the ideas can also apply to a pacemaker composed of many oscillators, like the SCN (Daan & Berde, 1978; Pittendrigh, 1974). The period of the pacemaker's overall rhythm is related to the periods of the component oscillators and, critically, it is affected by their coupling relations. When a previously free-running (non-24.0 h) system is synchronized to a 24 h period (by a lighting cycle or by daily melatonin treatments), the coupling relations among component oscillators change as a result of adopting a 24.0 h rhythm.

When the entraining agent is removed, this altered pattern of coupling among the oscillators is often retained for a few (or many) cycles before the individual oscillators gradually drift back toward their previous coupling arrangement, and the pacemaker system again approaches its original free-running period (**Figure 9.16**) (Pittendrigh & Daan, 1976a).

Retention of the imposed changes in the coupling relations among pacemaker components can account for persistent period changes illustrated in **Figure 9.7**. The slow approach to restoring the original free-running period indicates that these altered coupling relations are lost only gradually. Similarly, the amplitude of the output rhythm generated by the pacemaker will depend on the degree of coherence among its component oscillators. Thus, altered coupling relations among these components can also explain changes in the amplitude of circadian sleep–wake rhythms during melatonin treatments and their persistence after treatments end.

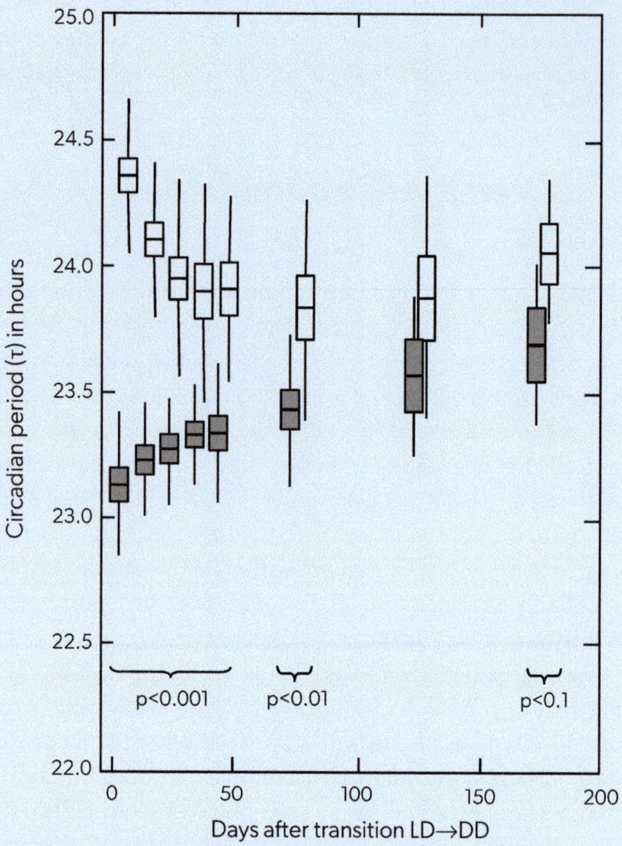

Figure 9.16 Average free-running periods in constant darkness (Y axis) of groups of mice after entrainment to light–dark cycles with periods of 28 h (white bars) or 20 h (grey bars). The average periods in the two groups differed significantly (p values shown at bottom) immediately after the mice were released from their different entrainment conditions to constant darkness on Day 0 and for over 150 days after the transition. These after-effects, and the length of time required to converge toward a common free-running period in DD, are modeled as the result of the slow process of reorganization of phase relations among constituent oscillators in the circadian pacemaker. These oscillators had been forced into different temporal relations by the 20 h and 28 h entrainment experiences and rebounded only slowly to reestablish their usual phase relations (and therefore circadian periods) in constant darkness. Reprinted with permission from Pittendrigh, C.S. & Daan, S. (1976) A functional analysis of circadian pacemakers in nocturnal rodents. I. The stability and lability of spontaneous frequency. *J Comp Physiol A* 106:223–252. © Springer:Nature (1976). doi: 10.1007/BF01417856.

Evidence from clinical studies supports the idea of long-lasting after-effects of melatonin treatments. Children and adolescents with autism spectrum disorder who showed improvements in sleep during a 2-year trial continued to show partially improved sleep features during a subsequent 2-week placebo period, suggesting some persistent benefits (Malow et al., 2021).

In patients with REM sleep behavior disorder (REMBD), the normal atonia of REM sleep is reduced or lost, resulting in individuals acting out often vigorous (and sometimes violent) activities during REM sleep (Boeve et al., 2007; Schenck et al., 1986); see Section 10.7.2. Nightly treatment with melatonin increased the amount of REM sleep and the degree of atonia during REM sleep, thereby reducing the abnormal motor symptoms (Boeve, 2003; Kunz & Mahlberg, 2010). The beneficial effects of melatonin treatments in REMBD patients persisted during a subsequent 4-week period of blinded placebo treatments. This benefit was not a "placebo response" because placebos given to patients (also blinded) *before* melatonin treatments did not improve REMBD symptoms, but subsequent melatonin treatments did (Kunz & Mahlberg, 2010).

The reduction in REMBD symptoms probably reflects the involvement of melatonin in regulating REM sleep expression (Cajochen et al., 1997; Chang et al., 2015) (see **Figure 9.3 B**) and the central role of the circadian system in regulating the expression of REM sleep (Dijk & Czeisler, 1995). The continuation of these benefits for weeks suggests that melatonin treatments had a reorganizing effect on some of the mechanisms that regulate REM sleep expression.

9.7.3 Summary

Several lines of evidence support the interpretation that the sleep benefits of melatonin treatments in many studies result from its effects on the SCN; in particular, its reinforcement of the amplitude of oscillation of the SCN and perhaps other circadian system components. The reported benefits of melatonin for sleep in aging and dementia tend to emerge slowly over weeks or months of treatment, which are unlikely to result from the immediate effects of melatonin in promoting earlier sleep onset.

This interpretation is supported by evidence that the effects of melatonin on circadian and sleep rhythms in people and rodents persisted for days or weeks after treatments ended, and its immediate pharmacological effects were long-since gone. Similarly, melatonin treatments given only during the luteal phase to women with PDD modified sleep parameters throughout their menstrual cycles, indicating persistent effects over days or weeks.

A role for the pineal and melatonin in regulating SCN rhythmicity was supported by evidence that pinealectomized rats lost behavioral rhythmicity much faster than controls when exposed to constant bright light. Similarly, the in vitro amplitude of the firing-rate rhythms of SCN cells from previously pinealectomized hamsters was lower than the rhythms from intact hamsters.

Amplifying SCN oscillation with exogenous melatonin could result from gradual resynchronization of a disrupted population of circadian component oscillators and/or increased oscillation amplitude of individual neurons in response to daily pulses of melatonin. The benefits for sleep would be an indirect result of more robust circadian modulation of rhythms of sleep–wake propensity, although direct effects on some aspects of sleep (e.g., REM sleep production) are also possible. Similar persistent effects occur when rhythm amplitude is increased using other methods. For example, the effects on SCN rhythm amplitude of exposing diurnal rodents to bright light during the daytime persisted in continuous darkness and were reflected in higher amplitude firing-rate rhythms of SCN neurons in vitro.

These findings imply that responses to repeated melatonin treatments depend on a combination of the circadian system's plasticity in response to altered inputs and the persistence of induced changes, which are well-documented features of multi-oscillator systems. Immediate changes in circadian periods induced by extreme photoperiods or acute exposure to light or other entraining/phase-shifting agents persist as long-lasting after-effects on the circadian system's period (see **Figure 9.16**).

9.8 Cautions in the use of melatonin

There is strong evidence that melatonin at low doses promotes earlier sleep onset under appropriate conditions, at least in some clinical populations, and that it has minimal or no toxicity even at extremely high doses.[6] There are also several other potential targets for melatonin treatments that have been suggested by many studies using cell lines or animal models, based on its function in antagonizing oxidative stress, and other properties (Galano et al., 2018). These studies have suggested that it might be beneficial as an adjunctive therapy for a variety of clinical conditions, including brain damage, cardiovascular disease, and cancer. Some clinical trials in which it was used as an adjunct in cancer treatments identified benefits (Li et al., 2017), but a meta-analysis of cancer trials reported little benefit for quality of life, including sleep quality (Fan et al., 2022). Demonstration of melatonin's usefulness in treating conditions other than circadian and sleep disorders will require additional rigorous clinical testing.

The available literature indicates that melatonin is generally a safe substance that could be used widely to treat delayed or disturbed sleep–wake patterns and could potentially be evaluated for treating other conditions, but some caution is also

[6] Among the few side effects that have been reported for melatonin treatments (besides drowsiness), one long-term study found an increase in negative mood (despite some benefits for sleep) in elderly participants living in group homes. These effects were seen in those treated with melatonin alone, but were not present if it was combined with daytime bright-light treatment (Riemersma-van der Lek et al., 2008).

appropriate. Melatonin is a naturally occurring hormone that cannot be patented and is available OTC in many countries. As a result, the composition of products labeled melatonin is not regulated rigorously by government agencies in all jurisdictions, so the purity and consistency of melatonin products can vary. One study of the composition of 31 OTC melatonin formulations found that they varied greatly in actual melatonin content relative to labeled amounts as well as between batches of the same product. In addition, about a quarter of these products contained some amount of serotonin, which was not listed on the labels and is a controlled substance that can be potentially dangerous (Erland & Saxena, 2017). As a result, self-treatment with OTC melatonin could produce inconsistent results, even for treating conditions for which it is effective in research studies that typically use a pharmaceutical grade product. This situation has contributed to an interest in developing patentable melatonin formulations (e.g., timed-release versions) and analogs and the identification of other drugs that act on melatonin receptors (Stein et al., 2020).

Melatonin is also a potent hormone that has well-characterized effects on the reproductive systems of many mammals, including affecting the timing of puberty and seasonal reproduction in several species. The data for humans are less compelling than for other species because of the absence of experimental studies, but several lines of evidence also link melatonin to human sexual development. Melatonin concentrations are high in children and normally decrease during puberty. Its levels are closely related to the stage of pubertal development, not to chronological age (Crowley et al., 2012; Salti et al., 2000; Silman et al., 1979) (**Figure 9.17**).

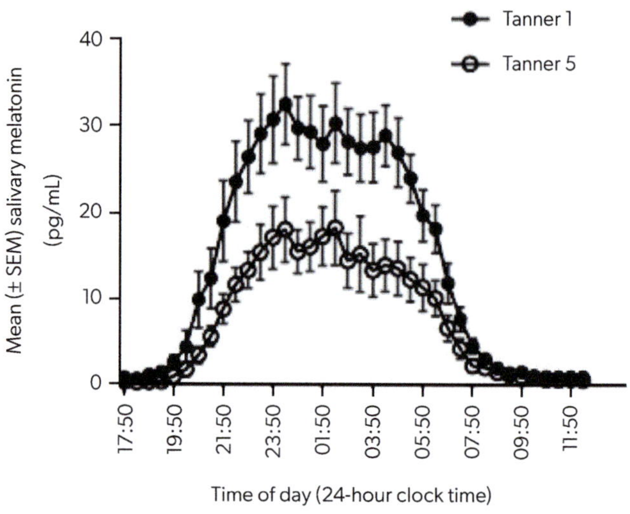

Figure 9.17 Salivary melatonin levels (Y axis) plotted against time of day (X axis) in children at different stages of pubertal development. The "Tanner" stage refers to the standard criteria for staging human pubertal development. Tanner stage 1 (black symbols) represents a prepubertal condition, while Tanner stage 5 (white symbols) represents completion of sexual maturation based on both primary and secondary external sexual characteristics. Reprinted with permission of John Wiley & Sons from Crowley S.J. et al. (2011) Human puberty: salivary melatonin profiles in constant conditions. *Dev Psychobiol* 54:468–473, 2012. © Wiley Periodicals, Inc. (2011) doi: 10.1002/dev.20605.

This correlational evidence does not prove that a decline in melatonin levels is involved in triggering puberty. An alternative interpretation is that these correlations reflect a decline in melatonin levels in response to changes in steroid hormone levels during puberty (Boafo et al., 2019). This idea is supported by evidence that high estrogen levels reduce melatonin production in both women and female rats (Okatani et al., 1998; Okatani et al., 2000). On the other hand, there are also scattered clinical observations that support a causal role for melatonin in relation to puberty in people. Several reports concluded that destructive tumors that damage pineal cells and reduce melatonin levels accelerate puberty onset, while proliferative pineal tumors that increase melatonin levels delay puberty (Kitay, 1954; Macchi & Bruce, 2004).

Melatonin levels have also been reported to change in relation to the timing of menopause in women, although these findings are inconsistent. One report described an increase in melatonin levels associated with decreasing estrogen levels during the transitional perimenopause, followed by decreasing melatonin levels after menopause (Okatani et al., 2000). However, another study comparing pre- to postmenopausal women found a shift in timing but little change in the amplitude of the melatonin secretion rhythm (Walters et al., 2005). In addition, there are reports that melatonin levels decline in both sexes in late middle age, during which there is less change in reproductive physiology in men (Reiter, 1998).

Changes in peak melatonin levels during aging may reflect a combination of responses to changing levels of reproductive hormones, aging of the pineal gland itself (including calcification), and a general reduction in the amplitude of circadian rhythms (including the SCN signals that drive pineal rhythms) rather than to an involvement of the pineal gland in the timing of menopause.

The more substantial clinical evidence that melatonin may play a role in timing pubertal development is consistent with evidence in other species that changes in melatonin secretion patterns trigger transitions between reproductive states (see Section 9.3). However, the relevance of melatonin-mediated reproductive changes in seasonally breeding species to humans is uncertain. People adjust their sleep–wake and other rhythms when exposed to different laboratory photoperiods (Wehr et al., 1993), and there are seasonal variations in many physiological and behavioral functions in people, including timing of births (for references see Roenneberg & Aschoff, 1990). But there is no substantial evidence that patterns of human reproduction are related to photoperiodic mechanisms (Roenneberg & Aschoff, 1990).

Studies of long-term effects of melatonin treatments on endocrine functions in children are limited in number and quality; for a review, see Kennaway, 2015. A recent, placebo-controlled trial in children and adolescents with autism spectrum disorder and impaired sleep used nightly treatments with a sustained-release melatonin formulation, resulting in improvements in sleep-onset latency, sleep duration, and parental satisfaction. The study was extended past the controlled phase for up to a 2-year period of treatments for 80 participants. The benefits for sleep were sustained throughout the study, and there was no indication of abnormal timing of puberty in this group (Malow et al., 2021). Nevertheless, there remains a need for larger, longer-term treatment studies to evaluate whether there are effects on the timing of any aspect of pubertal development. Pending such studies, there is probably a need for caution and close monitoring when providing long-term melatonin treatments in children and adolescents (Kennaway, 2015).

Studies of the acute effects of melatonin on glucose tolerance (i.e., how efficiently insulin can clear elevated glucose levels from the circulation) raised another concern about its use. Postmenopausal women who were treated with 1 mg of melatonin in the morning after an overnight fast showed reduced glucose tolerance and insulin sensitivity (Cagnacci et al., 2001).[7] Another study found impaired glucose tolerance in healthy young women immediately after acute treatment with 5 mg melatonin in either the morning or evening (Rubio-Sastre et al., 2014). These results suggest caution in taking melatonin close to mealtimes when it might prolong the normal post-meal increase in blood glucose levels.

In contrast to these results, a study of the effects of a sustained-release form of melatonin (2 mg) given nightly for 3 weeks in older patients with insomnia and Type 2 diabetes (i.e., with already impaired glucose metabolism), reported improvements in some sleep features and no change in glucose metabolism. Continued treatment for 5 months resulted instead in improvement in a marker of glucose metabolism (Garfinkel et al., 2011), an effect that may be an indirect outcome of improved sleep (see Section 14.6). It is unclear whether the formulation of melatonin, the timing or length of treatment, and/or the different populations studied produced these contrasting results.

A recent, long-term population-based study involving nearly 160,000 people examined whether adult male and female health care workers who either did or did not self-report use of melatonin differed in whether they developed Type 2 diabetes or cardiovascular disease over a follow-up period of up to 23 years. There were no differences between these groups in the hazard ratios for either condition. A subgroup analysis of female nurses who worked long-term (>5 years) on night shifts, however, found a decreased risk of cardiovascular disease among those reporting melatonin use (Li et al., 2024). This difference may be related to the utility of melatonin in improving sleep or strengthening circadian rhythms that may be disrupted by chronic night shift work (see Sections 13.9 and 13.10.

9.8.1 Summary

There is experimental evidence suggesting the potential for a variety of health benefits of melatonin use, related in part to its role as a scavenger of free oxygen radicals. However, the only functions for which there is substantial clinical evidence from well-controlled studies are related to effects on circadian rhythms and sleep. There is substantial evidence that melatonin can advance the phase of sleep onset in appropriate conditions and phase shift or entrain circadian rhythms in people. There is more limited evidence for its involvement in the regulation of REM sleep and for effects on total sleep amounts.

The short-term use of melatonin to modify sleep and circadian rhythms in some populations is justified based on the available evidence demonstrating benefits and the absence of significant side effects or risks. However, melatonin is an OTC medication in many jurisdictions, so product quality may be an issue because it is not regulated as rigorously as prescription medicines. Patented formulations of melatonin and of agonists acting on melatonin receptors have been developed to address this issue and to increase its duration of action, since melatonin itself is very rapidly metabolized.

One reason for caution in recommending the widespread use of melatonin, especially longer-term in children and adolescents, is the possibility of effects on regulation of reproductive and other endocrine functions, as in some other mammals. Observational clinical reports indicate that tumors that increase or decrease melatonin production are correlated with changes in the timing of pubertal development in children, but it remains unclear whether these observations represent causal relations. Larger, longer-term studies are needed to assess the potential risks associated with melatonin treatments, but the very limited information available did not indicate that lengthy melatonin treatments had detectable effects on reproductive physiology in children.

Treatment protocols using melatonin should also take account of the potential for effects on glucose metabolism in healthy people and in those with diabetes because there is

[7] Increased glucose levels cause increased release of insulin, which facilitates uptake and utilization of the excess glucose by peripheral tissues. Reduced insulin sensitivity allows increased blood glucose levels to circulate, which can be a precursor to metabolic abnormalities, including, in the extreme case, development of type 2 diabetes. See Section 14.6.2 and **Box 14.3**.

evidence indicating that it may have either potentially harmful or beneficial effects, although these remain to be confirmed. A large, prospective cohort study of health care workers found no difference in the occurrence of cardiovascular disease or Type 2 diabetes among those reporting use of melatonin or not. Among a subgroup of female nurses who worked night shifts over >5 years, those reporting melatonin use actually showed a reduced risk of developing cardiovascular disease.

Literature cited

Acuña-Castroviejo, D., Escames, G., Venegas, C., Díaz-Casado, M. E., Lima-Cabello, E., López, L. C., … Reiter, R. J. (2014). Extrapineal melatonin: sources, regulation, and potential functions. *Cell Mol Life Sci, 71*(16), 2997–3025. doi: 10.1007/s00018-014-1579-2

Ahuja, A. S., Arendt, J., Wallis, M., & Miles, P. J. (2006). Rapid responses to Buscemi et al. 2006. *Br Med J, 332*, 385–393.

Alam, M. N., McGinty, D., & Szymusiak, R. (1995a). Neuronal discharge of preoptic/anterior hypothalamic thermosensitive neurons: relation to NREM sleep. *Am J Physiol, 269*(5), R1240–R1249.

Alam, M. N., McGinty, D., & Szymusiak, R. (1995b). Preoptic/anterior hypothalamic neurons: thermosensitivity in rapid eye movement sleep. *Am J Physiol, 269*, R1250–R1257.

Aldhous, M., Franey, C., Wright, J., & Arendt, J. (1985). Plasma concentrations of melatonin in man following oral absorption of different preparations. *Br J Clin Pharmacol, 19*, 517–521.

Aoki, H., Ozeki, Y., & Yamada, N. (2009). Hypersensitivity of melatonin suppression in response to light in patients with delayed sleep phase syndrome. *Chronobiol Int, 18*(2), 263–271. doi: 10.1081/cbi-100103190

Arbon, E. L., Knurowska, M., & Dijk, D. J. (2015). Randomised clinical trial of the effects of prolonged-release melatonin, temazepam and zolpidem on slow-wave activity during sleep in healthy people. *J Psychopharmacol, 29*(7), 764–776. doi: 10.1177/0269881115581963

Arendt, J., & Skene, D. J. (2005). Melatonin as a chronobiotic. *Sleep Med Rev, 9*(1), 25–39. doi: 10.1016/j.smrv.2004.05.002

Arendt, J., Skene, D. J., Middleton, B., Lockley, S. W., & Deacon, S. (1997). Efficacy of melatonin treatment in jet lag, shift work, and blindness. *J Biol Rhythms, 12*, 604–617.

Armstrong, S. M., Cassone, V. M., Chesworth, M. J., Redman, J. R., & Short, R. V. (1986). Synchronization of mammalian circadian rhythms by melatonin. *J Neur Transm, 21*, 375–394.

Atkin, T., Comai, S., & Gobbi, G. (2018). Drugs for insomnia beyond benzodiazepines: pharmacology, clinical applications, and discovery. *Pharmacol Rev, 70*(2), 197–245. doi: 10.1124/pr.117.014381

Axelrod, J., & Wurtman, R. J. (1966). The formation, metabolism and some actions of melatonin, a pineal gland substance. *Res Publ Assoc Res Nerv Ment Dis, 43*, 200–211.

Balsalobre, A., Brown, S., Marcacci, L., Tronche, F., Kellendonk, C., Reichardt, H., Schütz, G., & Schibler, U. (2000). Resetting of circadian time in peripheral tissues by glucocorticoid signaling. *Science, 289*, 2344–2347.

Bano-Otalora, B., Martial, F., Harding, C., Bechtold, D. A., Allen, A. E., Brown, T. M., … Lucas, R. J. (2021). Bright daytime light enhances circadian amplitude in a diurnal mammal. *Proc Natl Acad Sci U S A, 118*(22), e2100094118. doi:10.1073/pnas.2100094118

Bartness, T. J., Goldman, B. D., & Bittman, E. L. (1991). SCN lesions block responses to systemic melatonin infusions in Siberian hamsters. *Am J Physiol, 260*, R102–R112.

Bartness, T. J., Powers, J. B., Hastings, M. H., Bittman, E. L., & Goldman, B. D. (1993). The timed infusion paradigm for melatonin delivery: what has it taught us about the melatonin signal, its reception, and the photoperiodic control of seasonal responses? *J Pineal Res, 15*, 161–190.

Bering, T., Blancas-Velazquez, A. S., & Rath, M. F. (2023). Circadian clock genes are regulated by rhythmic corticosterone at physiological levels in the rat hippocampus. *Neuroendocrinology, 113*(10), 1076–1090. doi: 10.1159/000533151

Boafo, A., Greenham, S., Alenezi, S., Robillard, R., Pajer, K., Tavakoli, P., & De Koninck, J. (2019). Could long-term administration of melatonin to prepubertal children affect timing of puberty? A clinician's perspective. *Nat Sci Sleep, 11*, 1–10. doi: 10.2147/NSS.S181365

Boeve, B. (2003). Melatonin for treatment of REM sleep behavior disorder in neurologic disorders: results in 14 patients. *Sleep Med, 4*(4), 281–284. doi: 10.1016/s1389-9457(03)00072-8

Boeve, B. F., Silber, M. H., Saper, C. B., Ferman, T. J., Dickson, D., Parisi, J., … Braak, H. (2007). Pathophysiology of REM sleep behaviour disorder and relevance to neurodegenerative disease. *Brain, 130*, 2770–2788.

Bothorel, B., Barassin, S., Saboureau, M., Perreau, S., Vivien-Roels, B., Malan, A., & Pévet, P. (2002). In the rat, exogenous melatonin increases the amplitude of pineal melatonin secretion by a direct action on the circadian clock. *Eur J Neurosci, 16*(6), 1090–1098. doi: 10.1046/j.1460-9568.2002.02176.x

Boulant, J. A. (2000). Role of the preoptic-anterior hypothalamus in thermoregulation and fever. *Clin Infec Dis, 31*, S157–S161.

Braam, W., Didden, R., Smits, M., & Curfs, L. (2008). Melatonin treatment in individuals with intellectual disability and chronic insomnia: a randomized placebo-controlled study. *J Intell Disabil Res, 52*(3), 256–264. doi: 10.1111/j.1365-2788.2007.01016.x

Braam, W., Smits, M. G., Didden, R., Korzilius, H., Geijlswijk, I. M. V., & Curfs, L. M. G. (2009). Exogenous melatonin for sleep problems in individuals with intellectual disability: a meta-analysis. *Dev Med Child Neurol, 51*(5), 340–349. doi: 10.1111/j.1469-8749.2008.03244.x

Breslow, E. R., Phillips, A. J., Huang, J. M., St Hilaire, M. A., & Klerman, E. B. (2013). A mathematical model of the circadian phase-shifting effects of exogenous melatonin. *J Biol Rhythms, 28*(1), 79–89. doi: 10.1177/0748730412468081

Bruni, O., Alonso-Alconada, D., Besag, F., Biran, V., Braam, W., Cortese, S., … Curatolo, P. (2015). Current role of melatonin in pediatric neurology: clinical recommendations. *Eur J Paediatr Neurol, 19*(2), 122–133. doi: 10.1016/j.ejpn.2014.12.007

Burgess, H. J., Revell, V. L., Molina, T. A., & Eastman, C. I. (2010). Human phase response curves to three days of daily melatonin: 0.5 mg versus 3.0 mg. *J Clin Endocr Metab, 95*(7), 3325–3331. doi: 10.1210/jc.2009-2590

Buscemi, N., Vandermeer, B., Hooton, N., Pandya, R., Tjosvold, L., Hartling, L., Baker, G., Klassen, T. P., & Vohra, S. (2005). The efficacy and safety of exogenous melatonin for primary sleep disorders. A meta-analysis. *J Gen Intern Med, 20*(12), 1151–1158. doi: 10.1111/j.1525-1497.2005.0243.x

Buscemi, N., Vandermeer, B., Hooton, N., Pandya, R., Tjosvold, L., Hartling, L., Vohra, S., Klassen, T., & Baker, G. (2006). Efficacy and safety of exogenous melatonin for secondary sleep disorders and sleep disorders accompanying sleep restriction: meta-analysis. *Br Med J, 332*(7538), 385–393. doi: 10.1136/bmj.38731.532766.F6

Cagnacci, A., Arangino, S., Renzi, A., Paoletti, A. M., Melis, G., Cagnacci, P., & Volpe, A. (2001). Influence of melatonin administration on glucose tolerance and insulin sensitivity of postmenopausal women. *Clin Endocrinol, 54*, 339–346.

Cagnacci, A., Elliott, J. A., & Yen, S. S. C. (1992). Melatonin: a major regulator of the circadian rhythm of core temperature in humans. *J Clin Endocr Metab, 75*(2), 447–452.

Cagnacci, A., Soldani, R., Laughlin, G. A., & Yen, S. S. C. (1996). Modification of circadian body temperature rhythm during the luteal menstrual phase: role of melatonin. *J Appl Physiol, 80*(1), 25–29.

Cagnacci, A., Soldani, R., & Yen, S. S. C. (1993). The effect of light on core body temperature is mediated by melatonin in women. *J Clin Endocr Metab, 76*, 1036–1038.

Cain, S. W., Dennison, C. F., Zeitzer, J. M., Guzik, A. M., Khalsa, S. B. S., Santhi, N., … Duffy, J. F. (2010). Sex differences in phase angle of entrainment and melatonin amplitude in humans. *J Biol Rhythms, 25*(4), 288–296. doi: 10.1177/0748730410374943

Cajochen, C., Frey, S., Anders, D., Spati, J., Bues, M., Pross, A., … Stefani, O. (2011). Evening exposure to a light emitting diodes (LED)-backlit computer screen affects circadian physiology and cognitive performance. *J Appl Physiol, 110*(5), 1432–1438. doi: 10.1152/japplphysiol.00165.2011

Cajochen, C., Kräuchi, K., Möri, D., Graw, P., & Wirz-Justice, A. (1997). Melatonin and S-20098 increase REM sleep and wake-up propensity without modifying NREM sleep homeostasis. *Am J Physiol Regul Integr Comp Physiol, 272*, R1189–R1196.

Cardinali, D. P., & Ritta, M. N. (1983). The role of prostaglandins in neuroendocrine junctions: studies in the pineal gland and the hypothalamus. *Neuroendocrinology, 36*(2), 152–160. doi: 10.1159/000123452

Carr, R., Wasdell, M., Hamilton, D., Weiss, M., Freeman, R., Tai, J., … Jan, J. (2007). Long-term effectiveness outcome of melatonin therapy in children with treatment-resistant circadian rhythm sleep disorders. *J Pineal Res, 43*(4), 351–359. doi: 10.1111/jpi.2007.43.issue-4

Carter, B., Rees, P., Hale, L., Bhattacharjee, D., & Paradkar, M. S. (2016). Association between portable screen-based media device access or use and sleep outcomes: a systematic review and meta-analysis. *JAMA Pediatr, 170*(12), 1202–1208. doi: 10.1001/jamapediatrics.2016.2341

Cassone, V. M. (1992). The pineal gland influences rat circadian activity rhythms in constant light. *J Biol Rhythms, 7*, 27–40.

Cassone, V. M., Chesworth, H. J., & Armstrong, S. M. (1986a). Entrainment of rat circadian rhythms by daily injection of melatonin depends upon the hypothalamic suprachiasmatic nuclei. *Physiol Behav, 36*, 1111–1121.

Cassone, V. M., Chesworth, M. J., & Armstrong, S. M. (1986b). Dose-dependent entrainment of rat circadian rhythms by daily injection of melatonin. *J Biol Rhythms, 1*, 219–229.

Cassone, V. M., Warren, W. S., Brooks, D. S., & Lu, J. (1993). Melatonin, the pineal gland, and circadian rhythms. *J Biol Rhythms, 8*, s73–s81.

Castanho, A., Bothorel, B., Seguin, L., Mocaër, E., & Pévet, P. (2014). Like melatonin, agomelatine (S20098) increases the amplitude of oscillations of two clock outputs: melatonin and temperature rhythms. *Chronobiol Int, 31*(3), 371–381. doi: 0.3109/07420528.2013.860457

Chang, A. M., Aeschbach, D., Duffy, J. F., & Czeisler, C. A. (2015). Evening use of light-emitting eReaders negatively affects sleep, circadian timing, and next-morning alertness. *Proc Natl Acad Sci U S A, 112*(4), 1232–1237. doi: 10.1073/pnas.1418490112

Chesworth, M. J., Cassone, V. M., & Armstrong, S. M. (1987). Effects of daily melatonin injections on activity rhythms of rats in constant light. *Am J Physiol, 253*, R101–R107.

Comai, S., Ochoa-Sanchez, R., Dominguez-Lopez, S., Bambico, F. R., & Gobbi, G. (2015). Melancholic-like behaviors and circadian neurobiological abnormalities in melatonin MT1 receptor knockout mice. *Int J Neuropsychopharmacol, 18*(3), pyu075. doi: 10.1093/ijnp/pyu075

Comai, S., Ochoa-Sanchez, R., & Gobbi, G. (2013). Sleep-wake characterization of double MT(1)/MT(2) receptor knockout mice and comparison with MT(1) and MT(2) receptor knockout mice. *Behav Brain Res, 243*, 231–238. doi: 10.1016/j.bbr.2013.01.008

Costello, R., Lentino, C., Boyd, C. C., O'Connell, M., Crawford, C., Sprengel, M., & Deuster, P. A. (2014). The effectiveness of melatonin for promoting healthy sleep: a rapid evidence assessment of the literature. *Nutr J, 13*, 106. doi: 10.1186/1475-2891-13-106

Crowley, S. J., Acebo, C., & Carskadon, M. A. (2012). Human puberty: salivary melatonin profiles in constant conditions. *Dev Psychobiol, 54*(4), 468–473. doi: 10.1002/dev.20605

Csernai, M., Borbély, S., Kocsis, K., Burka, D., Fekete, Z., Balogh, V., … Barthó, P. (2019). Dynamics of sleep oscillations is coupled to brain temperature on multiple scales. *J Physiol, 597*(15), 4069–4086. doi: 10.1113/JP277664

Cui, L. N., Coderre, E., & Renaud, L. P. (2001). Glutamate and GABA mediate suprachiasmatic nucleus inputs to spinal-projecting paraventricular neurons. *Am J Physiol, 281*, R1283–R1289.

Cunningham, J. E. A., & Shapiro, C. M. (2018). Cognitive Behavioural Therapy for Insomnia (CBT-I) to treat depression: a systematic review. *J Psychosom Res, 106*, 1–12. doi: 10.1016/j.jpsychores.2017.12.012

Czeisler, C. A., Shanahan, T. L., Klerman, E. B., Martens, H., Brotman, D. J., Emens, J. S., … Rizzo, J. F., III. (1995). Suppression of melatonin secretion in some blind patients by exposure to bright light. *New Engl J Med, 332*, 6–11.

Czeisler, C. A., Weitzman, E. D., Moore-Ede, M. C., Zimmerman, J. C., & Knauer, R. S. (1980). Human sleep: its duration and organization depend on its circadian phase. *Science, 210*, 1264–1267.

Daan, S., & Berde, C. (1978). Two coupled oscillators: simulations of the circadian pacemaker in mammalian activity rhythms. *J Theor Biol, 70*, 297–313.

Deacon, S., & Arendt, J. (1995). Melatonin-induced temperature suppression and its acute phase-shifting effects correlate in a dose-dependent manner in humans. *Brain Res, 688*, 77–85.

Dijk, D. J., & Czeisler, C. A. (1994). Paradoxical timing of the circadian rhythm of sleep propensity serves to consolidate sleep and wakefulness in humans. *Neurosci Lett, 166*, 63–68.

Dijk, D. J., & Czeisler, C. A. (1995). Contribution of the circadian pacemaker and the sleep homeostat to sleep propensity, sleep structure, electroencephalographic slow waves, and sleep spindle activity in humans. *J Neurosci, 15*, 3526–3538.

Dijk, D. J., Shanahan, T. L., Duffy, J., Ronda, J., & Czeisler, C. (1997). Variation of electroencephalographic activity during non-rapid eye movement and rapid eye movement sleep with phase of circadian melatonin rhythm in humans. *J Physiol, 505*(3), 851–858.

Dodge, N., & Wilson, G. (2001). Melatonin for treatment of sleep disorders in children with developmental disabilities. *J Child Neurol, 16*, 581–584.

Dollins, A. B., Zhdanova, I. V., Wurtman, R. J., Lynch, H. J., & Deng, M. H. (1994). Effect of inducing nocturnal serum melatonin concentrations in daytime on sleep, mood, body temperature, and performance. *Proc Natl Acad Sci USA, 91*, 1824–1828.

Dubocovich, M. L., Hudson, R. L., Sumaya, I. C., Masana, M. I., & Manna, E. (2005). Effect of MT1 melatonin receptor deletion on melatonin-mediated phase shift of circadian rhythms in the C57BL/6 mouse. *J Pineal Res, 39*(2), 113–120. doi: 10.1111/j.1600-079X.2005.00230.x

Eastman, C. I., & Burgess, H. J. (2009). How to travel the world without jet lag. *Sleep Med Clin, 4*(2), 241–255. doi: 10.1016/j.jsmc.2009.02.006

Edgar, D. M., Seidel, W. F., Martin, C. E., Sayeski, P. P., & Dement, W. C. (1991). Triazolam fails to induce sleep in suprachiasmatic nucleus-lesioned rats. *Neurosci Lett, 125*, 125–128.

Erland, L. A. E., & Saxena, P. K. (2017). Melatonin natural health products and supplements - presence of serotonin and variability of melatonin content. *J Clin Sleep Med, 13*(2), 275–281. doi: jc-00370-16

Etzioni, A., Luboshitzky, R., Tiosano, D., Ben-Harush, M., Goldsher, D., & Lavie, P. (1996). Melatonin replacement corrects sleep disturbances in a child with pineal tumor. *Neurology, 46*, 261–263.

Fan, R., Bu, X., Yang, S., Tan, Y., Wang, T., Chen, H., & Li, X. (2022). Effect of melatonin on quality of life and symptoms in patients with cancer: a systematic review and meta-analysis of randomised controlled trials. *Br Med J Open, 12*(9), e060912. doi:10.1136/bmjopen-2022-060912

Fisher, S. P., & Sugden, D. (2010). Endogenous melatonin is not obligatory for the regulation of the rat sleep-wake cycle. *Sleep, 33*(6), 833–840.

Flower, N. (Ed.). (1932). *The Journals of Arnold Bennett 1911–1921*. London: Cassell.

Franks, N. P. (2008). General anaesthesia: from molecular targets to neuronal pathways of sleep and arousal. *Nat Rev Neurosci, 9*(5), 370–386. doi: 10.1038/nrn2372

Galano, A., Tan, D. X., & Reiter, R. J. (2018). Melatonin: a versatile protector against oxidative DNA damage. *Molecules, 23*(3), 530. doi:10.3390/molecules23030530

Garfinkel, D., Zorin, M., Wainstein, J., Matas, Z., Laudon, M., & Zisapel, I. (2011). Efficacy and safety of prolonged-release melatonin in insomnia patients with diabetes: a randomized, double-blind, crossover study. *Diabetes Metab Syndr Obes, 4*, 307–313. doi: 0.2147/DMSO.S23904

Gibbs, J., Ince, L., Matthews, L., Mei, J., Bell, T., Yang, N., … Loudon, A. (2014). An epithelial circadian clock controls pulmonary inflammation and glucocorticoid action. *Nat Med, 20*(8), 919–926. doi: 10.1038/nm.3599

Gilbert, S. S., van den Heuvel, C. J., Ferguson, S. A., & Dawson, D. (2004). Thermoregulation as a sleep signalling system. *Sleep Med Rev, 8*(2), 81–93. doi: 10.1016/s1087-0792(03)00023-6

Glotzbach, S. F., & Heller, H. (1976). Central nervous regulation of body temperature during sleep. *Science, 194*(4264), 537–539.

Goldman, B. (2001). Mammalian photoperiodic system: formal properties and neuroendocrine mechanisms of photoperiodic time measurement. *J Biol Rhythms, 16*(4), 283–301.

Gooley, J. J., Chamberlain, K., Smith, K. A., Khalsa, S. B. S., Rajaratnam, S. M. W., Van Reen, E., … Lockley, S. W. (2011). Exposure to room light before bedtime suppresses melatonin onset and shortens melatonin duration in humans. *J Clin Endocr Metab, 96*, E463–E472. doi: 10.1210/jc.2010-2098

Gooneratne, N. S., Edwards, A. Y., Zhou, C., Cuellar, N., Grandner, M. A., & Barrett, J. S. (2012). Melatonin pharmacokinetics following two different oral surge-sustained release doses in older adults. *J Pineal Res, 52*(4), 437–445. doi: 10.1111/j.1600-079X.2011.00958.x

Green, A., Cohen-Zion, M., Haim, A., & Dagan, Y. (2017). Evening light exposure to computer screens disrupts human sleep, biological rhythms, and attention abilities. *Chronobiol Int, 34*(7), 855–865. doi: 10.1080/07420528.2017.1324878

Gringras, P., Gamble, C., Jones, A. P., Wiggs, L., Williamson, P. R., Sutcliffe, A., … MENDS Study Group. (2012). Melatonin for sleep problems in children with neurodevelopmental disorders: randomised double masked placebo controlled trial. *Br Med J, 345*, e6664. doi: 10.1136/bmj.e6664

Gringras, P., Nir, T., Breddy, J., Frydman-Marom, A., & Findling, R. L. (2017). Efficacy and safety of pediatric prolonged-release melatonin for insomnia in children with autism spectrum disorder. *J Am Acad Child Adolesc Psychiatry, 56*(11), 948–957 e944. doi: 10.1016/j.jaac.2017.09.414

Guardiola-Lemaitre, B., De Bodinat, C., Delagrange, P., Millan, M. J., Munoz, C., & Mocaer, E. (2014). Agomelatine: mechanism of action and pharmacological

profile in relation to antidepressant properties. *Br J Pharmacol, 171*(15), 3604–3619. doi: 10.1111/bph.12720
Hardeland, R. (2010). Investigational melatonin receptor agonists. *Expert Opin Investig Drugs, 19*(6), 747–764. doi: 10.1517/13543784.2010.482926
Hardeland, R. (2013). Chronobiology of melatonin beyond the feedback to the suprachiasmatic nucleus-consequences to melatonin dysfunction. *Int J Mol Sci, 14*(3), 5817–5841. doi: 10.3390/ijms14035817
Haskell, E., Palca, J., Walker, J., Berger, R., & Heller, H. (1981). The effects of high and low ambient temperatures on human sleep stages. *Electroencephalogr Clin Neurophysiol, 51*, 494–501.
Hastings, M. H., Herbert, J., Martensz, N. D., & Roberts, A. C. (1985). Annual reproductive rhythms in mammals: mechanisms of light synchronization. *Ann NY Acad Sci, 453*, 182–204.
Hayakawa, T., Uchiyama, M., Kamei, Y., Shibui, K., Tagaya, H., Asada, T., ... Takahashi, K. (2005). Clinical analyses of sighted patients with non-24-hour sleep-wake syndrome: a study of 57 consecutively diagnosed cases. *Sleep, 28*(8), 945–952.
Hermes, M. L. H. J., Coderre, E. M., Buijs, R. M., & Renaud, L. P. (1996). GABA and glutamate mediate rapid neurotransmission from suprachiasmatic nucleus to hypothalamic paraventricular nucleus in rat. *J Physiol (Lond), 496*, 749–757.
Huber, R., Deboer, T., Schwierin, B., & Tobler, I. (1998). Effect of melatonin on sleep and brain temperature in the Djungarian hamster and the rat. *Physiol Behav, 65*(1), 77–82.
Hughes, R. J., & Badia, P. (1997). Sleep-promoting and hypothermic effects of daytime melatonin administration in humans. *Sleep, 20*(2), 124–131.
Jan, J. E., & O'Donnell, M. E. (1996). Use of melatonin in the treatment of paediatric sleep disorders. *J Pineal Res, 21*, 193–199.
Jiao, Y. Y., Lee, T. M., & Rusak, B. (1999). Photic responses of suprachiasmatic area neurons in diurnal degus (*Octodon degus)* and nocturnal rats (*Rattus norvegicus*). *Brain Res, 817*(1-2), 93–103. doi: 10.1016/s0006-8993(98)01218-9
Kamara, D., & Beauchaine, T. P. (2020). A review of sleep disturbances among infants and children with neurodevelopmental disorders. *Rev J Autism Dev Disord*. doi: 10.1007/s40489-019-00193-8
Kawamura, H., & Sawyer, C. (1965). Elevation in brain temperature during paradoxical sleep. *Science, 150*(3698), 912–913.
Kennaway, D., Lushington, K., Dawson, D., Lack, L., van den Heuvel, C., & Rogers, N. (1999). Urinary 6-sulfatoxymelatonin excretion and aging: new results and a critical review of the literature. *J Pineal Res, 27*, 210–220.
Kennaway, D. J. (2015). Potential safety issues in the use of the hormone melatonin in paediatrics. *J Paediatr Child Health, 51*(6), 584–589. doi: 10.1111/jpc.12840
Kim, S., Benloucif, S., Reid, K., Weintraub, S., Kennedy, N., Wolfe, L., & Zee, P. (2014). Phase-shifting response to light in older adults. *J Physiol, 592*(1), 189–202. doi: 0.1113/jphysiol.2013.262899
Kitay, J. I. (1954). Pineal lesions and precocious puberty: a review. *Endocrinology, 14*, 622–625.
Klein, D. C., & Moore, R. Y. (1979). Pineal N-acetyltransferase and hydroxyindole-O-methyl-transferase: control by the retinohypothalamic tract and the suprachiasmatic nucleus. *Brain Res, 174*, 245–262.
Klein, D. C., Smoot, R., Weller, J. L., Higa, S., Markley, S. P., Creed, G. J., & Jacobowitz, D. M. (1983). Lesions of the paraventricular nucleus area of the hypothalamus disrupt the suprachiasmatic→ spinal cord circuit in the melatonin rhythm generating system. *Brain Res Bull, 10*(5), 647–652. doi: 10.1016/0361-9230(83)90033-3
Klein, T., Martens, H., Dijk, D. J., Kronauer, R. E., Seely, E. W., & Czeisler, C. A. (1993). Circadian sleep regulation in the absence of light perception: Chronic non-24-hour circadian rhythm sleep disorder in a blind man with a regular 24-hour sleep-wake schedule. *Sleep, 16*, 333–343.
Kräuchi, K., Cajochen, C., Werth, E., & Wirz-Justice, A. (2000). Functional link between distal vasodilation and sleep-onset latency? *Am J Physiol Regul Integr Comp Physiol, 278*(3), R741–748.
Kunz, D., & Mahlberg, R. (2010). A two-part, double-blind, placebo-controlled trial of exogenous melatonin in REM sleep behaviour disorder. *J Sleep Res, 19*(4), 591–596. doi: 10.1111/j.1365-2869.2010.00848.x
Labyak, S. E., Turek, F. W., Wallen, E. P., & Zee, P. C. (1998). Effects of bright light on age-related changes in the locomotor activity of Syrian hamsters. *Am J Physiol Regul Integr Comp Physiol, 43*, 830–839.
Lavie, P. (1997). Melatonin: role in gating nocturnal rise in sleep propensity. *J Biol Rhythms, 12*(6), 657–665.
Leitner, C., & Bartness, T. J. (2010). Distributed forebrain sites mediate melatonin-induced short-day responses in Siberian hamsters. *Endocrinology, 151*(7), 3133–3140. doi: 10.1210/en.2010-0002
Leliavski, A., Dumbell, R., Ott, V., & Oster, H. (2015). Adrenal clocks and the role of adrenal hormones in the regulation of circadian physiology. *J Biol Rhythms, 30*(1), 20–34. doi: 10.1177/0748730414553971
Lerner, A., & Nordlund, J. (1978). Melatonin: clinical pharmacology. *J Neur Transm, Supplement 13*, 339–347.
Leu-Semenescu, S., Arnulf, I., Decaix, C., Moussa, F., Clot, F., Boniol, C., ... Roze, E. (2010). Sleep and rhythm consequences of a genetically induced loss of serotonin. *Sleep, 33*(3), 307–314.
Lewy, A., Tetsuo, M., Markey, S. P., Goodwin, F. K., & Kopin, I. (1980). Pinealectomy abolishes plasma melatonin in the rat. *J Clin Endocr Metab, 50*(1), 204–205.
Lewy, A. J., Ahmed, S., Jackson, J. M., & Sack, R. L. (1992). Melatonin shifts human circadian rhythms according to a phase-response curve. *Chronobiol Int, 9*, 380–392.
Lewy, A. J., Emens, J. S., Sack, R. L., Hasler, B. P., & Bernert, R. A. (2002). Low, but not high, doses of melatonin entrained a free-running blind person with a long circadian period. *Chronobiol Int, 19*(3), 649–658. doi: 10.1081/cbi-120004546
Lewy, A. J., & Sack, R. L. (1989). The dim light melatonin onset as a marker for circadian phase position. *Chronobiol Int, 6*(1), 93–102.
Lewy, A. J., Wehr, T. A., Goodwin, F. K., Newsome, D. A., & Markey, S. P. (1980). Light suppresses melatonin secretion in humans. *Science, 210*, 1267–1269.
Li, Y., Huang, T., Redline, S., Willett, W. C., Manson, J. E., Schernhammer, E. S., & Hu, F. (2024). Use of melatonin supplements and risk of type 2 diabetes and cardiovascular diseases in the USA: insights from three prospective cohort studies. *Lancet Diabet Endocrinol, 12*(6), 404–413. doi: 10.1016/S2213-8587(24)00096-2
Li, Y., Zhou, Y., Meng, X., Zhang, J.-J., Xu, D.-P., & Li, H.-B. (2017). Melatonin for the prevention and treatment of cancer. *Oncotarget, 8*(24), 39895–39921.
Liu, C., Weaver, D. R., Jin, X., Shearman, L. P., Pieschi, R. L., Gribkoff, V. K., & Reppert, S. M. (1997). Molecular dissection of two distinct acctions of melatonin on the suprachiasmatic circadian clock. *Neuron, 19*, 91–102.
Lockley, S. W., Brainard, G. C., & Czeisler, C. A. (2003). High sensitivity of the human circadian melatonin rhythm to resetting by short wavelength light. *J Clin Endocrinol Metab, 88*(9), 4502–4505. doi: 10.1210/jc.2003-030570
Lockley, S. W., Dressman, M. A., Licamele, L., Xiao, C., Fisher, D. M., Flynn-Evans, E. E., ... Polymeropoulos, M. H. (2015). Tasimelteon for non-24-hour sleep–wake disorder in totally blind people (SET and RESET): two multicentre, randomised, double-masked, placebo-controlled phase 3 trials. *Lancet, 386*(10005), 1754–1764. doi: 10.1016/s0140-6736(15)60031-9
Lockley, S. W., Skene, D. J., Arendt, J., Tabandeh, H., Bird, A. C., & Defrance, R. (1997). Relationship between melatonin rhythms and visual loss in the blind. *J Clin Endocr Metab, 82*, 3763–3770.
Lokhorst, G. J. (2021). Descartes and the pineal gland. In E. N. Zalta (Ed.), *The Stanford Encyclopedia of Philosophy* (Winter, 2021 ed.): Metaphysics Research Lab, Stanford University. Retrieved from https://plato.stanford.edu/archives/win2021/entries/pineal-gland/.
Lokhorst, G. J., & Kaitaro, T. T. (2001). The originality of Descartes' theory about the pineal gland. *J Hist Neurosci, 10*(1), 6–18. doi: 10.1076/jhin.10.1.6.5629
Macchi, M. M., & Bruce, J. N. (2004). Human pineal physiology and functional significance of melatonin. *Front Neuroendocrinol, 25*(3–4), 177–195. doi: 10.1016/j.yfrne.2004.08.001
Magri, F., Sarra, S., Cinchetti, W., Guazzoni, V., Floravanti, M., Cravello, L., & Ferrari, E. (2004). Qualitative and quantitative changes in melatonin levels in physiological and pathological aging and in centenarians. *J Pineal Res, 36*(4), 256–261. doi: 10.1111/j.1600-079X.2004.00125.x
Mahlberg, R., Kienast, T., Hadel, S., Heidenreich, J. O., Schmitz, S., & Kunz, D. (2009). Degree of pineal calcification (DOC) is associated with polysomnographic sleep measures in primary insomnia patients. *Sleep Med, 10*(4), 439–445. doi: 10.1016/j.sleep.2008.05.003
Mahlberg, R., Tilmann, A., Salewski, L., & Kunz, D. (2006). Normative data on the daily profile of urinary 6-sulfatoxymelatonin in healthy subjects between the ages of 20 and 84. *Psychoneuroendocrinology, 31*(5), 634–641. doi: 10.1016/j.psyneuen.2006.01.009
Malow, B. A., Findling, R. L., Schroder, C. M., Maras, A., Breddy, J., Nir, T., ... Gringras, P. (2021). Sleep, growth, and puberty after 2 years of prolonged-release melatonin in children with autism spectrum disorder. *J Am Acad Child Adolesc Psychiatry, 60*(2), 252–261.e253. doi: 10.1016/j.jaac.2019.12.007
Mason, R., & Brooks, A. (1988). The electrophysiological effects of melatonin and a putative melatonin antagonist (N-acetyltryptamine) on rat suprachiasmatic neurones in vitro. *Neurosci Lett, 92*, 102–107.
McArthur, A. J., Gillette, M. U., & Prosser, R. A. (1991). Melatonin directly resets the rat suprachiasmatic circadian clock in vitro. *Brain Res, 565*, 158–161.

McArthur, A. J., Lewy, A. J., & Sack, R. L. (1996). Non-24-hour sleep-wake syndrome in a sighted man: circadian rhythm studies and efficacy of melatonin treatment. *Sleep, 19*(7), 544–553.

Meijer, J. H., Groos, G. A., & Rusak, B. (1986). Luminance coding in a circadian pacemaker: The suprachiasmatic nucleus of the rat and the hamster. *Brain Res, 382*, 109–118.

Meijer, J. H., Rusak, B., & Harrington, M. E. (1989). Photically responsive neurons in the hypothalamus of a diurnal ground squirrel. *Brain Res, 501*, 315–323.

Miano, S., & Ferri, R. (2010). Epidemiology and management of insomnia in children with autism spectrum disorders. *Pediatr Drugs, 12*(2), 75–84.

Miles, L. E. M., Raynal, D. M., & Wilson, M. A. (1977). Blind man living in normal society has circadian rhythms of 24.9 hours. *Science, 198*, 421–423.

Moderie, C., Boudreau, P., Shechter, A., Lesperance, P., & Boivin, D. B. (2021). Effects of exogenous melatonin on sleep and circadian rhythms In women with premenstrual dysphoric disorder. *Sleep, 44*(12), zsab171. doi:10.1093/sleep/zsab171

Moore, R. (1996). Neural control of the pineal gland. *Behav Brain Res, 73*, 125–130.

Moore, R. Y., & Eichler, V. B. (1972). Loss of circadian adrenal corticosterone rhythm following suprachiasmatic lesions in the rat. *Brain Res, 42*, 201–206.

Moore, R. Y., & Klein, D. C. (1974). Visual pathways and the central neural control of a circadian rhythm in pineal serotonin N-acetyltransferase activity. *Brain Res, 71*, 17–33.

Moore, R. Y., & Speh, J. C. (1993). GABA is the principal neurotransmitter of the circadian system. *Neurosci Lett, 150*, 112–116.

Morgan, P. J., Barrett, P., Howell, H. E., & Helliwell, R. (1994). Melatonin receptors: localization, molecular pharmacology and physiological significance. *Neurochem Int, 24*, 101–146.

Nelson, R. J., Badura, L. L., & Goldman, B. D. (1990). Mechanisms of seasonal cycles of behavior. *Annu Rev Psychol, 41*, 81–108.

Nelson, R. J., Demas, G. E., Klein, S. L., & Kriegsfeld, L. J. (1995). The influence of season, photoperiod, and pineal melatonin on immune function. *J Pineal Res, 19*, 149–165.

Ochoa-Sanchez, R., Comai, S., Lacoste, B., Bambico, F. R., Dominguez-Lopez, S., Spadoni, G., ... Gobbi, G. (2011). Promotion of non-rapid eye movement sleep and activation of reticular thalamic neurons by a novel MT2 melatonin receptor ligand. *J Neurosci, 31*(50), 18439–18452. doi: 10.1523/JNEUROSCI.2676-11.2011

Okatani, Y., Hayashi, K., Watanabe, K., Morioka, N., & Sagara, S. (1998). Estrogen modulates the nocturnal synthesis of melatonin in peripubertal female rats. *J Pineal Res, 24*, 224–229.

Okatani, Y., Morioka, N., & Wakatsuki, A. (2000). Changes in nocturnal melatonin secretion in perimenopausal women: correlation with endogenous estrogen concentrations. *J Pineal Res, 28*, 111–118.

Ortiz-Tudela, E., Martinez-Nicolas, A., Albares, J., Segarra, F., Campos, M., Estivill, E., ... Madrid, J. A. (2014). Ambulatory circadian monitoring (ACM) based on thermometry, motor activity and body position (TAP): a comparison with polysomnography. *Physiol Behav, 126*, 30–38. doi: 10.1016/j.physbeh.2013.12.009

Owens, J., Rosen, C., Mindell, J., & Kirchner, H. (2010). Use of pharmacotherapy for insomnia in child psychiatry practice: a national survey. *Sleep Med, 11*, 692–700. doi: 0.1016/j.sleep.2009.11.015

Parmeggiani, P. L. (2007). REM sleep related increase in brain temperature: a physiologic problem. *Arch Ital Biol, 145*, 13–21.

Parry, B. L., Berga, S. L., Mostofi, N., Klauber, M. R., & Resnick, A. (1997). Plasma melatonin circadian rhythms during the menstrual cycle and after light therapy in premenstrual dysphoric disorder and normal control subjects. *J Biol Rhythms, 12*, 47–64.

Perreau-Lenz, S., Kalsbeek, A., Garidou, M.-L., Wortel, J., Van Der Vliet, J., Van Heijningen, C., ... Buijs, R. M. (2003). Suprachiasmatic control of melatonin synthesis in rats: inhibitory and stimulatory mechanisms. *Eur J Neurosci, 17*(2), 221–228. doi: 10.1046/j.1460-9568.2003.02442.x

Perreau-Lenz, S., Kalsbeek, A., Pévet, P., & Buijs, R. (2004). Glutamatergic clock output stimulates melatonin synthesis at night. *Eur J Neurosci, 19*(2), 318–324.

Phillips, A. J. K., Vidafar, P., Burns, A. C., McGlashan, E. M., Anderson, C., Rajaratnam, S. M. W., ... Cain, S. W. (2019). High sensitivity and interindividual variability in the response of the human circadian system to evening light. *Proc Natl Acad Sci U S A, 116*(24), 12019–12024. doi: 10.1073/pnas.1901824116

Pittendrigh, C. (1974). Circadian oscillations in cells and the circadian organization of multicellular systems. In F. Schmitt & F. Worden (Eds.), *The Neurosciences: Third Study Program* (pp. 437–458). Cambridge: MIT Press.

Pittendrigh, C. S., & Daan, S. (1976a). A functional analysis of circadian pacemakers in nocturnal rodents. I. The stability and lability of spontaneous frequency. *J Comp Physiol A, 106*, 223–252.

Pittendrigh, C. S., & Daan, S. (1976b). A functional analysis of circadian pacemakers in nocturnal rodents. V. Pacemaker structure: a clock for all seasons. *J Comp Physiol A, 106*, 333–335.

Raymann, R. J. E. M., Swaab, D. F., & Van Someren, E. J. W. (2008). Skin deep: enhanced sleep depth by cutaneous temperature manipulation. *Brain, 131*(2), 500–513. doi: 10.1093/brain/awm315

Redman, J., Armstrong, S., & Ng, K. T. (1983). Free-running activity rhythms in the rat: Entrainment by melatonin. *Science, 219*, 1089–1091.

Reiter, R. J. (1998). Melatonin and human reproduction. *Ann Med, 30*(1), 103–108.

Reiter, R. J., Melchiorri, D., Sewerynek, E., Poeggeler, B., Barlow-Walden, L., Chuang, J., ... Acuña-Castroviejo, D. (1995). A review of the evidence supporting melatonin's role as an antioxidant. *J Pineal Res, 18*, 1–11.

Reppert, S. M., Weaver, D. R., Rivkees, S. A., & Stopa, E. G. (1988). Putative melatonin receptors in a human biological clock. *Science, 242*, 78–81.

Reynoldson, J. N., Elliott, E., Sr., & Nelson, L. A. (2008). Ramelteon: a novel approach in the treatment of insomnia. *Ann Pharmacother, 42*(9), 1262–1271. doi: 10.1345/aph.1K676

Riemersma-van der Lek, R. F., Swaab, D. F., Twisk, J., Hol, E. M., Hoogendijk, W. J. G., & Van Someren, E. J. W. (2008). Effect of bright light and melatonin on cognitive and non-cognitive function in elderly residents of group care facilities: a randomized controlled trial. *JAMA, 299*(22), 2642–2655. doi: 10.1001/jama.299.22.2642)

Roenneberg, T., & Aschoff, J. (1990). Annual rhythm of human reproduction: II. environmental correlations. *J Biol Rhythms, 5*, 217–239.

Rolling, J., Rabot, J., & Schroder, C. M. (2022). Melatonin treatment for pediatric patients with insomnia: is there a place for it? *Nat Sci Sleep, 14*, 1927–1944. doi: 10.2147/nss.S340944

Roth, T., Nir, T., & Zisapel, N. (2015). Prolonged release melatonin for improving sleep in totally blind subjects: a pilot placebo-controlled multicenter trial. *Nat Sci Sleep, 7*, 13–23. doi: 10.2147/NSS.S71838

Rubio-Sastre, P., Scheer, F. A., Gomez-Abellan, P., Madrid, J. A., & Garaulet, M. (2014). Acute melatonin administration in humans impairs glucose tolerance in both the morning and evening. *Sleep, 37*(10), 1715–1719. doi: 10.5665/sleep.4088

Rusak, B., Guido, M. E., Jiao, Y. Y., & Song, X. (2001). Light and the rodent circadian system: molecular, cellular and systemic effects. In K. Honma & S. Honma (Eds.), *Zeitgebers, Entrainment and Masking of the Circadian System* (pp. 131–146). Sapporo: Hokkaido University Press.

Rusak, B., & Morin, L. P. (1976). Testicular responses to photoperiod are blocked by lesions of the suprachiasmatic nuclei in golden hamsters. *Biol Reprod, 15*, 366–374.

Rusak, B., & Yu, G. D. (1993). Regulation of melatonin sensitivity and firing-rate rhythms in hamster suprachiasmatic nucleus neurons: effects of pinealectomy. *Brain Res, 602*, 200–204.

Sack, R., Brandes, R., Kendall, A., & Lewy, A. (2000). Entrainment of free-running circadian rhythms by melatonin in blind people. *New Engl J Med, 343*(15), 1070–1077.

Sack, R., Lewy, A., Erb, D., Vollmer, W., & Singer, C. (1986). Human melatonin production decreases with age. *J Pineal Res, 3*, 379–388.

Sack, R. L., & Lewy, A. J. (1997). Melatonin as a chronobiotic: Treatment of circadian desynchrony in night workers and the blind. *J Biol Rhythms, 12*, 595–603.

Sack, R. L., Lewy, A. J., Blood, M. L., Stevenson, J., & Keith, L. D. (1991). Melatonin administration to blind people: phase advances and entrainment. *J Biol Rhythms, 6*, 249–261.

Saksvik-Lehouillier, I., Harrison, S. L., Marshall, L. M., Tranah, G. J., Ensrud, K., Ancoli-Israel, S., ... Osteoporotic Fractures in Men Study Group. (2015). Association of urinary 6-sulfatoxymelatonin (aMT6s) levels and objective and subjective sleep measures in older men: the MrOS sleep study. *J Gerontol A Biol Sci Med Sci, 70*(12), 1569–1577. doi: 10.1093/gerona/glv088

Salti, R., Galluzzi, F., Bindi, G., Perfetto, F., Tarquini, R., Halberg, F., & Cornélissen, G. (2000). Nocturnal melatonin patterns in children. *J Clin Endocr Metab, 85*, 2137–2144.

Scheer, F. A. J. L., Morris, C. J., Garcia, J. I., Smales, C., Kelly, E. E., Marks, J., ... Shea, S. A. (2012). Repeated melatonin supplementation improves sleep in hypertensive patients treated with beta-blockers: a randomized controlled trial. *Sleep, 35*(10), 1395–1402. doi: 10.5665/sleep.2122

Scheer, F. A. J. L., Van Montfrans, G. A., van Someren, E. J. W., Mairuhu, G., & Buijs, R. M. (2004). Daily nighttime melatonin reduces blood pressure in male patients with essential hypertension. *Hypertension, 43*(2), 192–197. doi: 10.1161/01.HYP.0000113293.15186.3b

Schenck, C., Bundlie, S., Ettinger, M., & Mahowald, W. (1986). Chronic behavioral disorders of REM sleep: a new category of parasomnia. *Sleep, 9*(2), 293–308.

Schmidek, W., Hoshino, K., Schmidek, M., & Timo-Iaria, C. (1972). Influence of environmental temperature on the sleep-wakefulness cycle in the rat. *Physiol Behav, 8*, 363–371.

Schoonderwoerd, R. A., de Rover, M., Janse, J. A. M., Hirschler, L., Willemse, C. R., Scholten, L., … Meijer, J. H. (2022). The photobiology of the human circadian clock. *Proc Natl Acad Sci U S A, 119*(13), e2118803119. doi: 10.1073/pnas.2118803119

Schoonderwoerd, R. A., de Torres Gutierrez, P., Blommers, R., van Beurden, A. W., Coenen, T. C. J. J., Klett, N. J., … Meijer, J. H. (2022). Inhibitory responses to retinohypothalamic tract stimulation in the circadian clock of the diurnal rodent *Rhabdomys pumilio*. *FASEB J, 36*(8), e22415. doi: 10.1096/fj.202200477R

Schroder, C. M., Malow, B. A., Maras, A., Melmed, R. D., Findling, R. L., Breddy, J., … Gringras, P. (2019). Pediatric prolonged-release melatonin for sleep in children with autism spectrum disorder: impact on child behavior and caregiver's quality of life. *J Autism Dev Disord, 49*(8), 3218–3230. doi: 10.1007/s10803-019-04046-5

Schwichtenberg, A. J., & Malow, B. A. (2015). Melatonin treatment in children with developmental disabilities. *Sleep Med Clin, 10*(2), 181–187. doi: 10.1016/j.jsmc.2015.02.008

Shechter, A., Lesperance, P., Ng Ying Kin, N. M., & Boivin, D. B. (2012). Nocturnal polysomnographic sleep across the menstrual cycle in premenstrual dysphoric disorder. *Sleep Med, 13*(8), 1071–1078. doi: 10.1016/j.sleep.2012.05.012

Shibata, S., Cassone, V. M., & Moore, R. Y. (1989). Effects of melatonin on neuronal activity in the rat suprachiasmatic nucleus in vitro. *Neurosci Lett, 97*, 140–144.

Shochat, T., Luboshitzky, R., & Lavie, P. (1997). Nocturnal melatonin onset is phase locked to the primary sleep gate. *Am J Physiol, 273*(R364–R370).

Shoja, M. M., Hoepfner, L. D., Agutter, P. S., Singh, R., & Tubbs, R. S. (2016). History of the pineal gland. *Childs Nerv Syst, 32*(4), 583–586. doi: 10.1007/s00381-015-2636-3

Sigurdardottir, L. G., Markt, S. C., Sigurdsson, S., Aspelund, T., Fall, K., Schernhammer, E., … Mucci, L. A. (2016). Pineal gland volume assessed by MRI and its correlation with 6-sulfatoxymelatonin levels among older men. *J Biol Rhythms, 31*(5), 461–469. doi: 10.1177/0748730416656948

Silman, R. E., Leone, R., & Hooper, R. (1979). Melatonin, the pineal gland and human puberty. *Nature, 282*, 301–303.

Singer, C., Tractenberg, R., Kaye, J., Schafer, K., Gamst, A., Grundman, M., … Thal, L. (2003). A multicenter, placebo-controlled trial of melatonin for sleep disturbance in Alzheimer's disease. *Sleep, 26*(7), 893–901.

Slawik, H., Stoffel, M., Riedl, L., Vesely, Z., Behr, M., Lehmberg, J., … Krieg, S. M. (2016). Prospective study on salivary evening melatonin and sleep before and after pinealectomy in humans. *J Biol Rhythms, 31*(1), 82–93. doi: 10.1177/0748730415616678

Smith, M. R., & Eastman, C. I. (2012). Shift work: health, performance and safety problems, traditional countermeasures, and innovative management strategies to reduce circadian misalignment. *Nat Sci Sleep, 4*, 111–132. doi: 10.2147/NSS.S10372

Stehle, J., Vanecek, J., & Vollrath, L. (1989). Effects of melatonin on spontaneous electrical activity of neurons in rat suprachiasmatic nuclei: an in vitro iontophoretic study. *J Neur Transm, 78*, 173–177.

Stein, R. M., Kang, H. J., McCorvy, J. D., Glatfelter, G. C., Jones, A. J., Che, T., … Dubocovich, M. L. (2020). Virtual discovery of melatonin receptor ligands to modulate circadian rhythms. *Nature, 579*(7800), 609–614. doi: 10.1038/s41586-020-2027-0

St. Hilaire, M. A., & Lockley, S. W. (2015). Caffeine does not entrain the circadian clock but improves daytime alertness in blind patients with non-24-hour rhythms. *Sleep Med, 16*(6), 800–804. doi: 10.1016/j.sleep.2015.01.018

Sun, X., Whitefield, S., Rusak, B., & Semba, K. (2001). Electrophysiological analysis of suprachiasmatic nucleus projections to the ventrolateral preoptic area in the rat. *Eur J Neurosci, 14*, 1257–1274.

Szymusiak, R., & McGinty, D. (2008). Hypothalamic regulation of sleep and arousal. *Ann NY Acad Sci, 1129*(1), 275–286. doi: 10.1196/annals.1417.027

Takahashi, J., & Menaker, M. (1982a). Role of the suprachiasmatic nuclei in the circadian system of the house sparrow, *Passer domesticus*. *J Neurosci, 2*(6), 815–828.

Takahashi, J. S., Hamm, H., & Menaker, M. (1980). Circadian rhythms of melatonin release from individual superfused chicken pineal glands in vitro *Proc Natl Acad Sci USA, 77*, 2319–2322.

Takahashi, J. S., & Menaker, M. (1982b). Entrainment of the circadian system of the house sparrow: A population of oscillators in pinealectomized birds. *J Comp Physiol A, 146*, 245–253.

Takasu, N. N., Hashimoto, S., Yamanaka, Y., Tanahashi, Y., Yamazaki, A., Honma, S., & Honma, K. (2006). Repeated exposures to daytime bright light increase nocturnal melatonin rise and maintain circadian phase in young subjects under fixed sleep schedule. *Am J Physiol Regul Integr Comp Physiol, 291*(6), R1799–R1807. doi: 10.1152/ajpregu.00211.2006

Trachsel, L., Edgar, D., WF, S., Heller, H., & Dement, W. (1992). Sleep homeostasis in suprachiasmatic-lesions rats: effects of sleep deprivation and triazolam administration. *Brain Res, 589*, 253–261.

Tzischinsky, O., & Lavie, P. (1994). Melatonin possesses time-dependent hypnotic effects. *Sleep, 17*, 638–645.

Underwood, H. (1986). Circadian rhythms in lizards: Phase response curve for melatonin. *J Pineal Res, 3*, 187–196.

Utiger, R. D. (1992). Melatonin -the hormone of darkness. *New Engl J Med, 327*(19), 1377–1379.

Vandenheuvel, C., Ferguson, S., Milamacchi, M., & Dawson, D. (2005). Melatonin as a hypnotic: Con. *Sleep Med Rev, 9*(1), 71–80. doi: 10.1016/j.smrv.2004.07.001

Vanecek, J., Pavljk, A., & Illnerov, H. (1987). Hypothalamic melatonin receptor sites revealed by autoradiography. *Brain Res, 435*, 359–362.

van Geijlswijk, I. M., Korzilius, H., & Smits, M. (2010). The use of exogenous melatonin in delayed sleep phase disorder: a meta-analysis. *Sleep, 33*(12), 1605–1614.

van Geijlswijk, I. M., van der Heijden, K. B., Egberts, A. C., Korzilius, H. P., & Smits, M. G. (2010). Dose finding of melatonin for chronic idiopathic childhood sleep onset insomnia: an RCT. *Psychopharmacology (Berl), 212*(3), 379–391. doi: 10.1007/s00213-010-1962-0

van Maanen, A., Meijer, A. M., Smits, M. G., van der Heijden, K. B., & Oort, F. J. (2017). Effects of melatonin and bright light treatment in childhood chronic sleep onset insomnia with late melatonin onset: a randomized controlled study. *Sleep, 40*(2). doi: 10.1093/sleep/zsw038

von Gall, C., & Weaver, D. R. (2008). Loss of responsiveness to melatonin in the aging mouse suprachiasmatic nucleus. *Neurobiol Aging, 29*(3), 464–470. doi: 10.1016/j.neurobiolaging.2006.10.015

Wade, A., Ford, I., Crawford, G., McConnachie, A., Nir, T., Laudon, M., & Zisapel, I. (2010). Nightly treatment of primary insomnia with prolonged release melatonin for 6 months: a randomized placebo controlled trial on age and endogenous melatonin as predictors of efficacy and safety. *BMC Med, 8*(51). doi: 0.1186/1741-7015-8-51

Wagley, J. N., Rybarczyk, B., Nay, W. T., Danish, S., & Lund, H. G. (2013). Effectiveness of abbreviated CBT for insomnia in psychiatric outpatients: sleep and depression outcomes. *J Clin Psychol, 69*(10), 1043–1055. doi: 10.1002/jclp.21927

Walters, J. F., Hampton, S. M., Ferns, G. A., & Skene, D. J. (2005). Effect of menopause on melatonin and alertness rhythms investigated in constant routine conditions. *Chronobiol Int, 22*(5), 859–872. doi: 10.1080/07420520500263193

Wasdell, M., Jan, J., Bomben, M., Freeman, R., Rietveld, W., Tai, J., Hamilton, D., & Weiss, M. (2008). A randomized, placebo-controlled trial of controlled release melatonin treatment of delayed sleep phase syndrome and impaired sleep maintenance in children with neurodevelopmental disabilities. *J Pineal Res, 44*, 57–64.

Watanabe, N., Furukawa, T., Shimodera, S., Morokuma, I., Katsuki, F., Fujita, H., Sasaki, M., Kawamura, C., & Perlis, M. (2011). Brief behavioral therapy for refractory insomnia in residual depression: an assessor-blind, randomized control trial. *J Clin Psychiatry, 72*(12), 1651–1658. doi: 10.4088/JCP.10m06130gry

Watson, L. A., Phillips, A. J. K., Hosken, I. T., McGlashan, E. M., Anderson, C., Lack, L. C., Lockley, S. W., Rajaratnam, S. M. W., & Cain, S. W. (2018). Increased sensitivity of the circadian system to light in delayed sleep-wake phase disorder. *J Physiol, 596*(24), 6249–6261. doi: 10.1113/JP275917

Weaver, D. R., Rivkees, S. A., & Reppert, S. M. (1989). Localization and characterization of melatonin receptors in rodent brain by in vitro autoradiography. *J Neurosci, 9*, 2581–2590.

Weaver, D. R., Stehle, J. H., Stopa, E. G., & Reppert, S. M. (1993). Melatonin receptors in human hypothalamus and pituitary: Implications for circadian and reproductive responses to melatonin. *J Clin Endocr Metab, 76*, 295–301.

Wehr, T., Aeschbach, D., & Duncan, W. J. (2001). Evidence for a biological dawn and dusk in the human circadian timing system. *J Physiol, 535*(3), 937–951.

Wehr, T. A., Moul, D. E., Barbato, G., Giesen, H. A., Seidel, J. A., Barker, C., & Bender, C. (1993). Conservation of photoperiod-responsive mechanisms in humans. *Am J Physiol, 265*(4 Pt 2), R846–R857.

Wei, S., Smits, M. G., Tang, X., Kuang, L., Meng, H., Ni, S., Xiao, M., & Zhou, X. (2020). Efficacy and safety of melatonin for sleep onset insomnia in children and adolescents: a meta-analysis of randomized controlled trials. *Sleep Med, 68*, 1–8. doi: 10.1016/j.sleep.2019.02.017

Wirojanan, J., Jacquemont, S., Diaz, R., Bacalman, S., Anders, T., Hagerman, R., & Goodlin-Jones, B. (2009). The efficacy of melatonin for sleep problems in children with autism, fragile X syndrome, or autism and fragile X syndrome. *J Clin Sleep Med, 5*(2), 145–150.

Witting, W., Mirmiran, M., Bos, N. P. A., & Swaab, D. F. (1993). Effect of light intensity on diurnal sleep-wake distribution in young and old rats. *Brain Res Bull, 30*, 157–162.

Wu, Y.-H., Zhou, J.-N., Van Heerikhuize, J., Jockers, R., & Swaab, D. (2007). Decreased MT1 melatonin receptor expression in the suprachiasmatic nucleus in aging and Alzheimer's disease. *Neurobiol Aging, 28*, 1239–1247. doi: 0.1016/j.neurobiolaging.2006.06.002

Xu, J., Wang, L. L., Dammer, E. B., Li, C. B., Xu, G., Chen, S. D., & Wang, G. (2015). Melatonin for sleep disorders and cognition in dementia: a meta-analysis of randomized controlled trials. *Am J Alzheimers Dis Other Demen, 30*(5), 439–447. doi: 10.1177/1533317514568005

Yang, J., Jin, H. J., Mocaer, E., Seguin, L., Zhao, H., & Rusak, B. (2016). Agomelatine affects rat suprachiasmatic nucleus neurons via melatonin and serotonin receptors. *Life Sci, 155*, 147–154. doi: 10.1016/j.lfs.2016.04.035

Ying, S.-W., Rusak, B., Delagrange, P., Mocaër, E., Renard, P., & Gaurdiola-Lemaître, B. (1996). Melatonin analogues as agonists and antagonists in the circadian system and other brain areas *Eur J Pharmacol, 296*, 33–42.

Zeitzer, J. M., Daniels, J. E., Duffy, J. F., Klerman, E. B., Shanahan, T. L., Dijk, D.-J., & Czeisler, C. A. (1999). Do plasma melatonin concentrations decline with age? *Am J Med, 107*, 432–436.

Zhao, Z.-Y., Xie, Y., Fu, Y.-R., Bogdan, A., & Touitou, Y. (2002). Aging and the circadian rhythm of melatonin: a cross-sectional study of Chinese subjects 30–110 yr of age. *Chronobiol Int, 19*(6), 1171–1182. doi: 0.1081/CBI-120015958

Zhdanova, I. (2005). Melatonin as a hypnotic: Pro. *Sleep Med Rev, 9*(1), 51–65. doi: 10.1016/j.smrv.2004.04.003

Zimmerman, N. H., & Menaker, M. (1979). The pineal gland: A pacemaker within the circadian system of the house sparrow. *Proc Natl Acad Sci USA, 76*, 999–1003.

CHAPTER 10

Brainstem Regulation of Sleep and Waking

10.1 OVERVIEW

Chapters 10–12 review the principal neural systems, neurotransmitters, and other physiological mechanisms that regulate sleep and waking in mammals. There are many systems involved, distributed across much of the central nervous system. These mechanisms interact in complex ways to generate the patterns of neural activity, behavior, and states of consciousness that comprise the states of sleep and waking. Chapter 10 reviews systems in the brainstem (medulla, pons, and midbrain) and their associated neurotransmitters that are involved in sleep regulation. Chapter 11 deals with forebrain systems in the hypothalamus, preoptic area, and basal forebrain. Chapter 12 reviews the involvement of the thalamus and cortex in producing the electrophysiological and behavioral characteristics of different stages of sleep and waking.

Our knowledge of systems involved in sleep–wake regulation has grown rapidly in recent years because of the application of newer research methods. These include genetic manipulations (including optogenetic and chemogenetic methods) that selectively delete or reversibly inactivate or activate specific cell types in localized brain regions. See (Gompf & Anaclet, 2020; Venner et al., 2019) for discussions of some of these recent developments and their potential clinical applications. Because of the timing of preparation of these chapters, not all of these recent developments have been included.

10.2 States of arousal

10.2.1 Regulation of arousal

"Arousal" refers to the general state of activation of an individual; it is not equivalent to being awake. A person or animal that is awake can be in different arousal states ranging from extreme drowsiness to intense excitement or fear. The ability to modify levels of arousal from moment to moment while awake allows an organism to generate appropriate behaviors in response to changing conditions. A moderate level of arousal is necessary, for example, to engage in motivated behaviors (eating, courting, nest-building, hunting, etc.). Organisms must also be able to respond with more intense arousal and immediate behavioral activation in an emergency situation that may be life-threatening (e.g., a mouse approached by a person, or a person approached by a lion). But they must also be able to return to a lower level of arousal when the threat is removed; continued maintenance of intense arousal in the absence of an immediate threat wastes energy and causes physiological damage.

Gradations in arousal have an impact on adaptive behaviors, as illustrated by the "inverted-U"-shaped function (⌒) that represents a typical relationship between level of arousal and quality of behavioral performance on difficult tasks.[1] An example that would be familiar to students is how performance on a test is affected by the level of arousal. If a person is too sleepy or indifferent to be motivated to perform well, or too anxious and panicked to focus on the test material, performance would likely be poor. Optimal test performance results from an intermediate level of arousal that provides enough activation to perform well but is not intense enough to lead to complete behavioral disorganization.

Given the importance of appropriate arousal levels to performance, it is not surprising that the brain has numerous, overlapping regulatory mechanisms that continuously modulate the level of arousal. These mechanisms are also involved in

[1] This relationship was originally demonstrated experimentally as the impact on mice of different intensities of electric shock (and the resulting different levels of arousal) specifically on learning a difficult task (Yerkes & Dodson, 1908). The observed relationship is often cited incorrectly as representing the effect of arousal on performance of any task without regard to the task's level of difficulty (Diamond et al., 2007).

BOX 10.1 Day Hamsters and Night Hamsters

As a graduate student in Berkeley, California, I did research with golden hamsters (*Mesocricetus auratus*) and usually interacted with them during the day, their circadian rest phase. Daytime hamsters are typically curled up in their nesting material, so deeply asleep that one can sometimes move the cage, take hold of one by the loose fur around its shoulders and remove it gently from the cage before it wakes up. Even when awake, a daytime hamster that is already habituated to handling will tend to sniff half-heartedly and scan its environment in a sluggish manner; grooming and going back to sleep are its main priorities.

In their native, Middle Eastern territory, hamsters are reputed to spend their days in underground burrows, so I set up an apparatus including an "above-ground" open field and an attached artificial burrow below it, in which the hamster curled up to sleep during the day. I was curious to see where it would go and how it would behave when night fell. I slipped into the darkened room just before the night phase began inside the apparatus and waited. Shortly after the lights went out, the hamster emerged, stretched and groomed, and began to explore its environment. Within minutes, it began to behave like a different species from the one I was used to studying: it ran enthusiastically around the apparatus, exploring every corner. Any slight movement or sound I made from several feet away attracted intense scrutiny, and the hamster moved with a speed and focused intensity that I had never encountered in the daytime version of this species.

These striking differences in the level of arousal and the intensity of engagement with the external environment illustrate the sharp distinction between the rest and activity phases of circadian cycles, which is also reflected in the patterns of activity produced by animals housed in running wheels (e.g., in **Figure 3.1**).

regulating the changes in arousal level that occur during transitions between sleep and waking states. Just as very low arousal levels are not appropriate for dealing with a predatory attack or an examination, high arousal levels are incompatible with trying to transition to sleep.

In addition to environmental conditions that dictate moment-to-moment regulation of the level of arousal, there is also a gradual, programmed modulation of background arousal levels dictated by the circadian system, as discussed in Chapters 3 and 8. Circadian modulation ensures that nocturnal animals are more aroused and active during the night, while diurnal humans are more aroused and actively engaged with the environment during the day (see **Box 10.1**). Embedded within this circadian envelope of arousal modulation are cycles of sleep and waking and, within sleep, the higher frequency alternation between NREM and REM sleep, which also involves changes in levels of physiological arousal.

As reviewed in Chapter 1, the Ascending Reticular Activating System (ARAS) was originally described as a set of diffuse projections from the brainstem that combine collateral sensory input to regulate activation of the thalamus and cortex (Moruzzi & Magoun, 1949; see **Figure 1.1**). Our understanding of this system has since been refined by the identification of specific neural projections and neurotransmitters within the ARAS, which were the subject of a recent review (Jones, 2020).

A dorsal branch of the ARAS activates midline thalamic nuclei, which project to the cortex and cause diffuse cortical arousal. A more ventral branch runs through the medial forebrain bundle to innervate parts of the hypothalamus (e.g., the posterior and lateral hypothalamus) and eventually reach basal forebrain nuclei (e.g., the substantia innominata), which also project to the cortex (for reviews, see Brown et al., 2012; Jones, 2005; Jones, 2020). These projections contain several neurotransmitters that are discussed in this chapter.

10.2.2 Neurotransmitters and arousal

Most neurons in the mammalian brain contain one of three small-molecule, amino acid neurotransmitters: glutamate, its derivative γ-aminobutyric acid (GABA), and glycine. Another small-molecule neurotransmitter, formed from choline and acetyl coenzyme A, is acetylcholine (ACh), which is widely distributed in the brain and also serves as a neurotransmitter at the neuromuscular junction and in many parts of the autonomic nervous system (both sympathetic and parasympathetic). It functions as both a fast-acting neurotransmitter and as a neuromodulator (see Section 10.3.2) by acting on nicotinic and muscarinic receptors.

Neurotransmitters in the brain are released from presynaptic axon terminals (and in some cases from other parts of axons) and bind to one or more subtypes of receptors on postsynaptic target membranes, and/or on presynaptic axon terminals.[2] These receptors may be ionotropic or metabotropic. Ionotropic receptors respond to binding of the neurotransmitter molecule by opening an ion channel. The movement of ions through open channels results in a rapid change in membrane potential and thus in the excitability of the target neuron. Metabotropic

[2] Some neurotransmitters can also cross the membrane of target neurons and affect a variety of internal receptors and other mechanisms, the function of which is not well understood (Andrews et al., 2022).

receptors respond to neurotransmitter binding by slower processes involving activation of one or more second messenger cascades that can alter cell physiology in several ways: by indirectly affecting ion channels, by modifying aspects of cellular metabolism, or by changing patterns of gene expression.

Amino acid neurotransmitters have characteristic effects on the excitability of target neurons, at least in the adult brain. Glutamate is the principal excitatory neurotransmitter in the brain, GABA is the principal inhibitory neurotransmitter, and glycine is also an inhibitory neurotransmitter, especially in the spinal cord. The typical effects of these neurotransmitters are related to how they interact with their receptors, rather than to intrinsic properties of the molecules themselves. A single type of neurotransmitter can bind to several receptor subtypes that are linked to different kinds of ion channels and second messenger systems, resulting in different, even opposite, effects on the excitability of its target neurons (McCormick, 1992). As a result, the effects of the release of a single neurotransmitter from an axon terminal differ depending on the availability of different types of receptors in specific target regions.

Glutamate, for example, binds to several types of ionotropic and metabotropic receptors, resulting in different effects on target cells. Glycine is inhibitory at most of its targets, but it also binds to one class of glutamate receptors where its presence permits glutamate to have excitatory effects. GABA is usually inhibitory in adult mammals, but it is generally excitatory in early infancy; under some conditions, it can retain excitatory properties in specific brain regions even in adults[3] (e.g., Farajnia et al., 2014; Obrietan & van den Pol, 1995).

Many neurons in the ARAS, as well as the long-distance projection neurons of the thalamus and cortex, are glutamatergic (i.e., they release glutamate as a neurotransmitter). Glutamate, acting through its ionotropic receptors, rapidly depolarizes target neurons and increases their excitability. Glutamatergic neurons play a critical role in maintaining arousal and waking and in cortical activation during REM sleep, in concert with other types of ARAS neurons (Jones, 2020); they are also involved in rapid transmission and processing of information. ACh plays an important role in promoting cortical activation during both waking and REM sleep, among other functions.

GABA, acting through its ionotropic $GABA_A$ receptors, typically hyperpolarizes neurons and reduces their excitability (in adults). Activation of GABA receptors has the opposite effect of glutamate: reducing neuronal excitability and promoting sleep.[4] Most commonly used prescription sleep aids (and other sedating drugs, e.g., ethanol, barbiturates), anti-seizure medications, and anxiolytics (anxiety-reducing drugs) act as agonists at $GABA_A$ receptors (i.e., they mimic or strengthen the inhibitory actions of GABA on target neurons) (Davies, 2003).

The balance between small-molecule excitatory and inhibitory neurotransmitters is important in determining the tonic level of arousal. But their impact is modified by several other agents, which can have slower and broader modulatory effects on their targets, and are therefore sometimes called neuromodulators (McCormick, 1992; van den Pol, 2012). These include gases (e.g., nitric oxide), a large and growing number of identified neuroactive peptides and steroids, ACh, and monoamines (see Section 10.3). Most of the available information related to the neural regulation of sleep and waking involves the roles of amino acid neurotransmitters, ACh, monoamines, and peptides.

Many different methods have been used to assess the involvement of neurotransmitters in the regulation of sleep stages and waking. Appendix C contains a listing and brief description of some of the experimental approaches that have been used in studies of sleep physiology, including some comments and cautions about their use and interpretation. Readers who are less familiar with neuroscience methods should refer to these short summaries to better understand the results of studies that are discussed in the following sections and chapters.

Chapters 10 and 11 are organized around specific neurotransmitters and the brain nuclei in which they are concentrated, an approach that reflects the usual methods used to study these systems (ablation or stimulation studies, and pharmacological or genetic manipulations of neurotransmitter systems). However, the regulation of any stage of sleep or waking is not the product of a single neurotransmitter system or nucleus.

Production of the features of REM sleep, for example, is controlled by multiple interacting structures and neurotransmitters in several parts of the nervous system. Some neurons involved in REM sleep regulation are concentrated in well-defined brainstem nuclei, while others are scattered among populations of neurons with different characteristics and functions (see, e.g., Section 10.7). As a result, manipulating one component of a regulatory system can produce results that are complex, influenced by a variety of technical aspects of the research, and sometimes subject to different interpretations. The following sections provide summaries of broadly accepted views about the neural regulation of sleep and waking as well as acknowledging some alternative interpretations.

---

[3] Binding of GABA to $GABA_A$ receptors opens chloride ion channels in the cell membrane so that chloride ions flow from high to low concentrations. The switch from excitatory to inhibitory effects of $GABA_A$ receptor activation is determined by a developmental change in the resting transmembrane gradient of chloride ions. This gradient change during development results in a reversal of the direction of chloride ion flow when the channels open, thereby switching from depolarizing to hyperpolarizing target neurons (Obrietan & van den Pol, 1995).

[4] Note, however, that this depends on the "wiring diagram." Some GABAergic projections from basal forebrain neurons cause cortical *arousal* by inhibiting inhibitory GABAergic interneurons in the cortex, resulting in disinhibition (excitation) of the cortical pyramidal neurons to which the interneurons project. This mechanism is discussed in Section 11.5.

10.2.3 Summary

The three principal states of consciousness—waking, NREM sleep, and REM sleep—are characterized by different levels of arousal. Common mechanisms contribute to differences in arousal between waking and sleep and to the continuum of arousal regulation while awake. These mechanisms include the principal excitatory neurotransmitter in the adult mammalian brain, glutamate, the principal inhibitory neurotransmitter, GABA, and glycine, which is not only inhibitory in the spinal cord but also facilitates some glutamatergic neurotransmission. These amino acids act through ionotropic receptors to produce rapid changes in excitability of their target neurons as well as through more slowly acting metabotropic receptors.

ACh is another small-molecule neurotransmitter that is not only responsible for rapid signaling in some parts of the nervous system but also functions as a neuromodulator to influence cortical activation. Wakefulness depends on tonic cortical activation by glutamate and ACh (among other neuromodulators discussed in the following sections and in Chapter 11), while the transition to NREM sleep involves increased GABAergic neurotransmission and inhibition of glutamatergic and cholinergic systems. Drugs that strengthen GABAergic neurotransmission are commonly used to promote sleep.

The state of cortical arousal depends largely on the balance among glutamate, ACh, and GABA activity in the cortex. But the effects of these core neurotransmitters are modulated by several kinds of agents, including gases (e.g., nitric oxide), peptides, and monoamines. Much of what is known about the physiological regulation of sleep and waking relates to the actions of these neurochemicals.

10.3 Norepinephrine

10.3.1 Organization of monoamine neurons

Monoamines are neurochemicals derived from simple amino acids. The principal monoamines in the mammalian nervous system are dopamine (DA) and its derivative norepinephrine (NE, also called noradrenaline); histamine (HA); and serotonin (5-hydroxytryptamine, 5-HT). All are derived biochemically from aromatic[5] amino acids: DA and NE from tyrosine; 5-HT from tryptophan; and histamine from histidine. The neurons producing and releasing these neurotransmitters are organized anatomically in a generally similar way. Most of the cell bodies (somata) of NE, DA, and 5-HT neurons are found in relatively small clusters (nuclei) principally in the brainstem (medulla, pons, and midbrain); while HA neurons are found in part of the posterior hypothalamus (see Chapter 11). The elaborate axonal projections from cells in these nuclei reach most other brain regions and are widely distributed across the cerebral cortex.

Brain nuclei that are anatomically distinctive because they contain high levels of a particular neurotransmitter often include many neurons that use different neurotransmitters and project to different target regions (see, e.g., Kroeger et al., 2022; Luquin et al., 2018). Thus, a nucleus labeled as "noradrenergic," because NE is produced by many of its neurons, can also contain different kinds of neurons that play different functional roles. The discussions that follow about specific nuclei relate to the involvement of their principal neurotransmitters or neuromodulators in regulation of sleep and waking.

10.3.2 Role of norepinephrine

NE is synthesized from dopamine by clusters of neurons in the tegmentum of the pons and the reticular formation of the medulla. An important group of noradrenergic cell bodies that project broadly throughout the brain and spinal cord (except the striatum) is found in the locus coeruleus (LC; **Figure 10.1**)[6]

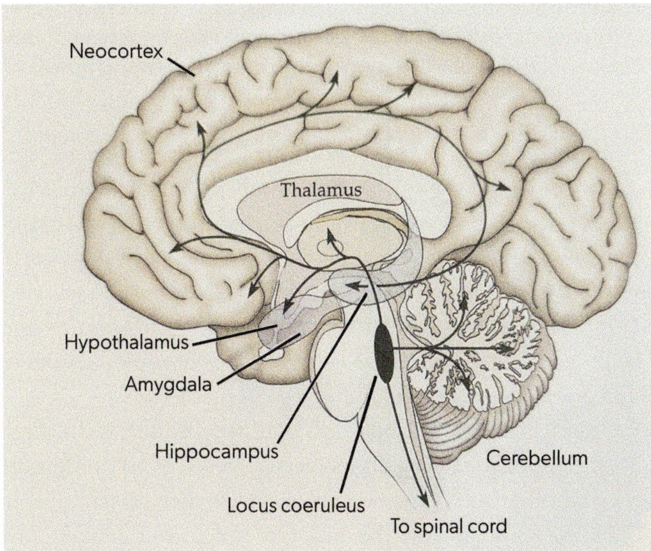

Figure 10.1 Norepinephrine (NE) neurons are concentrated in the pontine locus coeruleus (dark oval) and project to many structures in the brain (arrows), including most cortical regions, the cerebellum, hippocampus, amygdala, and hypothalamus. Reprinted with permission from Nicholls, J.G. et al. *From Neuron to Brain*, 5th Edition, 2012. Sinauer Associates; Sunderland, Massachusetts. © Oxford University Press (2012).

---

5 The term "aromatic" refers to a class of chemicals with specific structural and electrical properties and is unrelated to having an "aroma."

6 This name is Latin for "blue spot" because of its appearance in unstained tissue; "coeruleus" appears to be a misspelling of "caeruleus" (relating to the sky, "caelum" in Latin), which is also used by some authors. The misspelling is so common that it is unlikely to disappear. Some researchers avoid both troublesome diphthongs and use "ceruleus."

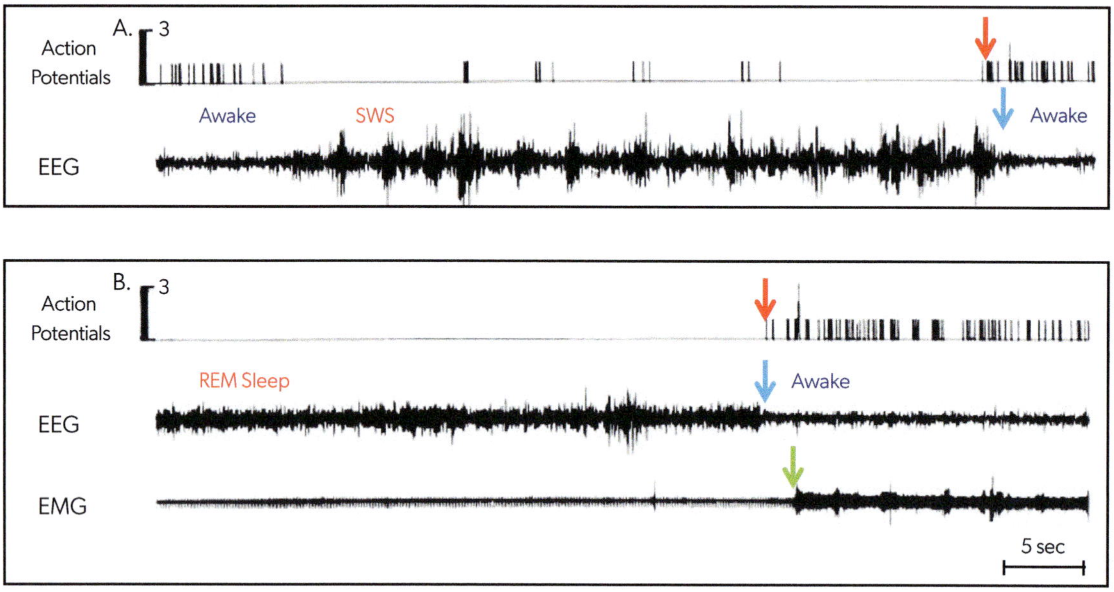

Figure 10.2 **A.** Top line: Action potentials recorded from a single locus coeruleus neuron (presumably noradrenergic) in a freely behaving rat. The Y axis shows a maximum of three spikes per unit time. Bottom line: The cortical EEG recording shows the transition from low-voltage activity when the rat is awake to high-voltage activity during slow-wave sleep (SWS), and back to low-voltage activity when awake again. The neuron fires at a high rate during waking and at a reduced rate during SWS; the firing rate increases again (red arrow) slightly before the rat wakes up (blue arrow). **B**. Top and middle lines: Locus coeruleus single-unit firing and EEG recordings during REM sleep and waking. Bottom line: Electromyogram (EMG) recording. The neuron is completely silent during REM sleep, characterized by an EMG showing atonia. Neuronal firing (red arrow) resumes just as the EEG changes to a low-voltage waking pattern (blue arrow), but 2–3 sec before atonia is reversed and muscle tone is restored (green arrow). Adapted with permission from Aston-Jones G. & Bloom F.E. (1981) Activity of norepinephrine-containing locus coeruleus neurons in behaving rats anticipates fluctuations in the sleep-waking cycle. *J Neurosci* 1:876–886. © Society for Neuroscience (1981). doi: 10.1523/JNEUROSCI.01-08-00876.1981.

and in nearby nuclei in the pons, including the nucleus subcoeruleus (Moore & Bloom, 1979; Swanson & Hartman, 1975). NE is released both synaptically and more broadly via extrasynaptic axonal sites—a characteristic also shared by dopamine, serotonin, and histamine projections (Beaudet & Descarries, 1978; Takagi et al., 1986). Consistent with their release through volume transmission, these agents act as neuromodulators to influence large regions of their target structures.

Firing rates of NE neurons recorded in the LC are high during waking, causing an increased release of NE in the cortex and other forebrain regions to which they project. Firing rates decrease during the onset of sleep and remain low throughout NREM sleep (**Figure 10.2 A**). These neurons typically decrease firing rates even further and become virtually silent during REM sleep; they are therefore considered "REM-Off" neurons (Aston-Jones & Bloom, 1981). An increase of LC neuronal activity accompanies the transition to waking at the end of a NREM sleep period or the end of a REM sleep episode (**Figure 10.2 B**).

LC neurons play an important role in the network involved in regulating the timing of REM sleep; see Section 10.7.2 (Hobson et al., 1975). The LC also projects to brainstem cholinergic and serotonergic cell groups involved in sleep regulation and to nuclei involved in regulation of the autonomic nervous system. Activation of these LC projections promotes increased sympathetic and decreased parasympathetic activity, which has arousing, alerting, and energy-mobilizing effects (Samuels & Szabadi, 2008).

When NE is released onto cortical or thalamic neurons, it causes EEG activation by increasing neural firing rates and decreasing the tendency to generate high-voltage, slow oscillations characteristic of NREM sleep (**Figure 10.2 A**). NE also enhances the responsiveness of cortical neurons to other excitatory inputs, for example, by amplifying the activation of cortical astrocytes in response to sensory inputs, which can indirectly facilitate neuronal activation (Paukert et al., 2014). (See Section 11.6.1 for a discussion of a possible role for astrocytes in sleep regulation.) Thus, NE promotes EEG activation, cortical arousal, and increased responsiveness to sensory inputs, which facilitate attention and information processing while awake (Aston-Jones et al., 1999). Activation of LC neurons and the resulting increase in cortical arousal during the daily active phase depends on indirect input from the suprachiasmatic nuclei (SCN) that is conveyed via the dorsomedial hypothalamic nuclei (Aston-Jones et al., 2001).

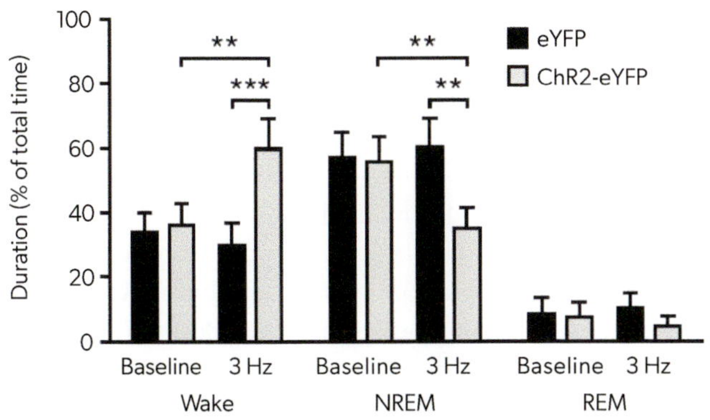

Figure 10.3 Effects of selective optogenetic activation of locus coeruleus (LC) neurons. Black columns represent control, wild-type mice (eYFP) who could not respond to optogenetic stimulation in the LC; and gray columns represent transgenic mice (ChR2-eYFP) that responded to illumination of the LC with increased activity of NE neurons. Pulses of light stimulation in the LC at 3 Hz increased the percentage of time spent awake and decreased the time spent in NREM sleep. There were no significant changes induced in REM sleep amounts or in episode lengths by either activation or suppression of LC neurons. ** $p<0.001$; *** $p<0.0001$. Reprinted with permission from Carter, M.E. et al. (2010) Tuning arousal with optogenetic modulation of locus coeruleus neurons. *Nat Neurosci* 13:1526–1535. © Springer: Nature (2010). doi: 10.1038/nn.2682.

Selective activation of LC neurons that contain NE using optogenetic methods (see Appendix C) caused sleeping mice during the daily light phase to immediately transition to waking and to reduce the total time spent in NREM sleep, as expected for a mechanism involved in promoting arousal (**Figure 10.3**). Selective inhibition of NE neurons during the dark phase had the opposite effect: shortening wake episodes and increasing the total amount of NREM sleep (Carter et al., 2010).

Widespread NE projections from the LC promote cortical desynchronization and waking by directly activating cortical neurons and other neural systems that support wakefulness, as well as by inhibiting sleep-promoting systems. Thus, NE is a key neurotransmitter triggering and sustaining wakefulness as well as promoting increased arousal and attention to environmental stimuli while awake. NE neurons are also involved in regulating transitions between NREM and REM sleep, as discussed in Section 10.7.

10.3.3 Summary

The monoamines are a family of small-molecule neurotransmitters derived from different amino acids; dopamine (DA) and norepinephrine (NE) are derived from tyrosine. Somata of NE neurons are located in nuclei in the pons and medulla and project to many subcortical and cortical regions. The locus coeruleus (LC) is a nucleus in the pontine tegmentum containing noradrenergic neurons that project broadly throughout the brain.

LC neurons fire at high rates during waking, show strongly suppressed activity during NREM sleep, and are essentially silent during REM sleep. The timing of changes in LC neuronal firing in anticipation of transitions in sleep–wake states (see **Figure 10.2A**) indicate that the release of NE plays a role in promoting waking. Optogenetic studies showed that activating NE neurons in the LC in sleeping mice caused immediate waking, while suppressing their firing in mice that were awake reduced the time spent awake and increased the time spent in NREM sleep.

NE is a key neurotransmitter involved in activating cortical regions and reducing the slow oscillations characteristic of NREM sleep. It also stimulates the activity of the sympathetic nervous system to increase arousal, alert wakefulness, and energy mobilization, as well as being involved in the regulation of NREM/REM sleep cycling.

10.4 Dopamine

10.4.1 Role of DA in regulation of sleep and waking

Dopamine (DA) is synthesized by groups of neurons in several parts of the brainstem and hypothalamus. Those most closely linked to regulation of sleep and waking are found in the mesencephalon, specifically in the substantia nigra ("black substance," so-named because of its dark appearance relative to surrounding tissue), and the ventral tegmental area (VTA) (**Figure 10.4**). Substantia nigra neurons project to the striatum (comprising the caudate and putamen), which plays a critical role in regulation of motor activity, and to a part of the thalamus involved in the production of cortical sleep spindles (see Section 12.2.3) (Freeman et al., 2001; Govindaiah et al., 2010). Degeneration of the nigrostriatal projection (also called the mesostriatal projection) leads to the development of the motor symptoms of Parkinson's disease, including tremor and motor retardation.

VTA dopaminergic neurons project broadly to the cortex in primates, contribute to the projection to the striatum, and reach parts of the limbic system, including the nucleus accumbens, amygdala, septum, and nearby structures (Aransay et al., 2015; Björklund & Dunnett, 2007). The brain regions that receive these mesocorticolimbic projections are involved in motivation, reward, motor activity, addictive behaviors, and other functions (Berke, 2018; Berridge, 2007; Björklund & Dunnett, 2007). Projections from both the VTA and the substantia nigra also reach several cholinergic nuclei in the basal forebrain (Gaykema & Zaborsky, 1996), which play an important role in promoting waking and cortical activation (see Chapter 11).

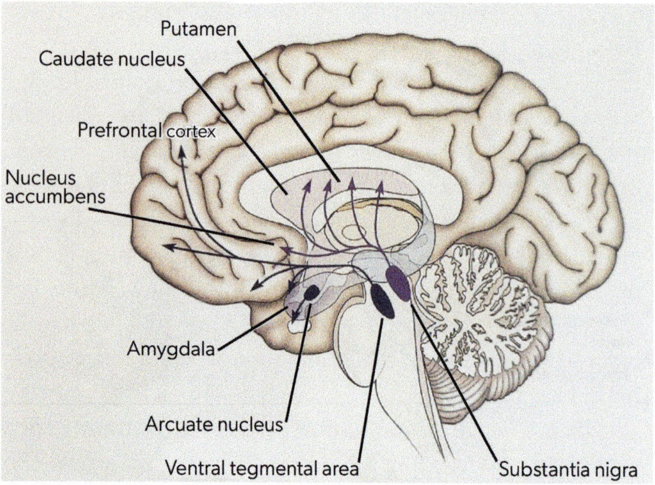

Figure 10.4 Projections in the brain containing dopamine (DA) originate in clusters of neurons found primarily in the midbrain. Dopaminergic neurons in the substantia nigra (SN) project primarily to the striatum, and those in the ventral tegmental area (VTA) project to several limbic structures (septum, amygdala, nucleus accumbens, hypothalamus) and to prefrontal and insular (limbic) cortex. Some areas receive projections from both the VTA and SN. Reprinted with permission from Nicholls, J.G. et al. (2012) *From Neuron to Brain*, 5th Edition, 2012. Sinauer Associates; Sunderland, Massachusetts. © Oxford University Press (2012).

Single DA neurons in both the substantia nigra and VTA tend to fire at relatively low rates during all arousal states, but at marginally higher rates during waking, and in bursts during waking motor activity and REM sleep (Trulson & Preussler, 1984; Trulson et al., 1981); for a review, see Datta & MacLean, 2007. The range of variation in firing rates across sleep–wake states is much smaller than for most other systems involved in sleep–wake regulation, such as the previously discussed NE neurons, or serotonergic neurons in the raphe nuclei (Trulson & Jacobs, 1979); see Section 10.5.

Despite limited changes in average firing rates across states of arousal, levels of DA in the prefrontal cortex are twice as high during waking as during SWS, and are also higher during REM sleep, implying involvement of DA in promoting both waking and REM sleep. Discrepancies between overall firing rates and DA levels may be related to the greater effectiveness of burst firing during waking in releasing DA (Léna et al., 2005), and/or to altered activity of the dopamine transporter (Ferris et al., 2014).[7] Other methods used to measure activity of the VTA also showed reduced activity during NREM sleep relative to waking (Eban-Rothschild et al., 2016).

A third population of dopaminergic neurons is scattered throughout the ventral periaqueductal gray (vPAG), a region close to the dorsal raphe nuclei and VTA. These neurons are reciprocally connected to many sleep–wake regulatory centers in both forebrain and brainstem. They are more active during waking than during sleep, as indicated by increased c-Fos gene expression during waking, and their destruction leads to increased sleep and reduced waking (Lu, Jhou, et al., 2006); see Appendix C for a discussion of c-Fos expression as a marker of neuronal activation.

DA neurons in the vPAG are involved in promoting waking. Injection of the neurotoxin 6-hydroxydopamine into this region selectively destroyed these DA neurons and caused a significant decrease in waking and increase in sleep duration over 24 h. The largest decrease in waking/increase in sleep was seen in those animals that had lost the largest proportion of DA neurons in the vPAG, indicating that the lesions damaged a major wake-promoting system (Lu, Jhou, et al., 2006) (**Figure 10.5**).

VTA DA neurons have also been reported to play an important role in promoting waking, as shown in studies in mice that

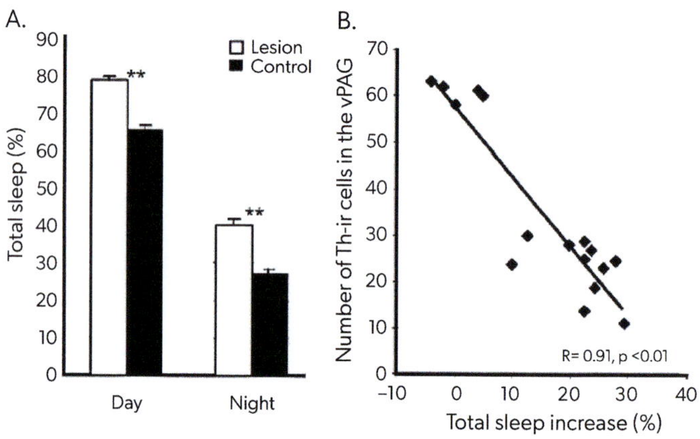

Figure 10.5 Effects of lesions in the rat ventral periaqueductal gray (vPAG) that decreased waking and increased sleep durations. Lesions were made using the toxin 6-hydroxydopamine, which selectively destroys dopaminergic cells. **A.** White columns show the significant increase in sleep during both day and night recordings after lesions of dopaminergic cells in the vPAG, relative to control animals (black columns). **B.** The regression line reflects a robust negative correlation between the number of surviving dopaminergic cells in the vPAG (Y axis) and the extent of sleep increase (X axis). Surviving dopaminergic cells were identified as those immunoreactive for tyrosine hydroxylase (TH-ir), an enzyme involved in the synthesis of dopamine. The fewer TH-ir cells that survived the lesion treatment, the greater the increase in total sleep time. Reprinted with permission from Lu, J. et al. (2006) Identification of wake-active dopaminergic neurons in the ventral periaqueductal gray matter. *J Neurosci* 26:193–202. © Society for Neuroscience (2006). doi: 10.1523/JNEUROSCI.2244-05.2006.

[7] Transporters are molecules on the presynaptic side of the synapse that transport released neurotransmitters from the synaptic cleft back into the presynaptic neuron (reuptake). Reuptake reduces the amount of neurotransmitter available to affect target (postsynaptic) neurons. Inhibiting reuptake results in higher concentrations of a neurotransmitter in the synapse and therefore stronger effects on postsynaptic neurons.

selectively manipulated the activity of these neurons. Activating VTA neurons promoted transitions to waking from NREM sleep, while suppressing their activity led to preparations for sleeping (nest-building) followed by sleep onset. Manipulation of specific VTA projection paths implicated the DA projection to the nucleus accumbens, one of the basal forebrain nuclei (see Section 11.5), in promoting waking (Eban-Rothschild et al., 2016). The VTA also contains inhibitory GABAergic interneurons that locally modulate the activity of dopaminergic (and glutamatergic) VTA projection neurons (Soden et al., 2020). Inhibiting GABAergic interneurons resulted in increased waking, probably as a result of disinhibiting these VTA projection neurons that promote waking (Cai et al., 2022).

Pharmacological evidence is also consistent with the conclusion that DA and its receptors are involved in increasing waking. A variety of stimulant drugs that promote wakefulness exert their effects principally via the dopaminergic system (Kanbayashi et al., 2000; Wisor et al., 2001). These include cocaine, amphetamine, modafinil, and methylphenidate (e.g., Ritalin™, Concerta™), which act in large part by inhibiting the reuptake activity of the DA transporter, resulting in increases in synaptic DA levels. In the case of cocaine, the direction of DA transport at the presynaptic membrane (normally involved in reducing synaptic DA levels) may even be reversed. Thus, cocaine can cause increased release of DA into the synapse as well as reducing its rate of removal by reuptake (Jones et al., 1998; Qu et al., 2008; Qu et al., 2010; Turner et al., 2014; Wisor, 2013).

Consistent with a role for DA in affecting sleep and waking, genetic analyses in a large human population sample linked polymorphisms in two dopamine-related genes to variations in habitual sleep durations (Rhodes et al., 2018).

Given the wide distribution of DA projections in the brain, its effects on sleep and waking are likely mediated at several levels, including by actions on the cortex, basal forebrain nuclei, hypothalamus, and thalamus (Björklund & Dunnett, 2007; Eban-Rothschild et al., 2016; Freeman et al., 2001; Gaykema & Zaborsky, 1996; Govindaiah et al., 2010; Lu, Jhou, et al., 2006). A novel mechanism by which DA could also affect sleep is by acting in the pineal gland to inhibit production and release of melatonin, which facilitates the transition to sleep (see Chapter 9) (González et al., 2012).

Cocaine and amphetamines have been used both medically and recreationally to reduce sleepiness and increase activation. Their usefulness, however, is limited by their potent reinforcing and addictive properties and the resulting serious potential for both abuse and addiction. At high doses, these drugs can also trigger hallucinations. Modafinil and methylphenidate have less abuse potential but may be correspondingly less potent as wake promoters. These drugs may also have different impacts on sleep homeostasis. Both modafinil and amphetamine increased waking in rats during the hours after treatment, but the later rebound increases in NREM sleep differed in pattern and timing for the two drugs (Edgar & Seidel, 1997; Wisor et al., 2006).

In addition to the classic motor symptoms that result from the loss of DA projections to the striatum, patients with Parkinson's disease (PD) also have many non-motor symptoms, including daytime sleepiness and disrupted sleep at night. These sleep symptoms probably result from loss of dopaminergic neurons that project to wake-promoting cholinergic neurons in the basal forebrain (Gaykema & Zaborsky, 1996) and to the striatum, as well as from loss of DA neurons in the vPAG (Lu, Jhou, et al., 2006).

This hypothesis is supported by evidence from a study that used a DA neurotoxin to produce a model of Parkinson's disease in macaque monkeys (*Macaca fascicularis*), a diurnal species. The development of Parkinsonian motor symptoms was accompanied by very large increases (from ~12 to ~92 min) in light NREM sleep during the 12 h day phase, decreases in REM sleep, and more disrupted sleep at night. It is unclear whether greater instability of sleep at night resulted from a reduced homeostatic sleep drive because of increased daytime sleep or from other effects of the neuronal damage.

Treatment with the DA precursor levodopa (L-dopa, which is used clinically to treat motor symptoms in PD patients) mostly reversed the increase in daytime sleepiness, increased REM sleep, and helped consolidate nighttime sleep (Belaid et al., 2014). Thus, damage to DA systems in a diurnal primate is associated with decreased REM sleep, increased daytime sleepiness, and disrupted nighttime sleep, recapitulating symptoms often seen in PD patients; augmenting dopaminergic activity improved these symptoms.

10.4.2 Dopamine, REM sleep, dreams, and hallucinations

As previously discussed, destruction of DA neurons in monkeys reduced REM sleep amounts, and increasing DA levels restored REM sleep (Belaid et al., 2014). Similarly, chemical depletion of DA levels in intact mice drastically reduced REM sleep, and pharmacological activation of a DA receptor subtype restored REM sleep. Mice that were genetically engineered to knock out the DA transporter (and therefore increase DA synaptic levels) showed abnormal intrusions into waking of mixed REM-like EEG states when they were exposed to a novel environment (presumably a mild stressor) (Dzirasa et al., 2006). Because gene knockouts and systemic drug treatments affect all DA systems, it is not clear which of several DA projections mediated these effects on REM sleep. The interpretation that DA increases REM sleep is consistent with evidence for higher DA levels in the prefrontal cortex during REM sleep (Léna et al., 2005).

There are other, more indirect, indications of links between DA regulation and aspects of REM sleep. Although dreaming can occur in other sleep stages (see Appendix A), people awakened from REM sleep have the highest probability of reporting dreams. The mechanisms responsible for dream production during REM sleep are poorly understood, but several neural systems have been proposed to be involved (Nir & Tononi, 2010; Solms, 2011), including a specific role for midbrain dopaminergic projections to the cortex. People who suffered bilateral damage to this DA pathway near the ventral part of the frontal lobes showed reduced or absent dream reports, even though they continued to produce EEG-defined REM sleep (Solms, 2000; Solms, 2011).

This same cortical region was likely damaged by some prefrontal lobotomies (lobe removal) and leucotomies (cutting fiber tracts) (Solms, 2000; Solms, 2011). These controversial surgical procedures were used during the middle of the 20th century in attempts to treat a variety of psychiatric conditions, including schizophrenia. In addition to other reported negative effects of these surgical procedures, they caused a reduction in dream reports, with no loss of PSG-defined REM sleep, as compared to patients with schizophrenia who had not undergone lobotomies (Jus et al., 1973).

These findings suggest that DA projections to the prefrontal cortex are involved in triggering dream production during REM sleep, although the narrative content of dreams depends on broader cortical activity (Nir & Tononi, 2010). The preservation of PSG features of REM sleep despite loss or reduction of dream reports is consistent with the generation of these PSG features by structures in the pons that would be unaffected by these surgical procedures (see Section 10.7). A recent publication, however, also reported evidence that a different dopaminergic projection also plays a role in triggering REM sleep features (Hasegawa et al., 2022).[8]

As discussed in Appendix A, there is no independent, objective way to verify the number and nature of dreams experienced by a research participant; studies of dreaming rely on self-reports by participants of their pre-awakening mental activity. This fact enforces caution in interpreting the effects of prefrontal cortical damage on dream reports. It is possible, for example, that the damage did not reduce the occurrence of dreams but rather impaired peoples' ability or motivation to either remember or report dreams.

People with schizophrenia and other psychotic disorders commonly report hallucinations while awake (most often auditory or visual). These have often been compared to the experience of dreams during sleep (Gottesmann, 2006); "[d]reaming is, after all, a psychotic state" (Solms, 2011, p. 528). The two phenomena are similar in that people experience dreams and hallucinations as real while they occur, even though the subjective experience is unrelated to objective reality. But that shared characteristic does not prove that they have a common underlying mechanism. Concluding that dreams and hallucinations are linked causally, rather than only metaphorically, requires evidence that they share a common neural substrate. DA neurotransmission may represent this common substrate.

Several findings discussed above link cortical DA levels with dreams and the REM sleep stage in which they most often occur. DA levels in the cortex are high during REM sleep, and loss of DA neurons reduces REM sleep amounts. Damage to a prefrontal cortical region that receives DA projections also reduces reports of dream content. There are also multiple lines of evidence supporting the idea that excess dopaminergic activity contributes to the production of hallucinations. Many of the "positive" symptoms of schizophrenia (i.e., hallucinations, delusions, and disordered thoughts) (Howes & Kapur, 2009) have been linked to increased presynaptic production and release of DA in the striatum.[9] This link may depend on indirectly activating the frontal cortex as a result of DA action in the striatum (Saunders et al., 2015). Most importantly, the effectiveness of different antipsychotic drugs in treating positive symptoms of schizophrenia closely parallels their effectiveness in reducing dopaminergic activity (Howes & Kapur, 2009; Seeman et al., 2006).[10]

Some doses of drugs of abuse can trigger hallucinations and drug-induced psychoses (e.g., cocaine and amphetamines), and can block—and even reverse—the function of the DA transporter, thereby increasing dopaminergic drive onto target systems. Similarly, hallucinations and intense, bizarre dreams (Solms, 2011) are a common side effect of treating the motor symptoms of PD with L-dopa, which is

[8] The study found that activation of a dopaminergic projection from the VTA to the basolateral nucleus of the amygdala triggered onset of REM sleep but with a surprisingly long latency (Hasegawa et al., 2022). A series of commentaries related to this publication (Fraigne et al., 2023) indicated that this projection appears to exert an indirect modulatory influence on the pontine mechanisms that are directly involved in initiating REM sleep; see Section 10.7.2. But the connection from the amygdala to these mechanisms remains to be determined.

[9] There is also evidence supporting a role for glutamatergic neurotransmission (linked in some cases to DA or to serotonin neurotransmission) in generating these symptoms (Aghajanian & Marek, 2000; Jauhar et al., 2018; Kantrowitz & Javitt, 2010).

[10] The "negative" symptoms of schizophrenia include reductions in motivation, emotional responsiveness, social interactions, speech, and movement (Andreasen & Olsen, 1982). These symptoms are usually not much improved by antipsychotic drugs, suggesting that they are not likely to be related directly to excess DA neurotransmission.

converted into DA in the brain. The occurrence of hallucinations may require reductions in the doses of L-dopa that are used (Diederich et al., 2009).

Thus, increased dopaminergic activity is linked to hallucinations while awake, and to REM sleep while asleep. Reducing dopaminergic activity can reduce hallucinations, and damaging dopaminergic projections can reduce the experience of dreaming.

10.4.3 Summary

The major sources of DA in the brain are the substantia nigra, which projects to the striatum, and the ventral tegmental area (VTA), which projects broadly to the cortex and to several limbic system structures. There are also DA neurons in the ventral periaqueductal gray (vPAG) that are involved in regulating sleep amounts.

Firing rates of DA neurons do not change dramatically across stages of sleep or waking. Nevertheless, DA levels in the prefrontal cortex are higher during waking and REM sleep than during NREM sleep. These changes may relate to reduced activity of the DA transporter or to the presence of burst firing patterns that more effectively increase DA release. vPAG neurons are also more active during REM sleep and waking than during NREM sleep, as measured by levels of c-Fos expression.

These hints that DA levels contribute to waking are supported by evidence that selectively activating VTA DA neurons promotes waking, while suppressing their activity triggers behavioral preparations for, and onset of, sleep. The vPAG is connected to other sleep-regulating systems in both forebrain and brainstem regions; destruction of dopaminergic neurons in this structure also decreases waking and increases sleep.

A variety of DA agonists, including several drugs of abuse (e.g., cocaine, amphetamines), sustain wakefulness and disrupt sleep. DA is also linked to both hallucinations and REM sleep dreaming. Damage to frontal cortical white matter pathways that interrupts DA projections reduces or eliminates dream reports, without affecting electrophysiological features of REM sleep, which are controlled by pontine systems. High doses of DA agonists can trigger hallucinations and psychotic episodes, while drugs that reduce the positive symptoms of schizophrenia (especially hallucinations) do so to the degree that they reduce dopaminergic drive. These links imply an important role for DA in generating the experience of waking hallucinations as well as in triggering dreams during sleep.

Taken together, the evidence strongly supports a role for DA in contributing to wake maintenance and in triggering dreams during sleep as well as hallucinations while awake.

10.5 Serotonin

10.5.1 Role of serotonin in regulation of sleep and waking

Serotonin (5-HT) is synthesized by neurons with somata located in a string of raphe nuclei stretching through the central part of the brainstem reticular formation, from the medulla through the pons and midbrain (**Figure 10.6**). Serotonergic projections from these nuclei collectively reach most of the nervous system. The more caudal raphe nuclei generally project toward the spinal cord and brainstem while the more rostral nuclei, especially the dorsal raphe nucleus (DRN), project to several parts of the forebrain, including most of the cerebral cortex.

Early research using animal models, along with some clinical data, indicated that lesion damage to the raphe nuclei or chemical depletion of 5-HT levels led to continuous arousal, agitation, and sleeplessness. Combined with other evidence suggesting that 5-HT promoted sleep, these findings led to the hypothesis that increased 5-HT levels were involved in initiating and maintaining sleep, especially NREM sleep (Jouvet, 1969). Contrary to what this hypothesis would predict, however,

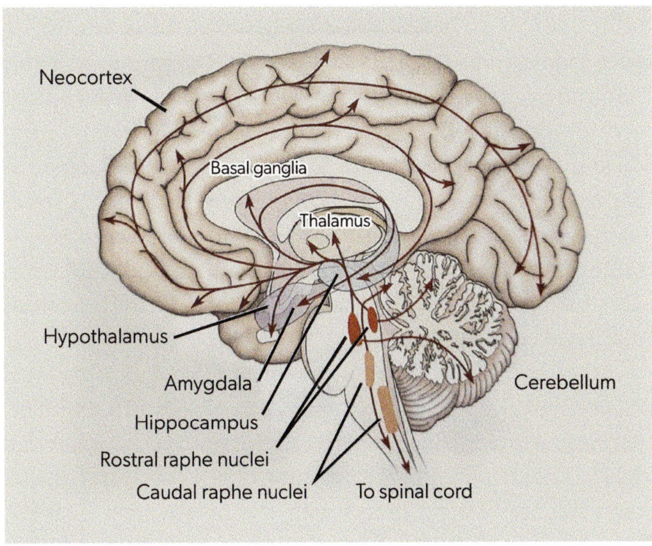

Figure 10.6 Serotonergic projections originate in a string of brainstem nuclei (raphe nuclei) located in the midline regions of the medulla, pons, and midbrain; these projections reach most of the brain. Cells in the median and dorsal raphe nuclei (the rostral raphe nuclei, red ovals) project broadly to the forebrain, including the cortex and hippocampus, and to the cerebellum, while those in the caudal raphe nuclei (orange ovals) project to the brainstem and spinal cord. Reprinted with permission from Nicholls, J.G. et al. (2012) *From Neuron to Brain*, 5th Edition. Sinauer Associates; Sunderland, Massachusetts. © Oxford University Press (2012).

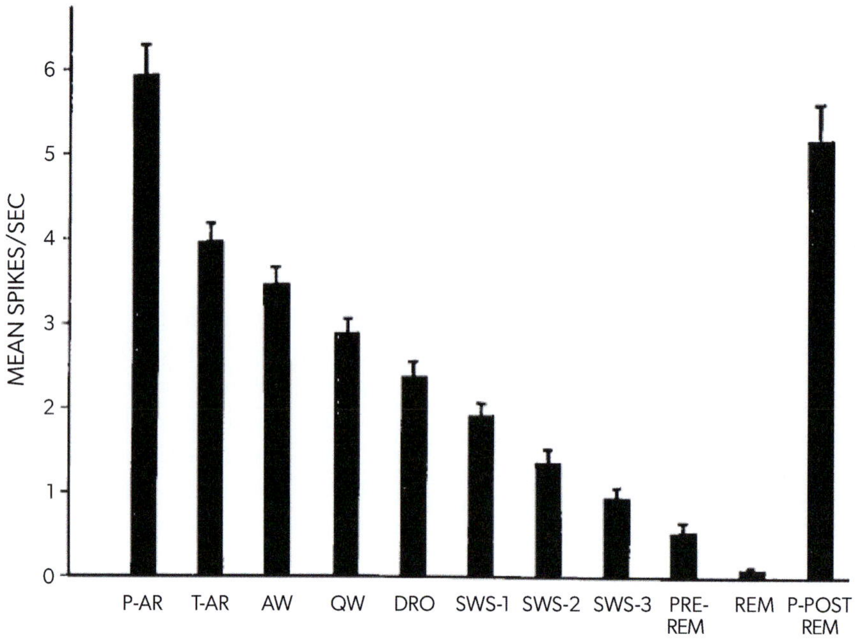

Figure 10.7 Average firing rates of raphe neurons in a cat recorded during different states of arousal. From left to right, these included very high firing rates during an arousal response to a click noise (phasic arousal, P-AR) and during the subsequent transient arousal period (T-AR). Firing rates were also high during active waking (AW) and fell progressively during quiet waking (QW) and when the cat was drowsy (DRO), and during early to late phases of a slow-wave sleep episode (SWS-1–3). Firing rates were very low in the minute before REM sleep onset (PRE-REM) and fell to zero during REM sleep (REM). There was also a sharp increase in firing immediately after waking from a REM sleep episode (P-POST REM). Reprinted with permission of Elsevier Ltd. from Trulson M.E. & Jacobs B.L. Raphe unit activity in freely moving cats: correlation with level of behavioral arousal. *Brain Res* 163:135–150. © Elsevier (1979). doi: 10.1016/0006-8993(79)90157-4.

later studies found that individual DRN neurons (probably serotonergic) fire most rapidly during waking, reduce their activity during NREM sleep, and become virtually silent during REM sleep (McGinty & Harper, 1976; Oikonomou et al., 2019; Trulson & Jacobs, 1979) (**Figure 10.7**). 5-HT levels in the cortex changed in parallel to these firing-rate changes, falling to low levels in NREM and very low levels in REM sleep. This pattern parallels the changes in activity of NE neurons discussed earlier (Section 10.3).

These results, combined with evidence that there is eventual recovery of sleep long after raphe ablations (which undoubtedly also damaged fibers of passage), led to the conclusion that 5-HT is not involved in the initiation of NREM sleep. Instead, the evidence was consistent with the involvement of 5-HT projections to the cortex in producing cortical arousal during waking, paralleling the role of NE; for a review, see Jones, 2005.

Another function of 5-HT that is generally accepted is its involvement in regulation of REM sleep. High firing rates of 5-HT (and NE) neurons during waking inhibit the pontine mechanisms that trigger REM sleep. A gradual decline in 5-HT/NE activity during NREM sleep leads ultimately to disinhibition of these pontine mechanisms, onset of REM sleep, and the virtual silence of 5-HT/NE neurons during REM sleep (see **Figure 10.7** and Section 10.7.3). These conclusions were supported by recordings from populations of DRN neurons across sleep–wake states and evidence that optogenetic silencing of DRN neurons permitted the emergence of REM sleep, while their activation during REM sleep triggered waking (Kato et al., 2022).

In contrast to claims that 5-HT promotes either waking or sleep, there is evidence for a more subtle role for one 5-HT projection in regulating arousal and activity. Neurons in the lateral hypothalamus that produce the peptide hypocretin are involved in triggering and maintaining wakefulness (see Section 11.3.1), and they are reciprocally connected to 5-HT neurons. Since both systems are proposed to support wakefulness, it is surprising that 5-HT input to hypocretin neurons is inhibitory (Muraki et al., 2004), while hypocretin input to 5-HT neurons is excitatory (Tsunematsu et al., 2011). Later research suggested that during the early daily dark phase, when hypocretin drive is strongest and mice are most active, 5-HT inhibition of hypocretin neurons provides a modest "braking" effect on their activity. Thus, 5-HT in this circuit does not specifically promote either sleep or waking. Rather, 5-HT provides feedback to an arousal mechanism that helps to fine-tune activation to an appropriate level during one phase of the circadian cycle (Tabuchi et al., 2013).

Other studies have involved administering 5-HT receptor agonists and antagonists (see Appendix C) to assess the role of 5-HT in sleep regulation. This approach, however, is complicated by the number, functional diversity, and widespread distribution of 5-HT receptors. Among mammalian species, there are at least 14 different 5-HT receptor subtypes. These are located postsynaptically, presynaptically, or both, and are linked to different second messenger systems that promote either neuronal activation or inhibition (Barnes & Sharp, 1999).

For example, postsynaptic 5-HT_{1A} receptors mediate inhibitory effects of 5-HT on many target neurons, including in parts of the cortex (Barnes & Sharp, 1999; Puig et al., 2005).[11] But 5-HT_{1A} receptors (autoreceptors) are also found on the somata of serotonergic raphe neurons. When raphe neurons are active, they can release 5-HT not only on distant target cells but also near their own somata through recurrent axon collaterals. When these neurons fire at high rates, the local release of 5-HT activates these inhibitory autoreceptors, which reduces the neuron's own firing. In turn, this limits the further release of 5-HT at inhibitory synapses on distant target neurons (e.g., in the cortex), which can reduce their inhibitory effects via 5-HT_{1A} receptors and/or their excitatory effects via 5-HT_{2A} receptors (Blier et al., 1998; Wang & Aghajanian, 1978).[12]

As a result, a 5-HT_{1A} receptor agonist could have unpredictable effects on cortical neurons, depending on how it is administered. Treating an animal systemically with this agonist could directly inhibit target neurons in the cortex. But its inhibitory effects on autoreceptors in the raphe nuclei would reduce firing of 5-HT projection neurons and the release of 5-HT in the cortex, resulting in disinhibition (excitation) of cortical neurons. The dynamic balance of these inhibitory and excitatory effects would determine the net effect on cortical arousal of systemic administration of a 5-HT_{1A} receptor agonist, which might differ among species.

One set of pharmacological results illustrates some of the complexity involved in these analyses. Ritanserin is an antagonist at the excitatory 5-HT_2 receptor. In cats, ritanserin reduced sleep (consistent with a sleep-promoting role for 5-HT), while in rats and people it increased sleep (Sommerfelt & Ursin, 1993). One possibility is that these differences could be related to ritanserin having additional effects on other 5-HT receptor subtypes, which could be differentially present in different species.

[11] Some cortical regions also have high levels of 5-HT_{2A} receptors. 5-HT acting on these receptors increases the release of glutamate and therefore has an indirect excitatory effect on cortical neurons (Aghajanian & Marek, 2000).

[12] There are alternative models of the mechanisms that underlie 5-HT autoinhibition (see Andrade et al., 2015).

Another potential source of information about the effects of 5-HT on sleep is the widespread use of antidepressant drugs that affect serotonergic activity. Many antidepressants affect serotonergic neurotransmission by inhibiting 5-HT reuptake and thereby increasing its synaptic availability. These include both classic tricyclic antidepressants and newer, more selective, 5-HT reuptake inhibitors (SSRIs; e.g., fluoxetine (Prozac™) and related drugs).

SSRIs have been reported to increase daytime drowsiness, delay REM sleep onset, reduce total REM sleep amounts, and disrupt sleep continuity. These changes are most pronounced initially and usually diminish over the course of treatment (Wilson & Argyropoulos, 2005). A likely contributor to these early effects is increased serotonergic inhibition of cholinergic mechanisms that contribute to both daytime alertness and the onset of REM sleep (see Section 10.7.2). Since sleep problems are a common symptom of untreated depression (see Section 15.3.2), improvement in sleep features during the course of treatment could reflect both improvements in depression symptoms generally and gradual adaptation to some pharmacological effects of increased 5-HT.

Experimental studies and clinical observations of the effects of systemic manipulations of 5-HT activity do not provide a clear picture of its role in sleep–wake regulation. The roles ascribed to 5-HT have evolved in part not only because of the application of different methods to study the issue but also because of growing knowledge of the complexity of the target receptor populations and second messenger systems affected by 5-HT projections. Systemic treatments could affect many functionally different receptor subtypes that vary in their distribution across brain regions (Beliveau et al., 2017). Similarly, there is evidence from single-unit recordings of putative 5-HT neurons in the DRN that there is great diversity in firing patterns associated with different behaviors and sleep–wake states, presumably reflecting different functional roles of individual 5-HT neurons (Sakai & Crochet, 2001).

Although there is considerable evidence consistent with a role for 5-HT in promoting waking (and inhibiting REM sleep onset), there is no agreement on why acute depletion of 5-HT and raphe ablations increase waking and decrease sleep. Some proposals that address these contradictory observations are discussed in Section 10.5.2. These proposed explanations focus on different findings related to 5-HT: the complexities associated with multiple 5-HT receptor subtypes; the existence of a subclass of apparently serotonergic neurons in the raphe nuclei whose activity is not related to waking; a role for 5-HT in motor activity; effects of 5-HT damage on body temperature regulation; and a role for 5-HT neurons in accumulating information about wake durations (Imeri & Opp, 2009; Jouvet, 1999; McGinty & Harper, 1976; Monti, 2011; Sakai & Crochet, 2001)

10.5.2 Questioning the role of 5-HT in cortical arousal

The original observations of decreased sleep and increased activity after chemical depletion of 5-HT (Jouvet, 1969; Mouret et al., 1967) led to the proposal that 5-HT is involved in triggering NREM sleep. Other experimental results were more consistent with the idea that 5-HT contributes to cortical arousal (see, e.g., **Figure 10.7**). A variety of pharmacological and lesion studies reported contradictory results supporting one or the other hypothesis (for a summary, see Oikonomou et al., 2019).

One attempt to resolve these differences focused on the possibility that the effects of 5-HT depletion on sleep are a consequence of its effects on body temperature regulation. Chemical depletion of 5-HT in mice caused a loss of capacity for thermoregulation at low ambient temperatures (4° C) and impaired thermoregulation, even at typical laboratory room temperatures (~20° C). Depletion of 5-HT caused mice housed at these temperatures to reduce sleep and become hyperactive in order to increase body temperature to its normal range. When 5-HT-depleted mice were instead housed in warm environments (33° C, which is thermoneutral for mice), they maintained normal body temperatures without increased activity levels and showed normal sleep patterns and durations (Murray et al., 2015).

Another study used a genetic method to ablate only the rostral raphe nuclei, based on evidence that the caudal raphe nuclei (in the medulla) are the system involved in thermoregulation. Chemical depletion of 5-HT in earlier studies would have affected neurons in both rostral and caudal raphe nuclei. Mice lacking only the rostral raphe nuclei showed reduced sleep amounts and impaired homeostatic increases after sleep deprivation, supporting the role of 5-HT originating in these nuclei as a sleep promoter (Oikonomou et al., 2019).

These results and those of other studies using several kinds of selective genetic lesions and optogenetic stimulation of raphe 5-HT neurons in both larval zebrafish and mice were consistent with the activity of 5-HT neurons promoting NREM sleep, not waking. These studies found that slow, regular optogenetic stimulation of 5-HT raphe neurons in mice at night promoted increased sleep, while burst stimulation during the day promoted waking. The effects of tonic optogenetic stimulation (or of the resulting spontaneous slow firing) of 5-HT raphe neurons were proposed to reflect the accumulation of homeostatic sleep pressure during waking, resulting in later increases in NREM sleep (Oikonomou et al., 2019).

This conclusion is consistent with an earlier proposal that attempted to resolve the apparent contradiction between the high firing rates of raphe neurons during waking and reductions in sleep after loss of 5-HT. It suggested that the slow, clock-like firing of serotonergic neurons releases 5-HT at forebrain targets at a constant pace, thereby providing a cumulative record of the length of waking, which in turn drives the need for later sleep (Jouvet, 1999). This account does not explain why burst stimulation of raphe neurons during the circadian rest phase promoted waking in mice. That result may be related to a broader release of 5-HT from extra-synaptic sites in the burst-firing mode or to recruitment of multiple subsets of raphe neurons, which may be functionally different from each other (Oikonomou et al., 2019).

There are other questions about the generality of the link between high cortical 5-HT levels and wakefulness. As discussed in Chapter 7, Northern fur seals (*Callorhinus ursinus*) are an amphibious species. While on land, they show mostly bihemispheric SWS (both hemispheres asleep or awake simultaneously) and rarely unihemispheric SWS. But in the water, they show mostly unihemispheric SWS. During unihemispheric SWS, the left and right cortices sleep in alternation, which is also the typical pattern in cetaceans, which are fully aquatic (see **Figures 7.9** and **7.10**).

When fur seals generated bihemispheric SWS, levels of both ACh and 5-HT were low in each hemisphere, consistent with the idea that both promote cortical arousal (Lapierre et al., 2013; Lapierre et al., 2007) (**Figures 7.14** and **10.8**). Also consistent with this hypothesis, during unihemispheric sleep, levels of ACh were high in the cortex of the waking hemisphere and low in the cortex of the sleeping hemisphere (**Figure 7.14**). A similar finding might be predicted for 5-HT, but instead, 5-HT levels were moderately and similarly reduced in both hemispheres during unihemispheric sleep, regardless of which hemisphere was asleep or awake (**Figure 10.8**). Although the awake hemisphere had slightly higher levels of 5-HT than the sleeping hemisphere, it was not at the level seen in quiet, bilateral waking. Nor did the sleeping hemisphere show as large a reduction in 5-HT as during bihemispheric SWS.

Thus, levels of 5-HT in the cortex (unlike levels of ACh) were not strongly correlated with the sleep–wake state of each hemisphere in seals during asymmetric sleep. The lowest cortical 5-HT levels were found during REM sleep and the highest levels when the seals were engaged in pleasurable, active waking behaviors, such as being fed or hosed down (**AW** in **Figure 10.8**) (Lapierre et al., 2013). The best correlate of cortical 5-HT levels appeared to be the intensity of motor activity shown by the seals: very low 5-HT levels during REM sleep atonia and progressively increasing levels through bihemispheric SWS, unihemispheric SWS, quiet waking, and active waking.

Since cortical EEG activation, motor activity, and sleep–wake state normally change together in species showing only bihemispheric sleep, it is difficult to evaluate whether 5-HT levels are linked to one or all of these variables. In fur seals, however, these variables are dissociated during unihemispheric

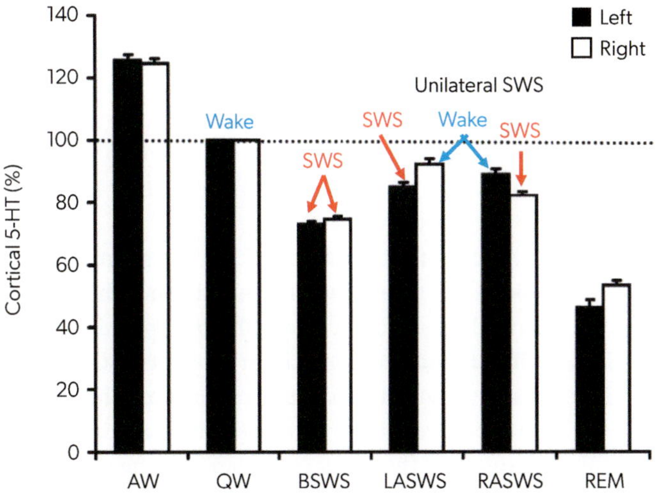

Figure 10.8 Levels of cortical serotonin (Y axis) in fur seals during different states of arousal, relative to levels during quiet wakefulness (QW), set at 100% (horizontal dotted line). During active waking (feeding, being hosed down, AW), 5-HT levels were elevated in both hemispheres. During REM sleep (REM), levels were reduced to about 50% of waking levels. Levels were also moderately reduced during bihemispheric SWS (BSWS) and somewhat less so during unilateral SWS. During unilateral SWS, regardless of whether the left (LASWS) or right (RASWS) hemisphere showed SWS, both hemispheres showed a similar small reduction relative to quiet waking. These results contrast to the robustly asymmetric levels of acetylcholine in the two hemispheres during unihemispheric sleep, as shown in **Figure 7.14**. Adapted with permission of the Society for Neuroscience under a Creative Commons Attribution License (CC-BY-NC-SA) from Lapierre, J. et al. (2013) Symmetrical serotonin release during asymmetrical slow-wave sleep: implications for the neurochemistry of sleep-waking states. *J Neurosci* 33:2555–2561. © The Authors (2013). doi: 10.1523/JNEUROSCI.2603-12.2013.

sleep, and 5-HT levels do not clearly reflect each hemisphere's sleep–wake state. These results are compatible with the hypothesis that one function of the serotonergic system is the facilitation of motor activity (Jacobs & Fornal, 1999), with especially high 5-HT levels in the cortex during strong behavioral activation, whether under pleasurable or stressful circumstances (Lapierre et al., 2013); see **Box 10.2**. The results are also consistent with the proposal that burst firing (and presumed high release of 5-HT) during stressful or highly arousing activities while awake support cortical activation (Oikonomou et al., 2019).

There were also no asymmetries during unihemispheric sleep in cortical levels of other neurotransmitters that have been linked to promoting waking (NE and histamine; see Sections 10.3, and 11.2) (Lyamin et al., 2016). Thus, NE, histamine, and 5-HT are not linked robustly to the production of waking EEG patterns during unihemispheric sleep in fur seals, while ACh levels closely track the degree of cortical activation.

BOX 10.2 Exercise, Serotonin, and Depression

The finding that serotonin levels in seals were closely linked to the intensity of motor activity led to the suggestion that the 5-HT-enhancing effect of exercise could be harnessed to improve outcomes in patients being treated for depression (Jacobs & Fornal, 1999). As discussed in the preceding section, many drugs currently used to treat depression enhance serotonergic neurotransmission, sometimes in combination with effects on other systems.

There have been dozens of trials conducted on the effects of increased physical activity on mood disorders (among other conditions). The superficial conclusion from most of these trials is that exercise has at least moderate benefits in improving symptoms of depression on its own or in conjunction with other treatments. Some recent meta-analyses of these studies concluded that there is substantial evidence that exercise of the appropriate kind and duration can reduce depressive symptoms (e.g., Kvam et al., 2016; Schuch et al., 2016). Other reviews concluded that, despite some supportive evidence, deficiencies in these studies did not allow the conclusion that exercise improves depression. Issues that were noted included a risk of bias in the design of some of the positive studies, evidence of publication bias, and evidence that the apparent benefits were lost in larger studies and in those that lasted longer (Krogh et al., 2017). Nevertheless, a recent meta-analysis of 41 clinical trials that accounted for some of these deficiencies still found significant benefits of several kinds of exercise intervention in reducing depressive symptoms. It also noted, however, that few studies addressed longer-term effects of exercise, and that benefits were weaker in longer trials (Heissel et al., 2023).

Despite sometimes reaching different conclusions, most reviews agreed that there is a need for larger-scale, better-designed studies to address this question. The underlying mechanism involved (if there is an effect) remains to be established. Exercise could work through multiple physiological or behavioral mechanisms to reduce depression symptoms; altering 5-HT neurotransmission could be one of them.

It is unclear whether these results can be generalized to other mammals or reflect a specialized adaptation in a species that can sleep unihemispherically. In terrestrial mammals, which sleep symmetrically, all of these neurotransmitters appear to contribute to EEG activation during waking, and high levels are incompatible with NREM sleep. It is interesting to note, however, that only ACh contributes to EEG activation during REM sleep in terrestrial mammals (see Section 10.7.1) and that it is selectively increased in the waking hemisphere in fur seals. These results suggest that ACh is unique in serving a universal role in contributing to cortical activation in mammals, regardless of the organization of their sleep patterns, but the results are ambiguous with respect to the role of 5-HT in cortical arousal.

10.5.3 Summary

Our understanding of the involvement of 5-HT in sleep regulation has changed considerably over the years, and some aspects of its role remain uncertain. An initial hypothesis, based on decreased sleep after depletion of 5-HT or damage to the raphe nuclei, was that 5-HT is involved in promoting NREM sleep. This idea was challenged in several ways. It seemed inconsistent with evidence that 5-HT neurons are most active during waking, less active during NREM sleep, and silent during REM sleep. The silence of 5-HT neurons during REM sleep is consistent with other evidence that their activity inhibits the transition to REM sleep (see Section 10.7.2).

The high activity of raphe neurons during waking supported the view that 5-HT acts as a neuromodulator that promotes cortical activation and waking, but there are findings that contradict this interpretation. For example, 5-HT inhibits hypocretin neurons in the mouse hypothalamus, acting as a brake on their wake-promoting effects at one circadian phase. In addition, unlike ACh, levels of 5-HT are not strongly asymmetric in the two cortices of fur seals when they are showing asymmetric cortical sleep and waking.

In fur seals, the best correlate of 5-HT levels was the intensity of motor activity being produced, ranging from the atonia of REM sleep (low 5-HT levels) to the moderate muscle tone of NREM sleep (intermediate level), and up to the intense activity associated with pleasurable activities (peak 5-HT levels). The fact that different sleep–wake states are characterized by different intensities of motor activity makes it uncertain whether it is the sleep–wake state or the activity level that is linked to 5-HT.

The increased activity and reduced sleep that follow depletion of 5-HT in mice were attributed to their need to be intensely active in order to maintain their body temperature when exposed to typical laboratory temperatures. At thermoneutral temperatures, these effects of 5-HT depletion did not appear. These results suggested that the apparent involvement of 5-HT in promoting sleep was an indirect effect of the need to increase activity to make up for the thermoregulatory deficit resulting from a loss of serotonergic activity.

However, these effects may in turn be linked to the use of global depletion of 5-HT, which includes raphe neurons in the medulla that are involved in thermoregulation. Other lines of evidence from genetic lesion and optogenetic stimulation studies supported a role for rostral raphe 5-HT neurons in accumulating sleep need during waking and promoting homeostatic increases in NREM sleep. These studies indicated that stimulating slow, regular firing of raphe neurons led to increased sleep need and more NREM sleep, but stimulating high rates of burst firing promoted waking.

Determining the functional role of 5-HT in sleep and waking is complicated by several factors. These include the number and functional diversity of receptor subtypes on which it acts; the possibility of species differences in receptor distributions; the breadth and variety of serotonergic projections throughout the brain and spinal cord; the heterogeneity of firing patterns of raphe neurons and the impact of different firing modes; the presence of inhibitory autoreceptors on raphe neurons, whose activation by local release of 5-HT modulates the release of 5-HT on forebrain targets; and the possibility of different subsets of serotonergic raphe neurons being recruited for different functions.

10.6 Brainstem glutamate and GABA systems

10.6.1 Parabrachial region

A region in the rostral pons was shown to project to the basal forebrain nuclei that play important roles in cortical arousal. The largest numbers of cells projecting to the basal forebrain were in the parabrachial nucleus and the adjacent precoeruleus region (near the locus coeruleus). Chemical lesions of these regions in rats caused the gradual development of a coma-like state with continuous slow EEG rhythms, a lack of spontaneous waking, and little c-Fos expression in the cortex in response to gentle handling. The neurons in these pontine regions that project to the basal forebrain were shown to be glutamatergic and to act on AMPA receptors (a subtype of glutamate receptor) in the basal forebrain to activate wake-promoting systems (Anaclet et al., 2014).

These results indicate that parabrachial and precoeruleus regions of the rostral pons send critical, excitatory (glutamatergic) inputs to the nuclei of the basal forebrain, which in turn provide input to the cortex that is essential for generating cortical activation and waking behavior.

10.6.2 Parafacial zone

With the exception of a possible role for the activity of 5-HT neurons in the raphe nuclei in helping to prepare the brain for onset of NREM sleep (see Section 10.5.2), the other brainstem neurotransmitter systems discussed so far are involved in promoting waking. Forebrain systems in the preoptic area and hypothalamus that are discussed in Chapter 11 have been the principal mechanisms identified as promoting NREM sleep. However, a series of studies have implicated a neural mechanism deep in the brainstem that plays an important role in the regulation of NREM sleep.

This region, called the parafacial zone, is in the medulla near the facial nerve. Neurons in this region were identified as projecting to the parabrachial nucleus in rats, which (as discussed in the preceding section) plays a critical role in activating forebrain arousal systems. Parafacial neurons, however, were found to be most active during sleep, based on c-Fos expression levels after sleep versus after waking. A large proportion of these neurons projecting to the parabrachial region were shown to be inhibitory and to use GABA.

Consistent with evidence that parafacial zone inputs inhibit a system that promotes arousal and waking, ablation of parafacial zone neurons caused very large increases in time awake, as did chemogenetic ablation of GABAergic neurotransmission by these cells (Anaclet et al., 2012). Optogenetic activation of parafacial zone neurons instead caused large increases in time in NREM sleep and decreases in both waking and REM sleep amounts (Anaclet et al., 2014).

Recordings from parafacial region neurons identified a large proportion that were moderately more active during NREM sleep than waking, increased activity before NREM onset, and showed a stably higher firing rate during NREM episodes, as well as some that were active during REM sleep (Alam et al., 2018). These results were consistent with a role for parafacial neurons in promoting NREM sleep, which is shared by the ventrolateral preoptic (VLPO) area and median preoptic nucleus (MnPO) (see Section 11.4). However, the firing-rate patterns of parafacial neurons differed from those of preoptic neurons in that they sustained their firing rates during NREM episodes. Preoptic neurons show decreasing firing rates as NREM episodes progress, suggesting sensitivity to gradual changes in homeostatic sleep need (Alam et al., 2018).

In addition, VLPO ablation decreased NREM sleep primarily by reducing the length of NREM episodes, but blocking input from the parafacial zone to the parabrachial region decreased NREM sleep by reducing the number of NREM episodes (Anaclet et al., 2012). These differences may indicate that parafacial neurons are more involved in initiating NREM sleep (Anaclet et al., 2014), while the VLPO may be involved in modulating NREM sleep in relation to the strength of the homeostatic sleep drive.

10.6.3 Summary

A region in the pons called the parabrachial nucleus and nearby structures project to the basal forebrain nuclei that are critical to producing cortical activation and waking. Parabrachial glutamatergic projections activate the basal forebrain and promote waking. Damage to, or inhibition of, this projection leads to a profound coma-like state. This system appears to be a critical route for producing waking and cortical activation.

A medullary region called the parafacial zone sends inhibitory GABAergic projections to the parabrachial region, terminating on neurons that form the projection to the basal forebrain. Inhibition of the parabrachial GABAergic projection leads to increased waking, and its optogenetic activation strongly promotes NREM sleep while decreasing waking and REM sleep. Firing rates of many parafacial neurons are elevated in anticipation of, and during, NREM sleep. Together these results demonstrate that the parafacial zone is an important promoter of NREM sleep that probably works in conjunction with preoptic area neurons that are known to be involved in production of NREM sleep.

10.7 Pontine acetylcholine

10.7.1 Regulation of waking and REM sleep

Somata of neurons that synthesize acetylcholine (ACh) are found in two brain regions: the basal forebrain, rostral to the hypothalamus, and parts of the brainstem reticular formation. As indicated in the preceding section, the basal forebrain system is critically involved in producing cortical activation and waking (see Chapter 11). Brainstem cholinergic neurons are found in the tegmentum of the mesencephalon (midbrain) and pons, collectively called the mesopontine tegmentum. They are concentrated in two structures, the laterodorsal (LDT) and pedunculopontine tegmental (PPT) nuclei. These neurons project rostrally to the thalamus, parts of the hypothalamus, and the basal forebrain as well as caudally to the nearby pontine reticular formation. Basal forebrain neurons project primarily to the cortex, hippocampus, and olfactory structures (**Figure 10.9**). Both forebrain and mesopontine "cholinergic" nuclei also contain many cells that use GABA and glutamate as neurotransmitters and do not contain ACh; cholinergic neurons are actually in the minority in the LDT and PPT (Ford et al., 1995; Kroeger et al., 2017; Luquin et al., 2018; Wang & Morales, 2009).

Some neurons in the LDT and PPT that project to the thalamus are active and release ACh during both waking and REM sleep, and show reduced activity and reduced ACh release during NREM sleep (Williams et al., 1994). This pattern is characteristic of most cholinergic neurons in both nuclei (**Figure 10.10**) (Cissé et al., 2018; Datta & Siwek, 2002;

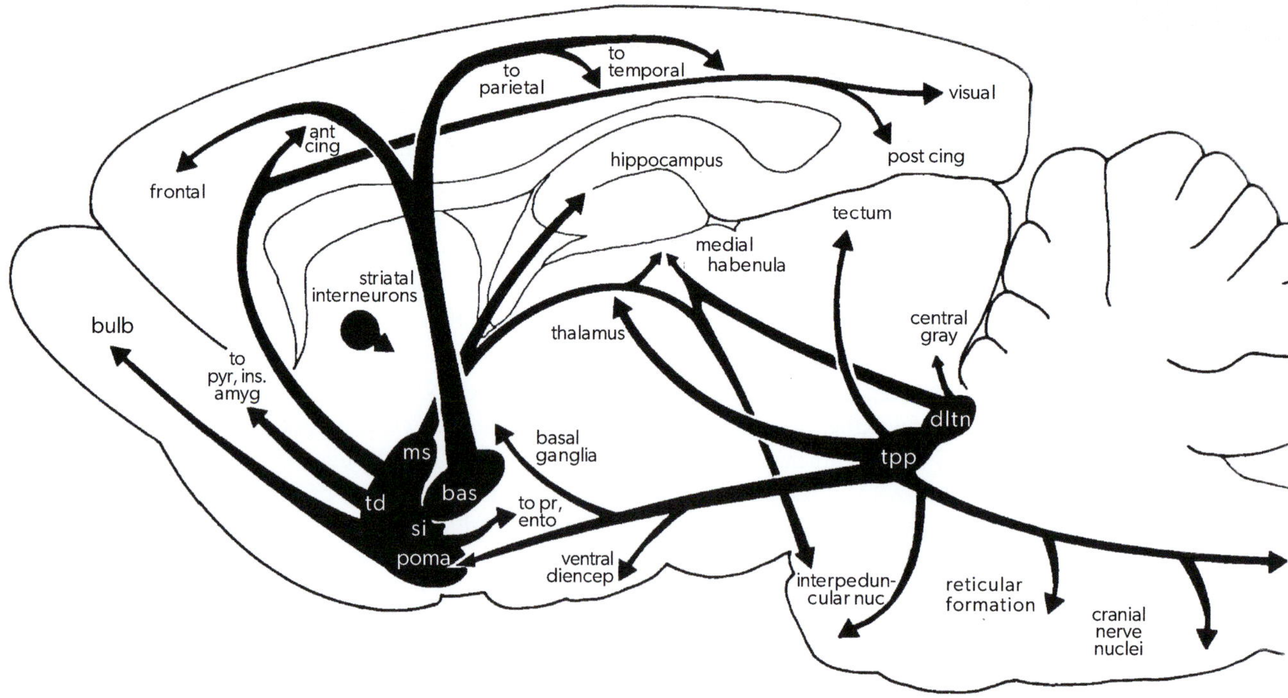

Figure 10.9 Acetylcholine (ACh)-containing cell clusters and their projections in the rat brain. The pedunculopontine (PPT, here labeled tpp) and laterodorsal tegmental nuclei (LDT, labeled dltn) in the mesopontine tegmentum project widely to the thalamus, hypothalamus, basal forebrain, pontine reticular formation, medulla, thalamus, and habenula. Forebrain cholinergic neurons are located in the medial septum (ms) as well as in the ventral and horizontal limbs of the diagonal band of Broca (td), the nucleus basalis (bas) and substantia innominata (si) which comprise the basal forebrain nuclei. Basal forebrain nuclei project principally to the cerebral cortex, hippocampus, and olfactory structures, as well as to the reticular nucleus of the thalamus. Reprinted with permission of Elsevier, Ltd. from Butcher, L.L. & Woolf, N.J. (1986) Central cholinergic systems: synopsis of anatomy and overview of physiology and pathology. In Scheibel, A.B. & Wechsel, A.F. (Eds.) *The Biological Substrates of Alzheimer's Disease*, pp.73–86. New York, Academic Press, 1986. © Elsevier (1986).

Ford et al., 1995). These neurons start to increase their firing rates during NREM sleep ~20–60 sec before cortical activation that marks a transition to either waking or REM sleep. Similarly, they decrease their firing rates during quiet waking ~10–20 sec before cortical synchronization signals the onset of NREM sleep (Steriade et al., 1990). Cholinergic LDT/PPT neurons also project to and activate neurons in the basal forebrain nuclei (including cholinergic neurons), which project directly

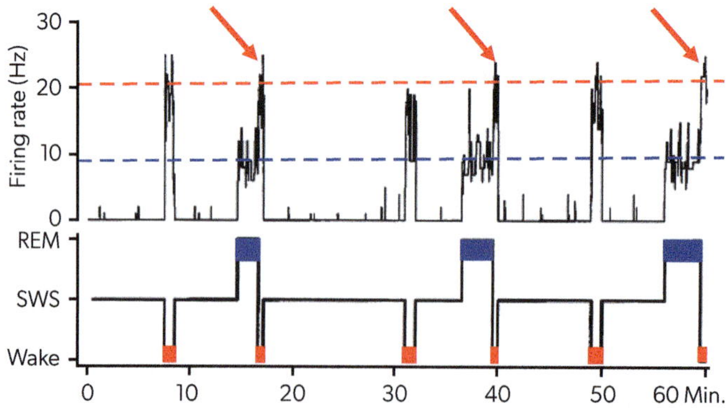

Figure 10.10 Firing-rate histograms showing the activity of a neuron in the pedunculopontine tegmental nucleus (PPT) (top panel) (presumed to be cholinergic) during different sleep stages (bottom panel) in a rat. This neuron was active during both REM sleep (blue rectangles) and waking (red rectangles) and showed very low firing rates during SWS. A moderate firing rate (blue dashed line) was associated with REM sleep episodes and a high firing rate (red dashed line) was associated with waking episodes. During transient arousals to wakefulness at the end of each REM sleep episode, the neuron showed a spike in firing rate above its characteristic REM sleep firing rate to the higher rate seen in other waking episodes (red arrows). Adapted with permission of John Wiley and Sons from Datta, S. & Siwek, D.F. (2002) Single cell activity patterns of pedunculopontine tegmentum neurons across the sleep–wake cycle in the freely moving rats. *J Neurosci Res* 70:611–621. © Wiley-Liss (2002). doi: 10.1002/jnr.10405.

to the cortex (see Chapter 11). Thus, one function of LDT/PPT neurons is to contribute indirectly to cortical activation during both waking and REM sleep by their effects on the thalamus and the basal forebrain (Datta & Siwek, 2002).

A subset of LDT/PPT neurons are highly active only during REM sleep and others only during waking, but these do not appear to be cholinergic. Juxtacellular recording/labeling can demonstrate both the electrophysiological activity and the neurotransmitter phenotype of a cell being recorded (see Appendix C). LDT/PPT neurons that were active during waking, and even more active during REM sleep, were cholinergic. Those neurons showing increased activity only during REM sleep were glutamatergic or GABAergic, and those that were active only during waking were glutamatergic (Boucetta et al., 2014). Consistent with that evidence, selective activation of glutamatergic PPT neurons using a chemogenetic method promoted sustained waking (Kroeger et al., 2017).

Activating cholinergic neurons in the LDT/PPT in mice using optogenetic methods resulted in transitions from NREM to REM sleep; damaging this region reduced REM sleep amounts (Van Dort et al., 2015). Although these findings are consistent with involvement of these cells in triggering REM sleep, a study using chemogenetic activation of PPT neurons found that activating cholinergic neurons alone during NREM sleep only reduced slow EEG activity and lightened NREM sleep, but did not directly increase REM sleep (Kroeger et al., 2017). Reducing slow-wave activity, however, could facilitate ending a NREM sleep episode and thereby promote a transition into either waking or REM sleep.

Despite some differences in results from studies using different methods, these studies generally agree that LDT/PPT cholinergic neurons act together with GABAergic and glutamatergic PPT neurons to support cortical activation. These effects increase the probability of waking and, in some studies, promote the transition to REM sleep.

Brainstem ACh, NE, and 5-HT neurons are highly active during waking and relatively inactive during NREM sleep. But during REM sleep, when NE and 5-HT neurons reduce firing to below even the low rates shown in NREM sleep (see **Figures 10.2** and **10.7**), cholinergic neurons become very active (**Figures 10.10** and **10.11**). Thus, ACh, NE, 5-HT,

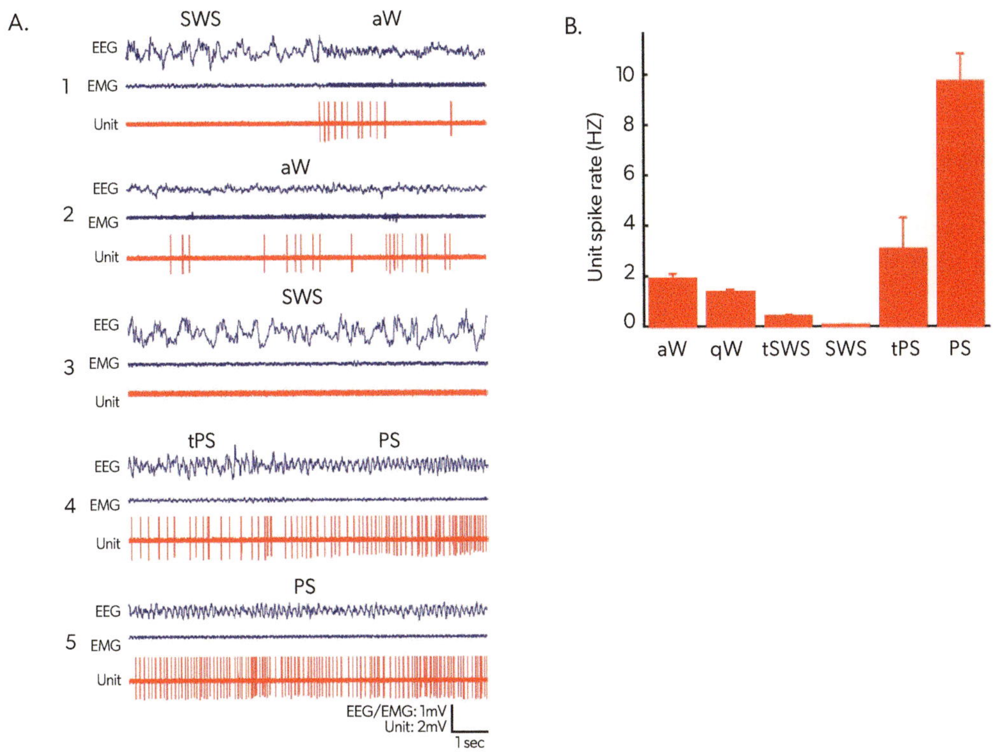

Figure 10.11 **A.** Firing-rate record (red) of a laterodorsal tegmental (LTD) neuron identified as cholinergic using juxtacellular labeling and the EEG (blue, top line) and EMG (black) records recorded simultaneously. **A. 1–3:** The cell was silent during slow-wave sleep (SWS), fired during active waking (aW) and was again silent when SWS occurred again. **A. 4 & 5:** The cell showed an increasing firing rate during the transition from SWS to REM (paradoxical) sleep (tPS), and very intense firing during REM sleep (PS). **B.** The average firing rates of this cholinergic cell during active wake, quiet wake (qW), transition to SWS (tSWS), SWS, transition to REM sleep (tPS), and during REM sleep (PS), demonstrating virtual silence during SWS, higher activity during waking, and very high activity during REM sleep. Reprinted with permission of the Society for Neuroscience under a Creative Commons Attribution License (CC-BY-NC-SA) from Boucetta, S. et al. (2014) Discharge profiles across the sleep-waking cycle of identified cholinergic, GABAergic, and glutamatergic neurons in the pontomesencephalic tegmentum of the rat. *J Neurosci* 34:4708–4727. © The Authors (2014). doi: 10.1523/JNEUROSCI.2617-13.2014.

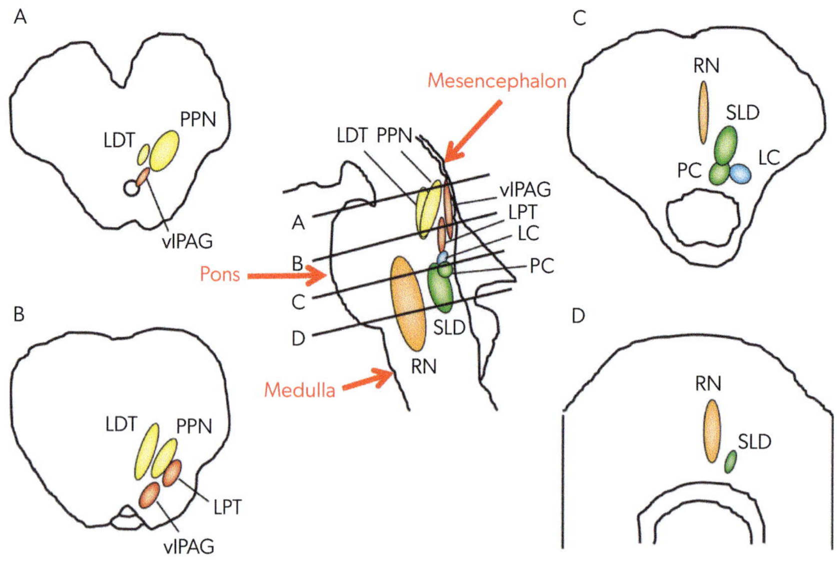

Figure 10.12 Proposed REM sleep regulatory mechanisms in the human brain, based primarily on results obtained from studies on cats and rats. Letters represent cross-sectional views at different levels through the brainstem (shown as a sagittal section in the center), with **A** corresponding to the junction of the mesencephalon and pons, **B** to the upper/mid pons, **C** to lower/mid pons and **D** to a region just rostral to the junction of the pons and medulla. The REM-off region is represented by the vlPAG and LPT in red, and the REM-on region is represented by the PC and SLD in green. The cholinergic LDT and PPN are in yellow and the raphe nuclei in orange. LC = locus coeruleus, LDT = laterodorsal tegmental nucleus, LPT = lateral pontine tegmentum, PC = pre-coeruleus, PPN = pedunculopontine nucleus (= PPT in the text), RN = raphe nuclei, SLD = sublaterodorsal nucleus, vlPAG = ventrolateral part of the periaqueductal gray matter. Adapted with permission from Boeve, B.F. et al. (2007) Pathophysiology of REM sleep behaviour disorder and relevance to neurodegenerative disease. *Brain* 130:2770–2788. © Oxford University Press (2007). doi: 10.1093/brain/awm056.

and DA projections act together (along with glutamate, histamine, and hypocretin; see Chapter 11) to sustain cortical activation during waking. But ACh projections also activate the cortex during REM sleep, during which 5-HT and NE neurons are silent.

Other features of REM sleep are also regulated by the LDT/PPT (for reviews, see Brown et al., 2012; Hobson et al., 1998). Some neurons in the LDT/PPT become active only seconds before onset of REM sleep and maintain high firing rates during REM sleep ("REM-On" neurons). These neurons project to a REM sleep induction zone in the tegmentum of the pontine reticular formation near the locus coeruleus, called the sublaterodorsal tegmental nucleus (SLD) (see **Figure 10.12**).[13] Some models propose that cholinergic inputs from the LDT/PPT to the SLD trigger it to initiate several components of REM sleep, including muscle atonia, rapid eye movements, and autonomic activation (Boeve & Saper, 2006; Boeve et al., 2007; Brown et al., 2012; Chase & Morales, 1990; Fuller et al., 2007; Weng et al., 2014). In addition, LDT/PPT projections to the thalamus trigger the ponto-geniculo-occipital (PGO) spikes seen during REM sleep (Datta, 1997).

There is also evidence that mechanisms in addition to cholinergic input to the SLD contribute to initiation of REM sleep. For example, REM sleep can be triggered without cholinergic involvement through interactions between glutamatergic and GABAergic mechanisms that link other pontine regions to the SLD (Fuller et al., 2007; Grace et al., 2014; Luppi et al., 2006), including by reducing inhibitory GABAergic input to the SLD (Pollock & Mistlberger, 2003). Other important regulators of REM sleep include a set of neurons in the lateral hypothalamus that contain the peptide melanin-concentrating hormone (MCH) (see Section 11.3.5), and dopaminergic projections from the VTA to the basolateral amygdala. The route by which the amygdala influences the pontine mechanisms involved in REM sleep production remains to be determined (Fraigne et al., 2023; Hasegawa et al., 2022).

Different conclusions about whether cholinergic input to the SLD is critical to REM sleep initiation probably relate to species differences and the use of different methods in these studies (e.g., lesions, application of agonists or antagonists, optogenetic or chemogenetic activation/inactivation). Nevertheless, the proposed mechanisms generally converge on a key role for increased activation of SLD neurons. This activation contributes to producing several components of

[13] The terminology used for this pontine region is not consistent across publications (including, e.g., "subcoeruleus," "(peri-)locus coeruleus α," "medial pontine reticular formation") in part because the region may be organized somewhat differently in rats and cats, the two species in which most relevant studies have been done. We will refer to it as the SLD.

REM sleep, including descending inhibition of spinal motor neurons, resulting in atonia. Consistent with this conclusion, studies of brain damage in people with disrupted REM sleep atonia tentatively point to damage in the human equivalent of the SLD as being involved (Boeve et al., 2007) (see Section 10.8).

10.7.2 Control of NREM-REM cycles

A prominent feature of mammalian sleep is the alternation between NREM and REM sleep episodes. A "reciprocal interaction" model, derived largely from research on cats, was developed to account for this rhythmic alternation as the result of interactions between two sets of neural mechanisms (Hobson et al., 1975; McCarley & Hobson, 1975). These mechanisms are the ACh neurons in the LDT/PPT that are key to initiating REM sleep via the SLD, and NE and 5-HT neurons (in the locus coeruleus and raphe nuclei) that inhibit the LDT/PPT (**Figure 10.13** A). Later research indicated that regulation of REM sleep also involves glutamatergic and GABAergic neurons, for example, in the midbrain PAG (Fuller et al., 2007; Kaur et al., 2009; Lu, Jhou, et al., 2006; Lu, Sherman, et al., 2006; Luppi et al., 2006; Nitz & Siegel, 1997; Sapin et al., 2009) as well as MCH neurons in the lateral hypothalamus (Hassani et al., 2009; Konadhode et al., 2013; Verret et al., 2003) and dopaminergic neurons in the VTA (Hasegawa et al., 2022).

The framework of the original reciprocal interaction model has been preserved in more recent versions that also incorporate the involvement of GABA and glutamate neurons interacting with the SLD to initiate or terminate REM sleep (Boeve et al., 2007; Brown et al., 2012; Hobson et al., 1998), as in **Figure 10.13 B**. GABA neurons are proposed to inhibit SLD neurons during wake and NREM sleep and to be reciprocally inhibited by the SLD during REM sleep.

The core features of the model are based on evidence that 5-HT and NE neurons are highly active during waking (e.g., **Figures 10.2** and **10.7**), contributing to cortical activation but sending inhibitory projections to the LDT/PPT (in particular to cholinergic REM-On neurons) (*point 1*, **Figure 10.13 B**),[14] thereby preventing the release of ACh onto the REM sleep-initiating neurons of the SLD, labeled "PRF" (pontine reticular formation) in **Figure 10.13 B**. The REM-On system in the SLD/PRF is also inhibited by GABAergic REM-Off neurons. During the transition from waking to NREM sleep, firing rates of 5-HT and NE neurons decline, in part because of self-inhibition. Decreased activity of these monoamine neurons reduces cortical activation and reduces their inhibition of LDT/PPT neurons.

[14] Numbered "points" in the following paragraphs all refer to **Figure 10.13 B**.

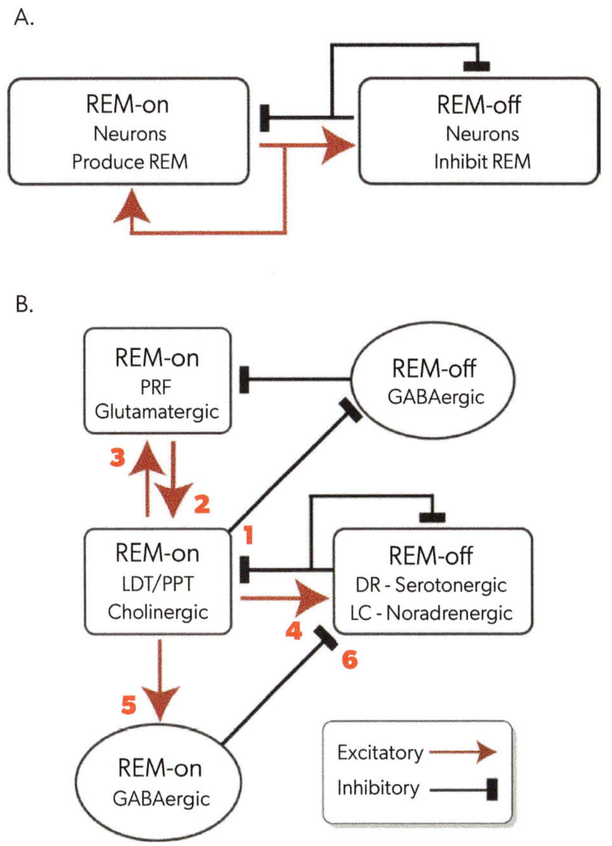

Figure 10.13 **A.** A summary of the principal relations among systems in the original reciprocal interaction model of McCarley and Hobson (1975). The REM-off neurons in this model are NE and 5-HT neurons that are most active during waking, reduce activity during NREM sleep, and become virtually silent in REM sleep. Auto-inhibition (black bars) contributes to their declining firing rate during NREM sleep, which disinhibits REM-on neurons and permits them to become active. Activated REM-On neurons feed excitation back on themselves, but also feed back excitation (red arrows) to the NE and 5-HT systems, facilitating the gradual transition back to NREM sleep or waking. **B.** An updated version of the model shows the neural structures and neurotransmitters involved in this reciprocal relationship as well as additional regulatory inputs involving GABAergic and glutamatergic projections. See the text for an explanation of the proposed functional relations among these structures, referring to the points numbered in red. PRF: pontine reticular formation (referred to as SLD in the text); LDT/PPT: laterodorsal and pendunculopontine tegmental nuclei; DR: dorsal raphe; LC: locus coeruleus. Both panels are adapted with permission from Brown, R.E. et al. (2012) Control of sleep and wakefulness. *Physiol Rev* 92:1087–1187; © American Physiological Society (2012); permission conveyed through Copyright Clearance Center, Inc. doi: 10.1152/physrev.00032.2011. Panel A was based with permission on a figure in McCarley, R.W. & Hobson, J.A. (1975) Neuronal excitability modulation over the sleep cycle: a structural and mathematical model. *Science* 189:58–60. © AAAS (1975). Panel B was based with permission of Elsevier, Ltd. on a figure in McCarley, R.W. (2007) Neurobiology of REM and NREM sleep. *Sleep Med* 8(4):302–330; © Elsevier (2007).

As cholinergic LDT/PPT neurons are gradually released from inhibition during NREM sleep, they begin to fire more rapidly and to increase their release of ACh, which activates SLD neurons (*point 3*). SLD neurons also feed activation back to the LDT/PPT, (*point 2*) and to REM-On GABAergic neurons (*point 5*), which accelerate the process of activating the SLD by inhibiting REM-Off GABAergic neurons (*point 6*). These feedback loops of excitation and disinhibition result in an accelerating increase in the firing rates of REM-On neurons, until the resulting activation causes the SLD to trigger a transition to REM sleep. Projections from the SLD activate GABA and glycine neurons in the medulla that project to and inhibit spinal motor neurons, resulting in postural atonia. Projections from the LDT/PPT also influence the thalamus and basal forebrain nuclei to contribute to cortical activation during REM sleep.

An important feature of the original model sounds somewhat counterintuitive: during REM sleep, REM-On cholinergic neurons in the LDT/PPT provide *activation* to the monoaminergic REM-Off neurons in the raphe nuclei and locus coeruleus (*point 4*). Because REM-On cells in the LDT/PPT are active continuously during REM sleep, this excitatory input contributes to a gradual increase in the activity of raphe and locus coeruleus neurons. As these REM-Off (5-HT/NE) neurons become progressively more active, their inhibitory input to cholinergic LDT/PPT neurons increases (*point 1*) until it eventually suppresses LDT/PPT and SLD activity, and the REM sleep episode ends (**Figure 10.13 B**).

Other mechanisms in the ventral medulla and the lateral hypothalamus (specifically melanin-concentrating hormone (MCH) neurons) can regulate the activity of GABAergic PAG neurons and thereby also exert potent effects on triggering and maintaining REM sleep (Clément et al., 2012; Kaur et al., 2009; Scammell et al., 2017; Weber et al., 2015) (see Section 11.3.5).

An attractive feature of the reciprocal interaction model is that it includes a mechanism, inherent in the relations between REM-On cholinergic and REM-Off monoaminergic systems, that can account for the cyclic alternation between NREM and REM sleep (Brown et al., 2012; Hobson et al., 1998). This mechanism allows for the observed alternation of states without requiring a third "supervisory" mechanism to time the switches or shift the balance between REM sleep-promoting and -inhibiting systems. Other models account for these features in different ways. Future research will need to develop an integrated model of how the many mechanisms that affect REM sleep expression interact to generate NREM–REM sleep cycles (see discussion in Fraigne et al., 2023).

10.7.3 Summary

There are two main clusters of ACh-containing neurons in the mammalian brain, located in the mesopontine tegmentum and the basal forebrain (discussed in Chapter 11). Mesopontine ACh neurons are concentrated in two nuclei, the laterodorsal and pedunculopontine tegmental nuclei (LDT and PPT), which also contain many glutamatergic and GABAergic neurons.

Like NE and 5-HT neurons, ACh neurons are more active during waking than during NREM sleep, but NE and 5-HT neurons are virtually silent during REM sleep, while ACh neurons remain highly active. The high firing rates of ACh neurons contribute to activation of the cortex during REM sleep, directly in the case of basal forebrain neurons that project to the cortex, and indirectly in the case of mesopontine ACh neurons. Activation of LDT/PPT ACh neurons increases the probability of a transition from NREM to REM sleep. This conclusion is supported by evidence that selective damage to LDT/PPT ACh neurons reduces REM sleep amounts.

ACh neurons in the LDT/PPT influence REM sleep by activating the nearby SLD, which in turn controls the expression of atonia and other features of REM sleep. LDT/PPT neurons also act via projections to the forebrain to increase cortical activation during REM sleep. Glutamatergic and GABAergic systems in the PAG and pontine regions also influence the expression of REM sleep by affecting SLD activity. Damage to the probable human analog of the SLD has been linked to the occurrence of REM sleep behavior disorder (REMBD), a condition in which there is a reduction or absence of atonia during REM sleep; see Section 10.8.2.

The original reciprocal interaction model proposed that high monoaminergic (NE, 5-HT) activity suppresses ACh neural activity in the LDT/PPT during waking; the decline of this activity during NREM sleep eventually permits ACh neurons to become active and to trigger REM sleep components through the SLD. Activation fed back to these monoamine systems from the LDT/PPT gradually leads to reductions in cholinergic activity, bringing the REM sleep episode to an end. This model provides an explanation for the alternation of NREM and REM sleep episodes during a sleep period. Newer versions of the model incorporate GABAergic REM-On and REM-Off neurons that contribute to both triggering and terminating REM sleep episodes. In addition, there is evidence that neurons in the lateral hypothalamus regulate the expression of REM sleep by acting on GABAergic mechanisms in the brainstem, and that DAergic neurons in the VTA modulate REM sleep expression.

10.8 Acting out one's dreams

10.8.1 Animal models

The neural mechanisms involved in REM sleep regulation, and in particular in the regulation of atonia, are of great interest in part because of the existence of two clinical disorders in which these mechanisms are disrupted. One is a condition in which atonia intrudes inappropriately during waking, namely, narcolepsy (see Section 11.3.2). The other is a condition in which atonia fails to occur during REM sleep, that is, REM sleep behavior disorder (REMBD).

Early research on REM sleep regulation demonstrated that lesions near the locus coeruleus in the pons of cats prevented the expression of components of REM sleep, especially atonia (Henley & Morrison, 1974; Jouvet & Delorme, 1965). Some dramatic demonstrations involved cats with these lesions that would fall asleep apparently normally and cycle through NREM sleep stages into REM sleep. At REM sleep onset that was marked by typical EEG activation, however, they did not show the atonia and body posture characteristic of this stage but would instead stand up while still asleep. In some cases, they would begin to show stalking and pouncing, snarling, fearful expressions, or attacking and biting behaviors directed at unseen objects. These observations showed that focal brain damage could cause the loss of a single component of REM sleep, atonia, while preserving other characteristics, such as cortical EEG activation. This finding implied that the features of REM sleep can be regulated by discrete regions of the pons at least somewhat independently of each other.

It appeared that damage to one pontine region caused the cats to lose the postural atonia that normally accompanies REM sleep, allowing them to generate behaviors that presumably reflected their subjective dream experiences (hunting, fear, fighting). REM sleep atonia normally ensures that responses to the content of dreams are expressed in the safety of the theater of the mind and not in the external world. This interpretation raises the question of whether this protective function is what drove the evolution of REM sleep atonia or whether it is an incidental consequence of a different function that has yet to be identified.

It is difficult to observe these extraordinary behaviors in a sleeping cat without concluding that it is acting out the contents of its dreams. These studies therefore come close to obtaining an indirect form of dream report from a nonhuman species. They provide at least semi-objective evidence of the dream-experience of another organism, a phenomenon that is otherwise restricted to science fiction stories. The evidence remains "semi-objective" because we cannot experience or observe the dream directly but must infer what the cat is experiencing based on its behavior.

10.8.2 REM sleep behavior disorder (REMBD)

A clinical counterpart in people to REM sleep without atonia is known as REMBD. Patients who come to medical attention with this condition (often middle-aged and older men) are typically reported by bed partners to show unusual motor activity during sleep. These behaviors turn out to occur during REM sleep and are accompanied by substantial or total loss of the atonia that normally occurs during this stage (Boeve et al., 2007; Schenck et al., 1986).

The actual prevalence of REMBD may not differ greatly between men and women (Haba-Rubio et al., 2017), but more vigorous behaviors that are associated with violent dreams may bring men to clinical attention more often. These behaviors often include strong kicking or rhythmic leg movements, striking out with their fists, and even getting out of bed and engaging in vigorous, sometimes violent, complex physical actions. Examples might include pushing a dresser across the room or striking at or near their bed partners, all while apparently sound asleep with eyes closed. REMBD is a different condition from sleepwalking, which typically begins during N3 sleep and is related to incomplete or abnormal arousals out of that stage (Broughton, 1968; Schenck et al., 1998; Zadra et al., 2004).

The inference that these actions reflect subjective dream content is supported by verbal reports from people awakened from these states. They might indicate that they were dreaming about playing football and blocking an opponent (pushing a dresser) or defending their family members against violent home invaders (kicking or punching at or near a bed partner). Whether the dream content gives rise to the behavior, or, alternatively, whether feedback from generating the behavior triggers the mental narrative, is an interesting, but unanswered question (Boeve et al., 2007).

Rare instances of REMBD symptoms may arise from injury or surgical damage to the pons, but most cases are idiopathic (i.e., spontaneous and with no obvious cause). People with idiopathic REMBD have a high probability of a subsequent diagnosis of Parkinson's disease (PD) or another neurodegenerative condition (e.g., Lewy body dementia), within 10–15 years of a diagnosis of REMBD. For those who live long enough, the conversion rate to PD may be as high as 80–90% (Howell & Schenck, 2015; Postuma et al., 2010; Yao et al., 2018).

As discussed in relation to the role of DA in sleep, PD is a progressive neurodegenerative disease, the motor symptoms of which are related to loss of dopaminergic projections from the substantia nigra to the striatum. It is a "synucleinopathy" that involves the deposition and spread of the protein synuclein progressively throughout the brain. The characteristic motor impairments are typically observed only late in the course of the disease, and are often preceded or accompanied by sleep disruption (including REMBD), loss of olfactory function, cognitive problems, autonomic disorders, and other symptoms (Berg et al., 2021; Haehner et al., 2007).

Brain imaging studies of REMBD patients who did not yet show the motor symptoms of PD found evidence of early damage to the integrity of projection pathways in the pons, substantia nigra, and basal ganglia (Pyatigorskaya et al., 2017; Rolinski et al., 2016; Unger et al., 2010). These results are consistent with the idea that many patients with REMBD are in the early stages of a neurodegenerative disease that has affected the integrity of the SLD or related pathways in the pons, which are responsible for triggering atonia during REM sleep (Boeve et al., 2007). Later motor and other symptoms of PD presumably reflect disease progression that affects dopaminergic projections to the striatum and other systems.

Treatment with either the long-acting benzodiazepine clonazepam or with melatonin has been reported to reduce these symptoms and restore more normal atonia during REM sleep (Boeve, 2003; Kunz & Mahlberg, 2010; Kunz et al., 2021). According to the results of a large clinical series, the benefits of melatonin treatment developed only gradually over days or weeks and depended on the regular timing of doses near bedtime. The benefits were also reported to persist after treatment had stopped in patients who had undergone a lengthy course of treatment (Kunz et al., 2021).

These features of gradual onset and long-term persistence of benefits, if confirmed in well-controlled clinical trials, would resemble the long-lasting effects of melatonin treatments on circadian rhythms in other clinical conditions (see discussion in Section 9.7.2). Whether melatonin acts only on the expression of symptoms of REMBD or exerts a lasting neuroprotective effect that influences disease progression remains to be determined.

Symptoms superficially resembling REMBD can also be seen in other sleep disorders. For example, some patients with severe periodic limb movements (PLMs)[15] show violent kicking, vocalizations, and other behaviors and have memories of aggressive dream content following PLM episodes. These symptoms, however, appear during confusional, partial arousals, mostly out of NREM sleep. Treatment with dopaminergic agents reduced the frequency of these incidents, suggesting a possible origin in parts of the motor system (Gaig et al., 2017).

10.8.3 Summary

Pontine lesions near the locus coeruleus in cats produced a syndrome in which cats entered REM sleep according to EEG criteria but did not develop atonia and instead produced apparently motivated behaviors related to predatory or aggressive interactions. These observations appear to represent the acting out of dream content in the absence of REM sleep atonia. They also indicate that different elements of REM sleep can be dissociated, presumably because they are regulated by separable neural mechanisms.

A human clinical analog of this phenomenon is REMBD, in which patients produce intense, often violent, behaviors during REM sleep, which, according to their later verbal reports, also match the content of their dreams. REMBD appears to result from brainstem neurological damage and often progresses to development of PD or a related synucleinopathy. Treatments that can reduce REMBD symptoms include the benzodiazepine, clonazepam, and melatonin. It is unclear whether melatonin treatments influence only the overt symptoms of REMBD or exert a neuroprotective effect that influences the progression of this neurodegenerative condition.

Literature cited

Aghajanian, G. K., & Marek, G. J. (2000). Serotonin model of schizophrenia: emerging role of glutamate mechanisms. *Brain Res Rev, 31*, 302–312.

Alam, M. A., Kostin, A., Siegel, J., McGinty, D., Szymusiak, R., & Alam, M. N. (2018). Characteristics of sleep-active neurons in the medullary parafacial zone in rats. *Sleep, 41*(10), zsy130. doi:10.1093/sleep/zsy130

Anaclet, C., Ferrari, L., Arrigoni, E., Bass, C. E., Saper, C. B., Lu, J., & Fuller, P. M. (2014). The GABAergic parafacial zone is a medullary slow wave sleep-promoting center. *Nat Neurosci, 17*(9), 1217–1224. doi: 10.1038/nn.3789

Anaclet, C., Lin, J. S., Vetrivelan, R., Krenzer, M., Vong, L., Fuller, P. M., & Lu, J. (2012). Identification and characterization of a sleep-active cell group in the rostral medullary brainstem. *J Neurosci, 32*(50), 17970–17976. doi: 10.1523/JNEUROSCI.0620-12.2012

Andrade, R., Huereca, D., Lyons, J. G., Andrade, E. M., & McGregor, K. M. (2015). 5-HT1A receptor-mediated autoinhibition and the control of serotonergic cell firing. *ACS Chem Neurosci, 6*(7), 1110–1115. doi: 10.1021/acschemneuro.5b00034

Andreasen, N. C., & Olsen, S. J. (1982). Negative *v* positive schizophrenia. *Arch Gen Psychiatr, 39*, 789–794.

Andrews, P. W., Bosyj, C., Brenton, L., Green, L., Gasser, P. J., Lowry, C. A., & Pickel, V. M. (2022). All the brain's a stage for serotonin: the forgotten story of serotonin diffusion across cell membranes. *Proc Roy Soc Lon B, 289*, 1–11. doi:10.1098/rspb.2022.1565

Aransay, A., Rodriguez-Lopez, C., Garcia-Amado, M., Clasca, F., & Prensa, L. (2015). Long-range projection neurons of the mouse ventral tegmental area: a single-cell axon tracing analysis. *Front Neuroanat, 9*, 59. doi: 10.3389/fnana.2015.00059

Aston-Jones, G., & Bloom, F. E. (1981). Activity of norepinephrine-containing locus coeruleus neurons in behaving rats anticipates fluctuations in the sleep-waking cycle. *J Neurosci, 1*, 876–886.

Aston-Jones, G., Chen, S., Zhu, Y., & Oshinsky, M. (2001). A neural circuit for circadian regulation of arousal. *Nat Neurosci, 4*(7), 732–738.

Aston-Jones, G., Rajkowski, J., & Cohen, J. (1999). Role of locus coeruleus in attention and behavioral flexibility. *Biol Psychiatry, 46*, 1309–1320.

Barnes, N. M., & Sharp, T. (1999). A review of central 5-HT receptors and their function. *Neuropharmacology, 38*, 1083–1152.

Beaudet, A., & Descarries, L. (1978). The monoamine innervation of rat cerebral cortex: synaptic and nonsynaptic axon terminals. *Neuroscience, 3*(10), 851–860. doi: 10.1016/0306-4522(78)90115-x

Belaid, H., Adrien, J., Laffrat, E., Tande, D., Karachi, C., Grabli, D., ... Francois, C. (2014). Sleep disorders in Parkinsonian macaques: effects of L-dopa treatment and pedunculopontine nucleus lesion. *J Neurosci, 34*(27), 9124–9133. doi: 10.1523/JNEUROSCI.0181-14.2014

Beliveau, V., Ganz, M., Feng, L., Ozenne, B., Hojgaard, L., Fisher, P. M., ... Knudsen, G. M. (2017). A high-resolution in vivo atlas of the human brain's serotonin system. *J Neurosci, 37*(1), 120–128. doi: 10.1523/JNEUROSCI.2830-16.2016

[15] These are vigorous, rhythmic movements of the legs and/or arms during sleep, which can occur in many sleep disorders, including in patients with REMBD (Fantini et al., 2002).

Berg, D., Borghammer, P., Fereshtehnejad, S. M., Heinzel, S., Horsager, J., Schaeffer, E., & Postuma, R. B. (2021). Prodromal Parkinson disease subtypes - key to understanding heterogeneity. *Nat Rev Neurol, 17*(6), 349–361. doi: 10.1038/s41582-021-00486-9

Berke, J. D. (2018). What does dopamine mean? *Nat Neurosci, 21*(6), 787–793. doi: 10.1038/s41593-018-0152-y

Berridge, K. C. (2007). The debate over dopamine's role in reward: the case for incentive salience. *Psychopharmacology (Berl), 191*(3), 391–431. doi: 10.1007/s00213-006-0578-x

Björklund, A., & Dunnett, S. B. (2007). Dopamine neuron systems in the brain: an update. *Trends Neurosci, 30*(5), 194–202. doi: 10.1016/j.tins.2007.03.006

Blier, P., Piñeyro, G., El Mansari, M., Bergeron, R. J., & de Montigny, C. (1998). Role of somatodendritic 5-HT autoreceptors in modulating 5-HT neurotransmission. *Ann NY Acad Sci, 861*, 204–216.

Boeve, B. (2003). Melatonin for treatment of REM sleep behavior disorder in neurologic disorders: results in 14 patients. *Sleep Med, 4*(4), 281–284. doi: 10.1016/s1389-9457(03)00072-8

Boeve, B. F., & Saper, C. B. (2006). REM sleep behavior disorder: a possible early marker for synucleinopathies. *Neurology, 66*(6), 796–797. doi: 10.1212/01.wnl.0000209264.61035.bb

Boeve, B. F., Silber, M. H., Saper, C. B., Ferman, T. J., Dickson, D., Parisi, J., … H. Braak, H. (2007). Pathophysiology of REM sleep behaviour disorder and relevance to neurodegenerative disease. *Brain, 130*, 2770–2788.

Boucetta, S., Cisse, Y., Mainville, L., Morales, M., & Jones, B. E. (2014). Discharge profiles across the sleep-waking cycle of identified cholinergic, GABAergic, and glutamatergic neurons in the pontomesencephalic tegmentum of the rat. *J Neurosci, 34*(13), 4708–4727. doi: 10.1523/JNEUROSCI.2617-13.2014

Broughton, R. (1968). Sleep disorders: disorders of arousal? *Science, 159*(3819), 1070–1078.

Brown, R. E., Basheer, R., McKenna, J. T., Strecker, R. E., & McCarley, R. W. (2012). Control of sleep and wakefulness. *Physiol Rev, 92*(3), 1087–1187. doi: 10.1152/physrev.00032.2011

Cai, P., Wang, F. D., Yao, J., Wang, W. F., Hu, Y. D., Liu, R. F., … Chen, L. (2022). Regulation of wakefulness by GABAergic DRN-VTA pathway. *Sleep, 45*(12), zsac235. doi:10.1093/sleep/zsac235

Carter, M. E., Yizhar, O., Chikahisa, S., Nguyen, H., Adamantidis, A., Nishino, S., … de Lecea, L. (2010). Tuning arousal with optogenetic modulation of locus coeruleus neurons. *Nat Neurosci, 13*(12), 1526–1533. doi: 10.1038/nn.2682

Chase, M., & Morales, F. (1990). The atonia and myoclonia of active (REM) sleep. *Annu Rev Psychol, 41*, 557–584.

Cissé, Y., Toossi, H., Ishibashi, M., Mainville, L., Leonard, C. S., Adamantidis, A., & Jones, B. E. (2018). Discharge and role of acetylcholine pontomesencephalic neurons in cortical activity and sleep-wake states examined by optogenetics and juxtacellular recording in mice. *eNeuro, 5*(4), 1–27. doi: 10.1523/ENEURO.0270-18.2018

Clément, O., Sapin, E., Libourel, P. A., Arthaud, S., Brischoux, F., Fort, P., & Luppi, P. H. (2012). The lateral hypothalamic area controls paradoxical (REM) sleep by means of descending projections to brainstem GABAergic neurons. *J Neurosci, 32*(47), 16763–16774. doi: 10.1523/JNEUROSCI.1885-12.2012

Datta, S. (1997). Cellular basis of pontine ponto-geniculo-occipital wave generation and modulation. *Cell Mol Neurobiol, 17*(3), 341–365.

Datta, S., & MacLean, R. (2007). Neurobiological mechanisms for the regulation of mammalian sleep-wake behavior: reinterpretation of historical evidence and inclusion of contemporary cellular and molecular evidence. *Neurosci Biobehav Rev, 31*(5), 775–824.

Datta, S., & Siwek, D. F. (2002). Single cell activity patterns of pedunculopontine tegmentum neurons across the sleep-wake cycle in the freely moving rats. *J Neurosci Res, 70*(4), 611–621. doi: 10.1002/jnr.10405

Davies, M. (2003). The role of $GABA_A$ receptors in mediating the effects of alcohol in the central nervous system. *J Psychiatr Neurosci, 28*(4), 263–274.

Diamond, D. M., Campbell, A. M., Park, C. R., Halonen, J., & Zoladz, P. R. (2007). The temporal dynamics model of emotional memory processing: a synthesis on the neurobiological basis of stress-induced amnesia, flashbulb and traumatic memories, and the Yerkes-Dodson law. *Neural Plast, 2007*, 1–33. doi: 10.1155/2007/60803

Diederich, N. J., Fenelon, G., Stebbins, G., & Goetz, C. G. (2009). Hallucinations in Parkinson disease. *Nat Rev Neurol, 5*(6), 331–342. doi: 10.1038/nrneurol.2009.62

Dzirasa, K., Ribeiro, S., Costa, R., Santos, L. M., Lin, S. C., Grosmark, A., … Nicolelis, M. A. L. (2006). Dopaminergic control of sleep-wake states. *J Neurosci, 26*(41), 10577–10589. doi: 10.1523/jneurosci.1767-06.2006

Eban-Rothschild, A., Rothschild, G., Giardino, W. J., Jones, J. R., & de Lecea, L. (2016). VTA dopaminergic neurons regulate ethologically relevant sleep-wake behaviors. *Nat Neurosci, 19*(10), 1356–1366. doi: 10.1038/nn.4377

Edgar, D., & Seidel, W. (1997). Modafinil induces wakefulness without intensifying motor activity or subsequent rebound hypersomnolence in the rat. *J Pharmacol Exp Ther, 283*(2), 757–769.

Fantini, M. L., Michaud, M., Gosselin, N., Lavigne, G., & Montplaisir, J. (2002). Periodic leg movements in REM sleep behavior disorder and related autonomic and EEG activation. *Neurology, 59*, 1889–1894.

Farajnia, S., van Westering, T. L., Meijer, J. H., & Michel, S. (2014). Seasonal induction of GABAergic excitation in the central mammalian clock. *Proc Natl Acad Sci USA, 111*(26), 9627–9632. doi: 10.1073/pnas.1319820111

Ferris, M. J., Espana, R. A., Locke, J. L., Konstantopoulos, J. K., Rose, J. H., Chen, R., & Jones, S. R. (2014). Dopamine transporters govern diurnal variation in extracellular dopamine tone. *Proc Natl Acad Sci USA, 111*(26), E2751–2759. doi: 10.1073/pnas.1407935111

Ford, B., Holmes, C., Mainville, L., & Jones, B. (1995). GABAergic neurons in the rat pontomesencephalic tegmentum: distribution with cholinergic and other tegmental neurons projecting to the posterior lateral hypothalamus. *J Comp Neurol, 363*, 177–196.

Fraigne, J. J., Luppi, P. H., Mahoney, C. E., De Luca, R., Shiromani, P. J., Weber, F., … Peever, J. (2023). Dopamine neurons in the ventral tegmental area modulate REM sleep. *Sleep, 46*(8), zsad024. doi:10.1093/sleep/zsad024

Freeman, A., Ciliax, B., Bakay, R., Daley, J., Miller, R. D., Keating, G., … Rye, D. (2001). Nigrostriatal collaterals to thalamus degenerate in parkinsonian animal models. *Ann Neurol, 50*(3), 321–329. doi: 10.1002/ana.1119

Fuller, P. M., Saper, C. B., & Lu, J. (2007). The pontine REM switch: past and present. *J Physiol, 584*(Pt 3), 735–741. doi: 10.1113/jphysiol.2007.140160

Gaig, C., Iranzo, A., Pujol, M., Perez, H., & Santamaria, J. (2017). Periodic limb movements during sleep mimicking REM sleep behavior disorder: a new form of periodic limb movement disorder. *Sleep, 40*(3). doi: 10.1093/sleep/zsw063

Gaykema, R., & Zaborsky, L. (1996). Direct catecholaminergic-cholinergic interactions in the basal forebrain. II. Substantia nigra-central tegmental area projections to cholinergic neurons. *J Comp Neurol, 374*, 555–577.

Gompf, H. S., & Anaclet, C. (2020). The neuroanatomy and neurochemistry of sleep-wake control. *Curr Opin Physiol, 15*, 143–151. doi: 10.1016/j.cophys.2019.12.012

González, S., Moreno-Delgado, D., Moreno, E., Peréz-Capote, K., Franco, R., Mallol, J., … McCormick, P. J. (2012). Circadian-related heteromerization of adrenergic and dopamine D(4) receptors modulates melatonin synthesis and release in the pineal gland. *PLoS Biol, 10*(6), e1001347. doi: 10.1371/journal.pbio.1001347

Gottesmann, C. (2006). The dreaming sleep stage: a new neurobiological model of schizophrenia? *Neuroscience, 140*(4), 1105–1115. doi: 10.1016/j.neuroscience.2006.02.082

Govindaiah, G., Wang, T., Gillette, M. U., Crandall, S. R., & Cox, C. L. (2010). Regulation of inhibitory synapses by presynaptic D(4) dopamine receptors in thalamus. *J Neurophysiol, 104*(5), 2757–2765. doi: 10.1152/jn.00361.2010

Grace, K., Vanstone, L., & Horner, R. (2014). Endogenous cholinergic input to the pontine REM sleep generator is not required for REM sleep to occur. *J Neurosci, 34*(3), 14198–14209.

Haba-Rubio, J., Frauscher, B., Marques-Vidal, P., Toriel, J., Tobback, N., Andries, D., … Heinzer, R. (2017). Prevalence and determinants of REM sleep behavior disorder in the general population. *Sleep, 41*(2), zsx197. doi:10.1093/sleep/zsx197

Haehner, A., Hummel, T., Hummel, C., Sommer, U., Junghanns, S., & Reichmann, H. (2007). Olfactory loss may be a first sign of idiopathic Parkinson's disease. *Mov Disord, 22*(6), 839–842. doi: 10.1002/mds.21413

Hasegawa, E., Miyasaka, A., Sakurai, K., Cherasse, Y., Li, Y., & Sakurai, T. (2022). Rapid eye movement sleep is initiated by basolateral amygdala dopamine signaling in mice. *Science, 375*, 994–1000.

Hassani, O. K., Lee, M. G., & Jones, B. (2009). Melanin-concentrating hormone neurons discharge in a reciprocal manner to orexin neurons across the sleep-wake cycle. *Proc Natl Acad Sci USA, 106*(7), 2418–2422. doi: 10.1073/pnas.0811400106

Heissel, A., Heinen, D., Brokmeier, L. L., Skarabis, N., Kangas, M., Vancampfort, D., … Schuch, F. (2023). Exercise as medicine for depressive symptoms? A systematic review and meta-analysis with meta-regression. *Br J Sports Med, 57*(16), 1049–1057. doi: 10.1136/bjsports-2022-106282

Henley, K., & Morrison, A. (1974). A re-evaluation of the effects of lesions of the pontine tegmentum and locus coeruleus on phenomena of paradoxical sleep in the cat. *Acta Neurobiol Exp, 34*, 215–232.

Hobson, J., Stickgold, R., & Pace-Schott, E. F. (1998). The neuropsychology of REM sleep dreaming. *NeuroReport, 9*, R1–R14.

Hobson, J. A., McCarley, R. W., & Wyzinski, P. W. (1975). Sleep cycle oscillation: reciprocal discharge by two brainstem neuronal groups. *Science, 189*, 55–58.

Howell, M. J., & Schenck, C. H. (2015). Rapid eye movement sleep behavior disorder and neurodegenerative disease. *JAMA Neurol, 72*(6), 707–712. doi: 10.1001/jamaneurol.2014.4563

Howes, O. D., & Kapur, S. (2009). The dopamine hypothesis of schizophrenia: version III--the final common pathway. *Schizophrenia Bull, 35*(3), 549–562. doi: 10.1093/schbul/sbp006

Imeri, L., & Opp, M. R. (2009). How (and why) the immune system makes us sleep. *Nat Rev Neurosci, 10*(3), 199–210. doi: 10.1038/nrn2576

Jacobs, B., & Fornal, C. (1999). Activity of serotonergic neurons in behaving animals. *Neuropsychopharmacology, 21*(25), 9S–15S.

Jauhar, S., McCutcheon, R., Borgan, F., Veronese, M., Nour, M., Pepper, F., … Howes, O. (2018). The relationship between cortical glutamate and striatal dopamine in first-episode psychosis: a cross-sectional multimodal PET and magnetic resonance spectroscopy imaging study. *Lancet, 5*, 816–823. doi: 10.1016/S2215-0366(18)30268-2

Jones, B. E. (2005). From waking to sleeping: neuronal and chemical substrates. *Trends Pharmacol Sci, 26*(11), 578–586. doi: 10.1016/j.tips.2005.09.009

Jones, B. E. (2020). Arousal and sleep circuits. *Neuropsychopharmacology, 45*(1), 6–20. doi: 10.1038/s41386-019-0444-2

Jones, S., Gainetdinov, R., Wightman, R., & Caron, M. (1998). Mechanisms of amphetamine action revealed in mice lacking the dopamine transporter. *J Neurosci, 18*(6), 1979–1986.

Jouvet, M. (1969). Biogenic amines and the states of sleep. *Science, 163*(3862), 32–41.

Jouvet, M. (1999). Sleep and serotonin: an unfinished story. *Neuropsychopharmacology, 21*, 24S–27S.

Jouvet, M., & Delorme, F. (1965). Locus coeruleus et sommeil paradoxal. *C R Seances Soc Biol Fil, 159*, 895–899.

Jus, A., Jus, K., Villeneuve, A., Pires, A., Lachance, R., Fortier, J., & Villeneuve, R. (1973). Studies on dream recall in chronic schizophrenic patients after prefrontal lobotomy. *Biol Psychiatry, 6*(3), 275–293.

Kanbayashi, T., Honda, K., Kodama, T., Mignot, E., & Nishino, S. (2000). Implication of dopaminergic mechanisms in the wake-promoting effects of amphetamine: a study of D- and L-derivatives in canine narcolepsy. *Neuroscience, 99*(4), 651–659.

Kantrowitz, J. T., & Javitt, D. C. (2010). Thinking glutamatergically: changing concepts of schizophrenia based upon changing neurochemical models. *Clin Schizophr Relat Psychoses, 4*(3), 189–200. doi: 10.3371/CSRP.4.3.6

Kato, T., Mitsukura, Y., Yoshida, K., Mimura, M., Takata, N., & Tanaka, K. F. (2022). Oscillatory population-level activity of dorsal raphe serotonergic neurons is inscribed in sleep structure. *J Neurosci, 42*(38), 7244–7255. doi: 10.1523/JNEUROSCI.2288-21.2022

Kaur, S., Thankachan, S., Begum, S., Liu, M., Blanco-Centurion, C., & Shiromani, P. J. (2009). Hypocretin-2 saporin lesions of the ventrolateral periaquaductal gray (vlPAG) increase REM sleep in hypocretin knockout mice. *PLoS One, 4*(7), e6346. doi: 10.1371/journal.pone.0006346

Konadhode, R. R., Pelluru, D., Blanco-Centurion, C., Zayachkivsky, A., Liu, M., Uhde, T., … Shiromani, P. J. (2013). Optogenetic stimulation of MCH neurons increases sleep. *J Neurosci, 33*(25), 10257–10263. doi: 10.1523/JNEUROSCI.1225-13.2013

Kroeger, D., Ferrari, L. L., Petit, G., Mahoney, C. E., Fuller, P. M., Arrigoni, E., & Scammell, T. E. (2017). Cholinergic, glutamatergic, and GABAergic neurons of the pedunculopontine tegmental nucleus have distinct effects on sleep/wake behavior in mice. *J Neurosci, 37*(5), 1352–1366. doi: 10.1523/JNEUROSCI.1405-16.2016

Kroeger, D., Thundercliffe, J., Phung, A., De Luca, R., Geraci, C., Bragg, S., … Scammell, T. E. (2022). Glutamatergic PPT neurons control wakefulness and locomotion via distinct axonal projections. *Sleep, 45*(12), zsac242. doi:10.1093/sleep/zsac242

Krogh, J., Hjorthoj, C., Speyer, H., Gluud, C., & Nordentoft, M. (2017). Exercise for patients with major depression: a systematic review with meta-analysis and trial sequential analysis. *Br Med J Open, 7*(9), e014820. doi: 10.1136/bmjopen-2016-014820

Kunz, D., & Mahlberg, R. (2010). A two-part, double-blind, placebo-controlled trial of exogenous melatonin in REM sleep behaviour disorder. *J Sleep Res, 19*(4), 591–596. doi: 10.1111/j.1365-2869.2010.00848.x

Kunz, D., Stotz, S., & Bes, F. (2021). Treatment of isolated REM sleep behavior disorder using melatonin as a chronobiotic. *J Pineal Res*, 1–9. doi:10.1111/jpi.12759

Kvam, S., Kleppe, C. L., Nordhus, I. H., & Hovland, A. (2016). Exercise as a treatment for depression: a meta-analysis. *J Affect Disord, 202*, 67–86. doi: 10.1016/j.jad.2016.03.063

Lapierre, J., Kosenko, P., Kodama, T., Peever, J., Mukhametov, L., Lyamin, O., & Siegel, J. (2013). Symmetrical serotonin release during asymmetrical slow-wave sleep: implications for the neurochemistry of sleep-waking states. *J Neurosci, 33*(6), 2555–2561. doi: 0.1523/JNEUROSCI.2603-12.2013

Lapierre, J. L., Kosenko, P. O., Lyamin, O. I., Kodama, T., Mukhametov, L. M., & Siegel, J. M. (2007). Cortical acetylcholine release is lateralized during asymmetrical slow-wave sleep in northern fur seals. *J Neurosci, 27*(44), 11999–12006. doi: 10.1523/jneurosci.2968-07.2007

Léna, I., Parrot, S., Deschaux, O., Muffat-Joly, S., Sauvinet, V., Renaud, B., … Gottesmann, C. (2005). Variations in extracellular levels of dopamine, noradrenaline, glutamate, and aspartate across the sleep-wake cycle in the medial prefrontal cortex and nucleus accumbens of freely moving rats. *J Neurosci Res, 81*(6), 891–899. doi: 10.1002/jnr.20602

Lu, J., Jhou, T. C., & Saper, C. B. (2006). Identification of wake-active dopaminergic neurons in the ventral periaqueductal gray matter. *J Neurosci, 26*(1), 193–202.

Lu, J., Sherman, D., Devor, M., & Saper, C. B. (2006). A putative flip-flop switch for control of REM sleep. *Nature, 441*(7093), 589–594. doi: 10.1038/nature04767

Luppi, P. H., Gervasoni, D., Verret, L., Goutagny, R., Peyron, C., Salvert, D., … Fort, P. (2006). Paradoxical (REM) sleep genesis: the switch from an aminergic-cholinergic to a GABAergic-glutamatergic hypothesis. *J Physiol Paris, 100*(5-6), 271–283. doi: 10.1016/j.jphysparis.2007.05.006

Luquin, E., Huerta, I., Aymerich, M. S., & Mengual, E. (2018). Stereological estimates of glutamatergic, GABAergic, and cholinergic neurons in the pedunculopontine and laterodorsal tegmental nuclei in the rat. *Front Neuroanat, 12*, 1–19. doi:10.3389/fnana.2018.00034

Lyamin, O. I., Lapierre, J. L., Kosenko, P. O., Kodama, T., Bhagwandin, A., Korneva, S. M., … Siegel, J. M. (2016). Monoamine release during unihemispheric sleep and unihemispheric waking in the fur seal. *Sleep, 39*(3), 625–636. doi: 10.5665/sleep.5540

McCarley, R. W., & Hobson, J. A. (1975). Neuronal excitability modulation over the sleep cycle: a structural and mathematical model. *Science, 189*, 58–60.

McCormick, D. (1992). Neurotransmitter actions in the thalamus and cerebral cortex. *J Clin Neurophysiol, 9*(2), 212–223.

McGinty, D., & Harper, R. (1976). Dorsal raphe neurons: depression of firing during sleep in cats. *Brain Res, 101*, 569–575.

Monti, J. M. (2011). Serotonin control of sleep-wake behavior. *Sleep Med Rev, 15*(4), 269–281. doi: 10.1016/j.smrv.2010.11.003

Moore, R., & Bloom, F. (1979). Central catecholamine neuron systems: anatomy and physiology of the norepinephrine and epinephrine systems. *Annu Rev Neurosci, 2*, 113–168.

Moruzzi, G., & Magoun, H. (1949). The brain stem reticular formation and activation of the EEG. *Electroencephalogr Clin Neurophysiol, 1*(4), 455–473.

Mouret, J., Bobillier, P., & Jouvet, M. (1967). Effets de la parachlorophénylalanine sur le sommeil du rat. *C R Séances Soc Biol, 161*, 1600–1603.

Muraki, Y., Yamanaka, A., Tsujino, N., Kilduff, T. S., Goto, K., & Sakurai, T. (2004). Serotonergic regulation of the orexin/hypocretin neurons through the 5-HT1A receptor. *J Neurosci, 24*(32), 7159–7166. doi: 10.1523/JNEUROSCI.1027-04.2004

Murray, N. M., Buchanan, G. F., & Richerson, G. B. (2015). Insomnia caused by serotonin depletion is due to hypothermia. *Sleep, 38*(12), 1985–1993. doi: 10.5665/sleep.5256

Nir, Y., & Tononi, G. (2010). Dreaming and the brain: from phenomenology to neurophysiology. *Trends Cogn Sci, 14*(2), 88–100. doi: 10.1016/j.tics.2009.12.001

Nitz, D., & Siegel, J. (1997). GABA release in the dorsal raphe nucleus: role in the control of REM sleep. *Am J Physiol, 273*, R451–R455.

Obrietan, K., & van den Pol, A. N. (1995). GABA neurotransmission in the hypothalamus: developmental reversal from Ca2+ elevating to depressing. *J Neurosci, 15*(7), 5065–5077.

Oikonomou, G., Altermatt, M., Zhang, R. W., Coughlin, G. M., Montz, C., Gradinaru, V., & Prober, D. A. (2019). The serotonergic raphe promote sleep in zebrafish and mice. *Neuron, 103*(4), 686–701 e688. doi: 10.1016/j.neuron.2019.05.038

Paukert, M., Agarwal, A., Cha, J., Doze, V. A., Kang, J. U., & Bergles, D. E. (2014). Norepinephrine controls astroglial responsiveness to local circuit activity. *Neuron, 82*(6), 1263–1270. doi: 10.1016/j.neuron.2014.04.038

Pollock, M., & Mistlberger, R. (2003). Rapid eye movement sleep induction by microinjection of the GABA-A antagonist bicuculline into the dorsal subcoeruleus area of the rat. *Brain Res, 962*, 68–77.

Postuma, R., Gagnon, J., Rompré, S., & Montplaisir, J. (2010). Severity of REM atonia loss predicts PD in idiopathic REM sleep behavior disorder predicts Parkinson disease. *Neurology, 73*, 239–244.

Puig, M. V., Artigas, F., & Celada, P. (2005). Modulation of the activity of pyramidal neurons in the rat prefrontal cortex by raphe stimulation *in vivo*: involvement of serotonin and GABA. *Cereb Cortex, 15*, 1–14.

Pyatigorskaya, N., Gaurav, R., Arnaldi, D., Leu-Semenescu, S., Yahia-Cherif, L., Valabregue, R., … Lehericy, S. (2017). Magnetic resonance imaging biomarkers to assess substantia nigra damage in idiopathic rapid eye movement sleep behavior disorder. *Sleep, 40*(11). doi: 10.1093/sleep/zsx149

Qu, W. M., Huang, Z. L., Xu, X. H., Matsumoto, N., & Urade, Y. (2008). Dopaminergic D1 and D2 receptors are essential for the arousal effect of modafinil. *J Neurosci, 28*(34), 8462–8469. doi: 10.1523/jneurosci.1819-08.2008

Qu, W. M., Xu, X. H., Yan, M. M., Wang, Y. Q., Urade, Y., & Huang, Z. L. (2010). Essential role of dopamine D2 receptor in the maintenance of wakefulness, but not in homeostatic regulation of sleep, in mice. *J Neurosci, 30*(12), 4382–4389. doi: 10.1523/JNEUROSCI.4936-09.2010

Rhodes, J. A., Lane, J. M., Vlasac, I. M., Rutter, M. K., Czeisler, C., & Saxena, R. (2018). Association of DAT1 genetic variants with habitual sleep duration in the UK Biobank. *Sleep, 42*(1), zsy193. doi: 10.1093/sleep/zsy193

Rolinski, M., Griffanti, L., Piccini, P., Roussakis, A. A., Szewczyk-Krolikowski, K., Menke, R. A., … Hu, M. T. (2016). Basal ganglia dysfunction in idiopathic REM sleep behaviour disorder parallels that in early Parkinson's disease. *Brain, 139*(Pt 8), 2224–2234. doi: 10.1093/brain/aww124

Sakai, K., & Crochet, S. (2001). Differentiation of presumed serotonergic dorsal raphe neurons in relation to behavior and wake-sleep states. *Neuroscience, 104*(4), 1141–1155.

Samuels, E., & Szabadi, E. (2008). Functional neuroanatomy of the noradrenergic locus coeruleus: its roles in the regulation of arousal and autonomic function part I: principles of functional organisation. *Curr Neuropharmacol, 6*, 235–253.

Sapin, E., Lapray, D., Berod, A., Goutagny, R., Leger, L., Ravassard, P., … Luppi, P. H. (2009). Localization of the brainstem GABAergic neurons controlling paradoxical (REM) sleep. *PLoS One, 4*(1), e4272. doi: 10.1371/journal.pone.0004272

Saunders, A., Oldenburg, I., Berezovskii, V., Johnson, C., Kingery, N., Elliott, H., … Sabatini, B. (2015). A direct GABAergic output from the basal ganglia to frontal cortex. *Nature, 521*(7550), 85–89. doi: 0.1038/nature14179

Scammell, T. E., Arrigoni, E., & Lipton, J. O. (2017). Neural circuitry of wakefulness and sleep. *Neuron, 93*(4), 747–765. doi: 10.1016/j.neuron.2017.01.014

Schenck, C., Bundlie, S., Ettinger, M., & Mahowald, W. (1986). Chronic behavioral disorders of REM sleep: a new category of parasomnia. *Sleep, 9*(2), 293–308.

Schenck, C., Pareja, J., Patterson, A., & Mahowald, M. (1998). Analysis of polysomnographic events surrounding 252 slow-wave sleep arousals in thirty-eight adults with injurious sleepwalking and sleep terrors. *J Clin Neurophysiol, 15*(2), 159–166.

Schuch, F. B., Vancampfort, D., Richards, J., Rosenbaum, S., Ward, P. B., & Stubbs, B. (2016). Exercise as a treatment for depression: a meta-analysis adjusting for publication bias. *J Psychiatr Res, 77*, 42–51. doi: 10.1016/j.jpsychires.2016.02.023

Seeman, P., Schwarz, J., Chen, J. F., Szechtman, H., Perreault, M., McKnight, G. S., … Sumiyoshi, T. (2006). Psychosis pathways converge via D2high dopamine receptors. *Synapse, 60*(4), 319–346. doi: 10.1002/syn.20303

Soden, M. E., Chung, A. S., Cuevas, B., Resnick, J. M., Awatramani, R., & Zweifel, L. S. (2020). Anatomic resolution of neurotransmitter-specific projections to the VTA reveals diversity of GABAergic inputs. *Nat Neurosci, 23*(8), 968–980. doi: 10.1038/s41593-020-0657-z

Solms, M. (2000). Dreaming and REM sleep are controlled by different brain mechanisms. *Behav Brain Sci, 23*, 843–850.

Solms, M. (2011). Neurobiology and the neurological basis of dreaming. In P. Montagna & S. Chokroverty (Eds.), *Handbook of Clinical Neurology, Sleep Disorders, Part 1* (Vol. 98, pp. 519–544). Elsevier B.V.

Sommerfelt, L., & Ursin, R. (1993). The 5-HT_2 antagonist ritanserin decreases sleep in cats. *Sleep, 16*(1), 15–22.

Steriade, M., Datta, S., Paré, D., Oakson, G., & Curró Dossi, R. (1990). Neuronal activities in brain-stem cholinergic nuclei related to tonic activation processes in thalamocortical systems. *J Neurosci, 10*(8), 2541–2559.

Swanson, L., & Hartman, B. (1975). The central adrenergic system. An immunofluorescence study of the location of cell bodies and their efferent connections in the rat utilizing dopamine-b-hydroxylase as a marker. *J Comp Neurol, 163*, 467–506.

Tabuchi, S., Tsunematsu, T., Kilduff, T. S., Sugio, S., Xu, M., Tanaka, K. F., … Yamanaka, A. (2013). Influence of inhibitory serotonergic inputs to orexin/hypocretin neurons on the diurnal rhythm of sleep and wakefulness. *Sleep, 36*(9), 1391–1404. doi: 10.5665/sleep.2972

Takagi, H., Morishima, Y., Matsuyama, T., Hayashi, H., Watanabe, T., & Wada, H. (1986). Histaminergic axons in the neostriatum and cerebral cortex of the rat: a correlated light and electron microscopic immunosytochemical study using histidine decarboxylase as a marker. *Brain Res, 364*, 114–123.

Trulson, M., & Preussler, D. (1984). Dopamine-containing ventral tegmental area neurons in freely moving cats: activity during the sleep-waking cycle and effects of stress. *Exp Neurol, 83*, 367–377.

Trulson, M. E., & Jacobs, B. L. (1979). Raphe unit activity in freely moving cats: correlation with level of behavioral arousal. *Brain Res, 163*, 135–150.

Trulson, M. E., Preussler, D. W., & Howell, G. A. (1981). Activity of substantia nigra units across the sleep-waking cycle in freely moving cats. *Neurosci Lett, 26*, 183–188.

Tsunematsu, T., Kilduff, T. S., Boyden, E. S., Takahashi, S., Tominaga, M., & Yamanaka, A. (2011). Acute optogenetic silencing of orexin/hypocretin neurons induces slow-wave sleep in mice. *J Neurosci, 31*(29), 10529–10539. doi: 10.1523/jneurosci.0784-11.2011

Turner, C., Belyavin, A. J., & Nicholson, A. N. (2014). Duration of activity and mode of action of modafinil: Studies on sleep and wakefulness in humans. *J Psychopharmacol, 28*(7), 643–654. doi: 10.1177/0269881113508173

Unger, M., Belke, M., Menzler, K., Heverhagen, J., Keil, B., Stiasny-Kolster, K., … Knake, S. (2010). Diffusion tensor imaging in idiopathic REM sleep behavior disorder reveals microstructural changes in the brainstem, substantia nigra, olfactory region, and other brain regions. *Sleep, 33*(6), 767–773.

van den Pol, A. N. (2012). Neuropeptide transmission in brain circuits. *Neuron, 76*(1), 98–115. doi: 10.1016/j.neuron.2012.09.014

Van Dort, C., Zachs, D., Kenny, J., Zheng, S., Goldblum, R., Gelwan, N., … Brown, E. (2015). Optogenetic activation of cholinergic neurons in the PPT or LDT induces REM sleep. *Proc Natl Acad Sci USA, 112*(2), 584–589. doi: 10.1073/pnas.1423136112

Venner, A., Todd, W. D., Fraigne, J., Bowrey, H., Eban-Rothschild, A., Kaur, S., & Anaclet, C. (2019). Newly identified sleep-wake and circadian circuits as potential therapeutic targets. *Sleep, 42*(5). doi: 10.1093/sleep/zsz023

Verret, L., Goutany, R., Fort, P., Cagnon, L., Salvert, D., Léger, L., … Luppi, P.-H. (2003). A role of melanin-concentrating hormone producing neurons in the central regulation of paradoxical sleep. *BMC Neurosci, 4*(19), 1–10.

Wang, H. L., & Morales, M. (2009). Pedunculopontine and laterodorsal tegmental nuclei contain distinct populations of cholinergic, glutamatergic and GABAergic neurons in the rat. *Eur J Neurosci, 29*(2), 340–358. doi: 10.1111/j.1460-9568.2008.06576.x

Wang, R., & Aghajanian, G. K. (1978). Collateral inhibition of serotonergic neurones in the rat dorsal raphe nucleus: pharmacological evidence. *Neuropharmacology, 17*(10), 819–825.

Weber, F., Chung, S., Beier, K. T., Xu, M., Luo, L., & Dan, Y. (2015). Control of REM sleep by ventral medulla GABAergic neurons. *Nature, 526*(7573), 435–438. doi: 10.1038/nature14979

Weng, F. J., Williams, R. H., Hawryluk, J. M., Lu, J., Scammell, T. E., Saper, C. B., & Arrigoni, E. (2014). Carbachol excites sublaterodorsal nucleus neurons projecting to the spinal cord. *J Physiol, 592*(7), 1601–1617. doi: 10.1113/jphysiol.2013.261800

Williams, J., Comisarow, J., Day, J., Fibiger, H. C., & Reiner, P. (1994). State-dependent release of acetylcholine in rat thalamus measured by *in vivo* microdialysis. *J Neurosci, 14*(9), 5236–5242.

Wilson, S., & Argyropoulos, S. (2005). Antidepressants and sleep: a qualitative review of the literature. *Drugs, 65*(7), 927–947.

Wisor, J. (2013). Modafinil as a catecholaminergic agent: empirical evidence and unanswered questions. *Front Neurol, 4*, 139. doi: 10.3389/fneur.2013.00139

Wisor, J., Nishino, S., Sora, I., Uhl, G., Mignot, E., & Edgar, D. (2001). Dopaminergic role in stimulant-induced wakefulness. *J Neurosci, 21*(5), 1787–1794.

Wisor, J. P., Dement, W. C., Aimone, L., Williams, M., & Bozyczko-Coyne, D. (2006). Armodafinil, the R-enantiomer of modafinil: wake-promoting effects and pharmacokinetic profile in the rat. *Pharmacol Biochem Behav, 85*(3), 492–499. doi: 10.1016/j.pbb.2006.09.018

Yao, C., Fereshtehnejad, S. M., Dawson, B. K., Pelletier, A., Gan-Or, Z., Gagnon, J. F., … Postuma, R. B. (2018). Longstanding disease-free survival in idiopathic REM sleep behavior disorder: Is neurodegeneration inevitable? *Parkinsonism Relat Disord, 54*, 99–102. doi: 10.1016/j.parkreldis.2018.04.010

Yerkes, R., & Dodson, J. (1908). The relation of strength of stimulus to rapidity of habit formation. *J Comp Neurol Psychol, 18*, 459–482.

Zadra, A., Pilon, M., Joncas, S., Rompré, S., & Montplaisir, J. (2004). Analysis of postarousal EEG activity during somnambulistic episodes. *J Sleep Res, 13*, 279–284.

CHAPTER 11

Forebrain Regulation of Sleep and Waking

11.1 OVERVIEW

This chapter continues the review begun in Chapter 10 of the neural systems that regulate sleep and waking. It focuses on neurotransmitters and other neurochemicals in several forebrain nuclei that are involved in regulating waking, NREM sleep, and REM sleep. These structures include the tuberomammillary nucleus (TMN) of the posterior hypothalamus (PH), the lateral hypothalamic area (LH), parts of the preoptic area, including the ventrolateral and median preoptic nuclei (VLPO and MnPO), and several nuclei anterior to the hypothalamus that comprise the basal forebrain nuclei.

11.2 Tuberomammillary nucleus and histamine

11.2.1 Anatomy of the histamine system

The posterior hypothalamic region (PH) was one of the first structures identified as playing a role in maintaining wakefulness when von Economo showed that localized brain damage to this region in people was associated with pathological sleepiness (von Economo, 1930) (see Section 1.3). Later studies used experimental ablations in animals to confirm that damage to the PH caused sustained sleepiness (Nauta, 1946). A more recent clinical case that was studied using PSG involved a woman with bilateral PH damage of unknown origin who slept for ~17.6 h during a 24 h recording session (Eisensehr et al., 2003).[1]

The PH region includes the tuberomammillary nucleus (TMN), which is the only brain structure containing neurons that synthesize histamine. Histaminergic neurons in the TMN project widely throughout the human cerebral cortex (Haas et al., 2008) (**Figure 11.1**), where release of histamine can depolarize target neurons directly or facilitate activation by increasing glutamate release (Bekkers, 1993; Reiner & Kamondi, 1994). In humans, the greatest number of histamine-1 (H_1) receptors are found in the frontal cortex, with large numbers also in parietal, cingulate, and temporal cortices as well as in parts of the limbic system, including the hippocampus and amygdala (Chang et al., 1979; Kanba & Richelson, 1984). Among other mammalian species that have been studied, there are pronounced differences in the distribution of histamine binding sites, with some species showing much lower levels of cortical binding than humans (Chang et al., 1979; Reiner & Kamondi, 1994).

In addition to direct cortical projections, histamine neurons project to other parts of the hypothalamus, to cholinergic neurons in the basal forebrain and brainstem, and to glutamatergic neurons in the thalamus, which in turn activate the cortex directly or indirectly (Zant et al., 2012). Histamine neurons form few synaptic connections but appear to release histamine mostly at extra-synaptic sites (which also characterizes other monoaminergic neurons (see Section 10.3.2) (Beaudet & Descarries, 1978; Takagi et al., 1986). This feature indicates that histamine neurons tend to modulate the general activity level of brain regions rather than transmitting specific information to its neuronal targets.

11.2.2 Histamine as a wake-promoting neuromodulator

Several lines of evidence link histamine to waking. Histamine neurons fire at highest rates during waking and are progressively less active in NREM and REM sleep (Vanni-Mercier et al., 1984). Levels of histamine in several brain regions (cortex, basal forebrain, preoptic/anterior hypothalamus) are also high

[1] It is important to recognize that damage caused by disease or injury would be unlikely to include only the PH. Damage could also impinge, for example, on part of the nearby lateral hypothalamus (see Section 11.3) that includes other wake-promoting systems, along with fibers of passage from brainstem structures.

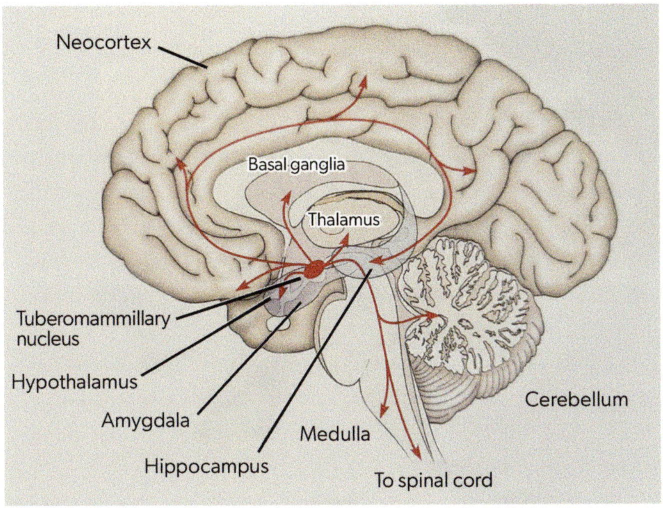

Figure 11.1 The location of neuronal somata that produce histamine (red oval) in the tuberomammillary nucleus of the posterior hypothalamus and their projection routes in a human brain. Histamine projections reach most parts of the cortex, the thalamus, the cerebellum, the hippocampus, the amygdala, and other parts of the hypothalamus. Reprinted with permission from Nicholls, J.G. et al. (2012) *From Neuron to Brain*, 5th Edition. Sinauer Associates; Sunderland, Massachusetts. © Oxford University Press (2012).

during the active phase and during forced activity in rats and cats, and are lower during NREM and REM sleep (Chu et al., 2004; Mochizuki et al., 1992; Strecker et al., 2002; Zant et al., 2012) (**Figure 11.2**). Consistent with this evidence, applications of histamine excited cortical neurons (Bekkers, 1993; Reiner & Kamondi, 1994) and infusions of histamine into the basal forebrain or the posterior hypothalamus increased waking (Lin et al., 1986; Zant et al., 2012).

Infusing an H_1 receptor antagonist into the basal forebrain reduced cortical activation and wakefulness. The activating effects of histamine infusion into the basal forebrain were also lost after selective neurotoxic lesions of cholinergic neurons in this region. These results implicate histaminergic activation of basal forebrain cholinergic neurons which, in turn, activate the cortex, as an important route by which histamine increases waking (Zant et al., 2012).

In contrast, decreasing histaminergic activity is important for transitioning to and maintaining sleep. Manipulations that decrease histamine levels, either by reducing its synthesis or inhibiting the activity of histamine neurons, acutely lengthen sleep durations (Lin et al., 1986; Saper et al., 2010; Takahashi et al., 2006). Similarly, antihistamines that readily cross the blood-brain barrier and act on H_1 receptors have potent sedating and

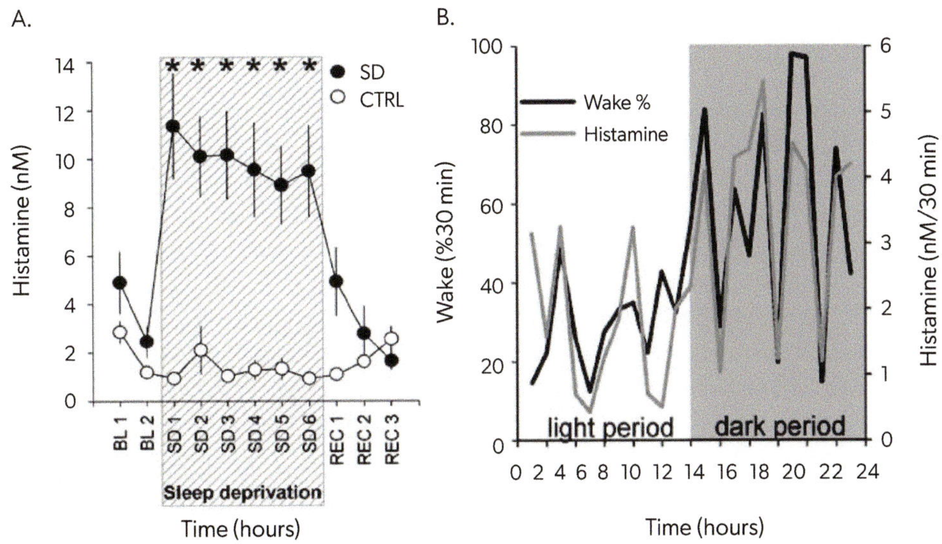

Figure 11.2 **A.** Levels of histamine in the basal forebrain (measured using microdialysis) in rats during two baseline hours (BL 1–2), during 6 h of sleep deprivation (SD 1–6, hatched region) using "gentle handling", and during a 3 h recovery sleep opportunity (REC 1–3). Data from sleep-deprived rats are shown as black symbols and those from unhandled controls as white symbols. **B.** Histamine levels measured every 30 min (gray line and right Y axis, plotted in nanomoles of histamine per 30 min sample) in the basal forebrain of rats in relation to the % time awake every 30 min (black line and left Y axis) during a 24 h period (X axis) of spontaneous sleep-wake cycles. There is a close correspondence between time awake and amount of histamine present in the basal forebrain across multiple, ultradian sleep-wake cycles. Ultradian sleep-wake cycles occur throughout the 24 h day, but there is more waking during the dark period (shaded) and a corresponding higher level of histamine in the basal forebrain. Reprinted with permission of the Society for Neuroscience under a Creative Commons Attribution License (CC-BY-NC-SA) from Zant, J.C. et al. (2012) Histamine release in the basal forebrain mediates cortical activation through cholinergic neurons. *J Neurosci* 32:13244–13254. © The Authors (2012). doi: 10.1523/JNEUROSCI.5933-11.2012.

BOX 11.1 Impact of Antihistamines on Sleep

In addition to its role as a neuromodulator in the brain, histamine is also found in other body tissues. Outside the brain, histamine is produced by cells that are part of the immune system (mast cells and basophils). It acts on peripheral tissues to activate immune responses, including allergic reactions, and in the digestive system to increase acid secretion, as well as having important effects on cardiorespiratory, endocrine, and thermoregulatory systems, among other functions (Schwartz et al., 1991; Simons, 2004).

Excess peripheral histamine release leads to uncomfortable allergic responses, including itching, sneezing, and swollen membranes that can be treated with antihistamines.[a] Older antihistamines that reduce peripheral allergic reactions, also readily cross the blood-brain barrier. As a result, these drugs (e.g., chlorpheniramine (Chlor-Tripolon™), diphenhydramine (Benadryl™)) also cause sleepiness by reducing the activity of H_1 histamine receptors in the brain that mediate wake-promoting effects. Similarly, many antidepressant and antipsychotic drugs increase sleepiness in part because they have antihistaminergic side effects at some dosage levels (Krystal et al., 2013).

Because of their potent effects in facilitating sleep onset in people, antihistamines are sold over the counter as sleep aids, sometimes in combination with an analgesic like acetaminophen (e.g., Nytol™, Sominex™, Tylenol PM™). Antihistamines are the drug treatment most commonly recommended by psychiatrists for insomnia in children with neurological or psychiatric disorders (Owens et al., 2010). Although they are effective in promoting sleep, several factors limit their long-term use as sleep aids: their anticholinergic side effects (including effects on bladder and cardiac function); their daytime sedation and cognitive effects; and the possibility of rapid development of tolerance (Richardson et al., 2002; Simons, 2004). These effects led to concerns about the regular use of first-generation antihistamines to treat either allergies or sleep problems.

Second-generation antihistamines that do not readily cross the blood-brain barrier are advertised as non-sedating allergy treatments (e.g., terfenadine (Seldane™), loratadine (Claritin™)), because typical therapeutic doses have little effect on brain H_1 receptors in most people. Antihistamines that act selectively on H_2 receptors are used to reduce stomach hyperacidity (e.g., cimetidine, ranitidine). Because these have little effect on H_1 receptors and do not readily cross the blood-brain barrier, they are also unlikely to increase sleepiness.

[a]These drugs are usually considered "inverse agonists," which are agents that bind to constitutively active receptors and stabilize them in an inactive state, thereby reducing their activity. This designation is in contrast to antagonists, which prevent agonists from binding to a receptor (Simons, 2004).

sleep-promoting effects in people (see **Box 11.1**) (Lin et al., 1986; Melville, 1973; Nicholson et al., 1985; Roth et al., 1987).

The TMN is a convergence point for several regulatory systems that promote both sleep and waking. Histamine neurons in the TMN are activated by hypocretin projections from the LH, which play an important role in increasing arousal (see Section 11.3.1) (Schone et al., 2012). They are also inhibited by, and send inhibition to, systems involved in initiating sleep, such as GABAergic neurons in the LH and in the preoptic area (see Sections 11.3.1 and 11.4), and are inhibited by the neurochemical adenosine, which is a key sleep-promoting agent (see Section 11.6.1) (Liu et al., 2010; Oishi et al., 2008).

Most research findings are consistent with the idea that reducing histamine levels is important for transitioning to sleep, but it is unclear whether high histamine levels are more important for initiating or maintaining waking. A study in freely moving cats found that most histamine neurons increased their activity a few seconds before the occurrence of EEG signs indicating a transition from sleep to waking, suggesting their involvement in triggering waking (Vanni-Mercier et al., 2003). In head-restrained mice, however, there was a significant delay between signs of a sleep/wake transition and onset of increased firing of histamine neurons (Takahashi et al., 2006). These differences may be attributable to the methods used or the species studied. It is unclear whether increased histaminergic activity in people is related to onset or maintenance of waking, or both.

Many neurons use more than one neurotransmitter or neuromodulator (Tritsch et al., 2016). TMN neurons, which activate their target neurons through the release of histamine, also contain and release the inhibitory neurotransmitter GABA (Takagi et al., 1986). The co-release of an inhibitory neurotransmitter along with histamine, which activates target neurons, seems counterintuitive. However, there is evidence in mice that histamine and GABA released from single TMN neurons in the prefrontal cortex exert their effects on different cortical cell types, with histamine affecting interneurons and GABA affecting pyramidal cells (principal input/output neurons). These combined effects were proposed to increase both the precision and synchrony of neuronal responses in the prefrontal cortex (Lucaci et al., 2023).

Knock-out mice that were genetically engineered to prevent the release of GABA selectively from histamine-producing neurons showed altered sleep patterns (**Figure 11.3**). They slept similarly to controls during the daily light phase but showed

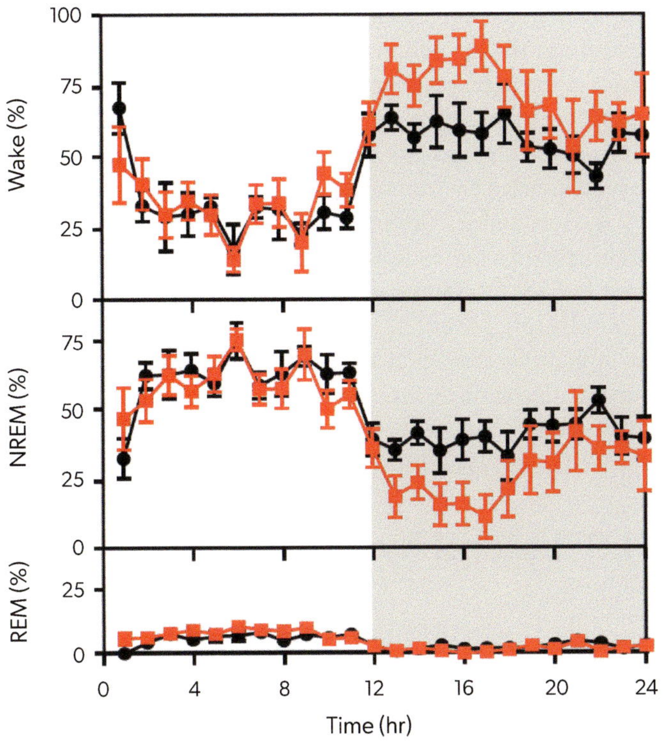

Figure 11.3 Mice that were genetically engineered to be incapable of releasing GABA selectively from histaminergic neurons (red symbols) spent a higher percentage of time awake (top panel) and lower percentage of time in NREM sleep (middle panel) compared to control mice (black symbols). This difference appeared only during the daily dark phase (shaded area), and especially during the early dark phase when mice are normally most active. There was no change in REM sleep percentage (bottom panel) at any phase. Reprinted with permission under a CC-BY license (http://creativecommons.org/licenses/by/4.0/) from Yu, X. et al. (2015) Wakefulness is governed by GABA and histamine cotransmission. *Neuron* 87:164–178. © 2015 The Authors; published by Elsevier Ltd. doi: 10.1016/j.neuron.2015.06.003.

reduced NREM sleep and large increases in wake time during the daily dark phase. Thus, GABA co-release with histamine in normal mice provided a brake on its potent arousing effects, especially during the first half of the dark phase when these neurons and other systems promote waking most strongly (Yu et al., 2015).

These knock-out mice also did not recover lost sleep as quickly as control mice after a period of sleep deprivation. This result suggests that they either had less drive to recover lost sleep or less capacity to suppress waking and permit recovery sleep. Thus, the balance of release of histamine and GABA from TMN neurons appears to be important for modulating the intensity of arousal and for suppressing waking to permit rebound sleep increases after sleep loss.

Given the clear involvement of histamine in promoting waking and of H_1 receptor antagonism in generating sleep (Monti, 1993), it might be expected that without histamine, there would be increased sleep and major changes in sleep–wake regulation, as in the woman with PH damage who was extremely somnolent (Eisensehr et al., 2003). It is surprising, therefore, that there was little change in the daily sleep–wake patterns of mice when chemogenetic methods were used to dramatically change the activity of TMN neurons either directly or by reducing or augmenting GABAergic input to them (Venner, Mochizuki, et al., 2019; Zecharia et al., 2012). Similarly, sleep–wake patterns in rats were minimally affected by lesions that eliminated most histaminergic neurons (Gerashchenko et al., 2004).

Mice that lacked histamine because of a genetic knock-out of the enzyme responsible for its synthesis (histidine decarboxylase) also did not show persistent somnolence but showed some changes in sleep–wake patterns. They had increased REM sleep during the daily light phase and decreased waking and more NREM sleep specifically during the hours centered on the light–dark transition, the beginning of their daily active phase (Anaclet et al., 2009; Parmentier et al., 2002).

There are several possible reasons for these mixed effects of reducing histaminergic activity using different methods. One potential explanation is that there are many other wake-promoting systems that could compensate for loss of histaminergic activity in some of these preparations. Another is that the effects of loss of histamine would be most apparent only at circadian phases when there are normally high spontaneous histamine levels (Krystal et al., 2013), namely, during the daily active phase (Haas et al., 2008; Mochizuki et al., 1992). Species differences may also be important, since the distribution of H_1 receptors differs among species, implying different potential roles for histamine (Chang et al., 1979; Reiner & Kamondi, 1994). Finally, technical aspects of how some studies were conducted could have played a role in generating different outcomes (see discussion in Lucaci et al., 2023). For example, some chemogenetic methods used to change histaminergic activity may result in "off-target" effects; i.e., effects outside the targeted histaminergic system (Naganuma et al., 2021).

Another perspective on the function of histamine emerged from the effects of modifying histaminergic activity in mice on their responses to environmental events. Preventing production of histamine in mice by knocking out the gene for histamine decarboxylase significantly reduced activation in response to several environmental events that normally disturb and arouse mice: cage changes, simulated injections, and exposure to novel environments (Parmentier et al., 2002). Enhancing histaminergic activity instead significantly increased the duration of activation and waking in response to cage changes, as well as enhancing aggressive responses to territorial intruders (Naganuma et al., 2021; Venner, Mochizuki, et al., 2019; Zecharia et al., 2012).

Taken together, these results indicate that histamine neurons play several important roles. Their inhibition is necessary to allow other systems to initiate a transition from wake to sleep (at least at times when histamine levels are normally high). In addition, histamine is involved in increasing activation in response to disturbing environmental stimuli. There is mixed evidence about histamine's involvement in sustaining alert wakefulness, perhaps because other arousal-related system can counteract their loss in ablation studies. These conclusions suggest that antihistamines promote sleep in people (see **Box 11.1**) both because they reduce global cortical activation and because they reduce the sleep-disrupting effects of arousing stimuli.

Arousing stimuli may be external events (e.g., cage or lighting changes for mice or environmental noise for people). Or they may be internal events, such as disturbing thoughts. For example, high levels of cognitive arousal in people predicted long latencies to fall asleep and longer wake episodes during the sleep period. This finding applied both to people diagnosed with insomnia and to otherwise good sleepers (Kalmbach et al., 2020). Antihistamines may accelerate sleep onset in people with chronic insomnia, anxiety, or mood disorders in part by reducing the level of cortical arousal and alertness triggered by persistent negative thoughts and worries ("rumination"), which is a common feature in these conditions.

11.2.3 Summary

The finding that damage to the posterior part of the hypothalamus increases sleepiness can be attributed to the fact that this region includes the TMN. The TMN is the brain's only source of histamine, with neurons that project throughout the cortex and to the thalamus, basal forebrain, and mesopontine cholinergic nuclei. TMN neurons do not generally form classical synapses but release histamine by volume conduction in target regions, where it depolarizes neurons and increases their activity. Histaminergic neurons are activated by other systems that increase arousal and are inhibited by those that promote sleep.

The involvement of histamine in sustaining waking is supported by evidence that suppressing the activity of TMN neurons or blocking histamine receptors promotes the transition to sleep. TMN neurons also contain the inhibitory neurotransmitter GABA. This feature may provide a braking effect on the activation resulting from histamine release at specific circadian phases, perhaps by varying the extent of co-release of histamine and GABA at different times.

Despite the clear evidence that histamine increases waking, several manipulations that augmented or depressed histaminergic activity had little impact on the overall sleep–wake patterns of mice and rats. One exception was a study in which mice lacking histamine showed increased REM sleep during the light phase and reduced waking around the light–dark transition. The blunted increase in waking in response to the onset of the night phase may reflect a more general reduction in responsiveness to other arousing stimuli. Mice lacking histamine also showed less sustained activation in response to several kinds of environmental disturbances.

Antihistamines (inverse agonists at H_1 receptors in the brain) are effective in inducing sleep in people and are often used as over-the-counter sleep aids; other drugs that have antihistaminergic side effects are also sedating. Their effectiveness in promoting sleep probably depends on decreasing global cortical activation by inactivating H_1 receptors, and on reducing responses to potentially arousing stimuli, including both external events and disturbing thoughts.

11.3 Lateral hypothalamus

11.3.1 Hypocretin/orexin and arousal regulation

In 1998, a novel brain peptide was identified that changed our views of both the regulation of normal sleep and the causes of the sleep disorder, narcolepsy. This peptide was named orexin by one research group (Sakurai et al., 1998) (from *orexis*, the Greek/Latin word for appetite or desire) and hypocretin by another group (de Lecea et al., 1998) (apparently because it is located in the *hypo*thalamus and is structurally related to the gut peptide hormone se*cretin*). Neurons immunoreactive for hypocretin are clustered in the posterior hypothalamus (PH) and in the caudal lateral hypothalamus (LH) near the fornix[2] as it passes through this region, which is often referred to as the perifornical (pf)LH (**Figure 11.4**).

There are two forms of hypocretin that are derived from a common precursor molecule: hypocretin-1 and -2 which bind to two subtypes of receptors ($HCRTR_{1/2}$); hypocretin-1 binds to both subtypes and hypocretin-2 only to $HCRTR_2$. Hypocretin generally depolarizes (excites) neurons through a number of different second messenger mechanisms (Hagan et al., 1999; Kukkonen & Leonard, 2014; Liu et al., 2002).

The small population of pfLH hypocretin cells projects very broadly throughout the nervous system. The estimates of hypocretin cell numbers range from <7,000 neurons in rats (Modirrousta et al., 2005) to 15–20,000 (Peyron et al., 2000) or ~70,000 (Thannickal et al., 2000) in people. Rostral hypocretin projections reach the thalamus and most of the cortex, and caudal projections reach the brainstem and spinal cord. There

[2] The fornix is a large fiber tract that passes through the lateral hypothalamus. It connects the hippocampus with several structures, including the septum, thalamus, and mammillary bodies (Senova et al., 2020).

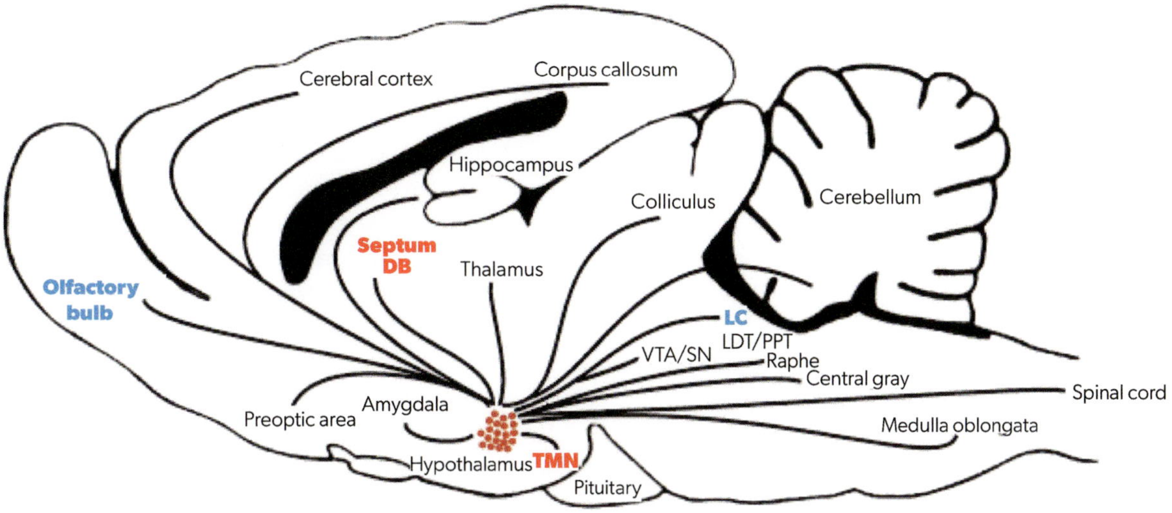

Figure 11.4 Hypocretin (Hcrt)/orexin neuronal somata are shown as a cluster of red dots in the lateral hypothalamic/perifornical area in a rodent brain. Their widespread projections reach structures from the olfactory bulbs and cerebral cortex to the spinal cord. Structures with Hcrt1 receptors (locus coeruleus [LC] and olfactory bulb) are labeled in blue. Those with Hcrt2 receptors (tuberomammillary nucleus [TMN], septum, and diagonal band [DB]) are labeled in red. Other structures that are labeled in black contain both types of receptors. LC: locus coeruleus; LDT/PPT: laterodorsal and pedunculopontine tegmental nuclei; VTA/SN: ventral tegmental area/substantia nigra; DB: diagonal band of Broca. Reprinted with permission of John Wiley and Sons from Hungs, M. & Mignot, E. (2001) Hypocretin/orexin, sleep and narcolepsy. *Bioessays* 23(5) 397–408. © John Wiley and Sons, Inc. (2001). doi: 10.1002/bies.1058; permission conveyed through Copyright Clearance Center, Inc.

are especially robust projections to structures involved in the regulation of sleep and waking in both animal models and people: TMN, locus coeruleus, ventral tegmental area, raphe nuclei, and basal forebrain (see **Figure 11.4**) (Moore et al., 2001; Sakurai, 2007).

Hypocretin neurons are virtually silent during sleep. They increase firing rates in anticipation of waking, show higher rates during quiet waking, and the highest rates during intense activity, often associated with motivated behaviors (Lee et al., 2005; Mileykovskiy et al., 2005). Consistent with these results, hypocretin levels in the cerebrospinal fluid (CSF) were elevated during the day in diurnally active squirrel monkeys (*Saimiri sciureus*) (Zeitzer et al., 2003) and at night in nocturnal rats (Deboer et al., 2004; Zhang et al., 2004).

CSF levels of hypocretin in monkeys rose during the wake phase to peak during the last third of the day (Zeitzer et al., 2003), when the length of previous waking would produce strong homeostatic pressure to initiate sleep (see Chapter 5). The nocturnal increase in hypocretin levels in rats was eliminated by lesions of the suprachiasmatic nuclei (SCN) (Deboer et al., 2004; Zhang et al., 2004). These results suggest that the increase in hypocretin levels late in the daily active phase of diurnal species (the wake-maintenance zone) (Zeitzer et al., 2003) may be an important mechanism by which the SCN opposes homeostatic sleep pressure to maintain long, consolidated wake periods in primates, including people.

This hypothesis is supported by evidence from patients with narcolepsy (who have a hypocretin deficiency; see Section 11.3.2). Narcolepsy patients and healthy controls were given 30 min sleep opportunities every 90 min over a 72 h period; they were instructed to try to sleep during each opportunity. Healthy controls showed the expected decrease in sleep amounts and lengthened sleep onset latencies during the evening wake-maintenance zone. Patients with narcolepsy showed relatively stable sleep amounts and latencies to fall asleep at all times of day, with only slight modulation of sleep-onset latencies. Nevertheless, the two groups had similar robust circadian body-temperature rhythms and similar rhythms of subjective sleepiness (Dantz et al., 1994). These results imply a specific role for circadian regulation of hypocretin levels in sustaining waking late in the circadian active phase in people.

Since hypocretin neurons project to many regions involved in activating the cortex during waking and in regulating REM sleep, it is not surprising that hypocretin also plays an important role in these processes. Selectively silencing hypocretin neurons in mice during their active phase (night) reduced waking and increased SWS amounts. Silencing hypocretin neurons during the day, when mice already showed high levels of SWS, caused no further increase (**Figure 11.5**) (Tsunematsu et al., 2013).

Infusion of hypocretin into the lateral ventricles or directly into the TMN resulted in increased time awake and reductions in NREM and REM sleep. The effects of hypocretin injections directly into the TMN were absent in mice lacking H_1 receptors. This finding suggests that one route by which hypocretin promotes waking is by stimulating local release in the TMN of

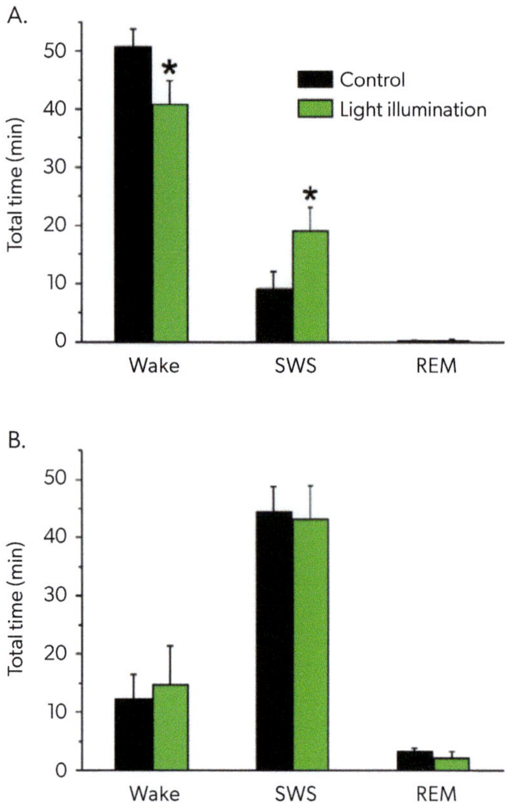

Figure 11.5 Optogenetic silencing of hypocretin neurons had different effects at different times of day. A light-sensitive molecule that hyperpolarizes neurons when it is activated was incorporated genetically into neurons that express the mRNA for hypocretin. A fiber-optic lead was implanted to terminate above the hypocretin neuronal population in the perifornical lateral hypothalamus of mice. Illumination of these cells through the fiber-optic lead inhibited these neurons and blocked release of hypocretin. **A.** Silencing hypocretin neurons for a 1 h period during the dark phase increased the amount of slow-wave sleep at the expense of time spent awake (green bars), compared to control mice (black bars). **B.** The same treatment during the light phase had no significant effects. These results support a role for hypocretin in sustaining waking during the daily active phase in mice. Reprinted with permission of Elsevier, Ltd. under CC BY-NC-ND open access license from Tsunematsu, T. et al. (2013) Long-lasting silencing of orexin/hypocretin neurons using archaerhodopsin induces slow-wave sleep in mice. *Behav Brain Res* 255:64–74. © The Authors (2013). doi: 10.1016/j.bbr.2013.05.021.

histamine (Huang et al., 2001), which acts on H_1 receptors to exert potent wake-promoting effects (see Section 11.2.2).

However, there are other routes for hypocretin effects, since optogenetic activation of hypocretin neurons still induced waking in mice that lacked the enzyme (histidine decarboxylase) needed to produce histamine (Carter et al., 2009). One mechanism involves activation by hypocretin/glutamate neurons of GABAergic neurons in the VLPO which, in turn, inhibit GABA/galanin neurons that are critical to the initiation of sleep (De Luca et al., 2022) (see Section 11.4). The effects of optogenetic stimulation of hypocretin neurons may also be mediated by release of hypocretin directly in the cortex or by hypocretin activation of other neurotransmitter systems that promote arousal during the daily active phase.

Hypocretin also decreased the probability of transitioning from NREM to REM sleep, apparently by activating monoaminergic systems (REM-Off cells) that oppose cholinergic triggering of REM sleep or by acting directly on the pontine mechanisms that trigger REM sleep features (see discussion in Section 10.6.2) (Adamantidis et al., 2010; Bourgin et al., 2000; Xi & Chase, 2010).

Although these results support the idea that hypocretin is a wake-promoting peptide, that is too simple a summary of its role. It is involved, for example, in many non-sleep related functions (see **Box 11.2**), and its role in sleep–wake regulation is also more complicated than only promoting waking. A fuller

BOX 11.2 Non-Sleep Related Functions of Hypocretin

Since hypocretin neurons project very widely throughout the central nervous system, it is not surprising that hypocretin has been demonstrated or hypothesized to play a role in many functions in addition to sleep regulation. These include regulation of food intake/energy balance (hence, the alternative name, orexin), learning, regulation of several hormones, stress responses, addictions, and reward. Anatomically defined subsets of hypocretin neurons (e.g., based on their different projection targets) have been proposed to be involved selectively in these different kinds of motivated behaviors (Mahler et al., 2014), but this suggestion remains to be proven.

Some of these functions may depend on hypocretin because it regulates structures involved in reinforcement of behavior (Mahler et al., 2014; Thannickal et al., 2018) or in achieving sufficient arousal to allow the vigorous expression of motivated behaviors aimed at adaptive goals (Carter et al., 2009; España et al., 2002; Mahler et al., 2014).

Hypocretin neurons maintained in vitro, for example, responded to low glucose levels by increasing firing rates, which in a hungry, intact animal would presumably reduce sleep and promote waking activities that increase the chances of finding food. Consistent with that idea, intact wild-type mice that were food-deprived increased waking during their rest phase and increased exploratory behavior, but transgenic mice with genetic ablation of hypocretin did not show either response to food deprivation (Yamanaka et al., 2003). Thus, hypocretin may have the specific function of responding to energy deficits with more waking and activity as well as a general function of increasing arousal to permit important motivated behaviors.

understanding of its regulatory roles depends in part on information about its involvement in the clinical sleep disorder narcolepsy. Before further addressing the normal physiological role of hypocretin in sleep–wake regulation, we will first discuss the nature of narcolepsy and the evidence demonstrating the critical role of hypocretin deficiency in the development of this condition.

11.3.2 The nature of narcolepsy

Narcolepsy is a neurological disorder that is characterized by a cluster of four classic symptoms (the narcoleptic tetrad): excessive daytime sleepiness, cataplexy, sleep-associated hallucinations, and sleep paralysis (Dauvilliers et al., 2007).

The most characteristic, and often most difficult to treat, symptom of narcolepsy is excessive daytime sleepiness (EDS) (Broughton et al., 1986), which usually develops gradually during the teen years or in young adulthood (Plazzi et al., 2018). Because daytime sleepiness is a common symptom related to many behavioral and physiological causes, a correct diagnosis can be delayed for many years as symptoms are ignored or alternative diagnoses and treatments are evaluated. In addition, children with narcolepsy may show unusual features not seen in older patients, which can further delay diagnosis (Dahl et al., 1994; Plazzi et al., 2018).

Sleepiness in narcolepsy can be extreme, so that individuals suffer irresistible daytime "sleep attacks" with little or no warning, despite having apparently adequate sleep durations at night. Sleep onset can occur in boring, sedentary situations in which anyone might fall asleep but it can also occur unpredictably at other times. Because the significance of early EDS symptoms is often unrecognized, those affected may not be aware of their condition until they experience a first sleep attack in a dangerous situation, such as while driving or operating machinery.

A second characteristic symptom of narcolepsy is cataplexy. This is a sudden reduction in muscle tone, which may be mild and localized to only some muscle groups (e.g., drooping facial musculature or loss of neck muscle tone), or it may be severe and involve loss of postural muscle tone, causing a person to fall to the ground. Typically, these attacks do not involve loss of consciousness, so the individual can be fully awake but paralyzed and unable to move or speak. Cataplexy is often triggered by experiencing a strong emotion, typically a positive emotion such as joy or a pleasant surprise; less frequently, a negative emotion like grief, shock, or anger may be a trigger. Narcolepsy is usually diagnosed as either a "classic" Type 1 form, which includes cataplexy, or a Type 2 form, which does not (Plazzi et al., 2018).

The other core symptoms are the experience of hallucinations while awake, typically while falling asleep (hypnagogic) or waking up (hypnopompic), and sleep paralysis. Individuals with sleep paralysis can become fully conscious as they wake up but be unable to speak or move for a period of time. A person falling asleep at night can have a similar experience, and sleep paralysis at either time may be accompanied by visual hallucinations.

Other characteristic features of narcolepsy can only be detected during sleep studies involving EEG recordings. These include disruption of nocturnal sleep continuity, especially continuity of REM sleep; early onset of REM sleep during the night; and sleep-onset REM episodes during daytime nap opportunities (i.e., without a preceding period of NREM sleep).

Disrupted REM sleep at night suggests a link between narcolepsy and REM sleep regulation that is reinforced by the nature of the symptoms in the classic tetrad. Cataplexy and sleep paralysis resemble the REM sleep feature of atonia but occur outside the context of REM sleep. Hallucinations while awake echo the vivid dreams that are typical of REM sleep. Normally these features occur together during REM sleep, and their expression is gated by the prior occurrence of NREM sleep. In those with narcolepsy, these elements of REM sleep can emerge directly out of waking and may be expressed independently (e.g., cataplexy on its own, or hallucinations together with sleep paralysis).

Patients with narcolepsy, especially those with cataplexy, show an increased number of transitions between wake and sleep, and between NREM and REM sleep during the night, indicating a general instability of state regulation (Broughton et al., 1986; Sorensen et al., 2013). Taken together, these symptoms suggest that patients with narcolepsy suffer from disruption of the mechanisms involved in regulating the expression and coordination of the components of REM sleep and in maintaining the stability of all states (i.e., wakefulness, NREM, and REM sleep).

11.3.3 The role of hypocretin in narcolepsy

Early studies showed that discrete pontine lesions could selectively prevent the expression of atonia during REM sleep (see Section 10.8.1). This finding suggested that the features of REM sleep are regulated relatively independently of each other by different pontine nuclei. An early hypothesis, therefore, was that the symptoms of narcolepsy could reflect damage to regions of the pons that control REM sleep elements, such as atonia, resulting in their expression at inappropriate times and disruption of their usual coordination.

Later research related to the genetics of narcolepsy led to a different hypothesis about its cause, linking it instead to the functions of hypocretin neurons in the pfLH. A genetic contribution to narcolepsy was implied by several observations.

Virtually everyone who develops classic narcolepsy with cataplexy has a particular allele of a gene (DQB1) that is part of the human leukocyte antigen (HLA) complex, a key component of the immune system. This allele is referred to as DQB1*06:02; other alleles of this gene are instead associated with a reduced risk of developing narcolepsy (Mignot, 2004). There are also very rare instances (probably ~1% of cases) of people who develop narcolepsy but do not have the 06:02 allele (Han, Lin, et al., 2014).

The presence of the 06:02 allele does not ensure that an individual will develop narcolepsy but, like genetic predispositions for other conditions, it increases the risk. The idea that there is a genetic predisposition involved is supported by evidence that the prevalence of narcolepsy varies with ethnicity. It affects up to ~1/2000 people (.025–.05% of the population) in the United States and Western Europe, but it is more common in some nationalities (e.g., in Japan (.16%) and China (.28%)) and very rare in others (e.g., among Israeli Jews and in Saudi Arabia (.01%)) (Lavie & Peled, 1987; Plazzi et al., 2018). The interpretation that there is a genetic contribution to narcolepsy is also supported by its occurrence in family clusters and the presence of increased risk if a genetically identical twin has narcolepsy.

Narcolepsy also occurs in other mammals, including in some dog breeds. Researchers at Stanford University (led by William Dement and Emmanuel Mignot) used selective breeding to generate canine lineages that had a high likelihood of developing narcolepsy in order to study the genetics and physiology of the condition. They eventually identified a gene linked to the occurrence of narcolepsy symptoms in dogs, which turned out to be responsible for the production of a receptor for the recently identified brain peptide hypocretin (Lin et al., 1999).

At the same time, another group observed that knocking out the gene in mice that codes for production of hypocretin caused symptoms similar to those shown by humans or dogs with narcolepsy. The mice showed inappropriate behavioral arrest during social encounters (resembling cataplexy) and abnormal regulation of REM sleep (Chemelli et al., 1999; Mochizuki et al., 2004). Subsequent studies confirmed that the loss of hypocretin was critical to the appearance of these symptoms. Infusions of hypocretin into the brain, or gene transfers that restored hypocretin production in knockout mice with narcolepsy-like symptoms, reduced both cataplexy symptoms and intrusions of sleep episodes into waking (Blanco-Centurion et al., 2013; Kantor et al., 2013; Mieda et al., 2004).

Studies of the levels of hypocretin in human patients with narcolepsy demonstrated that it is virtually undetectable in the CSF of almost all narcoleptic patients, particularly those with the classic form involving cataplexy (**Figure 11.6**). In contrast, most patients with excessive daytime sleepiness (hypersomnia) resulting from other causes had normal hypocretin levels. A small subset of patients with classic narcolepsy, however, were shown to have normal hypocretin levels, suggesting that there is a rare alternative mechanism that can generate human narcolepsy, such as reduced hypocretin receptor numbers or other damage to sleep-regulatory systems (Hungs & Mignot, 2001; Krahn et al., 2002; Mignot et al., 2002; Nishino et al., 2000; Ripley et al., 2001).

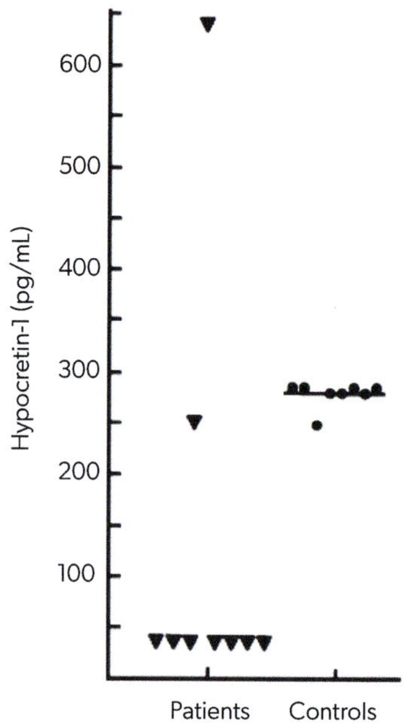

Figure 11.6 An early study examined levels of hypocretin in cerebrospinal fluid from controls (circles) and from patients with narcolepsy with cataplexy (triangles). Seven of nine patients with narcolepsy had levels below the detection limit of the assay (<40 pg/ml). One patient had normal levels, as also reported for ~10% of narcolepsy patients in larger studies. In contrast, patients with hypersomnia unrelated to narcolepsy typically had normal hypocretin levels (>200 pg/ml) (Ripley B. et al. *Neurology* 57:2253–3358, 2001). One patient had very high levels (>600 ng/mL) but was clinically indistinguishable from other patients, except for having the longest sleep onset latencies during nap tests in this group (Nishino et al. *Lancet* 355(9197):31–40, 2000). The subset of narcolepsy patients with normal or elevated hypocretin levels may have damage to systems on which hypocretin normally acts (e.g., loss of hypocretin receptors). Reprinted with permission from Hungs, M. & Mignot, E. (2001) Hypocretin/orexin, sleep and narcolepsy. *Bioessays* 23(5) 397–408. © John Wiley & Sons, Inc. (2001). doi: 10.1002/bies.1058; permission conveyed through Copyright Clearance Center, Inc.

Although disrupted hypocretin neurotransmission led to similar symptoms in three species (narcoleptic humans, dogs bred selectively to show narcolepsy symptoms, and hypocretin-gene knockout mice), the mechanisms involved were different in each case. In gene knockout mice, hypocretin production was prevented, presumably without affecting the survival of neurons that normally produce hypocretin.

In narcoleptic dogs, the deficit that led to symptoms was a genetic abnormality that eliminated a receptor for hypocretin. Neither of these is the mechanism responsible for most cases of narcolepsy with cataplexy in people. If the genes responsible for producing either hypocretin or its receptors were absent in people, symptoms would presumably be present from birth rather than developing gradually and appearing typically during adolescence or early adulthood. Instead, the evidence indicates that narcolepsy in most people is caused by a gradual loss over the course of development of the cells that produce hypocretin.[3]

Brains of deceased narcoleptic patients showed very large reductions in immunohistochemical staining for hypocretin (85–95% reduction relative to controls); although there was no loss of staining for another group of neurons in the pfLH—those containing melanin-concentrating hormone (MCH) (see Section 11.3.5). In addition, there was evidence of an increased number of glial cells (which are involved in responding to degeneration) in the pfLH, but not in a control brain region. These results indicated that there had been selective cell loss in the pfLH of hypocretin-immunoreactive (-ir) neurons. In dogs selectively bred to show narcolepsy, there was no loss of hypocretin-ir neurons at the time of onset of symptoms, consistent with the conclusion that the cause of narcolepsy in these animals was the loss of hypocretin receptors. Human narcolepsy in most cases appears instead to be the result of a neurodegenerative process that gradually and selectively destroys hypocretin neurons in the pfLH during development (Thannickal et al., 2000) (**Figure 11.7**).

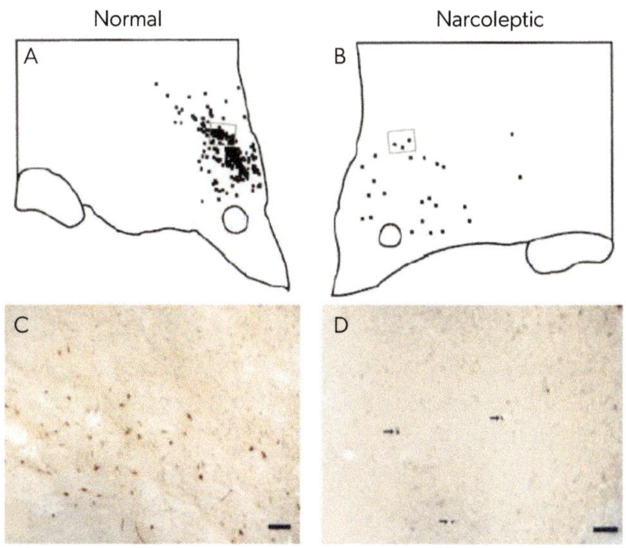

Figure 11.7 Drawings of the perifornical region in postmortem tissue from a person with no history of a neurological disease (**A**) and from one who had narcolepsy since age 20 (**B**; died at age 63). **C & D:** Actual tissue staining for hypocretin in the small, gray boxes outlined in **A** and **B**. The brown staining visible in **C** indicates the presence of many hypocretin-immunoreactive neurons. Three small arrows in **D** point to cells verified at higher magnification to be hypocretin-immunoreactive neurons. The average number of neurons immunoreactive for hypocretin was dramatically reduced in the brains of patients who suffered from narcolepsy, to about 7% of control levels. Adapted with permission of Elsevier, Ltd. from Thannickal, T.C. et al. (2000) Reduced number of hypocretin neurons in human narcolepsy. *Neuron* 27:469–474. © Elsevier (2000). doi: 10.1016/s0896-6273(00)00058-1.

It is also possible that reduced production of hypocretin by surviving pfLH neurons plays a role. Support for this idea comes from the serendipitous observation that a human brain studied postmortem contained much larger numbers of hypocretin-ir cells than is typical. This individual turned out to have been addicted to heroin. Studies of this brain and of others who had been addicted to heroin confirmed a ~50% increase in hypocretin-ir neurons, along with a reduction of neuron size (Thannickal et al., 2018).

The link between opiates and hypocretin was confirmed in mice undergoing long-term treatments with a related opioid, morphine. They showed increased hypocretin-ir but without signs of accompanying neurogenesis, suggesting that existing neurons were being triggered to produce increased hypocretin amounts. Similarly, in a mouse model of narcolepsy with reduced hypocretin-ir cell numbers and symptoms of cataplexy, treatment with morphine restored baseline numbers of hypocretin-ir neurons and greatly reduced the frequency of cataplexy. These results indicate that chronic opiate exposure can boost levels of hypocretin production from surviving neurons, resulting in reduced narcolepsy symptoms (Thannickal et al., 2018). Thus, it is possible that the dramatic reductions in hypocretin-ir in patients with narcolepsy result from both the loss of hypocretin neurons and a reduction of hypocretin production by surviving neurons.

Human infants have large numbers of hypocretin-ir neurons; numbers decrease into young adulthood and then further into old age in the absence of narcolepsy symptoms. These losses are relatively minor (~23% reduction over the lifespan but somewhat greater in the core pfLH region than in the adjacent hypothalamus) (Hunt et al., 2015) compared to the ~90% reduction in patients with narcolepsy, even at a younger age (Thannickal et al., 2000). Nevertheless, age-related reductions in hypocretin in some older people might contribute (along with other changes; see Section 8.4) to less stable sleep and wake states, resulting in more daytime sleepiness and more disrupted sleep at night.

[3] There is one reported human case of a spontaneous genetic abnormality that prevented the production of hypocretin. As might be predicted, this individual had shown symptoms of narcolepsy, including severe cataplexy triggered by laughter, as early as 6 months of age (Peyron et al., 2000).

The generally accepted view of the cause of the classic form of narcolepsy in people is based on the following features:

- it is rare (but not unknown) in children;
- it typically has an insidious onset with major overt symptoms appearing in adolescence or early adulthood;
- the DQB1*06:02 allele (part of the HLA complex) is present in the vast majority of people with classic narcolepsy with cataplexy (but also in others who do not develop narcolepsy);
- the great majority of patients with an established diagnosis of narcolepsy have very low or undetectable hypocretin levels in the CSF and very low levels of detectable hypocretin-ir neurons in the pfLH.

These characteristics can be accounted for by the hypothesis that narcolepsy is a genetically influenced neurodegenerative disorder affecting pfLH hypocretin neurons and, possibly, the ability of surviving neurons to produce hypocretin. Its gradual emergence during childhood and adolescence appears to reflect an autoimmune process (i.e., damage resulting from the activity of a person's own immune system) that destroys these neurons (Thannickal et al., 2000) or disables their production of hypocretin (Thannickal et al., 2018). The presence of the 06:02 allele of the DQB1 gene may make these neurons susceptible to damage from some aspect of immune system activation, which may be triggered by infections during childhood and adolescence. See Appendix D for a discussion of immune system activation and early onset of narcolepsy.

A puzzling feature of narcolepsy is the fact that cataplexy is often triggered by a strong emotion, usually a positive emotion like joy or laughter. One proposed explanation involves the amygdala, a component of the limbic system that plays a central role in the regulation of emotions. GABAergic neurons in the central nucleus of the amygdala (CeA) are activated by emotional states. They project to, and inhibit, brainstem regions that produce 5-HT and NE which normally oppose the initiation of REM sleep (see Section 10.7.2). Hypocretin neurons also project to some of these same areas, but their input is excitatory.

The proposed model states that when a positive emotion occurs, it activates both the inhibitory CeA and excitatory hypocretin neurons, resulting in balanced inhibitory/excitatory input to 5-HT and NE systems. In patients with narcolepsy, however, when positive emotions activate the amygdala, its inhibitory input to the brainstem is unopposed by excitatory hypocretin input, resulting in reduced catecholamine levels. This reduction in catecholamines would disinhibit cholinergic systems and allow them to trigger REM sleep components (e.g., atonia) while awake (Burgess et al., 2013) (**Figure 11.8**).

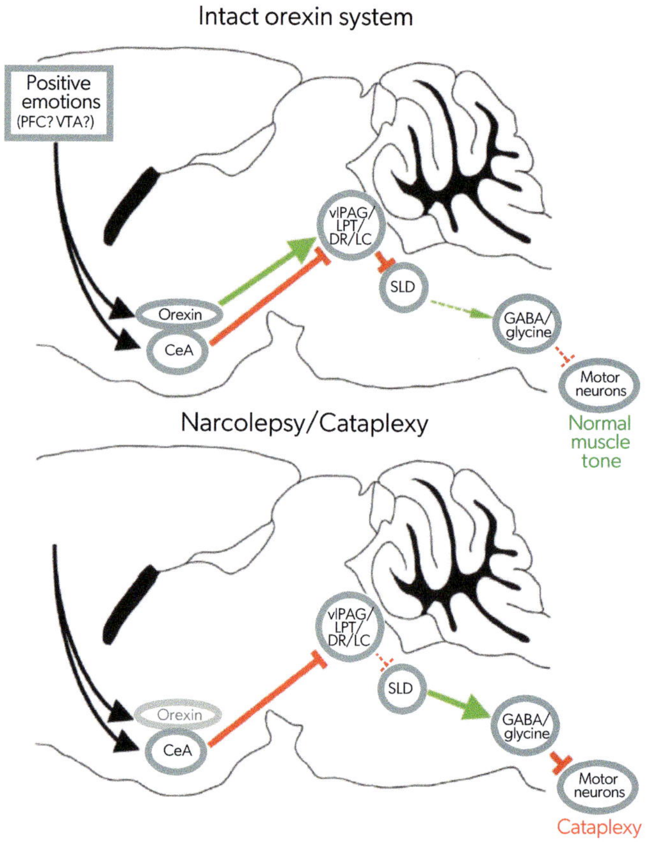

Figure 11.8 A model of interactions between hypocretin (orexin) neurons and the output of the central nucleus of the amygdala (CeA) in the regulation of muscle tone. The top panel shows the normal response to positive emotions which activate projections from both hypocretin neurons (excitatory, green) and CeA neurons (inhibitory, red) to the ventrolateral periaqueductal gray (vlPAG), the laterodorsal pedunculopontine nucleus (LPT), dorsal raphe (DR), and locus coeruleus (LC). Projections from these structures inhibit the sublaterodorsal nucleus (SLD) so it does not activate neurons that release GABA and glycine to inhibit motor neurons in the spinal cord. As a result of this balanced input, normal muscle tone is maintained during an emotional event. The bottom panel shows the same system in the absence of hypocretin neurons, which allows CeA inhibition to act during an emotional event without the opposing excitatory input from hypocretin, resulting in reduced inhibitory input to the SLD (dotted red line). As a result, SLD activity is disinhibited, which allows it to activate downstream systems that inhibit motor neurons (solid red line). The profound suppression of activity in spinal motor neurons is manifest as cataplexy emerging out of waking during emotional activation. Reprinted with permission of the Society for Neuroscience under a Creative Commons Attribution License (CC-BY-NC-SA) from Burgess, C.R. et al. (2013) Amygdala lesions reduce cataplexy in orexin knock-out mice. *J Neurosci* 33:9734–9742. © The Authors (2013). doi: 10.1523/JNEUROSCI.5632-12.2013.

The components of this model are supported by several lines of evidence. Epilepsy patients with microdialysis probes implanted into the amygdala showed high hypocretin levels when awake, but even higher levels during positive emotional experiences, indicating a strong elevation of hypocretin release during positive experiences (Blouin et al., 2013). A study of dogs with narcolepsy found that activity of neurons in the CeA was elevated both immediately before and during spontaneous cataplectic attacks (Gulyani et al., 2002). In mice lacking hypocretin, activating GABAergic neurons in the CeA triggered cataplexy (Snow et al., 2017). Finally, lesions of the amygdala in these mice reduced cataplectic symptoms in response to pleasurable stimuli (access to a running wheel or to chocolate) (Burgess et al., 2013).

In summary, the model proposes that positive emotions both activate the amygdala and increase hypocretin release, resulting in opposing effects on pontine systems. In patients with narcolepsy experiencing a strong emotion, their reduced hypocretin levels cannot oppose amygdala outputs that inhibit 5-HT and NE systems. The resulting reduction in 5-HT and NE levels allows cholinergic neurons to activate the systems responsible for REM sleep atonia and produce cataplectic symptoms (Burgess et al., 2013).

11.3.4 The role of hypocretin in sleep–wake regulation

The evidence linking the loss of hypocretin in people to the symptoms of narcolepsy provides the background for a better understanding of the role of hypocretin in normal sleep regulation. Although hypocretin contributes to arousal, it is clear that features of narcolepsy, other than excessive daytime sleepiness, cannot be explained by the loss of a wake-promoting system alone. Studies in mouse models of narcolepsy also showed that abnormalities in homeostatic or circadian regulation of sleep do not explain their symptoms (Mochizuki et al., 2004). Rather, the symptoms of narcolepsy are proposed to reflect the loss of a system critical to maintaining state stability, resulting in disrupted organization of REM sleep, NREM sleep, and waking, including the inappropriate intrusion of REM sleep components into waking (Broughton et al., 1986; Mochizuki et al., 2004).

This hypothesis about the role of hypocretin is based on the idea that there are multiple, mutually opposed mechanisms that promote waking, NREM, and REM sleep. Homeostatic, circadian, and other factors shift the current balance among these systems so that each state is maintained stably for a species-appropriate duration before altered inputs (e.g., satisfying a homeostatic drive, or entering a different circadian phase) shift the balance among these mechanisms to a different stable state.

The abruptness of switches among these states has been modeled as similar to the actions of a "flip-flop" mechanism that generates rapid, complete switches between states and enforces stability of state once a switch has occurred. Hypocretin is hypothesized to contribute to maintaining these states and to allowing orderly transitions among them. In the absence of hypocretin, small shifts in balance among these mutually opposed mechanisms result in state instability, manifest as fragmented wakefulness (i.e., unpredictable daytime sleepiness) and fragmented sleep (wake after sleep onset) (Fulcher et al., 2014; Saper et al., 2005).

The separate components of REM sleep are regulated by different neural mechanisms, as demonstrated by the selective loss of atonia but not of other features of REM sleep after small pontine lesions (see Section 10.8.1). Hypocretin appears to regulate these neural systems to ensure the synchronous emergence of REM sleep features after an appropriate duration of NREM sleep. Without hypocretin, the components of REM sleep may be expressed individually and at inappropriate times (i.e., appearing during waking rather than following NREM sleep).

The results of a study in cats are consistent with a role for hypocretin in both gating state changes and maintaining state stability. Hypocretin injections into the nucleus pontis oralis (the REM sleep initiation region of the pons in cats, equivalent to the SLD; see Section 10.7.1) during quiet sleep (NREM) caused a rapid transition to REM sleep and an increase in its duration at the expense of waking. However, when injected into the same region during waking, hypocretin tended to prolong and sustain waking at the expense of both REM and NREM sleep (**Figure 11.9**) (Xi & Chase, 2010). These effects indicate that hypocretin does not trigger a specific stage of sleep or waking, but rather that it regulates the timing of transitions among these states.

Most drugs used to reduce the frequency of cataplectic attacks in people or dogs act as agonists of NE and/or 5-HT

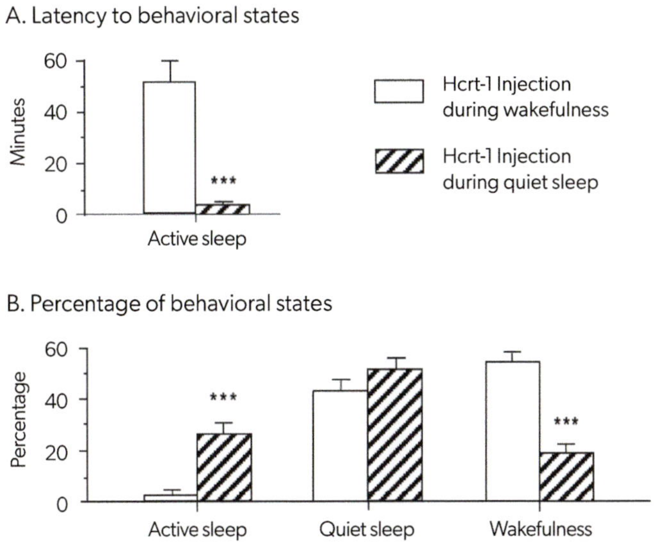

Figures 11.9 Effects of injections of hypocretin-1 into the nucleus pontis oralis (equivalent to SLD) in cats. **A.** In the hour after an injection during NREM sleep (hatched column), cats showed a very short latency (Y axis) to enter active (REM) sleep. But, when injected while awake (white column), they stayed awake, showing very long latencies to onset of REM sleep. **B.** The percentage (Y axis) of REM and NREM sleep (active and quiet sleep) and wakefulness shown during the hour after an injection depended on the cats' state when they were injected. If injected during NREM sleep (hatched columns), they either stayed in NREM sleep or transitioned to REM (active) sleep but were less likely to transition to waking. When injected during waking (white columns), they either stayed awake or entered NREM (quiet) sleep, but rarely transitioned to REM (active) sleep. ***$p < 0.001$ for comparisons between states at the time of injections. Reprinted with permission of Oxford University Press from Xi, M. & Chase, M.H. (2010) The injection of hypocretin-1 into the nucleus pontis oralis induces either active sleep or wakefulness depending on the behavioral state when it is administered. *Sleep* 33:1236–1243. © Sleep Research Society (2010). doi:10.1093/sleep/33.9.1236.

BOX 11.3 Insomnia Treatments

Benzodiazepines were the most commonly used prescription sleep aids for many years. They act as agonists at $GABA_A$ receptors and are very effective in increasing sleep amounts, but they also modify sleep parameters, for example, by reducing SWA (Borbély et al., 1991). Their long-term use has the potential for abuse, development of tolerance (requiring dose increases), dependence, and increased daytime somnolence. The newer "z-drugs" (zolpidem, (es)zopiclone, zaleplon) also act as $GABA_A$ receptor agonists, but at a different site on the receptor complex. To varying degrees, they have less pronounced risks associated with their use, although they can have side effects, including daytime sleepiness, reduced SWS (in some studies but not others), and potential for abuse (Arbon et al., 2015; Buscemi et al., 2007; Schifano et al., 2019).[a]

Because hypocretin antagonists act via a different mechanism, they reportedly have little effect on sleep EEG characteristics, except for possibly accelerating REM sleep onset during the night (Bettica, Squassante, Groeger, et al., 2012; Bettica, Squassante, Zamuner, et al., 2012; Fox et al., 2013), and they may not have significant abuse potential. They may be especially useful for treating some types of insomnia (Zheng et al., 2020), but, as with most sleep aids, there is also a risk of unwanted persistence of sleepiness into daytime, depending on dosage.

Because the loss of hypocretin in patients with narcolepsy leads to cataplexy, it is important to know whether blocking hypocretin receptors with drugs has similar effects. In a mouse study, two drugs that antagonize both hypocretin receptors increased the incidence of cataplexy when mice were given access to a sweet reward (chocolate) during their active phase (Mahoney et al., 2019). In another study, chronic treatment in mice with suvorexant reduced hypocretin levels and increased hypocretin receptor numbers. Following a washout period, acute suvorexant treatment resulted in narcoleptic-like symptoms, which were made worse by providing access to chocolate[b] (Kaushik et al., 2021). However, clinical trials in people have reported only very rare cataplexy-like side effects, so it remains to be seen whether side effects will become an issue if hypocretin receptor antagonists are used as sleep aids over longer periods of time in more patients.

An alternative approach to treating chronic insomnia is Cognitive Behavioral Therapy for Insomnia (CBT-I), which involves a combination of psychological and behavioral interventions. This treatment has no known side effects and is generally effective in producing lasting reductions in key insomnia symptoms (Morin et al., 2006; Trauer et al., 2015). Although access to skilled professionals who can deliver CBT-I was a limiting factor in the past, there is increasing evidence that CBT-I can be delivered successfully over the internet (Cheng et al., 2019; Zachariae et al., 2016) and therefore can be accessed more widely.

[a]The use of melatonin and melatonin receptor agonists as sleep aids is discussed in Sections 9.5 and 9.6. For a comprehensive set of reviews related to the nature of insomnia and options for its treatment, see a recent issue of the *Journal of Sleep Research* 32(6), December 2023.

[b]These results reflect the mechanism discussed earlier (see Section 11.3.3 and **Figure 11.8**) by which positive emotions activate GABAergic amygdala neurons, resulting ultimately in disinhibition of REM sleep features in the absence of the counterbalancing effects of activation of hypocretin receptors.

neurotransmission as well as having anticholinergic effects (Dauvilliers et al., 2014; Mignot et al., 1993). NE and 5-HT normally promote cortical activation and inhibit the transition to REM sleep, while ACh triggers REM sleep features, including atonia; see Section 10.7.2. Thus, these drugs are likely effective because they increase NE/5-HT activity and reduce cholinergic activity. Hypocretin neurons project to all of the sleep-regulatory systems that use these neurotransmitters (see **Figure 11.4**). Reductions in hypocretin amounts in narcolepsy appear to shift the balance among these systems toward promoting cholinergic activity, allowing the breakthrough expression of cataplexy and other REM sleep features into waking.[4]

In addition to its other regulatory functions, hypocretin is involved in producing arousal and wakefulness in people. For example, activation of the hypocretin system mediates waking up from anesthesia (Kelz et al., 2008), and a mutation in the *DEC2* gene that increases levels of hypocretin (Hirano et al., 2018) is associated with unusually short sleep in people and mice (He et al., 2009).

As a result, antagonists acting on hypocretin receptors have been developed as potential sleep aids. In both rats and humans, antagonists to the two subtypes of hypocretin receptors accelerate sleep onset and help maintain sleep, including in patients with a diagnosis of insomnia (Bettica, Squassante, Groeger, et al., 2012; Bettica, Squassante, Zamuner, et al., 2012; Fox et al., 2013). Dual hypocretin receptor antagonists have been approved for sale as sleep aids by the US Food and Drug Administration since 2014 (e.g., suvorexant (Belsomra™), lemborexant (Dayvigo™), and others are under development; see **Box 11.3**).

[4] Another drug used in the treatment of narcolepsy is gamma-hydroxybutyrate (GHB or Xyrem™), which has a very different mode of action. It promotes sustained sleep at night and reduces the risk of daytime sleepiness and cataplexy (US Xyrem Multicenter Study Group 2004; Mayer et al., 2018). Despite several attractive hypotheses, its mechanisms of action in improving narcolepsy symptoms remain uncertain (Kilduff, 2023).

11.3.5 Melanin-concentrating hormone

Intermingled among the hypocretin neurons within and near the pfLH are neurons that are immunoreactive for another peptide, melanin-concentrating hormone (MCH) (Konadhode et al., 2013; Modirrousta et al., 2005) (**Figure 11.10**). MCH, like hypocretin, has been linked to regulation of food intake, energy balance, and sleep. MCH neurons also project widely throughout the nervous system, including to regions involved in sleep regulation. MCH neurons, and other LH neurons that contain neither hypocretin nor MCH, contain GABA (Elias et al., 1998).

MCH neurons are implicated in the regulation of REM sleep and in sleep homeostasis. During recovery REM sleep after selective REM sleep deprivation, MCH neurons showed increased levels of the immediate-early gene product c-Fos, a marker of neuronal activation (Verret et al., 2003). They also accumulated c-Fos during recovery sleep after total sleep deprivation, in contrast to hypocretin neurons, which showed highest levels at the end of a period of sleep deprivation, that is, while rats were still awake and had not been allowed to begin recovery sleep (Modirrousta et al., 2005) (**Figure 11.11**). Greater activation of MCH neurons during recovery sleep is probably related to increases in both NREM and REM sleep, since injection of MCH into the lateral ventricles increased both stages, although the effects on REM sleep were more robust (Verret et al., 2003).

Juxtacellular recording/labeling was used to identify the neurochemical phenotype of LH neurons that were active during different stages of sleep and waking. MCH neurons were inactive during waking, showed some activity during NREM sleep, and very high firing rates during REM sleep. These patterns of activation and silence are generally opposite to those shown by hypocretin neurons (**Figure 11.12**) (Hassani et al., 2009).

Selective, brief activation of MCH neurons using optogenetic methods suppressed the activity of arousal-promoting histamine neurons in the TMN and lengthened episodes of REM, but not NREM, sleep (Jego et al., 2013). Optogenetic activation of MCH neurons over 24 h periods in mice and rats increased both NREM and REM sleep amounts during the night phase, when they would normally be most active, and also increased REM sleep during the day in rats (Blanco-Centurion et al., 2016; Konadhode et al., 2013). A role for MCH in increasing sleep is consistent with evidence that levels of MCH in the amygdala of human epilepsy patients were high at sleep onset and decreased after waking (Blouin et al., 2013).

These findings support the conclusion that MCH neurons in the LH are involved in regulating onset and maintenance of REM sleep as well as promoting NREM sleep. Activation of MCH neurons in nocturnal rodents promoted sleep onset even during the night when their influence would be opposed by several wake-promoting systems that are most active during that circadian phase (Blanco-Centurion et al., 2016; Clément et al., 2012; Hassani et al., 2009; Konadhode et al., 2013; Torterolo et al., 2011).

Other LH GABAergic neurons that do not contain either hypocretin or MCH are also activated during REM sleep (Hassani et al., 2010; Sapin et al., 2010). One mechanism by which these neurons, along with GABA-containing MCH neurons, promote sleep onset is by inhibiting the

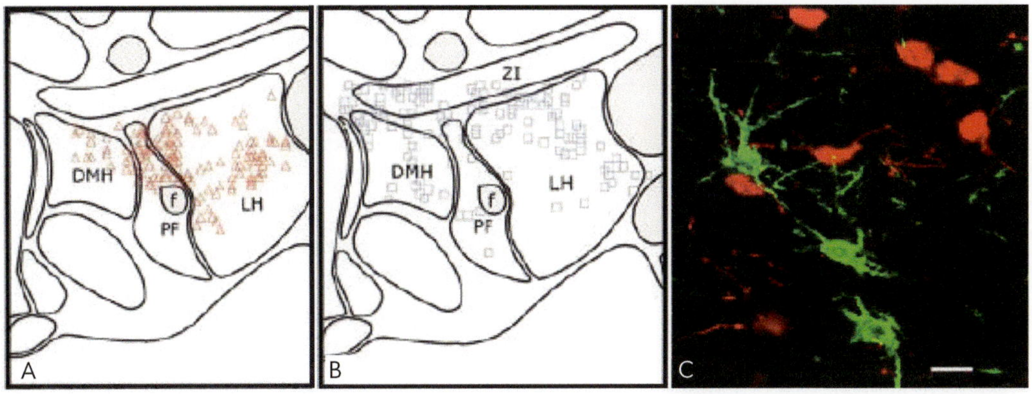

Figure 11.10 **A & B.** The locations of neurons containing hypocretin (triangles) and melanin-concentrating hormone (MCH) (squares) in the perifornical region of the rat hypothalamus. LH: lateral hypothalamus; ZI: zona incerta; DMH: dorsomedial hypothalamic nucleus; f: fornix; PF: perifornical region. Reprinted with permission from Modirrousta, M. et al. (2005) Orexin and MCH neurons express c-Fos differently after sleep deprivation vs. recovery and bear different adrenergic receptors. *Eur J Neurosci* 21:2807–2816. © Federation of European Neuroscience Societies (2005). Journal Compilation © John Wiley and Sons. doi: 10.1111/j.1460-9568.2005.04104.x. **C.** Intermingling of hypocretin (red) and MCH (green) neurons in the posterior hypothalamus of a mouse; scale bar = 25 μm. Reprinted with permission of the Society for Neuroscience under a Creative Commons Attribution License (CC-BY-NC-SA) from Konadhode, R.R. et al. (2013) Optogenetic stimulation of MCH neurons increases sleep. *J Neurosci* 33:10257–10263. © The Authors (2013). doi: 10.1523/JNEUROSCI.1225-13.2013.

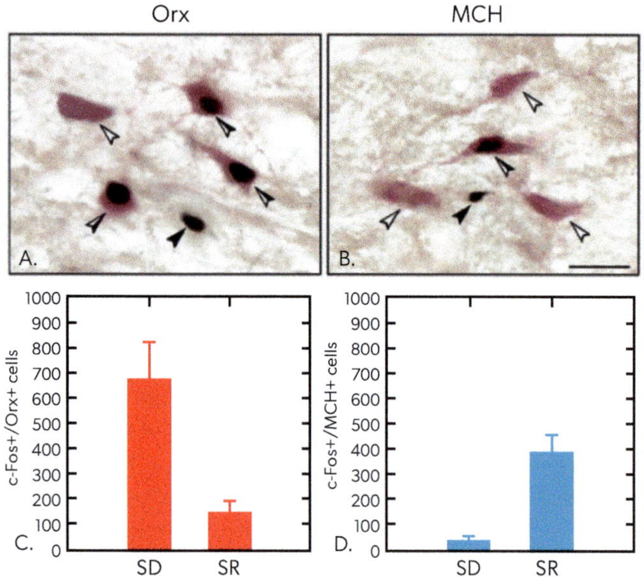

Figure 11.11 Expression of the nuclear activity marker c-Fos in hypocretin (orexin, Orx) neurons and melanin-concentrating hormone (MCH) neurons in the perifornical lateral hypothalamic area occurred at different times during sleep loss and recovery sleep. Hypocretin neurons were selectively activated during sleep deprivation, while MCH neurons were selectively activated during recovery sleep. **A**. The effects of sleep deprivation. Cells include a hypocretin neuron with no c-Fos immunoreactivity in the nucleus (pink soma; white arrowhead); a non-hypocretin neuron with c-Fos labeling (black nucleus with unstained soma; black arrowhead); and double-labeled cells (pink somata with black nuclei; black & white arrowheads). Double-labeled cells are hypocretin neurons that were activated by sleep deprivation. **B.** The effects of recovery sleep. Cells include MCH neurons that were not activated (pink somata; white arrowheads); a non-MCH neuron that increased c-Fos immunoreactivity after recovery sleep (black nucleus, unstained soma; black arrowhead); an MCH neuron that was activated during recovery sleep (black nucleus and pink soma; black & white arrowhead). The scale bar is 20 μm. **C.** The number of double-labeled hypocretin neurons after sleep deprivation (SD) and after recovery sleep (SR). **D**. The number of double-labeled MCH neurons after sleep deprivation (SD) and after recovery sleep (SR). Reprinted with permission from Modirrousta, M. et al. (2005) Orexin and MCH neurons express c-Fos differently after sleep deprivation vs. recovery and bear different adrenergic receptors. *Eur J Neurosci* 21:2807–2816. © Federation of European Neuroscience Societies (2005). Published by John Wiley and Sons. doi: 10.1111/j.1460-9568.2005.04104.x.

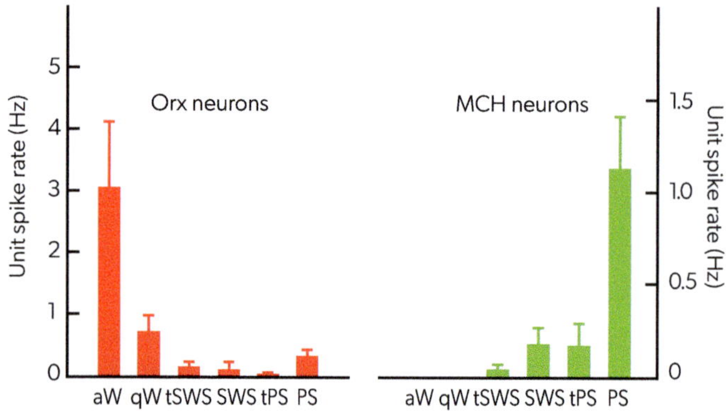

Figure 11.12 Firing rates of hypocretin (Orx; red) and MCH neurons (green) in the lateral hypothalamus of rats during different states of arousal. Hypocretin neurons were most active during active wake (aW), were less active during quiet wake (qW), and showed very low activity in other stages: transition to slow-wave sleep (tSWS), SWS, transition to paradoxical (REM) sleep (tPS), and REM sleep (PS). MCH neurons were silent during active and quiet waking, fired at low rates during tSWS, SWS, and tPS, and were most active during REM sleep (PS). Reprinted with permission from Hassani, O.K. et al. (2009) Melanin-concentrating hormone neurons discharge in a reciprocal manner to orexin neurons across the sleep–wake cycle. *PNAS* 106:2418–2422. © National Academy of Sciences USA (2009). doi: 10.1073/pnas.0811400106.

intermingled hypocretin neurons that promote waking when they are active (see **Figure 11.10**). These GABAergic neurons also project to the septum and TMN in the forebrain and to the midbrain ventrolateral PAG, which plays a role in triggering REM sleep (Clément et al., 2012; Jego et al., 2013; Sapin et al., 2010). In contrast to these sleep-promoting roles for LH GABAergic neurons, another subset of LH neurons project to the preoptic area where their inhibition of sleep-promoting systems (see Section 11.4) results in rapid awakening (Venner, De Luca, et al., 2019).

11.3.6 Summary

The pfLH and surrounding regions contain intermingled neurons that are immunoreactive for the peptides hypocretin or MCH. Both MCH neurons and others that are not immunoreactive for either of these peptides contain the inhibitory neurotransmitter GABA. Hypocretin neurons show highest activity during spontaneous active waking (and during forced waking), while MCH neurons are most active during sleep, especially during REM sleep, and after a period of recovery sleep following deprivation.

Although hypocretin plays a role in promoting alert wakefulness, it also has other functions, inferred especially from evidence of sleep behavior in the absence of hypocretin. It is involved in regulating transitions between states (waking, NREM, and REM sleep) and therefore in determining their characteristic durations. In patients with narcolepsy, there is a dramatic loss of hypocretin staining in the pfLH. This observation is interpreted as the result of progressive degeneration of hypocretin-producing neurons, caused by an autoimmune reaction in people with a genetic susceptibility (presence of the DQB1*06:02 allele of the HLA complex). There is, however, also evidence that hypocretin neurons survive but produce less hypocretin and might still retain the capacity to increase production in response to appropriate stimulation.

The symptoms of narcolepsy can be interpreted as reflecting the loss of coordination among normally synchronous elements of REM sleep in the absence of hypocretin, and the intrusion of these elements into waking. These elements include excessive daytime sleepiness, cataplexy, short latencies to onset of REM sleep, hypnogogic hallucinations, and sleep paralysis. The occurrence of cataplexy in response to positive emotions in patients with narcolepsy has been attributed to brainstem mechanisms that regulate the expression of REM atonia being activated indirectly by input from the amygdala that is not counterbalanced by opposing hypocretin input.

MCH neurons (and other GABAergic neurons) in the pfLH help to promote sleep onset by inhibiting adjacent hypocretin neurons and other wake-promoting systems, such as histamine neurons in the TMN. They also play an important role in the regulation of REM sleep, in part through projections to the ventrolateral PAG neurons that are involved in triggering REM sleep. In contrast to these roles, other GABAergic LH neurons promote rapid awakening when they are activated because they inhibit sleep-promoting neurons in preoptic nuclei.

11.4 Preoptic area

The preoptic area includes several nuclei in the anterior hypothalamic region near the optic chiasm. In parallel to Von Economo's analysis of the brains of patients with excessive sleep, he also found that those with reduced sleep (severe insomnia) had suffered damage to the anterior hypothalamic region, suggesting its involvement in promoting sleep (von Economo, 1930); see Section 1.3. This conclusion was reinforced by animal studies in which experimental ablations of the preoptic area led to profound reductions in sleep (Nauta, 1946). Complementary studies showed that electrical activation of the lateral preoptic area triggered EEG synchronization and sleep onset (Sterman & Clemente, 1962).

In contrast to the several brain regions that have been identified as promoting waking and regulating REM sleep, few regions have been shown to regulate NREM sleep. These include GABA/MCH neurons in the LH (Konadhode et al., 2013) and a region in the medulla called the parafacial zone (Anaclet et al., 2012); see Section 10.6.2. Most studies of NREM sleep regulation, however, have focused on the preoptic area.

Most neurons in the ventrolateral preoptic area (VLPO) and in the nearby median preoptic nucleus (MnPO) are more active during sleep, as demonstrated by increased accumulation of c-Fos protein (Gong et al., 2004; Sherin et al., 1996) (**Figure 11.13**) and increased firing rates (Alam et al., 2018; Suntsova et al., 2002; Szymusiak et al., 1998). The VLPO of rats includes a dense concentration of neurons that increase activity during both REM and NREM sleep (although to different extents), and an adjacent region of similar but more dispersed cells (the "extended VLPO") that is active primarily during REM sleep (Gaus et al., 2002; Lu et al., 2002). Inhibition of VLPO neurons by activation of GABAergic input from the lateral hypothalamus triggers rapid arousal from sleep (Venner, De Luca, et al., 2019).

Many neurons in the VLPO and MnPO that are sleep-active produce the inhibitory neurotransmitter GABA; VLPO (but not MnPO) neurons also contain the inhibitory peptide galanin (Gaus et al., 2002) (**Figure 11.13**). When VLPO and MnPO neurons fire at high rates, they release GABA (and galanin) onto several wake-promoting systems to which they project. The inhibition of these systems triggers sleep onset. The firing

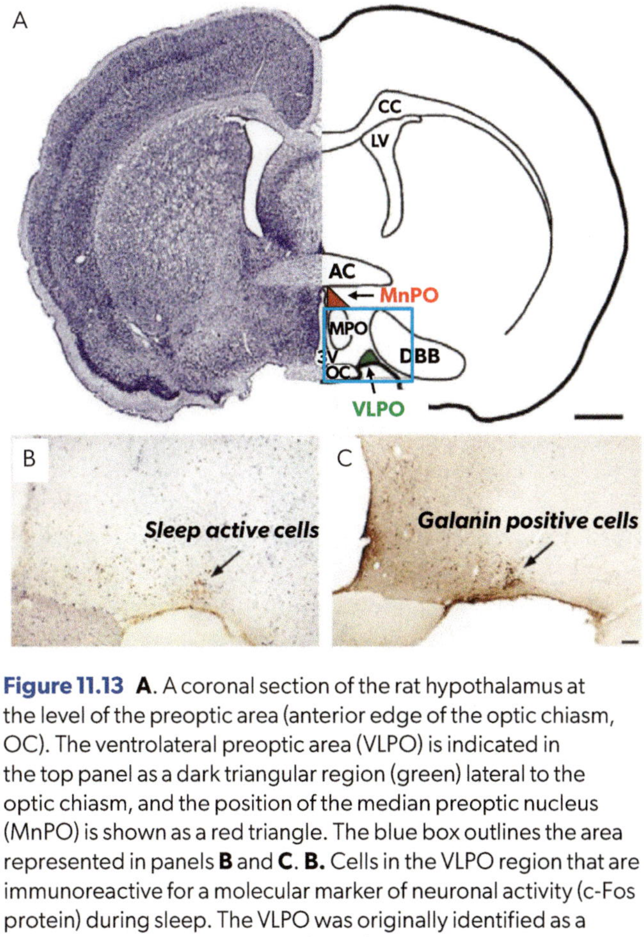

Figure 11.13 **A.** A coronal section of the rat hypothalamus at the level of the preoptic area (anterior edge of the optic chiasm, OC). The ventrolateral preoptic area (VLPO) is indicated in the top panel as a dark triangular region (green) lateral to the optic chiasm, and the position of the median preoptic nucleus (MnPO) is shown as a red triangle. The blue box outlines the area represented in panels **B** and **C**. **B.** Cells in the VLPO region that are immunoreactive for a molecular marker of neuronal activity (c-Fos protein) during sleep. The VLPO was originally identified as a cluster of sleep-active neurons (arrow). **C.** A similar section stained to show immunoreactivity for the inhibitory peptide galanin, which co-localizes with GABA in sleep-active neurons in the VLPO (arrow). CC: corpus callosum; LV: lateral ventricle; AC: anterior commissure; MPO: medial preoptic area; 3V: third ventricle; DBB: diagonal band of Broca. Scale bars are 1 mm for A and 100 μm for B and C. Adapted with permission of Elsevier, Ltd. from Gaus S.E. et al. (2002) Ventrolateral preoptic nucleus contains sleep-active, galaninergic neurons in multiple mammalian species. *Neuroscience* 115(1):285–294. © IBRO (2002). Published by Elsevier Science Ltd. doi: 10.1016/s0306-4522(02)00308-1.

rates of MnPO neurons increase in the seconds before sleep onset and increase further at sleep onset but fire at somewhat lower rates during continued NREM sleep. These neurons may be particularly important for transitioning to sleep (Alam et al., 2018; Suntsova et al., 2002). In addition, the higher firing rates at the onset of sleep compared to later in sleep episodes suggest a role in homeostatic responses to sleep need, which dissipates as sleep is produced.

MnPO neurons were most active during REM sleep and were especially responsive to increasing REM sleep pressure. GABAergic and non-GABAergic cells in the MnPO and VLPO showed high levels of accumulation of c-Fos protein after periods of sleep deprivation, especially after selective REM sleep deprivation (Gvilia, Turner, et al., 2006; Gvilia, Xu, et al., 2006). Among brain regions studied in rats, the medial preoptic area was unusual in showing increases in immediate-early gene expression that were responsive to the length of deprivation and affected by the circadian phase at which it occurred, suggesting a role for this region in integrating these regulatory influences (Semba et al., 2001). VLPO neurons showed high firing rates at sleep onset that were also related to the degree of sleep pressure (i.e., length of prior waking). These high rates were maintained throughout lengthy sleep episodes, implying an important role in initiating sleep in response to homeostatic needs as well as in maintenance of sleep episodes (Szymusiak & McGinty, 1986; Szymusiak & McGinty, 2008).

It is uncertain which structure in the human brain is functionally equivalent to the rat VLPO because galanin is found in several nuclei in the human preoptic region. There is, however, indirect support for the intermediate nucleus playing this role. Postmortem studies of the brains of patients with Alzheimer's disease (AD)[5] showed a reduction of galanin-ir neurons in this nucleus, relative to controls who died without AD. Both AD patients and controls had been studied using actigraphy before death. Those whose sleep/rest patterns had been more intact and consolidated before death had more galanin-containing neurons in the intermediate nucleus. These results are consistent with the hypothesis that galanin-positive neurons in the intermediate nucleus are important for maintaining sleep continuity (Lim et al., 2014).

The VLPO and MnPO project to key wake-promoting regions in both the forebrain and brainstem, including the TMN, the dorsal raphe nucleus, the locus coeruleus, and the pfLH. Preoptic projections inhibit these wake-promoting systems and help induce sleep onset. Some of these target regions also send direct or indirect inhibitory projections to the VLPO and MnPO (Steininger et al., 2001; Williams et al., 2014). For example, a projection from pfLH hypocretin/glutamate neurons to the VLPO activates a population of GABA neurons which, in turn, project to and inhibit sleep-promoting GABA/galanin neurons, resulting in increased arousal (De Luca et al., 2022). As discussed previously in relation to the role of hypocretin (Section 11.3.4), these mutual inhibitory relations between sleep-promoting preoptic nuclei and wake-promoting nuclei can facilitate bistability; that is, once the system enters a sleep or wake state, it tends to remain there stably for a prolonged period by suppressing opposing mechanisms (Saper et al., 2005).

An individual must, however, eventually transition from sleep to wake, or vice versa, so other mechanisms must be able to reverse the dominance of each system. Changing input from hypocretin neurons, which play a role in maintaining state stability, are likely involved (Saper et al., 2005). In addition, circadian and homeostatic mechanisms contribute to both maintaining state stability and ensuring the flexibility to switch states with appropriate timing. Projections from the circadian pacemaker in the SCN (see Chapter 8) reach neurons in the preoptic area and in the locus coeruleus both directly and indirectly (Aston-Jones et al., 2001; Chou et al., 2003; Deurveilher & Semba, 2005; Sun et al., 2001). These inputs, along with circadian modulation of many aspects of physiology (e.g., body temperature, endocrine activity, and autonomic activity), provide a sustained bias toward arousal and waking during part of the circadian cycle and toward sleep during the opposite phase. This circadian influence may be particularly important in species like humans and other primates that sustain lengthy, consolidated sleep and wake periods during different circadian phases.

The homeostatic system (see Chapter 5) also contributes to state maintenance. When sleep need (modeled as the level of substance S) is high, it promotes sleep onset, including by activating sleep-initiating mechanisms in the preoptic region. Neurons in the VLPO and MnPO increase firing rates (and therefore their inhibition of wake systems) in relation to the degree of sleep (or REM sleep) pressure, reflecting their role in the expression of sleep homeostasis. As the level of S falls during sleep, VLPO/MnPO activation is reduced, which allows wake-promoting systems to become disinhibited and to facilitate waking. In polyphasic sleepers like nocturnal rodents (see, e.g., **Figures 7.10** and **11.2 B**), this buildup of sleep need and its satisfaction during sleep occurs repeatedly during both day and night, with a circadian bias toward more sleep during the day.

Changing metabolic needs can also affect the interaction between the VLPO and wake-promoting systems like pfLH hypocretin neurons. Low blood glucose levels activated hypocretin neurons and inhibited VLPO neurons (Yamanaka et

---

[5] AD is a neurodegenerative disease that is best known for its debilitating effects on cognitive functions. In many patients with AD, there are also disruptions of daily rhythms and of sleep, especially in late stages of the illness (see Section 15.5).

al., 2003), resulting in more waking and activity. Hunger would presumably activate this system to increase arousal and activity levels in order to facilitate finding food. High-calorie meals that raise blood glucose levels would have the opposite effect, activating the VLPO and increasing sleepiness (Varin et al., 2015).

Evidence that glutamatergic input to the lateral preoptic area (LPO) is involved in sleep promotion by activating GABA neurons came from a study in which a transgene was inserted locally in the LPO to eliminate an essential subunit of NMDA (glutamate) receptors on GABAergic neurons. Mice lacking functional NMDA receptors on GABAergic neurons in this subregion showed disrupted NREM sleep and strongly reduced REM sleep amounts. These changes were attributed to reduced NMDA-mediated activation of sleep-promoting GABAergic neurons in the LPO (Miracca et al., 2022), and are consistent with a key role for the activity of GABA-containing neurons in the preoptic area in promoting sleep.

Another study, however, identified a role for glutamatergic neurons spread across a broad region of the preoptic area in promoting waking. Selective chemogenetic activation of glutamatergic neurons in this region reduced and disrupted NREM sleep, increased waking, and almost completely suppressed REM sleep production. The same treatments also reduced body temperature, which suggests the possibility that low body temperatures might trigger behavioral activation and reduce sleep in order to increase body temperature; see Section 10.5.2. However, activation of glutamatergic neurons selectively in the MnPO had similar effects in lowering body temperature but did not alter sleep characteristics. These results suggest that the effects of activation of glutamatergic neurons in the broader preoptic region in disrupting sleep were unlikely to be related primarily to an impact on body temperature (Mondino et al., 2021).

Both of these studies found disrupted NREM and strongly reduced REM sleep as a result of manipulations of glutamatergic activity. However, in one study loss of glutamatergic input to GABAergic neurons was involved (Miracca et al., 2022), and in the other study, activation of glutamatergic cells housed in the LPO was responsible (Mondino et al., 2021). It will be important to identify the routes and connections by which the activity of glutamatergic cells in the preoptic area disrupt sleep, and the sources of glutamatergic inputs to this region that act on GABAergic neurons to facilitate sleep in order to clarify the implications of these findings.

11.4.1 Summary

Clusters of neurons in the preoptic area of rats are active in different patterns during sleep. A large proportion of VLPO neurons are most active during NREM sleep and maintain high firing rates during sleep in proportion to cumulative sleep need. These neurons contain GABA and the inhibitory peptide galanin. Many MnPO neurons are most active early in sleep episodes and show highest firing rates during REM sleep, as do those in the extended VLPO. The VLPO and MnPO/extended VLPO play key roles in promoting the onset of NREM and REM sleep, respectively, and may be involved in mediating homeostatic regulation of sleep durations. Inhibition of neural activity in the VLPO results in rapid arousal.

The human preoptic area has several galanin-containing regions. The number of galanin-ir neurons in one of these areas (the intermediate nucleus) in postmortem brain tissue of AD patients was positively correlated with the stability of their sleep–wake states before death, suggesting that this nucleus serves a function similar to that of the VLPO in other species.

Neurons in both the VLPO and MnPO send inhibitory projections to several wake-promoting regions. The preoptic nuclei and wake-promoting systems form a mutually inhibitory (flip-flop) system that allows for transitions to sleep and waking and the stable maintenance of these states for appropriate durations. Circadian and homeostatic inputs interact with this flip-flop mechanism to ensure species-characteristic timing and durations of sleep and wake that are modulated by sleep need.

Metabolic needs also affect VLPO activity: low blood glucose levels inhibit VLPO activity and promote increased hypocretin neural activity, which may serve the function of reducing sleep and activating starving animals to find food. High-calorie meals tend to have the opposite effect, resulting in increased sleep.

Recent studies implicated glutamatergic neurotransmission in a broad preoptic area in regulation of both NREM and REM sleep but in different ways. Further studies are needed to determine the specific preoptic regions, input systems, and neural circuits that are involved in producing glutamate-related changes in sleep.

These findings emphasize the complexity of the neural circuitry responsible for sleep regulation that is being revealed by newer research methods. In particular, they emphasize the fact that brain regions with one well-characterized role in sleep regulation often contain a mixture of cell types that are involved in different ways in other aspects of sleep regulation, as was discussed in relation to the roles of different cell types in "cholinergic" pontine nuclei in Section 10.6.1.

11.5 Basal forebrain nuclei and acetylcholine

Surrounding and rostral to the anterior hypothalamus are the nuclei of the basal forebrain (BF), which play a key role in cortical activation. The nuclei composing the BF can be defined

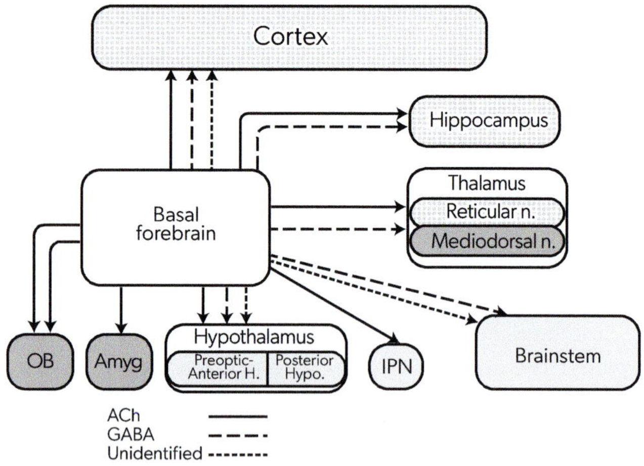

Figure 11.14 Efferent projections from basal forebrain nuclei, grouped by the functions of their target systems. Targets primarily involved in cognition are shown as stippled boxes (cortex, hippocampus, thalamic reticular nucleus). Those involved in motivation and emotion regulation are shown in dark shading (olfactory bulb, amygdala, thalamic mediodorsal nucleus). Those involved in regulation of sleep–wake and autonomic functions are shown in light shading (preoptic/anterior hypothalamus, posterior hypothalamus, interpeduncular nucleus (IPN), brainstem nuclei). Neurotransmitters involved are coded by different arrow styles: ACh (solid), GABA (dashed), unidentified (dotted). Reprinted with permission of Elsevier, Ltd. from Semba, K. Multiple output pathways of the basal forebrain: organization, chemical heterogeneity, and roles in vigilance. *Behav Brain Res* 115:117–141. © Elsevier (2000). doi: 10.1016/s0166-4328(00)00254-0.

somewhat differently, but they generally include the nucleus accumbens, nucleus basalis, substantia innominata, nucleus of the diagonal band, and medial septum. These are heterogeneous structures that are involved in different processes, but all contain cholinergic neurons, which are found among neurons containing other neurotransmitters, including glutamate, GABA, and peptides, including galanin. These neurons collectively project to all of the cerebral cortex, but also to other brain regions, including the hippocampus and thalamus. Different efferent projections reach brain regions involved in cognition, motivation, sleep, and autonomic regulation (**Figures 10.9** and **11.14**) (Semba, 2000; Woolf, 1991).

Increased firing of cholinergic neurons in the basal forebrain produces higher ACh levels in the cortex during waking and REM sleep relative to NREM sleep (Jasper & Tessier, 1971; Kanai & Szerb, 1965). A small projection from the basal forebrain to the suprachiasmatic nuclei links this cholinergic system to the circadian system, which may help to coordinate their joint regulation of sleep–wake cyclicity (Bina et al., 1993).

Basal forebrain cholinergic inputs are key to generating the cortical EEG activation that characterizes both waking and REM sleep (Détári et al., 1999; Han, Shi, et al., 2014; Jones, 2005; Semba, 2004). Cholinergic neurons differ from other arousal-related systems that use norepinephrine, serotonin, histamine, or hypocretin, which are active during waking but not during REM sleep. The unique role served by ACh is emphasized by the finding in fur seals that during unihemispheric sleep, the waking hemisphere has high acetylcholine levels, and the sleeping hemisphere has low levels (Lapierre et al., 2007) (see **Figure 7.14**). In contrast, other excitatory neurotransmitters do not show markedly asymmetric levels in the two cortices during unihemispheric sleep (Lapierre et al., 2013; Lyamin et al., 2016) (see **Figure 10.8**).

Cholinergic projections promote global cortical activation, which is necessary to sustain waking and to facilitate some cognitive functions of the awake cortex (see, e.g., Kukolja et al., 2009); damage to the cholinergic system is associated with cognitive deficits (see **Box 11.4**). Similar cortical arousal during REM sleep likely facilitates the expression of complex cognitions experienced as dreams (Sarter & Bruno, 2000). A familiar cholinergic agonist, nicotine, derived from tobacco plants, acts as an agonist for one class of ACh receptors (nicotinic) and increases alertness and attention (Myers et al., 2013). But in addition to the role of ACh in global cortical arousal, basal forebrain inputs and ACh provide precise information to cortical targets related to behavior and cognition, for example, learning about reward timing (Liu et al., 2015).

The activating effects of ACh are terminated by the enzyme acetylcholinesterase (AChE), which catabolizes ACh. Blocking AChE activity with an inhibitor results in increased arousal and cortical activation by prolonging the synaptic action of ACh. The AChE inhibitor physostigmine has different effects on sleep depending on the initial state of the individual. Given systemically to people during NREM sleep, it induces a transition to REM sleep (consistent with the role of ACh in triggering REM sleep; see Section 10.7.2); but if given during REM sleep, it triggers waking (Sitaram et al., 1976).

Basal forebrain cholinergic (and other) neurons contribute to cortical activation and cognition via direct projections to the cortex, hippocampus, amygdala, and other structures (Semba, 2000; Woolf, 1991). Cholinergic projections from the mesopontine ACh nuclei (PPT and LDT), which do not reach the cortex, promote cortical activation indirectly by their input to basal forebrain and thalamic systems that project to the cortex; see **Figure 10.9**. These indirect projections may be especially important in helping to activate the cortex during REM sleep, in the absence of activating inputs from monoamine and peptide systems. Consistent with this idea, ACh levels in the basal forebrain rise higher during REM sleep than during waking (Vazquez & Baghdoyan, 2001). These levels probably reflect a combination of cholinergic input from the PPT/LDT along with local release of ACh from basal forebrain cholinergic neurons.

BOX 11.4 Cognition, Cholinergic Activity and "Cognitive Enhancement"

Mild memory impairment in aging has been linked to a reduced function of cholinergic neurons projecting to the cortex and hippocampus. More extensive degeneration of these neurons is related to EEG slowing and the severe loss of cognitive function (and disruption of sleep–wake rhythms) seen in dementing conditions such as Alzheimer's disease (AD) (Hut & Van der Zee, 2011; Montplaisir et al., 1998; Schliebs & Arendt, 2010). High cortical ACh levels during waking may be essential for acquiring new information (Kukolja et al., 2009), and decreased levels during NREM sleep may be important for later consolidating newly acquired memories (Conner et al., 2003; Gais & Born, 2004; Hasselmo, 2006); see Section 18.13. As a result, disruption of cholinergic functions can cause deficits in the processes of learning and consolidating memory.

Reversible AChE inhibitors (e.g., donepezil (Aricept™)), which prolong ACh-mediated neurotransmission, can improve memory and other cognitive functions in patients with AD (Bond et al., 2012) and may slow progression of cognitive symptoms. These drugs do not, however, target the underlying neural degeneration; instead, they improve function by compensating in part for the downstream cholinergic deficits that result from the disease process.

The idea that AChE inhibitors can also produce "cognitive enhancement" in healthy individuals has become quite popular, but it appears to be based on very little evidence relevant to the general population, rather than to AD patients (Repantis et al., 2010). This may not be surprising, since the benefits of AChE inhibitors in AD patients is related to partially reversing a demonstrated cholinergic deficit. It does not necessarily follow that the same drugs would benefit healthy people who have intact cholinergic systems.

The growth and dissemination of the idea of cholinergic-based cognitive enhancement in healthy people has been studied by neuroethicists as an example of how very limited and ambiguous research findings can be exaggerated and distorted in commercial communications aimed at the general public (Wade et al., 2014).

The idea that local release of ACh within the basal forebrain is important for cortical arousal is supported by studies using optogenetic activation. Selectively activating basal forebrain cholinergic neurons increased waking and reduced sleep, but this effect was blocked by injecting a cholinergic antagonist *locally* into the basal forebrain at the same time. This finding indicates that cortical activation depended on the release of ACh within the basal forebrain, which in turn activated other basal forebrain neurons (e.g., glutamatergic and GABAergic neurons) that project to the cortex (Zant et al., 2016).

Some GABAergic neurons in the basal forebrain that project to the cortex promote cortical synchrony and sleep, as might be expected for an inhibitory neurotransmitter (Xu et al., 2015). However, other GABAergic projections from these nuclei that reach both the cortex and thalamus (Gritti et al., 1997; Gritti et al., 1998) instead promote cortical activation and waking (Brown & McKenna, 2015; Jones, 2017).

Increasing cortical activation by the release of GABA in the cortex requires an intervening step. That step is inhibition by GABA of cortical (and perhaps thalamic) GABAergic interneurons, resulting in disinhibition (excitation) of cortical pyramidal neurons (Freund & Meskenaite, 1992). The importance of this mechanism was demonstrated by evidence that neurochemical injections into the basal forebrain that selectively ablated GABAergic neurons, but largely spared cholinergic cells, reduced cortical arousal and deepened sleep. By removing inhibitory input from the basal forebrain to cortical GABAergic interneurons, these lesions allowed them to more strongly hyperpolarize cortical pyramidal neurons and increase the amount of delta-band activity during sleep (Kaur et al., 2008).

Basal forebrain cholinergic neurons are also involved in mediating the homeostatic increases in NREM sleep that occur after sleep loss. Relatively selective cholinergic lesions of this region in rats reduced rebound increases in NREM sleep after 6 h of sleep deprivation. Neurotoxic lesions of the same region that selectively spared cholinergic neurons had much less effect on NREM sleep rebound (Kaur et al., 2008) (**Figure 11.15**). As discussed in Section 11.6, these results are consistent with a specific role for basal forebrain cholinergic neurons in mediating the effects of adenosine, which signals homeostatic sleep need through its accumulation in the basal forebrain (Basheer et al., 2004; Kalinchuk et al., 2011).

11.5.1 Summary

The basal forebrain nuclei comprise a mixture of cells that include ACh, GABA, and glutamate. These neurons project to the cortex, hippocampus, and other brain regions involved in the regulation of cognition, motivation/emotion, and sleep/waking. Basal forebrain cholinergic neurons are active during waking and REM sleep, unlike other wake-promoting systems that contribute to cortical activation only during waking. Brainstem cholinergic neurons (PPT/LDT) contribute to cortical activation indirectly via their projections to the basal forebrain and thalamus.

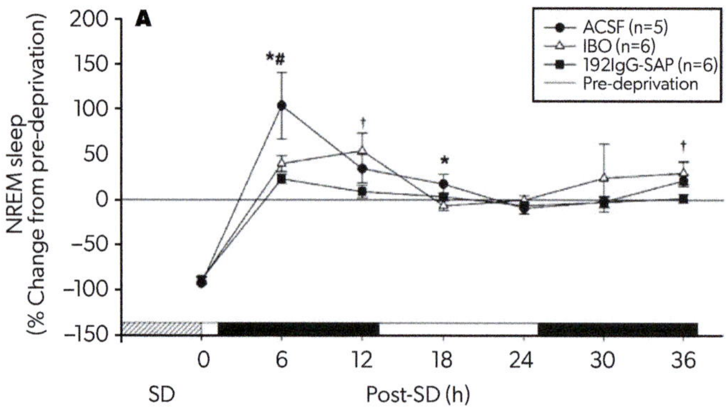

Figure 11.15 Percentage rebound increases in NREM sleep amounts in rats during 36 h of free sleep (0–36 h) after 6 h of sleep deprivation (SD), relative to pre-deprivation baseline levels (set at 0) (Y axis). Treatment groups included: control rats injected with artificial cerebrospinal fluid vehicle (ACSF; black circles) into the basal forebrain; rats that received similar injections containing the excitatory neurotoxin ibotenic acid (IBO; white triangles), which kills other cells but largely spares ACh neurons; and rats that received similar injections containing 192IgG-saporin (192IgG-SAP; black squares), which selectively kills ACh neurons. Saporin-treated rats accumulated a significantly smaller rebound increase in NREM sleep than controls after 6 h of recovery sleep (#) and significantly less than ibotenic acid-treated rats after 12 and 36 h (†); ibotenic acid-treated rats showed less increase than controls by 6 and 18 h of recovery sleep (*). The hatched area on the X axis shows the period of sleep deprivation (SD) and the white and black areas show the light–dark cycle. Loss of cholinergic neurons after saporin lesions most strongly suppressed rebound NREM sleep increases after deprivation. Reprinted with permission from Kaur, S. et al. (2008) Effects of ibotenate and 192IgG-saporin lesions of the nucleus basalis magnocellularis/substantia innominata on spontaneous sleep and wake states and on recovery sleep after sleep deprivation in rats. *J Neurosci* 28:491–504. © Society for Neuroscience (2008). doi: 10.1523/JNEUROSCI.1585-07.2008.

In addition to cholinergic and glutamatergic projections to the cortex, GABAergic neurons in the basal forebrain also activate the cortex by inhibiting GABAergic interneurons and thereby disinhibiting cortical pyramidal neurons. Local release of ACh by neurons within the basal forebrain nuclei is important for maintaining waking. This effect was demonstrated by injecting a cholinergic antagonist locally into the basal forebrain nuclei, which blocked the increased waking that would otherwise follow optogenetic activation of basal forebrain ACh neurons.

Cholinergic mechanisms in the basal forebrain also contribute to the homeostatic regulation of sleep. Rebound increases in sleep after deprivation were strongly reduced by neurochemical lesions in the basal forebrain that specifically targeted cholinergic neurons. Lesions that affected other neuronal types, but largely spared cholinergic neurons, were less effective.

Thus, cholinergic neurons (as well as glutamatergic and GABAergic neurons) in the basal forebrain are involved in maintaining alert wakefulness, activating the cortex during REM sleep, and contributing to the homeostatic regulation of sleep.

11.6 Adenosine, astrocytes, and sleep homeostasis

11.6.1 Adenosine

Adenosine is a nucleoside composed of an adenine molecule and a sugar. Combined with three phosphate groups, it forms the molecule adenosine triphosphate (ATP), which is the principal energy source for cellular metabolic activity. Combining adenosine with one or two phosphate groups forms AMP and ADP (adenosine mono- and diphosphate), respectively. Adenosine is transported into cells and incorporated into ATP using energy derived from the oxidation (metabolism) of glucose. This process results in the formation of high-energy bonds between the adenosine molecule and the three phosphate groups. When cells are active, these bonds are broken, liberating energy that is used in many cellular processes and releasing free adenosine extracellularly. Free adenosine can also be formed extracellularly through enzymatic breakdown of ATP (or ADP, AMP) (Huang et al., 2014; Reichert et al., 2022).

As a result of neuronal metabolic activity, extracellular levels of adenosine increase in some brain regions (especially the basal forebrain and cortex) when cells are more active during waking than during sleep. Levels increase further during prolonged waking (i.e., sleep deprivation), and fall during recovery sleep (Porkka-Heiskanen & Kalinchuk, 2011; Porkka-Heiskanen et al., 2000) (**Figure 11.16**). Thus, the level of extracellular adenosine in these brain regions reflects the strength of the homeostatic sleep drive; high levels play an important role in triggering sleep onset. Cholinergic basal forebrain neurons are a major target for the effects of adenosine on sleep (Basheer et al., 2004; Strecker et al., 2000) and mediate homeostatic responses to sleep loss (Kalinchuk et al., 2008; Kaur et al., 2008).

Extracellular adenosine in the brain binds to two principal subtypes of membrane-bound receptors, A_1 and A_{2a}, which are linked to different cellular second messenger responses: inhibition via A_1 and excitation via A_{2a} (Huang et al., 2014). Activation of each receptor subtype in different brain regions promotes sleep onset but in different ways.

Adenosine acts postsynaptically via A_1 receptors to inhibit basal forebrain cholinergic neurons and presynaptically to inhibit glutamatergic inputs to these neurons. Together these effects reduce the firing rates of basal forebrain cholinergic

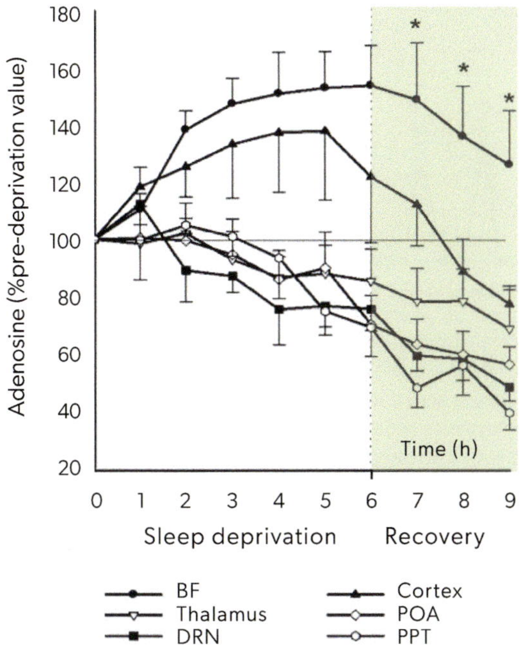

Figure 11.16 Impact of sleep deprivation and recovery sleep on changes in concentration of adenosine, relative to baseline values (= 100%, Y axis) in different brain regions of cats. Cats were sleep-deprived for 6 h (0-6) followed by a 3 h free-sleep recovery period (6-9). Adenosine levels increased in the cortex (black triangles) but even more strongly in the basal forebrain (BF; black circles) throughout the 6 h sleep deprivation period (hours 1-6). Other brain regions (thalamus, dorsal raphe nucleus (DRN), preoptic area (POA), and pedunculopontine tegmental nucleus (PPT)) showed no change or small decreases in adenosine levels. Adenosine levels fell throughout the 3 h recovery sleep period in all brain regions. Adapted with permission of Elsevier, Ltd. from Porkka-Heiskanen, T. et al. Brain site-specificity of extracellular adenosine concentration changes during sleep deprivation and spontaneous sleep: an in vivo microdialysis study. *Neuroscience* 99(3):507-517. © IBRO (2000). Published by Elsevier. doi: 10.1016/s0306-4522(00)00220-7.

neurons and reduce their wake-promoting effects on the cortex, thereby facilitating sleep onset (Basheer et al., 2004; Hawryluk et al., 2012; Strecker et al., 2000; Thakkar et al., 2003) (**Figure 11.17 A**). Adenosine also acts via A_1 receptors to promote onset of NREM sleep by inhibiting wake-promoting HA neurons in the TMN of the hypothalamus (Oishi et al., 2008) and hypocretin neurons in the lateral hypothalamus (Alam et al., 2009; Thakkar et al., 2008) (**Figure 11.17 B**).

Another route by which adenosine contributes to sleep onset is via excitatory A_{2a} receptors on sleep-promoting VLPO neurons (Gallopin et al., 2005) and neurons in the nucleus accumbens (part of the basal forebrain) (Lazarus et al., 2011), which send inhibitory projections to several wake-promoting systems (**Figure 11.17 C**); for a review, see Huang et al., 2014. Thus, adenosine acts directly and indirectly on several critical subcortical nuclei involved in regulation of sleep and waking. It reduces the activity of wake-promoting systems (basal forebrain, TMN, pfLH) and increases the activity of sleep-promoting systems (VLPO and nucleus accumbens).

Adenosine and its receptors are involved in homeostatic and allostatic responses to chronic sleep restriction (see Section 5.4.1); in particular, they are involved in the production of slow-wave activity (SWA) during slow-wave sleep (SWS). Mice that received injections into the cerebral ventricles of a highly selective A_1 receptor agonist showed large increases in SWA, and the frequency characteristics of their EEG closely resembled those of mice recovering from total sleep deprivation (Benington et al., 1995).

Mice with a conditional knockout that eliminated A_1 receptors from neurons showed similar sleep patterns to wild-type mice at baseline (except for a small decrease in SWA during SWS) and normal performance on a working memory task. During 48 h of continuous 6 h cycles of sleep restriction/recovery (4 h deprivation/2 h recovery), however, those lacking A_1

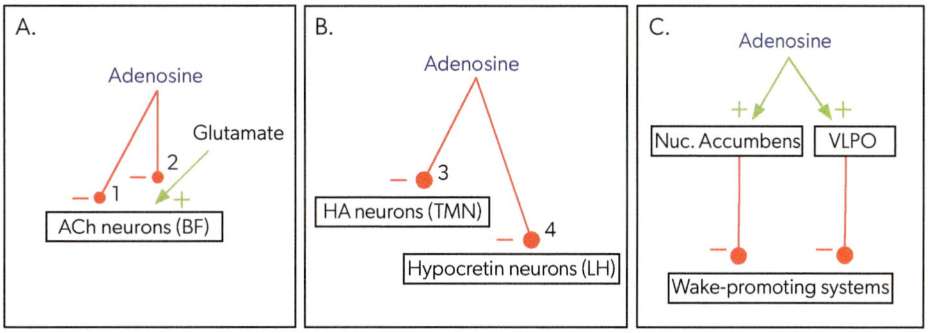

Figure 11.17 **A.** Adenosine acts via inhibitory A_1 receptors (–) to reduce firing of basal forebrain (BF) ACh neurons by direct (postsynaptic) inhibitory effects (1) and by inhibiting release of excitatory (+) glutamatergic input presynaptically (2). **B.** It also acts postsynaptically to inhibit histamine (HA) neurons in the tuberomammillary nucleus (TMN) (3) and hypocretin neurons in the perifornical lateral hypothalamus (LH) (4). Each of these effects would reduce release of neurotransmitters involved in maintaining waking and would therefore promote sleep onset. **C.** Adenosine also acts via excitatory A_{2a} receptors (+) to increase the activity of neurons in the nucleus accumbens (a basal forebrain nucleus) and the ventrolateral preoptic nucleus (VLPO), both of which send inhibitory projections to several wake-promoting systems. Adenosine binding to these receptors would therefore strengthen the inhibition of wake-promoting systems and promote sleep onset.

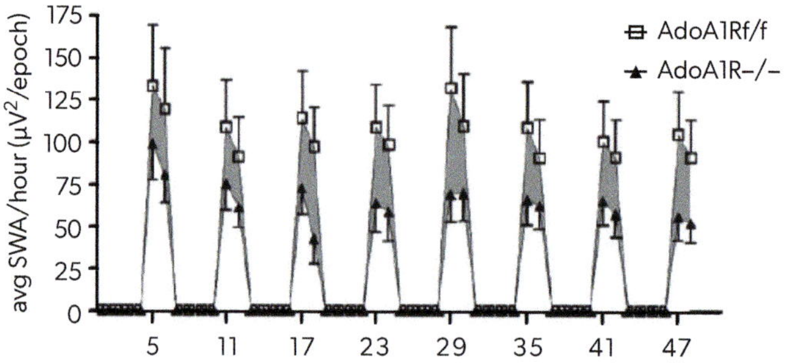

Figure 11.18 Slow-wave activity (SWA) within slow-wave sleep (SWS) in mice during 48 h of alternating periods of 4 h sleep deprivation (black bars on X axis) and 2 h free sleep; SWS occurred during the free sleep periods. The plot shows the average amount of SWA/h within SWS for control mice with functional A_1 receptors (white squares) and for mice with conditional knockout of the A_1 receptor gene (black triangles). The grey areas show the differences in amounts of SWA between these mouse strains at each time point. In the absence of A_1 receptors, there was much less compensatory increase in SWA after sleep loss, compared to mice with intact receptors. Reprinted with permission from Bjorness T.E. et al. (2009) Control and function of the homeostatic sleep response by A1 receptors. *J Neurosci* 29:1267–1276. © Society for Neuroscience (2009). doi: 10.1523/JNEUROSCI.2942-08.2009.

receptors showed greatly decreased expression of SWA in SWS during the recovery periods (**Figure 11.18**). In addition, the knockout mice showed cognitive deficits on the working memory task administered during the intervening 2 h wake periods after sleep deprivation. Thus, the loss of A_1 receptors reduced the amount of SWA shown during short recovery periods after sleep loss, and this reduction in SWA was associated with deficits in working memory performance. When allowed a full recovery day with free sleep, the knockout mice recovered their baseline working memory performance (Bjorness et al., 2009).

These findings reinforce the conclusion that A_1 receptors (and therefore adenosine) are specifically involved in modulating the production of SWA, especially following sleep loss. The fact that cognitive performance was restored in the knockout mice lacking A_1 receptors when allowed to sleep freely for 24 h indicates that other mechanisms can also contribute to homeostatic recovery from the effects of sleep loss but perhaps not within short recovery episodes (Bjorness et al., 2009).

In a study discussed in Section 5.4.1, mice that had a prior history of chronic sleep restriction responded to acute, total sleep loss with smaller rebound increases in sleep during a recovery period, compared to naïve controls. They also showed a smaller increase in adenosine levels, measured in hippocampal slices (Clasadonte et al., 2014) (see **Figure 5.10**). These results are consistent with the idea that higher adenosine levels promote homeostatic recovery sleep and suggest that changes in adenosine levels may be a component of allostatic adjustments made in response to chronic sleep loss (see also Kim et al., 2012).

11.6.2 Adenosine antagonists

Adenosine receptors are the targets on which methylxanthines act. These chemicals are the most commonly used psychoactive agents in the world, namely, caffeine, theobromine, and (to a lesser extent) theophylline. They are the principal psychoactive agents in coffee beans, tea leaves, kola nuts, cocoa beans, and their products (including chocolate in its many forms) and in many soft drinks (Fredholm et al., 1999; Reyes & Cornelis, 2018). All of these chemicals act as antagonists at the adenosine A_1 and A_{2a} receptors (among other effects), thereby preventing adenosine from binding to these receptors and from affecting the neurons on which they are located.

By preventing adenosine from exerting its sleep-promoting actions, these drugs function as stimulants, wake promoters, and vigilance enhancers (Jacobson et al., 2020; Reichert et al., 2022). As a result, excess intake of tea, coffee, and many soft drinks, some of which consumers do not recognize as having high caffeine content, is a frequent contributor to sleep problems. These effects can be even more pronounced among those deliberately dosing themselves with high-caffeine "energy drinks" (e.g., Red Bull™, Monster™, and many others). The actual cellular "energy" source in these drinks is their very high sugar content; their caffeine content contributes only blockade of adenosine receptors.

Because caffeine antagonizes the action of adenosine at both A_1 and A_{2a} receptors, its wake-promoting (and sleep-disrupting) effects may be related to either or both receptor subtypes. One study demonstrated that knockout mice that could not produce A_1 receptors still showed a strong waking response to a moderate dose of caffeine, while those lacking A_{2a} receptors showed no increase in waking when given caffeine (Huang et al., 2005) (**Figure 11.19**). These results indicate a dominant role for the A_{2a} receptor in mediating caffeine's wake-promoting effects in mice (Huang et al., 2014; Lazarus et al., 2011). Although there may be differences among species, this finding is consistent with evidence that structural variations in the A_{2a} gene are related to how sensitive people are

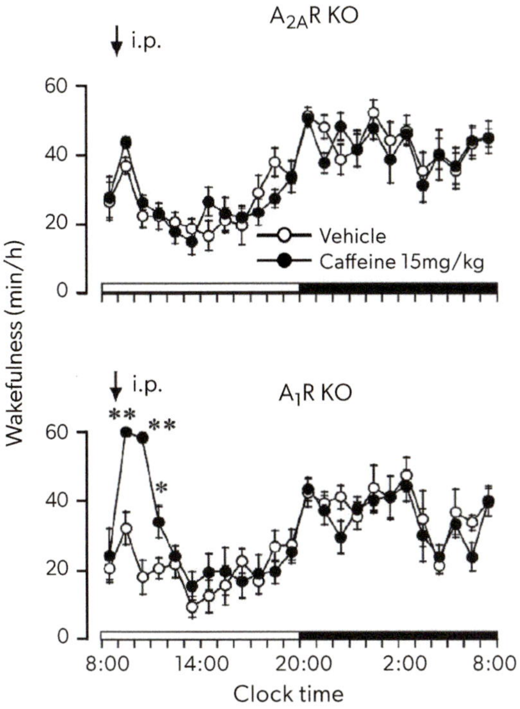

Figure 11.19 Top panel: Effects of injecting a single intraperitoneal dose (i.p., arrow) of 15 mg/kg caffeine (black circles) or control vehicle (white circles) in knockout mice lacking the A_{2A} receptor (A_{2A}R KO). Caffeine treatments did not alter the amount of hourly wakefulness (Y axis) shown over the next day, compared to vehicle controls. **Bottom panel:** A similar experiment using mice lacking the A_1 receptor (A_1R KO) resulted in a robust increase in wakefulness during the 2–3 h following treatment with caffeine. These results imply a critical role for the A_{2A} receptor subtype in mediating the wake-promoting effects of caffeine in mice. The X axis shows the light-dark cycle and clock time. Reprinted with permission from Huang, Z.L. et al. (2005) Adenosine A2A, but not A1, receptors mediate the arousal effect of caffeine. *Nat Neurosci* 8:858–859. © Springer:Nature (2005). doi: 10.1038/nn1491.

to the wake-promoting effects of caffeine (Byrne et al., 2012; Rétey et al., 2006; Rétey et al., 2007).

Caffeine consumption by people at night not only promotes waking but also delays and reduces the nocturnal rise in melatonin levels (Wright Jr et al., 1997). This finding can be explained by the ability of caffeine to delay the circadian rhythm of the SCN (Ding et al., 1998), which regulates melatonin secretion (see Section 9.2.2). Delaying the rise of melatonin would delay its sleep-promoting effect (see Section 9.5) and thus further prolong waking. This effect of caffeine is mediated by its antagonism at A_1 receptors, and through other cellular mechanisms (Burke et al., 2015; Ding et al., 1998). Caffeine also elevates nocturnal body temperature (Wright Jr et al., 1997), probably in part because it suppresses and delays the nocturnal rise of melatonin, which decreases body temperature (Cagnacci et al., 1992; Cagnacci et al., 1993) (see **Figure 9.12**).

Although subcortical centers involved in the system-level control of sleep and waking accumulate adenosine during waking, there is also more modest adenosine accumulation in the cortex while awake (see **Figure 11.16**) (Porkka-Heiskanen et al., 2000). This increase presumably reflects high metabolic rates of cortical cells during waking, resulting in an increased rate of free adenosine release (Benington et al., 1995). Cortical areas that are especially active during waking would be expected to generate higher local levels of extracellular adenosine, resulting in increased local cortical "sleepiness." In fact, experimental manipulations that selectively increased the activity of local cortical regions resulted in increased SWA in these areas during later sleep. These results indicate a stronger local sleep drive as a result of increased cortical activity (Kattler et al., 1994; Vyazovskiy et al., 2000). The phenomenon of localized cortical sleep is discussed further in Section 12.6.

These findings are consistent with the evidence that increased neural activity increases adenosine levels, which promotes SWA via A_1 receptors (Benington et al., 1995). They also suggest that caffeine (and other adenosine antagonists) may increase alertness in part by blocking adenosine's effects on cortical neurons as well as by acting on subcortical sleep-wake regulatory systems, such as the basal forebrain.

One study showed that activation of adenosine receptors in the prefrontal cortex of mice modulated ACh release, EEG delta power, and sleep indirectly by altering activity in a descending cortical projection to the pons (Van Dort et al., 2009). This finding closes the complex loop of sites at which adenosine may promote sleep. Adenosine can act on known subcortical sleep-regulatory systems (e.g., basal forebrain, VLPO, TMN); it can act locally in cortical regions that are active during waking; and it can affect cortical mechanisms that influence subcortical systems involved in sleep regulation.

11.6.3 Astrocytes

There is evidence that astrocytes, one of the major classes of glial cells in the brain, are an important source of adenosine and are involved in several aspects of sleep regulation. The following brief review of some aspects of the physiology of astrocytes provides background information related to this issue.

Astrocytes in the cortex occupy unique territories that create a kind of tiled mosaic, forming the substrate within which a number of neurons are embedded (Livet et al., 2007). This anatomical arrangement positions each astrocyte to influence large numbers of neurons in its local vicinity. Although astrocytes are not electrically excitable in the same way that neurons are, they are intimately involved in regulating neuronal metabolism, synaptic activity, and plasticity (Zorec et al., 2012).

Astrocytes contain the brain's supply of glycogen, which serves as its major energy reserve. Glycogen is metabolized within astrocytes to produce glucose and/or lactate, which are provided to neurons as their primary energy sources (Pellerin & Magistretti, 2012; Schurr, 2006). One hypothesis about the function of sleep is that it allows astrocytes to replenish glycogen stores, which are then used during waking as a neuronal energy source, thereby maintaining brain energy metabolism (Benington & Heller, 1995). Evidence supporting this hypothesis includes decreases in levels of stored glycogen during sleep deprivation and increases during recovery sleep (Kong et al., 2002). Similarly, there are changes in the expression of genes related to glycogen metabolism during the sleep–wake cycle and in response to sleep deprivation (Petit et al., 2010).

Astrocytes also engage in gliotransmission, the release into extracellular space of active substances that can affect neurons locally and, as a result of diffusion, probably more broadly. Astrocytes respond to neuronal signals and in turn release substances (including ATP, which is metabolized to release free adenosine) that affect neuronal regulation of sleep and waking (Bojarskaite et al., 2020; Ingiosi & Frank, 2022; Ingiosi et al., 2020; Pascual et al., 2005).

Mice that were genetically engineered so that their astrocytes could not release adenosine differed from wild-type mice in several ways. They showed less accumulation of sleep pressure during waking, as indexed by reduced SWA during spontaneous sleep and during recovery sleep after deprivation. They also showed fewer cognitive deficits after sleep loss, supporting the idea of reduced functional sleepiness. These mice also did not show a reduction in sleep time after pharmacological blockade of adenosine receptors, as wild-type mice do. These findings indicate that astrocytes are a source of increased extracellular adenosine that promotes sleepiness, and that preventing astrocytic release increases arousal and disrupts sleep homeostasis (Halassa et al., 2009; Schmitt et al., 2012).

This conclusion was questioned based on evidence that the approach used to block release of adenosine from astrocytes could also affect neurons (Fujita et al., 2014). However, there is other evidence supporting a role for astrocytes in sleep regulation. For example, an adenosine-regulating enzyme was shown to sense the metabolic state of glia and to act via a glial-neuronal circuit to regulate sleep homeostasis (Bjorness et al., 2016).

Other studies reported that calcium ion (Ca^{2+}) signaling in astrocytes is involved in several aspects of sleep–wake regulation, including SWS homeostasis and arousal from SWS (Bojarskaite et al., 2020; Cai et al., 2022; Ingiosi & Frank, 2022; Ingiosi et al., 2020). A chemogenetic (DREADD-based) approach (see Appendix C) was used in basal forebrain astrocytes of mice to activate G proteins that are linked to increasing astrocytic Ca^{2+} levels. This manipulation produced sustained waking during the light phase when mice normally show substantial sleep periods. The resulting decreases in both REM and NREM sleep did not induce a rebound increase in sleep amounts or NREM delta power during the subsequent dark phase.

In contrast, mice sleep-deprived by gentle handling during the same daily phase showed the expected increases in sleep and NREM delta power during the subsequent dark phase (Ingiosi et al., 2023). These results indicate that the astrocytic mechanisms involved in triggering wakefulness did not engage the usual homeostatic responses to sleep loss, at least within the 24 h period that was studied. They also imply that increased waking induced by glial activation did not trigger the full cascade of responses that follow sleep loss induced in other ways, suggesting that these responses, rather than waking itself, are responsible for homeostatic regulation of sleep amounts and quality. See (Ingiosi et al., 2023) for further discussion of the implications of these results.

11.6.4 Summary

Adenosine is a product of the catabolism of ATP (or ADP/AMP), the brain's principal source of cellular energy. During more intense neural activity, free adenosine accumulates extracellularly and binds to several classes of receptors, the most important of which for sleep are the inhibitory A_1 and excitatory A_{2a} receptors.

Adenosine reduces cortical activation in several ways. Via its A_1 receptors, it directly inhibits ACh neurons in the basal forebrain and reduces their activation by glutamatergic inputs. It also inhibits hypocretin and histamine neurons in the hypothalamus that contribute to cortical activation. Via its A_{2a} receptors, it activates neurons in the nucleus accumbens and VLPO, which provide inhibitory inputs to several wake-promoting systems. The effects of adenosine occur not only on subcortical regulatory mechanisms, like those in the basal forebrain, but also in the cortex where adenosine levels rise in response to increased neural activity related to local cortical functions. The net effect of increased adenosine is therefore to reduce cortical activation and to support sleep onset.

Activating A_1 receptors pharmacologically increased SWA, implying an important role for this subtype in sleep homeostasis. This conclusion was supported by studies of knockout mice lacking A_1 receptors. During cycles of sleep deprivation and recovery opportunities, these mice showed reduced homeostatic increases of SWA during their recovery sleep opportunities and resulting impairment of cognitive functions while awake.

The psychoactive substances most commonly used by people are those containing caffeine, including coffee, tea, kola nut-based, and other soft drinks, as well as cocoa in many forms. These all contain caffeine, theobromine, and other chemicals that are potent antagonists at adenosine receptors. In mice, caffeine acts by blocking A_{2a} receptors to promote waking, and variations in the A_{2a} gene in people are related to their caffeine sensitivity. Caffeine also affects sleep by delaying the onset of melatonin secretion and allowing body temperature to remain elevated, both of which would reduce the likelihood of sleep onset.

The means by which adenosine buildup triggers homeostatic increases in cortical SWA involve a glial sensing mechanism that interacts with neurons to hyperpolarize them and make them more likely to produce slow waves. Astrocytes are an important source of the extracellular adenosine that affects neurons and are involved in homeostatic responses to sleep loss. Increasing Ca^{2+} levels in basal forebrain astrocytes induced sustained waking that did not trigger immediate rebound increases in sleep/delta activity as does behavioral sleep deprivation. This finding indicates that inducing waking through astroglial activation did not trigger the same responses as waking that is induced behaviorally and leads to homeostatic increases in SWA. These results imply that homeostatic responses depend on other mechanisms being activated by sleep loss, and not only on the presence of excess waking.

11.7 Other physiological regulators of sleep

11.7.1 Prostaglandin D2

Prostaglandins are a family of lipid-containing chemicals that are secreted by cells in most parts of the body. Prostaglandins can be distinguished from hormones, which are secreted by organized endocrine glands in one site (e.g., adrenal or pituitary gland) and are distributed through the circulation to act broadly on distant tissues. Prostaglandins function mostly through paracrine action (i.e., they affect tissues locally where they are produced and secreted, although some may act more remotely). Prostaglandins serve a variety of local functions related to reproduction, circulation, respiration, immune responses, and most other physiological functions (Katz & Katz, 1974). Treatments that use natural or synthetic prostaglandins, or that regulate the cyclooxygenase enzymes (COX 1 & 2) that produce prostaglandins, are used in the treatment of many clinical conditions (Dannhardt & Kiefer, 2001).

One prostaglandin (PG), D_2, is produced principally in the pia-arachnoid meninges (membranes covering the brain) near the basal forebrain and in the ventricular choroid plexus, and is then secreted into the cerebrospinal fluid (CSF) (Cherasse et al., 2018; Urade & Hayaishi, 1999). It is the most abundant prostaglandin in the brain and has been implicated in sleep regulation by several lines of evidence (Huang et al., 2007).

Levels of the synthetic enzyme for PGD_2 measured in blood serum were highest in people during sleep at night, and the daily rhythm was disrupted during sleep deprivation (Jordan et al., 2004). In rats, the levels of PGD_2 in the CSF were instead higher during the daily light phase (Pandey et al., 1995) and increased with increasing length of sleep deprivation. Comparison of levels during sleep and wake at different times of day in rats showed highest levels during daytime sleep and lower levels during nighttime sleep. These results indicate that PGD_2 levels were regulated by both sleep-related and circadian factors (Ram et al., 1997).

Infusion of physiological amounts of PGD_2 into the CSF triggers a short-latency transition to polygraphically normal sleep in a number of species, including rhesus monkeys. The binding protein for PGD_2 is concentrated in the preoptic area (which includes the VLPO), and infusion of PGD_2 into the nearby third ventricle of monkeys is especially effective in triggering sleep (Onoe et al., 1988). Preventing production of PGD_2, or blocking the receptor on which it acts, prevents the homeostatic increases in sleep duration normally observed after sleep deprivation. In summary, PGD_2 increases in association with sleep, can stimulate onset of normal sleep and is involved in mediating homeostatic responses to sleep loss (Onoe et al., 1988; Urade & Hayaishi, 1999).

PGD_2 exerts these effects by stimulating the release of adenosine which binds to A_{2a} receptors to activate VLPO neurons. Activated VLPO projections then inhibit a number of wake-promoting systems (e.g., histamine neurons in the posterior hypothalamus) and trigger sleep onset (see **Figure 11.17 C**). Blocking A_{2a} receptors prevented the sleep-inducing effects of elevated PGD_2 (Huang et al., 2007; Huang et al., 2014).

11.7.2 Peptides and the immune system

For over more than a century, many different chemicals have been proposed to act as endogenous regulators of sleep. The first studies related to this topic demonstrated that blood from sleep-deprived animals could induce sleepiness in those that had not been sleep-deprived; for a review, see Kubota, 1989. Although other interpretations are possible, these results suggested that one or more chemicals circulating in the bloodstream are increased by sleep loss.

Several methods were applied to try to purify and identify circulating sleep factors, with varying degrees of success; for a review, see Borbély & Tobler, 1989. One of the successfully isolated substances, referred to initially as Factor S, was ultimately identified as a small peptide molecule containing muramic acid, one of a family of muramyl peptides (Borbély & Tobler, 1989; Krueger et al., 1978). Both muramyl peptides extracted from body fluids and a synthetic muramyl dipeptide have since been shown to cause increases in normal-appearing SWS when infused into animals' brains (Johannsen et al., 1989).

Muramyl peptides, however, unlike peptides discussed earlier in this chapter (hypocretin, MCH, galanin), are not produced by mammalian cells, but are components of bacterial cell walls. These peptides and other bacterial cell wall components evoke strong immune system responses when injected into mammals or when present in large amounts as a result of a bacterial infection. The immune system components that are up-regulated as a result of increased amounts of muramyl peptides have been shown to mediate their sleep-inducing effects.

It is a common observation that systemic acute infection or chronic tumor burden (cancer) are accompanied by increased lethargy and sleep, along with decreased food intake and activity; some of the mechanisms involved have been identified. While many immune system components can play a role, the best-studied and probably most potent agents are the pro-inflammatory cytokines interleukin (IL)-1β and tumor necrosis factor (TNF)α, which are among the cytokines produced by the immune system in response to infection (Imeri & Opp, 2009).

The effects of elevated levels of IL-1β include increased amounts of NREM sleep, but with disrupted sleep continuity, as well as reduced REM sleep amounts (Majde & Krueger, 2005). Some effects of IL-1β, as well as other pro-inflammatory cytokines, are mediated by activation of GABAergic neurons in the lateral hypothalamus, which, in turn, inhibit hypocretin neurons. Because hypocretin neurons play an important role in generating cortical arousal (see Section 11.3.4), their inhibition increases sleepiness and reduces cortical activation. This mechanism has been shown to be involved in producing the lethargy characteristic of animals suffering from infection or bearing tumors (Grossberg et al., 2011).

Changes in sleep and activity in response to infection, mediated by immune system components, likely improve defense against infection. Decreased energy expenditure as a result of reduced activity and increased NREM sleep could offset the increase in energy costs involved in responding to an infection. Energy is needed, for example, to increase production of immune system components and to generate shivering to raise body temperature (i.e., cause fever). Higher body temperatures improve immune system function but make bacterial replication less efficient (Imeri & Opp, 2009).

The sleep changes observed during infection support these functions. Disrupting NREM sleep continuity blunts the decreases in body temperature typical of NREM sleep, which would interfere with sustaining a fever. Similarly, during REM sleep, thermoregulation is disrupted and shivering is absent, so reducing REM sleep amounts could also help sustain fever (Imeri & Opp, 2009).

A remaining question is whether immune system components and bacterial products are also involved in the regulation of normal sleep outside of situations of acute infection. The healthy human body, particularly the digestive system, is inhabited by large numbers of bacteria of many different species. Variations in gut bacterial populations have been implicated in conditions ranging from obesity and digestive diseases to psychiatric disorders (Foster et al., 2016). However, the strength of the evidence supporting these proposed roles has been questioned because findings have been weak, inconsistent, and typically correlational (Walker & Hoyles, 2023).

Nevertheless, there is robust evidence that muramyl peptides of bacterial origin exert potent effects on sleep regulation. Although older estimates of bacterial cell numbers were even higher, a reevaluation indicated that an average human body contains roughly equal numbers of human and bacterial cells (Sender et al., 2016). The continuous turnover of this large bacterial biomass would ensure that there is an ongoing supply of muramyl peptides in the body. Their function in relation to sleep regulation in healthy individuals remains to be established.

There has also been increasing interest recently in the role of hormones and neurohormones in the regulation of sleep. One peptide, growth hormone releasing hormone (GHRH), for example, has been shown to trigger NREM sleep, in addition to its more familiar role in regulating the release of growth hormone from the pituitary gland (Obal & Krueger, 2004). GHRH exerts its effects on sleep by acting on GABAergic neurons in parts of the preoptic area that are known to be involved in mediating homeostatic regulation of sleep (Peterfi et al., 2010). This dual role of GHRH in promoting both growth and sleep is consistent with the timing of the release of growth hormone near the onset of N3 sleep (Redwine, 2000).

11.7.3 Nitric oxide

The gaseous neuromodulator nitric oxide (NO) is synthesized in many brain regions, including structures involved in the regulation of sleep and waking. NO is produced by the action of several enzymes and may serve different functions depending on where and how its production and release occur. One function that has been demonstrated is the role of NO in homeostatic responses to sleep loss. NO production increased during sleep deprivation, and blocking NO production in the basal forebrain region prevented rebound sleep increases after sleep deprivation (Cespuglio et al., 2012; Kalinchuk et al., 2011).

This finding is related to the fact that adenosine accumulation in the basal forebrain during prolonged waking is a trigger for sleep onset, as discussed in Section 11.6. NO is a key mediator of the production of adenosine during sleep deprivation. When NO synthesis was prevented specifically in the basal forebrain, no increase in adenosine was detected during sleep loss, and consequently there was no rebound NREM sleep increase. In addition, the sleep increase that would otherwise be stimulated by higher NO levels could be blocked by antagonists of adenosine receptors (Kalinchuk et al., 2006). Taken together, these results indicate that NO release during sleep loss is critical to initiating the cascade that results in increasing adenosine in the basal forebrain and inhibiting cholinergic activity in this region, resulting in increased sleep amounts (Cespuglio et al., 2012; Kalinchuk et al., 2011).

The link between NO and cholinergic system activation extends to the pontine cholinergic systems involved in regulating the onset of REM sleep (see Section 10.7.2). Increasing NO levels locally in the region of the medial pontine reticular formation of cats (= SLD) boosted REM sleep amounts by increasing cholinergic activity, while blocking NO production locally in this region decreased REM sleep amounts (Leonard & Lydic, 1997). Higher NO levels have also been linked to rebound increases in REM sleep amounts after sleep deprivation (Cespuglio et al., 2012). Thus, NO is involved in the regulation of normal sleep–wake patterns as well as in the sequence of events leading to compensatory increases in sleep duration after sleep loss.

11.7.4 Summary

Levels of the prostaglandin PGD_2 are elevated during the sleep phase. Injection of PGD_2 near the VLPO caused rapid onset of sleep, while preventing its production impaired homeostatic responses to sleep loss. The effects of increased PGD_2 on sleep are mediated by increases in adenosine levels and are absent if adenosine receptors are blocked.

Muramyl peptides are produced by bacteria, and levels therefore increase during bacterial infections. They are also a breakdown product of the large volume of bacteria that normally live in the human digestive system. Both naturally occurring and synthetic muramyl peptides alter human sleep. These peptides can increase total NREM sleep amounts but decrease its continuity as well as decrease the amount of REM sleep. Their effects are mediated by increases in cytokines, especially IL-1β and TNFα, which are part of the immune system response to infection or tumor burden. These changes in sleep are likely adaptive because they help preserve the capacity to maintain fevers, which could be disrupted by REM sleep, and avoid the temperature decrease characteristic of sustained SWS. Fevers are beneficial in dealing with infections because they benefit the immune system and impair bacterial replication. Several other peptides that are not bacterial products (e.g., GHRH) have also been shown to promote sleep.

Nitric oxide (NO) is generated in many regions of the brain and functions as a neuromodulator. It acts on cholinergic systems in the basal forebrain and pons to affect the expression of NREM and REM sleep. NO mediates the effects of extended waking on adenosine accumulation in the basal forebrain and therefore on adenosine receptor-mediated increases in rebound sleep. NO in the basal forebrain is ineffective if adenosine receptors are blocked. Pontine injections of NO affect the REM initiation mechanism in the SLD by increasing cholinergic drive, resulting in increased REM sleep amounts and contributing to compensatory REM sleep increases following sleep loss.

11.8 Overview of forebrain systems involved in sleep regulation

Several neural mechanisms in the forebrain are involved in regulating sleep and waking. Waking and cortical activation depend on inputs from the following systems: thalamus (glutamate), pfLH (hypocretin), TMN (histamine), and basal forebrain (ACh, glutamate, and GABA, the latter acting via inhibitory interneurons). These systems receive direct or indirect excitatory inputs from brainstem activating systems, some of which also act directly on the cortex: locus coeruleus (NE), VTA/substantia nigra (dopamine), pontine tegmentum (ACh), and raphe nuclei (5-HT).

The forebrain contains a few key systems that promote falling asleep, principally the VLPO and MnPO that use GABA (and galanin in the VLPO) to inhibit wake-promoting systems. These systems interact with medullary GABAergic neurons in the parafacial zone that promote NREM sleep by their inhibition of glutamatergic neurons in the pontine parabrachial region. The parabrachial projections to the basal forebrain activate its cortical arousal system, so inhibition of parabrachial neurons promotes sleep onset.

Lateral hypothalamic hypocretin neurons promote waking in part by inhibiting sleep-promoting VLPO neurons. MCH neurons in the lateral hypothalamus inhibit hypocretin neurons and act on a number of other forebrain targets to reduce arousal and promote NREM sleep onset. Other GABAergic neurons in the LH instead promote waking by inhibiting preoptic sleep-promoting mechanisms.

During REM sleep, only a handful of mechanisms are involved in producing cortical activation, particularly cholinergic, GABAergic, and other inputs from basal forebrain nuclei to the cortex. MCH and other GABAergic neurons in the lateral hypothalamus also act via projections to the septum and TMN in the forebrain and to the midbrain periaqueductal gray to influence pontine mechanisms that trigger REM sleep. Neurons in the MCH and the MnPO are involved in REM sleep regulation, including in responding to sleep loss with homeostatic increases in REM sleep amounts.

Adenosine is a key mediator of sleep-promoting effects and therefore of NREM sleep homeostasis. It is released from cells (in an NO-dependent manner), including astrocytes, and accumulates in both basal forebrain (nucleus accumbens) and preoptic structures (VLPO), where it acts via A_{2a} receptors to activate these sleep-promoting systems. It also acts via A_1 receptors on cells in the cholinergic basal forebrain, TMN, and lateral hypothalamus to inhibit wake-promoting systems and facilitate sleep onset.

Adenosine also acts locally to increase SWA in parts of the cortex that have been unusually active during waking. Dynamic changes in adenosine levels in the basal forebrain parallel the homeostatic buildup and dissipation of sleep need. Adenosine also mediates the effects of the prostaglandin PGD_2 on sleep homeostasis. The involvement of astrocytes in the regulation of adenosine amounts gives these cells an important role in NREM sleep homeostasis.

Literature cited

Adamantidis, A., Carter, M., & De Lecea, L. (2010). Optogenetic deconstruction of sleep-wake circuitry in the brain. *Front Mol Neurosci, 2*(31), 1–9. doi: 10.3389/neuro.02.031.2009

Alam, M. A., Kostin, A., Siegel, J., McGinty, D., Szymusiak, R., & Alam, M. N. (2018). Characteristics of sleep-active neurons in the medullary parafacial zone in rats. *Sleep, 41*(10), zsy130. doi:10.1093/sleep/zsy130

Alam, M. N., Kumar, S., Rai, S., Methippara, M., Szymusiak, R., & McGinty, D. (2009). Role of adenosine A(1) receptor in the perifornical-lateral hypothalamic area in sleep-wake regulation in rats. *Brain Res, 1304*, 96–104. doi: 10.1016/j.brainres.2009.09.066

Anaclet, C., Lin, J. S., Vetrivelan, R., Krenzer, M., Vong, L., Fuller, P. M., & Lu, J. (2012). Identification and characterization of a sleep-active cell group in the rostral medullary brainstem. *J Neurosci, 32*(50), 17970–17976. doi: 10.1523/JNEUROSCI.0620-12.2012

Anaclet, C., Parmentier, R., Ouk, K., Guidon, G., Buda, C., Sastre, J. P., ... Lin, J. S. (2009). Orexin/hypocretin and histamine: distinct roles in the control of wakefulness demonstrated using knock-out mouse models. *J Neurosci, 29*(46), 14423–14438. doi: 10.1523/jneurosci.2604-09.2009

Arbon, E. L., Knurowska, M., & Dijk, D. J. (2015). Randomised clinical trial of the effects of prolonged-release melatonin, temazepam and zolpidem on slow-wave activity during sleep in healthy people. *J Psychopharmacol, 29*(7), 764–776. doi: 10.1177/0269881115581963

Aston-Jones, G., Chen, S., Zhu, Y., & Oshinsky, M. (2001). A neural circuit for circadian regulation of arousal. *Nat Neurosci, 4*(7), 732–738.

Basheer, R., Strecker, R., Thakkar, M., & McCarley, R. (2004). Adenosine and sleep/wake regulation. *Prog Neurobiol, 73*(6), 379–396. doi: 10.1016/j.pneurobio.2004.06.004

Beaudet, A., & Descarries, L. (1978). The monoamine innervation of rat cerebral cortex: synaptic and nonsynaptic axon terminals. *Neuroscience, 3*(10), 851–860. doi: 10.1016/0306-4522(78)90115-x

Bekkers, J. M. (1993). Enhancement by histamine of NMDA-mediated synaptic transmission in the hippocampus. *Science, 261*, 104–106.

Benington, J., & Heller, H. (1995). Restoration of brain energy metabolism as the function of sleep. *Prog Neurobiol, 45*, 347–360.

Benington, J. H., Kodali, S. K., & Heller, H. C. (1995). Stimulation of A1 adenosine receptors mimics the electroencephalographic effects of sleep deprivation. *Brain Res, 692*, 79–85.

Bettica, P., Squassante, L., Groeger, B., Gennery, B., Winsky-Sommerer, R., & Dijk, D.-J. (2012). Differential effects of a dual orexin receptor antagonist (SB-649868) and zolpidem on sleep initiation and consolidation, SWS, REM sleep, and EEG power spectra in a model of situational insomnia. *Neuropsychopharmacology, 37*, 1224–1233. doi: 0.1038/npp.2011.310

Bettica, P., Squassante, L., Zamuner, S., Nucci, G., Danker-Hopfe, H., & Ratti, E. (2012). The orexin antagonist SB-649868 promotes and maintains sleep in men with primary insomnia. *Sleep, 35*(8), 1097–1104. doi: 10.5665/sleep.1996

Bina, K. G., Semba, K., & Rusak, B. (1993). Localization of cholinergic neurons projecting to the suprachiasmatic nucleus of the rat. *J Comp Neurol, 335*(2), 295–307.

Bjorness, T., Kelly, C., Gao, T., Poffenberger, V., & Greene, R. (2009). Control and function of the homeostatic sleep response by A1 receptors. *J Neurosci, 29*(5), 1267–1276. doi: 0.1523/JNEUROSCI.2942-08.2009

Bjorness, T. E., Dale, N., Mettlach, G., Sonneborn, A., Sahin, B., Fienberg, A. A., Yanagisawa, M., Bibb, J. A., & Greene, R. W. (2016). An adenosine-mediated glial-neuronal circuit for homeostatic sleep. *J Neurosci, 36*(13), 3709–3721. doi: 10.1523/JNEUROSCI.3906-15.2016

Blanco-Centurion, C., Liu, M., Konadhode, R., Pelluru, D., & Shiromani, P. J. (2013). Effects of orexin gene transfer in the dorsolateral pons in orexin knockout mice. *Sleep, 36*(1), 31–40. doi: 10.5665/sleep.2296

Blanco-Centurion, C., Liu, M., Konadhode, R. P., Zhang, X., Pelluru, D., van den Pol, A. N., & Shiromani, P. J. (2016). Optogenetic activation of melanin-concentrating hormone neurons increases non-rapid eye movement and rapid eye movement sleep during the night in rats. *Eur J Neurosci, 44*(10), 2846–2857. doi: 10.1111/ejn.13410

Blouin, A. M., Fried, I., Wilson, C. L., Staba, R. J., Behnke, E. J., Lam, H. A., ... Siegel, J. M. (2013). Human hypocretin and melanin-concentrating hormone levels are linked to emotion and social interaction. *Nat Commun, 4*, 1547. doi: 10.1038/ncomms2461

Bojarskaite, L., Bjornstad, D. M., Pettersen, K. H., Cunen, C., Hermansen, G. H., Abjorsbraten, K. S., ... Nagelhus, E. A. (2020). Astrocytic Ca(2+) signaling is reduced during sleep and is involved in the regulation of slow wave sleep. *Nat Commun, 11*(1), 3240. doi: 10.1038/s41467-020-17062-2

Bond, M., Rogers, G., Peters, J., Anderson, R., Hoyle, M., Miners, A., ... Hyde, C. (2012). The effectiveness and cost-effectiveness of donepezil, galantamine, rivastigmine and memantine for the treatment of Alzheimer's disease (review of Technology Appraisal No. 111): a systematic review and economic model. *Health Technol Assess, 16*(21), 1–470. doi: 10.3310/hta16210

Borbély, A., & Tobler, I. (1989). Endogenous sleep-promoting substances and sleep regulation. *Physiol Rev, 69*(2), 605–670.

Borbély, A. A., Åkerstedt, T., Benoit, O., Holsboer, F., & Oswald, I. (1991). Hypnotics and sleep physiology: a consensus report. *Eur Arch Psychiatry Clin Neurosci, 241*, 13–21.

Bourgin, P., Hultrón-Reséndiz, S., Spier, A., Fabre, V., Morte, B., Criado, J., ... de Lecea, L. (2000). Hypocretin-1 modulates rapid eye movement sleep through activation of locus coeruleus neurons. *J Neurosci, 20*(20), 7760–7765.

Broughton, R., Valley, V., Aguirre, M., Roberts, J., Suwalski, W., & Dunham, W. (1986). Excessive daytime sleepiness and the pathophysiology of narcolepsy-cataplexy: a laboratory perspective. *Sleep*, *9*(1), 205–215.

Brown, R. E., & McKenna, J. T. (2015). Turning a negative into a positive: ascending GABAergic control of cortical activation and arousal. *Front Neurol*, *6*, 135. doi: 10.3389/fneur.2015.00135

Burgess, C. R., Oishi, Y., Mochizuki, T., Peever, J. H., & Scammell, T. E. (2013). Amygdala lesions reduce cataplexy in orexin knock-out mice. *J Neurosci*, *33*(23), 9734–9742. doi: 10.1523/JNEUROSCI.5632-12.2013

Burke, T., Markwald, R., McHill, A., Chinoy, E., Snider, J., Bessman, S., … Wright Jr, K. P. (2015). Effects of caffeine on the human circadian clock *in vivo* and *in vitro*. *Sci Transl Med*, *7*(305), 305ra146. doi: 10.1126/scitranslmed.aac5125

Buscemi, N., Vandermeer, B., Friesen, C., Bialy, L., Tubman, M., Ospina, M., … Witmans, M. (2007). The efficacy and safety of drug treatments for chronic insomnia in adults: a meta-analysis of RCTs. *J Gen Intern Med*, *22*(9), 1335–1350. doi: 10.1007/s11606-007-0251-z

Byrne, E. M., Johnson, J., McRae, A. F., Nyholt, D. R., Medland, S. E., Gehrman, P. R., … Martin, N. G. (2012). A genome-wide association study of caffeine-related sleep disturbance: confirmation of a role for a common variant in the adenosine receptor. *Sleep*, *35*(7), 967–975. doi: 10.5665/sleep.1962

Cagnacci, A., Elliott, J. A., & Yen, S. S. C. (1992). Melatonin: a major regulator of the circadian rhythm of core temperature in humans. *J Clin Endocr Metab*, *75*(2), 447–452.

Cagnacci, A., Soldani, R., & Yen, S. S. C. (1993). The effect of light on core body temperature is mediated by melatonin in women. *J Clin Endocr Metab*, *76*, 1036–1038.

Cai, P., Huang, S. N., Lin, Z. H., Wang, Z., Liu, R. F., Xiao, W. H., … Wang, W. X. (2022). Regulation of wakefulness by astrocytes in the lateral hypothalamus. *Neuropharmacology*, *221*, 109275. doi:10.1016/j.neuropharm.2022.109275

Carter, M. E., Adamantidis, A., Ohtsu, H., Deisseroth, K., & de Lecea, L. (2009). Sleep homeostasis modulates hypocretin-mediated sleep-to-wake transitions. *J Neurosci*, *29*(35), 10939–10949. doi: 10.1523/jneurosci.1205-09.2009

Cespuglio, R., Amrouni, D., Meiller, A., Buguet, A., & Gautier-Sauvigné, S. (2012). Nitric oxide in the regulation of the sleep-wake states. *Sleep Med Rev*, *16*(3), 265–279. doi: 10.1016/j.smrv.2012.01.006

Chang, R. S. L., Tran, V. T., & Snyder, S. H. (1979). Heterogeneity of histamine H_1-receptors: species variations in [^{3}H]mepyramine binding of brain membranes. *J Neurochem*, *32*, 1653–1663.

Chemelli, R., Willie, J., Sinton, C., Elmquist, J., Scammell, T., Lee, C., … Yanagisawa, M. (1999). Narcolepsy in *orexin* knockout mice: molecular genetics of sleep regulation. *Cell*, *98*, 437–451.

Cheng, P., Kalmbach, D. A., Tallent, G., Joseph, C. L., Espie, C. A., & Drake, C. L. (2019). Depression prevention via digital cognitive behavioral therapy for insomnia: a randomized controlled trial. *Sleep*, *42*(10), zsz150. doi: 10.1093/sleep/zsz150

Cherasse, Y., Aritake, K., Oishi, Y., Kaushik, M. K., Korkutata, M., & Urade, Y. (2018). The leptomeninges produce prostaglandin D2 involved in sleep regulation in mice. *Front Cell Neurosci*, *12*, 1–8. doi:10.3389/fncel.2018.00357

Chou, T. C., Scammell, T. E., Gooley, J. J., Gaus, S. E., Saper, C. B., & Lu, J. (2003). Critical role of dorsomedial hypothalamic nucleus in a wide range of behavioral circadian rhythms. *J Neurosci*, *23*(33), 10691–10702.

Chu, M., Huang, Z.-L., Qu, W.-M., Eguchi, N., Yao, M.-H., & Urade, Y. (2004). Extracellular histamine level in the frontal cortex is positively correlated with the amount of wakefulness in rats. *Neurosci Res*, *49*, 417–420. doi: 0.1016/j.neures.2004.05.001

Clasadonte, J., McIver, S. R., Schmitt, L. I., Halassa, M. M., & Haydon, P. G. (2014). Chronic sleep restriction disrupts sleep homeostasis and behavioral sensitivity to alcohol by reducing the extracellular accumulation of adenosine. *J Neurosci*, *34*(5), 1879–1891. doi: 10.1523/JNEUROSCI.2870-12.2014

Clément, O., Sapin, E., Libourel, P. A., Arthaud, S., Brischoux, F., Fort, P., & Luppi, P. H. (2012). The lateral hypothalamic area controls paradoxical (REM) sleep by means of descending projections to brainstem GABAergic neurons. *J Neurosci*, *32*(47), 16763–16774. doi: 10.1523/JNEUROSCI.1885-12.2012

Conner, J., Culberson, A., Packowski, C., Chiba, A., & Tuszynski, M. (2003). Lesions of the basal forebrain cholinergic system impair task acquisition and abolish cortical plasticity associated with motor skill learning. *Neuron*, *38*, 819–829.

Dahl, R., Holttum, J., & Trubnick, L. (1994). A clinical picture of child and adolescent narcolepsy. *J Am Acad Child Adolesc Psychiatry*, *33*(6), 834–841.

Dannhardt, G., & Kiefer, W. (2001). Cyclooxygenase inhibitors- current status and future prospects. *Eur J Med Chem*, *36*, 109–126.

Dantz, B., Edgar, D. M., & Dement, W. C. (1994). Circadian rhythms in narcolepsy: studies on a 90 minute day. *Electroencephalogr Clin Neurophysiol*, *90*, 24–35.

Dauvilliers, Y., Arnulf, I., & Mignot, E. (2007). Narcolepsy with cataplexy. *Lancet*, *369*(9560), 499–511. doi: 10.1016/s0140-6736(07)60237-2

Dauvilliers, Y., Siegel, J. M., Lopez, R., Torontali, Z. A., & Peever, J. H. (2014). Cataplexy--clinical aspects, pathophysiology and management strategy. *Nat Rev Neurol*, *10*(7), 386–395. doi: 10.1038/nrneurol.2014.97

Deboer, T., Overeem, S., Visser, N. A., Duindam, H., Frolich, M., Lammers, G. J., & Meijer, J. H. (2004). Convergence of circadian and sleep regulatory mechanisms on hypocretin-1. *Neuroscience*, *129*(3), 727–732. doi: 10.1016/j.neuroscience.2004.07.049

de Lecea, L., Kilduff, T., Peyron, C., Gao, X.-B., Foye, P., Danielson, P. E., Fukuhara, C., Battenberg, E., … Sutcliffe, J. (1998). The hypocretins: hypothalamus-specific peptides with neuroexcitatory activity. *Proc Natl Acad Sci USA*, *95*, 322–327.

De Luca, R., Nardone, S., Grace, K. P., Venner, A., Cristofolini, M., Bandaru, S. S., Sohn, L. T., Kong, D., . . . Arrigoni, E. (2022). Orexin neurons inhibit sleep to promote arousal. *Nat Commun*, *13*(1), 4163. doi:10.1038/s41467-022-31591-y

Détári, L., Rasmusson, D., & Semba, K. (1999). The role of basal forebrain neurons in tonic and phasic activation of the cerebral cortex. *Prog Neurobiol*, *58*, 249–277.

Deurveilher, S., & Semba, K. (2005). Indirect projections from the suprachiasmatic nucleus to major arousal-promoting cell groups in rat: implications for the circadian control of behavioural state. *Neuroscience*, *130*(1), 165–183. doi: 10.1016/j.neuroscience.2004.08.030

Ding, J., Buchanan, G. F., Tischkau, S., Chen, D., Kuriashklina, L., Faiman, L. E., … Gillette, M. U. (1998). A neuronal ryanodine receptor mediates light-induced phase delays of the circadian clock. *Nature*, *394*(381–384).

Eisensehr, I., Noachtar, S., von Schlippenbach, C., Uttner, I., Kleine, J., Seelos, K., & Helmchen, C. (2003). Hypersomnia associated with bilateral posterior hypothalamic lesion. *Eur Neurol*, *49*(3), 169–172. doi: 10.1159/000069088

Elias, C. F., Saper, C. B., Maratos-Flier, E., Tritos, N. A., Lee, C., Kelly, J., … Elmquist, J. K. (1998). Chemically defined projections linking the mediobasal hypothalamus and the lateral hypothalamic area. *J Comp Neurol*, *402*(4), 442–459.

España, R., Plahn, S., & Berridge, C. (2002). Circadian-dependent and circadian-independent behavioral actions of hypocretin/orexin. *Brain Res*, *943*, 224–236.

Foster, J. A., Lyte, M., Meyer, E., & Cryan, J. F. (2016). Gut microbiota and brain function: an evolving field in neuroscience. *Int J Neuropsychopharmacol*, *19*(5). doi: 10.1093/ijnp/pyv114

Fox, S. V., Gotter, A. L., Tye, S. J., Garson, S. L., Savitz, A. T., Uslaner, J. M., … Renger, J. J. (2013). Quantitative electroencephalography within sleep/wake states differentiates GABAA modulators eszopiclone and zolpidem from dual orexin receptor antagonists in rats. *Neuropsychopharmacology*, *38*(12), 2401–2408. doi: 10.1038/npp.2013.139

Fredholm, B. B., Bättig, K., Holmén, J., Nehlig, A., & Zvartau, E. E. (1999). Actions of caffeine in the brain with special reference to factors that contribute to its widespread use. *Pharmacol Rev*, *51*(1), 83–133.

Freund, T. F., & Meskenaite, V. (1992). γ-Aminobutyric acid-containing basal forebrain neurons innervate inhibitory interneurons in the neocortex. *Proc Natl Acad Sci USA*, *89*, 738–742.

Fujita, T., Chen, M. J., Li, B., Smith, N. A., Peng, W., Sun, W., … Nedergaard, M. (2014). Neuronal transgene expression in dominant-negative SNARE mice. *J Neurosci*, *34*(50), 16594–16604. doi: 10.1523/JNEUROSCI.2585-14.2014

Fulcher, B. D., Phillips, A. J., Postnova, S., & Robinson, P. A. (2014). A physiologically based model of orexinergic stabilization of sleep and wake. *PLoS One*, *9*(3), e91982. doi: 10.1371/journal.pone.0091982

Gais, S., & Born, J. (2004). Low acetylcholine during slow-wave sleep is critical for declarative memory consolidation. *Proc Natl Acad Sci USA*, *101*(7), 2140–2144. doi: 10.1073/pnas.0305404101

Gallopin, T., Luppi, P. H., Cauli, B., Urade, Y., Rossier, J., Hayaishi, O., … Fort, P. (2005). The endogenous somnogen adenosine excites a subset of sleep-promoting neurons via A2A receptors in the ventrolateral preoptic nucleus. *Neuroscience*, *134*(4), 1377–1390. doi: 10.1016/j.neuroscience.2005.05.045

Gaus, S. E., Strecker, R. E., Tate, B. A., Parker, R. A., & Saper, C. B. (2002). Ventrolateral preoptic nucleus contains sleep-active, galaninergic neurons in multiple mammalian species. *Neuroscience*, *115*(1), 285–294.

Gerashchenko, D., Chou, T. C., Blanco-Centurion, C. A., Saper, C. B., & Shiromani, P. J. (2004). Effects of lesions of the histaminergic tuberomammillary nucleus on spontaneous sleep in rats. *Sleep*, *27*(7), 1275–1281.

Gong, H., McGinty, D., Guzman-Marin, R., Chew, K. T., Stewart, D., & Szymusiak, R. (2004). Activation of c-fos in GABAergic neurones in the preoptic area during sleep and in response to sleep deprivation. *J Physiol, 556*(Pt 3), 935–946. doi: 10.1113/jphysiol.2003.056622

Gritti, I., Mainville, L., Mancia, M., & Jones, B. (1997). GABAergic and other noncholinergic basal forebrain neurons, together with cholinergic neurons, project to the mesocortex and isocortex in the rat. *J Comp Neurol, 383*, 163–177.

Gritti, I., Mariotti, M., & Mancia, M. (1998). GABAergic and cholinergic basal forebrain and preoptic-anterior hypothalamic projections to the mediodorsal nucleus of the thalamus in the cat. *Neuroscience, 85*(1), 149–178.

Grossberg, A. J., Zhu, X., Leinninger, G. M., Levasseur, P. R., Braun, T. P., Myers, M. G., & Marks, D. L. (2011). Inflammation-induced lethargy is mediated by suppression of orexin neuron activity. *J Neurosci, 31*(31), 11376–11386. doi: 10.1523/jneurosci.2311-11.2011

Gulyani, S., Wu, M.-F., Nienhuis, R., John, J., & Siegel, J. (2002). Cataplexy-related neurons in the amygdala of the narcoleptic dog. *Neuroscience, 112*(2), 355–365.

Gvilia, I., Turner, A., McGinty, D., & Szymusiak, R. (2006). Preoptic area neurons and the homeostatic regulation of rapid eye movement sleep. *J Neurosci, 26*(11), 3037–3044. doi: 10.1523/jneurosci.4827-05.2006

Gvilia, I., Xu, F., McGinty, D., & Szymusiak, R. (2006). Homeostatic regulation of sleep: a role for preoptic area neurons. *J Neurosci, 26*(37), 9426–9433. doi: 10.1523/jneurosci.2012-06.2006

Haas, H., Sergeeva, O. A., & Selbach, O. (2008). Histamine in the nervous system. *Physiol Rev, 88*, 1183–1241. doi: 10.1152/physrev.00043.2007

Hagan, J., Leslie, R., Patel, S., Evans, M., Wattam, T., Holmes, S., … Upton, N. (1999). Orexin A activates locus coeruleus cell firing and increases arousal in the rat. *Proc Natl Acad Sci USA, 96*, 10911–10915.

Halassa, M. M., Florian, C., Fellin, T., Munoz, J. R., Lee, S.-Y., Abel, T., … Frank, M. G. (2009). Astrocytic modulation of sleep homeostasis and cognitive consequences of sleep loss. *Neuron, 61*(2), 213–219. doi: 10.1016/j.neuron.2008.11.024

Han, F., Lin, L., Schormair, B., Pizza, F., Plazzi, G., Ollila, H. M., … Mignot, E. (2014). HLA DQB1*06:02 negative narcolepsy with hypocretin/orexin deficiency. *Sleep, 37*(10), 1601–1608. doi: 10.5665/sleep.4066

Han, Y., Shi, Y. F., Xi, W., Zhou, R., Tan, Z. B., Wang, H., … Yu, Y. Q. (2014). Selective activation of cholinergic basal forebrain neurons induces immediate sleep-wake transitions. *Curr Biol, 24*(6), 693–698. doi: 10.1016/j.cub.2014.02.011

Hassani, O. K., Henny, P., Lee, M. G., & Jones, B. E. (2010). GABAergic neurons intermingled with orexin and MCH neurons in the lateral hypothalamus discharge maximally during sleep. *Eur J Neurosci, 32*(3), 448–457. doi: 10.1111/j.1460-9568.2010.07295.x

Hassani, O. K., Lee, M. G., & Jones, B. (2009). Melanin-concentrating hormone neurons discharge in a reciprocal manner to orexin neurons across the sleep–wake cycle. *Proc Natl Acad Sci USA, 106*(7), 2418–2422. doi: 10.1073/pnas.0811400106

Hasselmo, M. E. (2006). The role of acetylcholine in learning and memory. *Curr Opin Neurobiol, 16*(6), 710–715. doi: 10.1016/j.conb.2006.09.002

Hawryluk, J. M., Ferrari, L. L., Keating, S. A., & Arrigoni, E. (2012). Adenosine inhibits glutamatergic input to basal forebrain cholinergic neurons. *J Neurophysiol, 107*(10), 2769–2781. doi: 10.1152/jn.00528.2011

He, Y., Jones, C., Fujiki, N., Xu, Y., Guo, B., Holder, J., … Fu, Y. (2009). The transcriptional repressor DEC2 regulates sleep length in mammals. *Science, 325*(5942), 866–870. doi: 10.1126/science.1174443

Hirano, A., Hsu, P. K., Zhang, L., Xing, L., McMahon, T., Yamazaki, M., … Fu, Y. H. (2018). DEC2 modulates orexin expression and regulates sleep. *Proc Natl Acad Sci USA, 115*(13), 3434–3439. doi: 10.1073/pnas.1801693115

Huang, Z., Urade, Y., & Hayaishi, O. (2007). Prostaglandins and adenosine in the regulation of sleep and wakefulness. *Curr Opin Pharmacol, 7*(1), 33–38. doi: 10.1016/j.coph.2006.09.004

Huang, Z. L., Qu, W. M., Eguchi, N., Chen, J. F., Schwarzschild, M. A., Fredholm, B. B., … Hayaishi, O. (2005). Adenosine A2A, but not A1, receptors mediate the arousal effect of caffeine. *Nat Neurosci, 8*(7), 858–859. doi: 10.1038/nn1491

Huang, Z.-L., Qu, W.-M., Li, W.-D., Mochizuki, T., Eguchi, E., Watanabe, T., … Hayaishi, O. (2001). Arousal effect of orexin A depends on activation of the histaminergic system. *Proc Natl Acad Sci USA, 98*(17), 9965–9970. doi: 10.1073/pnas.181330998

Huang, Z. L., Zhang, Z., & Qu, W. M. (2014). Roles of adenosine and its receptors in sleep–wake regulation. *Int Rev Neurobiol, 119*, 349–371. doi: 10.1016/B978-0-12-801022-8.00014-3

Hungs, M., & Mignot, E. (2001). Hypocretin/orexin, sleep and narcolepsy. *Bioessays, 23*(5), 397–408. doi: 10.1002/bies.1058

Hunt, N., Rodriguez, M., Waters, K., & Machaalani, R. (2015). Changes in orexin (hypocretin) neuronal expression with normal aging in the human hypothalamus. *Neurobiol Aging, 36*, 292–300. doi: 0.1016/j.neurobiolaging.2014.08.010

Hut, R. A., & Van der Zee, E. A. (2011). The cholinergic system, circadian rhythmicity, and time memory. *Behav Brain Res, 221*(2), 466–480. doi: 10.1016/j.bbr.2010.11.039

Imeri, L., & Opp, M. R. (2009). How (and why) the immune system makes us sleep. *Nat Rev Neurosci, 10*(3), 199–210. doi: 10.1038/nrn2576

Ingiosi, A. M., & Frank, M. G. (2022). Goodnight, astrocyte: waking up to astroglial mechanisms in sleep. *FEBS J, 290*(10), 2553–2564. doi: 10.1111/febs.16424

Ingiosi, A. M., Hayworth, C. R., & Frank, M. G. (2023). Activation of basal forebrain astrocytes induces wakefulness without compensatory changes in sleep drive. *J Neurosci, 43*(32), 5792–5809. doi: 10.1523/JNEUROSCI.0163-23.2023

Ingiosi, A. M., Hayworth, C. R., Harvey, D. O., Singletary, K. G., Rempe, M. J., Wisor, J. P., & Frank, M. G. (2020). A role for astroglial calcium in mammalian sleep and sleep regulation. *Curr Biol.* doi: 10.1016/j.cub.2020.08.052

Jacobson, K. A., Gao, Z. G., Matricon, P., Eddy, M. T., & Carlsson, J. (2020). Adenosine A2A receptor antagonists: from caffeine to selective non-xanthines. *Br J Pharmacol, 179*(14), 3496–3511. doi:10.1111/bph.15103

Jasper, H., & Tessier, J. (1971). Acetylcholine liberation from cerebral cortex during paradoxical (REM) sleep. *Science, 172*(3983), 601–602.

Jego, S., Glasgow, S. D., Herrera, C. G., Ekstrand, M., Reed, S. J., Boyce, R., … Adamantidis, A. R. (2013). Optogenetic identification of a rapid eye movement sleep modulatory circuit in the hypothalamus. *Nat Neurosci, 16*(11), 1637–1643. doi: 10.1038/nn.3522

Johannsen, L., Rosenthal, R. S., Martin, S. A., Cady, A. B., Obal Jr., F., Guinard, M., & Krueger, J. M. (1989). Somnogenic activity of O-acetylated and dimeric muamyl peptides. *Infect Immun, 57*(9), 2726–2732.

Jones, B. E. (2005). From waking to sleeping: neuronal and chemical substrates. *Trends Pharmacol Sci, 26*(11), 578–586. doi: 10.1016/j.tips.2005.09.009

Jones, B. E. (2017). Principal cell types of sleep-wake regulatory circuits. *Curr Opin Neurobiol, 44*, 101–109. doi: 10.1016/j.conb.2017.03.018

Jordan, W., Tumani, H., Cohrs, S., Eggert, S., Rodenbeck, A., Brunner, E., … Hajak, G. (2004). Prostaglandin D synthase (ß-trace) in healthy human sleep. *Sleep, 27*(5), 867–874.

Kalinchuk, A. V., Lu, Y., Stenberg, D., Rosenberg, P. A., & Porkka-Heiskanen, T. (2006). Nitric oxide production in the basal forebrain is required for recovery sleep. *J Neurochem, 99*(2), 483–498. doi: 10.1111/j.1471-4159.2006.04077.x

Kalinchuk, A. V., McCarley, R. W., Porkka-Heiskanen, T., & Basheer, R. (2011). The time course of adenosine, nitric oxide (NO) and inducible NO synthase changes in the brain with sleep loss and their role in the non-rapid eye movement sleep homeostatic cascade. *J Neurochem, 116*(2), 260–272. doi: 10.1111/j.1471-4159.2010.07100.x

Kalinchuk, A. V., McCarley, R. W., Stenberg, D., Porkka-Heiskanen, T., & Basheer, R. (2008). The role of cholinergic basal forebrain neurons in adenosine-mediated homeostatic control of sleep: lessons from 192 IgG-saporin lesions. *Neuroscience, 157*(1), 238–253. doi: 10.1016/j.neuroscience.2008.08.040

Kalmbach, D. A., Buysse, D. J., Cheng, P., Roth, T., Yang, A., & Drake, C. L. (2020). Nocturnal cognitive arousal is associated with objective sleep disturbance and indicators of physiologic hyperarousal in good sleepers and individuals with insomnia disorder. *Sleep Med, 71*, 151–160. doi: 10.1016/j.sleep.2019.11.1184

Kanai, T., & Szerb, J. (1965). Mesencephalic reticular activating system and cortical acetylcholine output. *Nature, 205*(4966), 80–82.

Kanba, S., & Richelson, E. (1984). Histamine H_1 receptors in human brain labelled with [^{3}H]doxepin. *Brain Res, 304*(1), 1–7. doi: 10.1016/0006-8993(84)90856-4

Kantor, S., Mochizuki, T., Lops, S. N., Ko, B., Clain, E., Clark, E., … Scammell, T. E. (2013). Orexin gene therapy restores the timing and maintenance of wakefulness in narcoleptic mice. *Sleep, 36*(8), 1129–1138. doi: 10.5665/sleep.2870

Kattler, H., Dijk, D.-J., & Borbély, A. (1994). Effect of unilateral somatosensory stimulation prior to sleep on the sleep EEG in humans. *J Sleep Res, 3*, 159–164.

Katz, R. L., & Katz, G. J. (1974). Prostaglandins - basic and clinical considerations. *Anesthesiology, 40*(5), 471–493.

Kaur, S., Junek, A., Black, M. A., & Semba, K. (2008). Effects of ibotenate and 192IgG-saporin lesions of the nucleus basalis magnocellularis/substantia innominata on spontaneous sleep and wake states and on recovery sleep after sleep deprivation in rats. *J Neurosci, 28*(2), 491–504. doi: 10.1523/JNEUROSCI.1585-07.2008

Kaushik, M. K., Aritake, K., Cherasse, Y., Imanishi, A., Kanbayashi, T., Urade, Y., & Yanagisawa, M. (2021). Induction of narcolepsy-like symptoms by orexin receptor antagonists in mice. *Sleep, 44*(8), zsab043. doi:10.1093/sleep/zsab043

Kelz, M. B., Sun, Y., Chen, J., Cheng Meng, Q., Moore, J. T., Veasey, S. C., … Yanagisawa, M. (2008). An essential role for orexins in emergence from general anesthesia. *Proc Natl Acad Sci USA, 105*(4), 1309–1314. doi: 10.1073/pnas.0707146105

Kilduff, T. S. (2023). The mystery of gamma-hydoxybutyrate efficacy in narcolepsy type 1. *Sleep, 46*(9), zsad156. doi:10.1093/sleep/zsad156

Kim, Y., Bolortuya, Y., Chen, L., Basheer, R., McCarley, R. W., & Strecker, R. E. (2012). Decoupling of sleepiness from sleep time and intensity during chronic sleep restriction: evidence for a role of the adenosine system. *Sleep, 35*(6), 861–869. doi: 10.5665/sleep.1890

Konadhode, R. R., Pelluru, D., Blanco-Centurion, C., Zayachkivsky, A., Liu, M., Uhde, T., ... Shiromani, P. J. (2013). Optogenetic stimulation of MCH neurons increases sleep. *J Neurosci, 33*(25), 10257–10263. doi: 10.1523/JNEUROSCI.1225-13.2013

Kong, J., Shepel, P., Holden, C., Mackiewicz, M., Pack, A., & Geiger, J. (2002). Brain glycogen decreases with increased periods of wakefulness: implications for homeostatic drive to sleep. *J Neurosci, 22*(13), 5581–5587.

Krahn, L. E., Pankratz, S., Oliver, L., Boeve, B. F., & Silber, M. H. (2002). Hypocretin (orexin) levels in cerebrospinal fluid of patients with narcolepsy: relationship to cataplexy and HLA DQB1*0602 status. *Sleep, 25*(7), 733–736.

Krueger, J., Pappenheimer, J., & Karnovsky, M. (1978). Sleep-promoting factor S: purification and properties. *Proc Natl Acad Sci USA, 75*(10), 5235–5238.

Krystal, A. D., Richelson, E., & Roth, T. (2013). Review of the histamine system and the clinical effects of H_1 antagonists: basis for a new model for understanding the effects of insomnia medications. *Sleep Med Rev, 17*, 263–272.

Kubota, K. (1989). Kuniomi Ishimori and the first discovery of sleep-inducing substances in the brain. *Neurosci Res, 6*, 497–518.

Kukkonen, J., & Leonard, C. (2014). Orexin/hypocretin receptor signaling cascades. *Br J Pharmacol, 171*, 314–331. doi: 0.1111/bph.2014.171.issue-2

Kukolja, J., Thiel, C. M., & Fink, G. R. (2009). Cholinergic stimulation enhances neural activity associated with encoding but reduces neural activity associated with retrieval in humans. *J Neurosci, 29*(25), 8119–8128. doi: 10.1523/JNEUROSCI.0203-09.2009

Lapierre, J., Kosenko, P., Kodama, T., Peever, J., Mukhametov, L., Lyamin, O., & Siegel, J. (2013). Symmetrical serotonin release during asymmetrical slow-wave sleep: implications for the neurochemistry of sleep-waking states. *J Neurosci, 33*(6), 2555–2561. doi: 0.1523/JNEUROSCI.2603-12.2013

Lapierre, J. L., Kosenko, P. O., Lyamin, O. I., Kodama, T., Mukhametov, L. M., & Siegel, J. M. (2007). Cortical acetylcholine release is lateralized during asymmetrical slow-wave sleep in northern fur seals. *J Neurosci, 27*(44), 11999–12006. doi: 10.1523/jneurosci.2968-07.2007

Lavie, P., & Peled, R. (1987). Narcolepsy is a rare disease in Israel. *Sleep, 10*(6), 608–609.

Lazarus, M., Shen, H. Y., Cherasse, Y., Qu, W. M., Huang, Z. L., Bass, C. E., ... Chen, J. F. (2011). Arousal effect of caffeine depends on adenosine A2A receptors in the shell of the nucleus accumbens. *J Neurosci, 31*(27), 10067–10075. doi: 10.1523/JNEUROSCI.6730-10.2011

Lee, M. G., Hassani, O. K., & Jones, B. E. (2005). Discharge of identified orexin/hypocretin neurons across the sleep-waking cycle. *J Neurosci, 25*(28), 6716–6720. doi: 10.1523/JNEUROSCI.1887-05.2005

Leonard, T. O., & Lydic, R. (1997). Pontine nitric oxide modulates acetylcholine release, rapid eye movement sleep generation, and respiratory rate. *J Neurosci, 17*(2), 774–785.

Lim, A. S., Ellison, B. A., Wang, J. L., Yu, L., Schneider, J. A., Buchman, A. S., ... Saper, C. B. (2014). Sleep is related to neuron numbers in the ventrolateral preoptic/intermediate nucleus in older adults with and without Alzheimer's disease. *Brain, 137*(Pt 10), 2847–2861. doi: 10.1093/brain/awu222

Lin, J.-S., Sakai, K., & Jouvet, M. (1986). Rôle des systèmes histaminergiques hypothalamiques dans la régulation des états de vigilance chez le chat. *C R Acad Sci Paris 303*(11), 469–474.

Lin, L., Faraco, J., Li, R., Kadotani, H., Rogers, W., Lin, X., ... Mignot, E. (1999). The sleep disorder canine narcolepsy is caused by a mutation in the *Hypocretin (Orexin) Receptor 2* gene. *Cell, 98*, 365–376.

Liu, C. H., Coleman, J. E., Davoudi, H., Zhang, K., & Hussain Shuler, M. G. (2015). Selective activation of a putative reinforcement signal conditions cued interval timing in primary visual cortex. *Curr Biol, 25*(12), 1551–1561. doi: 10.1016/j.cub.2015.04.028

Liu, R.-J., van den Pol, A., & Aghajanian, G. K. (2002). Hypocretins (orexins) regulate serotonin neurons in the dorsal raphe nucleus by excitatory direct and inhibitory indirect actions. *J Neurosci, 22*(21), 9453–9464.

Liu, Y. W., Li, J., & Ye, J. H. (2010). Histamine regulates activities of neurons in the ventrolateral preoptic nucleus. *J Physiol, 588*(21), 4103–4116. doi: 10.1113/jphysiol.2010.193904

Livet, J., Weissman, T. A., Kang, H., Draft, R. W., Lu, J., Bennis, R. A., ... Lichtman, J. W. (2007). Transgenic strategies for combinatorial expression of fluorescent proteins in the nervous system. *Nature, 450*(7166), 56–62. doi: 10.1038/nature06293

Lu, J., Bjorkum, A., Xu, M., Gaus, S., Shiromani, P., & Saper, C. (2002). Selective activation of the extended ventrolateral preoptic nucleus during rapid eye movement sleep. *J Neurosci, 22*(11), 4568–4576.

Lucaci, D., Yu, X., Chadderton, P., Wisden, W., & Brickley, S. G. (2023). Histamine release in the prefrontal cortex excites fast-spiking interneurons while GABA released from the same axons inhibits pyramidal cells. *J Neurosci, 43*(2), 187–198. doi: 10.1523/jneurosci.0936-22.2022

Lyamin, O. I., Lapierre, J. L., Kosenko, P. O., Kodama, T., Bhagwandin, A., Korneva, S. M., ... Siegel, J. M. (2016). Monoamine release during unihemispheric sleep and unihemispheric waking in the fur seal. *Sleep, 39*(3), 625–636. doi: 10.5665/sleep.5540

Mahler, S. V., Moorman, D. E., Smith, R. J., James, M. H., & Aston-Jones, G. (2014). Motivational activation: a unifying hypothesis of orexin/hypocretin function. *Nat Neurosci, 17*(10), 1298–1303. doi: 10.1038/nn.3810

Mahoney, C. E., Mochizuki, T., & Scammell, T. E. (2019). Dual orexin receptor antagonists increase sleep and cataplexy in wild type mice. *Sleep, 43*(6), zsz302. doi: 10.1093/sleep/zsz302

Majde, J. A., & Krueger, J. M. (2005). Links between the innate immune system and sleep. *J Allergy Clin Immunol, 116*(6), 1188–1198. doi: 10.1016/j.jaci.2005.08.005

Mayer, G., Plazzi, G., Iranzo, A., Ortega-Albas, J., Quinnell, T., Pesch, H., ... Bentz, J. W. G. (2018). Long-term compliances, safety, and tolerability of sodium oxybate treatment in patients with narcolepsy type 1: a post-authorization, non-interventional surveillance study. *Sleep, 41*(9), zsy128. doi: 10.1093/sleep/zsy128

Melville, K. I. (1973). Antihistamine drugs. In M. Schachter (Ed.), *Histamine and Antihistamines* (pp. 127–171). Oxford: Pergamon Press.

Mieda, M., Willie, J. T., Hara, J., Sinton, C. M., Sakurai, T., & Yanagisawa, M. (2004). Orexin peptides prevent cataplexy and improve wakefulness in an orexin neuron-ablated model of narcolepsy in mice. *Proc Natl Acad Sci USA, 101*(13), 4649–4654. doi: 10.1073/pnas.0400590101

Mignot, E. (2004). Sleep, sleep disorders and hypocretin (orexin). *Sleep Med, 5*(Suppl. 1), S2–S8. doi: 10.1016/j.sleep.2004.04.000

Mignot, E., Lammers, G., Ripley, B., Okun, M. L., Nevsimalova, S., Overeem, S., ... Nishino, S. (2002). The role of cerebrospinal fluid hypocretin measurement in the diagnosis of narcolepsy and other hypersomnias. *Arch Neurol, 59*(10), 1553–1562. doi: 10.1001/archneur.59.10.1553

Mignot, E., Renaud, A., Nishino, S., Arrigoni, J., Guilleminault, C., & Dement, W. (1993). Canine cataplexy is preferentially controlled by adrenergic mechanisms: evidence using monoamine selective uptake inhibitors and release enhancers. *Psychopharmacology, 113*, 76–82.

Mileykovskiy, B. Y., Kiyashchenko, L. I., & Siegel, J. M. (2005). Behavioral correlates of activity in identified hypocretin/orexin neurons. *Neuron, 46*(5), 787–798. doi: 10.1016/j.neuron.2005.04.035

Miracca, G., Anuncibay-Soto, B., Tossell, K., Yustos, R., Vyssotski, A. L., Franks, N. P., & Wisden, W. (2022). NMDA receptors in the lateral preoptic hypothalamus are essential for sustaining NREM and REM sleep. *J Neurosci, 42*(27), 5389–5409. doi: 10.1523/JNEUROSCI.0350-21.2022

Mochizuki, T., Crocker, A., McCormack, S., Yanagisawa, M., Sakurai, T., & Scammell, T. E. (2004). Behavioral state instability in orexin knock-out mice. *J Neurosci, 24*(28), 6291–6300. doi: 10.1523/JNEUROSCI.0586-04.2004

Mochizuki, T., Yamatodani, A., Okakura, K., Horii, A., Inagaki, N., & Wada, H. (1992). Circadian rhythm of histamine release from the hypothalamus of freely moving rats. *Physiol Behav, 51*, 391–394.

Modirrousta, M., Mainville, L., & Jones, B. E. (2005). Orexin and MCH neurons express c-Fos differently after sleep deprivation vs. recovery and bear different adrenergic receptors. *Eur J Neurosci, 21*, 2807–2816. doi: 0.1111/j.1460-9568.2005.04104.x

Mondino, A., Hambrecht-Wiedbusch, V., Li, D., York, A. K., Pal, D., Gonzalez, J., ... Vanini, G. (2021). Glutamatergic neurons in the preoptic hypothalamus promote wakefulness, destabilize NREM sleep, suppress REM sleep, and regulate cortical dynamics. *J Neurosci, 41*(15), 3462–3478. doi: 10.1523/JNEUROSCI.2718-20.2021

Monti, J. M. (1993). Involvement of histamine in the control of the waking state. *Life Sci, 53*, 1331–1338.

Montplaisir, J., Petit, D., Gauthier, S., Gaudreau, H., & Décary, A. (1998). Sleep disturbance and EEG slowing in Alzheimer's disease. *Sleep Res Online, 1*(4), 147–151.

Moore, R. Y., Abrahamson, E. A., & van den Pol, A. (2001). The hypocretin neuron system: an arousal system in the human brain. *Arch Ital Biol, 139*, 195–205.

Morin, C. M., Bootzin, R. R., Buysse, D. J., Edinger, J. D., Espie, C. A., & Lichstein, K. L. (2006). Psychological and behavioral treatment of insomnia: update of the recent evidence (1998–2004). *Sleep, 29*(11), 1398–1414.

Myers, C. S., Taylor, R. C., Salmeron, B. J., Water, A. J., & Heishman, S. J. (2013). Nicotine enhances alerting, but not executive, attention in smokers and non-smokers. *Nicot Tobac Res*, *15*(1), 277–281.

Naganuma, F., Nakamura, T., Kuroyanagi, H., Tanaka, M., Yoshikawa, T., Yanai, K., & Okamura, N. (2021). Chemogenetic modulation of histaminergic neurons in the tuberomamillary nucleus alters territorial aggression and wakefulness. *Sci Rep*, *11*(1), 17935. doi: 10.1038/s41598-021-95497-3

Nauta, W. J. H. (1946). Hypothalamic regulation of sleep in rats. An experimental study. *J Neurophysiol*, *9*, 285–315.

Nicholson, A. N., Pascoe, P. A., & Stone, B. M. (1985). Histaminergic systems and sleep. Studies in man with H1 and H2 antagonists. *Neuropharmacology*, *24*(3), 245–250. doi: 10.1016/0028-3908(85)90081-4

Nishino, S., Ripley, B., Overeem, S., Lammers, G. J., & Mignot, E. (2000). Hypocretin (orexin) deficiency in human narcolepsy. *Lancet*, *355*(9197), 39–40. doi: 10.1016/S0140-6736(99)05582-8

Obal, F., Jr., & Krueger, J. M. (2004). GHRH and sleep. *Sleep Med Rev*, *8*(5), 367–377. doi: 10.1016/j.smrv.2004.03.005

Oishi, Y., Huang, Z. L., Fredholm, B. B., Urade, Y., & Hayaishi, O. (2008). Adenosine in the tuberomammillary nucleus inhibits the histaminergic system via A1 receptors and promotes non-rapid eye movement sleep. *Proc Natl Acad Sci USA*, *105*(50), 19992–19997. doi: 10.1073/pnas.0810926105

Onoe, H., Ueno, R., Fujita, I., Nishino, H., & Oomura, Y. (1988). Prostaglandin D2, a cerebral sleep-inducing substance in monkeys. *Proc Natl Acad Sci USA*, *85*, 4082–4086.

Owens, J., Rosen, C., Mindell, J., & Kirchner, H. (2010). Use of pharmacotherapy for insomnia in child psychiatry practice: a national survey. *Sleep Med*, *11*, 692–700. doi: 0.1016/j.sleep.2009.11.015

Pandey, H. P., Ram, A., Matsumura, H., & Hayaishi, O. (1995). Concentration of prostaglandin D2 in cerebrospinal fluid exhibits a circadian alteration in conscious rats. *Biochem Mol Biol Int*, *37*(3), 431–437.

Parmentier, R., Ohtsu, H., Djebbara-Hannas, Z., Valatx, J.-L., Watanabe, T., & Lin, J.-S. (2002). Anatomical, physiological, and pharmacological characteristics of histidine decarboxylase knock-out mice: evidence for the role of brain histamine in behavioral and sleep-wake control. *J Neurosci*, *22*(17), 7695–7711.

Pascual, O., Casper, K. B., Kubera, C., Zhang, J., Revilla-Sanchez, R., Sul, J.-Y., ... Haydon, P. G. (2005). Astrocytic purinergic signaling coordinates synaptic networks. *Science*, *310*(5745), 113–116.

Pellerin, L., & Magistretti, P. J. (2012). Sweet sixteen for ANLS. *J Cereb Blood Flow Metab*, *32*(7), 1152–1166. doi: 10.1038/jcbfm.2011.149

Peterfi, Z., McGinty, D., Sarai, E., & Szymusiak, R. (2010). Growth hormone-releasing hormone activates sleep regulatory neurons of the rat preoptic hypothalamus. *Am J Physiol Regul Integr Comp Physiol*, *298*(1), R147–156. doi: 10.1152/ajpregu.00494.2009

Petit, J.-M., Tobler, I., Kopp, C., Morgenthaler, F., Borbély, A., & Magistretti, P. J. (2010). Metabolic response of the cerebral cortex following gentle sleep deprivation and modafinil administration. *Sleep*, *33*(7), 901–908.

Peyron, C., Faraco, J., Rogers, W., Ripley, B., Overeem, S., Charnay, Y., ... Mignot, E. (2000). A mutation in a case of early onset narcolepsy and a generalized absence of hypocretin peptides in human narcoleptic brains. *Nat Med*, *6*(9), 991–997.

Plazzi, G., Clawges, H. M., & Owens, J. A. (2018). Clinical characteristics and burden of illness in pediatric patients with narcolepsy. *Pediatr Neurol*, *85*, 21–32. doi: 10.1016/j.pediatrneurol.2018.06.008

Porkka-Heiskanen, T., & Kalinchuk, A. V. (2011). Adenosine, energy metabolism and sleep homeostasis. *Sleep Med Rev*, *15*(2), 123–135. doi: 10.1016/j.smrv.2010.06.005

Porkka-Heiskanen, T., Strecker, R. E., & McCarley, R. W. (2000). Brain site-specificity of extracellular adenosine concentration changes during sleep deprivation and spontaneous sleep: an *in vivo* microdialysis study. *Neuroscience*, *99*(3), 507–517.

Ram, A., Pandey, H. P., Matsumura, H., Kasahara-Orita, K., Nakajima, T., Takahata, R., ... Hayaishi, O. (1997). CSF levels of prostaglandins, especially the level of prostaglandin D2, are correlated with increasing propensity towards sleep in rats. *Brain Res*, *751*, 81–89.

Redwine, L. (2000). Effects of sleep and sleep deprivation on interleukin-6, growth hormone, cortisol, and melatonin levels in humans. *J Clin Endocr Metab*, *85*(10), 3597–3603. doi: 10.1210/jc.85.10.3597

Reichert, C. F., Deboer, T., & Landolt, H. P. (2022). Adenosine, caffeine, and sleep-wake regulation: state of the science and perspectives. *J Sleep Res*, *31*(4), e13597. doi:10.1111/jsr.13597

Reiner, P. B., & Kamondi, A. (1994). Mechanisms of antihistamine-induced sedation in the human brain: H1 receptor activation reduces a background leakage potassium current. *Neuroscience*, *59*(3), 579–588.

Repantis, D., Laisney, O., & Heuser, I. (2010). Acetylcholinesterase inhibitors and memantine for neuroenhancement in healthy individuals: a systematic review. *Pharmacol Res*, *61*(6), 473–481. doi: 10.1016/j.phrs.2010.02.009

Rétey, J. V., Adam, M., Gottselig, J. M., Khatami, R., Durr, R., Achermann, P., & Landolt, H. P. (2006). Adenosinergic mechanisms contribute to individual differences in sleep deprivation-induced changes in neurobehavioral function and brain rhythmic activity. *J Neurosci*, *26*(41), 10472–10479. doi: 10.1523/jneurosci.1538-06.2006

Rétey, J. V., Adam, M., Khatami, R., Luhmann, U. F., Jung, H. H., Berger, W., & Landolt, H. P. (2007). A genetic variation in the adenosine A2A receptor gene (ADORA2A) contributes to individual sensitivity to caffeine effects on sleep. *Clin Pharmacol Ther*, *81*(5), 692–698. doi: 10.1038/sj.clpt.6100102

Reyes, C. M., & Cornelis, M. C. (2018). Caffeine in the diet: country-level consumption and guidelines. *Nutrients*, *10*(11), 1–34. doi:10.3390/nu10111772

Richardson, G., Roehrs, T., Rosenthal, L., Koshorek, G., & Roth, T. (2002). Tolerance to daytime sedative effects of H1 antihistamines *J Clin Psychopharm*, *22*(5), 511–515. doi: 10.1097/01.jcp.0000033406.43191.e8

Ripley, B., Overeem, S., Fujiki, N., Nevsimalova, S., Uchino, M., Yesavage, J., ... Nishino, S. (2001). CSF hypocretin/orexin levels in narcolepsy and other neurological disorders. *Neurology*, *57*, 2253–2258.

Roth, T., Roehrs, T., Koshorek, G., Sicklesteel, J., & Zorick, F. (1987). Sedative effects of antihistamines. *J Allergy Clin Immunol*, *80*(1), 94–98. doi: 10.1016/s0091-6749(87)80197-5

Sakurai, T. (2007). The neural circuit of orexin (hypocretin): maintaining sleep and wakefulness. *Nat Rev Neurosci*, *8*(3), 171–181. doi: 10.1038/nrn2092

Sakurai, T., Amemiya, A., Ishii, M., Matsuzaki, I., Chemelli, R. M., Tanaka, H., ... Yanagisawa, M. (1998). Orexins and orexin receptors: a family of hypothalamic neuropeptides and G protein-coupled receptors that regulate feeding behavior. *Cell*, *92*(4), 573–585.

Saper, C. B., Fuller, P. M., Pedersen, N. P., Lu, J., & Scammell, T. E. (2010). Sleep state switching. *Neuron*, *68*(6), 1023–1042. doi: 10.1016/j.neuron.2010.11.032

Saper, C. B., Scammell, T. E., & Lu, J. (2005). Hypothalamic regulation of sleep and circadian rhythms. *Nature*, *437*(7063), 1257–1263. doi: 10.1038/nature04284

Sapin, E., Berod, A., Leger, L., Herman, P. A., Luppi, P. H., & Peyron, C. (2010). A very large number of GABAergic neurons are activated in the tuberal hypothalamus during paradoxical (REM) sleep hypersomnia. *PLoS One*, *5*(7), e11766. doi: 10.1371/journal.pone.0011766

Sarter, M., & Bruno, J. P. (2000). Cortical cholinergic inputs mediating arousal, attentional processing and dreaming: differential afferent regulation of the basal forebrain by telencephalic and brainstem afferents. *Neuroscience*, *95*(4), 933–952.

Schifano, F., Chiappini, S., Corkery, J. M., & Guirguis, A. (2019). An insight into Z-drug abuse and dependence: an examination of reports to the European Medicines Agency Database of Suspected Adverse Drug Reactions. *Int J Neuropsychopharmacol*, *22*(4), 270–277. doi: 10.1093/ijnp/pyz007

Schliebs, R., & Arendt, T. (2010). The cholinergic system in aging and neuronal degeneration. Behav Brain Res. doi: 10.1016/j.bbr.2010.11.058

Schmitt, L. I., Sims, R. E., Dale, N., & Haydon, P. G. (2012). Wakefulness affects synaptic and network activity by increasing extracellular astrocyte-derived adenosine. *J Neurosci*, *32*(13), 4417–4425. doi: 10.1523/jneurosci.5689-11.2012

Schone, C., Cao, Z. F., Apergis-Schoute, J., Adamantidis, A., Sakurai, T., & Burdakov, D. (2012). Optogenetic probing of fast glutamatergic transmission from hypocretin/orexin to histamine neurons in situ. *J Neurosci*, *32*(36), 12437–12443. doi: 10.1523/JNEUROSCI.0706-12.2012

Schurr, A. (2006). Lactate: the ultimate cerebral oxidative energy substrate? *J Cereb Blood Flow Metab*, *26*(1), 142–152. doi: 10.1038/sj.jcbfm.9600174

Schwartz, J.-C., Arrang, J.-M., Garbarg, M., Pollard, H., & Ruat, M. (1991). Histaminergic transmission in the mammalian brain. *Physiol Rev*, *71*(1), 1–51.

Semba, K. (2000). Multiple output pathways of the basal forebrain: organization, chemical heterogeneity, and roles in vigilance. *Behav Brain Res*, *115*, 117–141.

Semba, K. (2004). Phylogenetic and ontogenetic aspects of the basal forebrain cholinergic neurons and their innervation of the cerebral cortex. *Prog Brain Res*, *145*, 3–43.

Semba, K., Pastorius, J., Wilkinson, M., & Rusak, B. (2001). Sleep deprivation-induced c-fos and junB expression in the rat brain: effects of duration and timing. *Behav Brain Res*, *120*, 75–86.

Sender, R., Fuchs, S., & Milo, R. (2016). Revised estimates for the number of human and bacteria cells in the body. *PLoS Biol*, *14(8): e1002533*(8). doi: 10.1371/journal.pbio.1002533

Senova, S., Fomenko, A., Gondard, E., & Lozano, A. M. (2020). Anatomy and function of the fornix in the context of its potential as a therapeutic target. *J Neurol Neurosurg Psychiatry*, *91*(5), 547–559. doi: 10.1136/jnnp-2019-322375

Sherin, J., Shiromani, P., McCarley, R., & Saper, C. (1996). Activation of ventrolateral preoptic neurons during sleep. *Science*, *271*(5246), 216–219.

Simons, F. E. R. (2004). Advances in H_1-antihistamines. *New Engl J Med, 351*, 2203–2217.

Sitaram, N., Wyatt, J., Dawson, S., & Gillin, J. (1976). Sleep induction by physostigmine infusion during sleep. *Science, 191*(4233), 1281–1283.

Snow, M. B., Fraigne, J. J., Thibault-Messier, G., Chuen, V. L., Thomasian, A., Horner, R. L., & Peever, J. (2017). GABA cells in the central nucleus of the amygdala promote cataplexy. *J Neurosci, 37*(15), 4007–4022. doi: 0.1523/JNEUROSCI.4070-15.2017

Sorensen, G. L., Knudsen, S., & Jennum, P. (2013). Sleep transitions in hypocretin-deficient narcolepsy. *Sleep, 36*(8), 1173–1177. doi: 10.5665/sleep.2880

Steininger, T. L., Gong, H., McGinty, D., & Szymusiak, R. (2001). Subregional organization of preoptic area/anterior hypothalamic projections to arousal-related monoaminergic cell groups. *J Comp Neurol, 429*(4), 638–653.

Sterman, M., & Clemente, C. (1962). Forebrain inhibitory mechanisms: cortical synchronization induced by basal forebrain stimulation. *Exp Neurol, 6*, 91–102.

Strecker, R. E., Morairty, S., Thakkar, M. M., Porkka-Heiskanen, T., Basheer, R., Dauphin, L. J., ... McCarley, R. W. (2000). Adenosinergic modulation of basal forebrain and preoptic: anterior hypothalamic neuronal activity in the control of behavioral state. *Behav Brain Res, 115*(2), 183–204. doi: 10.1016/s0166-4328(00)00258-8

Strecker, R. E., Nalwalk, J., Dauphin, L. J., Thakkar, M. M., Chen, Y., Ramesh, V., ... McCarley, R. W. (2002). Extracellular histamine levels in the feline preoptic anterior hypothalamic area during natural sleep–wakefulness and prolonged wakefulness: an *in vivo* microdialysis study. *Neuroscience, 113*(3), 663–670.

Sun, X., Whitefield, S., Rusak, B., & Semba, K. (2001). Electrophysiological analysis of suprachiasmatic nucleus projections to the ventrolateral preoptic area in the rat. *Eur J Neurosci, 14*, 1257–1274.

Suntsova, N., Szymusiak, R., Md. Alam, N., Guzman-Marin, R., & McGinty, D. (2002). Sleep-waking discharge patterns of median preoptic nucleus neurons in rats. *J Physiol, 543*(2), 665–677. doi: 10.1113/jphysiol.2002.023085

Szymusiak, R., Alam, N., Steininger, T., & McGinty, D. (1998). Sleep–waking discharge patterns of ventrolateral preoptic/anterior hypothalamic neurons in rats. *Brain Res, 803*, 178–188.

Szymusiak, R., & McGinty, D. (1986). Sleep-related discharge in the basal forebrain of cats. *Brain Res, 370*, 82–92.

Szymusiak, R., & McGinty, D. (2008). Hypothalamic regulation of sleep and arousal. *Ann NY Acad Sci, 1129*(1), 275–286. doi: 10.1196/annals.1417.027

Takagi, H., Morishima, Y., Matsuyama, T., Hayashi, H., Watanabe, T., & Wada, H. (1986). Histaminergic axons in the neostriatum and cerebral cortex of the rat: a correlated light and electron microscopic immunocytochemical study using histidine decarboxylase as a marker. *Brain Res, 364*, 114–123.

Takahashi, K., Lin, J. S., & Sakai, K. (2006). Neuronal activity of histaminergic tuberomammillary neurons during wake-sleep states in the mouse. *J Neurosci, 26*(40), 10292–10298. doi: 10.1523/JNEUROSCI.2341-06.2006

Thakkar, M., Delgiacco, R., Strecker, R., & McCarley, R. (2003). Adenosinergic inhibition of basal forebrain wakefulness-active neurons: a simultaneous unit recording and microdialysis study in freely behaving cats. *Neuroscience, 122*, 1107–1113. doi: 10.1016/S0306-4522(03)00634-1

Thakkar, M. M., Engemann, S. C., Walsh, K. M., & Sahota, P. K. (2008). Adenosine and the homeostatic control of sleep: effects of A1 receptor blockade in the perifornical lateral hypothalamus on sleep-wakefulness. *Neuroscience, 153*(4), 875–880. doi: 10.1016/j.neuroscience.2008.01.017

Thannickal, T. C., John, J., Shan, L., Swaab, D. F., Wu, M.-F., Ramanathan, L., ... Siegel, J. M. (2018). Opiates increase the number of hypocretin-producing cells in human and mouse brain and reverse cataplexy in a mouse model of narcolepsy. *Sci Transl Med, 10*(447), eaao4953. doi: 10.1126/scitranslmed.aao4953

Thannickal, T. C., Moore, R. Y., Nienhuis, R., Ramanathan, L., Gulyani, S., Aldrich, M. S., ... Siegel, J. M. (2000). Reduced number of hypocretin neurons in human narcolepsy. *Neuron, 27*(September), 469–474.

Torterolo, P., Lagos, P., & Monti, J. M. (2011). Melanin-concentrating hormone: a new sleep factor? *Front Neurol, 2*, 14. doi: 10.3389/fneur.2011.00014

Trauer, J. M., Qian, M. Y., Doyle, J. S., Rajaratnam, S. M., & Cunnington, D. (2015). Cognitive behavioral therapy for chronic insomnia: a systematic review and meta-analysis. *Ann Intern Med, 163*(3), 191–204. doi: 10.7326/M14-2841

Tritsch, N. X., Granger, A. J., & Sabatini, B. L. (2016). Mechanisms and functions of GABA co-release. *Nat Rev Neurosci, 17*(3), 139–145. doi: 10.1038/nrn.2015.21

Tsunematsu, T., Tabuchi, S., Tanaka, K. F., Boyden, E. S., Tominaga, M., & Yamanaka, A. (2013). Long-lasting silencing of orexin/hypocretin neurons using archaerhodopsin induces slow-wave sleep in mice. *Behav Brain Res, 255*, 64–74. doi: 10.1016/j.bbr.2013.05.021

Urade, Y., & Hayaishi, O. (1999). Prostaglandin D2 and sleep regulation. *Biochem Biophys Acta, 1436*, 606–615.

U.S. Xyrem Multicenter Study Group. (2004). Sodium oxybate demonstrates long-term efficacy for the treatment of cataplexy in patients with narcolepsy. *Sleep Med, 5*(2), 119–123. doi: 10.1016/j.sleep.2003.11.002

Van Dort, C. J., Baghdoyan, H. A., & Lydic, R. (2009). Adenosine A1 and A2A receptors in mouse prefrontal cortex modulate acetylcholine release and behavioral arousal. *J Neurosci, 29*(3), 871–881. doi: 10.1523/jneurosci.4111-08.2009

Vanni-Mercier, G., Gigout, S., Debilly, G., & Lin, J. S. (2003). Waking selective neurons in the posterior hypothalamus and their response to histamine H_3-receptor ligands: an electrophysiological study in freely moving cats. *Behav Brain Res, 144*(1-2), 227–241. doi: 10.1016/s0166-4328(03)00091-3

Vanni-Mercier, G., Sakai, K., & Jouvet, M. (1984). Neurones spécifiques de l'éveil dans l'hypothalamus postérieur du chat ["Waking-state specific" neurons in the caudal hypothalamus of the cat]. *C R Acad Sci III, 298*(7), 195–200.

Varin, C., Rancillac, A., Geoffroy, H., Arthaud, S., Fort, P., & Gallopin, T. (2015). Glucose induces slow-wave sleep by exciting the sleep-promoting neurons in the ventrolateral preoptic nucleus: a new link between sleep and metabolism. *J Neurosci, 35*(27), 9900–9911. doi: 10.1523/JNEUROSCI.0609-15.2015

Vazquez, J., & Baghdoyan, H. (2001). Basal forebrain acetylcholine release during REM sleep is significantly greater than during waking. *Am J Physiol, 280*, R598–R601. doi: 10.1152/ajpregu.2001.280.2.R598

Venner, A., De Luca, R., Sohn, L. T., Bandaru, S. S., Verstegen, A. M. J., Arrigoni, E., & Fuller, P. M. (2019). An inhibitory lateral hypothalamic-preoptic circuit mediates rapid arousals from sleep. *Curr Biol, 29*(24), 4155–4168 e4155. doi: 10.1016/j.cub.2019.10.026

Venner, A., Mochizuki, T., De Luca, R., Anaclet, C., Scammell, T. E., Saper, C. B., Arrigoni, E., & Fuller, P. M. (2019). Reassessing the role of histaminergic tuberomammillary neurons in arousal control. *J Neurosci, 39*(45), 8929–8939. doi: 10.1523/JNEUROSCI.1032-19.2019

Verret, L., Goutany, R., Fort, P., Cagnon, L., Salvert, D., Léger, L., ... Luppi, P.-H. (2003). A role of melanin-concentrating hormone producing neurons in the central regulation of paradoxical sleep. *BMC Neurosci, 4*(19), 1–10.

von Economo, C. (1930). Sleep as a problem of localization. *J Nerv Ment Dis, 71*(3), 249–259.

Vyazovskiy, V., Borbély, A. A., & Tobler, I. (2000). Unilateral vibrissae stimulation during waking induces interhemispheric EEG asymmetry during subsequent sleep in the rat. *J Sleep Res, 9*, 367–371.

Wade, L., Forlini, C., & Racine, E. (2014). Generating genius: how an Alzheimer's drug became considered a "cognitive enhancer" for healthy individuals. *BMC Med Ethics, 15*(37), 1–14.

Walker, A. W., & Hoyles, L. (2023). Human microbiome myths and misconceptions. *Nature Microbiology, 8*(8), 1392–1396. doi: 10.1038/s41564-023-01426-7

Williams, R. H., Chee, M. J., Kroeger, D., Ferrari, L. L., Maratos-Flier, E., Scammell, T. E., & Arrigoni, E. (2014). Optogenetic-mediated release of histamine reveals distal and autoregulatory mechanisms for controlling arousal. *J Neurosci, 34*(17), 6023–6029. doi: 10.1523/JNEUROSCI.4838-13.2014

Woolf, N. J. (1991). Cholinergic systems in mammalian brain and spinal cord. *Prog Neurobiol, 37*(6), 475–524.

Wright Jr, K. P., Badia, P., Myers, B., Plenzler, S., & Hakel, M. (1997). Caffeine and light effects on nighttime melatonin and temperature levels in sleep-deprived humans. *Brain Res, 747*, 78–84.

Xi, M., & Chase, M. H. (2010). The injection of hypocretin-1 into the nucleus pontis oralis induces either active sleep or wakefulness depending on the behavioral state when it is administered. *Sleep, 33*(9), 1236–1243.

Xu, M., Chung, S., Zhang, S., Zhong, P., Ma, C., Chang, W. C., ... Dan, Y. (2015). Basal forebrain circuit for sleep-wake control. *Nat Neurosci, 18*(11), 1641–1647. doi: 10.1038/nn.4143

Yamanaka, A., Beuckmann, C., Willie, J., Hara, J., Tsujino, N., Mieda, M., ... Sakurai, T. (2003). Hypothalamic orexin neurons regulate arousal according to energy balance in mice. *Neuron, 38*, 701–713.

Yu, X., Ye, Z., Houston, C. M., Zecharia, A. Y., Ma, Y., Zhang, Z., ... Wisden, W. (2015). Wakefulness is governed by GABA and histamine cotransmission. *Neuron, 87*(1), 164–178. doi: 10.1016/j.neuron.2015.06.003

Zachariae, R., Lyby, M. S., Ritterband, L. M., & O'Toole, M. S. (2016). Efficacy of internet-delivered cognitive-behavioral therapy for insomnia: a systematic review and meta-analysis of randomized controlled trials. *Sleep Med Rev, 30*, 1–10. doi: 10.1016/j.smrv.2015.10.004

Zant, J. C., Kim, T., Prokai, L., Szarka, S., McNally, J., McKenna, J. T., ... Basheer, R. (2016). Cholinergic neurons in the basal forebrain promote wakefulness by actions on neighboring non-cholinergic neurons: an opto-dialysis study. *J Neurosci, 36*(6), 2057–2067. doi: 10.1523/JNEUROSCI.3318-15.2016

Zant, J. C., Rozov, S., Wigren, H. K., Panula, P., & Porkka-Heiskanen, T. (2012). Histamine release in the basal forebrain mediates cortical activation through cholinergic neurons. *J Neurosci*, *32*(38), 13244–13254. doi: 10.1523/JNEUROSCI.5933-11.2012

Zecharia, A. Y., Yu, X., Götz, T., Ye, Z., Carr, D. R., Wulff, P., ... Wisden, W. (2012). GABAergic inhibition of histaminergic neurons regulates active waking but not the sleep-wake switch or propofol-induced loss of consciousness. *J Neurosci*, *32*(38), 13062–13075. doi: 0.1523/JNEUROSCI.2931-12.2012

Zeitzer, J. M., Buckmaster, C. L., Parker, K. J., Hauck, C. M., Lyons, D. M., & Mignot, E. (2003). Circadian and homeostatic regulation of hypocretin in a primate model: implications for the consolidation of wakefulness. *J Neurosci*, *23*(8), 3555–3560.

Zhang, S., Zeitzer, J., Yoshida, Y., Wisor, J., Nishino, S., Edgar, D., & Mignot, E. (2004). Lesions of the suprachiasmatic nucleus eliminate the daily rhythm of hypocretin-1 release. *Sleep*, *27*(4), 619–627.

Zheng, X., He, Y., Yin, F., Liu, H., Li, Y., Zheng, Q., & Li, L. (2020). Pharmacological interventions for the treatment of insomnia: quantitative comparison of drug efficacy. *Sleep Med*, *72*, 41–49. doi: 10.1016/j.sleep.2020.03.022

Zorec, R., Araque, A., Carmignoto, G., Haydon, P. G., Verkhratsky, A., & Parpura, V. (2012). Astroglial excitability and gliotransmission: an appraisal of Ca2+ as a signalling route. *ASN Neuro*, *4*(2), e00080. doi:10.1042/AN20110061

CHAPTER 12

Thalamocortical Mechanisms

12.1 OVERVIEW

The cerebral cortex is the main source of electrophysiological information about sleep states; it is also the structure responsible for changes in responsiveness and in mental experiences that occur during sleep. The thalamus is the principal structure conveying information to and from the cortex. This chapter reviews how the cortex and thalamus interact to generate the characteristic electrical patterns, changes in consciousness, and responsiveness to external stimuli that occur during different sleep stages.

It also reviews how features of NREM sleep (K complexes, sleep spindles, delta waves and slow oscillations (SOs)) are generated and discusses the effects of these features and of sleep stages on responsiveness to environmental stimuli. The general loss of conscious awareness of the environment is a defining characteristic of sleep. Yet, people can evaluate and respond selectively to environmental stimuli while asleep. The author Margaret Atwood described this paradoxical vigilance: "It's as if there is a part of me that never sleeps at all, but keeps one eye a little open . . ." (Atwood, 1996, p. 313).[1] The evidence addressing which part of a person never sleeps at all is discussed in Sections 12.3 and 12.4 in relation to how the cortex and thalamus interact to process and evaluate sensory information during NREM and REM sleep. This chapter also discusses the idea that slow-wave activity (SWA) is regulated not only globally but also locally in the cortex in response to waking experiences.

[1] Excerpt from *Alias Grace* by Margaret Atwood, copyright © 1996 by O. W. Toad Ltd. Reprinted by permission of Emblem/McClelland & Stewart, a division of Penguin Random House Canada Limited. Used by permission of Doubleday, an imprint of the Knopf Doubleday Publishing Group, a division of Penguin Random House LLC, and Bloomsbury Publishing Plc. All rights reserved. Any third party use of this material, outside of this publication, is prohibited. Interested parties must apply directly to Penguin Random House Canada Limited for permission.

12.2 Generating cortical rhythms

12.2.1 Thalamic inputs to the cortex

In Chapter 2, we described the distinctive electrical features and rhythms of the EEG that are associated with waking and with the stages of sleep. These electrical patterns are recorded from surface electrodes on the scalp of people or from electrodes implanted directly into the cerebral cortex of animals (and sometimes directly from the brains of people). Chapters 10 and 11 reviewed the roles of several subcortical structures, neurotransmitters, and other mechanisms in controlling the occurrence and timing of waking and sleep stages. But we have yet to address the mechanisms involved in generating the EEG patterns that are the critical markers of sleep stages. Understanding how these rhythms arise depends on understanding the interaction of two structures: the cerebral cortex itself and the thalamus.

Thalamic relay nuclei are the final gateway through which most sensory and motor-related information reaches the cortex. Some nuclei receive and process information from sensory systems (except the olfactory system), several components of the motor system, and the limbic system, and convey their output via glutamatergic projections to specific, primary cortical regions. These nuclei also receive reciprocal inputs from the cortical regions to which they project, and may convey this input to other cortical areas, forming complex cortico-thalamocortical processing loops. Other thalamic relay nuclei project more broadly to reach sensory and motor areas of cortex as well as association cortical areas. Association cortices are large cortical regions that do not receive primary sensory inputs directly or generate motor outputs.

Among the most often studied thalamic relay nuclei are the lateral and medial geniculate nuclei (LGN and MGN). These structures receive and process information about many aspects of vision and audition, respectively, and convey this information through precisely mapped (topographic) projections that reach visual and auditory cortical regions. Despite their importance in the history of brain research, these are relatively small thalamic relay nuclei in humans.

Other groups of thalamic nuclei include midline and intralaminar nuclei (e.g., the central medial nucleus, central lateral nucleus, reuniens nucleus, pulvinar, and several others). They receive input from a broad range of structures, including the reticular formation, hypothalamus, striatum, cerebellum, and hippocampus. They are involved in several aspects of arousal, motivation, memory, and executive function. Although they have highly organized and complex input and output projections, they are sometimes referred to as "nonspecific" nuclei, because they do not project in the precise topographic patterns of primary relay nuclei.

Some nonspecific nuclei project broadly to many cortical regions (as well as to subcortical systems) and have been proposed to regulate cortical "tone" or level of arousal and to maintain consciousness (Blumenfeld, 2016; Vertes et al., 2022). However, their projections to cortex have a degree of anatomical specificity. As a result, although these nuclei together regulate global cortical arousal, different subsets are most active in relation to specific sensory, motor, or cognitive functions (Van der Werf et al., 2002).

Thalamic relay and nonspecific nuclei differ functionally in part because they contain different ratios of two cell types that project in different patterns. "Core" cells are the dominant cell type in thalamic relay nuclei. They contain the protein parvalbumin and form restricted projections to middle layers (i.e., layers III and IV of the six cortical layers) of functionally distinct cortical regions, such as visual, auditory, or somatosensory cortex (Jones, 2001).

"Matrix" cells containing the protein calbindin are found in all thalamic nuclei but are especially concentrated in the nonspecific nuclei. Matrix cells receive broader subcortical inputs, and their projections terminate more widely across the cortex in its superficial layers. Thus, core cells are able to provide specific information to primary sensory and motor cortical regions, while matrix cells are better positioned to regulate the overall level of cortical activity through their more diffuse projections (Jones, 2001).

12.2.2 Cortical slow rhythms

The defining features of NREM sleep include slow cortical EEG rhythms, loss of conscious awareness of the environment, and a reduction of cortical (and thus behavioral) responsiveness to sensory inputs. Since the thalamus is the principal structure that conveys information to the cortex, changes in thalamic input are likely to play a major role in modifying cortical EEG patterns and influencing awareness of, and responsiveness to, the environment.

Core contributions to understanding the cellular mechanisms in the thalamus and cortex that generate sleep EEG patterns were made through electrophysiological studies in

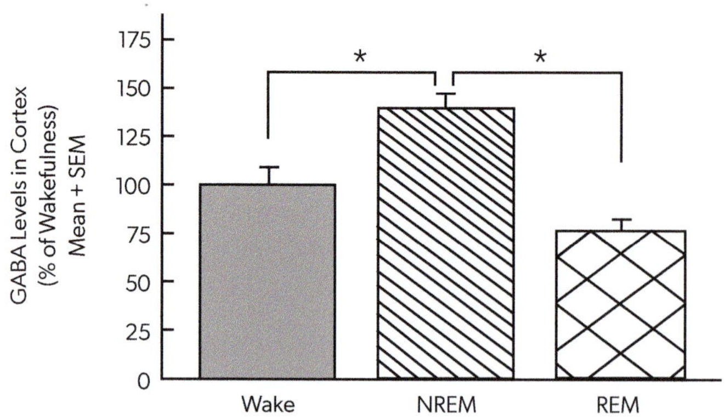

Figure 12.1 Average GABA levels in cat cortex measured using microdialysis and expressed as a percentage relative to levels during Wake (=100%). Average levels were significantly higher during NREM sleep than either wakefulness or REM sleep. These averages, however, obscure both temporal and anatomical variations in GABA levels; e.g., GABA levels rose during prolonged waking and fell gradually during NREM sleep. Levels in each state, therefore, depended on when a sample was taken; e.g., beginning vs. end of a NREM sleep episode. High GABA levels do not imply that all cortical neurons are inhibited during NREM sleep. For example, GABAergic interneurons involved in local circuits that help regulate low-frequency oscillations in cortex may be very active during NREM sleep. Reprinted with permission of Oxford University Press from Vanini, G. et al. (2012) GABA-to-ACh ratio in basal forebrain and cerebral cortex varies significantly during sleep. *Sleep* 35:1325–1334. © Sleep Research Society (2012). doi: 10.5665/sleep.2106.

Mircea Steriade's laboratory (Steriade, 2000). During waking, excitatory inputs to both thalamus and cortex (e.g., glutamate, acetylcholine, norepinephrine, hypocretin, histamine) promote thalamic and cortical activation by depolarizing their target neurons. During the transition from waking to NREM sleep, levels of these neurotransmitters in the forebrain fall while levels of the inhibitory neurotransmitter GABA become elevated in the cortex (Vanini et al., 2012) (**Figure 12.1**).

The combination of reduced subcortical excitatory input and increased GABAergic levels causes both thalamic and cortical neurons to become hyperpolarized.[2] Electrophysiological evidence from intracellular recordings of cortical neurons in unanesthetized cats supports a primary role for decreased excitatory input in this process (Steriade et al., 2001). The hyperpolarization of thalamic neurons is reinforced because they receive less excitatory glutamatergic input from the hyperpolarized cortex. As a result of these reciprocal relations,

[2] As discussed in Section 11.5, not all GABAergic input results in cortical hyperpolarization. Some basal forebrain GABAergic projections to cortex instead promote cortical activation by selectively inhibiting cortical GABAergic interneurons, resulting in disinhibition (activation) of the cortex's principal pyramidal neurons (Freund & Meskenaite, 1992).

thalamocortical relay neurons are among the first cells to show strong membrane hyperpolarization during the transition to NREM sleep (Steriade, 2000).

The consequences of cortical/thalamic hyperpolarization are related to a key characteristic shared by both thalamic relay and cortical neurons, particularly the large pyramidal output neurons in layer V of cortex. These neurons operate in two distinct modes, depending on their membrane potential. When they are at their resting membrane potential during waking, they respond to inputs with changes in firing rates that track the balance of excitation and inhibition they receive. In this mode, neurons are responding faithfully to incoming information, processing it, and conveying the information to other brain regions.

These neurons function in a different mode, however, when they are hyperpolarized. They contain a class of voltage-sensitive calcium (Ca^{2+}) channels that are activated by strong hyperpolarization. These channels interact with other membrane channels and with local neuronal circuits to generate slow, spontaneous rhythms in membrane potential. These slow rhythms are composed of alternating, brief depolarized Up states (also called "On"), during which these neurons fire in bursts, often as rapidly as during waking, and hyperpolarized Down states ("Off"), during which they are essentially silent (Steriade et al., 2001).

A complex balance of recurrent excitatory and inhibitory interactions involving pyramidal cells and interneurons within the cortex sustains the resulting cortical slow rhythms (Crunelli et al., 2015; Haider et al., 2006). Because of these interactions, cortical neurons generate spontaneous rhythms of membrane potential that appear in human scalp recordings as delta waves with large amplitudes (75–140 μV) and slow frequencies in the range of ~1–4.5 Hz.

Loss of excitatory input and tonic hyperpolarization of the cortex does not simply make cortical neurons inactive, but rather triggers their intrinsic capacity to alternate between burst-firing On and silent Off phases (Steriade, 1994). Activation of a class of cortical inhibitory interneurons that contain the peptide somatostatin triggers the Off states; inhibition of these neurons permits the appearance of On states (Funk et al., 2017). When cortical and thalamic neurons are in this alternating burst-firing/silent mode, their activity is being driven primarily by their intrinsic membrane properties and local circuits rather than by external excitatory or inhibitory inputs from sensory and other systems. As a result, these intrinsic oscillations tend to isolate the cortex from most external inputs, and thus reduce its capacity during NREM sleep to respond to environmental events or to generate awareness of them (Steriade, 2000); but see the discussion in Section 12.3.

Oscillations in the delta frequency range arise independently in both cortex and thalamus when neurons in these structures are hyperpolarized (Amzica & Steriade, 1998). Their independent origins are confirmed by their occurrence both in intact organisms and when each structure is studied in isolation in vitro, and in the cortex after large thalamic lesions (Amzica & Steriade, 2000).[3] In an intact organism, however, delta rhythms occur relatively synchronously across large cortical regions and are also integrated between the thalamus and cortex by feedback between them (see next section), resulting in a common pattern of low-frequency, high-amplitude oscillations in membrane potential across both structures.

One cortical structure has been proposed to play an important role in synchronizing this slow-wave activity (SWA) pattern across the cortex. The claustrum is a thin cellular layer between the cingulate cortex and the basal ganglia that is connected reciprocally to most cortical regions. Targeted optogenetic activation of the claustrum promoted broad silencing of cortical neural activity (Off states), and genetic ablation of the claustrum reduced SWA in frontal cortical regions (Narikiyo et al., 2020).

Early in the transition to NREM sleep, thalamocortical relay neurons become strongly hyperpolarized (Steriade, 2000). In mice, changes in electrical activity in the central medial thalamic nucleus, which projects broadly to cortical regions, preceded those in the cortex (Baker et al., 2014). A study involving electrophysiological recordings directly from the brains of people undergoing presurgical assessments for treatment of epilepsy found similar results. During spontaneous sleep onsets, slowing frequencies in thalamic nuclei preceded parallel changes in cortical regions by up to a few minutes, so the two structures could be transiently at different phases of the transition into sleep (Magnin et al., 2010). The hippocampus and neocortex in rats have also been shown to transiently express sleep–wake states asynchronously, especially during state transitions (Emrick et al., 2016).

Onset of sleep features in the thalamus and hippocampus for short periods, while the cortex continues to generate a waking EEG pattern, may contribute to unusual perceptual experiences during transitions to sleep. In these conditions, EEG activity in the cortex typical of normal waking occurs while sensory input from the thalamus is reduced or altered because it has entered a hyperpolarized, rhythmic sleep mode. Ongoing, internally generated cortical activity during this transiently dissociated state may be misinterpreted by the still-awake cortex as the product of external sensory input. These conditions may form the basis of unusual experiences while falling asleep, e.g., hypnagogic hallucinations, such as seeing or "sensing" someone in the room.

[3] Steriade distinguished two components contributing to delta rhythms in the thalamus, one which is intrinsic to the thalamus and one which is dependent on cortical input (Amzica & Steriade, 2000).

Much more common experiences during REM sleep may also depend on functional disconnections among neural systems. In this case, loss of normal functional connections among cortical regions, especially between frontal and other regions, may contribute to an uncritical acceptance by a dreamer of impossible elements in dream narratives (Horovitz et al., 2009; Maquet et al., 1996; Muzur et al., 2002); see discussion in Appendix A, Section A.2.

Although slow EEG waves are typically associated with NREM sleep, oscillations in the delta frequency range also appear less frequently during REM sleep and waking. High-density EEG studies in people during REM sleep identified waves at the fast end of the delta range (2–4 Hz) in several parts of the cortex in association with rapid eye movements. Slower waves (<2 Hz) were recorded in other cortical regions that were not associated with eye movements (Bernardi et al., 2019). Similar waves were also observed during REM sleep in the pons of a human patient during presurgical mapping studies (Lim et al., 2007); see discussion in Section 12.2.6. Although classic ponto-geniculo-occipital (PGO) waves that are commonly recorded in cats and other mammals during REM sleep (often associated with eye movements) are not readily detected in people, these observations suggest that some slow EEG waves during REM sleep in people may be analogs of PGO waves (Gott et al., 2017; Nelson et al., 1983).

In mice, low-amplitude SWA was recorded during REM sleep locally in primary visual, motor, and somatosensory cortices, and in association with phasic REM sleep phenomena (twitching of the vibrissal [whisker] muscles). These observations suggest that the prominent Off phases of these waves could play a role in inhibiting cortical responses to sensory inputs during REM sleep (Bernardi et al., 2019; Funk et al., 2016); see Section 12.3.3.

12.2.3 Thalamic reticular nucleus

The thalamic reticular nucleus (TRN) in humans consists of a thin band of tissue on the lateral edge of the thalamus, essentially wrapped around much larger, adjacent thalamic nuclei (**Figure 12.2**). It is responsible for modulating the flow of information in both directions between thalamic relay nuclei and the cortex (Fuentealba & Steriade, 2005; Steriade, 2000). The TRN is unique for several reasons. Unlike other thalamic nuclei, it does not contain glutamatergic neurons, nor does it project to the cortex. Instead, TRN neurons send inhibitory GABAergic projections to other thalamic nuclei; the TRN itself receives excitatory glutamatergic input from both cortical and thalamic neurons (**Figure 12.3**).

Because of these unique functional relations among the TRN, other thalamic nuclei, and the cortex, the TRN plays an important role in regulating features of the cortical EEG across sleep–wake states, in particular in generating sleep spindles (see the next section). Activating the TRN triggered cortical spindles, typical of NREM sleep, and increased the amount of NREM sleep (Halassa et al., 2011; Kim et al., 2012; Thankachan et al., 2019). Conversely, indirect inhibition of one class of TRN neurons reduced cortical spindle density and increased waking (Thankachan et al., 2019). Selective, brief activation of a targeted portion of the TRN generated an increase in delta waves in a restricted cortical region, similar to the occurrence of "local sleep" events that are discussed in Section 12.6 (Lewis et al., 2015).

In addition to its role in generating EEG features during sleep, the TRN is also involved in regulating waking behavior. It can affect the quality of performance in cognitive tasks by influencing attentional mechanisms, modulating arousal, and selectively regulating the flow of sensory inputs from thalamic relay nuclei to the cortex (Halassa et al., 2014; Wimmer et al., 2015). One mechanism that may be involved is the TRN's role

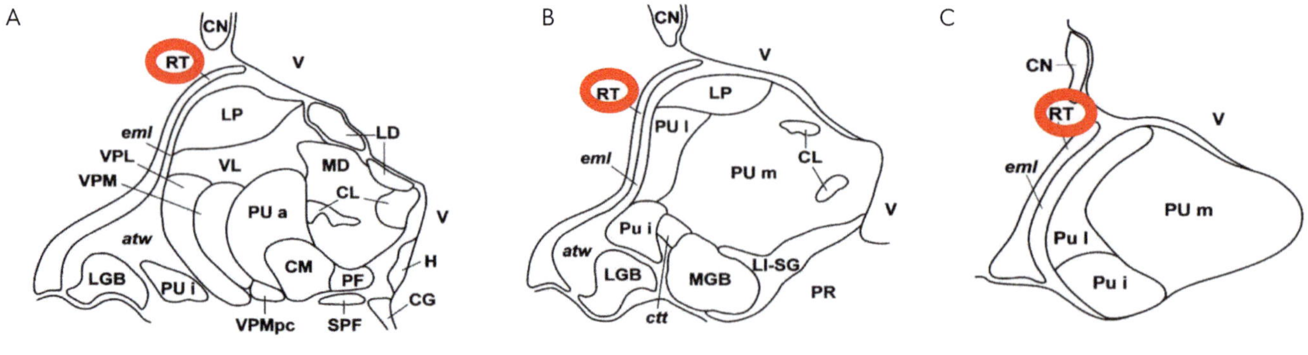

Figure 12.2 Drawings of frontal sections at three levels of the caudal thalamus of humans (**A–C**) (with **C** representing the caudal pole of the thalamus) illustrating parts of numerous thalamic nuclei, including the thalamic reticular nucleus (RT, red circles), which is a thin layer of cells at the lateral edge of the thalamus. RT neurons project not to cortex, but to other thalamic nuclei, and they receive projections from both cortex and other thalamic nuclei. Adapted with permission from Rüb U. et al. (2003) Thalamic involvement in a spinocerebellar ataxia type 2 (SCA2) and a spinocerebellar ataxia type 3 (SCA3) patient, and its clinical relevance. *Brain* 126:2257–2272. © Guarantors of Brain (2003). Published by Oxford University Press. doi: 10.1093/brain/awg234.

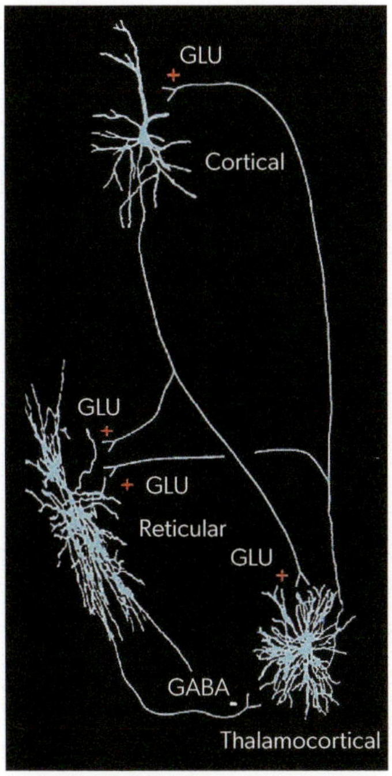

Figure 12.3 Thalamic reticular nucleus neurons ("Reticular" or TRN neurons) project to other thalamic nuclei, releasing the inhibitory (-) neurotransmitter GABA. Thalamacortical relay neurons release the excitatory neurotransmitter glutamate (+ GLU) on both TRN and cortical neurons. Cortical projections to both the TRN and to thalamic relay nuclei are also glutamatergic and excitatory (+). This circuit is involved in gating the exchange of information between thalamus and cortex and in generating bursts of electrical activity in the cortex (sleep spindles) that characterize N2/N3 sleep. Reprinted with permission from Steriade M. (2001) The GABAergic reticular nucleus: a preferential target of corticothalamic projections. *PNAS* 98:3625–3627. © National Academy of Sciences, USA (2001). doi: 10.1073/pnas.071051998.

as a pacemaker for gamma-range (~40 Hz) oscillations that have been implicated in a variety of cognitive functions (Pinault & Deschênes, 1992; Steriade et al., 1996). The TRN also projects to a region of the pontine reticular activating system, giving it the capacity to influence global activation of the thalamocortical system (Parent & Steriade, 1984).

12.2.4 Sleep spindles

The appearance of sleep spindles in the cortical EEG marks entry into N2 sleep. Sleep spindles are bursts of higher frequency electrical activity that appear against the slower background oscillation between Off and On states seen in N2 and N3 sleep (see Section 2.3.2 and **Figures 1.4** and **2.4**). They occur in most cortical regions and to some extent in the hippocampus. Sleep spindles are triggered by the TRN indirectly through its inhibitory input to thalamic relay neurons that influence cortical activity (**Figure 12.3**), and their appearance is modulated by cortical input to the thalamus.

During waking, the cortex provides tonic excitatory input to the thalamus and TRN. During cortical hyperpolarized Off states in N2, this input is reduced, which helps promote hyperpolarization of these structures. Like other thalamic and cortical neurons when moderately hyperpolarized, TRN neurons also enter a burst-firing mode because of activation of their voltage-gated Ca^{2+} and other ion channels. This tendency for TRN neurons to produce bursts of action potentials is further strengthened because cortical and thalamic relay neurons in their own On phases convey bursts of transient excitatory input to the TRN.

As a result, inhibitory GABAergic neurons in the TRN fire in bursts, resulting in the periodic release of GABA onto thalamocortical relay neurons. GABA transiently inhibits (hyperpolarizes) these thalamocortical neurons, which respond to a release from inhibition with a parallel burst of post-inhibitory rebound action potentials. These action potentials cause the release of glutamate onto cortical neurons, with a similar temporal pattern. Thus, a burst of inhibitory input from the TRN to thalamocortical neurons indirectly results in a parallel burst of excitatory input to cortical neurons. Pyramidal neurons in the cortex respond to this depolarizing input with bursts of firing, generating the characteristic frequencies (~12–16 Hz) and patterns of sleep spindles recorded in the EEG (Fuentealba & Steriade, 2005; Lüthi, 2014; Mak-McCully et al., 2017).[4]

Spindles are typically triggered in the TRN at the low point of cortical Off phases. Because of the circuitry involved, this timing results in their appearance in the cortex during the following On phase (Andrillon et al., 2011; Mak-McCully et al., 2017). See Section 18.6.2 for a discussion of the importance of the timing of sleep spindles relative to cortical EEG oscillations for memory consolidation during sleep.

Spindling in the TRN is triggered when the thalamus is moderately hyperpolarized (N2 sleep), but stronger, tonic hyperpolarization (as in N3 sleep) makes spindling less likely (Amzica & Steriade, 2000). There are also more large-amplitude slow waves during N3 sleep, which may make it more difficult to detect spindles in scalp recordings. As a result, the density of measurable sleep spindles in human NREM sleep increases over the course of the night in parallel to increasing amounts of N2 and decreasing amounts of N3 sleep (De Gennaro & Ferrara, 2003; Dijk et al., 1993). Within single NREM sleep episodes, the dynamics are more complex, with parallel changes in the number of spindles and delta waves at the start and end of an episode, but fewer spindles during the middle when delta waves are most frequent (Dijk et al., 1993; Uchida et al., 1994).

---

[4] Several membrane conductances, as well as local-circuit activity in the thalamus and cortex, contribute to the generation of rebound bursts of firing in response to hyperpolarization (Grenier et al., 1998).

In human epilepsy patients undergoing presurgical assessments, intracortical electrodes were able to detect sleep spindles in N3 (and "early" sleep, which would be dominated by N3) (Andrillon et al., 2011; Nir et al., 2011; Peter-Derex et al., 2012). However, spindles were much less frequent during deepest NREM sleep, when SWA was at its peak (Andrillon et al., 2011).

One study that used recordings from scalp electrodes in people detected many spindles during deeper NREM sleep produced during 2 h afternoon naps after partial overnight sleep restriction (Cox et al., 2012). These results suggest that either circadian phase or prior sleep loss increased the number of spindles usually recorded during nighttime N3 sleep. A role for circadian modulation seems most likely because sleep loss generally decreases, rather than increases, spindle activity, as would be predicted by the large amounts of N3 sleep typically seen immediately after starting to recover from sleep deprivation (Dijk et al., 1993). This conclusion is supported by other evidence that there is a spontaneous circadian-controlled peak of fast sleep spindle activity in the afternoon (Dijk et al., 1997).

Spindle production is also affected by other inputs. A very rare neurological condition called auto-activation deficit (AAD) is caused by damage to the basal ganglia. Patients with this condition showed a syndrome involving a combination of "mental emptiness" and a lack of spontaneously generated behavior, but reasonably intact responsiveness to external prompts for behavior. In a study of 13 of these patients, 6 did not generate sleep spindles during NREM sleep, while the remaining patients produced spindles with abnormal frequencies (Leu-Semenescu et al., 2013). These subgroups did not differ in terms of their degree of mental emptiness while awake (Dr. Isabelle Arnulf, personal communication, 2013).

Since the thalamus was largely or completely intact in most patients who did not generate spindles, this loss of spindles appeared to be unrelated to TRN or other thalamic damage, suggesting that the basal ganglia contribute to the regulation of thalamocortical interactions that generate spindle activity. This hypothesis is supported by evidence that thalamic nuclei that receive projections from the basal ganglia are active at the time spindles are triggered (Ushimaru et al., 2012). The impact of AAD on dreaming is discussed in Appendix A.

Selective genetic disruption of TRN function impaired attention and disrupted sleep organization in a mouse model system, suggesting links to conditions like attention deficit hyperactivity disorder (ADHD) and some forms of autism that are characterized by changes in attentional mechanisms and sleep (Wells et al., 2016). A study involving children and adolescents with autism spectrum disorder (ASD) found altered timing of sleep spindles relative to slow oscillations (SOs) during N2 sleep and fewer spindles in N3 sleep than in controls. In addition, there was a negative correlation between spindle numbers in N3 sleep and performance on a spatial memory task, while typically developing controls showed a positive correlation (see Chapters 17 and 18 for discussions of the role of sleep in memory consolidation). These results suggest that some children with ASD undergo a developmental change in thalamocortical circuitry linked to altered TRN function, which can affect both attentional and learning mechanisms (Mylonas et al., 2022). See Section 15.4.2 for a discussion of changes in sleep spindles in patients with schizophrenia.

12.2.5 Slow oscillations and K complexes

Slow oscillations (SOs) are defined as very large amplitude EEG waves (>140 μV in human scalp recordings), typically with both On- and Off-phase components. They have frequencies of <1 Hz (averaging ~0.7–0.8 Hz but can be much slower in anesthetized animal preparations), which are below the range of delta rhythms (1.0–4.5 Hz); see "Stage IV" in **Figure 1.4**. The number of SOs increases when neurons are more hyperpolarized (as in N3 sleep). Reductions of cholinergic and noradrenergic inputs to the cortex associated with NREM sleep are permissive for the expression of SOs (Steriade, Amzica, et al., 1993). Most single pyramidal neurons recorded intracellularly in the cortex of cats were both hyperpolarized (and silent) and then depolarized (and burst firing) during SOs (**Figure 12.4**), but some

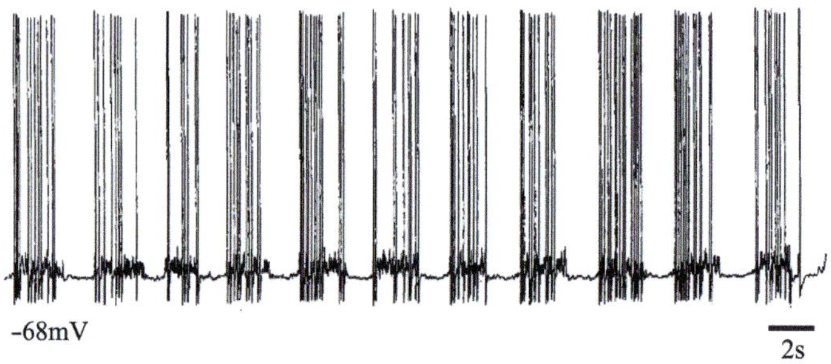

Figure 12.4 Intracellular single-unit recording under anesthesia from one neuron in the cat primary visual cortex, demonstrating a burst pattern of firing with intervening periods of inhibition, similar to that seen in deep stages of NREM sleep. Depth EEG recordings from a nearby electrode demonstrated that the firing bursts corresponded to transient cortical depolarizations during On phases of slow oscillations (SOs). Time scale bar = 2 sec. Intervals between burst onsets varied around 3–4 sec, implying a frequency of oscillation near 0.3 Hz, a typical frequency for SOs under anesthesia; SO frequencies during normal sleep average 0.7–0.8 Hz. Reprinted with permission of the Society for Neuroscience from Steriade, M. et al. (1993) A novel slow (<1 Hz) oscillation of neocortical neurons in vivo: depolarizing and hyperpolarizing component. *J Neurosci* 13:3252–3265. © Society for Neuroscience (1993). doi:10.1523/JNEUROSCI.13-08-03252.1993.

oscillated instead between strong hyperpolarization and resting membrane potential levels (Steriade, Nuñez, et al., 1993b).

In addition to differences in amplitude and frequency, SOs have also been distinguished from delta waves by other characteristics. Cortical delta waves are strongly influenced by diffuse projections from the thalamus that reach large regions of the cortex, so they tend to occur relatively synchronously across the cortex. Slow oscillations do not occur diffusely throughout the cortex, but are expressed locally, so that some cortical regions show SOs while nearby regions do not, as confirmed by intracortical recordings from people (Nir et al., 2011).

Some reports indicated that SOs recorded from scalp electrodes originated in several frontal neocortical regions and usually propagated caudally, often via the cingulate cortical area. Frontal and association cortices were more likely than sensory cortices to propagate the oscillations (Massimini et al., 2004; Murphy et al., 2009). Another study instead identified localized sources for SOs in the ventral "limbic cortex," including the anterior medial temporal lobe and orbitofrontal lobe, especially on the left side (Morgan et al., 2021).

SOs arise only in the cortex and continue to occur when the thalamus is inactivated or ablated or when the cortex is studied in vitro (Steriade, Nuñez, et al., 1993a), but thalamic input can modify their characteristics. Thalamocortical projections time the onset of SOs in intact organisms as well as increasing their frequency and synchrony across cortical columns. Loss of thalamic input transiently reduces SOs, but they recover in the absence of the thalamus and are then expressed at a lower frequency (David et al., 2013; Lemieux et al., 2014; Neske, 2016).

Other evidence distinguishes the physiology of delta waves and SOs. In an fMRI study of large-scale brain regional activity during SWS, there were increases in activity of different brain regions (relative to background activity during SWS) coincident with the occurrence of delta waves and SOs. SOs were associated with increased activity in hippocampal and parahippocampal regions, the cerebellum, and the brainstem. The occurrence of delta waves was associated more with increased activity in frontal and cingulate brain regions (Dang-Vu et al., 2008).

Delta waves and SOs are also affected differently by homeostatic mechanisms. Amounts of SWA, defined as EEG power in the 0.75–4.5 Hz range, peak at the start of a night's sleep and decline during the sleep phase (Achermann et al., 1993); see **Figures 5.2** and **5.3**. This range includes both delta rhythms (1.0–4.5 Hz) and SOs (<1.0 Hz), so it is unclear whether both respond similarly. Other studies found that EEG power in the 1.9–5.0 Hz range (only delta activity) declined from the first to the second nightly NREM sleep episode. This observation is consistent with the idea that delta power reflects the strength of the current homeostatic sleep drive, which decreases as one sleeps and produces SWA. EEG power in the SO range (<1 Hz, centered on 0.75 Hz), however, did not decline, and even increased slightly, from the first to the second NREM sleep episode. As a result, SO frequencies made up an increasing proportion of the <3 Hz frequency band over a night's first three NREM sleep episodes, as the amount of delta-band activity declined (Achermann & Borbély, 1997; Borbély et al., 1981; Church et al., 1975; Hubbard et al., 2020).

This evidence for differences in homeostatic regulation is supported by studies of the effects of sleep loss. Total overnight sleep deprivation increased power in the delta frequency range during later recovery sleep (see **Figure 5.3**), consistent with homeostatic regulation, but it *decreased* power in the SO range (Borbély et al., 1981). There is, therefore, no evidence for homeostatic regulation of SO numbers, either within a typical night's sleep or after sleep loss, in contrast to delta waves. These results are consistent with the interpretation that delta range activity and SOs are different phenomena regulated by different mechanisms.

K complexes are also large-amplitude voltage changes, but they occur as isolated events during NREM sleep. They typically include a high-amplitude, negative half-wave (Off phase), sometimes followed by a slower positive half-wave (On phase). They have a duration of >0.5 sec and occur at a rate of 1–3 per minute rather than appearing in a continuous series, as SOs often do. K complexes appear first in N2 sleep but persist with similar features through N3 sleep (Gonzalez et al., 2018). A K complex in N2 is often associated with a following sleep spindle (see **Figure 2.4**), which starts near the Off-On transition phase of the K complex. This timing relates to the impact on the TRN of receiving increasing excitatory input from cortical neurons that are starting to become depolarized at that phase (Amzica & Steriade, 1997; Andrillon et al., 2011; Cash et al., 2009; Gonzalez et al., 2018; Ushimaru et al., 2012).

One interpretation is that K complexes are examples of isolated SOs, although sometimes lacking the typical On phase. An alternative interpretation is that they are a different phenomenon but are strongly influenced by underlying SOs. Fourier analysis of human K complexes suggested that they are the product of a slow oscillation interacting with ongoing delta waves (Amzica & Steriade, 1997). In addition to their spontaneous occurrence, K complexes can also be evoked by external stimuli during sleep, as discussed in Section 12.4.2.

Studies have examined the pattern of appearance of K complexes during intracortical recordings from patients with epilepsy. They were reported to arise independently in many cortical regions and to propagate in different directions. There was only a very small bias toward an anterior-posterior direction of propagation (Gonzalez et al., 2018; Mak-McCully et al., 2015). These presurgical studies are aimed at only limited brain regions because they are intended primarily to obtain clinically relevant information about the sources of seizures.

It is unclear, therefore, whether the reported differences in the origins and propagation patterns of SOs and K complexes are characteristic of these features or are influenced by the type of participants being studied or the recording sites and methods used.

The several rhythmic EEG patterns seen in the cortex during NREM sleep are not expressed independently of each other. Rather, SOs' high-amplitude cycles of depolarization and hyperpolarization influence the amplitude and phase coupling across local cortical regions of other rhythmic features (delta waves, K complexes, and sleep spindles) as well as patterns of neural activity in multiple brain regions (Cox et al., 2014; Dang-Vu et al., 2008; Steriade, Nuñez, et al., 1993a). The resulting temporal relations between, for example, sleep spindles and other NREM EEG features are functionally important for responsiveness to external stimuli (see Section 12.4.2) and for memory consolidation (see Chapter 18) (Csercsa et al., 2010; Helfrich et al., 2018; Latchoumane et al., 2017; Steriade, Nuñez, et al., 1993a).

12.2.6 Cortical activation

The thalamus plays a central role in generating the cortical EEG features of waking and REM sleep, as well as of NREM sleep. The mechanisms contributing to the cortical EEG patterns shown during waking and REM sleep were addressed in part in other chapters (Sections 10.2–10.7, and 11.5). To summarize, neurons in several brainstem nuclei project to the midline thalamus and to basal forebrain nuclei, which in turn project to the cortex; a subset of these brainstem neuromodulatory systems (see Chapter 10) and projections from hypothalamic regions (see Chapter 11) also reach the cortex directly. Glutamate and ACh from the basal forebrain and glutamate from the thalamus play a central role in activating cortical neurons during both waking and REM sleep. ACh (and other neurotransmitters) from pontine projections that activate the thalamus and basal forebrain are also involved in activating the cortex indirectly.

The use of optogenetic and chemogenetic approaches to activating and silencing neuronal groups has identified several other hypothalamic and brainstem neurons that can promote waking when they are activated; see Chapter 11. How their activity fits into the sequence of events that trigger cortical activation remains to be determined (Gompf & Anaclet, 2020).

Other neuromodulators (NE, 5-HT, histamine, and hypocretin) that contribute to cortical activation during waking differ from ACh because they do not contribute to activation during REM sleep. Dopamine may be an exception because its levels in the cortex are higher during both waking and REM sleep than during NREM sleep, and a subset of dopaminergic neurons are proposed to be involved in triggering dreaming, which occurs most often during REM sleep (see Sections 10.4.1 and 10.4.2). Some GABAergic projections from basal forebrain nuclei also promote cortical activation by inhibiting GABAergic cortical interneurons that inhibit pyramidal neurons (Brown et al., 2012; Jones, 2020; Steriade et al., 1984); see Chapters 10 and 11 for more details.

Brainstem activating systems that project to the thalamus mostly reach nonspecific nuclei that are involved in triggering and sustaining cortical activation across large cortical regions. In rats, individual neurons in one midline thalamic nucleus (nucleus reuniens) were most active during either, or both, waking and REM sleep (Viena et al., 2021). In mice, optogenetic activation of another nonspecific thalamic nucleus (ventromedial nucleus) caused rapid waking from NREM sleep (Honjoh et al., 2018).

Cortical activation involves expression of a range of higher frequencies in the EEG, including gamma-range frequencies (~40 Hz). These frequencies may also be driven in part by nonspecific thalamic input. Firing rates of neurons in one intralaminar thalamic nucleus (centrolateral nucleus) in cats fell into this frequency range during waking and REM sleep. During NREM sleep, these cells instead produced bursts of firing in the spindle frequency range (Steriade, Curró Dossi, et al., 1993).

PGO waves are a characteristic feature of REM sleep, which can be recorded with macroelectrodes from the pons, lateral geniculate nucleus of the thalamus, and visual cortex of cats and other species. These ascending bursts of neural activity are strongly associated with rapid eye movements during REM sleep (Callaway et al., 1987; Datta, 1997; Sakai & Cespuglio, 1974). Their presence in people has been less clear, but studies using scalp recordings provided suggestive evidence that PGO-like waves (usually called P-waves, because their functional equivalence to PGO waves in cats is uncertain) also occur during human REM sleep (McCarley et al., 1983).

Depth recordings from the pons of a human patient with Parkinson's disease confirmed the presence of P-waves that were structurally similar to PGO waves immediately before and during REM sleep. About 41% of rapid eye movements were associated with P-waves in this individual (Lim et al., 2007), while in cats ~80% were associated with PGO waves (Sakai & Cespuglio, 1974).

12.2.7 Summary

The thalamus conveys both specific sensory/motor information and nonspecific activation to the cortex. Sensory and motor relay nuclei (that include many parvalbumin-containing neurons) project to middle cortical layers in modality-specific regions of cortex. Midline and intralaminar thalamic nuclei (containing many calbindin neurons) receive input from brainstem components of the reticular activating system and project more broadly to superficial cortical layers, including to association cortices.

When cortical and thalamic neurons are hyperpolarized (by increased GABA and reduced excitatory neuromodulators), they develop slow waves of alternating silent (Off) and burst-firing (On) states in the frequency range of 1–4.5 Hz (delta range). During sleep onset, some thalamic neurons tend to enter this slow oscillatory mode before the cortex. Temporal gaps between onset of delta waves in different brain regions may contribute to some sensory misperceptions during wake–sleep transitions. Slow EEG waves can also occur in some cortical layers and regions during human REM sleep and waking. These features may represent human analogs of PGO waves seen in other mammals and may contribute to the suppression of sensory input during REM sleep.

The thalamic reticular nucleus (TRN) is a thin structure that wraps around other thalamic nuclei. It sends inhibitory input to other thalamic nuclei but does not project to the cortex; it receives excitatory input from both thalamic relay nuclei and the cortex. The TRN also projects to part of the pontine reticular activating system and is involved in regulating sensory input and in attentional processes during waking. It triggers the electrical patterns that appear as EEG spindles in the cortex during sleep. Spindles are most common in N2 sleep, and therefore during the second half of a night's sleep, but appear less frequently in N3 sleep early in the night.

Slow cortical waves can be divided into delta waves (1–4.5 Hz) and SOs (<1 Hz, averaging.7–.8 Hz). K complexes, which may be isolated components of SOs, are especially characteristic of N2 sleep. The distinction between delta waves and SOs is based on several features in addition to their frequencies and amplitudes. Delta oscillations originate in both thalamus and cortex. Slow oscillations originate in the cortex, although there are different views as to whether they originate primarily in frontal neocortex or in ventral limbic paleocortex. SOs occur during deeper states of neuronal hyperpolarization and propagate across cortical regions but avoid primary sensory areas. They organize higher-frequency oscillations, so that delta waves and sleep spindles often cluster within specific phases of SOs.

Delta waves tend to appear more synchronously across cortical regions (and in the thalamus), and are broadly distributed, probably because of the influence of diffuse thalamocortical inputs. Delta waves are a marker of sleep need, so they increase in number during recovery sleep after sleep deprivation, while power in the SO frequency range decreases during recovery sleep. Delta wave activity also decreases during NREM sleep episodes over the course of the night, as sleep need is gradually satisfied. In contrast, SOs do not appear to be homeostatically regulated, and their number does not decrease after the first NREM sleep episode.

Cortical activation during waking and REM sleep is produced by glutamate from nonspecific thalamic nuclei and glutamate, ACh, and GABA projections from basal forebrain nuclei. These structure are in turn activated by glutamatergic and cholinergic projections from several brainstem nuclei. Cortical activation during waking is also supported by direct projections to the cortex from brainstem and hypothalamic nuclei that use several neuromodulators (including NE, 5-HT, dopamine, histamine, and hypocretin).

As in waking, during REM sleep, brainstem neurons act on midline thalamic nuclei to produce cortical activation. Brainstem cholinergic projections to the basal forebrain contribute to activation by triggering cholinergic, glutamatergic, and GABAergic neurons that project to the cortex. Except for DA, levels of other neuromodulators that promote cortical arousal during waking by projections to the cortex are strongly reduced during REM sleep relative to waking. Pontine generators trigger PGO waves during REM sleep in cats and other species, and probably also in people. PGO waves are conveyed to the cortex via the LGN and are strongly linked to the occurrence of rapid eye movements in cats, and, with lower probability, in people.

12.3 Information processing during sleep

12.3.1 Sensory input during sleep

Sleep is defined in part by the loss of conscious awareness of most external events and by the objective evidence of reduced or absent responsiveness to these events. But environmental stimuli that are intrusive and important enough (e.g., those signaling danger) are usually able to awaken a person quickly. Both of these features are defining characteristics of sleep—it is a rapidly reversible state of unconsciousness.

Responsiveness to some but not other stimuli raises the question of how, and on the basis of what information, a sleeping brain decides that an external event is important. How much information about external events does the sleeping brain receive and process while remaining "unconscious"? In addition, since sleep stages are characterized by significant differences in patterns of activity in thalamocortical and other systems, a secondary question is the extent to which processing of environmental information differs among sleep stages.

Audition is the sense that is usually studied in relation to information processing about potential danger during sleep. Among our senses, vision, touch, nociception (pain perception), and taste are not useful for providing early warnings of danger. By the time something unpleasant or dangerous is touching or hurting you (or in your mouth!), it is likely to be too late. Although our visual system is exquisitely adapted for gathering environmental information at a distance, vision is essentially useless as an early-warning system with eyes closed in the darkness of night.

Olfaction is relatively poorly developed in humans and depends on a slowly moving chemical stimulus, although it may be useful for detecting some strong stimuli at a short distance (e.g., the odor of smoke). However, tests of people's ability to detect and respond to a strong olfactory cue found few or no responses during sleep stages beyond N1, in contrast to auditory signals (Carskadon & Herz, 2004). It is no accident that electronic smoke and carbon monoxide detectors are designed to convert subtle signals of danger to a loud auditory alarm. For people, audition is the only sense that functions over relatively long distances, conveys information quickly, is unaffected by darkness, and is not physically obstructed during sleep (i.e., we have no "earlids").

An early hypothesis suggested that the "sentinel" function required to monitor the environment during sleep was served by REM sleep. The evidence that led to this idea included the fact that cortical EEG patterns during REM sleep resemble those of waking, so the brain appears more prepared to respond to an auditory warning by reverting to full alertness. In fact, those deliberately awakened from REM sleep are more alert and functional than those awakened from NREM, especially N3, sleep (Dement & Kleitman, 1957). In addition, many REM sleep episodes are followed by transient cortical arousals to waking (Snyder, 1966). This phenomenon in a rat is illustrated in **Figure 10.12**; but note that this rat also showed arousals out of NREM sleep that did not immediately follow REM sleep. As discussed in the following sections, the evidence does not suggest a special role for REM sleep in environmental monitoring.

The ability to process and respond to different categories of auditory information during sleep has been studied for decades. These studies examined the kinds of stimuli that do or do not trigger arousal, whether responses vary across sleep stages, and how motivation and familiarity affect responsiveness.

Several different methods have been used to present stimuli and to evaluate responsiveness. In some studies, a series of identical sounds were repeated, and the latency until the sleeper responded was recorded. Other studies involved measuring the threshold intensity at which a stimulus evoked a response by regularly increasing its intensity until it triggered a response. In others, a variety of different sounds were presented to assess whether responsiveness varied depending on the characteristics of the sounds. Another method used was presenting a monotonous series of identical stimuli, interrupted by one different stimulus ("oddball" paradigm) to assess whether the sleeper detected and responded to the change in stimulus parameters.

12.3.2 Impact of meaning, motivation, and novelty

An obvious intuition about noise is that louder sounds are more likely to wake sleepers than quieter sounds. In fact, evidence that noise at night disrupts sleep and produces adverse health effects led the World Health Organization to develop guidelines for acceptable intensities of noise at night (Hume et al., 2012). However, there are also anecdotal reports and research findings indicating that low-intensity sounds that are novel or personally important can wake people up, even when louder, familiar sounds do not.

An often cited, anecdotal example of the importance of meaning and motivation is that parents of young infants can be wakened by a relatively weak cry from their infant in the next room, but do not respond to familiar, louder noises (James, 1890).[5] A similar anecdote, but in this case based on a clinician's experience and documented with published EEG records, relates to a woman with narcolepsy. She had episodes of deep sleep from which she could not be awakened by banging a bucket with a hammer next to her ear or pinching her. But she woke immediately to the sound of her own name being spoken softly (Jasper et al., 1952).

A similar expression of the role of motivation and meaning in determining responsiveness appeared in a recent novel: "What woke me was the metallic click of the rifle's safety being released. No soldier in battle could ever miss that sound, even in a deep sleep" (Murakami, 1994, 1995, p. 151).[6] If these anecdotes are correct, and it is not only the volume but also the meaning of a sound that is important, then people must be performing a quite sophisticated, ongoing analysis of the meaning of external stimuli while they remain asleep, despite an apparent general lack of conscious awareness of the environment.

Experimental studies in several species have evaluated this idea and tested the degree of sensitivity to meaningful sounds

---

[5] In his foundational volume *The Principles of Psychology*, William James described the phenomenon and a hypothetical mental mechanism to explain it: "The mother who is asleep to every sound but the stirrings of her babe, evidently has the babe-portion of her auditory sensibility systematically awake. Relatively to that, the rest of her mind is in a state of systematized anaesthesia. That department, split off and disconnected from the sleeping part, can none the less wake the latter up in case of need." (James, 1890, v.1, p. 213).

[6] Excerpt from *The Wind-Up Bird Chronicle* by Haruki Murakami, translated by Jay Rubin, copyright ©1994, 1995 by Haruki Murakami Archival Labyrinth. Used by permission of Alfred A. Knopf, an imprint of the Knopf Doubleday Publishing Group, a division of Penguin Random House LLC and by permission of Harukimurakami Archival Labyrinth. All rights reserved.

in different sleep stages. Cats conditioned to expect milk after hearing a series of clicks responded to the clicks by waking out of NREM sleep, but were less likely to do so out of REM sleep, unless the sound intensity was increased (Siegel & Langley, 1965). Rats trained to expect a foot shock after a tone woke out of NREM sleep with high probability in response to the tone, but rarely out of REM sleep when presented at the same intensity (Van Twyver & Garrett, 1972).

People in an early study were instructed to clench a fist and wake up if they heard their own name or another target (control) name. A long series of names were played while they slept. They responded with higher probability to their own name than to the targeted control name or to other names; they also generated K complexes most frequently to their own name (Oswald et al., 1960). When participants in another study were offered "extra payment" for waking fully from sleep to two particular sounds from among many others, there was a large increase in the proportion of waking responses selectively to the targeted sounds (Zung & Wilson, 1961). One study of young women, both late in pregnancy and shortly after childbirth, reported that they had a lower threshold to waken in response to a recording of a baby crying, or to the voice of a woman stating that a baby is crying, than to a recording of meaningless human speech sounds (Poitras et al., 1973).

The role of motivation has even been addressed in fruit flies. Drosophila that had been quiescent for at least 5 min (presumed to be sleeping) were exposed to the odor of acetic acid at a concentration that flies find attractive. They became active in response to that cue with higher probability than in response to a control puff of air or to a higher concentration of acetic acid that is aversive. Deprivation of food also increased responses to food-related odors more than to non-food odors (French et al., 2021).

In summary, for several species, the meaning of auditory stimuli (and smells in fruit flies) was important in determining whether a sleeping individual would respond. The threshold for responding in mammals was typically lower during NREM sleep than during REM sleep.

Factors other than meaning also influence responsiveness to sounds during sleep. People sleeping in an unfamiliar laboratory environment for the first time were classified as demonstrating a "first-night effect"[7] if they showed a lengthened sleep-onset latency. During their first sleep study, these participants produced less SWA, and they showed more EEG responses during NREM sleep to an unexpected sound (oddball stimulus), but only when delivered to the left hemisphere (Tamaki et al., 2016). The hemispheric difference in responding to the oddball stimulus disappeared during a second sleep study when the environment was familiar and the "first-night effect" on sleep-onset latency was gone (Tamaki et al., 2016). (See Section 7.5.3 for more discussion of this phenomenon and other examples of brain asymmetries during sleep.)

The idea that familiarity reduces sensitivity to sounds was supported by a study in which young people were exposed to loud recordings of street noises nightly for a week. These noises disturbed sleep and reduced sleep efficiency during the first few nights, but these effects diminished during the last nights of the study (Saletu et al., 1989). The basis for this change in responsiveness is not clear. One possibility is that the novel noise initially disturbed sleep until it became familiar and non-threatening, allowing sleep to be maintained. Alternatively, losing sleep over the first nights of the study could have increased homeostatic sleep pressure and the depth of recovery sleep during later nights (see Chapter 5). Increased EEG delta activity during recovery sleep after deprivation in both people and rats has been shown to reduce both behavioral and electrophysiological responsiveness to sounds (Frederickson & Rechtschaffen, 1978; Williams et al., 1964).

12.3.3 Assessing responsiveness during different sleep stages

The measures used to test whether a sleeper has detected and responded to a stimulus have varied across studies. Responses have included: waking up, as defined by the usual EEG criteria; alterations in EEG patterns that indicate detection of the stimulus, but without waking (e.g., generating a burst of EEG alpha rhythm); specific features in stimulus-evoked EEG potentials (event-related potentials (ERPs)); vascular changes indicating arousal; and participants producing a prearranged verbal or motor response to a particular class of stimuli. Not surprisingly, these different measures can produce different results.

Studies that compared responses across sleep stages typically found that it is more difficult to evoke a response to sounds as one goes from lighter to deeper stages of NREM sleep (Zung & Wilson, 1961). It is less clear where REM sleep fits relative to NREM stages. In the early animal conditioning studies discussed in Section 12.3.2, louder sounds were needed to trigger responses from REM than NREM sleep (Oswald et al., 1960; Siegel & Langley, 1965). In people, thresholds to produce a behavioral response to a noise during REM sleep were similar to the very high thresholds in Stage 4 NREM sleep. In contrast, a vascular response to noise (constriction of a peripheral blood vessel) was easiest to evoke in REM sleep and most difficult to evoke in Stage 4 NREM sleep (Williams et al., 1964).

[7] This typical terminology for the effects of sleeping in an unfamiliar place was used in this report. The studies discussed were actually conducted during a 90 min daytime nap, so it might better be described as a "novel environment" effect.

Another study had participants respond by pressing a switch to indicate they were awake when they heard a recording of their own name or of a meaningless sound (their own name played backwards). It found that participants responded somewhat more quickly during REM sleep than N2 sleep, but there was no difference in latency for occipital alpha to appear as a marker of waking. By either measure, participants responded more quickly to their own name than to the meaningless sound (Langford et al., 1974).

Sleep stage differences in responsiveness could relate to differences at some or all phases of the response process: detection of a stimulus, interpretation of its meaning, or production of a response. For example, the higher level of background autonomic arousal during REM sleep could make it easier to generate a vascular response mediated by the autonomic system, as compared to during NREM sleep (Williams et al., 1964).

The degree of sleep inertia also differs after waking from different sleep stages and could affect how quickly a participant could produce a required motor response. Those waking out of REM sleep tend to be alert and well oriented to their environment; while those waking out of N3 show sleep inertia, including disorientation and confusion (Broughton, 1968; Dement & Kleitman, 1957; Tassi & Muzet, 2000). Thus, different response latencies could result from differences in the ability to produce a response, even if there were no differences in detecting stimuli or in processing and interpreting their content.

Another important issue in these studies is that different conclusions about responsiveness to stimuli during REM sleep can result from conducting studies without reference to different REM sleep substages, namely, tonic and phasic REM sleep. Tonic REM sleep is characterized by sustained EEG desynchronization, low EMG, and suppressed thermoregulation (present throughout REM sleep). Phasic REM sleep is marked by transient bursts of rapid eye movements, PGO waves (or P-waves in people), and rapid respiration (see **Figure 2.6**).

In studies in which participants used switch closures to indicate that they had detected a sound, response thresholds were high during Stage 4 sleep, but even slightly higher during phasic REM sleep. Response thresholds during tonic REM sleep, however, were considerably lower and resembled those in N2 sleep (**Figure 12.5A**) (Ermis et al., 2010; Price & Kremen, 1980). Similarly, there was a higher probability of showing cortical activation or waking in response to mildly painful heat from a laser during tonic REM sleep (~34% of trials) than during phasic REM sleep (~6% of trials) (Bastuji et al., 2008). Consistent with these behavioral effects, cortical evoked responses to tones presented during waking and REM sleep substages were smallest in phasic REM sleep and largest during waking (Sallinen et al., 1996).

These differences in response thresholds could be related to the inhibitory effects of phasic events (e.g., neural activity

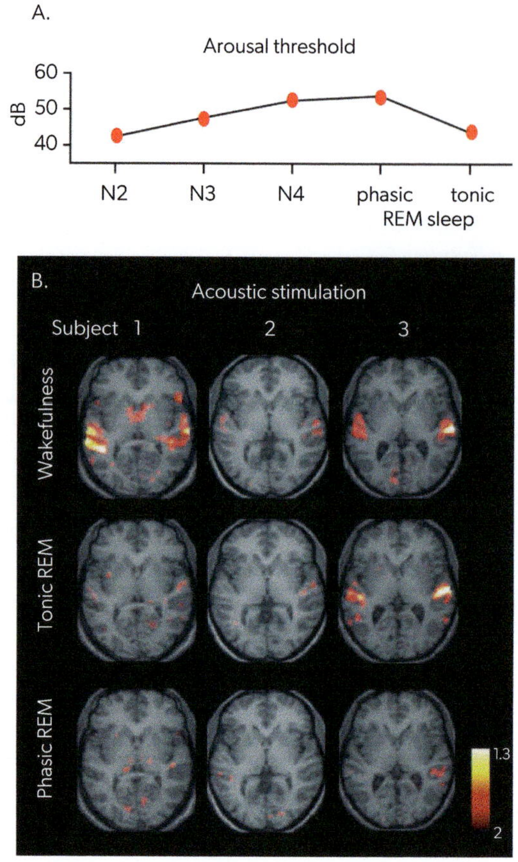

Figure 12.5 **A:** Thresholds of sound intensity (given in decibels, dB, Y axis) required in different sleep stages to awaken participants sufficiently to press a response button. Progressively louder sounds were required to awaken people from sleep going from NREM stages N2 to N4. REM sleep was divided into scoring periods that included phasic events (e.g., rapid eye movements) and those that included only the tonic features of REM sleep (atonia, EEG activation). The highest intensity stimuli were required to awaken people from N4 and phasic REM sleep, both of which were characterized by high levels of delta power in the EEG. Thresholds were lower during tonic REM sleep and were similar to those in N2 sleep. The differences appear small on this compressed scale but note that dBs are plotted on a logarithmic scale. A 50 dB sound is roughly 10 times louder than a 40 dB sound. Adapted with permission of John Wiley and Sons from Ermis et al. (2010) *J Sleep Res* 19:400–406. Journal Compilation © European Sleep Research Society (2010) and John Wiley and Sons. doi: 10.1111/j.1365-2869.2010.00831.x. **B:** fMRI responses to brief auditory stimuli in three participants (Subjects 1, 2 & 3) while awake (Top), during tonic REM sleep (Middle), and during phasic REM sleep (Bottom). Cortical responses were reduced during REM sleep relative to waking, and during phasic compared to tonic REM sleep. Bright yellow/white indicates the most intense activation, as shown on the scale at the bottom right. Reprinted with permission of John Wiley and Sons from Wehrle et al. (2007) Functional microstates within human REM sleep: first evidence from fMRI of a thalamocortical network specific for phasic REM periods. *Eur J Neurosci* 25:863–871. © The Authors (2007). Journal Compilation © Federation of European Neuroscience Societies and Blackwell Publishing Ltd. doi:10.1111/j.1460-9568.2007.05314.x.

that drives eye movements) on stimulus processing. Slow EEG events during REM sleep may be interpreted as resembling either PGO waves or delta waves. In both mice and people, these events occur more frequently during phasic than tonic REM sleep (defined by the number of rapid eye movements or muscle twitches present). Phasic REM sleep also includes less EEG high-frequency activity and more delta-band power than tonic REM sleep (Bernardi et al., 2019; Ermis et al., 2010; Funk et al., 2016).

Other contributing factors were identified in an fMRI study that showed increased thalamocortical synchrony and decreased responses of auditory brain regions to sounds during phasic relative to tonic REM sleep (**Figure 12.5 B**). Higher thalamocortical synchrony was attributed to internally generated loops of activity between the cortex and thalamus that were unrelated to external sensory inputs and would presumably make detection of these events more difficult (Wehrle et al., 2007).

Recordings directly from the anterior thalamus and from electrodes on the scalp in people undergoing surgery also found highest levels of synchrony in the delta-frequency band between thalamic and cortical rhythms during phasic REM sleep (Simor et al., 2021). Both recurrent thalamocortical activity that is independent of external inputs and reduced auditory system responses during phasic REM sleep could contribute to effectively isolating the cortex from the impact of external events, resulting in very high response thresholds during this substage (Wehrle et al., 2007).

Another way to assess information processing during sleep is to study the event-related potentials (ERPs) generated by auditory stimuli during different sleep stages; for a review, see Coenen, 2024. ERPs are averaged EEG responses that occur in the first few hundred milliseconds after stimuli are presented. Different features of ERP waveforms are known to reflect specific early stages of the brain's processing of stimuli while awake, including detecting physical features of sounds, such as frequency and intensity, or the meaning (semantic content) of sounds. An advantage of ERP studies is that they do not depend on the slower and more complex sequences of neural events required to generate a measurable motor output, such as a button press or verbal response, which could be influenced by many intervening factors.

One study of ERPs provided a surprising exception to the several studies that showed decreased responsiveness to external stimuli during phasic, relative to tonic, REM sleep. It was a study of the influence of the novel-environment effect during a daytime nap. This study focused on the P2 ERP component (a positive component at 200 msec latency) that is responsive to deviant tones (oddball stimuli) presented in an otherwise identical series. It first replicated the demonstration (Tamaki et al., 2016) of increased vigilance during NREM sleep to oddball stimuli presented to the left, versus the right, hemisphere, during the first session in a sleep laboratory, a so-called first-night effect; see Sections 7.5.3 and 12.3.2. However, during REM sleep there was no hemispheric asymmetry in responsiveness and no difference in the size of the P2 ERP between phasic and tonic REM sleep (Tamaki & Sasaki, 2019).

During a second sleep session, when participants were habituated to the novel environment, the hemispheric asymmetry in responses during NREM sleep was lost, confirming an earlier observation (Tamaki et al., 2016). In addition, the usual difference in responsiveness between REM sleep substages was restored by a reduction in the size of the P2 component during phasic REM sleep but not during tonic REM sleep (Tamaki & Sasaki, 2019) (**Figure 12.6**). These results indicate that increased vigilance when sleeping in a new environment selectively enhanced responsiveness to a deviant stimulus during phasic REM sleep. As a result, the typical difference in responsiveness during REM sleep substages was lost in a novel sleep environment and restored when participants were accustomed to the situation (Tamaki & Sasaki, 2019). These

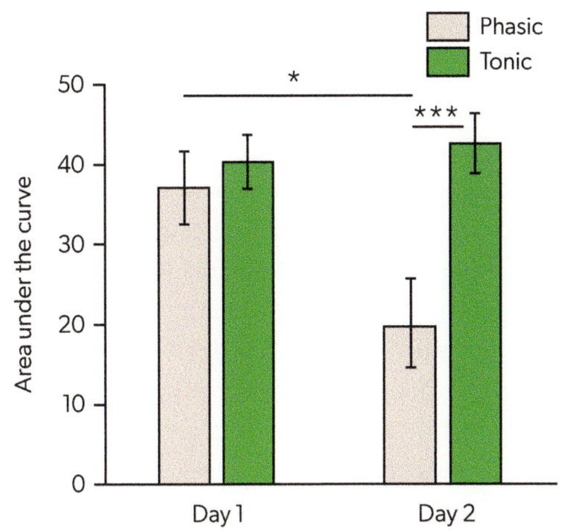

Figure 12.6 The area under the curve (Y axis) of the P2 evoked response in a central cortical region in response to an "oddball" sound during REM sleep. The participants experienced a "first-night effect" (novel-environment effect) on Day 1 and had become accustomed to the sleep environment by Day 2 (a week later). The Day 2 amplitudes of the P2 wave are consistent with most studies showing more responsiveness to the environment during tonic vs. phasic REM sleep. The Day 1 responses, however, show that the presumed increased vigilance associated with the novelty of the experience increased responsiveness during phasic REM sleep, so it was equivalent to that shown during tonic REM sleep. * $p < 0.05$ for the comparison of responses on the two days during phasic REM sleep. *** $p < 0.001$ for the comparison of responses in the two REM sleep substages on Day 2. Reprinted with permission under a Creative Commons Attribution License (CC-BY) from Tamaki, M. & Sasaki, Y. (2019) Surveillance during REM sleep for the first-night effect. *Front Neurosci* 13: doi:10.3389/fnins.2019.01161. © M. Tamaki & Y. Sasaki (2019).

results imply that differences in responsiveness to environmental stimuli between sleep stages can be altered by factors that affect individuals' motivational state.

Despite the advantages of using a direct measure of brain responsiveness (e.g., ERPs), there are limitations. Interpretation of ERPs collected during different sleep stages is complicated by the difficulty of comparing averaged signals that are extracted from different background EEG patterns. ERP features may show different latencies, patterns, and distributions because of differences in the background EEG and in cortical functional organization during different sleep stages (Colrain & Campbell, 2007; Hennevin et al., 2007). In addition, different test procedures and analytic techniques have been applied in different ERP studies, making it difficult to compare their results.

For example, one study reported that the personal relevance of a sound (a participant's own name vs. unfamiliar names) was reflected in ERPs during both N2 and REM sleep, as in waking, indicating that the semantic content of the stimulus was recognized in both sleep stages (Perrin et al., 1999). A study using different methods, however, concluded that this kind of personal salience affected ERPs during N2 sleep but not during N3 or REM sleep. Instead, ERPs during REM sleep were interpreted as reflecting physical differences between stimuli rather than their semantic content (Pratt et al., 1999).

An alternative approach that also avoids the complexities related to overt motor responses is measuring the EEG activity that occurs during preparations to produce a motor response. Examples include training participants while awake to press a button with one hand when they heard one category of words (animals) and with the other hand for a different category (objects) or to use different hands to respond to words and nonword sounds. While a stimulus was presented, EEG activity was monitored over the motor and premotor cortical areas of the brain to assess whether there was increased activity on the appropriate side (contralateral to the correct hand) in preparation for generating a response. Preparing the correct motor response required first having to detect the stimulus and then to decode its meaning (animals or objects, real words or meaningless syllables).

When these tests were conducted during either N1 or N2 sleep, but not during REM or deep NREM sleep, stimuli evoked an asymmetric response preparation signal on the side of the motor cortex that was appropriate for each category. Later control testing showed that participants were unaware of which items had been presented during sleep, indicating that they had not processed the stimuli during a brief, undetected waking event. Thus, during lighter NREM sleep stages, but not during REM or deep NREM sleep, the sleeping brain recognized the meaning of a spoken word and prepared an appropriate response, even though participants were not consciously aware of having heard the words (Andrillon et al., 2016; Kouider et al., 2014).

12.3.4 Summary

Most tests of information processing during sleep involve presenting auditory stimuli, both for technical convenience and because this modality is most likely to provide an early warning to sleepers of potential danger or other relevant information. While louder stimuli are obviously more likely to waken people, there is both anecdotal and experimental evidence that the subjective importance of stimuli is also relevant.

This conclusion implies that some degree of processing of external information continues during sleep. In fact, a surprisingly sophisticated evaluation of auditory stimuli can occur, especially in lighter NREM stages and sometimes in REM sleep. The extent to which differences in information processing among sleep stages were observed depended on several features of studies: the nature of the stimuli used; the response requirements involved; how sleep (sub)stages were defined; whether participants were sleep deprived; the test environment; and how motivated participants were to detect and respond to specific stimuli.

One consistent conclusion is that it is difficult to detect and/or respond to stimuli during N3 sleep (or Stage 4 when that classification is used). This result probably indicates that continuous, internally generated slow-wave EEG oscillations (and accompanying changes in cortical connectivity; see Section 12.4.1) are incompatible with detecting and responding to most auditory inputs. The very high response thresholds during phasic, relative to tonic, REM sleep reflect several characteristics of this substage: increased delta-band activity, perhaps including P-waves, despite the overall activated cortical pattern; internally generated synchronous looping of activity in thalamocortical circuits; and reduced spread of activation in the cortex beyond the auditory cortex (see Section 12.4.1). Nevertheless, responsiveness during this substage was increased in those experiencing a novel sleep environment, indicating a degree of motivation-related plasticity in the mechanisms affecting stimulus processing during sleep.

Although sleep is often characterized as involving a loss of conscious awareness of the external world, it is clear that the loss is only partial. The most extreme disconnection from external events occurs in the deepest levels of N3 sleep and during phasic REM sleep. In lighter NREM and tonic REM sleep, participants are more capable of detecting auditory inputs, evaluating their importance, and deciding whether and how to respond. These actions imply both awareness of the stimuli at some neural level and a sophisticated assessment of their significance. The existence of these abilities raises the question of where and how these assessments occur, and why they sometimes result in continued sleep and, at other times, trigger waking and a return to full consciousness. These issues are the focus of the following sections.

12.4 Sleep protection and information processing in NREM sleep

12.4.1 Thalamocortical connectivity during sleep

The thalamus is likely to be involved in determining responsiveness during sleep because it functions as a gateway to the cortex, conveying both specific sensory and motor information, and nonspecific arousing input. It also becomes hyperpolarized and shows synchronized slow waves before the cortex during the transition to NREM sleep (Magnin et al., 2010). Because of its synchronization and reduced metabolic activity during NREM sleep (Nofzinger et al., 2002), the thalamus is presumably less able to convey information to the cortex (Steriade, 2000), even though some information clearly does get through.

As reviewed in the preceding section, auditory input during sleep can be evaluated based on the strength of the signal, its relation to an individual's personal history, its potential monetary value, its semantic content, and its relevance as a warning signal. It is improbable that thalamic circuitry alone could generate the necessary judgments about these features. Nor is it likely that on the basis of those judgments the thalamus alone would determine whether inputs should be blocked or allowed to reach the cortex and trigger a response. Cortical processing must be involved in this sophisticated evaluation of sensory inputs.

Sounds are conveyed to the auditory cortex via the medial geniculate nucleus (MGN) of the thalamus. In the absence of sound stimuli, the spontaneous firing rates of most neurons in the MGN of guinea pigs (*Cavia porcellus*) were reduced during SWS, but not during REM sleep, relative to waking. Responses of MGN neurons to sounds, however, were reduced in amplitude, slower, and more variable during both SWS and REM sleep. Nevertheless, selective tuning of neurons to specific sound frequencies remained intact (Edeline et al., 2000). Thus, information related to the content of sounds (frequency characteristics) was preserved during sleep at the level of the thalamus, but neural responses were smaller, slower, and more variable.

In the auditory cortex of rats, single neurons responded to sounds with only minor changes during all sleep stages (Nir et al., 2015; Sela et al., 2016). In marmosets (*Callithrix jacchus*, a small South American monkey), average responses of individual neurons in layers of the auditory cortex beyond those that receive direct thalamic input were not changed systematically during sleep (Issa & Wang, 2011). Despite small changes in the amplitude and consistency of responses to sounds among MGN neurons during sleep, there was generally intact transmission of the characteristics of sounds to the auditory cortex.

A study in rats compared how sleep depth affected both evoked responses to auditory input (tones) at the level of the MGN and cortical desynchronization responses. To manipulate sleep depth, rats were studied before and after periods of sleep deprivation, intended to produce deeper SWS during a recovery opportunity. Auditory evoked potentials in the MGN were similar during SWS before and after sleep deprivation. However, during recovery sleep, more intense sounds were needed to trigger cortical EEG desynchronization. Despite similar responses at the level of the MGN, deeper or more-sustained SWS after deprivation increased the threshold for broad cortical activation in response to thalamic input. In contrast to these differences, cortical desynchronization responses to electrical stimulation of the trigeminal nerve were unaffected by prior sleep loss (Frederickson & Rechtschaffen, 1978).

These results indicate that processing of a neutral auditory stimulus beyond the level of the MGN was affected by depth of sleep, while a stimulus that engaged the trigeminal nerve, which normally processes somatosensory and painful inputs, was not. A suggestion as to where beyond the MGN this processing occurs comes from a study in rats of single-unit responses to auditory stimuli in two regions of cortex. Consistent with earlier studies, average neuronal responses at the level of the auditory cortex (which receives MGN input) were minimally affected by the stages of sleep and waking. However, responses of neurons in the perirhinal cortex, a region that functions as a higher-order integrator of sensory and other input, were differentially affected by sleep stages. Most neurons in the perirhinal cortex showed strongly attenuated responses during NREM sleep and moderately attenuated responses during REM sleep (Sela et al., 2020).

An important difference between the auditory and perirhinal cortices in this study was that most neuronal response latencies in the auditory cortex were very short, but most response latencies in the perirhinal cortex were longer. A measure of response latencies combined across all neurons recorded in both structures proved to be a stronger predictor of the degree of attenuation of responses during SWS and REM sleep than the particular cortical region being recorded. Long latency responses were strongly attenuated while short-latency responses were minimally affected in both the auditory and perirhinal cortices. The perirhinal cortex appeared to be more affected by sleep stages because it included more cells with long response latencies (Sela et al., 2020).

One potential explanation for these results is that longer latencies may be a marker for neurons that are further removed from the input. Reductions during sleep of cortical effective connectivity might result in a subset of neurons being functionally more disconnected from the initial auditory input stage (Massimini et al., 2005); see Section 12.5. It is also possible that late-responding neurons were those that received input after an intervening, sleep-related, filtering process that determined whether the stimuli were important.

Studies using fMRI in people found that sounds continued to activate the thalamus, auditory cortex, and caudate nucleus during NREM sleep. Activation in the thalamus, however, was reduced, as was activation of nonauditory regions, such as the frontal, cingulate, and left parietal cortices (Portas et al., 2000; Schabus et al., 2012). Similarly, sounds activated fewer cortical regions outside the auditory cortex during tonic REM sleep, and even fewer during phasic REM sleep (Wehrle et al., 2007); see **Figure 12.5 B**.

One contributor to reduced cortical spread of auditory input during sleep is altered connectivity between some thalamic nuclei and the cortex. An fMRI study assessed the strength of functional connectivity between the lateral geniculate nucleus (LGN; the visual relay nucleus in the thalamus) and the visual cortex. There was no change in LGN-visual cortex connectivity strength between waking and either N2 or N3 sleep, indicating preserved connectively during sleep in a direct sensory processing stream. However, during both N2 and N3 sleep, functional connectivity was reduced between the centromedian thalamic nucleus (a nonspecific midline nucleus projecting broadly to the cortex) and several association cortical regions (Picchioni et al., 2014). Generalizing from the visual to the auditory pathway, it may be that reduced activating input from nonspecific thalamic nuclei to association cortical regions contributes to these regions showing muted responses to auditory input.

The responses in primary sensory cortices indicated that there was preserved functional connectivity with their respective thalamic relay nuclei during sleep, despite relatively minor changes in signal quality and amplitude. Beyond the auditory cortex, however, cortical responses to auditory stimuli were diminished and showed more restricted spread. These effects may be attributable to a reduction in activating input from nonspecific thalamic nuclei to association cortical regions. As discussed in Section 12.5, the effects of altered thalamic input may be further reinforced by reduced coherence and functional connectivity among cortical regions.

Thalamocortical interactions during sleep are also modulated by other systems. An fMRI study involving moderate sedation induced by the anesthetic propofol indicated a role for the corpus striatum (a part of the basal ganglia that includes the putamen and caudate nucleus) in regulating thalamocortical interactions. Loss of responsiveness to external events during sedation was associated with loss of functional connectivity between the putamen and other brain regions, including the thalamus and cortex. This loss of connectivity occurred earlier and was more profound than the loss of direct functional connectivity between thalamus and cortex (Mhuircheartaigh et al., 2010). A study using positron emission tomography (PET) also found that changes in blood flow (reflecting intensity of neural activity) were more dramatic in the striatum than in most other brain structures during the transitions from waking to NREM sleep and from NREM to REM sleep (Braun et al., 1997).

Sedation and sleep both involve slow cortical oscillations and loss of consciousness, but they also differ in a number of ways, so the results obtained from studies using sedation should be applied cautiously to natural sleep. Nevertheless, these findings indicate an influence of the striatum on thalamocortical interactions and responsiveness to external inputs. Other evidence also supports a role for interactions among the cortex, thalamus, and basal ganglia in regulating state transitions and the changes in consciousness that characterize them (Braun et al., 1997; Leu-Semenescu et al., 2013; Mhuircheartaigh et al., 2010); see Appendix A and Section 12.2.4.

12.4.2 Role of K complexes and sleep spindles

Sleep has been proposed to affect the processing of information about sounds in several ways. These include both general effects, such as by influencing the amplitude and fidelity of responses in the auditory pathway and by determining the extent of activation and information spread to cortical regions beyond the auditory cortex. Some studies have also proposed specific effects on processing auditory inputs in relation to the timing of features of NREM sleep, including cortical SOs/K complexes and sleep spindles (Dang-Vu et al., 2011; Schabus et al., 2012).

As described in Section 12.2.5, a K complex is similar to a cortical slow oscillation in structure, but it may include only the Off component and typically appears as an isolated, transient event. In addition to their spontaneous appearance in the absence of specific external inputs, K complexes can also be evoked by sensory stimuli during sleep (Halász, 2005). K complexes and sleep spindles often occur sequentially in response to external stimuli, suggesting that both may be involved in responding to these events. Historically, there have been different views about the functions these features perform in relation to sensory input. One view is that one or both of them reflect cortical processing of the information content of an auditory stimulus; another view is that they instead play a role in suppressing processing and conscious awareness of a stimulus.

A study of ERPs generated during N2 sleep in response to pure tones found that the loudest, most intrusive stimuli triggered ERPs that included features related to inhibition of information processing, accompanied by an apparent late K complex. The most robust changes relative to waking ERPs were observed when a sleep spindle also followed the stimulus presentation (Campbell, 2010; Cote et al., 2000). These findings implied that the evoked K complex and its linked sleep spindle were involved in preserving NREM sleep in the face of disturbing noise rather than in processing the information content of a stimulus.

When auditory stimuli evoked cortical K complexes, they also triggered robust activity in cortical regions that probably represent cycles of activation within corticothalamic loops (Dang-Vu et al., 2011; Schabus et al., 2012). These results suggest that auditory stimuli during NREM sleep trigger a cortical process (reflected in modified ERPs, K complexes, and activation of thalamocortical loops) that modulates neural responses to that input and thereby helps to reduce the probability of waking.

This conclusion is supported by the results of a study in people that used recorded environmental noises (traffic or wind-farm noises). It found that the number of K complexes in N2/N3 sleep increased when these noises were presented, especially at louder volumes and in participants who self-reported high noise sensitivity. Although louder volumes increased the probability of arousal from sleep, it was very rare for a noise presentation that evoked a K complex to be followed by an arousal (Lechat et al., 2021).

These findings suggest that K complexes are part of a filtering response that reduces the probability of waking to an unimportant stimulus. However, it is not clear at what level the filtering or response inhibition occur. One electrophysiological study found that low-volume auditory stimuli reaching the auditory cortex of rats during the Off phase of large amplitude "slow waves" in NREM sleep evoked weaker responses than outside this phase, but that responses to louder stimuli during this phase were not attenuated, and to very loud stimuli, were actually enhanced (Sela et al., 2016). The fact that the type of response generated depended on the stimulus intensity makes it difficult to compare results across studies that may have been effectively studying different parts of the intensity range.

Sleep spindles that sometimes follow K complexes may be a downstream result of cortical-TRN-thalamocortical activity that is triggered by the initial filtering process. Spindles may further reduce the probability of waking in response to the stimulus (Cote et al., 2000). Consistent with the interpretation that sleep spindles reduce the probability of waking, people who spontaneously generated larger numbers of sleep spindles were more resistant to being awakened by external noises (Dang-Vu et al., 2010).

The idea that sleep spindles act as filters to prevent auditory stimuli from disturbing sleep has, however, been challenged by studies in people and rats. One human study found that auditory stimuli presented during spontaneous sleep spindles evoked robust cortical and cardiovascular responses (Church et al., 1978). A study in rats found that there was little or no change in the responses of auditory cortex neurons, assessed either from single neurons or as multiunit or field responses, to auditory stimuli presented during spindles (Sela et al., 2016). An fMRI study in people also reported that auditory stimuli presented during spindles activated both brainstem and cortical auditory structures. However, responses assessed using fMRI were reported to be more inconsistent, smaller, and less likely to reach the cortex when stimuli occurred during, rather than outside, spindles (Dang-Vu et al., 2011).

These studies involved different methods: multiunit neural recordings, single-unit recordings, evoked EEG responses, and fMRI responses, as well as different species. These methods may be differentially sensitive to specific stages of the flow of auditory information, which could contribute to reaching different conclusions. Thus, one could emphasize either that auditory information at the level of the auditory cortex is not blocked when presented during spindles, or that there are changes in the quality and consistency of the information flow. The intensity-dependence of effects elicited during large slow waves, ranging from decreasing to augmenting responses (Sela et al., 2016), also raises the question of how comparable the auditory stimuli were among these studies.

The positive correlation between spindle numbers and resistance to waking in response to sounds (Dang-Vu et al., 2010) could reflect several mechanisms that support sleep continuity. First, sounds occurring during spontaneous spindles often reach the auditory cortex but (according to some studies) in attenuated form, reducing the probability of detection that leads to broader cortical activation and waking. Second, stimuli occurring outside spindles can trigger K complexes and activity in corticothalamic loops that help to preserve sleep. A downstream consequence of this corticothalamic activity may then be the generation of a sleep spindle (Cote et al., 2000). Spindles might not preserve sleep by reducing transmission to the auditory cortex but may be a secondary result of triggering a K complex and may then influence further processing of the stimulus.

The cortical effects of sounds occurring during spindles, K complexes, and SOs are superimposed on the general changes characteristic of N2/N3 sleep. These include less activating input from nonspecific thalamic nuclei, higher cortical GABA levels, and decreased EEG phase coherence between association and sensory cortical regions (Bastuji et al., 2021; Picchioni et al., 2014; Vanini et al., 2012). These background changes would tend to make the broad spread of activation across the cortex less likely, whether the information arriving at the auditory cortex is fully intact or partially degraded.

Any role for sleep spindles in modulating responses to sensory input would involve the TRN, which is key to spindle production. During waking, TRN circuits play a role in switching attention among different sources of input reaching the thalamocortical system, as well as modulating arousal systems (Halassa et al., 2014). Based on these functions during waking, it is possible to suggest a mechanism for the involvement of the TRN in processing input during sleep. Incoming auditory stimuli may arrive intact (or partially degraded) in the auditory cortex and be evaluated at that level. Depending on the nature of the stimulus, the cortex could then generate output to the TRN which triggers spindle activity (Fuentealba & Steriade, 2005). Spindle activity would regulate the TRN's filtering function to determine whether information flow from thalamic relay nuclei should be modified, as well as influencing whether attentional mechanisms and broader cortical arousal would be recruited.

The TRN may be involved in either nonspecific or selective effects on thalamic relay neurons. Inhibition that is selective for the input that initially triggered cortical-TRN production of a spindle would be useful in reducing processing of repetitive, uninformative inputs (e.g., persistent traffic noises during the night). In support of the idea of selectivity, there is evidence in awake rats that the TRN is involved in responding to novel auditory stimuli occurring in the midst of an otherwise repetitive series. Differential responses of MGN neurons to a deviant stimulus were blocked by inactivating the TRN (Yu et al., 2009). This interpretation of the role of the TRN is consistent with an earlier theoretical suggestion that the TRN functions as the guardian that controls the thalamic gateway for input to the cortex (Crick, 1984).

The effects of sleep stages on responses to stimuli in senses other than audition have also been evaluated. Painful stimuli were reported in some studies to provoke waking differentially across sleep stages. However, these studies tended to use relatively short-lasting stimuli that are, for example, not characteristic of the kinds of somatic pain experienced by chronic pain patients, which often disrupts their sleep, that is, triggers waking; for a review, see Lavigne et al., 2004. In contrast, painful, longer-lasting stimuli (hypertonic saline injection into a muscle) triggered awakening in people similarly across all sleep stages (Lavigne et al., 2004).

Waking responses to a series of laser pulses that created heat sensations on the skin were also similar across NREM and REM sleep stages, although responses were reduced during phasic REM sleep relative to tonic REM sleep (Bastuji et al., 2008). Heat pulses also had similar effects on electrical responses in the cortex and thalamus when they were delivered within or outside sleep spindles in N2/N3 sleep (Claude et al., 2015). As indicated earlier, in rat studies, electrical stimulation of the trigeminal nerve, which conveys pain information, also evoked similar cortical desynchronization regardless of sleep depth (Frederickson & Rechtschaffen, 1978).

Thus, filtering with respect to painful stimuli varied depending on stimulus intensity and duration, with sleep stages influencing responsiveness mostly for short, less intense stimuli. Longer-lasting and more intense painful stimuli were equally effective in triggering responses across sleep stages and regardless of the co-occurrence of sleep spindles. Although these results contrast to the sleep stage differences often reported for sounds, this apparent difference may be related to the typical sound intensities used in these studies. Sleep stage dependence for responses to sounds can also be overcome to a large extent by increasing stimulus intensity (Siegel & Langley, 1965; Van Twyver & Garrett, 1972). Thus, differential responses across sleep stages may be most prominent for relatively weaker stimuli across sensory modalities.

Reduced responsiveness to sensory input has been attributed to the slow background EEG, large-amplitude oscillations, and spindles of NREM sleep. But responses to sounds are also attenuated during REM sleep, especially during phasic REM sleep, which mostly lacks these features. Several factors likely contribute to these effects. Levels of most activating neuromodulators that reach the cortex during waking are reduced during REM sleep, except for acetylcholine (Datta & Siwek, 2002) and dopamine (Léna et al., 2005). Despite the activated appearance of the cortical EEG during REM sleep, spectral analysis shows that there is an increase in low-frequency EEG activity, especially during phasic REM sleep (Bernardi et al., 2019; Lim et al., 2007). This low-level slow activity and the loss of other neuromodulators may reduce the capacity to further increase cortical activation or trigger waking in response to sensory input.

Functional connectivity between frontal and other cortical regions is also reduced during REM sleep (Horovitz et al., 2009; Maquet et al., 1996; Muzur et al., 2002), which would diminish the spread of information from the auditory cortex to association cortices. Phasic REM sleep also includes transient events (PGO or P-waves) that, like spindle patterns, may interfere with processing external inputs (Gott et al., 2017; Nelson et al., 1983). Taken together, these REM sleep features could reduce responsiveness by reducing the degree of cortical activation and the extent of spread outside the auditory cortex, especially during phasic REM sleep (Wehrle et al., 2007).

12.4.3 Summary

Responsiveness during NREM sleep to sensory input has been studied mostly in relation to audition. The evidence relating to how different parts of the auditory system respond to sounds during sleep is complex. Individual neurons in the brainstem and thalamus (MGN) respond to the frequency features of sounds similarly during different sleep stages and waking. Some studies also found largely intact transmission to the primary auditory cortex during sleep, and others reported small changes in the consistency of input.

Some studies reported reduced responses to stimuli that coincided with spontaneous sleep spindles, but others did not. Low intensity sounds that occurred during the Off phase of large slow waves in NREM sleep were reported to elicit smaller responses in the auditory cortex, but for louder sounds, responses were intact or even increased. However, beyond the primary auditory cortex, responses to auditory stimuli in multimodal or association cortices were clearly reduced during sleep.

Spontaneous K complexes and sleep spindles may not block auditory inputs, but those that are evoked by sounds may represent part of a response that inhibits further processing and spread of information beyond the level of the auditory cortex. fMRI studies identified cortico-thalamocortical loops of activity triggered by sounds, which may inhibit further processing of incoming stimuli.

The effects of sleep on the breadth of cortical activation may be critical to determining whether or not a stimulus provokes waking. During NREM sleep, input from nonspecific nuclei to association cortices is strongly reduced, so these regions tend to be less activated and responsive to input. Communication and EEG coherence among cortical regions is also reduced, probably because of increased GABA levels during NREM sleep stages. Together, these features reduce the likelihood that stimuli activating the auditory cortex will also spread activation to other cortical regions, which may be essential to triggering waking.

People who produce the most spontaneous sleep spindles are least likely to be awakened by noise during sleep. One interpretation of this finding is that sounds that are evaluated locally in the auditory cortex as being unimportant result in the production of K complexes and sleep spindles that inhibit further cortical responses and further reduce the likelihood of spread of activation.

These effects may be relevant only to sounds of moderate intensity. Very loud sounds, especially if they are novel, can break through these filtering mechanisms. Responses to painful stimuli that are brief and of moderate intensity differed across sleep stages, but longer-lasting and more intensely painful stimuli were equally effective in evoking waking across sleep stages.

Despite the background activation of the cortex during REM sleep and the absence of SOs and spindles, REM sleep characteristics also result in reduced spread of auditory activation from the auditory cortex to other regions, especially during phasic REM sleep. These include reduced connectivity across the cortex, increased EEG background activity in the delta band, reduced levels of most excitatory neuromodulators, and phasic events (P-waves) that may affect processing of sensory inputs.

12.5 Modulation of awareness during sleep

The previous section reviewed evidence that some sounds do not enter conscious awareness or wake people from sleep. Other sounds (typically those that are loud, unusual, or personally meaningful) can provoke a range of overt responses: cortical or autonomic activation, selective motor preparatory responses, waking, and appropriate behavioral responses. These findings raise the question of how the process of receiving a sensory input, evaluating its significance, and selecting an appropriate response can occur without initial conscious awareness of the stimulus.

Answering that question fully would require first addressing what consciousness is, and how neural mechanisms generate this fundamental human experience.[8] Much has been written on these difficult questions, expressing a variety of views that we will not attempt to summarize here (for references, see Raccah et al., 2021). But most scientists would at least agree that cortical neural activity is correlated with, and forms the basis of, conscious awareness. If so, why do we not become consciously aware of most sensory stimuli that occur during sleep and affect the cortex?

A review of a few relevant findings provides a partial answer to this question. One common view is that activity in thalamocortical circuitry is part of the mechanism that permits consciousness (Blumenfeld, 2016; Tononi, 2004); consciousness can be severely impaired by quite restricted damage to regions of the thalamus (Schiff, 2008). Anything that modifies reciprocal communication between the thalamus and cortex, especially affecting multimodal association cortical areas, could affect conscious awareness, including the reduced and altered flow of communication between the thalamus and cortex that

[8] In 1998, a neuroscientist (Christof Koch) reportedly bet a philosopher (David Chalmers) that the neural basis of consciousness would be identified within 25 years. In 2023, a set of studies that pitted two competing neural models of consciousness against each other were completed. The results were not completely consistent with either set of predicted outcomes, indicating that neither model of consciousness was accurate nor complete. Dr. Koch announced the results of the studies and conceded the bet, which involved a case of wine being delivered to Dr. Chalmers (https://tinyurl.com/2rahpn5s). They, and other colleagues, have since initiated an adversarial collaborative research project that will pit contrasting models of visual consciousness against each other (Melloni et al., 2023).

occurs during sleep (Dang-Vu et al., 2011; Picchioni et al., 2014; Spoormaker et al., 2010).

Nonspecific (especially intralaminar) thalamic projections to cortex may be essential to maintaining waking consciousness (Blumenfeld, 2016); for example, stimulating one nonspecific thalamic nucleus in mice caused rapid waking from NREM sleep (Honjoh et al., 2018). The relations that exist between these thalamic nuclei and the cortex during waking change during sleep. The alert, waking cortex produces high-gamma range activity (~40 Hz), which in cats was generated by neurons in an intralaminar thalamic nucleus during both waking and REM sleep. The same neurons instead fired in bursts in the low sigma (spindle frequency) range during NREM sleep (Steriade, Curró Dossi, et al., 1993). fMRI imaging studies also demonstrated a reduction during NREM sleep relative to waking in functional connectivity between the thalamus and multimodal (association) cortices in people (Picchioni et al., 2014).

Some models of conscious awareness of external events propose that it depends on the spread of activation from a cortical region that receives sensory input to multiple other regions. According to these models, consciousness depends on the integration of information processing across cortical regions rather than on activity within a single region (Baars, 2005; Sämann et al., 2011; Tononi, 2004). Other models propose that conscious awareness of an event depends on selective, sustained activity of linked neuronal components across prefrontal-parietal-cingulate cortical regions, forming part of a "global neuronal workspace," along with thalamocortical circuit activation (Dehaene & Changeux, 2011).

These ideas are relevant because of the changes that occur during NREM sleep, including increased GABA levels, decreased input to the cortex from most activating neuromodulatory systems, and reduced activity of midline and intralaminar (nonspecific) thalamic nuclei. As discussed in Section 12.4, the result of these changes is that activation of the auditory cortex produces little or no spread of activation to association cortical regions during some sleep stages (see **Figures 12.5** and **12.7**).

Studies of brain metabolism and blood flow during sleep are consistent with the conclusion that a major change in information processing during sleep is the loss of integration across the cortex. A PET imaging study showed functional dissociations during sleep between activity in primary sensory and association cortices. Association cortices showed large decreases in blood flow during NREM sleep and further reductions during REM sleep, while primary sensory regions did not (Braun et al., 1997). These effects were especially prominent in frontal and parietal association regions, which are among a few key regions involved in generating conscious awareness (Blumenfeld, 2016; Dehaene & Changeux, 2011; Li et al., 2014).

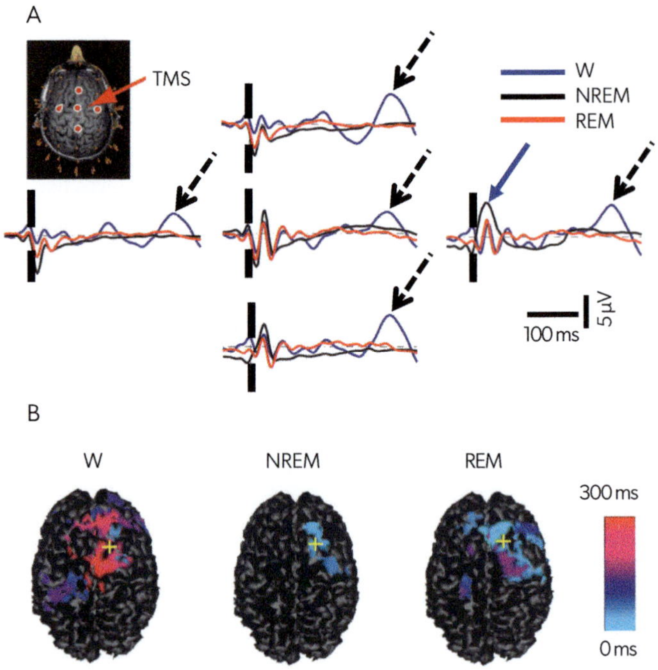

Figure 12.7 **A.** Location of transcranial magnetic stimulation (TMS; red arrow) and recording sites of responses (red dots). The waveforms of TMS-evoked responses over time at each location are displayed in a spatial pattern that matches the relative locations of the 5 recording sites (most rostral site on top). Responses are shown during waking (W, blue line), NREM sleep (black), and REM sleep (red) to stimuli presented at the time of the vertical, black dashed lines. Although initial responses to TMS were visible at all locations (and largest near the stimulation site during waking [right-most waveform], indicated by the solid blue arrow), these responses damped out rapidly during both NREM and REM sleep, while large-amplitude responses were still detectable after 300 ms during waking (W) in all locations (dashed black arrows). **B.** The timing of significant activity increases after stimulation is color-coded so that green-blue indicates an immediate response and red indicates the most delayed responses (300 ms later; see dashed black arrows in **A**). During NREM sleep, responses were localized to the region where TMS was applied (yellow cross) and were short-lived (blue only). Responses were more anatomically extensive and somewhat longer-lasting (blue and purple) during REM sleep, but widespread middle and late responses occurred only during waking (W) (purple and red areas). Adapted with permission of Dr. Marcello Massimini and Informa UK from Massimini, M. et al. (2010) Cortical reactivity and effective connectivity during REM sleep in humans. *Cogn Neurosci* 1:176–183. © Psychology Press/Informa UK Ltd. (2010). doi:10.1080/17588921003731578.

Studies using fMRI, EEG, or measures of metabolic activity also reported reduced activity during NREM sleep in association cortices, including frontal and parietal regions (Baars, 2005; Nofzinger et al., 2002). These methods also identified a loss of integration of activity across cortical regions, especially between primary sensory and association regions during NREM sleep (Chow et al., 2013; Horovitz et al., 2009;

Spoormaker et al., 2010). The loss of spatial integration within the cortex during sleep was accompanied by loss of long-range temporal integration of metabolic activity across the cortex (Tagliazucchi et al., 2013), and loss of EEG temporal coherence between sensory and association cortices (Bastuji et al., 2021).

These findings of reduced integration between primary sensory and association cortices can explain why patterns of brain activity in response to sensory inputs differ strongly among sleep stages. One study used transcranial magnetic stimulation (TMS) to model the nature of brain responses to sensory inputs. Localized TMS produced focal activation in one cortical region during waking, NREM, and REM sleep. During waking, this local stimulation triggered a broad spread of activation from the targeted region to other cortical areas. When the same stimulation was repeated during NREM or REM sleep, there was still increased activity at the site of stimulation, but little or no spread of activation laterally to other cortical regions. In particular, late responses around 300 msec after the stimulation were essentially absent during NREM and REM sleep (Massimini et al., 2005; Massimini et al., 2010) (**Figure 12.7**). Studies of patients with variably reduced levels of consciousness after injury or stroke also demonstrated a correlation between levels of consciousness and the extent of long-range, complex interactions in the cortex triggered by similar stimulation (Gosseries et al., 2014; Rosanova et al., 2018).

A modeling study showed that a shift from activation toward inhibition in the cortex during NREM sleep, reflecting in part an increase in GABA levels, would effectively dampen the spread of activation from one cortical region to others (Esser et al., 2009). The presence of silent, Off states during slow cortical rhythms may also contribute to restricting activation to local regions (Camassa et al., 2022).

During REM sleep, however, cortical neurons are not hyperpolarized by GABA, and large, slow oscillations are absent. Nevertheless, frontal cortical regions are partially disconnected from other parts of cortex (Horovitz et al., 2009; Maquet et al., 1996; Muzur et al., 2002). TMS stimulation during REM sleep triggered immediate cortical responses near the stimulation site that shared some features with waking responses. However, the responses lacked the late components (~300 msec after stimulation) that were produced across large regions of the cortex by stimulation during waking (**Figure 12.7**) (Massimini et al., 2010). Thus, there was more spread of activation than during NREM sleep, but, compared to waking, it was restricted in both spatial and temporal extent.

Urethane anesthesia permits continued rhythmic alternation of cortical EEG patterns between activated and synchronized states (Whitten et al., 2009). A study of rats under urethane anesthesia found that during synchronized cortical activity (analogous to NREM sleep), cortical waves propagated more slowly and with altered trajectories through the cortex (Wanger et al., 2013). In a human study, an ERP feature that reflects detection of an oddball auditory stimulus in an otherwise uniform series was evoked during waking in both parietal and frontal regions. This feature did not appear in either region during N2 sleep, and it appeared in parietal but not in frontal cortex during REM sleep (Cote et al., 2001). These results are consistent with evidence of a functional disconnection among cortical regions and, specifically, of a reduction in connectivity between the frontal cortex and other brain regions during both N2 and REM sleep (Braun et al., 1997; Maquet et al., 1996; Massimini et al., 2010).

Coherence of oscillations in the gamma frequency band across cortical regions has been reported to be associated with complex cognitive processes, including the generation of conscious awareness of events (Melloni et al., 2007; Singer, 1993), although there is controversy about how such frequency coherence should be measured and interpreted (Buzsáki & Schomburg, 2015). Gamma frequency coherence was decreased during both SWS and REM sleep, relative to waking (Cantero et al., 2004), and temporal coupling between frontal association and primary sensory regions in the gamma frequency range was reduced specifically during REM sleep (Pérez-Garci et al., 2001). These results suggest that loss of gamma-band coherence across cortical regions, and reduced coherence between frontal and other regions during sleep, could contribute to a reduced capacity to engage in higher-level cognition, including achieving conscious awareness of sensory events.

A recent study required people to respond with contraction of different muscle groups in response to different categories of sounds (real words vs. meaningless pseudowords) during a daytime nap (during all sleep stages, but with limited data from N3 sleep). People performed the task above chance level, but their performance depended on the EEG pattern immediately preceding a stimulus presentation. Transiently higher frequencies and increased measures of complexity in the EEG typically preceded stimuli to which people responded correctly, while remaining asleep. These results were interpreted as indicating that there is an ongoing modulation of the depth of sleep and pattern of brain activity that opens cognitive "windows" periodically through which people can monitor and analyze external stimuli (Türker et al., 2023).

Despite the global changes in neural activity during sleep that impede activation and arousal in response to sensory input, there must also be a mechanism that evaluates stimuli to determine their importance and can restore waking and conscious awareness. This mechanism is not well understood, and it remains to be determined whether it depends on a stimulus occurring during specific EEG microstates, as described above. The question remains how sensory input reaching a limited area of cortex is processed and evaluated so that it either permits sleep to continue or intervenes to trigger waking, based on the intensity, meaning, novelty, etc. of the stimulus.

One component of the awakening response may involve activation of subcortical arousal mechanisms and association cortical regions. One study compared fMRI activation patterns during NREM sleep in response to meaningful and meaningless auditory stimuli. There was increased activation in the amygdala (a part of the limbic system involved in emotion regulation) and in the left prefrontal cortex in response to the sound of the participant's own name compared to a neutral tone (Portas et al., 2000).

Prefrontal cortical activation may be a key part of the process of responding to the stimulus. Projections from the prefrontal cortex reach many subcortical systems, including wake-promoting areas, such as the reticular formation, the basal forebrain, lateral hypothalamus, raphe nuclei, and locus coeruleus (Gaykema et al., 1991; Sesack et al., 1989). Other cortical regions also project to the midbrain reticular formation and intralaminar thalamic nuclei, among other structures (Jasper et al., 1952). Local electrical stimulation of these cortical regions in monkeys can produce broad cortical activation, presumably by activating descending projections to brainstem and thalamic structures that respond with widespread activating input to the cortex (Segundo et al., 1955).

A speculative account of events that could lead to waking might be as follows. During sleep, auditory input reaching the MGN is transmitted to neurons in the primary auditory cortex. Frequency tuning of these neurons is intact, and the amplitude of auditory input to this area is also preserved—or may be only somewhat weakened. Thus, the semantic content and other features of the stimulus reach the auditory cortex largely intact, and the input is presumably evaluated locally in this region. A decision that the content is important is transmitted to other cortical regions, including the prefrontal cortex and other association cortices.

Projections from the prefrontal, parietal, or temporal cortices could activate wake-promoting systems in the midbrain reticular formation and nonspecific thalamic nuclei and, through connections to the limbic system and hypothalamus, shift autonomic balance toward sympathetic activation. Activating thalamic input to the cortex would block production of slow EEG rhythms, restore the potential for gamma frequency activity, and facilitate communication and gamma-frequency coherence among cortical regions. These changes would permit the development of conscious awareness of the stimulus, as well as provoking partial or full awakening.[9]

This speculative account suggests a series of events that could link auditory stimuli during sleep to awakening and awareness. However, it leaves several important questions unanswered. A central question is what the nature and mechanism is of the critical analysis that is hypothesized to occur within the auditory cortex. This narrative is also vague about the mechanism by which a decision based on this analysis is transmitted to other cortical regions and promotes functional reorganization of cortical activity (increased regional and temporal integration, development of gamma frequency activity), and the emergence of awareness of the stimulus.

12.5.1 Summary

Hyperpolarization of cortical neurons and reduced thalamic activation of association cortices during NREM sleep restrict interactions among cortical regions, including loss of gamma-band activity and coherence across regions. This restriction of activation is evident in studies of local cortical stimulation using TMS. Auditory inputs that produced only local activation of auditory cortex during NREM sleep did not result in a spread of activation into association cortices (e.g., frontal, cingulate, and parietal regions). Restricted spread of activation across cortical regions is also characteristic of states of reduced consciousness following brain injury. Spread of activation across cortical regions and achieving coherence in gamma frequency activity are hypothesized to be necessary to achieve conscious awareness of stimuli that reach primary sensory cortices.

Although cortical neurons are not hyperpolarized during REM sleep, there is also decreased coherence of activity between sensory cortices and frontal cortical regions, and reduced spread of stimulus-evoked activation beyond the auditory cortex. As a result, many stimuli reaching the auditory cortex during REM sleep would not have enough impact

[9] A prescient summary was included in a 1937 lecture by Edgar Adrian (co-winner with Charles Sherrington of the 1932 Nobel Prize in Physiology for his work on neurophysiology): "A loud noise which has no importance for the sleeper affects the auditory nerve as usual but produces only a transient and localized response in the cortex. The cry of a child or a few words in a low voice will give a message of much smaller intensity, judged by the number of nerve impulses per second, yet the message will set the whole brain in action. It will do so presumably because it has a pattern which enables it to excite a system of neurones kept much nearer to the waking level of excitability and in close touch with other excitable systems of the same kind." (Adrian, 1937, p. 245). Reproduced with permission of Springer: Nature from Adrian, E.D. (1937) The physiology of sleep. *Irish Journal of Medical Science 12*(138), 237–248.

on association cortices to generate either waking or conscious awareness of the stimulus.

There is recent evidence of brief EEG "windows" occurring during sleep that have more of the characteristics of waking cortical functioning (higher frequency and more complexity), which may allow detection and evaluation of stimuli that occur during those events.

A hypothetical sequence that would lead to a return to conscious awareness during sleep would involve local processes in the auditory cortex determining that a stimulus was unusually loud, personally relevant, or potentially threatening. This information would be transmitted to frontal and other cortical regions. Outputs from these regions to association cortices and to subcortical wake-promoting systems (including regulators of the autonomic nervous system) would result in activation of broader cortical domains, integration of their information processing, and development of coherent gamma frequency activity. The resulting activation across broad cortical regions would trigger waking and permit conscious awareness of the stimulus.

12.6 Sleep as a local cortical phenomenon

12.6.1 Asymmetric sleep EEG features

EEG recordings during sleep typically show differences in the features recorded at different scalp (or brain) sites. In people, for example, theta frequencies are strongest in the occipital region, and low sigma frequencies (in the spindle range) are strongest in the midline vertex region (Achermann et al., 2001; Finelli et al., 2001) (**Figure 12.8**).

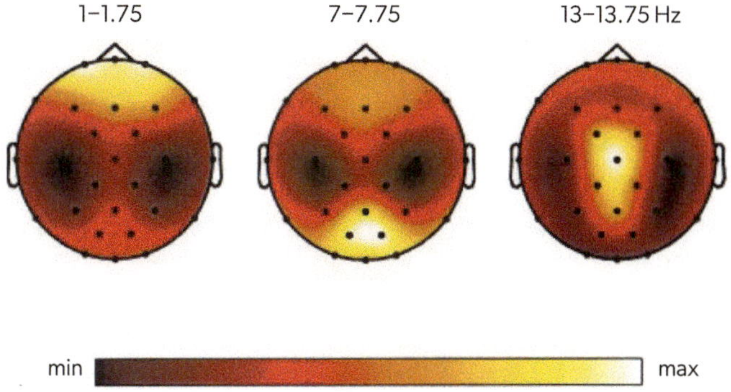

Figure 12.8 The intensity of different EEG frequencies expressed in the brain during overnight NREM sleep in healthy young men, shown in a "heat map" format for three different EEG frequencies. For orientation, symbols representing the nose and ears are shown at the top and sides of the model heads; each black dot represents the position of an EEG recording electrode. The brightest areas indicate the highest levels of the frequencies shown, and darkest areas show the lowest levels, as illustrated in the "min-max" intensity scale at the bottom. The values above each panel show the frequency band represented, including 1–1.75 Hz (low delta), 7–7.75 Hz (high theta), and 13–13.75 Hz (low sigma). Low frequencies were strongest in the frontal area, theta frequencies in the occipital area, and sigma frequencies in the midline vertex region. Reprinted with permission of John Wiley & Sons from Finelli, L.A. et al. (2001) Functional topography of the human nonREM sleep electroencephalogram. *Eur J Neurosci* 13:2282–2290. Journal Compilation © Federation of European Neuroscience Societies and John Wiley and Sons (2001). doi: 10.1046/j.0953-816x.2001.01597.x.

Frontal cortical regions also express more low-frequency (delta) EEG activity, especially early in the night (Werth et al., 1997). Sleep deprivation in people (Finelli et al., 2001), rats, and mice (Huber et al., 2000; Schwierin et al., 1999; Vyazovskiy et al., 2002) further strengthens low-frequency activity in frontal cortex and depresses spindle-frequency activity in the vertex region (Achermann et al., 2001; Finelli et al., 2001).

The amount of cortical theta-band activity while awake and delta-band activity during sleep reflect current sleep need (see Sections 5.3.2 and 5.7.3) (Cajochen et al., 1995), so the uneven distribution of activity in these frequency bands implies that different cortical regions have developed more or less sleep need. Thus, frontal cortical regions develop the highest sleep need, are most affected by sleep loss, and compensate most robustly with increased SWA during recovery sleep. These conclusions are consistent with evidence that cognitive tasks that rely on frontal cortical regions are strongly affected by sleep deprivation (see Section 13.7.2).

The idea of local cortical differences in sleep need and in recovery during sleep is consistent with PET and fMRI studies showing spontaneous differences in the extent to which different brain regions change their activity levels from waking to sleep (Kaufmann, 2006; Maquet et al., 1997). There is also evidence from intracortical recordings in sleeping patients of the transient, independent appearance of local SOs, accompanied by suppressed firing of nearby neurons, that are often undetectable using scalp electrodes (Nir et al., 2011). These scattered Off periods in different regions of cortex may be a response to local increases in sleep need.

Changes in response to sleep loss show a left–right asymmetry in some frequency bands, with the left hemisphere showing more power in the sigma band during NREM sleep, and the right hemisphere showing more theta power during NREM sleep and less during REM sleep than the left hemisphere (Roth et al., 1999). The increase in delta power after extended sleep loss in people is also much larger on the left than the right side of the frontal cortex (Achermann et al., 2001; Finelli et al., 2001).

12.6.2 Use-dependent changes in cortical EEG

Why do different cortical regions spontaneously show different levels of apparent sleep need and different degrees of increase in SWA during sleep? A strong possibility is that these phenomena are the result of regional differences in the intensity of cortical activity while awake. Levels of adenosine (a potent sleep-promoting agent) increase globally in the cortex during sleep deprivation and decrease during recovery sleep; see **Figure 11.16**. Local increases in activity would presumably result in local increases in adenosine and sleep need, reflected in increases in SWA during later recovery sleep. Thus, SWA amounts during NREM sleep are locally use-dependent: the more neurons are active, the more adenosine accumulates in the region, and the more neurons require SWA to recover from that activity.

The idea of use-dependence is supported by several lines of evidence. In one study, participants received sustained, localized somatosensory stimulation of their right hand while awake. During the first NREM sleep episode the next night, there was a selective increase in SWA over the corresponding left somatosensory cortex (Kattler et al., 1994).

Reducing neural activity has the opposite effect. Rats had their vibrissae (whiskers) removed from one side of their faces to reduce somatosensory stimulation unilaterally while they explored and interacted with novel objects during a 6 h sleep deprivation period. During a later sleep period, there was more low-frequency EEG power during NREM sleep in the cortical hemisphere that received normal vibrissal input while awake than in the hemisphere that was deprived of such input (Vyazovskiy et al., 2000) (**Figure 12.9**). Because results were expressed as a ratio of EEG power in the two hemispheres, this finding could reflect either (or both) reduced SWA on the deprived side or enhanced activity on the side receiving novel sensory input. Either interpretation supports the idea that the amount of SWA in a cortical region during sleep reflects its history of activation while awake.

Another study involved using a sling to immobilize one arm of human participants for a 12 h period during the day. Immobilization has two effects. It reduces the activity of motor systems that generate movements of that arm, and it reduces somatosensory input to the cortex from that arm. This input comes from surface touch receptors and movement-sensitive receptors in arm muscles and joints. During early NREM sleep after the immobilization period, regions of the somatosensory and motor cortices linked to the previously immobilized arm showed significantly reduced SWA relative to amounts shown in a control condition after a day of free use of both arms (**Figure 12.10**) (Huber et al., 2006).

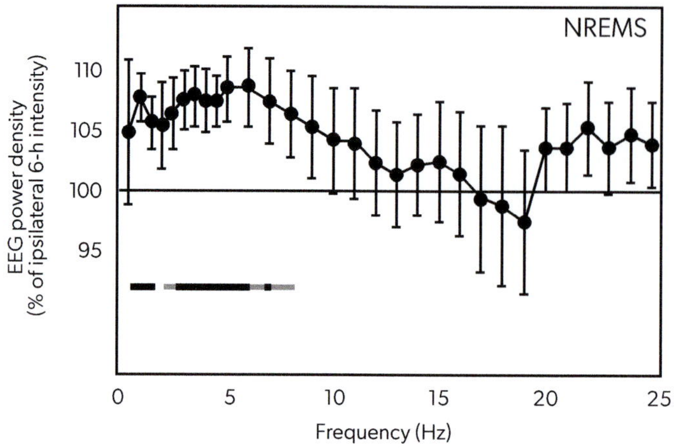

Figure 12.9 Mean differences (±SEM; Y axis) in EEG frequencies (X axis) expressed during NREM sleep over a 6 h period. The values shown are those from the cortical hemisphere of rats that previously received sensory input while awake, relative to the hemisphere that was deprived of input by removing the vibrissae (whiskers) on one side of the face (set at 100%). The bars below the data indicate that there was significantly more power in low EEG frequencies in the cortex that received stimulation from vibrissae than in the contralateral, deprived cortex (black, $p < 0.05$; gray, $p < 0.1$). Adapted with permission of John Wiley and Sons from Vyazovskiy, V.V. et al. (2000) Unilateral vibrissae stimulation during waking induces interhemispheric EEG asymmetry during subsequent sleep in the rat. *J Sleep Res* 9:367–371. Journal Compilation © European Sleep Research Society and John Wiley and Sons (2000). doi: 10.1046/j.1365-2869.2000.00230.x.

The mechanism underlying this change was studied using two methods involving evoked potentials. Evoked potentials were generated in the motor cortex by transcranial magnetic stimulation (TMS) and by electrical stimulation of the median nerve in the arm, which triggers evoked responses in the somatosensory cortex. Both sets of evoked potentials were reduced in amplitude on the side of the cortex opposite to the immobilized arm, relative to a control condition. The reduced amplitude was attributed to depression of synaptic activity in the motor and somatosensory regions of cortex linked to the immobilized arm. Participants also showed higher variability in the trajectories of movements using that arm during a simple motor task after immobilization. This effect was attributed to poorer coordination between joints as a result of reduced synaptic strength in the deprived cortical region (Huber et al., 2006).

There are different proposed mechanisms that could link synaptic depression to later reductions in SWA during sleep. One interpretation relates to the idea that the amplitude of slow waves depends on the degree of synchrony within a local

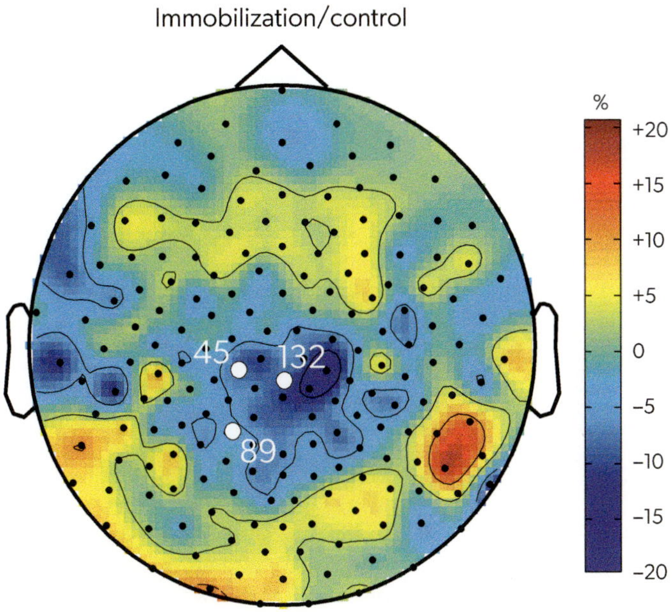

Figure 12.10 The intensity of slow-wave activity (SWA: 1–4.5 Hz) recorded by an array of electrodes (black & white dots) from people during the first 20 min of NREM sleep after one arm was immobilized in a sling for ~12 h, divided by the same measure after a control day during which the arm was used normally. The blue regions indicate areas in which SWA during sleep was reduced by prior arm immobilization and the three numbered white dots represent EEG electrode locations at which the decrease was statistically significant. Head orientation is indicated by symbols representing the nose and ears. The electrodes showing significant changes in SWA were positioned over the sensorimotor cortex (#s 45 and 132) and over a parietal cortex region involved in integrating sensorimotor information (#89). Recordings from electrode #132 showed the largest evoked responses at baseline in response to stimulating a nerve that innervates the wrist; there were significant reductions in the size of these evoked responses after immobilization. Reprinted with permission from Huber, R. et al. (2006) Arm immobilization causes cortical plastic changes and locally decreases sleep slow wave activity. *Nat Neurosci* 9: 1169–1176. © Springer:Nature (2006). doi: 10.1038/nn1758.

neural population. Decreased synaptic strengths as a result of disuse could produce reduced local synchrony among neurons, which would result in lower amplitude slow waves in that region. An alternative interpretation is that normal daily actions and sensory experiences continuously produce plastic changes in the neural circuits that are involved in producing those movements or sensations. SWA during sleep is a response to the processes involved in generating this neural plasticity, which would be greatly reduced by arm immobilization (Huber et al., 2006).

These studies in people and animals show that the degree of waking use (or disuse) of local regions of cortex predicts the amount of SWA produced during later sleep. These changes are interpreted as being use-dependent (i.e., related only to the level of activity of neural circuits, without a requirement for new learning). The concept of learning-dependent changes in the sleep EEG refers to modifications in sleep features that facilitate consolidation of newly acquired information or skills, a process in which slow waves play an important role (as discussed in Chapters 17 and 18). Although these mechanisms are conceptually different, both depend on forms of synaptic plasticity resulting from neural activity while awake. Some waking experiences that influence features of later sleep likely involve both higher intensity neural activity (use-dependence) and specific new learning (learning-dependence).

The functional and anatomical specificity of the effects of waking activity on sleep EEG parameters were demonstrated in a study in which human participants stayed awake for 24–36 h during two different sessions and engaged in very different activities for a total of 12 h during each session. During one session, they listened to audio books on a variety of topics, and during the other they practiced using a driving simulator. After 21 h awake and multiple sessions of either one task or the other, they showed increases in cortical theta-band activity (5–9 Hz), which is considered a marker of increasing sleep need that is detectable during waking (Cajochen et al., 1995; Hung et al., 2013); see Section 5.7.3 and (Finelli et al., 2000; Vyazovskiy & Tobler, 2005).

The increases in theta-band power and in theta-wave amplitude were specific to brain regions linked to the tasks participants had been performing. Listening to audio books increased theta activity in a left frontal region that is involved in language processing. Repeated driving simulator sessions instead increased theta activity in a posterior parietal region involved in sensorimotor processing (**Figure 12.11**). In addition, during later recovery sleep, there was increased EEG power in the 1–11 Hz range in the frontal region after audio book experiences and in the parietal region after simulated driving sessions (Hung et al., 2013).[10]

Intense use of a cortical region can also result in increased, localized "sleepiness" in the form of transient slow waves (Off periods) while awake that appear in cortical regions related to the activity; these transient events have functional consequences. Rats that had been trained to perform a skilled reaching task for a sugar reward were then tested after periods of sleep deprivation early in the daily light phase (when they would usually sleep). Recordings of cortical activity during

[10] It is unclear whether these changes were strictly use-dependent or whether knowledge or skills that were acquired or refined during the sessions also contributed learning-dependent effects.

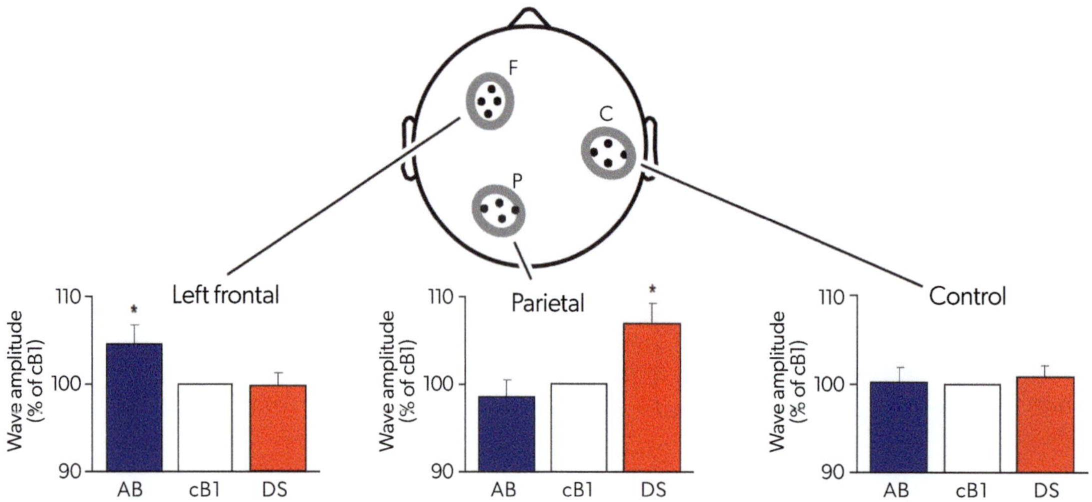

Figure 12.11 The peak amplitude of theta waves in different regions of the cortex of paritcipants after lengthy wakefulness involving two different kinds of sustained experiences. In one session, participants listened to audio books (AB; blue) on a variety of topics for a total of 12 h; and in the other session, they practiced on a driving simulator (DS, red) for the same duration. Theta-wave amplitude increased relative to control baseline levels (cB1, white) in a left frontal region of cortex (F) after the audio books experience (left chart), in a parietal region (P) after the driving simulator task (center chart), but not in a control region (C) after either task (right chart). There were corresponding, task-specific increases in theta energy over similar regions while awake and in low-mid frequency EEG power (1–11 Hz) during subsequent recovery sleep. Reprinted with permission of Oxford University Press from Hung et al. (2013) Local experience-dependent changes in the wake EEG after prolonged wakefulness. *Sleep* 36:59–72. © Sleep Research Society (2013). doi: 10.5665/sleep.2302.

testing showed localized, transient Off periods (i.e., times of reduced neuronal firing) in frontal and parietal cortices. The overall cortical EEG pattern and behavior of the rats indicated that, by the usual criteria, they remained awake and active during these local cortical events.

Cortical Off events (especially in the frontal cortex) were often followed a few hundred milliseconds later by failures to perform the learned task correctly (performance lapses). Successful trials were much less likely to be preceded by frontal Off periods (**Figure 12.12**). The frequency of Off events increased with the length of time awake while performing the task. These results were interpreted as showing that cortical circuits involved in performing the motor task repeatedly over an extended period developed high levels of use-dependent sleep need. As a result, these "overused" neural circuits periodically "slept," that is, generated brief, local episodes of reduced activity (Off events), that interfered with current task performance (Vyazovskiy et al., 2011).

Similar results were obtained in human studies. Both motor and sensory learning experiences increased localized theta activity in people, and these localized theta increases were reversed after sleeping but not after an equivalent period of waking rest. This localized sleepiness also impaired performance on tasks that relied specifically on the same cortical resources as the training tasks (Nelson et al., 2021; Ricci et al., 2021).

In summary, these and other lines of evidence for localized changes in the cortical EEG during sleep or extended waking as a result of previous use or disuse indicate that different cortical regions can acquire different degrees of sleep need and sleepiness. Sleepiness related to increased use is reflected in increased local theta activity while awake, an increased amount of SWA during sleep, and breakthrough episodes of localized inhibition (Off periods) while still awake (Huber, Esser, et al., 2007; Krueger et al., 2008; Rector et al., 2009).

12.6.3 Mechanisms of use-dependence

These findings are consistent with the view that SWA is a marker of homeostatic sleep need (process S in the two-process model; see Chapter 5) but in relation to local rather than global sleep need. NREM sleep (and especially SWA) is proposed to be involved in reversing the neuronal effects of waking. The need for this repair function is greater in brain regions that have engaged in unusually intense neural activity (Vyazovskiy et al., 2000).[11] This idea raises the

[11] An earlier hypothesis proposed that sleep might provide internally generated stimulation of neural circuits that had been *underutilized* during waking, in order to maintain the integrity of the underlying neural architecture (Krueger et al., 1995). This proposal, however, was related to overall neural activity during sleep and was not specific to the functions served by SWA during NREM sleep.

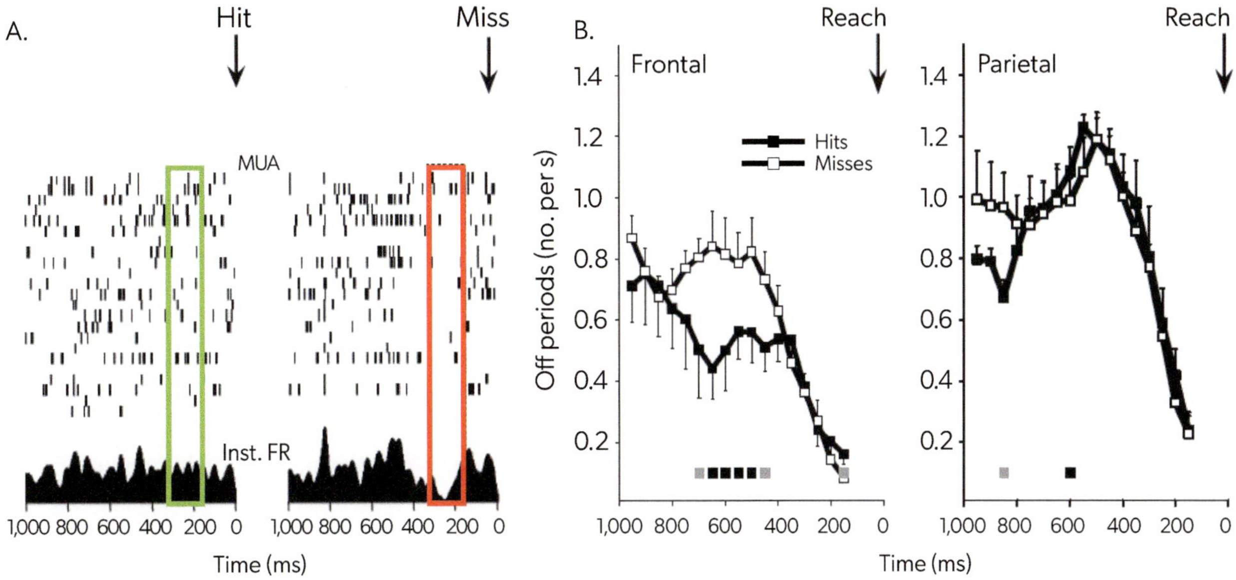

Figure 12.12 **A.** Rats were moderately sleep deprived and then performed a skilled reaching task for sugar pellet rewards. Raster plots show the firing of 20 frontal cortical neurons (multiple unit activity, MUA) in the second before a reaching trial that was successful (Hit) or unsuccessful (Miss). The red outlined region illustrates the low firing activity in a 200–300 msec Off period before an unsuccessful trial. The green outlined area shows the corresponding time window on a successful trial. The records at the bottom of the figure show the instantaneous firing rate (Inst. FR) of all recorded single neurons, showing the strong decrease in average firing just before unsuccessful trials, but not before successful trials. **B.** The number of Off periods per second in the frontal cortex (left) and parietal cortex (right) in the second before reaching trials that were successful (Hits, black symbols) and unsuccessful (Misses, white symbols). Boxes below the data indicate times at which the differences between Hit and Miss trials were statistically significant (black, $p < 0.05$) or approached significance (gray, $p < 0.1$). In the frontal cortex, but not the parietal cortex, Off periods occurred significantly more frequently during the second before Miss trials as compared to before Hit trials. Adapted with permission from Vyazovskiy, V.V. et al. (2011) Local sleep in awake rats. *Nature* 472: 443–472. © Springer: Nature (2011). doi: 10.1038/nature10009.

question of which physiological changes resulting from increased neural activity create the deficit that is reversed by later SWA.

One possibility is that the increased firing of neurons in an "overused" part of cortex creates a sleep need because the energy required for this activity is derived from the metabolism of ATP, resulting in the local release of free adenosine. As reviewed in Section 11.6, increased brain adenosine levels induce sleepiness, and blocking adenosine receptors (e.g., with caffeine) promotes waking and counteracts the behavioral effects of sleep loss.

There is, however, evidence that increased firing of neurons alone may not be sufficient to produce an increased need for SWA. Keeping mice awake for 6 h during the daily light phase by providing them with novel stimuli to explore (sometimes called gentle handling; see Section 14.2) resulted in increased cortical activity while awake. The mice also showed increased SWA and more frequent and longer Off periods during subsequent sleep. Other mice had clusters of neurons in regions of their frontal cortex stimulated optogenetically for 6 h during NREM sleep to achieve similar changes in firing rates. The activated cortical regions in these mice did not show increases in amounts of either SWA or Off periods during the following 2 h. These results indicate that changes in addition to higher firing rates were involved in producing later increases in neural sleepiness and in the need for SWA (Rodriguez et al., 2016).

To discuss what could have contributed to their increased neural sleepiness and local increases in SWA, we have to briefly introduce two topics. One is related to a hypothesis about the function of SWA and the other to the role of neurotrophins in both learning and sleep regulation.

The synaptic downscaling hypothesis proposes that the neural activity associated with ordinary experiences while awake causes strengthening of synaptic connections broadly across the cortex. Most of these strengthened synapses are not functionally important, and they create a metabolic burden because of the energetic costs of maintaining synapses. In addition, the process would tend over time to saturate available synaptic capacity, which would reduce the potential for plasticity that could serve later learning. The hypothesis proposes that SWA functions to reverse the "excess," incidental synaptic strengthening that occurs during waking by decreasing synaptic strengths overall (Cirelli et al., 2005; Tononi & Cirelli, 2006); see discussion in Section 18.15.

The mice that were kept awake in this study had many sensory and motor experiences as they explored novel objects.

They would have learned something about them: how they smell and feel and how they can be manipulated. Learning is generally assumed to depend on strengthening or growth of specific synaptic connections that are actively involved in the learning experience (Cooper, 2005; Hebb, 1949). In contrast, the mice that were induced to express similar levels of neuronal activity during sleep had no opportunities for new learning. As a result, any synaptic strengthening would have been associated only with the increased firing rates that were generated, and not with the additional neuronal effects of novel learning experiences.

Synaptic growth depends on neurochemical factors in the brain, which have also been linked to production of SWA. One of these is the neurotrophin, brain-derived neurotrophic factor (BDNF), which facilitates activity-dependent, plastic changes in synapses, including, for example, those occurring during long-term potentiation (see Section 18.2). Brain levels of BDNF increase during usual wake periods, increase further during sleep deprivation, and decrease during sleep. Previous studies showed that increasing exploratory behavior while rats are awake results in increases in gene expression for BDNF and other plasticity-related genes, as well as increases in SWA during later sleep (Huber, Tononi, et al., 2007).

The link between BDNF and sleep is also supported by evidence that injecting BDNF into one side of the cortex of rats while they were awake increased SWA selectively in the treated hemisphere during later NREM sleep. In contrast, injecting antibodies against BDNF into the cortex during waking reduced later SWA in the injected cortical region (Faraguna et al., 2008) (**Figure 12.13**). These results confirm that increased

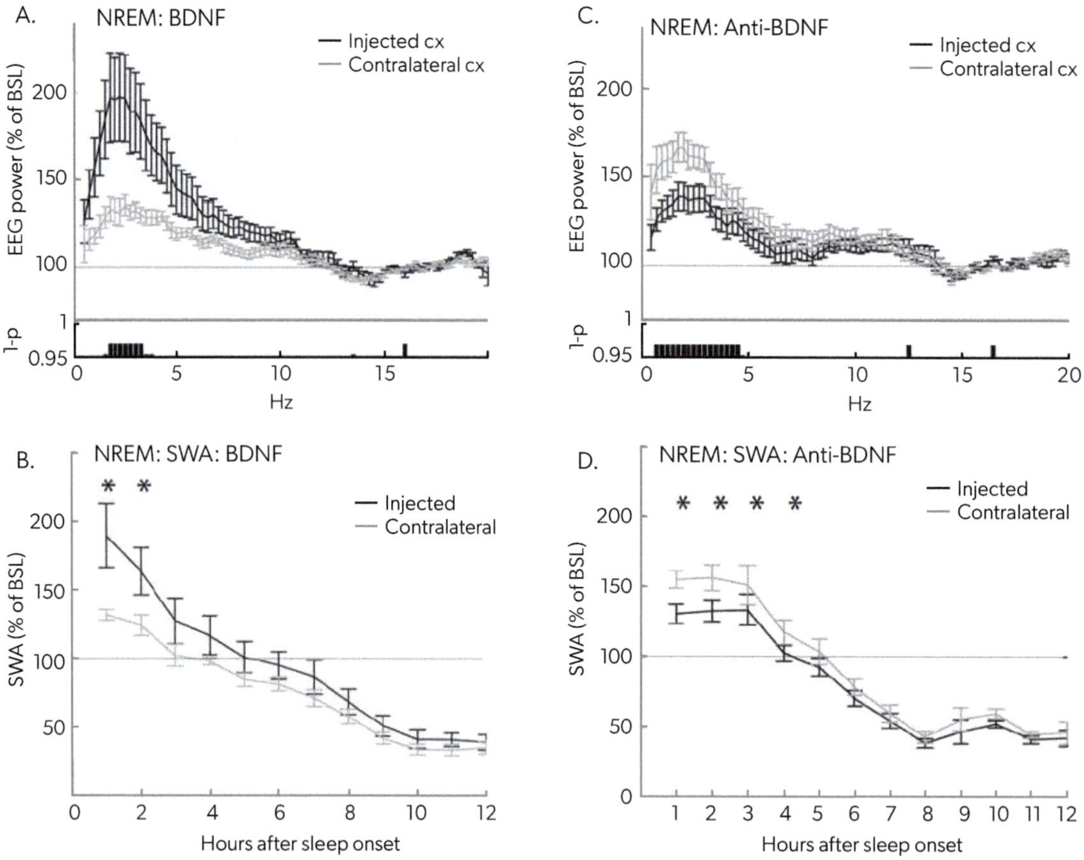

Figure 12.13 **A.** EEG power during 2 h of NREM sleep in the cortex of rats that received a unilateral injection of brain derived neurotrophic factor (BDNF) (black line) and in the uninjected contralateral cortex (gray line). The black box on the X axis indicates EEG frequency ranges with significantly more power in the injected cortex relative to the uninjected cortex. **B.** The time course of slow-wave activity (SWA: 0.5–4.0 Hz) during the hours after sleep onset relative to baseline levels (=100%). There was increased SWA during the first 2 h after sleep onset in the cortex that received a BDNF injection compared to the uninjected contralateral cortex (* indicates p <0.01). **C.** Labels as in panel **A**. Injection of an anti-BDNF antibody in one cortex (black line) resulted in significantly *less* EEG power in the SWA range relative to the uninjected cortex (gray line). **D.** Labels as in panel B. Injection of an anti-BDNF antibody into one cortex (black line) resulted in significantly (*) *reduced* power in the SWA range relative to the uninjected side (gray line) during the first 4 h after sleep onset. Reprinted with permission from Faraguna, U. et al. (2008) A causal role for brain-derived neurotrophic factor in the homeostatic regulation of sleep. *J Neurosci* 28(15): 4088–4095. © Society for Neuroscience (2008). doi:10.1523/jneurosci.5510-07.2008.

BDNF levels, which contribute to strengthening synaptic connections, also promote later increases in SWA.

The mice that received cortical stimulation while asleep not only had no opportunity to learn but their increased neural activity also occurred in a neural environment that does not favor synaptic plasticity. BDNF and norepinephrine (NE) levels in cortex are low during sleep and elevated during waking. NE promotes higher levels of gene expression for BDNF and other plasticity-related genes (Cirelli & Tononi, 2000). It is linked to increasing SWA by the finding that depletion of cortical NE before 6 h of sleep deprivation blunted the increase in SWA that usually occurs during later recovery sleep (Cirelli et al., 2005).

The mice kept awake and exploring novel stimuli would have had elevated NE and BDNF levels and would have undergone synaptic strengthening as a result of their experience. Another effect of strengthened synaptic connectivity within a local neural population is to make the activity of those neurons more synchronous, which would favor production of larger slow waves (Rodriguez et al., 2016). In addition, the increased energy costs of synaptic growth related to learning, above those associated with higher firing rates, would increase adenosine as a product of metabolism of ATP. Higher adenosine levels would further promote sleepiness and increased SWA.

Thus, increased SWA during later sleep in the mice that were kept awake can be explained by a combination of factors: increased neural firing during their waking activities (i.e., use-dependence); elevated NE and BDNF levels while awake and active; increased (BDNF-dependent) synaptic growth associated with both increased activity and learning; increased local neural synchrony as a result of synaptic growth; and increased adenosine levels as a product of metabolic activity involved in both synaptic growth and neural firing.

Mice receiving neural stimulation while sleeping would have had the benefits only of increased firing rates and the associated adenosine increases, but in the context of low BDNF and NE levels. These differences, together with the hypothesized role for SWA in downscaling synaptic strengths, can account for why mice that were stimulated during sleep subsequently showed less local SWA and fewer neural Off periods than mice that experienced similar levels of neural activity while actively exploring novel objects (Rodriguez et al., 2016).

12.6.4 Local and global regulation of sleep

The standard view of sleep regulation is that interactions among subcortical mechanisms (representing both homeostatic and circadian influences) create cyclically alternating states of waking, NREM, and REM sleep. These states are expressed as EEG-detectable changes in cortical neural activity and accompanying changes in consciousness. Specific subcortical regions (e.g., in the preoptic area and basal forebrain) monitor sleep need (perhaps in the form of adenosine buildup) and are primarily responsible for triggering sleep onset in response to that signal at an appropriate circadian phase.

An alternative hypothesis is that locally developed sleep need across cortical regions is summed to generate the need for global sleep (Krueger et al., 1995; Krueger et al., 2008). The idea that sleep need is regulated locally is supported by evidence of both spontaneous and use-dependent asymmetries in cortical sleep features in mammals (reviewed in Sections 12.6.1 and 12.6.2). Evidence that unihemispheric sleep occurs in some vertebrates and that sleep loss affecting one hemisphere is compensated by recovery sleep in that hemisphere with little effect on the contralateral side (Oleksenko et al., 1992) also supports the idea of local regulation of sleep need.

This apparent independence of the regulation of sleep need and its expression in restricted regions of the cortex (or in each hemisphere) does not support the idea that local cortical sleep needs are normally summed to generate a global sleep need. Nevertheless, there is also evidence from studies in people that locally induced EEG changes can influence the cortex more broadly. For example, SOs that were triggered in a local cortical region by external stimulation during sleep propagated across the cortex and led to deepened global sleep (Hathaway et al., 2021; Massimini et al., 2007). Similarly, rhythmic acoustic stimulation delivered unilaterally to one ear during naps enhanced low-frequency EEG oscillations in both cerebral hemispheres. This bilateral effect of unilateral inputs may be a product of either close coupling between cortical regions in both hemispheres or activation by auditory input of subcortical systems that influence both hemispheres (Simor et al., 2018).

Some observations, however, are more difficult to explain based on the hypothesis that local sleep need creates the drive for global sleep. For example, sleep-like states can appear under conditions that involve little cortical activity; encéphale isolé brains and animals anesthetized with urethane still alternate between cortical SWA and activation. Little in the way of significant activity or experience-dependent plasticity would occur locally in the cortex in those preparations that could cumulatively trigger a cortical state transition. The periodic emergence of sleep-like cortical states under those conditions seems more likely to be a product of interactions among intact subcortical regulatory systems that control the expression of global cycles of sleep and waking in the cortex, as discussed in Chapters 10 and 11.

12.6.5 Summary

The distribution of EEG frequencies during sleep varies spontaneously across brain regions (e.g., frontal regions show higher levels of SWA, and spindles occur more frequently in the midline vertex region). Deliberately increasing sensory or motor activity related to specific cortical regions can increase SWA in those regions during subsequent sleep; decreasing specific sensory/motor activity has the opposite effect. These are considered use-dependent changes. These results indicate that increased local neural activity during waking creates a homeostatic, local increase in sleep need; increased SWA in that region is part of a recovery process that satisfies that sleep need.

Similarly, sustained use of a specific neural circuit involved in performing a learned skill can lead to intrusions into waking of transient, local slow waves and Off states in cortical regions responsible for producing that behavior. These Off states are associated with brief lapses in performance of the learned skill, presumably reflecting transient silencing of overused neural circuits involved in their performance. While use-dependent and learning-dependent processes that affect EEG features during sleep can be distinguished, some situations probably contain elements of both processes.

Increased local sleep need could result from higher local levels of the sleep-promoting neurochemical adenosine, a product of increased metabolism of ATP that is used to support the energy costs of neuronal activity. Learning can generate growth of synaptic connections, requiring more energy usage and therefore also resulting in production of free adenosine. Strengthened synaptic connections among local neurons can also increase neural synchrony which would further increase the amplitude of slow waves in that region.

Artificially generating increased neuronal activity alone, especially during sleep, may not be sufficient to induce homeostatic increases in sleep need, in part because there would likely be little synaptic strengthening locally as a result of the increased firing rates. Synaptic strengthening depends on increased levels of plasticity-related neurochemicals, such as BDNF and NE, both of which are reduced in the cortex during sleep. The combination of increased neural activity during waking exploration and the synaptic plasticity induced by learning during these experiences may be necessary to promote more SWA during later sleep.

There is also evidence that locally generated changes in EEG activity during sleep can spread across cortical regions and influence the depth of global sleep. These effects, combined with other evidence for local, use-dependent changes in SWA and spontaneous regional differences in sleep features, suggest the possibility that global sleep represents the sum of local sleep needs in the cortex. However, there is evidence that under some conditions sleep-like states emerge periodically when little cortical plasticity seems possible. Local sleep need and its expression as increased SWA are more likely to modulate global patterns of sleep and waking that are controlled primarily by interacting subcortical mechanisms.

Literature cited

Achermann, P., & Borbély, A. (1997). Low frequency (<1 Hz) oscillations in the human sleep electroencephalogram. *Neuroscience, 81*(1), 213–222.

Achermann, P., Dijk, D. J., Brunner, D. P., & Borbély, A. A. (1993). A model of human sleep homeostasis based on EEG slow-wave activity: quantitative comparison of data and simulations. *Brain Res Bull, 31*, 97–113.

Achermann, P., Finelli, L. A., & Borbély, A. (2001). Unihemispheric enhancement of delta power in human frontal sleep EEG by prolonged wakefulness. *Brain Res, 913*, 220–223.

Adrian, E. D. (1937). The physiology of sleep. *Irish J Med Sci, 12*(138), 237–248.

Amzica, F., & Steriade, M. (1997). The K-complex: its slow (<1-Hz) rhythmicity and relation to delta waves. *Neurology, 49*(4), 952–959. doi: 10.1212/WNL.49.4.952<t>10.1212/WNL.49.4.952

Amzica, F., & Steriade, M. (1998). Electrophysiological correlates of sleep delta waves. *Electroencephalogr Clin Neurophysiol, 107*, 69–83.

Amzica, F., & Steriade, M. (2000). Integration of low-frequency sleep oscillations in corticothalamic networks. *Acta Neurobiol Exp, 60*, 229–245.

Andrillon, T., Nir, Y., Staba, R. J., Ferrarelli, F., Cirelli, C., Tononi, G., & Fried, I. (2011). Sleep spindles in humans: insights from intracranial EEG and unit recordings. *J Neurosci, 31*(49), 17821–17834. doi: 10.1523/JNEUROSCI.2604-11.2011

Andrillon, T., Poulsen, A. T., Hansen, L. K., Leger, D., & Kouider, S. (2016). Neural markers of responsiveness to the environment in human sleep. *J Neurosci, 36*(24), 6583–6596. doi: 10.1523/JNEUROSCI.0902-16.2016

Atwood, M. (1996). *Alias Grace*. Toronto: McClelland & Stewart.

Baars, B. J. (2005). Global workspace theory of consciousness: toward a cognitive neuroscience of human experience. *Prog Brain Res, 150*, 45–53. doi: 10.1016/s0079-6123(05)50004-9

Baker, R., Gent, T. C., Yang, Q., Parker, S., Vyssotski, A. L., Wisden, W., … Franks, N. P. (2014). Altered activity in the central medial thalamus precedes changes in the neocortex during transitions into both sleep and propofol anesthesia. *J Neurosci, 34*(40), 13326–13335. doi: 10.1523/JNEUROSCI.1519-14.2014

Bastuji, H., Cadic-Melchior, A., Magnin, M., & Garcia-Larrea, L. (2021). Intra-cortical functional connectivity predicts arousal to noxious stimuli during sleep in humans. *J Neurosci, 41*(23), 5115–5123. doi: 10.1523/JNEUROSCI.2935-20.2021

Bastuji, H., Perchet, C., Legrain, V., Montes, C., & Garcia-Larrea, L. (2008). Laser evoked responses to painful stimulation persist during sleep and predict subsequent arousals. *Pain, 137*(3), 589–599. doi: 10.1016/j.pain.2007.10.027

Bernardi, G., Betta, M., Ricciardi, E., Pietrini, P., Tononi, G., & Siclari, F. (2019). Regional delta waves in human rapid eye movement sleep. *J Neurosci, 39*(14), 2686–2697. doi: 10.1523/JNEUROSCI.2298-18.2019.

Blumenfeld, H. (2016). Neuroanatomical basis of consciousness. In S. Laureys, O. Gosseries & G. Tononi (Eds.), *The Neurology of Consciousness* (2nd ed., pp. 3–29). San Diego: Elsevier.

Borbély, A. A., Baumann, F., Brandeis, D., Strauch, I., & Lehmann, D. (1981). Sleep deprivation: effect on sleep stages and EEG power density in man. *Electroencephalogr Clin Neurophysiol, 51*, 483–493.

Braun, A., Balkin, T., Wesensten, N., Carson, R., Varga, M., Baldwin, P., … Herscovitch, P. (1997). Regional cerebral blood flow throughout the sleep–wake cycle: an $H_2^{15}O$ PET study. *Brain, 120*, 1173–1197.

Broughton, R. (1968). Sleep disorders: disorders of arousal? *Science, 159*(3819), 1070–1078.

Brown, R. E., Basheer, R., McKenna, J. T., Strecker, R. E., & McCarley, R. W. (2012). Control of sleep and wakefulness. *Physiol Rev, 92*(3), 1087–1187. doi: 10.1152/physrev.00032.2011

Buzsáki, G., & Schomburg, E. W. (2015). What does gamma coherence tell us about inter-regional neural communication? *Nat Neurosci, 18*(4), 484–489. doi: 10.1038/nn.3952

Cajochen, C., Brunner, D. P., Kräuchi, K., Graw, P., & Wirz-Justice, A. (1995). Power density in theta/alpha frequencies of the waking EEG progressively increases during sustained wakefulness. *Sleep, 18*(10), 890–894.

Callaway, C. W., Lydic, R., Baghdoyan, H. A., & Hobson, J. A. (1987). Pontogeniculooccipital waves: spontaneous visual system activity during rapid eye movement sleep. *Cell Mol Neurobiol, 7*, 105–149.

Camassa, A., Galluzzi, A., Mattia, M., & Sanchez-Vives, M. V. (2022). Deterministic and stochastic components of cortical down states: dynamics and modulation. *J Neurosci, 42*(50), 9387–9400. doi: 10.1523/JNEUROSCI.0914-22.2022

Campbell, K. (2010). Event-related potentials as a measure of sleep disturbance: a tutorial review. *Noise Health, 12*(47), 137–153. doi: 10.4103/1463-1741.63216

Cantero, J., Atienza, M., Madsen, J., & Stickgold, R. (2004). Gamma EEG dynamics in neocortex and hippocampus during human wakefulness and sleep. *Neuroimage, 22*(3), 1271–1280. doi: 10.1016/j.neuroimage.2004.03.014

Carskadon, M. A., & Herz, R. S. (2004). Minimal olfactory perception during sleep: why odor alarms will not work for humans. *Sleep, 27*(3), 402–405.

Cash, S. S., Halgren, E., Dehghani, N., Rossetti, A. O., Thesen, T., Wang, C., … Ulbert, I. (2009). The human K-complex represents an isolated cortical downstate. *Science, 324*(5930), 1084–1087. doi: 10.1126/science.1169626

Chow, H. M., Horovitz, S. G., Carr, W. S., Picchioni, D., Coddington, N., Fukunaga, M., … Braun, A. R. (2013). Rhythmic alternating patterns of brain activity distinguish rapid eye movement sleep from other states of consciousness. *Proc Natl Acad Sci U S A, 110*(25), 10300–10305. doi: 10.1073/pnas.1217691110

Church, M., Johnson, L., & Seales, D. (1978). Evoked K-complexes and cardiovascular responses to spindle-synchronous and spindle-asynchronous stimulus clicks during NREM sleep. *Electroencephalogr Clin Neurophysiol, 45*, 443–453.

Church, M. W., March, J. D., Hibi, S., Benson, K., Cavness, C., & Feinberg, I. (1975). Changes in frequency and amplitude of delta activity during sleep. *Electroencephalogr Clin Neurophysiol, 39*, 1–7.

Cirelli, C., Huber, R., Gopalakrishnan, A., Southard, T. L., & Tononi, G. (2005). Locus ceruleus control of slow-wave homeostasis. *J Neurosci, 25*(18), 4503–4511. doi: 10.1523/JNEUROSCI.4845-04.2005

Cirelli, C., & Tononi, G. (2000). Differential expression of plasticity-related genes in waking and sleep and their regulation by the noradrenergic system. *J Neurosci, 15*(2), 9187–9194.

Claude, L., Chouchou, F., Prados, G., Castro, M., De Blay, B., Perchet, C., … Bastuji, H. (2015). Sleep spindles and human cortical nociception: a surface and intracerebral electrophysiological study. *J Physiol, 593*(22), 4995–5008. doi: 10.1113/JP270941

Coenen, A. (2024). Sensory gating and gaining in sleep: the balance between the protection of sleep and the safeness of life (a review). *J Sleep Res, 33*(5). doi: 10.1111/jsr.14152

Colrain, I., & Campbell, K. (2007). The use of evoked potentials in sleep research. *Sleep Med Rev, 11*(4), 277–293. doi: 10.1016/j.smrv.2007.05.001

Cooper, S. J. (2005). Donald O. Hebb's synapse and learning rule: a history and commentary. *Neurosci Biobehav Rev, 28*(8), 851–874. doi: 10.1016/j.neubiorev.2004.09.009

Cote, K., Epps, T., & Campbell, K. (2000). The role of the spindle in human information processing of high-intensity stimuli during sleep. *J Sleep Res, 9*, 19–26.

Cote, K., Etienne, L., & Campbell, K. (2001). Neurophysiological evidence for the detection of external stimuli during sleep. *Sleep, 24*(7), 1–13.

Cox, R., Hofman, W. F., & Talamini, L. M. (2012). Involvement of spindles in memory consolidation is slow wave sleep-specific. *Learn Mem, 19*(7), 264–267. doi: 10.1101/lm.026252.112

Cox, R., van Driel, J., de Boer, M., & Talamini, L. M. (2014). Slow oscillations during sleep coordinate interregional communication in cortical networks. *J Neurosci, 34*(50), 16890–16901. doi: 10.1523/JNEUROSCI.1953-14.2014

Crick, F. (1984). Function of the thalamic reticular complex: the searchlight hypothesis. *Proc Natl Acad Sci USA, 81*, 4586–4590.

Crunelli, V., David, F., Lorincz, M. L., & Hughes, S. W. (2015). The thalamocortical network as a single slow wave-generating unit. *Curr Opin Neurobiol, 31*, 72–80. doi: 10.1016/j.conb.2014.09.001

Csercsa, R., Dombovari, B., Fabo, D., Wittner, L., Eross, L., Entz, L., … Ulbert, I. (2010). Laminar analysis of slow wave activity in humans. *Brain, 133*(9), 2814–2829. doi: 10.1093/brain/awq169

Dang-Vu, T., Bonjean, M., Schabus, M., Boly, M., Darsaud, A., Desseilles, M., … Maquet, P. (2011). Interplay between spontaneous and induced brain activity during human non-rapid eye movement sleep. *Proc Natl Acad Sci USA, 108*(37), 15438–15443.

Dang-Vu, T. T., McKinney, S. M., Buxton, O. M., Solet, J. M., & Ellenbogen, J. M. (2010). Spontaneous brain rhythms predict sleep stability in the face of noise. *Curr Biol, 20*(15), R626–R627. doi: 10.1016/j.cub.2010.06.032

Dang-Vu, T. T., Schabus, M., Desseilles, M., Albouy, G., Boly, M., Darsaud, A., … Maquet, P. (2008). Spontaneous neural activity during human slow wave sleep. *Proc Natl Acad Sci USA, 105*(39), 15160–15165. doi: 10.1073/pnas.0801819105

Datta, S. (1997). Cellular basis of pontine ponto-geniculo-occipital wave generation and modulation. *Cell Mol Neurobiol, 17*(3), 341–365.

Datta, S., & Siwek, D. F. (2002). Single cell activity patterns of pedunculopontine tegmentum neurons across the sleep-wake cycle in the freely moving rats. *J Neurosci Res, 70*(4), 611–621. doi: 10.1002/jnr.10405

David, F., Schmiedt, J. T., Taylor, H. L., Orban, G., Di Giovanni, G., Uebele, V. N., … Crunelli, V. (2013). Essential thalamic contribution to slow waves of natural sleep. *J Neurosci, 33*(50), 19599–19610. doi: 10.1523/JNEUROSCI.3169-13.2013

De Gennaro, L., & Ferrara, M. (2003). Sleep spindles: an overview. *Sleep Med Rev, 7*(5), 423–440. doi: 10.1016/S1087-0792(02)00116-8

Dehaene, S., & Changeux, J. P. (2011). Experimental and theoretical approaches to conscious processing. *Neuron, 70*(2), 200–227. doi: 10.1016/j.neuron.2011.03.018

Dement, W., & Kleitman, N. (1957). The relation of eye movements during sleep to dream activity: an objective method for the study of dreaming. *J Exp Psychol, 53*(5), 339–346.

Dijk, D.-J., Hayes, B., & Czeisler, C. A. (1993). Dynamics of electroencephalographic sleep spindles and slow wave activity in men: effect of sleep deprivation. *Brain Res, 626*, 190–199.

Dijk, D.-J., Shanahan, T. L., Duffy, J., Ronda, J., & Czeisler, C. (1997). Variation of electroencephalographic activity during non-rapid eye movement and rapid eye movement sleep with phase of circadian melatonin rhythm in humans. *J Physiol, 505*(3), 851–858.

Edeline, J.-M., Manunta, Y., & Hennevin, E. (2000). Auditory thalamus neurons during sleep: changes in frequency selectivity, threshold, and receptive field size. *J Neurophysiol, 84*, 934–952.

Emrick, J. J., Gross, B. A., Riley, B. T., & Poe, G. R. (2016). Different simultaneous sleep states in the hippocampus and neocortex. *Sleep, 39*(12), 2201–2209. doi: 10.5665/sleep.6326

Ermis, U., Krakow, K., & Voss, U. (2010). Arousal thresholds during human tonic and phasic REM sleep. *J Sleep Res, 19*(3), 400–406. doi: 10.1111/j.1365-2869.2010.00831.x

Esser, S., Hill, S., & Tononi, G. (2009). Breakdown of effective connectivity during slow wave sleep: investigating the mechanism underlying a cortical gate using large-scale modeling. *J Neurophysiol, 47*. doi: 10.1152/jn.00059.2009

Faraguna, U., Vyazovskiy, V. V., Nelson, A. B., Tononi, G., & Cirelli, C. (2008). A causal role for brain-derived neurotrophic factor in the homeostatic regulation of sleep. *J Neurosci, 28*(15), 4088–4095. doi: 10.1523/jneurosci.5510-07.2008

Finelli, L. A., Baumann, H., Borbély, A. A., & Achermann, P. (2000). Dual electroencephalogram markers of human sleep homeostasis: correlation between theta activity in waking and slow-wave activity in sleep. *Neuroscience, 101*(3), 523–529.

Finelli, L. A., Borbély, A., & Achermann, P. (2001). Functional topography of the human nonREM sleep electroencephalogram. *Eur J Neurosci, 13*, 2282–2290.

Frederickson, C., & Rechtschaffen, A. (1978). Effects of sleep deprivation on awakening thresholds and sensory evoked potentials in the rat. *Sleep, 1*, 69–82.

French, A. S., Geissmann, Q., Beckwith, E. J., & Gilestro, G. F. (2021). Sensory processing during sleep in *Drosophila melanogaster*. *Nature, 598*, 479–482. doi:10.1038/s41586-021-03954-w

Freund, T. F., & Meskenaite, V. (1992). γ-Aminobutyric acid-containing basal forebrain neurons innervate inhibitory interneurons in the neocortex. *Proc Natl Acad Sci USA, 89*, 738–742.

Fuentealba, P., & Steriade, M. (2005). The reticular nucleus revisited: intrinsic and network properties of a thalamic pacemaker. *Prog Neurobiol, 75*, 125–141. doi: 0.1016/j.pneurobio.2005.01.002

Funk, C., Honjoh, S., Rodriguez, A., Cirelli, C., & Tononi, G. (2016). Local slow waves in superficial layers of primary cortical areas during REM sleep. *Curr Biol, 6*, 396–403.

Funk, C. M., Peelman, K., Bellesi, M., Marshall, W., Cirelli, C., & Tononi, G. (2017). Role of somatostatin-positive cortical interneurons in the generation of sleep slow waves. *J Neurosci, 37*(38), 9132–9148. doi: 10.1523/JNEUROSCI.1303-17.2017

Gaykema, R., van Weeghel, R., Hersh, L. B., & Luiten, P. (1991). Prefrontal cortical projections to the cholinergic neurons in the basal forebrain. *J Comp Neurol, 303*(4), 563–583.

Gompf, H. S., & Anaclet, C. (2020). The neuroanatomy and neurochemistry of sleep-wake control. *Curr Opin Physiol, 15*, 143–151. doi: 10.1016/j.cophys.2019.12.012

Gonzalez, C. E., Mak-McCully, R. A., Rosen, B. Q., Cash, S. S., Chauvel, P. Y., Bastuji, H., … Halgren, E. (2018). Theta bursts precede, and spindles follow, cortical and thalamic downstates in human NREM sleep. *J Neurosci, 38*(46), 9989–10001. doi: 10.1523/JNEUROSCI.0476-18.2018

Gosseries, O., Thibaut, A., Boly, M., Rosanova, M., Massimini, M., & Laureys, S. (2014). Assessing consciousness in coma and related states using transcranial magnetic stimulation combined with electroencephalography. *Ann Fr Anesth Reanim*, *33*(2), 65–71. doi: 10.1016/j.annfar.2013.11.002

Gott, J. A., Liley, D. T., & Hobson, J. A. (2017). Towards a functional understanding of PGO waves. *Front Hum Neurosci*, *11*, 89. doi: 10.3389/fnhum.2017.00089

Grenier, F., Timofeev, I., & Steriade, M. (1998). Leading role of thalamic over cortical neurons during postinhibitory rebound excitation. *Proc Natl Acad Sci USA*, *95*, 13929–13934.

Haider, B., Duque, A., Hasentaub, A., & McCormick, D. (2006). Neocortical network activity *in vivo* is generated through a dynamic balance of excitation and inhibition. *J Neurosci*, *26*(27), 4535–4545.

Halassa, M. M., Chen, Z., Wimmer, R. D., Brunetti, P. M., Zhao, S., Zikopoulos, B., … Wilson, M. A. (2014). State-dependent architecture of thalamic reticular subnetworks. *Cell*, *158*(4), 808–821. doi: 10.1016/j.cell.2014.06.025

Halassa, M. M., Siegle, J. H., Ritt, J. T., Ting, J. T., Feng, G., & Moore, C. I. (2011). Selective optical drive of thalamic reticular nucleus generates thalamic bursts and cortical spindles. *Nat Neurosci*, *14*(9), 1118–1120. doi: 10.1038/nn.2880

Halász, P. (2005). K-complex, a reactive EEG graphoelement of NREM sleep: an old chap in a new garment. *Sleep Med Rev*, *9*, 391–412. doi: 0.1016/j.smrv.2005.04.003

Hathaway, E., Morgan, K., Carson, M. S., R., Fernandez-Corazza, M., Luu, P., & Tucker, D. M. (2021). Transcranial electrical stimulation targeting limbic cortex increases the duration of human deep sleep. *Sleep Med*, *81*, 350–357. doi: 10.1016/j.sleep.2021.03.001

Hebb, D. O. (1949). *The Organization of Behavior: A Neuropsychological Theory*. Oxford, England: Wiley.

Helfrich, R. F., Mander, B. A., Jagust, W. J., Knight, R. T., & Walker, M. P. (2018). Old brains come uncoupled in sleep: slow wave-spindle synchrony, brain atrophy, and forgetting. *Neuron*, *97*(1), 221–230. doi: 10.1016/j.neuron.2017.11.020

Hennevin, E., Huetz, C., & Edeline, J. (2007). Neural representations during sleep: from sensory processing to memory traces. *Neurobiol Learn Mem*, *87*(3), 416–440. doi: 10.1016/j.nlm.2006.10.006

Honjoh, S., Sasai, S., Schiereck, S. S., Nagai, H., Tononi, G., & Cirelli, C. (2018). Regulation of cortical activity and arousal by the matrix cells of the ventromedial thalamic nucleus. *Nat Commun*, *9*(1), 2100. doi: 10.1038/s41467-018-04497-x

Horovitz, S. G., Braun, A., Carr, W., Picchioni, D., Balkin, T., Fukunaga, M., & Duyn, J. H. (2009). Decoupling of the brain's default mode network during deep sleep. *Proc Natl Acad Sci USA*, *106*(27), 11376–11381.

Hubbard, J., Gent, T. C., Hoekstra, M. M. B., Emmenegger, Y., Mongrain, V., Landolt, H. P., … Franken, P. (2020). Rapid fast-delta decay following prolonged wakefulness marks a phase of wake-inertia in NREM sleep. *Nat Commun*, *11*(1), 1–16. doi: 10.1038/s41467-020-16915-0

Huber, R., Deboer, T., & Tobler, I. (2000). Topography of EEG dynamics after sleep deprivation in mice. *J Neurophysiol*, *84*(4), 1888–1893.

Huber, R., Esser, S. K., Ferrarelli, F., Massimini, M., Peterson, M. J., & Tononi, G. (2007). TMS-induced cortical potentiation during wakefulness locally increases slow wave activity during sleep. *PLoS One*, *2*(3), e276. doi: 10.1371/journal.pone.0000276

Huber, R., Ghilardi, M. F., Massimini, M., Ferrarelli, F., Riedner, B. A., Peterson, M. J., & Tononi, G. (2006). Arm immobilization causes cortical plastic changes and locally decreases sleep slow wave activity. *Nat Neurosci*, *9*(9), 1169–1176. doi: 10.1038/nn1758

Huber, R., Tononi, G., & Cirelli, C. (2007). Exploratory behavior, cortical BDNF expression, and sleep homeostasis. *Sleep*, *30*(2), 129–139.

Hume, K. I., Brink, M., & Basner, M. (2012). Effects of environmental noise on sleep. *Noise Health*, *14*(61), 297–302. doi: 10.4103/1463-1741.104897

Hung, C. S., Sarasso, S., Ferrarelli, F., Riedner, B., Ghilardi, M. F., Cirelli, C., & Tononi, G. (2013). Local experience-dependent changes in the wake EEG after prolonged wakefulness. *Sleep*, *36*(1), 59–72. doi: 10.5665/sleep.2302

Issa, E. B., & Wang, X. (2011). Altered neural responses to sounds in primate primary auditory cortex during slow-wave sleep. *J Neurosci*, *31*(8), 2965–2973. doi: 10.1523/jneurosci.4920-10.2011

James, W. (1890). *The Principles of Psychology* (Vol. 1). London: Macmillan.

Jasper, H., Ajmone-Marsan, C., & Stoll, J. (1952). Corticofugal projections to the brain stem. *AMA Arch Neurol Psychiatry*, *67*(2), 155–171. doi: 10.1001/archneurpsyc.1952.02320140023003

Jones, B. E. (2020). Arousal and sleep circuits. *Neuropsychopharmacology*, *45*(1), 6–20. doi: 10.1038/s41386-019-0444-2

Jones, E. G. (2001). The thalamic matrix and thalamocortical synchrony. *Trends Neurosci*, *24*(10), 595–601.

Kattler, H., Dijk, D.-J., & Borbély, A. (1994). Effect of unilateral somatosensory stimulation prior to sleep on the sleep EEG in humans. *J Sleep Res*, *3*, 159–164.

Kaufmann, C. (2006). Brain activation and hypothalamic functional connectivity during human non-rapid eye movement sleep: an EEG/fMRI study. *Brain*, *129*(3), 655–667. doi: 10.1093/brain/awh686

Kim, A., Latchoumane, C., Lee, S., Kim, G., Cheong, E., Augustine, G., & Shin, H.-S. (2012). Optogenetically induced sleep spindle rhythms alter sleep architectures in mice. *Proc Natl Acad Sci USA*, *109*(50), 20673–30678.

Kouider, S., Andrillon, T., Barbosa, L. S., Goupil, L., & Bekinschtein, T. A. (2014). Inducing task-relevant responses to speech in the sleeping brain. *Curr Biol*, *24*(18), 2208–2214. doi: 10.1016/j.cub.2014.08.016

Krueger, J., Obál, F. J., Kapás, L., & Fang, J. (1995). Brain organization and sleep function. *Behav Brain Res*, *69*, 177–185.

Krueger, J. M., Rector, D. M., Roy, S., Van Dongen, H. P. A., Belenky, G., & Panksepp, J. (2008). Sleep as a fundamental property of neuronal assemblies. *Nat Rev Neurosci*, *9*(12), 910–919. doi: 10.1038/nrn2521

Langford, G., Meddis, R., & Pearson, A. (1974). Awakening latency from sleep for meaningful and non-meaningful stimuli. *Psychophysiology*, *11*(1), 1–5.

Latchoumane, C. V., Ngo, H. V., Born, J., & Shin, H. S. (2017). Thalamic spindles promote memory formation during sleep through triple phase-locking of cortical, thalamic, and hippocampal rhythms. *Neuron*, *95*(2), 424–435. doi: 10.1016/j.neuron.2017.06.025

Lavigne, G., Brousseau, M., Kato, T., Mayer, P., Manzini, C., Guitard, F., & Montplaisir, J. (2004). Experimental pain perception remains equally active over all sleep stages. *Pain*, *110*, 646–655. doi: 0.1016/j.pain.2004.05.003

Lechat, B., Hansen, K., Micic, G., Decup, F., Dunbar, C., Liebich, T., … Zajamsek, B. (2021). K-complexes are a sensitive marker of noise-related sensory processing during sleep: a pilot study. *Sleep*, *44*(9), zsab065. doi:10.1093/sleep/zsab065

Lemieux, M., Chen, J. Y., Lonjers, P., Bazhenov, M., & Timofeev, I. (2014). The impact of cortical deafferentation on the neocortical slow oscillation. *J Neurosci*, *34*(16), 5689–5703. doi: 10.1523/JNEUROSCI.1156-13.2014

Léna, I., Parrot, S., Deschaux, O., Muffat-Joly, S., Sauvinet, V., Renaud, B., … Gottesmann, C. (2005). Variations in extracellular levels of dopamine, noradrenaline, glutamate, and aspartate across the sleep--wake cycle in the medial prefrontal cortex and nucleus accumbens of freely moving rats. *J Neurosci Res*, *81*(6), 891–899. doi: 10.1002/jnr.20602

Leu-Semenescu, S., Uguccioni, G., Golmard, J. L., Czernecki, V., Yelnik, J., Dubois, B., … Arnulf, I. (2013). Can we still dream when the mind is blank? Sleep and dream mentations in auto-activation deficit. *Brain*, *136*(Pt 10), 3076–3084. doi: 10.1093/brain/awt229

Lewis, L. D., Voigts, J., Flores, F. J., Schmitt, L. I., Wilson, M. A., Halassa, M. M., & Brown, E. N. (2015). Thalamic reticular nucleus induces fast and local modulation of arousal state. *Elife*, *4*, e08760. doi: 10.7554/eLife.08760

Li, Q., Hill, Z., & He, B. J. (2014). Spatiotemporal dissociation of brain activity underlying subjective awareness, objective performance and confidence. *J Neurosci*, *34*(12), 4382–4395. doi: 10.1523/JNEUROSCI.1820-13.2014

Lim, A., Lozano, A., Moro, E., Hamani, C., Hutchison, W., Dostrovsky, J., … Murray, B. (2007). Characterization of REM-sleep associated ponto-geniculo-occipital waves in the human pons. *Sleep*, *30*(7), 823–827.

Lüthi, A. (2014). Sleep spindles: where they come from, what they do. *Neuroscientist*, *20*(3), 243–256. doi: 10.1177/1073858413500854

Magnin, M., Rey, M., Bastuji, H., Guillemant, P., Mauguiere, F., & Garcia-Larrea, L. (2010). Thalamic deactivation at sleep onset precedes that of the cerebral cortex in humans. *Proc Natl Acad Sci U S A*, *107*(8), 3829–3833. doi: 10.1073/pnas.0909710107

Mak-McCully, R. A., Rolland, M., Sargsyan, A., Gonzalez, C., Magnin, M., Chauvel, P., … Halgren, E. (2017). Coordination of cortical and thalamic activity during non-REM sleep in humans. *Nat Commun*, *8*, 15499. doi:10.1038/ncomms15499

Mak-McCully, R. A., Rosen, B. Q., Rolland, M., Regis, J., Bartolomei, F., Rey, M., … Halgren, E. (2015). Distribution, amplitude, incidence, co-occurrence, and propagation of human K-complexes in focal transcortical recordings. *eNeuro*, *2*(4). doi: 10.1523/ENEURO.0028-15.2015

Maquet, P., Degueldre, C., Delfiore, G., Aerts, J., Péters, J.-M., Luxen, A., & Franck, G. (1997). Functional neuroanatomy of human slow wave sleep. *J Neurosci*, *17*(8), 2807–2812.

Maquet, P., Péters, J.-M., Aerts, J., Delfiore, G., Degueldre, C., Luxen, A., & Franck, G. (1996). Functional neuroanatomy of human rapid-eye-movement sleep and dreaming. *Nature*, *383*, 163–166.

Massimini, M., Ferrarelli, F., Esser, S. K., Riedner, B. A., Huber, R., Murphy, M., … Tononi, G. (2007). Triggering sleep slow waves by transcranial magnetic stimulation. *Proc Natl Acad Sci USA*, *104*(20), 8496–8501. doi: 10.1073/pnas.0702495104

Massimini, M., Ferrarelli, F., Huber, R., Esser, S., Singh, H., & Tononi, G. (2005). Breakdown of cortical effective connectivity during sleep. *Science*, *309*, 2228–2232.

Massimini, M., Ferrarelli, F., Murphy, M. J., Huber, R., Riedner, B. A., Casarotto, S., & Tononi, G. (2010). Cortical reactivity and effective connectivity during REM sleep in humans. *Cogn Neurosci, 1*(3), 176–183. doi: 10.1080/17588921003731578

Massimini, M., Huber, R., Ferrarelli, F., Hill, S., & Tononi, G. (2004). The sleep slow oscillation as a traveling wave. *J Neurosci, 24*(31), 6862–6870. doi: 10.1523/JNEUROSCI.1318-04.2004

McCarley, R. W., Nelson, J. W., & Duffy, F. H. (1983). Human cerebral potentials associated with REM sleep rapid eye movements: links to PGO waves and waking potentials. *Brain Res, 274*, 359–364.

Melloni, L., Molina, C., Pena, M., Torres, D., Singer, W., & Rodriguez, E. (2007). Synchronization of neural activity across cortical areas correlates with conscious perception. *J Neurosci, 27*(11), 2858–2865. doi: 10.1523/JNEUROSCI.4623-06.2007

Melloni, L., Mudrik, L., Pitts, M., Bendtz, K., Ferrante, O., Gorska, U., ... Tononi, G. (2023). An adversarial collaboration protocol for testing contrasting predictions of global neuronal workspace and integrated information theory. *PLoS One, 18*(2), e0268577. doi: 10.1371/journal.pone.0268577

Mhuircheartaigh, R., Rosenorn-Lanng, D., Wise, R., Jbabdi, S., Rogers, R., & Tracey, I. (2010). Cortical and subcortical connectivity changes during decreasing levels of consciousness in humans: a functional magnetic resonance imaging study using propofol. *J Neurosci, 30*(27), 9095–9102. doi: 10.1523/jneurosci.5516-09.2010

Morgan, K. K., Hathaway, E., Carson, M., Fernandez-Corazza, M., Shusterman, R., Luu, P., & Tucker, D. M. (2021). Focal limbic sources create the large slow oscillations of the EEG in human deep sleep. *Sleep Med, 85*, 291–302. doi: 10.1016/j.sleep.2021.07.028

Murakami, H. (1994, 1995). *The Wind-Up Bird Chronicle* (J. Rubin, Trans.). New York: Vintage International, Random House.

Murphy, M., Riedner, B. A., Huber, R., Massimini, M., Ferrarelli, F., & Tononi, G. (2009). Source modeling sleep slow waves. *Proc Natl Acad Sci USA, 106*(5), 1608–1613. doi: 10.1073/pnas.0807933106

Muzur, A., Pace-Schott, E. F., & Hobson, J. A. (2002). The prefrontal cortex in sleep. *Trends Cogn Sci, 6*(11), 475–481.

Mylonas, D., Machado, S., Larson, O., Patel, R., Cox, R., Vangel, M., ... Manoach, D. S. (2022). Dyscoordination of non-rapid eye movement sleep oscillations in autism spectrum disorder. *Sleep, 45*(3), 1–15. doi: 10.1093/sleep/zsac010

Narikiyo, K., Mizuguchi, R., Ajima, A., Shiozaki, M., Hamanaka, H., Johansen, J. P., ... Yoshihara, Y. (2020). The claustrum coordinates cortical slow-wave activity. *Nat Neurosci, 23*(6), 741–753. doi: 10.1038/s41593-020-0625-7

Nelson, A. B., Ricci, S., Tatti, E., Panday, P., Girau, E., Lin, J., ... Ghilardi, M. F. (2021). Neural fatigue due to intensive learning is reversed by a nap but not by quiet waking. *Sleep, 44*(1), zsaa143. doi: 10.1093/sleep/zsaa143

Nelson, J. P., McCarley, R. W., & Hobson, J. A. (1983). REM sleep burst neurons, PGO waves, and eye movement information. *J Neurophysiol, 50*, 784–797.

Neske, G. T. (2016). The slow oscillation in cortical and thalamic networks: mechanisms and functions. *Front Neural Circuits, 9*(88), 1–25. doi: 10.3389/fncir.2015.00088

Nir, Y., Staba, R. J., Andrillon, T., Vyazovskiy, V. V., Cirelli, C., Fried, I., & Tononi, G. (2011). Regional slow waves and spindles in human sleep. *Neuron, 70*(1), 153–169. doi: 10.1016/j.neuron.2011.02.043

Nir, Y., Vyazovskiy, V. V., Cirelli, C., Banks, M. I., & Tononi, G. (2015). Auditory responses and stimulus-specific adaptation in rat auditory cortex are preserved across NREM and REM sleep. *Cereb Cortex, 25*(5), 1362–1378. doi: 10.1093/cercor/bht328

Nofzinger, E., Buysse, D., Miewald, J. M., Meltzer, C., Price, J., Sembrat, R., ... Moore, R. (2002). Human regional cerebral glucose metabolism during non-rapid eye movement sleep in relation to waking. *Brain, 125*, 1105–1115.

Oleksenko, A., Mukhametov, L., Polyakova, I., Supin, A., & Kovalzon, V. (1992). Unihemispheric sleep deprivation in bottlenose dolphins. *J Sleep Res, 1*, 40–44.

Oswald, I., Taylor, A. M., & Treisman, M. (1960). Discriminative responses to stimulation during human sleep. *Brain, 83*, 440–453.

Parent, A., & Steriade, M. (1984). Midbrain tegmental projections of nucleus reticularis thalami of cat and monkey: a retrograde transport and antidromic invasion study. *J Comp Neurol, 229*(4), 548–558.

Pérez-Garci, E., del-Rio-Portilla, Y., Guevara, M., Arce, C., & Corsi-Cabrera, M. (2001). Paradoxical sleep is characterized by uncoupled gamma activity between frontal and perceptual cortical regions. *Sleep, 24*(1), 118–126.

Perrin, F., García-Larrea, L., Mauguière, F., & Bastuji, H. (1999). A differential brain response to the subject's own name persists during sleep. *Clin Neurophysiol, 110*, 2153–2164.

Peter-Derex, L., Comte, J.-C., Mauguière, F., & Salin, P. (2012). Density and frequency caudo-rostral gradients of sleep spindles recorded in the human cortex. *Sleep, 35*(1), 69–79. doi: 0.5665/sleep.1588

Picchioni, D., Pixa, M. L., Fukunaga, M., Carr, W. S., Horovitz, S. G., Braun, A. R., & Duyn, J. H. (2014). Decreased connectivity between the thalamus and the neocortex during human nonrapid eye movement sleep. *Sleep, 37*(2), 387–397. doi: 10.5665/sleep.3422

Pinault, D., & Deschênes, M. (1992). Voltage-dependent 40-Hz oscillations in rat reticular thalamic neurons in vivo. *Neuroscience, 51*(2), 245–258.

Poitras, A., Thorkildsen, A., Gagnon, M., & Naiman, J. (1973). Auditory stimulation during REM and non-REM sleep in women before and after delivery. *Can Psychiatr Assoc J, 18*(6), 519–526.

Portas, C., Krakow, K., Allen, P., Josephs, O., Armony, J. L., & Frith, C. (2000). Auditory processing across the sleep-wake cycle: simultaneous EEG and fMRI monitoring in humans. *Neuron, 28*, 991–999.

Pratt, H., Berlad, I., & Lavie, P. (1999). "Oddball" event-related potentials and information processing during REM and non-REM sleep. *Clin Neurophysiol, 110*, 53–61.

Price, L. J., & Kremen, I. (1980). Variations in behavioral response threshold within the REM period of human sleep. *Psychophysiology, 17*, 133–140.

Raccah, O., Block, N., & Fox, K. C. R. (2021). Does the prefrontal cortex play an essential role in consciousness? Insights from intracranial electrical stimulation of the human brain. *J Neurosci, 41*(10), 2076–2087. doi: 10.1523/JNEUROSCI.1141-20.2020

Rector, D. M., Schei, J. L., Van Dongen, H. P. A., Belenky, G., & Krueger, J. M. (2009). Physiological markers of local sleep. *Eur J Neurosci, 29*(9), 1771–1778. doi: 10.1111/j.1460-9568.2009.06717.x

Ricci, S., Tatti, E., Nelson, A. B., Panday, P., Chen, H., Tononi, G., ... Ghilardi, M. F. (2021). Extended visual sequence learning leaves a local trace in the spontaneous EEG. *Front Neurosci, 15*, 1–10. doi:10.3389/fnins.2021.707828

Rodriguez, A. V., Funk, C. M., Vyazovskiy, V. V., Nir, Y., Tononi, G., & Cirelli, C. (2016). Why does sleep slow-wave activity increase after extended wake? Assessing the effects of increased cortical firing during wake and sleep. *J Neurosci, 36*(49), 12436–12447. doi: 10.1523/JNEUROSCI.1614-16.2016

Rosanova, M., Fecchio, M., Casarotto, S., Sarasso, S., Casali, A. G., Pigorini, A., ... Massimini, M. (2018). Sleep-like cortical OFF-periods disrupt causality and complexity in the brain of unresponsive wakefulness syndrome patients. *Nat Commun, 9*(1), 4427. doi: 10.1038/s41467-018-06871-1

Roth, C., Achermann, P., & Borbély, A. (1999). Frequency and state specific hemispheric asymmetries in the human sleep EEG. *Neurosci Lett, 271*, 139–142.

Sakai, K., & Cespuglio, R. (1974). Evidence for the presence of eye movement potentials during paradoxical sleep in cats. *Electroencephalogr Clin Neurophysiol, 41*, 37–48.

Saletu, B., Frey, R., & Grünberger, J. (1989). [Street noise and sleep: whole-night somnopolygraphic, psychometric and psychophysiological studies in comparison with normal data]. *Wien Med Wochenschr, 139*(11), 257–263.

Sallinen, M., Kaartinen, J., & Lyytinen, H. (1996). Processing of auditory stimuli during tonic and phasic periods of REM sleep as revealed by event-related brain potentials. *J Sleep Res, 5*(4), 220–228. doi: 10.1111/j.1365-2869.1996.00220.x

Sämann, P. G., Wehrle, R., Hoehn, D., Spoormaker, V. I., Peters, H., Tully, C., ... Czisch, M. (2011). Development of the brain's default mode network from wakefulness to slow wave sleep. *Cereb Cortex, 21*(9), 2082–2093. doi: 10.1093/cercor/bhq295

Schabus, M., Dang-Vu, T. T., Heib, D. P. J., Boly, M., Desseilles, M., Vandewalle, G., ... Maquet, P. (2012). The fate of incoming stimuli during NREM sleep is determined by spindles and the phase of the slow oscillation. *Front Neurol, 3*(40). doi: 10.3389/fneur.2012.00040

Schiff, N. D. (2008). Central thalamic contributions to arousal regulation and neurological disorders of consciousness. *Ann NY Acad Sci, 1129*(1), 105–118. doi: 10.1196/annals.1417.029

Schwierin, B., Achermann, P., Deboer, T., Oleksenko, A., Borbély, A., & Tobler, I. (1999). Regional differences in the dynamics of the cortical EEG in the rat after sleep deprivation. *Clin Neurophysiol, 110*, 869–875.

Segundo, J. P., Naquet, R., & Buser, P. (1955). Effects of cortical stimulation on electrocortical activity in monkeys. *J Neurophysiol, 18*(3), 236–245. doi: 10.1152/jn.1955.18.3.236

Sela, Y., Krom, A. J., Bergman, L., Regev, N., & Nir, Y. (2020). Sleep differentially affects early and late neuronal responses to sounds in auditory and perirhinal cortices. *J Neurosci, 40*(14), 2895–2905. doi: 10.1523/JNEUROSCI.1186-19.2020

Sela, Y., Vyazovskiy, V. V., Cirelli, C., Tononi, G., & Nir, Y. (2016). Responses in rat core auditory cortex are preserved during sleep spindle oscillations. *Sleep, 39*(5), 1069–1082. doi: 10.5665/sleep.5758

Sesack, S., Deutch, A. Y., Roth, R., & Bunney, B. (1989). Topographical organization of the efferent projections of the medial prefrontal cortex in the rat:

an anterograde tract-tracing study with *Phaseolus vulgaris* leucoagglutinin. *J Comp Neurol, 290*, 213–242.

Siegel, J., & Langley, T. D. (1965). Arousal threshold in the cat as a function of sleep phase and stimulus significance. *Experientia, 21*, 740–741.

Simor, P., Steinbach, E., Nagy, T., Gilson, M., Farthouat, J., Schmitz, R., … Peigneux, P. (2018). Lateralized rhythmic acoustic stimulation during daytime NREM sleep enhances slow waves. *Sleep, 41*(12), zsy176. doi: 10.1093/sleep/zsy176

Simor, P., Szalardy, O., Gombos, F., Ujma, P. P., Jordan, Z., Halasz, L., … Bodizs, R. (2021). REM sleep microstates in the human anterior thalamus. *J Neurosci, 41*(26), 5677–5686. doi: 10.1523/JNEUROSCI.1899-20.2021

Singer, W. (1993). Synchronization of cortical activity and its putative role in information processing and learning. *Annu Rev Physiol, 55*, 349–374.

Snyder, F. (1966). Toward an evolutionary theory of dreaming. *Am J Psychiatry, 123*(2), 121–136.

Spoormaker, V. I., Schroter, M. S., Gleiser, P. M., Andrade, K. C., Dresler, M., Wehrle, R., … Czisch, M. (2010). Development of a large-scale functional brain network during human non-rapid eye movement sleep. *J Neurosci, 30*(34), 11379–11387. doi: 10.1523/JNEUROSCI.2015-10.2010

Steriade, M. (1994). Sleep oscillations and their blockage by activating systems. *J Psychiatr Neurosci, 19*(5), 354–358.

Steriade, M. (2000). Corticothalamic resonance, states of vigilance and mentation. *Neuroscience, 101*(2), 243–276.

Steriade, M., Amzica, F., & Contreras, D. (1996). Synchronization of fast (30–40 Hz) spontaneous cortical rhythms during brain activation. *J Neurosci, 16*, 392–417.

Steriade, M., Amzica, F., & Nuñez, A. (1993). Cholinergic and noradrenergic modulation of the slow (~0.3 Hz) oscillation in neocortical cells. *J Neurophysiol, 70*(4), 1385–1400.

Steriade, M., Curró Dossi, R., & Contreras, D. (1993). Electrophysiological properties of intralaminar thalamocortical cells discharging rhythmic (~40 Hz) spike-bursts at ~1000 Hz during waking and rapid eye movement sleep. *Neuroscience, 56*(1), 1–9.

Steriade, M., Nuñez, A., & Amzica, F. (1993a). Intracellular analysis of relations between the slow (<1 Hz) neocortical oscillation and other sleep rhythms of the electroencephalogram. *J Neurosci, 13*(8), 3266–3283.

Steriade, M., Nuñez, A., & Amzica, F. (1993b). A novel slow (<1 Hz) oscillation of neocortical neurons in vivo: depolarizing and hyperpolarizing components. *J Neurosci, 13*(8), 3252–3265.

Steriade, M., Sakai, K., & Jouvet, M. (1984). Bulbo-thalamic neurons related to thalamocortical activation processes during paradoxical sleep. *Exp Brain Res, 54*, 463–475.

Steriade, M., Timofeev, I., & Grenier, F. (2001). Natural waking and sleep states: a view from inside neocortical neurons. *J Neurophysiol, 85*, 1969–1985.

Tagliazucchi, E., von Wegner, F., Morzelewski, A., Brodbeck, V., Jahnke, K., & Laufs, H. (2013). Breakdown of long-range temporal dependence in default mode and attention networks during deep sleep. *Proc Natl Acad Sci U S A, 110*(38), 15419–15424. doi: 10.1073/pnas.1312848110

Tamaki, M., Bang, J. W., Watanabe, T., & Sasaki, Y. (2016). Night watch in one brain hemisphere during sleep associated with the first-night effect in humans. *Curr Biol, 26*(9), 1190–1194. doi: 10.1016/j.cub.2016.02.063

Tamaki, M., & Sasaki, Y. (2019). Surveillance during REM sleep for the first-night effect. *Front Neurosci, 13*. doi: 10.3389/fnins.2019.01161

Tassi, P., & Muzet, A. (2000). Sleep inertia. *Sleep Med Rev, 4*(4), 341–353. doi: 10.1053/smrv.2000.0098

Thankachan, S., Katsuki, F., McKenna, J. T., Yang, C., Shukla, C., Deisseroth, K., Uygun, D. S., Strecker, R. E., … Basheer, R. (2019). Thalamic reticular nucleus parvalbumin neurons regulate sleep spindles and electrophysiological aspects of schizophrenia in mice. *Sci Rep, 9*(1), 3607. doi: 10.1038/s41598-019-40398-9

Tononi, G. (2004). An information integration theory of consciousness. *BMC Neurosci, 5*, 42. doi: 10.1186/1471-2202-5-42

Tononi, G., & Cirelli, C. (2006). Sleep function and synaptic homeostasis. *Sleep Med Rev, 10*(1), 49–62. doi: 10.1016/j.smrv.2005.05.002

Türker, B., Musat, E. M., Chabani, E., Fonteix-Galet, A., Maranci, J. B., Wattiez, N., … Oudiette, D. (2023). Behavioral and brain responses to verbal stimuli reveal transient periods of cognitive integration of the external world during sleep. *Nat Neurosci, 26*(11), 1981–1993. doi:10.1038/s41593-023-01449-7

Uchida, S., Atsumi, Y., & Kojima, T. (1994). Dynamic relationships between sleep spindles and delta waves during a NREM period. *Brain Res Bull, 33*, 351–355.

Ushimaru, M., Ueta, Y., & Kawaguchi, Y. (2012). Differentiated participation of thalamocortical subnetworks in slow/spindle saves and desynchronization. *J Neurosci, 32*(5), 1730–1746. doi: 10.1523/jneurosci.4883-11.2012

Van der Werf, Y., Witter, M., & Groenewegen, H. (2002). The intralaminar and midline nuclei of the thalamus. Anatomical and functional evidence for participation in processes of arousal and awareness. *Brain Res Rev, 39*, 107–140.

Van Twyver, H., & Garrett, W. (1972). Arousal threshold in the rat determined by "meaningful" stimuli. *Behav Biol, 7*, 205–215.

Vanini, G., Lydic, R., & Baghdoyan, H. A. (2012). GABA-to-ACh ratio in basal forebrain and cerebral cortex varies significantly during sleep. *Sleep, 35*(10), 1325–1334. doi: 10.5665/sleep.2106

Vertes, R. P., Linley, S. B., & Rojas, A. K. P. (2022). Structural and functional organization of the midline and intralaminar nuclei of the thalamus. *Front Behav Neurosci, 16*, 964644. doi:10.3389/fnbeh.2022.964644

Viena, T. D., Vertes, R. P., & Linley, S. B. (2021). Discharge characteristics of neurons of nucleus reuniens across sleep-wake states in the behaving rat. *Behav Brain Res, 410*, 113325. doi:10.1016/j.bbr.2021.113325

Vyazovskiy, V., Borbély, A., & Tobler, I. (2002). Interhemispheric sleep EEG asymmetry in the rat is enhanced by sleep deprivation. *J Neurophysiol, 88*, 2280–2286. doi: 10.1152/jn.00304.2002

Vyazovskiy, V., Borbély, A. A., & Tobler, I. (2000). Unilateral vibrissae stimulation during waking induces interhemispheric EEG asymmetry during subsequent sleep in the rat. *J Sleep Res, 9*, 367–371.

Vyazovskiy, V. V., Olcese, U., Hanlon, E. C., Nir, Y., Cirelli, C., & Tononi, G. (2011). Local sleep in awake rats. *Nature, 472*(7344), 443–447. doi: 10.1038/nature10009

Vyazovskiy, V. V., & Tobler, I. (2005). Theta activity in the waking EEG is a marker of sleep propensity in the rat. *Brain Res, 1050*, 64–71. doi: 0.1016/j.brainres.2005.05.022

Wanger, T., Takagaki, K., Lippert, M. T., Goldschmidt, J., & Ohl, F. W. (2013). Wave propagation of cortical population activity under urethane anesthesia is state dependent. *BMC Neurosci, 14*, 78. doi: 10.1186/1471-2202-14-78

Wehrle, R., Kaufmann, C., Wetter, T. C., Holsboer, F., Auer, D. P., Pollmacher, T., & Czisch, M. (2007). Functional microstates within human REM sleep: first evidence from fMRI of a thalamocortical network specific for phasic REM periods. *Eur J Neurosci, 25*(3), 863–871. doi: 10.1111/j.1460-9568.2007.05314.x

Wells, M. F., Wimmer, R. D., Schmitt, L. I., Feng, G., & Halassa, M. M. (2016). Thalamic reticular impairment underlies attention deficit in Ptchd1(Y/-) mice. *Nature, 532*(7597), 58–63. doi: 10.1038/nature17427

Werth, E., Achermann, P., & Borbély, A. (1997). Fronto-occipital power gradients in human sleep. *J Sleep Res, 6*, 102–112.

Whitten, T. A., Martz, L. J., Guico, A., Gervais, N., & Dickson, C. T. (2009). Heat synch: inter- and independence of body-temperature fluctuations and brain-state alternations in urethane-anesthetized rats. *J Neurophysiol, 102*(3), 1647–1656. doi: 10.1152/jn.00374.2009

Williams, H. L., Hammack, J. T., Daly, R. L., Dement, W. C., & Lubin, A. (1964). Responses to auditory stimulation, sleep loss and the EEG stages of sleep. *Electroencephalogr Clin Neurophysiol, 16*, 269–279.

Wimmer, R. D., Schmitt, L. I., Davidson, T. J., Nakajima, M., Deisseroth, K., & Halassa, M. M. (2015). Thalamic control of sensory selection in divided attention. *Nature, 526*(7575), 705–709. doi: 10.1038/nature15398

Yu, X.-J., Xu, X.-X., He, S., & He, J. (2009). Change detection by thalamic reticular neurons. *Nat Neurosci, 12*(9), 1165–1170. doi: 10.1038/nn.2373

Zung, W., & Wilson, W. (1961). Response to auditory stimulation during sleep. *Arch Gen Psychiatr, 4*, 548–552.

D.

Impacts of Sleep Duration & Quality

CHAPTER 13

Behavioral Effects of Inadequate Sleep and Shift Work

13.1 OVERVIEW

Laboratory studies of how sleep restriction affects human performance and other aspects of behavior have been conducted for well over a century. There has also been research on how cognition, behavior, and health are affected by extended work durations, night shift work, and jet lag. These topics are of special interest because of the importance of adequate performance by people who work in protection services (military and civilian), health care, transportation, and other industries in which people are often required to work during the night or for extended lengths of time (adverse work schedules).

This chapter reviews how inadequate sleep, shift work, and jet lag affect cognition, performance, and emotional regulation and how individuals differ in their responses to these conditions. It discusses potential mechanisms underlying these effects, including the roles of sleep loss and of circadian factors in influencing job performance on adverse schedules. It also reviews a range of health risks that have been linked to long-term work on adverse schedules and the mechanisms that may be involved. Finally, it discusses why the problems associated with shift work are difficult to address.

13.2 How much sleep do you need?

13.2.1 Defining sleep need

In 2016, the Rand Corporation issued a report on the economic costs of inadequate sleep in five countries (United States, Japan, Germany, United Kingdom, and Canada). The estimated annual cost to these economies totaled over US$680 billion or about 2% of their combined gross domestic products (RAND, 2016). Extrapolated across the world and updated, the cost would easily amount to more than $1 trillion annually. Some of these costs reflect increased rates of illness and early mortality (see Chapters 14 and 15). Other costs were related to lost work productivity resulting from both impaired work performance and worker absenteeism. The focus of this section is on the cognitive, behavioral, and emotional consequences of insufficient sleep that contribute to these consequences.

The first published study of the effects of sleep loss on human cognition and performance involved 90 h of continuous waking (Patrick & Gilbert, 1896) (see Section 5.2). This report described deterioration of performance in three young men on several informal tests of letter reading, arithmetic, and memory during their extended time awake. Complete overnight (or longer) sleep deprivation in later laboratory studies has been a valuable tool for learning about the behavioral and physiological consequences of sleep loss and for helping to identify some functions of sleep. But few people undergo such extended deprivation on a regular basis. The more common phenomenon that accounts for most of the societal costs of sleep loss is chronic sleep restriction (i.e., sleeping less than is physiologically required over days, weeks, or longer).

This definition begs the question of whether there *is* a physiologically required duration of sleep. In clinical settings, the typical definition of "required sleep" is the amount of sleep a person needs to wake up feeling alert and refreshed, and to function well and without excessive sleepiness throughout the day. These criteria are partly subjective ("feeling alert and refreshed") and partly related to objective performance ("and function well"). This approach has the advantage of allowing somewhat different lengths of sleep to be considered normal and adequate for different individuals. It is likely that people vary in their sleep requirements, as they do in most physiological and behavioral parameters.

The clinical criteria for adequate sleep, however, do not provide a numerical answer to a question frequently asked of sleep clinicians and researchers. How many hours of sleep do I (or my children) need? An initiative was launched that brought together experts on this topic who surveyed the available literature and tried to develop "the best, most reasoned answer possible" to the question of how much sleep is sufficient to maintain optimal health (Watson et al., 2015). The answers they reached depended on the specific endpoints used (effects on general health, weight regulation, immune system function, mortality risk, etc.; see Chapters 14 and 15), but fell generally in the 7–9 h range for adults. The report also identified many gaps in our knowledge that made its conclusions tentative.

These suggested amounts can be contrasted to the results of a survey in which older American adults (55–84 years) reported sleeping an average of 7 h nightly on weeknights, and younger adults (18–54 years) only 6.7 h. Both groups reported sleeping somewhat longer on weekends. Since these are averages, many people reported sleeping less than the proposed 7 h minimum for adults: 34% in the older group and 41% in the younger group, while 6–7% reported sleeping more than 9 h (National Sleep Foundation, 2003). In a more recent (2017) representative national survey, 32.9% of American adults reported sleeping 6 h or less nightly, an increase from 27% a decade earlier (Sheehan et al., 2019).

The existence of large individual differences in reported sleep amounts raises the question of whether different people need more or less sleep, or whether they get different amounts, regardless of need. One analysis of studies correlating sleep length with metabolic and other health risks concluded that the physiological core sleep requirement for people is about 6 h nightly, and that sleep beyond this duration is optional and not physiologically necessary. Sleeping longer than 6 h was considered a product of acquired habits, or a pleasurable indulgence. This review noted that most of the negative effects attributed through survey results to sleeping "less than 7 h" were in fact driven by those sleeping ≤5 h (Horne, 2011). Evidence related to this hypothesis is discussed in Section 13.2.2, but this analysis makes the important point that how sleep duration categories are reported in different studies can influence the conclusions reached.

13.2.2 Experimental studies of sleep need

Studies have used methods other than surveys to assess whether people get the sleep they need. One approach is based on evidence that power in the EEG theta frequency band while awake is a marker of sleep need. Theta-band activity increases progressively during extended waking in both people and rats (Cajochen et al., 1995; Vyazovskiy & Tobler, 2005). In addition, the rate of increase in theta activity during waking predicts the later increase in delta-band activity (a measure of sleep intensity) during recovery sleep (Finelli et al., 2000). Theta-band activity while awake and delta-band activity during NREM sleep therefore reflect both the length of time awake and the resulting accumulated sleep debt (see discussion in Chapter 5).

A study of people who spontaneously slept <6 h nightly showed that they had more power in the theta and adjacent low-frequency alpha bands (5.25–9 Hz) during waking than those who habitually slept >9 h nightly. By this measure, habitual short sleepers carried a larger current sleep debt than long sleepers (Aeschbach et al., 2001). This study, however, did not address whether those sleeping <6 h differed from those sleeping the generally recommended 7–9 h. Another study did compare EEG patterns during 15 min of quiet rest of natural short sleepers (<6.5 h nightly) to those sleeping 7–9 h, as verified by 14 days of actigraphy and sleep diaries. It found evidence of increased drowsiness and microsleeps in the short sleepers, despite the fact that they also reported lower sleepiness ratings than the controls who slept the recommended durations (Curtis et al., 2024).

Another tool that has been used to assess whether people get as much sleep as they need is the Multiple Sleep Latency Test (MSLT; see Section 2.7 for a description of this method) (Carskadon et al., 1986; Roehrs & Roth, 1992). Results of MSLT studies are valuable because a variety of approaches have shown that shorter sleep onset latencies (SOLs) during these tests reflect increased cumulative sleep need. For example, participants were allowed different lengths of time in bed (TIB) (0–10 h) for a single night. The shorter the TIB, the shorter the SOLs during MSLT nap opportunities the next day, reflecting a stronger sleep drive (Carskadon & Dement, 1987). Similarly, when participants were allowed 5 h TIB nightly for 1–7 nights, those sleep-restricted for more nights had shorter SOLs during nap tests, implying greater cumulative sleep need (**Figure 13.1 A**) (Carskadon & Dement, 1981).

The results of studies using sleep extension also support the interpretation that shorter SOLs reflect increased sleep need. People who averaged ~7.3 h sleep when they had 8 h TIB increased sleep lengths to 8.5 h when allowed 10 h TIB, and also lengthened their SOLs during later nap tests (**Figure 13.1 B**), indicating that their baseline sleep amounts did not fully satisfy their sleep needs (Carskadon & Dement, 1982). Similarly, healthy participants with no sleep complaints (averaging ~7 h sleep nightly) were divided into those who were physiologically "sleepy" (defined as showing ≤6 min SOLs during daytime MSLTs) and those who were especially "alert" (≥16 min SOLs). When TIB was extended from 8 to 10 h for 6 nights, "sleepy" participants with short SOLs at baseline lengthened SOLs during daytime naps throughout the 6 nights of sleep extension. Those with long SOLs at baseline showed only a small increase in SOLs, and that appeared only after the last (6th) night of 10 h TIB (Roehrs et al., 1989).

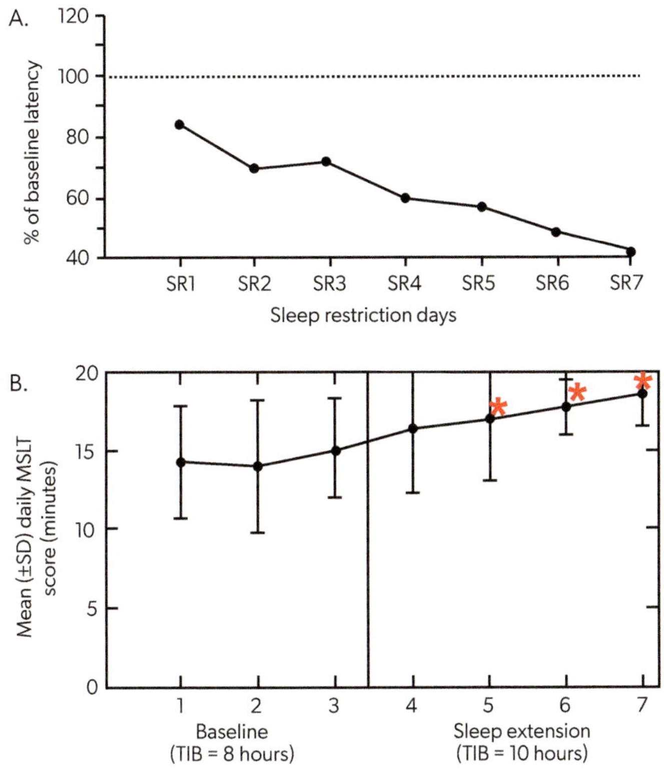

Figure 13.1 **A.** Average latency for participants to fall asleep during daytime Multiple Sleep Latency Tests (MSLTs) over 7 days (SR1–7) of sleep that was restricted to 5 h time in bed (TIB). Latencies are expressed as a percentage of the average baseline latency (=100%) on the last 3 days of 10 h TIB before sleep restriction began. There is a nearly linear decrease in sleep onset latency (SOL) with increasing number of days of sleep restriction. Reprinted with permission of John Wiley and Sons from Carskadon M.A. & Dement W.C. (1981) Cumulative effects of sleep restriction on daytime sleepiness. *Psychophysiology* 18:107–113. Journal Compilation © The Society for Psychophysiological Research, Inc. and John Wiley and Sons (1981). Permission conveyed through Copyright Clearance Center, Inc. doi: 10.1111/j.1469-8986.1981.tb02921.x. **B.** During baseline with 8 h TIB over 3 nights (left side), participants showed stable average SOLs during MSLTs. Latencies increased progressively during MSLTs when participants were given 10 h TIB for 4 nights (right side) (*= statistically significant increase), reflecting a reduction in daytime sleepiness. Average sleep durations increased from ~7.3 to 8.5 h nightly when TIB increased from 8 to 10 h. Adapted with permission of Oxford University Press from Carskadon, M.A. & Dement, W.C. (1982) Nocturnal determinants of daytime sleepiness. *Sleep* 5(Suppl.2):S73–S81. © Sleep Research Society (1982). doi: 10.1093/sleep/5.s2.s73.

A different sleep extension paradigm involved participants (18–32 years old) with habitual TIB of 6–10 h who were given 12 h TIB opportunities at night plus 4 h TIB during the day over 3 days. Self-reported spontaneous short sleepers (also confirmed by actigraphy) had very short SOLs during MSLTs at baseline (indicating high sleep drive), compared to long sleepers. They also dramatically lengthened their sleep durations during the extended sleep opportunities. Even after 3 days with greatly extended TIB, habitual short sleepers still slept for longer than habitual long sleepers. Participants also reported feeling more alert and less sleepy during the extension period (Klerman & Dijk, 2005).

The most informative result was the finding of a negative correlation showing that those with the shortest habitual sleep durations expressed the longest sleep durations when given extended sleep opportunities, especially clearly on the third extension night. These rebound increases in sleep duration reinforce the evidence from their short baseline SOLs that those with short spontaneous sleep durations were not satisfying their sleep needs (Klerman & Dijk, 2005).

An alternative interpretation is that sleep extension protocols demonstrate participants' capacity to generate "excess" sleep, not their need for sleep, which is already satisfied by their baseline sleep duration of at least 6 h (Horne, 2011). It is unclear, however, how this interpretation can account for those with the shortest baseline sleep durations (~6 h) showing the largest increases in sleep duration. If participants with the shortest sleep durations already met their sleep needs, why would additional TIB produce the largest increases in sleep durations? The straightforward interpretation of a correlation between shorter baseline sleep and longer durations during extended sleep opportunities is that many habitual short sleepers do not satisfy their physiological sleep needs.

Another approach to determining sleep need is to ask whether different habitual sleep lengths are linked to differences in daytime functioning. In a population-based study, cognitive performance was assessed in ~3,700 high school and college students. They were classified based on self-report as being short, intermediate, or long sleepers (averaging 5.8, 7.7, and 9.7 h, respectively). Short sleepers performed significantly worse than one or both other groups in three of four cognitive domains tested: verbal memory, visual memory, and reaction time. Short sleepers also reported more somatic, cognitive, and emotional complaints than those in the other groups (McClure et al., 2014). As with other correlational studies, however, these results do not establish the direction of causality.

A 2009 US survey (CDC, 2011) asked whether habitual sleep duration is related to daytime sleepiness. Adult participants reported on their experiences of falling asleep unintentionally during the day and while driving. Those reporting <7 h sleep daily (>35% of those surveyed) were much more likely than those sleeping ≥7 h to report unintentional sleep onsets,[1] implying a higher level of unmet sleep need (**Figure 13.2**). These results support the conclusion that spontaneous, chronic

[1] The risk of falling asleep while driving was smallest for those >65 years old (2.0%) and greatest for those 25–34 years old (7.2%) (CDC, 2011). These results are probably related to younger people being more likely than older people to be driving late at night as well as the fact that they experience stronger circadian pressure to sleep at night (see Section 8.5).

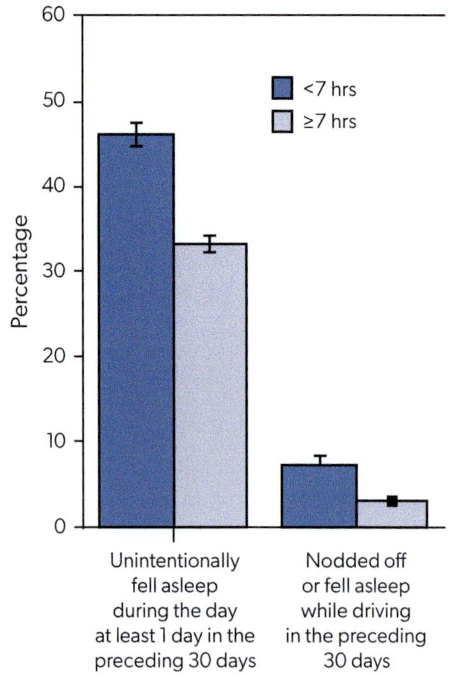

Figure 13.2 Results of a 2009 survey of respondents in 12 American states showing the probability of unintentionally falling asleep during the day at least once during the preceding 30 days (left columns) and falling asleep while driving (right columns). The columns represent those reporting average 24 h sleep totals of <7 h (dark blue) or ≥7 h (light blue). The error bars shown are 95% confidence intervals, so the differences between those sleeping <7 h and at least 7 h nightly are highly statistically significant. Adapted from Centers for Disease Control and Prevention (2011) Unhealthy sleep behaviors—12 states, 2009. Morbidity and Mortality Weekly Report 60:8, p.233-238, March 4, 2011 (https://stacks.cdc.gov/view/cdc/29020).

short sleep (<7 h) is not benign but is associated with daytime functional deficits that result from unmet sleep needs.

Over a third of Americans responding to this survey reported sleeping <7 h nightly, but this value conceals large geographic differences. In the results of a 2010 US census, the proportion of people reporting <7 h sleep varied in different regions from the lowest quintile (24.9–32.5%) to the highest quintile (38.5–47.3) of respondents (CDC, 2014) (**Figure 13.3**). This diversity suggests that environmental, demographic, economic, and other factors, beyond individual differences, play important roles in determining habitual sleep lengths.

13.2.3 Summary

There is no simple way of determining how much sleep people need; the answer depends on the outcome measures used and the way sleep durations are categorized. Surveys of how much sleep people currently get can establish a population average but cannot determine whether that amount of sleep is adequate or not. What surveys do demonstrate is that people vary a great deal in how much sleep they get. Based on the sleep durations that are associated with reduced risks for a variety of illnesses, the recommended durations for adults are in the 7–9 h range, with longer durations recommended for adolescents and children; see Box 4,1, Section 4.3. Many people regularly do not get these recommended amounts.

One measure that is sensitive to the length of sleep and the cumulative effect of restricting sleep is the latency to fall asleep (SOL) during the day, assessed using the MSLT (or the related Maintenance of Wakefulness Test). Results obtained from these tests and from studies of the resting EEG of short sleepers indicate that most people who are regular short sleepers are objectively sleepier than habitual average or long sleepers. Sleep extension studies also demonstrated that SOLs among short sleepers lengthen when they are allowed more time in bed. Critically, the largest increases were shown by those who were the shortest spontaneous sleepers at baseline.

Other evidence shows that habitual short sleep is associated with daytime functional deficits, including worse cognitive performance and increased likelihood of falling asleep unintentionally during the day or while driving. Whatever measure is used, individuals will vary in how much sleep they need to function optimally. But these lines of evidence converge on the conclusion that most adults need 7–9 h sleep nightly. Survey studies show large geographic differences within the United States in the proportion of adults getting adequate sleep, suggesting that cultural, environmental, economic, and other factors, in addition to personal choice, probably contribute to getting inadequate sleep amounts.

13.3 Sleep loss and sustained attention

Since many people occasionally or habitually do not get the recommended sleep amounts, it is important to understand the cognitive consequences of inadequate sleep. Experimental sleep restriction has been studied in relation to cognitive tasks ranging from simple reaction-time tasks to those involving language, decision making, or complex problem solving. The following sections review the impacts of short sleep on aspects of cognition that have been studied extensively, including vigilance, executive functions, and emotional regulation. Since shift work typically results in inadequate and shortened sleep for most workers, a final section discusses the impact of shift work on human performance and health.

13.3.1 The Psychomotor Vigilance Test

The Psychomotor Vigilance Test (PVT) and similar tasks (e.g., the Conners Continuous Performance Test) are reaction-time

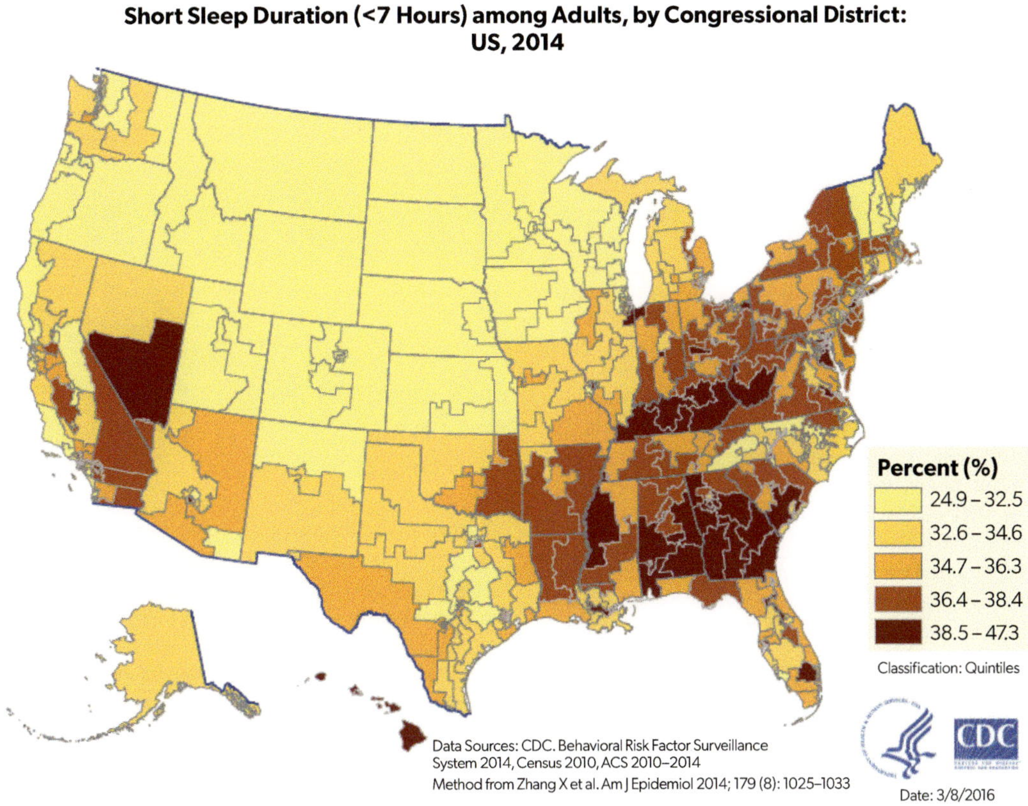

Figure 13.3 Distribution of short sleep (averaging <7 h in a 24 h period) in the American population plotted by congressional district, based on a 2010 census. There were large regional differences in reports of short sleep and the percent of the population reporting short sleep in some regions was as high as 38.5–47.3%. Retrieved December 12, 2022, from http://www.sleepresearchsociety.org/PDFs/SAE_CD113_2014_Sleep.pdf

tests that have been used frequently to assess the ability to sustain attention after sleep loss. The PVT requires participants to respond quickly (usually within 500 ms) with a button/key press to the appearance of a signal that occurs at irregular intervals, varying between 2–10 s. Among the outcome measures used are changes in the number of correct responses (hits), which are defined as occurring within 500 ms of the stimulus; response latencies of hits (i.e., average duration from stimulus onset to a successful hit); fastest (or slowest) e.g., 10% of hits; the number of misses (not responding, or taking longer than 500 ms to respond), reflecting lapses in attention performance; and premature responses (those occurring before the stimulus appears).

The PVT has several advantages as a tool for laboratory (and field) studies of vigilance. It is brief (most versions run for 5 or 10 min), easy to administer, and readily implemented on a smart phone, tablet, or computer. It requires essentially no learning after initial training, so it can be used repeatedly without concerns about accounting for learning-related improvements. It generates very reliable results on repeated testing in individuals and is also clearly and systematically sensitive to increasing sleep loss that is produced in different ways (Basner et al., 2018; Belenky et al., 2003; Lim & Dinges, 2008; Smith et al., 2021; Van Dongen et al., 2005).

A version of the PVT designed to be used with rats has also been developed. The performance of rats during sleep loss did not replicate all aspects of human results in parallel studies (e.g., performance recovered over days of sleep restriction, rather than progressively worsening as in most studies of people). But this model allowed for invasive studies of some of the neural correlates of changes in PVT performance (Christie, McKenna, et al., 2008; Deurveilher et al., 2015; Lim & Dinges, 2010; Oonk et al., 2015).

The PVT is clearly different from the more cognitively demanding tasks to which one would like to generalize, including those tasks that people regularly perform after inadequate sleep. However, by measuring the ability to maintain attention, the PVT taps into a basic requirement for many of the complicated, real-world jobs that may be affected by sleep loss (Lim & Dinges, 2010). Without the ability to sustain attention on a task, a person cannot effectively drive a vehicle, perform a surgical procedure, memorize a formula, or monitor air traffic radar in a control tower.

An influential set of studies investigated the effects on PVT performance, self-rated sleepiness, and later recovery sleep of restricting adult participants' TIB to durations of 3–9 h nightly over periods of 7 or 14 days (Belenky et al., 2003; Dinges et al.,

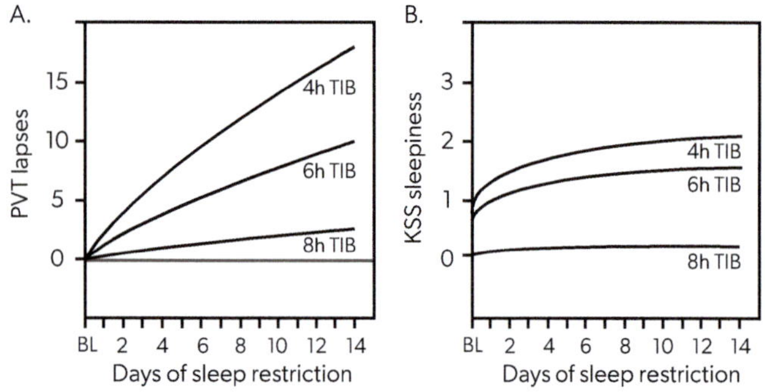

Figure 13.4 **A.** Effects of 14 days of restriction to 8, 6, or 4 h time in bed (TIB) on lapses in performance on the Psychomotor Vigilance Test (PVT). **B.** Similar effects on self-rated sleepiness assessed using the Karolinska Sleepiness Scale (KSS). There appears to be a slight, but nonsignificant, increase in lapses on the PVT over 14 days with 8 h TIB, while there are clear, progressive increases in lapses with 6 h and 4 h TIB. After an initial increase in subjective sleepiness when 6 or 4 h TIB were allowed, subjective sleepiness showed only very small increases over most of the 14 days, compared to the steep increases in PVT lapses over the same period. Adapted with permission of the American Academy of Sleep Medicine from Banks, S. & Dinges, D.F. (2007) Behavioral and physiological consequences of sleep restriction. *J Clin Sleep Med* 3(5): 519–528; © American Academy of Sleep Medicine (2007). PMID:17803017. Figure based on data reported in Van Dongen, H.P.A. et al. (2003) The cumulative cost of additional wakefulness: dose-response effects on neurobehavioral functions and sleep physiology from chronic sleep restriction and total sleep deprivation. *Sleep* 26:117–126. doi:10.1093/sleep/26.2.117. Permission conveyed through Copyright Clearance Center, Inc.

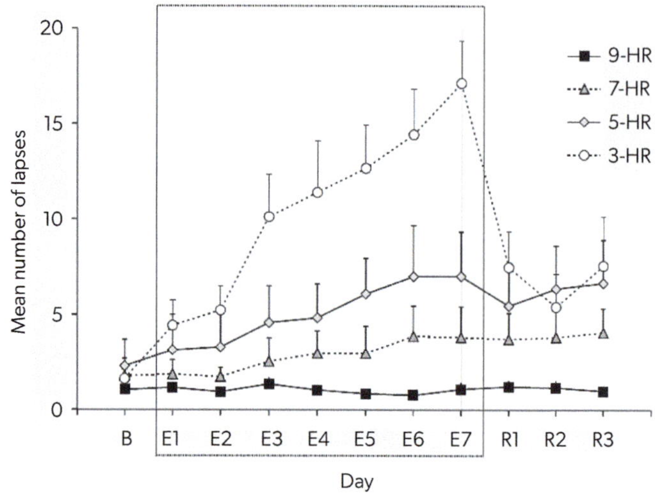

Figure 13.5 Impact of different durations of sleep opportunities on performance on the Psychomotor Vigilance Test (PVT), shown as the number of lapses per 10 min trial (failures to respond within the time allowed). Lapses increased over the 7-day period when sleep was restricted to time in bed (TIB) of 3 h (circles), 5 h (diamonds) and (slightly) even 7 h (triangles), but not when participants had 9 h TIB (squares). Recovery days (R1–R3) allowed 8 h TIB each. Reprinted with permission of John Wiley and Sons from Belenky, G. et al. (2003) Patterns of performance degradation and restoration during sleep restriction and subsequent recovery: a sleep dose-response study. *J Sleep Res* 12:1–12. Journal Compilation © European Sleep Research Society and John Wiley and Sons (2003). doi: 10.1046/j.1365-2869.2003.00337.x.

1997; Van Dongen et al., 2003). PVT performance got progressively worse over the days of sleep restriction, and the speed with which deficits emerged was related to the severity of the restriction (**Figures 13.4** and **13.5**). Deficits appeared rapidly in those allowed 3 or 4 h TIB but emerged more slowly over days in those allowed 5–7 h. Related studies that are discussed below provided information about the mechanisms by which sleep loss affects vigilance, how individuals differ in sensitivity to sleep loss, and how objective effects on performance are related to subjective feelings of sleepiness.

There are fewer studies of sleep duration effects on attention performance in children and adolescents. A meta-analysis of observational studies involving children did not report a significant correlation between spontaneous sleep durations and quality of performance on attention tasks (Astill et al., 2012). Studies of experimental sleep restriction reported mixed results: some found deficits in sustained attention after sleep restriction relative to baseline (Gruber et al., 2011; Louca & Short, 2014; Peters et al., 2009), but others did not (Fallone et al., 2001; Sadeh et al., 2003). One factor influencing these results is that sleep restriction was sometimes modest relative to that imposed in research with adults and in many studies did not extend over multiple nights, especially for younger children. Many parents are probably reluctant to have their school-aged children undergo severe or repeated sleep restriction.

There are also a few studies with older teenagers (16–18 years) that involved overnight total sleep deprivation. A meta-analysis of the effects of partial sleep restriction and total sleep deprivation in adolescents concluded that there was little effect of partial sleep restriction, but that overnight sleep deprivation impaired sustained attention performance (de Bruin et al., 2017).

Detecting effects of sleep restriction in children depends not only on the planned changes in sleep timing, but also on the control condition to which restricted sleep is compared; namely, baseline sleep or extended (or optimized) sleep. In one study, very modest sleep restriction (~30 min nightly over 3 nights)[2] did not impair performance relative to baseline sleep conditions.

[2] Manipulating children's home bedtimes by a certain amount does not guarantee equivalent changes in sleep duration. Children in this study were scheduled to go to bed 60 min later (restriction) or earlier (extension) than usual. However, the actual changes in sleep duration (monitored by actigraphy) were closer to 30 min in each direction. Going to bed later increases sleepiness, so sleep onset may occur more quickly, reducing the effective net sleep loss. Going to bed earlier may instead increase the latency to fall asleep, resulting in less increase in actual sleep time. In each case, the relatively small resulting changes in sleep duration are considerably less than intended.

But sleep extension by a similar amount improved performance on reaction time and short-term memory tasks relative to baseline (Sadeh et al., 2003). One interpretation of these results is that if children at baseline are getting inadequate sleep (as seems likely), adding a small amount of additional restriction may not significantly alter performance, but even modest sleep extension can produce improvements (Sadeh et al., 2003).

Compared to sleep-extended children, those who were sleep-restricted also showed poorer performance on tests of short-term memory, working memory, and divided attention, but not on sustained attention (Vriend et al., 2013). A meta-analysis concluded that there is some support for effects of sleep restriction on attention in children, but these are most evident among boys and older children, and are clearest when the comparison is to a sleep-extension condition rather than to a baseline sleep condition (Lundahl et al., 2015).

In addition to the impact of inadequate baseline sleep and the very limited sleep restriction imposed, studies in children sometimes include procedures that can mask potential deficits. For example, children are often encouraged to remain focused on the tasks and to continue performing them, which is not a common procedure with adults. It is also possible that children are more resilient than adults to the effects of partial sleep loss (Astill et al., 2012), but direct comparison studies that apply strictly identical procedures in adults and children would be needed to test this hypothesis.

In studies that did not find effects of partial sleep restriction on objective tests of sustained attention, parents, teachers, and experimenters often reported seeing signs of impaired attention among participants. These incidental observations suggest that observers noticed attentional problems that were not detected by the formal tests (Fallone et al., 2001; Fallone et al., 2005; Vriend et al., 2013). Similarly, in a study comparing a week of sleep extension to one of sleep restriction among adolescents with attention-deficit/hyperactivity disorder, both participants and their parents reported more inattentive and oppositional behaviors during restriction, but an objective test of attention showed no significant differences (Becker et al., 2019).

Thus, informal observations, self-reports, and reports from observers blinded to treatment conditions often indicate that sleep restriction affects attention in children, even when formal tests of attention do not capture these changes. Modified test procedures, more severe restriction, or more sensitive measures of attention may be needed to demonstrate effects of sleep loss on attention in children and adolescents.

13.3.2 How sleep loss affects vigilance

There are several mechanisms that could contribute to deterioration of vigilance performance after sleep loss in adults. One possibility relates to loss of N3/SWA/delta power. Reductions in these sleep features have been implicated in several aspects of physiological health, including regulation of glucose metabolism, blood pressure, and brain β-amyloid levels (see Chapters 14 and 15). The functional importance of N3 and SWA is also supported by evidence that they are recovered preferentially after total sleep deprivation in people (see Chapter 5).

The evidence, however, does not indicate a specific role for N3/SWA in regulation of attentional abilities. Restricting sleep to 4 h TIB nightly caused rapid deterioration in PVT performance (**Figure 13.4, left panel**) and increases in subjective sleepiness (**Figure 13.4, right panel**) as well as in tests of cognitive throughput and working memory. But these effects were unrelated to loss of N3 sleep, which was preferentially protected during sleep loss. Over 2 weeks of 4 h TIB, N3 was preserved near baseline durations (~1–1.5 h nightly) while other stages were shortened in proportion to the reduction of TIB (**Figure 13.6**; see similar results in Figure 5.11) (Banks & Dinges, 2007; Carskadon & Dement, 1981; Stenuit & Kerkhofs, 2005; Van Dongen et al., 2003); see Chapter 5.

Similarly, delta power summed across all NREM sleep stages hardly changed during 2 weeks of restriction to 4 or 6 h TIB, while cognitive performance deteriorated and subjective sleepiness increased (Van Dongen et al., 2003). There is, therefore, no correlation between changes in N3/SWA/delta power and changes in attentional performance or self-reported sleepiness. Other consequences of sleep restriction must be involved in producing attentional deficits.

An alternative explanation is that the total amount of sleep lost, rather than loss of any one stage or sleep feature, is what affects daytime performance. This idea is supported by evidence that shorter sleep opportunities result in faster and more severe deterioration in PVT performance (see **Figures 13.4 and 13.5**). Over a 2-week study, the rate at which lapses increased was related to the length of TIB (8, 6, or 4 h) (**Figure 13.4**). Given a baseline duration of ~8.2 h of sleep, participants in the three restriction conditions lost cumulative amounts of sleep ranging from near 0 to 56 h, and their performance deficits increased as a linear function of their cumulative sleep loss (Van Dongen et al., 2003).

However, the effects of total sleep deprivation over 1–3 days were not consistent with the idea that the amount of sleep lost determined the attention deficits. Deficits after 24, 48, and 72 h of continuous waking were much more severe than predicted by the number of hours of sleep lost during partial sleep restriction studies. Assuming ~8 h of sleep loss nightly, these groups would have lost 8, 16, and 24 h, respectively. Losing 8 h of sleep over 24 h had more potent effects on vigilance than losing the same amount over 2 nights (i.e., restricted to 4 h sleep nightly), or over 4 nights (i.e., restricted to 6 h sleep nightly). Instead, the

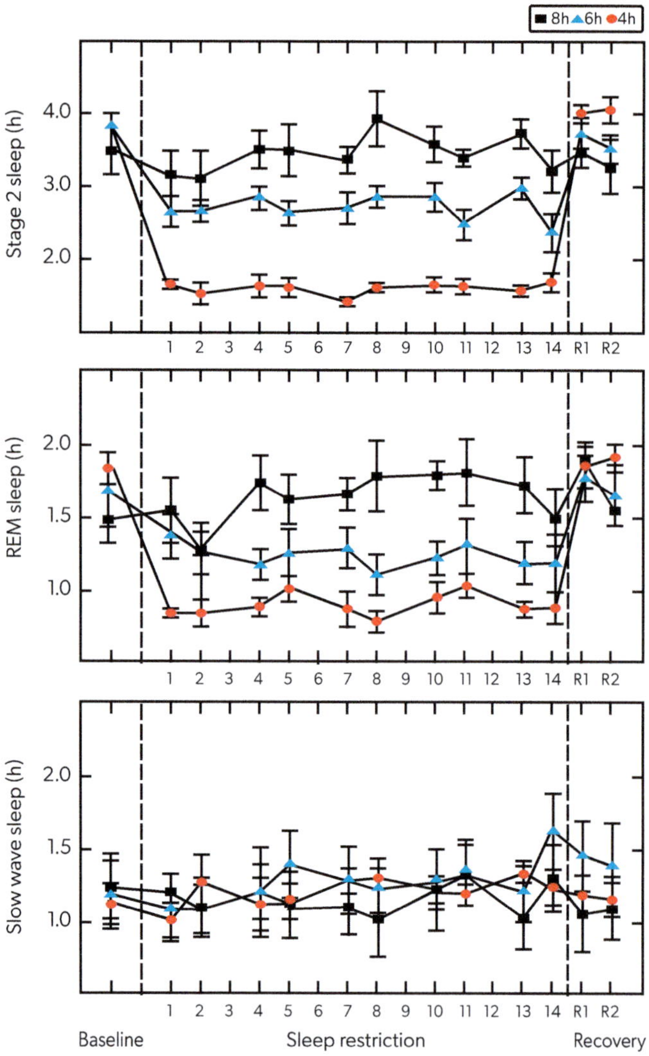

Figure 13.6 Duration of Stage 2 sleep (top), REM sleep (middle), and slow-wave sleep (bottom) during a baseline night, 14 nights (1–14) of restriction to time in bed (TIB) of 4 h (red circles), 6 h (blue triangles) or 8 h (black squares), and during 2 recovery sleep nights (R1–R2). Participants showed immediate and sustained reductions in REM sleep and Stage 2 sleep that were proportional to the reduction in total TIB, but slow-wave sleep duration was preserved throughout the restriction period, regardless of the length of TIB. Adapted with permission of American Academy of Sleep Medicine from Banks, S. & Dinges, D.F. (2007) Behavioral and physiological consequences of sleep restriction. *J Clin Sleep Med* 3(5): 519–528. © American Academy of Sleep Medicine (2007). PMID17803017. Based on data presented in Van Dongen, H.P.A. et al. (2003) The cumulative cost of additional wakefulness: dose-response effects on neurobehavioral functions and sleep physiology from chronic sleep restriction and total sleep deprivation. *Sleep* 26:117–112. doi:10.1093/sleep/26.2.117; permission conveyed through Copyright Clearance Center, Inc.

impact of 24 h awake was more similar to the effects of losing 32 h of sleep cumulatively over 14 nights.

An alternative interpretation that can account for the severity of the effects of continuous waking is that performance changes were related not to hours of sleep lost but to the accumulation of hours of waking. A model based on these findings indicated that the rate of lapses in PVT tests was proportional to the accumulation of hours awake, regardless of whether these hours were accumulated in a single block or gradually over multiple cycles (Van Dongen et al., 2003).

The question this conclusion raises is which neural changes associated with staying awake more than ~16 h continuously are involved in determining waking performance, and how do these interact with different patterns of sleep loss, continuous vs. cyclic. There are two likely mechanisms that can be proposed based on evidence of how waking and sleep affect the brain.

One hypothesis is that being awake for >16 h results in excessive levels of adenosine in the brain. The accumulation of adenosine, especially in key regions involved in sleep regulation, is an important determinant of sleepiness (Porkka-Heiskanen & Kalinchuk 2011). Levels of adenosine in the basal forebrain and cortex accumulate during continuous waking and fall during recovery sleep (Porkka-Heiskanen et al., 2000); see **Figure 11.16** and Section 11.6.1). The impact on vigilance performance of adenosine levels was studied in a rat model of PVT performance (Christie, McKenna, et al., 2008; Porkka-Heiskanen & Kalinchuk, 2011). Injections of adenosine into the basal forebrain of rats that were not sleep deprived resulted in patterns of lapses and slow responses similar to those shown by rats undergoing total sleep deprivation (Christie, Bolortuya, et al., 2008).

For participants in the study by (Van Dongen et al., 2003), adenosine levels would normally rise for ~16 h before starting to fall after sleep onset. When they stayed awake for 20 h during 2 successive days, adenosine levels would have risen even higher by the end of each 20 h wake period. During each 4 h sleep opportunity, however, there would be a partial fall in adenosine levels, which would result in reduced sleepiness and partial recovery of performance during the next day. But levels of adenosine would not have fallen to the usual baseline levels that would be achieved by ~8 h sleep opportunities. The next day would involve another cycle of substantially increasing levels (during 20 h) and partially decreasing levels (during 4 h), until participants would have lost a total of 8 h of sleep and accumulated 8 h worth of additional adenosine.

Staying awake for 24 h also results in a total of 8 h of additional wake time beyond 16 h, but the dynamics of adenosine accumulation would be quite different. Adenosine would accumulate throughout 24 h and there would be no opportunity to reverse the elevated levels. Thus, staying awake for 24 h would include a total of 8 h of "excess" waking beyond 16 h, during which adenosine levels could not fall. As a result, the effect of the additional wake time on adenosine levels would have been added to the accumulation of adenosine over 16 h, with no decrease possible. Thus, the effects on vigilance of "losing 8 h of sleep" for one night would be much worse than the effects of the same sleep loss over multiple sleep–wake cycles that included time for reversal of adenosine increases.

An alternative hypothesis relates to evidence that repeated cycles of sleep restriction that exceed the capacity for homeostatic compensation can trigger allostatic adjustments in the regulation of adenosine and its receptors. These changes allow participants to compensate in part for the effects of extended waking on performance (Grant & Van Dongen, 2013). Examples of such allostatic adjustments were discussed in Section 5.4.1. Mice with a history of repeated sleep restriction cycles who were then acutely sleep deprived showed smaller increases in hippocampal adenosine levels and less rebound increase in SWA than those naïve to sleep restriction (Clasadonte et al., 2014). In rats, repeated sleep restriction cycles caused changes in mRNA levels for two subtypes of adenosine receptors in the basal forebrain and frontal cortex (Kim et al., 2012; Kim et al., 2015). Thus, repeated cycles of sleep restriction resulted in modifications of adenosine physiology that may help buffer some of the effects of sleep loss, which may not be possible during a single session of continuous waking.

These hypotheses are not mutually exclusive. Larger performance deficits after continuous sleep loss, as compared to repeated sleep restriction, may relate to both the lack of an opportunity to partially reduce elevated adenosine levels and the lack of protective effects resulting from allostatic changes that emerge over cycles of sleep restriction.

Although these results are consistent with the idea that waking for >16 h is responsible for deficits in attention performance, there is also evidence that loss of sleep itself leads to attention performance decrements, even without extended wake durations. The relevant study was conducted using a forced internal desynchronization protocol (see Section 3.5.2) in which participants were given sleep opportunities on a non-circadian schedule (every 20 h). A control group had ~6.7 h sleep opportunities every 20 h (1:2 ratio of sleep to wake, analogous to 8 h sleep and 16 h waking), and an experimental group had ~4.7 h sleep opportunities every 20 h (1:3.3 ratio). Although the experimental group participants were not required to be awake for more than 15.33 h at any point in the study, they quickly began to show response lapses and slowed response times on PVT tests, while the control group did not. These effects appeared first, and were subsequently most pronounced, during the subjective night (McHill, Hull, et al., 2018). Taken together, the results of these studies indicate that the physiological consequences of insufficient sleep and excessive lengths of waking both contribute to producing attention deficits.

In the forced desynchronization study, there were large differences between treatment groups in the amounts of N2 and REM sleep obtained, while there were no differences in N3 sleep amounts (McHill, Hull, et al., 2018), as also seen in more traditional sleep restriction studies (Brunner et al., 1990; Stenuit & Kerkhofs, 2005; Webb & Agnew, 1965) (see Section 5.4.2). Despite the group differences in objective measures of vigilance and in production of some sleep stages, there were no group differences in self-reported sleepiness across the entire study (McHill, Hull, et al., 2018).

13.3.3 Recovery from sleep restriction

Another aspect of how chronic sleep restriction affects performance is the pattern of recovery shown by previously restricted participants when they were allowed adequate sleep for several nights. Participants in one study were allowed 3, 5, 7, or 9 h (= controls) TIB for 7 nights and were then allowed 8 h TIB for 3 nights during the recovery period. During recovery days with 8 h TIB, the 5 and 7 h TIB groups showed essentially no change in their rates of lapses (see **Figure 13.5**), nor in their overall speed of responding. The residual impairment in the 5 and 7 h TIB groups was relatively similar and significantly different from the performance of the 9 h TIB control group.

The 3 h TIB group, however, showed an initial, rapid improvement in both lapses and speed of performance after the first recovery night, but only to about the impaired level of the 5 and 7 h TIB groups (see **Figure 13.5**). Despite these persistent performance deficits, there were no significant differences among the four groups in self-rated sleepiness during the three recovery days (Belenky et al., 2003). These results indicate that full, functional recovery from chronic sleep restriction is a slow process that is not completed in a few nights of adequate sleep, and that self-evaluations of sleepiness are poor indicators of the extent of objective recovery from previous sleep restriction; see Section 13.3.5.

Another study compared the effects on PVT performance in two groups that underwent different sleep deprivation procedures. One group had 5 nights of 4 h TIB and the other underwent 36 h of acute sleep deprivation; both groups then had 4 recovery nights that included 12 h TIB. Speed of PVT performance recovered fully after a single night of 12 h TIB in the group that had been awake for 36 h. But in the group that underwent repeated sleep restriction cycles, speed of performance did not rebound to baseline levels even after 4 nights of 12 h TIB. In addition to continuing to show slower PVT response speeds, participants in the chronic restriction group were objectively sleepier, as shown by shorter sleep onset latencies during Maintenance of Wakefulness Tests on recovery days (Yamazaki et al., 2021).

It is possible that 3 nights of 8 h TIB in one study was insufficient to allow full recovery of performance after days of sleep restriction (Belenky et al., 2003), but a generous allowance of

12 h TIB over 4 nights seemed to have little more benefit after chronic sleep loss (Yamazaki et al., 2021). Perhaps even more recovery time was needed, but it is likely that allostatic adjustments in response to repeated restriction events were involved, making recovery sleep less effective in restoring vigilance functions. See the discussions in Section 13.10 and Chapters 14 and 15 of other evidence of long-lasting consequences of chronic, inadequate sleep.

Allostatic adjustments during chronic sleep restriction may be helpful in dealing with the immediate physiological challenges of repeated cycles of inadequate sleep but at the cost of longer-term effects on objective sleepiness and performance after restriction ends. The mechanism involved is unknown, but based on results from studies in rodents, it is likely to be related to changes in the regulation of adenosine and its receptors or of SWA (Clasadonte et al., 2014; Grant & Van Dongen, 2013; Kim et al., 2012; Kim et al., 2015).

It is noteworthy that subjective sleepiness ratings among groups did not differ during recovery days during which previously restricted participants continued to show performance deficits relative to controls (Belenky et al., 2003). Similar findings are discussed below in Section 13.4.4. These results suggest that chronically sleep-restricted participants had adapted subjectively to their degree of sleep loss and no longer recognized their residual sleepiness, despite the fact that objective tests of both sleepiness and performance showed continuing deficits (Belenky et al., 2003; Yamazaki et al., 2021). It is potentially important for real-world work situations to understand how long these effects of prior chronic sleep restriction persist.

13.3.4 Lapses and state instability

Gaps in attention (lapses) have been recognized as key to the deterioration of cognitive performance since the earliest studies of sleep deprivation. When Patrick & Gilbert asked a participant to memorize lists of numbers, they noted that performance began to fail because "[t]he attention could not be held upon the work. A kind of mental lapse would constantly undo the work done" (Patrick & Gilbert, 1896, p. 479). A number of effects of sleep loss may contribute to lapses, including reduced motivation to perform optimally. Most researchers, however, focus on the idea of state instability as the mechanism underlying lapses (see, e.g., Doran et al., 2001). State instability refers to the irregular occurrence of brief, inattentive states during which participants are slow to respond to stimuli or fail to respond within the time allowed (usually 500 msec on the PVT).

These inattentive states may be microsleeps involving intrusions of slow waves into the waking EEG, or other changes in neural networks involved in maintaining attention (see, e.g., Carskadon et al., 1981). An fMRI study during PVT performance found that there was increased activity in parts of the default mode network during slow responses (Drummond et al., 2005). This network comprises linked brain regions that are most active when people are *not* engaged in purposeful cognitive activity (sometimes described as functioning like a car idling in neutral; see discussion in Section 7.5.3). Increases in this network's activity during slow responses are consistent with the idea that participants are briefly disengaging from performing the PVT task. Lapses in attention have also been correlated with brief reductions in thalamic activity, which would reduce excitatory input to the cortex (Chee et al., 2008) and with reduced functional connectivity between the frontal cortex and both the thalamus and visual cortex (Cai et al., 2021).

In addition to these transient changes that occurred during lapses, sleep deprivation also caused a background reduction in activity in parietal cortical regions (involved in attention regulation) and in frontal regions. Surprisingly, sleep loss also caused an *increase* in background thalamic activity (Ma et al., 2015). Increased background activity in the thalamus may be an attempt to compensate for sleepiness by increasing tonic arousing input to the cortex (Krause et al., 2017; Ma et al., 2015). Acute decreases in thalamic activity and in frontal connectivity during lapses would then represent failures of this attempted compensation (Chee et al., 2008).

The increasing frequency of lapses during chronic sleep restriction parallels the changes observed in other objective measures of sleepiness, such as increases in slow eyelid closures and decreases in MSLT latencies (see **Figure 13.1**) (Carskadon & Dement, 1981; Dinges et al., 1997; Lim & Dinges, 2008). Even participants who were severely sleep deprived, however, responded within 500 msec to some stimuli presented during a PVT session, indicating that they continued to become alert periodically. But their average speed of responding successfully decreased with more sleep loss, and the number of lapses increased (see **Figures 13.4** and **13.5**).

In one study using 4 h TIB over 5 days, the fastest 10% of responses were reported to show no decrease over days among middle-aged men (average age, 50 years) (Philip et al., 2012). But a similar study of younger people (average age, 29 years, equal number of males and females) found steadily decreasing speeds for even the fastest 10% of responses (Banks et al., 2010). Similarly, the fastest 10% of responses became steadily slower over a week involving 5 h TIB and especially 3 h TIB in a group of men and women (average age, ~39 years) (Belenky et al., 2003). Whether differences among these studies in the extent of slowing over days of the fastest responses were related to the age or gender of participants would need to be tested in a study comparing these characteristics directly.

These results support the idea that sleep loss leads to both instability of alertness and overall slowing of responses to stimuli in most studies. Instability is reflected in periodic neural events that disengage attention from task performance, and in the occurrence of brief eye closures and microsleeps. During very long periods of sleep deprivation, microsleep durations may increase to 30 s or more, which would clearly be incompatible with detecting and responding to very briefly available stimuli (Lim & Dinges, 2008). The importance of this kind of state instability becomes clear if one translates these laboratory findings to real-world situations, such as when driving a vehicle or monitoring a radar screen. Under those conditions, slipping briefly and without warning from alertness into disengagement from the environment, or into seconds of overt sleep, can have disastrous consequences (see Section 13.9).

13.3.5 Objective vs. subjective sleepiness

An important practical question is whether people whose performance is impaired by sleep loss are aware of their impairment, which could allow them to take appropriate precautions. In some studies of PVT performance, participants were asked to rate their sleepiness using self-rating scales. The changes in PVT performance and in self-reported sleepiness did not follow the same pattern. For example, during days 10–14 of sleep restriction to 6 or 4 h TIB, there were steep increases in lapses on the PVT, but there were only slight changes in subjective sleepiness after the first day (Van Dongen et al., 2003) (see **Figure 13.4**).

In a similar study, those restricted to 3 h sleep for a week showed a steadily increasing number of lapses (see **Figure 13.5**) and decreasing average response speeds throughout the week. But for self-reported sleepiness, using a scale on which "7" represents the sleepiest possible feeling, average scores rose to 2.5 by day 2 and remained essentially unchanged until the study ended on day 7. As discussed above, despite persistent group differences in PVT performance during recovery days, subjective sleepiness ratings also did not differ among treatment groups (Belenky et al., 2003).

In a within-participant study of the benefits of prior sleep history, adult male participants had either extended (~10 h) or habitual (~8 h) sleep opportunities for 6 nights before they were totally sleep deprived for 21 h. In the sleep-extended condition, participants had fewer lapses on the PVT than during the habitual-sleep condition. They also showed better PVT performance and less evidence of objective sleepiness (using MSLTs) during the sleep deprivation period after the sleep-extended than after the habitual-sleep condition. Nevertheless, subjective sleepiness scores did not differ between treatment conditions (Arnal et al., 2015).

The neural correlates of subjective and objective measures of sleepiness are also different. In a 27 h constant routine study (for a description of the method, see Section 3.5.2), increases in subjective fatigue were positively correlated with less power in the EEG high alpha range, while slower responses on a reaction time task were positively correlated with more power in the high delta range (Leproult et al., 2003).

One factor that could contribute to unchanging sleepiness ratings despite increasing performance deficits during sleep loss is habituation. During chronic sleep restriction, people may come to experience their current state as "normal" and therefore not evaluate themselves as particularly sleepy. The driver of a semi-trailer, who drove long hours to compensate for dramatically increased fuel costs in 2008 and got only 2–3 h sleep a night, summed up his experience by indicating that it was hard, but that his body got used to it (Halifax Mail Star, July 5, 2008). Despite this common belief, people do not adapt functionally to chronic sleep restriction. Objective alertness deteriorates progressively as sleep restriction continues, regardless of how habituated people may become to their persistently sleepy state.

The dissociation between objective and subjective measures of sleepiness also occurs in the opposite direction. People were tested repeatedly using the PVT during 40 h of continuous wakefulness. After relatively stable performance for the first 16 h after waking up, they showed parallel increases in lapses on the PVT and increases in self-rated sleepiness during their subjective night phase (hours 16–24 awake). Despite not having any sleep, during hours 26–40 (their subjective day phase), performance improved (i.e., PVT lapses decreased) because of the alerting impact of circadian phase, but sleepiness self-ratings stayed relatively high and stable (Åkerstedt & Wright Jr., 2009) (**Figure 13.7**). In addition to the common dissociation between subjective and objective sleepiness measures, the structure of the study and participants' logical inference about sleepiness may have affected this result. Participants who remembered their previous sleepiness ratings and had still not slept might not have felt that it was reasonable to rate themselves as less sleepy, regardless of how they felt.

A retrospective review of clinical records related to adolescents (10–18 years old) with sleep disorders and other medical conditions provides a real-world example of these discrepancies. Patients rated their own daytime sleepiness and also underwent MSLT testing to establish objective evidence of daytime sleepiness. Nearly 50% showed discrepancies between these measures. The largest proportion of these adolescents self-reported daytime sleepiness but did not show evidence in MSLTs of excessive sleepiness, while a smaller proportion showed the opposite pattern (Munkhjargal et al., 2022).

Several factors may influence differences between subjective and objective measures of sleepiness. They are based on different categories of evidence—introspective cues vs.

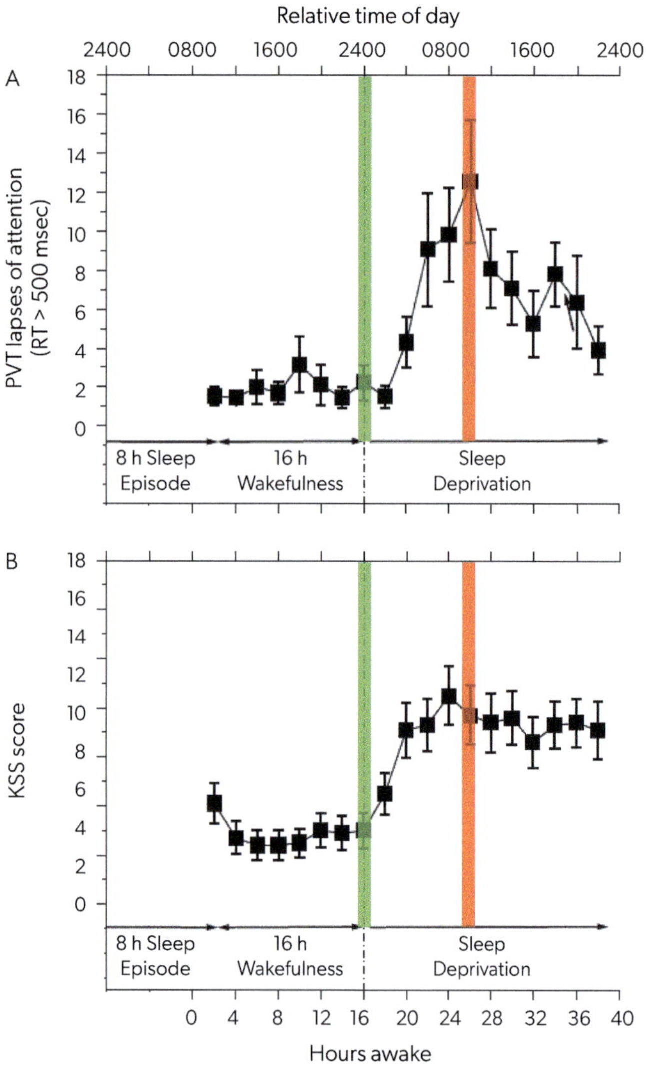

Figure 13.7 Participants were studied during continuous waking for 40 h in a constant routine procedure. **A.** The number of lapses on the Psychomotor Vigilance Test (PVT) during the 40 h study. **B.** Self-rated sleepiness on the Karolinska Sleepiness Scale (KSS) throughout the study. Note the steep increase in KSS scores and PVT lapses starting after ~16 h awake (green line), with PVT lapses peaking after about 26 h awake (red line). During the following subjective day, the number of PVT lapses fell, presumably because the circadian system promoted alertness during the daytime, while subjective sleepiness stabilized and did not decrease despite the reduction in PVT lapses. Adapted with permission of Elsevier, Ltd. from Åkerstedt, T. & Wright, K.P., Jr. (2009) Sleep loss and fatigue in shift work and shift work disorder. *Sleep Med Clin* 4:257–271. © Elsevier (2009). doi: 10.1016/j.jsmc.2009.03.001.

objective performance differences, and they may reflect different changes in EEG features. In addition, both habituation over time to ongoing sleepiness symptoms and awareness of previous self-ratings in studies with sequential self-ratings may also play a role. Whatever the mechanisms involved, subjective reports of sleepiness are not generally good predictors of objective performance on attention tests (see Section 13.4).[3] In addition, because of circadian effects, neither measure is a simple, linear function of the number of hours of prior waking.

13.3.6 Summary

The PVT is a convenient and useful tool for studying how sleep loss affects the ability to remain vigilant. Deficits in attention measured by the PVT increase with time awake beyond ~16 h and increase further with more severe restriction and when repeated over days. In addition, there is evidence that cumulative loss of sleep itself can cause deterioration of attention performance, even in the absence of extensions of wake time beyond 16 h.

Sleep loss during continuous waking (e.g., for 24 or 48 h) has more severe effects on vigilance performance than equal amounts of sleep loss during cycles of sleep restriction over several days. Effects of sleep restriction on PVT performance are best predicted by the cumulative length of waking beyond 16 h, rather than by hours of sleep lost. Excess waking affects PVT performance in large part by increasing the irregular occurrence of lapses, during which participants are either slow to respond, or fail to respond, to stimulus presentations. Some studies also found slowing of even the fastest correct responses, but this may depend on the age of participants or other factors.

One effect of sleep loss that could increase sleepiness and promote lapses is the increase in brain adenosine levels that occurs during waking. Short daily sleep periods may allow partial reversal of increases in adenosine levels and therefore reduce functional sleepiness, while sustained waking would not allow adenosine levels to fall. Repeated episodes of sleep restriction may also trigger allostatic adjustments that alter how adenosine and its receptors respond to sleep loss; a single period of sustained waking may not trigger similar changes.

In addition to the less severe immediate effects of cycles of sleep restriction when compared to total sleep deprivation, there are also different effects of recovery sleep in these conditions. There is incomplete recovery of baseline attention performance after cyclic sleep restriction even after several days of extended sleep opportunities, while there is rapid recovery after acute total sleep loss. Allostatic adjustments that help blunt the impact of cycles of sleep restriction may also have

[3] Modified test procedures in other studies improved the correlation between subjective ratings and some objective measures of performance. However, the number of lapses in vigilance tests remained uncorrelated with self-ratings of sleepiness (Horne & Burley, 2010; Yang et al., 2004). In a study of overnight sleep deprivation using different vigilance measures that included only overnight data, there was, however, a strong correlation between deteriorating vigilance performance and self-rated sleepiness (Gillberg et al., 1994), as is also shown for the overnight period in **Figure 13.7**.

residual effects (e.g., on adenosine and/or its receptors) that impede full recovery from sleep loss after restriction ends.

There is a tonic increase in thalamic activity during PVT testing after sleep loss, which may represent an attempt to stimulate the cortex to maintain vigilance. However, lapses of attention still occur, reflecting state instability which appears to be the result of several other changes in neural activity. These changes include periodic microsleeps (represented by slow waves intruding on the waking EEG); increased activity of the Default Mode Network; decreased activity in brain regions involved in attention (e.g., the parietal lobe); reduced frontal cortical connectivity to other systems; and transient reductions in thalamic activity.

Changes in participants' self-rated sleepiness during sleep restriction are not well correlated with changes in either performance on vigilance tests or objective measures of sleepiness (e.g., sleep onset latencies during MSLTs). During lengthy sleep deprivation or repeated cycles of restriction, participants do not rate themselves as getting progressively sleepier while their objective performance continues to deteriorate. Sleep deprived participants who improve attentional performance during the circadian day phase may also not rate themselves as becoming less sleepy. Differences between subjective and objective measures of sleepiness may reflect changes in different EEG features influencing these measures. Other factors may also affect subjective ratings, including habituation to the consequences of sleep loss and participants' expectations about what should affect their sleepiness.

13.4 Individual differences in response to sleep loss

13.4.1 Predictors of individual differences

Most studies report large individual differences among both people and animals in the degree to which sleep restriction impairs vigilance performance; some participants are vulnerable and others are resilient to sleep loss (Chua et al., 2014; Deurveilher et al., 2015; Van Dongen et al., 2004). When people were kept awake for 36 h and tested on the PVT, the average number of lapses they showed during tests over the last 24 h of waking ranged from 8 to 80. Three possible explanations for these individual differences were evaluated: 1. The results reflected random variability; i.e., the differences would not be consistent if the same individuals were retested. 2. Participants had different histories of recent sleep satiation or loss before participating in the study, which combined with the experimental sleep loss to produce different results. 3. These differences reflected stable characteristics of the individuals (e.g., their genetic makeup) and would be replicable in a repeated trial.

To test the second possibility, participants were either sleep-satiated (12 h TIB) or moderately sleep-restricted (6 h TIB) for a week before a 36 h sleep deprivation period. Their performance during sleep deprivation was unrelated to their sleep history during the preceding week, so the degree of baseline sleep satiation did not determine individual differences in performance. To test hypotheses 1 and 3, the participants who had experienced a week of 12 h TIB were retested weeks later under identical deprivation conditions, following another week of 12 h TIB. With few exceptions, individual participants showed very similar performance levels during the two tests. Thus, differences in vulnerability to sleep loss did not represent random variations but reflected stable, replicable traits of almost all participants (**Figure 13.8 A**) (Van Dongen et al., 2004).

Similarly, people who were tested while staying awake during two separate 27 h constant routines showed very similar patterns of both EEG changes and vigilance-test performance on the two tests (Leproult et al., 2003). This consistency also applies to different types of sleep loss. Participants who had shown the largest performance deficits during 63 h of continuous waking also showed the worst performance during a week with 3 h TIB nightly (Rupp et al., 2012). In a study that used several different patterns of sleep loss, the vigilance performance of participants was consistently resilient or vulnerable to the impact of reduced sleep (Yamazaki & Goel, 2020).

Self-rated sleepiness during sleep deprivation was also a stable feature of individuals across repeated tests under identical conditions, and like PVT performance, varied considerably among participants (**Figure 13.8 B**) (Van Dongen et al., 2004; Yamazaki & Goel, 2020). The stability of sleepiness self-ratings over repeated trials suggests that these ratings might identify the degree to which someone's performance would be affected by sleep loss. This would be valuable information for those who must sometimes work under conditions of limited sleep (e.g., health care providers, police, military personnel, and other shift workers).

As could be predicted based on the relative independence of changes in objective performance and subjective ratings (Section 13.3.4), self-reports of sleepiness after sleep loss were a poor guide to actual performance. Some participants with very low sleepiness self-ratings in one study (**Figure 13.8**, participants **T** and **E**, **red**) showed average or very high numbers of lapses. Similarly, those with consistently few lapses (participants **U, O, Q,** and **F**, **blue**)—the target group one would like to identify—gave sleepiness ratings that were either average (**U, O, Q**) or very high (**F**). Neither variable predicted the other. The independence of these measures was apparent even within individuals, as illustrated by participant **R** (**yellow**), who gave

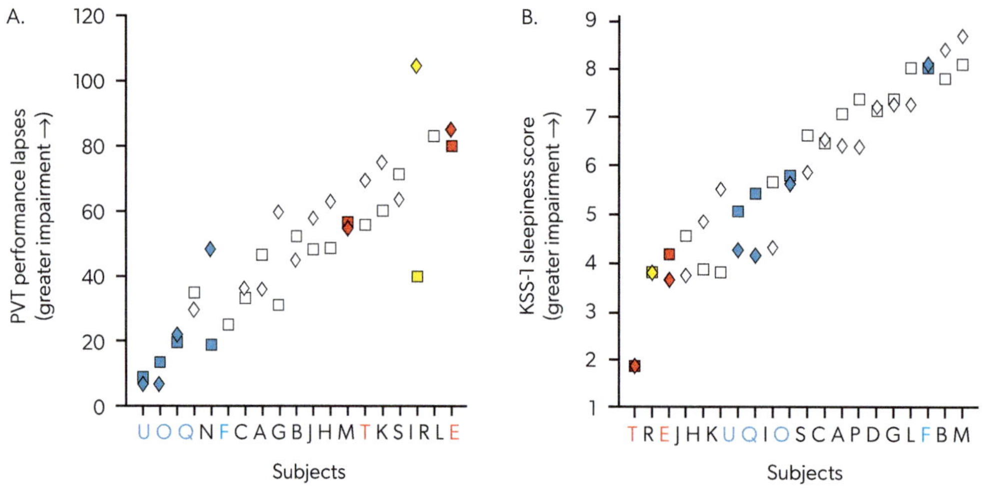

Figure 13.8 **A.** Psychomotor Vigilance Test (PVT) performance (number of lapses; Y axis) during the last 24 h of a 36 h sleep deprivation period for individual participants (letters on the X axis). A square represents an individual's performance during the first experience of this condition and a diamond represents the same individual's performance when identical conditions were repeated several weeks later. **B.** For the same participants, self-rated sleepiness on the Karolinska Sleepiness Scale (KSS-1) is plotted using the same symbols. Participants who showed few lapses (U, O, Q and F; blue symbols in panel **A**) reported medium or high levels of subjective sleepiness (blue symbols in panel **B**). Those self-reporting low sleepiness (T & E, red symbols in panel **B**) showed medium or very high numbers of lapses (red symbols in panel **A**). One individual reported relatively low sleepiness self-ratings that were identical on the two repeated trials (R, overlapping yellow symbols in panel **B**). The same individual showed the highest number of errors on the PVT during one trial (yellow diamond in panel **A**), but also the largest difference in performance between the two repetitions of the test (yellow diamond and square), despite reporting identical levels of sleepiness during the two tests. Adapted with permission of Oxford University Press from Van Dongen, H.P.A. et al. (2004) Systematic individual differences in neurobehavioral impairment from sleep loss: evidence of trait-like differential vulnerability. *Sleep* 27:423–433. © Sleep Research Society (2004). doi: 10.1093/sleep/27.3.423.

identical, low self-ratings of sleepiness during repeated testing but showed the largest discrepancy among participants in objective performance on the two tests (Van Dongen et al., 2004).

Studies of brain changes after sleep loss provide some insight into mechanisms underlying individual differences in performance. Participants who had 4 h sleep opportunities showed reduced blood flow in frontal and parietal brain regions involved in attention regulation and in a basal forebrain area involved in arousal regulation. Reductions were largest in those who were judged to be drowsiest (based on features of their eye movements). Those who were judged to be most alert showed increased blood flow in basal forebrain and cingulate regions that are associated with arousal (Poudel et al., 2012).

Other studies have identified differences in baseline performance and in brain activation as predictors of resilience to sleep loss. fMRI measures of brain activation were compared between participants who were selected as being either resilient or vulnerable to the performance effects of sleep loss on a working memory task. Vulnerable participants showed lower levels of brain activation during task performance at baseline before sleep restriction. These results suggest that the degree to which participants recruit the brain's arousal mechanisms during task performance predicts their responses to sleep deprivation (Mu et al., 2005).

Baseline sleep characteristics have also been examined as potential predictors of performance during sleep loss. One study divided participants into thirds based on their PVT performance during 26 h of waking; the lowest and highest performing thirds were considered, respectively, vulnerable and resilient to sleep loss. Those who turned out to be most vulnerable to sleep loss had habitually longer sleep, higher sleep efficiency, and more SWS at baseline. They also showed more variability in physiological measures related to the autonomic nervous system and more variability in reaction times while performing the PVT before sleep deprivation (Chua et al., 2014). Thus, people with higher homeostatic sleep need and more instability at baseline, both in performance and in autonomic function, were most sensitive to the effects of sleep loss.

In contrast to some of these results, another study reported a lack of correlation between a host of sleep, personality, and cognitive variables with resilience or vulnerability to sleep loss. The only reliable predictors of good PVT performance after sleep loss in this study were better baseline PVT performance before deprivation and long latencies to sleep onset in a Maintenance of Wakefulness Test (MWT). These results suggest that resilience to sleep loss is predicted by the ability of participants when they are sleep-satiated to recruit resources to remain alert during a repetitive task or in a sleep-promoting environment (as in the MWT). This evidence was interpreted as indicating that people who can maintain alert performance under different external demand conditions are most resilient to sleep loss (Galli et al., 2022).

13.4.2 Genetic factors affecting responses to sleep loss

Adenosine plays an important role in regulating sleepiness, and its receptors are a target of caffeine's alerting effects (Huang et al., 2005); see Section 11.6. A polymorphism in the gene that codes for the adenosine A_{2A} receptor has been linked to individual differences in performance after sleep loss and differences in responsiveness to caffeine treatment (Bodenmann et al., 2012; Rétey et al., 2007). Men who self-identified as being caffeine-sensitive (based on difficulty sleeping at night after afternoon caffeine intake) showed worse PVT performance during a 40 h sleep deprivation period than those who rated themselves as caffeine-insensitive (**Figure 13.9 A,B**). Considering all participants, those whose performance was most impaired by sleep loss also showed the largest improvement after a dose of caffeine at night, consistent with high caffeine sensitivity (**Figure 13.9 C**).

These results indicate that individual differences in adenosine accumulation or genetic differences in adenosine receptors are related to how vulnerable people are to extended waking, and how sensitive they are to the adenosine-blocking effects of caffeine (Bodenmann et al., 2012; Rétey et al., 2006). Consistent with the proposal that variation in the gene for the A_{2A} receptor is related to differences in the effects of sleep loss, studies comparing monozygotic (identical) and dizygotic twins found that responsiveness to sleep loss is a highly heritable trait (Kuna et al., 2012).

A different genetic factor affected subjective sleepiness during sleep loss. It was identified in a study comparing currently healthy carriers of the *DQB1*0602* gene allele (linked to an increased risk of developing narcolepsy; see Section 11.3.3) to controls without this allele. During chronic partial sleep restriction, carriers rated themselves as sleepier and more fatigued than controls lacking this allele, but their PVT performance under sleep restriction did not respond differently from controls (Goel et al., 2010). The results of this study, combined with those related to genes influencing adenosine physiology, suggest that variations in different genes may be linked differentially to objective performance deficits and subjective reports of sleepiness during sleep loss. Since these genetic variations presumably occur independently, they could contribute to the lack of strong positive correlations between subjective and objective measures of sleepiness in many studies.

Mutations in a gene known to be involved in circadian clock regulation (*DEC2*) were associated with naturally short sleep (~6 h) in a human family. Transgenic mice and fruit flies bred to express the same mutation also had shortened sleep durations (He et al., 2009). Other variants of the same gene were associated with both habitual short sleep and resistance to performance deterioration during sleep restriction (Pellegrino et al., 2014). Thus, variations in a gene that promotes habitual short sleep, presumably reflecting a slower rate of accumulation of homeostatic sleep need, were associated with a reduced impact of sleep loss on performance.

A variant of another gene involved in circadian rhythm regulation (*PER3*) was linked to poorer performance after sleep deprivation. People homozygous for a longer form of the *PER3* gene showed more theta activity when kept awake (a marker of increasing sleepiness), faster sleep onset, and more SWS. They also showed more deterioration in cognitive performance during sleep deprivation, especially on tasks related to executive functions (Dijk & Archer, 2010). These findings are consistent with the idea that the long form of the *PER3* gene is associated with a more rapid buildup of sleep need during waking, leading to a larger impact of sleep loss on cognitive performance. This conclusion is consistent with evidence discussed in Section 13.4.1 that poor performance during sleep loss is predicted by high homeostatic sleep need at baseline (Chua et al., 2014; Pellegrino et al., 2014).

13.4.3 Summary

Both performance on the PVT and subjective sleepiness during sleep loss are stable characteristics of individuals. But these two measures of how sleep loss affects people are not well correlated with each other. People with high levels of subjective sleepiness during deprivation do not necessarily perform poorly on the PVT, and people who perform poorly do not necessarily report high levels of sleepiness.

People who perform best on the PVT during sleep loss were found to recruit more activation in frontal and parietal cortical regions, the cingulate, and basal forebrain, which are linked to regulation of attention and arousal. Individual differences in sensitivity of performance to sleep loss are highly stable and heritable and appear to reflect a general ability to perform successfully under external demand conditions. Among the physiological mechanisms contributing to differential effects on performance are the rate of buildup of sleep need (linked to one form of the *PER3* gene); mutations in a gene linked to circadian regulation and to short sleep (*DEC2*); altered adenosine receptor function; and the amount of instability in physiological regulation and in PVT performance at baseline.

In contrast, the presence of an allele of the *DQB1* gene that is linked to susceptibility to developing narcolepsy predicted more subjective sleepiness and fatigue in healthy people during chronic sleep restriction. These participants did not, however,

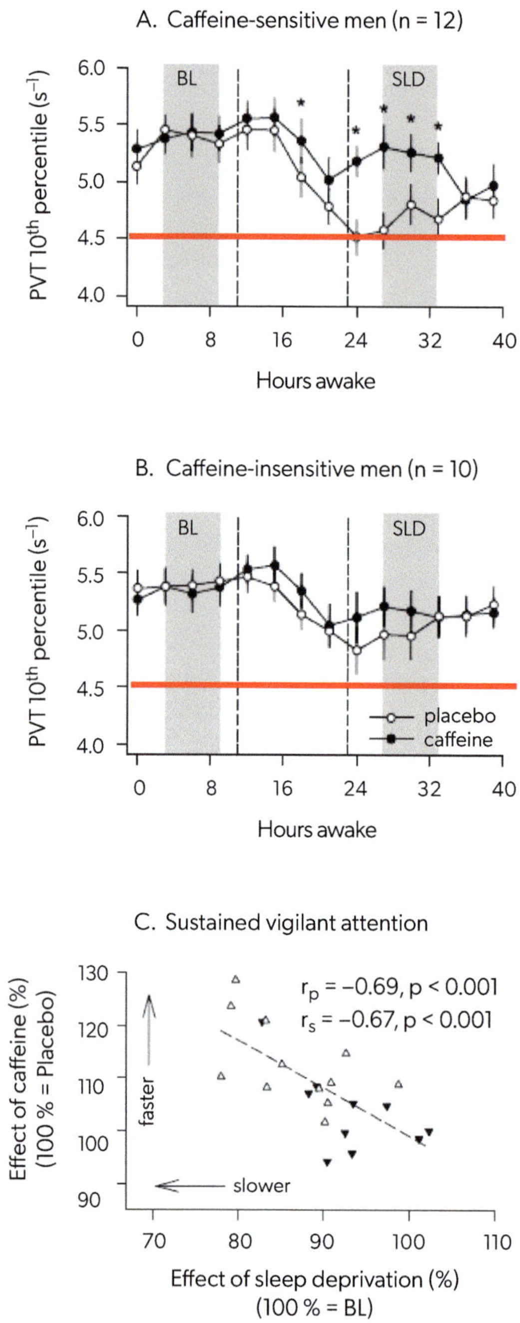

Figure 13.9 Responsiveness to the effects of caffeine on Psychomotor Vigilance Test (PVT) performance during sleep deprivation is related to self-reported caffeine sensitivity. **A.** Participants who reported that they were sensitive to caffeine (afternoon intake interfered with later sleep) showed deficits in optimal PVT performance (measured as their fastest 10% of responses) when kept awake during the night (white symbols, placebo treatment). These effects were larger than those shown by caffeine-insensitive participants (white symbols in panel **B**). The red lines reproduced in **A & B** indicate the trough of performance among caffeine-sensitive men in **A**. Treatment with 200 mg of caffeine (black symbols) at the times indicated by vertical dashed lines strongly improved performance in self-defined caffeine-sensitive men (**A**) but not in caffeine-insensitive men (**B**). The shaded areas indicate the clock times during which performance was compared between Baseline (BL) and Sleep Deprivation (SLD) conditions. There was a trough in performance in the placebo groups at 24 h of waking, but performance gradually improved during the following 16 daytime hours, despite continued sleep deprivation. **C.** There was a robust negative correlation (dashed diagonal line) between the degree to which sleep deprivation impaired performance (X axis) and the degree to which caffeine treatment improved performance (Y axis), indicating that sensitivity to caffeine and to sleep loss are linked. Black triangles represent caffeine insensitive and white triangles represent caffeine-sensitive men. This correlation probably reflects the impact of adenosine on sleepiness. Staying awake increases both adenosine levels and sleepiness, while caffeine blocks adenosine receptors and decreases sleepiness. Adapted with permission of Dr. Hans-Peter Landolt from Rétey, J.V. et al. (2006) Adenosinergic mechanisms contribute to individual differences in sleep deprivation-Induced changes in neurobehavioral function and brain rhythmic activity. *J Neurosci* 26:10472–10479. © Society for Neuroscience (2006). doi: 10.1523/JNEUROSCI.1538-06.2006.

differ from controls in their objective performance on the PVT or other cognitive tests.

Taken together, these results indicate that a faster buildup of homeostatic sleep need during the day (probably mediated via the adenosine system) predicts worse vigilance performance during extended waking. In contrast, habitual short sleep and genes that are linked to shorter sleep (presumably reflecting slower homeostatic buildup of sleep need) are associated with a reduced impact of sleep loss on performance. Other genes that do not affect performance during sleep restriction instead influence subjective sleepiness.

The fact that some genes involved in the molecular mechanism of the circadian clock also contribute to differences in sleep duration and sleep need reinforces the idea that homeostatic and circadian regulators of sleep are closely intertwined (Dijk & Archer, 2010; Franken & Dijk, 2009) (for other examples, see **Box 8.2** in Section 8.5.3).

13.5 **Sleep loss, circadian phase, and performance**

The results obtained in laboratory studies of simple vigilance are reinforced by results from studies of the effects of sleep loss on more complex sensory-motor skills, such as those involved in driving. Driving simulators have been used to study the effects of acute or chronic sleep restriction on deficits in driving skills (drifting across lane lines, failing to maintain appropriate speeds, delays in braking). The impact of fatigue resulting from the combination of sleep loss and the circadian phase during simulated driving has been confirmed by studies involving actual driving in instrumented cars (Filtness et al., 2014) and by population-based statistics related to road accidents. The latter studies have shown increased risk of accidents and near misses in those with conditions that increase sleepiness, including obstructive sleep apnea (see Appendix B), insomnia, and narcolepsy (George & Smiley, 1999; Liu et al., 2018), and extended work hours (see Section 13.9).

Impairments in driving performance during extended waking have been compared to the well-known deficits caused by high blood alcohol levels. In one study, people were tested for their performance on a simulated driving task starting soon after they woke up and repeatedly over the next 28 h (Dawson & Reid, 1997). After slight improvement during the morning hours, performance stabilized at a high level until 15–16 h after waking (**Figure 13.10**). Performance began to deteriorate after ~17 h awake and reached a low point after ~23 h. By ~17 h awake, performance was equivalent to that caused by a blood alcohol level of 0.05%, and after ~22 h awake, by a blood alcohol concentration of 0.08%. In many jurisdictions, these are levels at which drivers can have their licenses suspended immediately (0.05%) or can be convicted of driving while intoxicated (0.08%).

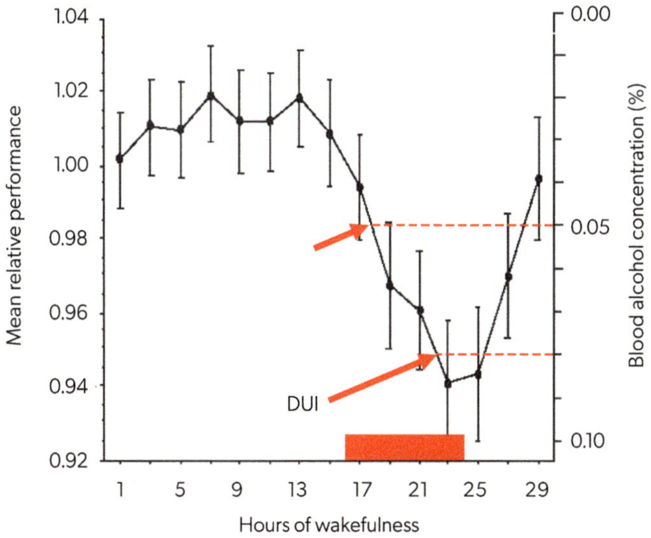

Figure 13.10 Effects of extended hours of waking and the time of day on performance during a simulated driving task; the red bar indicates the usual timing of a sleep phase. After initial improvement, performance relative to baseline (= 1.00) (left Y axis) was quite stable during the first 16 h awake but began to decline after that and fell to a low point 23–25 h after waking. Performance then improved during the next 5 h, presumably in response to circadian alerting effects, despite the continued lack of sleep. Participants were also assessed for their driving performance under the influence of different levels of blood alcohol, which are shown on the right Y axis. The upper dashed red line shows that driving performance after 17 h awake was equivalent to that of an individual with a 0.05% blood alcohol level. The lower dashed red line shows that driving performance after 22 h of waking was equivalent to that of an individual with a 0.08% blood alcohol level, considered to be DUI (driving under the influence = DWI, driving while intoxicated). Adapted with permission from Dawson, D. & Reid, K. (1997) Fatigue, alcohol and performance impairment. *Nature* 388:235. © Springer: Nature (1997). doi: 10.1038/40775.

To put these performance levels into context, if one woke up at 06:00, one would be awake for 17 h by 23:00, and for 22 h by 04:00. The results indicate that driving home from a party (at which one had consumed no intoxicating substances) any time after 23:00 would be as dangerous as doing so while legally intoxicated. Similar parallels between the effects of extended waking and chronic sleep restriction to those of alcohol intake were shown for several other motor performance and cognitive tasks (Lamond & Dawson, 1999; Powell et al., 2001; Williamson & Feyer, 2000). Other studies demonstrated the further deterioration of driving performance that results from adding even small doses of alcohol to the already significant impact of extended time awake (Horne et al., 2003).

It is important to note, however, that in studies that included testing during overnight sleep deprivation and into the following day, performance began to improve again, despite the lack of any recovery sleep (see **Figure 13.10**, hours 25–29 awake) (Dawson & Reid, 1997; Lamond & Dawson, 1999). This finding reflects the potent arousing effects exerted by the circadian system in the morning hours, despite increased homeostatic sleep pressure from extended waking. Similar effects of circadian phase were also shown for PVT performance in the morning hours after overnight sleep deprivation (**Figure 8.21**, young participants; **Figure 13.9,** placebo controls), and during waking for 40 h in a constant routine (**Figure 13.7**).

The length of time awake is confounded in these studies with the circadian phase of testing. Deteriorating nighttime performance in overnight sleep deprivation studies results from the combined effects of extended wake and testing during the circadian night phase, leading to the worst performance in the early morning hours. Because both factors contribute to impaired performance, it would be dangerous to be driving at 04:00 even without sleep loss, and very dangerous to be doing so while sleep deprived. The impact of this sleep-circadian confound on research in aging was discussed in Section 8.5.3.

The combined effect of extended waking and circadian phase was demonstrated clearly in a study of nurses commuting to and from work while working different shifts (day, evening, or night shifts). There was a strong interaction between circadian phase (assessed using a marker of melatonin secretion) and length of time awake in predicting sleepiness and driving-related hazards (e.g., long eye closures). Maximal sleepiness and risk of driving-related inattention or sleep events occurred during drives home in the early morning after night shifts. The most hazardous time to be driving was after being awake ≥16 h when that coincided with an interval centered on the peak of melatonin secretion, representing the middle of the circadian night phase (Mulhall et al., 2019) (**Figure 13.11**).

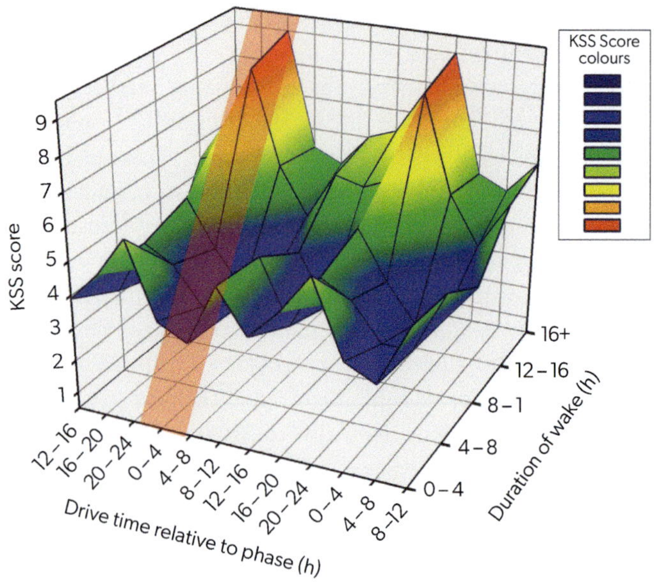

Figure 13.11 Interaction of the circadian phase of driving and the length of waking on subjective sleepiness. Duration of Wake is shown on the Z axis (right) and circadian phase of driving, based on melatonin secretion (Drive time relative to phase), is shown on the X axis (front). Subjective sleepiness (KSS Score: Karolinska Sleepiness Scale) is plotted on the Y axis. The study involved nurses driving home after shift work. The Drive Time axis is double plotted to show a 48 h period and allow better visualization of the shape of the curves. Peak sleepiness, represented by the "hot" colors (yellow, orange, red), was shown during drives occurring when >16 h of waking coincided with the peak of the daily melatonin secretion phase (labeled hour 0). The semi-transparent red bar is centered on the peak of the melatonin secretion rhythm, representing roughly +/− 3 h. There was also a peak in sleep-related events (e.g., long eye closures) during drives at those phases. Adapted with permission of Oxford University Press from Mulhall, M.D. et al. (2019) Sleepiness and driving events in shift workers: the impact of circadian and homeostatic factors. *Sleep* 42(6):1–13. © Sleep Research Society (2019). doi:10.1093/sleep/zsz074.

The importance of the circadian phase of testing was also demonstrated in a study that used a forced desynchronization protocol involving extremely non-circadian "days," each 42.85 h in length (see Section 3.5.2). Two groups of participants experienced different non-circadian sleep schedules, which were roughly equivalent to having a sleep opportunity of ~5.5 h/24 h (23% of each cycle, or moderate sleep restriction) vs. the equivalent of ~8 h/24 h (33% of each cycle, or adequate sleep).

Participants were tested using the PVT throughout the waking periods of each "day" cycle, resulting in performance testing at all possible phases of their unentrained circadian rhythms, which were monitored using measures of melatonin secretion. During weeks 2 and 3 on these schedules, those with the short sleep opportunities showed progressively worse PVT performance overall, especially as the length of time awake in each cycle increased (**row A, Figure 13.12**).

When performance of the short sleepers was compared at different circadian phases, however, it was generally good during the subjective day (indicated by the phase when melatonin levels were low; **row B**). However, performance during the circadian night phase (indicated by high melatonin levels; **row C**) deteriorated throughout the study, with performance deficits rising during each waking period. The performance effects during the subjective night were the main contributor to the overall effect of sleep restriction on performance summed across all circadian phases (**row A**). These findings demonstrate that observing the effects of chronic, moderate sleep restriction on attention depends critically on the circadian phase of testing (Cohen et al., 2010).

It is important to note that performance during the first few hours after waking up (2–6 h awake on the X axis) was excellent throughout all weeks of the study for the chronically sleep restricted, even during the circadian night phase (see weeks 2 and 3 in **row C, Figure 13.12**). Even the shorter

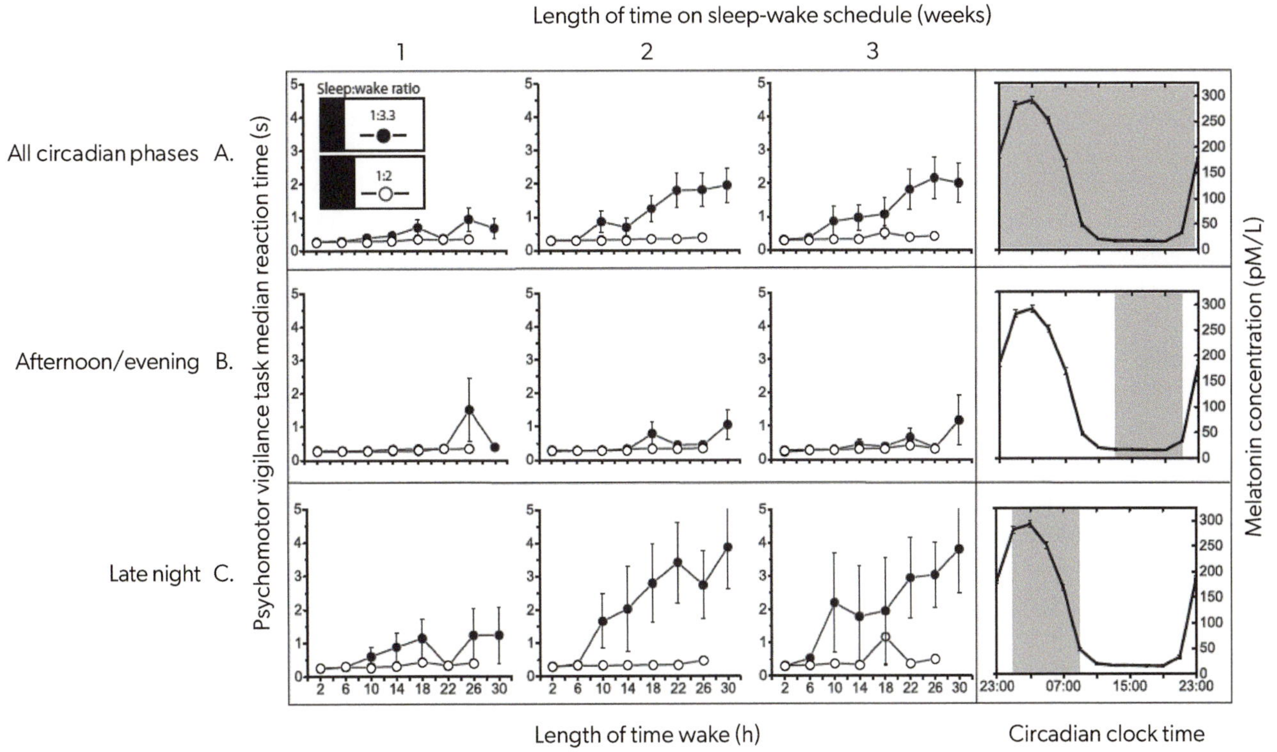

Figure 13.12 Participants in a temporal isolation environment were scheduled to sleep and wake within a cycle with a non-circadian period (42.85 h), resulting in forced internal desynchronization. They were permitted to sleep during either ~23% (black symbols) or 33% (white symbols) of each sleep-wake cycle (which would be equivalent to ~5.5 h vs. ~8 h sleep nightly on a 24 h schedule). The right-hand column shows circadian time indexed by the rhythm of melatonin concentration; high melatonin levels characterize the subjective night. The shaded region in the right-hand panels shows the part of the circadian cycle included in three different analyses of performance (**A**, **B**, and **C**). Performance on the Psychomotor Vigilance Task (PVT) (median reaction times on the Y axis) is shown on each X axis during repeated tests every 4 h during the waking phase for weeks **1**, **2**, and **3** of the study (left to right). **A**. Reaction times measured at all circadian phases (shaded area in the right-hand column) increased late in the waking episode for those on a restricted sleep schedule (equivalent to 5.5 h), particularly during weeks 2 and 3, but not for those on a sleep schedule equivalent to 8 h nightly. **B.** A similar plot of performance only during the subjective equivalent of the afternoon/early evening (shaded area on the right; low melatonin levels) showed essentially no effect of sleep restriction on performance during that circadian phase across all 3 weeks (except near the end of the longer wake phases). **C.** A similar plot of performance only during the circadian subjective night (shaded area on the right; high melatonin levels) showed that sleep restriction caused performance at that phase to deteriorate somewhat even during the first week, and very strongly during weeks 2 and 3 for those on restricted sleep, but not for those getting the equivalent of 8 h sleep opportunities during each cycle. The impact of moderate, chronic sleep restriction was robustly modulated by circadian phase, with essentially the full impact of sleep loss on performance occurring during the circadian (subjective) night phase. No error bars are shown for the control group, as these were all uniformly small. Reprinted with permission of AAAS from Cohen, D.A. et al. (2010) Uncovering residual effects of chronic sleep loss on human performance. *Sci Transl Med* Jan 13;2(14) 2:14ra3. © American Academy for the Advancement of Science (2010). doi: 10.1126/scitranslmed.3000458.

sleep opportunities allowed recovery from the acute effects of prior waking, probably by reversing the accumulation of adenosine (see Section 11.6). But after the first few hours awake, performance deteriorated steeply during the subjective night over the weeks of the study. Thus, sleep opportunities, despite their immediate benefits for performance, did not compensate for the chronic homeostatic deficit that accumulated during 3 weeks of sleep restriction, which was expressed almost exclusively during the circadian night phase (Cohen et al., 2010).

Although overall performance averaged over the first 2–6 h awake was excellent even for those undergoing sleep restriction, a finer-grained analysis in a study using a similar protocol revealed additional important details. In the first few minutes after waking from a sleep period, participants who had undergone chronic sleep restriction (equivalent to ~5.5 h/24 h) showed deficits in working memory performance, reflecting the effects of sleep inertia (see Section 2.3.3). These effects were present at all circadian phases during the third week of sleep restriction, but it was only during the circadian night phase that these transient deficits were sustained for as long as an hour after waking (McHill et al., 2019).

It is not uncommon for adults to get <6 h of sleep nightly, especially among shift workers. A history of chronic, moderate sleep restriction may only reveal its effects on cognition when people are called on to perform their jobs during the night shortly after being awakened. This is a situation that might occur frequently for emergency responders, military personnel, and some health care providers, all of whom may work at night or during extended shifts. It is also likely that people in this situation would not be aware of their own functional impairment. The research participants in this study who were showing impaired performance during the period of sleep inertia shortly after waking did not differ from controls in their subjective sleepiness ratings (McHill et al., 2019).

Participants in another study who were allowed 6 h TIB for one week showed deficits in attention but not in memory performance relative to controls with 10 h TIB. However, when they were then immediately tested during 40 h awake in a constant routine, the previously sleep-restricted participants showed more severe deterioration than controls on both sustained attention and working memory tasks. These effects were also strongly modulated by circadian phase (Lo et al., 2012). This evidence of hidden effects of long-term, modest sleep debt implies that even if workers' performance is not impaired immediately, they may show performance deficits when they are required to stay awake for an extended period, especially during their circadian night phase. As discussed in Section 13.6, there is other evidence that chronic changes in sleep amounts have long-lasting effects on performance.

13.5.1 Summary

Individuals tested on a complex sensory-motor skill, driving, showed a steep deterioration in performance beginning after ~16 h awake. When tested late in the night during an extended wake period, driving performance was equivalent to that of people who are legally intoxicated. If participants continued to stay awake into the next morning, however, performance recovered significantly. These results show that performance deficits late in the night are not attributable only to sleep loss. Studying people who are kept wake overnight confounds the interacting effects of time awake with the effects of circadian phase on performance.

The importance of the circadian phase of testing was demonstrated in a forced desynchronization study involving weeks of chronic, moderate sleep restriction on a non-circadian schedule. PVT performance deteriorated during the subjective night over the weeks of testing but showed little change during the subjective day. These results are consistent with other studies in showing that repeated sleep loss has cumulative, long-term effects on performance. They emphasize, however, that the circadian phase of testing is critical to revealing these effects.

A similar study found that cumulative sleep loss impaired working memory performance during short-lived periods of sleep inertia after waking up at all circadian phases, but these periods lasted for up to an hour only during the circadian night phase. Nevertheless, after this initial inertia, performance was very good during the first few hours of waking, even after weeks of sleep restriction. As waking was extended, however, performance during the subjective night deteriorated steeply.

13.6 Banking effects of sleep duration

As implied by the findings related to recovery from sleep restriction (discussed in Section 13.3.3), there is other evidence related to how a prior history of altered sleep amounts affects performance under current sleep conditions. One study examined the effects on PVT performance of two 5-day periods of sleep restriction (4 h of sleep nightly). The two restriction periods were interrupted by a single night with different sleep opportunities, ranging from 0 to 12 h TIB. Regardless of the length of the single recovery opportunity, performance decrements during the second restriction period followed trajectories continuous with that observed during the first 5-day restriction period. Despite immediate recovery of performance in those with the longer sleep opportunities during the intervening recovery night, subsequent performance during sleep restriction reflected their longer-term history of prior sleep restriction (Banks et al., 2023).

These findings imply the existence of long-term, homeostatic regulation of sleep need; other results are consistent with this idea. In one study, male participants (average age ~31 years) performed PVT tests during baseline waking periods, and then spent habitual TIB (~8 h) or extended TIB (~10 h) for 6 nights. They were then tested repeatedly during 38 h of sleep deprivation; participants experienced both sleep conditions in a random order. Both before and during the sleep deprivation period, participants had fewer lapses and faster response times after extended sleep periods. Prior sleep extension also reduced the frequency of unintentional microsleeps during sleep deprivation and increased latencies to fall asleep during MSLTs. Remarkably, the benefits for attention performance of the previous sleep extension days were still present after the 38 h sleep deprivation period and a following recovery night of 10 h TIB for all participants (Arnal et al., 2015).

Participants in another study (men and women, average age ~25 years) either slept their usual durations (averaging just over 7 h nightly) or had 10 h TIB (extended sleep opportunity) for a week. All participants then experienced 3 h TIB for a week followed by 5 days of recovery sleep (8 h TIB). The previously sleep-extended group showed better performance during the last day of sleep restriction on a serial response task (similar to the PVT). They also showed better performance on the task on 3 of 5 days and on a math processing task (involving short-term memory) on 4 of 5 days during the recovery period (Rupp et al., 2009).

The evidence from these studies indicates that prior extended sleep buffered participants against some of the effects of later sleep loss on performance, and that these benefits persisted over one or more recovery days involving a standard sleep duration. These results contrast to the absence of differential effects of prior 12 h and 6 h sleep opportunities in a study reviewed above (Section 13.3.2). It reported no benefit for PVT performance of "banking" more sleep before sleep deprivation, also using a within-participant design (Van Dongen et al., 2004). This difference from the results of (Arnal et al., 2015) may be related to order effects that were noted in the earlier study (Van Dongen et al., 2004), likely because of a shorter gap (2 weeks) between the 6 h and 12 h sleep conditions than the 6-week gap in (Arnal et al., 2015).

These several studies indicate that chronic increases or decreases in sleep relative to habitual durations have long-term performance effects that interact with the immediate effects of participants' current state of sleep satiation. Observing these banking effects may be sensitive to features of experimental designs because of the risk of carry-over effects of sleep history.

13.6.1 Summary

The costs and benefits of long-term differences in sleep amounts can be latent and revealed only under specific conditions. Chronic sleep restriction led to a similar pattern of increasing performance deterioration under subsequent sleep restriction regardless of whether participants had an intervening night of either extended or even more restricted sleep.

Chronic, moderate sleep restriction had hidden effects that were only revealed when people were later challenged by acute total sleep loss or by having to perform tasks at night, especially shortly after waking up. Conversely, "banking" sleep ahead of time can be beneficial, as revealed under some test conditions. Extended sleep durations over several days reduced deficits in people when they were later tested during total sleep deprivation or during sleep–wake cycles that severely restricted sleep.

The persistence of these effects for days after participants who had experienced both extended and habitual sleep were given adequate sleep opportunities indicates that these banking effects may be very long-lasting. These effects are parallel to those caused by chronic, moderate sleep loss, which may result in "banking" undetectable deficits in performance capacity that are only revealed during later periods of acute or chronic sleep loss.

13.7 Sleep loss and executive task performance

13.7.1 Sleep and executive functions in adults and children

Executive tasks assess higher cognitive abilities, which have usually been described as those requiring active cognitive control of behavior (Friedman & Robbins, 2022). These include planning, balancing conflicting demands of multiple tasks (e.g., shifting attention), monitoring consequences, and inhibiting planned responses, in order to achieve specific goals. A succinct summary of executive functioning is "the ability to initiate, monitor, and stop actions so as to achieve goals" (Tucker et al., 2010). It is often defined in contrast to lower-level cognitive mechanisms involved in performing simpler, more automatic tasks; e.g., sustained attention/reaction time tasks, such as the PVT. It remains controversial, however, whether executive tasks measure a unique set of abilities (Salthouse, 2005).

Studies involving experimental sleep restriction in adults found performance deficits on some tasks involving executive functions, but not others (Harrison et al., 2000; Jackson et al., 2013; Jones & Harrison, 2001; Pace-Schott et al., 2009); see (Tucker et al., 2010) for additional references. Reviews and meta-analyses of this literature concluded that sleep loss affected performance on some executive and memory tasks, but that these effects were relatively small compared to those on simple reaction time/attention tasks, and were inconsistent across studies (Lim & Dinges, 2010; Waters & Bucks, 2011).

Executive control is involved in more complex aspects of attention beyond simply maintaining vigilance and responding to events. These aspects include orienting (prioritizing attention to events based on their location or type), filtering to resolve response conflicts, or switching attention among different stimulus dimensions (Posner & Rothbart, 1998). The effects of sleep loss on these tasks depended on the extent and pattern of deprivation and on the specific tasks that were used. For example, one executive function (filtering visual stimuli in a working memory task) was impaired after complete overnight deprivation but not after several nights of partial sleep loss (Drummond et al., 2012). Women who underwent a single night of restricted sleep showed deficits in vigilance and in some executive functions (e.g., filtering and inhibiting responses) but not in others (e.g., dual task performance) (Cunningham et al., 2018).

Studies of preschool- and school-aged children have examined how sleep relates to expression of some of the symptoms seen in children with developmental neurological conditions, who are often reported to have sleep problems. Parental reports of sleep problems in children with neurological conditions (e.g., cerebral palsy, epilepsy, acquired brain injury) were correlated with deficits in executive aspects of verbal working memory tasks (McCann et al., 2018).

Other studies have addressed the relation of sleep features to attention, hyperactivity, language skills, and conduct disorders because these are often problem areas in children diagnosed with attention-deficit hyperactivity disorder (ADHD) and autism spectrum disorders (ASDs). Reviews of this literature indicate that few of these studies addressed executive functions (Davidson et al., 2019; Maski & Kothare, 2013; Reynaud et al., 2018).

One longitudinal study examined how parental sleep-diary reports for their 1-year-old infants correlated with children's general cognitive abilities and performance on specific executive tasks at 2 and 4 years of age. At both ages, total reported sleep amounts at 1 year were unrelated to either general cognition or executive functions. However, the proportion of total sleep that occurred at night at 1 year predicted executive task performance at both 2 and 4 years of age, but did not predict general cognitive abilities (Bernier et al., 2013; Bernier et al., 2010). Another study used actigraphy to monitor sleep in 3–5 year-olds. It reported that more nighttime sleep (or less daytime napping) was associated with reduced errors of commission (impulsive responses) on a Go/No-go task (a test of executive control) and better performance on tests of vocabulary and auditory attention span (Lam et al., 2011).

One interpretation of these findings is that aspects of the infant's social/physical environment promoted both earlier switching to more nocturnal sleep and better performance on executive tasks. An alternative interpretation is that the rate of achieving more mature nocturnality of sleep is a marker of other maturational processes in the brain that play a role in executive functioning. This interpretation is supported by the results of a study of ~6 year-old children, which reported a difference in hippocampal morphology between those who were still habitual nappers and those who had stopped napping. A developmental reduction in napping was associated with more mature features of hippocampal anatomy (Riggins & Spencer, 2020).

An observational study of 8–12 year-old children found that spontaneous higher sleep efficiency (measured by actigraphy) was related to faster completion of the Children's Color Trails-2 task (CCTT-2), which assesses some executive functions, including divided attention and inhibition–disinhibition (Vriend et al., 2012). An observational study of sleep duration measured by actigraphy in adolescents (average age ~13 years), combined with parental assessment of executive functions in daily life, found that shorter sleep was associated with poorer executive functioning, independent of insomnia symptoms (Gruber et al., 2023).

A longitudinal, observational study involved parental reports of children's sleep at several time points between ages 4 and 16. Both the presence of sleep problems (e.g., nightmares, less sleep, trouble sleeping) and the trajectory of changes in sleep problems over time were correlated with performance at age 17 on executive functions (including updating, category shifting, and inhibiting). Sleep problems at any specific age did not predict later executive test performance, but the trajectory of change was important: participants with a decreasing trajectory of sleep problems showed better executive task performance at age 17 (Friedman et al., 2009).

A study of parental reports of sleep duration and problems between 2 and 5 years of age found that shorter sleep overall predicted more parental reports of poor behavioral regulation at age 8 years. In addition, more decrease in sleep duration across ages 2–5 predicted more impulsive errors on a continuous performance task at age 8 years. Parental reports of poor sleep quality in this study did not, however, predict problems with behavioral regulation or impulse control (Nigro et al., 2023).

A study that obtained parental reports on children's nocturnal sleep durations between ages 2.5 to 6 years also obtained school performance reports at age 10. The trajectories of sleep change over these early years predicted academic performance at the later age. Children with sustained short sleep throughout the 2.5–6 year sampling period, and those with very short sleep at 2.5 years that normalized later in the period, had poorer academic performance than those with the recommended 10–11 h of sleep during the sampling period. Sleep duration at 10 years did not predict current academic performance (Petit et al., 2023).

A meta-analysis of observational studies in school-aged children reported a small, but significant, association of reduced sleep amounts with poorer performance on tasks involving executive functions, on multiple-domain cognitive problems, and on school performance (Astill et al., 2012).

There have been few experimental studies of the involvement of sleep specifically in relation to children's executive functions (Reynaud et al., 2018). Performance of 3–6 year-olds on a "flanker" task[4] designed to assess executive attention regulation was more accurate after an afternoon nap than after a similar quiet time spent awake. For one category of trials, responses were also faster for those with longer naps. The benefit observed was similar for habitual non-nappers and nappers. Given the interpretation discussed above that children who have given up habitual napping may be more cognitively mature (Bernier et al., 2013; Bernier et al., 2010), these results

[4] In this task, participants indicate the direction to which a central object is pointing as quickly as they can. The surrounding, identical objects may point in the same direction or the opposite direction, requiring executive control to filter out conflicting information and choose a correct response.

suggest that, even among these children, a nap can still have an immediate benefit for cognitive performance (Cremone et al., 2017), perhaps by reducing current accumulated sleep need.

Sleep restriction of 10–14 year-olds to 5 h TIB (vs. 11 h for controls) impaired performance on two tasks that tap into executive functions: a verbal creativity task and the Wisconsin Card Sorting Test (which requires adaptive switching between dimensions of classification; e.g., color or shape) (Randazzo et al., 1998). Tests of cognitive and emotional regulation were conducted among 8–12 year-old children with habitual sleep reduced by ~30 min for 4 nights compared to those with sleep increased by similar amounts. After the sleep restricted condition, children showed performance deficits in short-term memory, working memory, and the CCTT-2, relative to those in the extended-sleep condition (Vriend et al., 2013).

13.7.2 Possible brain mechanisms

Stroke or injury that damages prefrontal cortical regions impairs executive task performance, suggesting that these regions serve critical roles in executive aspects of cognition. Frontal cortical regions are also responsive to sleep and to sleep loss. Frontal and other association cortices showed especially large decreases in metabolism during sleep (Braun et al., 1997), larger increases in slow-wave energy (SWE)[5] than other regions during chronic sleep restriction (Skorucak et al., 2018), and the largest increases in low-frequency EEG activity during recovery sleep after deprivation (Cajochen et al., 1999)

The interpretation that SWA levels during recovery sleep reflect a buildup of homeostatic sleep need during waking was supported by evidence that the higher levels of SWA in frontal regions early in NREM sleep gradually diminished over the course of recovery sleep (Werth et al., 1997). Taken together, these results suggest that insufficient sleep could impair executive task performance by curtailing sleep-related recovery processes involving SWA in the prefrontal cortex (Beebe & Gozal, 2002; Horne, 1993; Reynaud et al., 2018).

It is, however, unclear whether performance deficits on tests of executive function are always related to changes in prefrontal brain mechanisms that are specifically involved in these functions. Overall performance on tests of executive functions depends on sensory, motor, and motivational subprocesses linked to many brain regions (Baddeley, 1998; Jones & Harrison, 2001; Tucker et al., 2010) (**Figure 13.13**). One study attempted to determine whether methods used to assess executive functions identify a unique set of specific, "executive" cognitive abilities. It concluded that the functions involved are quite general and closely related to other cognitive abilities, such as reasoning and perceptual speed (Salthouse, 2005).

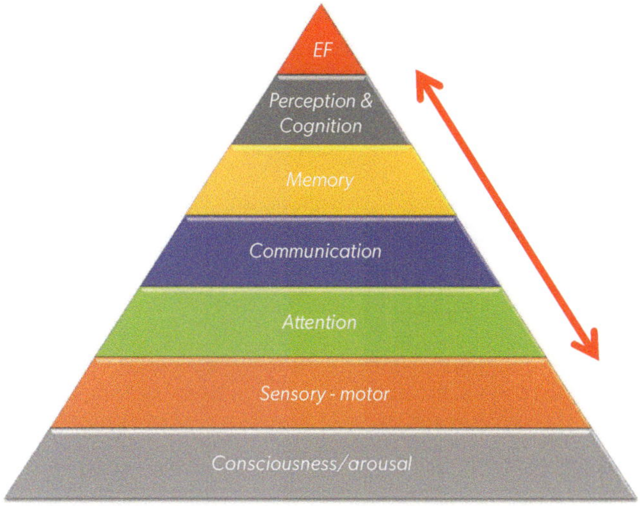

Figure 13.13 This image reflects a hierarchy of interacting cognitive functions; EF refers to Executive Functions. The double-headed arrow indicates the two-way relations among the different kinds of cognitive functioning. In the context of this discussion, it indicates that executive performance depends on a hierarchy of other kinds of cognitive functions. Impaired performance on executive tasks can arise at the executive level but can also result from impairments at any of the levels that feed up to the executive level. Thus, impaired arousal, attention, memory, etc. can result in impaired performance on an executive task, without implying that executive mechanisms are themselves impaired. Reprinted with permission from Dr. Gail Eskes, Dalhousie University.

Sleep loss could affect executive performance in several ways: by impairing prefrontal cortical functioning; by interfering with "lower-level" processes that provide input into executive mechanisms, such as stimulus detection or encoding (Jackson et al., 2013; Lim & Dinges, 2010); or by reducing motivation or arousal (Jones & Harrison, 2001). Some studies that were designed to assess the independent roles of executive processes and lower-level functions after sleep loss found that overall performance on executive *tasks* was clearly impaired, but that there were no deficits attributable specifically to the executive *processes* involved (Roca et al., 2012; Tucker et al., 2010). Instead, performance was impaired by other deficits that affected executive systems indirectly.

Brain imaging studies have found that performance of executive tasks after sleep deprivation increased activation in the same brain regions that are activated in sleep-satiated people, but also recruited activation in other regions. The more difficult and complex the task, the more robust was the additional activation (Chee & Choo, 2004; Drummond et al., 2004). These results suggest that one reason sleep loss causes relatively small or variable deficits in performance of difficult executive tasks

[5] SWE is a cumulative measure of SWA derived from multiplying the average SWA in NREM sleep epochs in 30 min recording segments by the number of NREM sleep epochs in each segment.

is that participants often recruit additional neural resources to compensate for their sleepiness. In contrast, repetitive, boring tasks such as the PVT may not trigger similar recruitment, resulting in larger performance deficits (Chee & Choo, 2004; Lim & Dinges, 2010).

13.7.3 Summary

Experimental sleep loss in adults can impair performance on some executive tasks, but usually less severely than performance on simple vigilance tasks. Most studies in children have been correlational, either cross-sectional or longitudinal. Their interpretation is limited by the frequent use of parental reports about "sleep problems," "poor sleep" or equivalent terms, which may have a variety of meanings.

Different studies have identified either poor sleep quality or short sleep early in development as predicting problems with impulse control or executive task performance in school-age children. There is also evidence that early or sustained inadequate sleep durations at young ages are associated with poorer academic performance in preadolescent children. It is not clear whether these longitudinal correlations reflect effects of early inadequate sleep on cognitive development or whether other variables influence both early sleep and later behavior and academic achievement.

There have been fewer studies of effects of experimental sleep restriction on executive task performance in children. However, these studies generally found that aspects of executive task performance were worse in children with reduced sleep. In addition, the extent of maturation of sleep in preschool age children, as indexed by longer nocturnal sleep and less napping, was associated with fewer executive task deficits.

Sleep loss appears to generate especially strong sleep need in frontal brain regions, and damage to these regions is known to impair executive functions. The observed deficits after sleep loss have, therefore, often been attributed to impaired frontal lobe functioning. Despite these links, the experimental evidence does not necessarily imply that sleep loss affects frontal executive mechanisms specifically. Performance deficits on executive tasks can result from disruption of lower-level functions, such as alertness, motivation, and stimulus encoding, on which executive functions depend.

Brain imaging studies show that executive tasks recruit more brain regions, including frontal cortical mechanisms, after sleep loss. More complex, difficult tasks increase brain activation more strongly and widely. This finding may explain why performance on challenging executive tasks is often less affected than performance on simple, repetitive reaction-time tests of attention, which are not likely to recruit additional neural resources to the same extent.

13.8 Effects of sleep loss on emotional regulation and perception

13.8.1 Studies in children

A review of observational studies involving preschoolers found that "sleep problems" (variously defined) were associated with emotional, behavioral, and cognitive problems, although results were often inconsistent among studies, especially among those with small numbers of participants (Reynaud et al., 2018). Among school-aged children and adolescents, both sleep problems earlier in development and current short sleep were associated with the presence of internalizing symptoms (e.g., anxiety, depression) and externalizing symptoms (hyperactivity, conduct problems) (Astill et al., 2012; Beebe, 2011; Foley & Weinraub, 2017; Gregory & O'Connor, 2002; Ojio et al., 2016). Persistent (in contrast to transient) insomnia symptoms during childhood predicted an increased incidence of anxiety and externalizing symptoms in late adolescence (Armstrong et al., 2014). Among adolescents (11–19 years), a large survey study linked worse sleep quality to reduced positive emotions and increased negative emotions (Shen et al., 2018).

As with other observational studies, these findings do not establish a causal relation between sleep problems and emotional or cognitive functioning. Stronger supportive evidence comes from longitudinal studies that showed associations between early sleep symptoms and later problems with emotional regulation.[6] It is likely that there are bidirectional relations between emotional and sleep problems, the nature of which will need to be established using larger studies and experimental approaches.

A "natural experiment" is the presence of obstructive sleep apnea (OSA; see Appendix B) in young children. This condition disrupts and shortens sleep and periodically reduces blood oxygenation. It is associated with a variety of behavioral and cognitive symptoms, including problems related to attention, emotional regulation, hyperactivity, and cognition. A similar range of symptoms are seen in children diagnosed with attention deficit/hyperactivity disorder (ADHD) (Fischman et al., 2015; Yu et al., 2017). Breathing disorders accompanied by short sleep in infants predicted cognitive deficits as early as 2 years of age (Smithson et al., 2018) as well as later symptoms of hyperactivity, emotional dysregulation, and conduct problems (Bonuck et al., 2012). Among adults with untreated OSA, there is also evidence for impairments in vigilance, executive functions, and motor coordination (Beebe et al., 2003).

[6] For a discussion of links between early sleep problems and a clinical mood disorder, see Section 15.3.3.

In young children, OSA is often the result of enlarged tonsils and/or adenoids impinging on the airway during sleep. This condition may be treated with surgical removal of the obstructing structures (adenotonsillectomy [ATX]). ATX in children with OSA (5–9 years old) resulted in improvements in breathing during sleep as well as in several domains of cognitive functioning 6–10 months after surgery (Friedman et al., 2003). In another study, approximately 28% (22/78) of children with OSA (5–13 years old) had behavioral profiles consistent with a diagnosis of ADHD, including high levels of hyperactivity and inattention. A year after ATX surgery that corrected their breathing symptoms, half of these children (11/22) no longer met diagnostic criteria for ADHD (Chervin et al., 2006).

These results are consistent with the idea that a significant proportion of cognitive and emotional regulatory problems in children with OSA result from their disrupted sleep and periodic blood deoxygenation. One estimate was that controlling snoring and sleep-related breathing disorders could eliminate ADHD symptoms in 25% of all children diagnosed with ADHD (Chervin et al., 1997).

A meta-analysis including 11 studies of children who had OSA reported that they had significant impairments relative to healthy controls in general intelligence, memory, attention-executive function, and verbal ability. Assessments 6–12 months after ATX showed normalized functions in the attention-executive and verbal ability domains, but not in general intelligence and memory (Yu et al., 2017). The persistent deficits could indicate that more recovery time was needed to approach control performance levels across all cognitive domains. Alternatively, a history of reduced blood oxygenation and disrupted sleep could have compromised developing neural mechanisms and produced long-lasting deficits. This idea is supported by evidence of continued cognitive deficits in adults even after successful treatment for OSA symptoms (Bédard et al., 1993; Lau et al., 2010).

Experimental studies in children also support a connection between sleep loss and emotional and behavioral dysregulation. Among school-age children and adolescents, sleep restriction ranging from modest to severe over a few days reduced positive affective responses, increased emotional lability, and, in some studies, increased negative emotions. These effects were assessed using a variety of measures that included parent or teacher ratings, self-reports, performance on formal tests, physiological measures, and observed behavior in the course of social interactions (Baum et al., 2014; Dagys et al., 2012; Gruber et al., 2012; McMakin et al., 2016; Talbot et al., 2010; Vriend et al., 2013).

The conclusion that reduced sleep results in negative effects on emotional regulation is supported by evidence that extending sleep has the opposite effect. Lengthening sleep in preteen children by less than 30 min nightly reduced emotional lability and restless-impulsive behaviors (Gruber et al., 2012), and extending nightly sleep in adolescents during school nights by an average of 73 min reduced symptoms of sleepiness and emotional dysregulation (Van Dyk et al., 2017).

Other findings related to the effects of short sleep on emotional regulation, school performance, health, and safety of adolescents were reviewed in Section 4.4.4, along with a discussion of the benefits of instituting later school start times to facilitate teens getting more adequate sleep amounts.

Reviews of the potential role of childhood sleep-related symptoms in the development of problems with emotional regulation and of psychiatric conditions later in life identified a number of methodological and analytic issues. Topics that were identified as needing additional focus included the following: how best to use objective and subjective measures of sleep; determining which sleep characteristics have predictive power, beyond broad terms like "sleep problems"; improving the validation of outcome measures; conducting more longitudinal studies; identifying mechanisms that link sleep developmentally to the outcomes of interest; and setting these analyses in the context of family conditions (Gregory & Sadeh, 2016; Lollies et al., 2022; Reynaud et al., 2018).

13.8.2 Studies in adults

Sleep loss in adults has been associated with increased negative moods. Sleep restriction increased confusion, tension, and total mood disturbance (Dinges et al., 1997) and led to more somatic complaints and symptoms of anxiety, depression, and paranoia (Kahn-Greene et al., 2007). Reducing total sleep amounts or repeatedly disrupting sleep continuity also increased negative or decreased positive mood self-ratings, with the latter effect being mediated by reductions in SWS (Finan et al., 2017; Finan et al., 2015).

Meta-analyses of the relations between sleep and emotional regulation across ages reported somewhat different results based on the inclusion of different sets of studies. One analysis reported large effects, especially of total sleep deprivation, in reducing positive emotions, and more modest effects of sleep loss in increasing negative emotions (Tomaso et al., 2021). An analysis that included more studies also found large effects of sleep loss or disruption in reducing positive affect, increasing anxiety, and blunting emotional responses. It noted mixed effects across studies of sleep loss on negative emotions, and an effect of loss of REM sleep, but little effect of loss of SWS sleep, on emotional responses to negative stimuli (Palmer et al., 2023).

Adult participants in one study rated the intensity of emotional expression of images of faces twice, once before and once after one group had a daytime nap opportunity and the other remained awake. The daytime naps (especially naps including REM sleep) reduced later ratings of the emotional intensity of faces portraying anger or fear relative to controls, indicating that sleep reduced the subjective intensity of negative emotional stimuli (Gujar, McDonald, et al., 2011).

Another approach to studying the impact of sleep and sleep loss on emotion-related stimuli is evaluating how well people recognize the nature of the emotion being portrayed in a facial image. Participants who had undergone sleep loss had a reduced ability to recognize the differences between neutral and emotional facial expressions and to discriminate the intensity of emotional expressions on faces (Ben Simon et al., 2015; Goldstein-Piekarski et al., 2015; van der Helm et al., 2010), although not necessarily for all emotions (Cote et al., 2014).

Stimuli used in most of these studies were static, often ambiguous, facial images. In contrast, overnight sleep deprivation did not impair the accuracy of discriminating emotions when these were portrayed in video clips by actors using rich visual and auditory cues[7] (Holding et al., 2017). These results suggest that more complex presentations of emotional stimuli can overcome the effects of sleep loss on the interpretation of static images.

However, the results obtained using static, information-poor images may be especially relevant to some real-world conditions. Law-enforcement personnel may have to make judgments about a person's emotional state and intentions under conditions that provide only ambiguous, degraded information about facial and other cues that reflect emotional states. These conditions can involve poorly lit locations at night and may be encountered by personnel who are themselves working with inadequate sleep; see Section 13.9.

Other studies related to emotions and sleep have examined its involvement in memory for emotional stimuli; this topic is discussed in Section 17.4.

Given the impacts of sleep loss on emotion regulation, it is not surprising that there are also effects on behavior and interpersonal relations. Self-rated poor sleep overnight in one member of a couple was associated with increased interpersonal conflict the next day and reduced capacity for conflict resolution (Gordon & Chen, 2014). In a prison population, short sleep was associated with increases in hostility, self-rated aggression, and impulsivity (Kamphuis et al., 2014). An online study reported that poor sleep quality was associated with increases in self-reported aggression, hostility, and stress. These effects were mediated in part by the influence of sleep quality on emotion regulation, and this mediation was strongest for physical aggression (Demichelis et al., 2022).

13.8.3 Mechanisms of sleep effects on emotion regulation

Studies have examined mechanisms that may contribute to the effects of sleep and sleep loss on evaluation of emotional stimuli. Sleep loss affected fMRI-based measures of neural activity in response to negative images. Staying awake for 35 h resulted in increased amygdala[8] activation, relative to controls, in response to emotionally aversive visual stimuli. This activation was also less strongly correlated with activity in the medial prefrontal cortex and more strongly correlated with activity in other brainstem structures that are involved in emotion regulation (Yoo et al., 2007). Similarly, sleep loss was reported to increase positive evaluations of positive emotional stimuli, with similar patterns of increased amygdala activation and altered functional connectivity with frontal cortical regions and parts of the limbic system (Gujar, Yoo, et al., 2011).

Animal studies support the idea that sleep loss strengthens positive emotional reactions. Sleep deprivation in mice increased later intake of an attractive sweet solution, in this case by reducing input from the frontal cortex to the nucleus accumbens, a structure that is involved in evaluating reward value (Liu et al., 2016). Sleep restriction also increased disinhibited eating and the selection of attractive, calorie-rich foods in people; see Section 14.7. These results are consistent with the idea that sleep loss impairs the modulatory function exerted by frontal cortical regions on both positive and negative emotional responses mediated by subcortical systems (Gujar, Yoo, et al., 2011; Yoo et al., 2007).

This interpretation may also account for the results of laboratory studies of risky decision making after sleep loss, typically measured using gambling tasks in people. Experimental sleep loss increased risky and impulsive gambling choices and reduced the ability to inhibit responses to negative stimuli, suggesting a decrease in emotional self-regulation (Anderson & Platten, 2011; Killgore et al., 2006; Womack et al., 2013). People reporting spontaneous short sleep, and those combining habitual short sleep with self-reported greater sleep need, also showed increased impulsivity and made riskier choices (Curtis et al., 2018; Lau et al., 2019). The patterns of risk-taking and disinhibition after sleep loss suggest an effect on evaluations of risk and reward, which have been linked to the activity of the ventromedial prefrontal cortex (vmPFC) (Libedinsky et al., 2011; Womack et al., 2013).

The vmPFC and a linked network, including part of the parietal lobe, have also been implicated in the regulation of social cognition and prosocial behaviors, such as making

[7] Auditory cues were meaningless syllables that allowed actors to express emotions vocally without using real words that would explicitly convey their intended emotional states.

[8] The amygdala is a temporal lobe structure that plays an important role in regulating emotions in combination with other brain regions. Its activation can be inhibited by projections from the prefrontal cortex.

charitable donations (Hare et al., 2010). Overnight sleep deprivation reduced charitable giving in a laboratory game situation and was associated with reduced activity in the medial PFC and components of the social cognition network, including the temporoparietal junction (TPJ), middle temporal gyrus, and inferior frontal gyrus (Ben Simon et al., 2022). A later study found that the extent of prosocial behavior in a laboratory task that involved making monetary donations was positively correlated with the amount of SWA that participants had shown in the TPJ region during the previous night's sleep (Studler et al., 2024).

13.8.4 Summary

Habitual short sleep and acute sleep loss have been associated with higher levels of anxiety, depression, impulsivity, hostility, and interpersonal conflict. Persistent insomnia during childhood predicted more anxiety and externalizing symptoms in late adolescence. Poorer sleep quality in adolescents increased negative and decreased positive emotions in young adulthood. A sleep-related breathing disorder (OSA) disrupts sleep continuity and reduces blood oxygenation during sleep; it was associated with hyperactivity and inattention in children, which can mimic symptoms of ADHD. Surgical correction of airway obstruction in children with OSA reduced these symptoms in many of these children. It also improved some, but not all, cognitive symptoms associated with OSA.

Sleep loss increased the intensity of both negative and positive emotional responses to stimuli with emotional content; but the strength of these effects varied, with more robust effects on positive emotions. These changes were linked to reduced inhibitory input from frontal cortical regions to brainstem motivational systems. Variable results among studies may be related to the measures used, the degree of sleep loss, the age of participants, and other experimental variables.

Sleep loss also impaired the accuracy of discriminating emotional states when these tests were based on viewing ambiguous, static images, which may be relevant to some real-world settings. Sleep loss did not alter discrimination of emotional states when more elaborate visual and auditory cues were used to represent these states. These results indicate that a rich array of relevant stimuli can overcome the deficits in discrimination of emotional states induced by sleep loss.

The idea that sleep loss disrupts frontal cortical regulation of brainstem motivational systems is supported by evidence that it impaired emotional and behavioral self-regulation (e.g., increased consumption of attractive, energy-rich foods in people and increased sucrose intake in mice). Impaired emotional self-regulation related to poor sleep quality was also associated with increased interpersonal conflict and, in a prison setting, with increased hostility and aggression. Reductions in prosocial behaviors after sleep loss were correlated with reduced activity in the prefrontal cortex and temporoparietal junction (TPJ), part of a social cognition network. The amount of spontaneously produced SWA in the TPJ during sleep predicted the extent of later prosocial behavior, consistent with the involvement of sleep in supporting prosocial behavior and sleep loss in various forms of antisocial behavior.

13.9 Adverse work hours and shift work

13.9.1 Shift work and sleep loss

Some of the interest in how sleep loss affects human performance is related to the fact that people who experience adverse work shifts (those that occur during the night or that result in staying awake for more than 16 h) are inevitably sleep deprived to some extent. Shift work involving adverse shifts is quite common. One estimate in 2014 was that 15–30% of the adult work force in industrialized nations are involved in shift work, and this proportion has probably increased since that time (Boivin & Boudreau, 2014).

Several elements contributed to the growth of shift work over the last 100+ years, including factories that could operate around the clock as a result of electrification late in the 19th century (see Chapter 6); the desire for continuous health and protection services (hospitals, ambulances, firefighters, police, military); and demands for rapid, long-distance transportation by road, sea, rail, and air. Another driver of increased shift work is the growth in many parts of the world of 24 h services (gas stations, convenience stores, casinos, pharmacies, restaurants, etc.), partly in response to the number of potential customers who are awake and active at all hours. More recently, the spread of internet access across the world has facilitated and encouraged around-the-clock international financial, communications, gaming, and entertainment activities (see **Box 13.1**). As a result, large portions of the population are now working, traveling, and playing at nontraditional hours.

Those working at night, or for long hours, typically sleep less (because their work extends into or through their usual sleep hours) or sleep at different times of day. As discussed in Chapter 5, sleep that occurs at an inappropriate circadian phase is usually shortened and disrupted, despite increased homeostatic sleep drive (Åkerstedt, 2003; Åkerstedt & Wright Jr., 2009). Critical care nurses, for example, slept less between two successive night shifts than between two successive day shifts (Hirsch Allen et al., 2014), and nurses that experienced more "quick returns" (<11 h) between shifts had an increased risk of experiencing pathological fatigue and shift-work disorder (Flo et al., 2014).

BOX 13.1 Technology Gives and Technology Takes Away

Electrification, the internet, and computer technology promoted work and play beyond the daytime, but computer-based automation can also reduce the number of people working on adverse schedules. This change has already occurred in manufacturing industries where robotic systems have replaced some humans in many routine factory jobs. More advanced robotic systems are now being used to drive vehicles without human assistance.

It is possible that in the future self-driving trucks, buses, trains, and taxis, guided by computers that have no circadian rhythms and need no sleep, could greatly reduce the number of people providing transportation services at night (and during the day), assuming related safety concerns are addressed. Self-driving vehicles have already operated in some locations and, at this moment, self-driving "robotaxis" are operating on the streets of San Francisco.

The safety benefits of not having sleepy humans in control of vehicles during the night are offset by concerns about the potential job losses involved. In the 2011 Canadian census, "transport truck driver" was the second largest employment category for men over age 15 (>253,000 men); another >82,000 men were delivery/courier drivers (http://tinyurl.com/l72kp7t). The combination of these two made up the largest employment category for adult men in Canada. It is challenging to think of where these drivers will find employment if self-driving vehicles become the norm. At least one company involved in these developments has countered that vehicles driving themselves for 24 h daily will need more frequent, at least partially human-supported, maintenance than standard vehicles, providing new employment opportunities for some workers.

Those working at night are also at a double disadvantage in their job performance because their circadian clocks are promoting sleep while at work and because inadequate daytime sleep adds homeostatic sleep drive to the impact of circadian phase. As a result, job performance during the night can deteriorate, as illustrated in many surveys and in the experimental studies that are discussed later in this chapter. There is, for example, a large literature documenting the deficits in performance and effects on personal health of physicians working long hours and adverse shifts (Anderson et al., 2012; Landrigan et al., 2004; McHill, Czeisler, et al., 2018; Philibert, 2005; Rollinson et al., 2003; Sharpe et al., 2010).

13.9.2 Sleepiness and public safety

There is no doubt that there is an increased tendency for workers to make errors at night and when sleep deprived, but it is more difficult to predict the effects of these errors in specific situations. Errors made by one member of a health care team may be noticed and corrected by others. A police officer may fall asleep in a parked vehicle at night but become rapidly alert in response to an emergency radio call. In fact, despite working adverse shifts on many occasions, an individual worker may not cause any serious problems.

This situation is analogous to jaywalking through traffic or riding in a vehicle without a seatbelt: although these behaviors are known to be unsafe, most such excursions do not result in accidents or injuries. Nevertheless, at a population level, not wearing a seatbelt when an accident does occur increases the risk of serious injury or death. In 2015, for example, the US National Highway Traffic Safety Administration (NHTSA) reported that ~11.5% of vehicle occupants in the United States were not restrained by seat belts or car seats, but they accounted for nearly 50% of those killed in traffic accidents (https://tinyurl.com/mw9d5fv).

Similarly, when accidents related to sleepiness occur, as they inevitably will, they can be catastrophic. The result is that there are frequent news reports of sleep-related accidents in transportation (e.g., cars going off the road under good driving conditions), resulting in the deaths of its occupants and others typically at night or during a long drive. Although falling asleep does not leave any physical evidence, its role in serious accidents or near misses is often readily inferred (see **Box 13.2**).

In a 2009 poll by the US National Sleep Foundation, 28% of respondents reported falling asleep while driving during the preceding year, and drowsy driving in the United States was estimated to cause ~100,000 accidents and >1,500 deaths annually. The National Highway Traffic Safety Administration reported that 42% of serious injury or fatal accidents caused by drifting out of the lane were the result of driver incapacitation. Half of those were incapacitated by drugs, alcohol, or illness; the other half were apparently asleep.

These may be underestimates since it is often difficult to establish the role of driver sleepiness in accidents. Given the large number of people reporting falling asleep while driving, it is perhaps surprising that the number of accidents is not larger. This may reflect the fact that disasters resulting from human error typically involve a combination of factors, each of which has a low probability: a car drifting toward your lane or a deer or pedestrian entering the roadway just as you experience a 2–3 sec microsleep. Hence, such accidents are statistically rare relative to the number of vehicles and of drowsy drivers on

BOX 13.2 Sleep and Circadian Phase in Transportation Accidents

In some cases, the role of sleep can be inferred from accident conditions. For example, news sources reported that a vehicle went off Interstate 25 in Colorado in June 2008 under good driving conditions at 04:30, killing all seven occupants. A family member suggested they must have fallen asleep after driving "day and night" to try to get home to Alberta.

Other accidents and potential accidents are demonstrably related to excess sleepiness and falling asleep:

- Researchers in Sweden, who accompanied drivers on trains overnight to study their behavior, observed drivers going straight through red stop signals without seeing or responding to them (Torsvall & Åkerstedt, 1987).
- In 2008, two pilots on a passenger plane flight in the morning failed to respond to a Hawaii control tower's repeated calls after they had overflown their destination; both were asleep (https://tinyurl.com/ybw9sw7k). The captain was diagnosed with severe obstructive sleep apnea, which disrupts sleep and leads to sometimes severe daytime sleepiness (see Appendix B).
- In 2011, two planes landed during the night at a Washington DC airport without control tower guidance because the one air traffic controller on duty in the tower had fallen asleep during his fourth consecutive night shift (https://tinyurl.com/y72f5h2r).
- In 2014, a train entering Chicago's O'Hare airport at 03:50 overshot the end of the line and drove partway up an escalator, resulting in 34 injuries and $6 million in damage. The driver admitted to falling asleep, as she had done the previous month, and indicated she had worked a lot of overtime recently (https://tinyurl.com/2ecxo3kt).

the road. But when these low-probability events coincide, the results are often tragic.

Despite the difficulty of demonstrating the cause of any one accident, the literature related to major catastrophes over recent decades strongly suggests a role for sleep loss and circadian phase as contributing factors. The partial meltdown of the nuclear power plant at Three Mile Island, Pennsylvania in 1979 occurred around 4 AM when workers failed to understand the nature of a mechanical problem and took inappropriate steps in trying to fix it (http://tinyurl.com/2j92yt). The catastrophic meltdown of the Chernobyl nuclear plant in Ukraine in 1986, resulting in thousands of deaths and many more illnesses, occurred when a poorly prepared work crew took over control of a dangerous test of the system during the night (https://en.wikipedia.org/wiki/Chernobyl_disaster).

Analyses of these incidents (and many others) include reports of individuals activating inappropriate systems, misinterpreting confusing information, and failing to resolve conflicting data. These are the kinds of cognitive errors to which both inadequate sleep and working at an adverse circadian phase can contribute. Reports on the causes of two major accidents involving US Naval vessels highlighted these features, as reported in the New York Times in 2017 (https://nyti.ms/2z34Xz5).

In the case of the USS Fitzgerald in June 2017, the accident was attributed to bridge officers failing to recognize how close they were to another ship and making poor decisions starting around 01:00, contributing to an accident that killed seven crew members. In the case of the USS John S. McCain in August 2017, the commanding officer had been on duty since 01:15 and was joined by his second in command at 04:30. Starting around 05:20, crew members made mistakes and misunderstood the condition of their steering and propulsion systems while attempting to respond to an imminent collision, resulting ultimately in an accident that caused 10 deaths. Among other responses, naval warships were subsequently ordered to increase crew sleep time and reduce workweeks to a maximum of 100 h.

13.9.3 Medical trainees

There is a long history of interest in the effects of extended work hours on physician performance, especially during the middle of the night. An example of an effect on performance of medical residents using a simulated patient during an extended wake period is shown in **Figure 13.14** (Sharpe et al., 2010). A well-known case involving an actual patient is that of Libby Zion, an undergraduate student who died in New York Hospital in 1984 in part because of errors and misjudgments during her treatment in the middle of the night. Legal proceedings and other investigations reached somewhat different conclusions about the factors that contributed to her avoidable death. One issue highlighted was that medical residents involved in her care were working 36 h duty shifts. Partly as a result of this incident, work shifts for residents were restricted to a maximum of 24 h and their workweek to 80 h, first in New York State and then nationally in the United States (in 2003). These limits have since been modified further and remain the object of intense debate (McHill, Czeisler, et al., 2018). Other jurisdictions have different limits; junior doctors in the European Union are limited to a 48 h workweek and must have 11 continuous hours off work per day, although there is a provision for opting out of these limits.

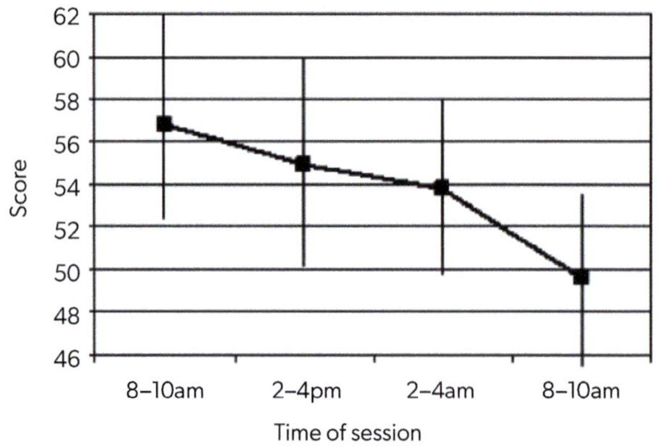

Figure 13.14 Performance ratings (Y axis) of internal medicine residents dealing with complex, critically ill patient scenarios (e.g., meningitis, massive pulmonary embolism) presented by a high-fidelity simulated patient during 26 h of continuous waking (X axis). The patient scenarios required complex analyses and decision making in order to identify the medical condition, review "patient" charts, and select appropriate interventions. The values shown are the mean scores (± SEM) of ratings made by experts of videotaped performance of the residents, without knowledge of the time of day. There was a significant, near-linear decline in ratings of performance as length of time awake increased overnight and into the next morning. Similarly, in other studies, deficits were reported during the latter part of night shifts in intubation procedure skills, vigilance performance, and fluid intelligence test scores. Reprinted with permission from Sharpe, R. et al. (2010) The impact of prolonged continuous wakefulness on resident clinical performance in the intensive care unit: a patient simulator study. *Crit Care Med* 38(3): 766–770. © 2010 by the Society of Critical Care Medicine and Lippincott Williams & Wilkins. doi: 10.1097/CCM.0b013e3181cd122a.

On-the-job performance is not the only issue for medical trainees; those working extended shifts are also at increased risk of motor vehicle accidents after work. In one study, interns who drove home after a shift of 24 h or longer (an "extended shift") were 5.9 times more likely to report a near-miss incident, and 2.3 times more likely to report an actual accident than after a <24 h shift. The same study compared interns who had or had not worked extended shifts in the last month. Those who had worked 1–4 or ≥5 extended shifts were, respectively, 1.7 and 3.7 times as likely to fall asleep while stopped at a red light than those with no extended shifts. Even worse, they were 1.8 and 2.4 times more likely to fall asleep while actually driving (Barger et al., 2005).

In other studies, resident physicians who had worked a heavy on-call schedule (80–90 h work per week), showed impaired vigilance and driving performance compared to their performance after a "light" schedule (~44 h work per week) (Arnedt et al., 2005), and repeated adverse work shifts had cumulative effects on performance (Anderson et al., 2012). Physicians are well aware of the effects of their work schedules on sleepiness and on their own and others' safety (see **Box 13.3** for one attempt at reducing the risk of sleepiness while driving).

BOX 13.3 An Unusual Countermeasure for Sleepiness

Because of the risks involved in sleepy driving, many kinds of countermeasures to sleepiness have been developed and tried (alerting drugs, loud music, cold air, and eye monitors that trigger an alarm when slow, drifting eye movements are detected). A few years ago, I had the pleasure of hosting Dr. Charles Czeisler, a leading expert on circadian rhythms and physician work hours, as a visiting speaker at Dalhousie University. During one of his presentations, he heard from an emergency room physician about a novel countermeasure to sleepiness.

She was acutely aware of how dangerously sleepy she might be in the morning after finishing an overnight shift at the hospital. Before she started her commute home, she put her long hair in a ponytail and closed her car's sunroof on the end of the ponytail, so that the closed window would tug at her hair if her head snapped forward as she fell asleep while driving. This creative countermeasure to sleepiness, along with many others that have been tried, probably had some net benefit, but none are as effective as getting adequate sleep.

Several observational and experimental studies examined the impact of regulations that restricted resident workweeks in the United States. Some studies found an improved sense of well-being among residents. But they also reported that residents were getting fewer educational opportunities because attending presentations during the day extended their time in the hospital beyond their allowed weekly limit; more senior residents were especially negative about their educational experience (Goitein et al., 2005). Shorter shifts also reduced the amount of overlap among caregivers in the hospital, resulting in more frequent transfers of care and the risk of less effective communication about patients. Because of these issues, many residents reported that they were less satisfied with their overall clinical and educational experience, despite reporting some reduction in their perceived risk of burnout (Goitein et al., 2005; Gopal et al., 2005).

After resident work hours were restricted in the United States, two studies were also designed to test whether 30 h work shifts actually increased risks to patient care. These studies required waiving the restriction that was in effect at the time, which limited first-year residents to maximum shift durations of 16 h. Publicity about the existence of these studies led to a heated debate about the ethics of exposing patients to potential risks as a result of their caregivers working 30 h shifts, weighed against the desire to establish empirically the true extent of these risks (Lenzer, 2015). Studies of the effects of reduced shift

Table 13.1 Factors Related to Work Hours of Resident Physicians

Problems related to extended work hours of residents
- Risk of medical errors and implications for current patient health and safety
- Risks of resident traffic accidents after adverse shifts
- Resident stress and burnout related to excess work hours
Problems related to reducing lengths of shifts and total work hours
- Communication issues during increased handovers of care
- Reduced extent and quality of education and hands-on training for residents
- Risk to quality of care for future patients if training is not adequate
- Requirement for additional staff, which increases costs for the health care system and the public that funds it

lengths for residents have produced mixed results in relation to both benefits and costs, and the risk of burnout among residents remains high (McHill, Czeisler, et al., 2018).

The issues related to resident work hours illustrate a few of the many complexities and trade-offs that bedevil trying to assess the impact of adverse work hours, and then to regulate them optimally, even in just this one profession (see **Table 13.1**). Similar issues have been debated in relation to work hours in other professions, including firefighters, police officers, nurses, pilots, air traffic controllers, military personnel, and others.

13.9.4 Summary

There is a wealth of evidence that cognitive performance deteriorates when people stay awake overnight. This deterioration reduces the ability of people driving cars, trucks, trains, and airplanes, as well as workers in many different industries, to do their work safely and effectively at night. These effects are compounded by being awake for more than 16 h at a time. Nevertheless, an increasing number of societal demands for 24 h safety, health, entertainment, and other services has led a large proportion of the workforce to be involved in working on adverse schedules (i.e., being awake for extended periods (>16 h) and/or working during the night).

Inadequate functioning because of sleepiness resulting from adverse work schedules have contributed regularly to accidents on the road, to errors in other transportation settings, to mistakes in health care and in other professions, and to some major disasters.

Physicians have traditionally worked long hours during their training in clinical settings. These training experiences are critical to their development of necessary skills, and they contribute importantly during these periods to the medical services available to the public. However, the extended work hours increase risks for both patients and physicians and are also a source of stress that increases the risk of burnout.

Attempts to address these problems have included legislated reductions in shift lengths and total weekly work hours allowed for residents during their training years. Some research shows that these changes resulted in reduced risk of burnout and improved self-assessed wellbeing. However, residents expressed concerns that limitations on work hours reduced their learning opportunities and reduced the quality of patient care, in part, because of increases in transfers of care. These handovers interrupt the continuity of care and increase the chances of miscommunication and missing patient information. Adding additional staff to replace the reduced work hours of physicians increases costs for the health care system and for society in general.

13.10 Physiological effects of jet lag and shift work

13.10.1 The nature of jet lag

Jet lag is a useful model to consider when trying to understand the impacts of shift work. Jet lag is the result of traveling rapidly across multiple time zones (transmeridian flights) and attempting to function at times that are shifted relative to a person's previous phase of circadian rhythm entrainment. It is not the geographical change that is relevant, but the speed with which it is achieved on a modern jet. Crossing four time zones by walking from Halifax to Vancouver would cause no circadian disruption. A person's circadian system would receive continually updated information from the changing timing of light exposure while traveling and would synchronize accordingly over the many days needed to complete the journey (~46 days of continuous walking, according to Google maps). Similarly, travel on horseback, by stagecoach, or overseas by boat, would allow time for local solar-day cues to gradually phase shift circadian systems (see Chapter 3).

It was only the advent of modern airplane travel that allowed people to cross multiple time zones over durations that are much shorter than the circadian system needs to adjust its phase—hence, the name of the disorder. The result is that our circadian system can find itself in an environment in which local cues about time of day (light–dark cycles, mealtimes, social interactions) may be up to 12 h out of phase with its own internally generated cycles. Adjusting to the new environmental time cues takes several days (the number depending on how many time zones were crossed), during which most people have trouble falling or staying asleep at night and experience digestive upsets and daytime sleepiness.

Animal models have revealed additional complexities in the physiology of phase-shifting that would make adaptation to a new time zone problematic. Mice were exposed to abrupt shifts of the external lighting cycle to mimic the effects of rapid transmeridian flights, and various organs were then dissected out and cultured in vitro, including the suprachiasmatic nuclei (SCN). Clock gene expression rhythms in the cultured tissues continued to oscillate, but rhythms in peripheral tissues shifted more slowly than those in the SCN, creating a state of internal desynchronization (Davidson et al., 2009; Yamazaki et al., 2000). The reliability of these results was questioned because of evidence that altered lighting conditions could make tissues sensitive to phase-shifting effects caused by the dissection procedures, which would complicate interpretation of the results (Leise et al., 2020).

An alternative approach involved measuring clock gene expression in different tissues in mice immediately after dissection at 4 h intervals for many days after a phase shift of the lighting cycle. This approach confirmed that rhythms of clock gene expression in the mouse SCN resynchronized to a shifted lighting cycle more quickly than rhythms of body temperature and of gene expression in peripheral organs (liver and kidney) (Yamaguchi et al., 2013). A similar approach was used to study the rates of phase-shifting of the dorsal and ventral halves of the rat SCN. Gene-expression rhythms in the retinorecipient ventral SCN shifted more rapidly than those in the dorsal SCN (Nagano et al., 2003), a finding that is consistent with in vitro evidence from the mouse SCN (Davidson et al., 2009).

These studies show that abrupt changes in the timing of lighting cycles cause desynchronization of circadian rhythmicity at several levels of physiological organization, implying major disruption of the usually harmonious organization of circadian physiology; for a review, see Nicholls et al., 2019. These results have implications for understanding some of the health consequences of a history of long-term shift work, as discussed in Section 13.10.3.

13.10.2 Why shift work is worse than jet lag

Shift work shares some of the features of jet lag but its consequences can be worse. Their shared features include trying to work, eat, and sleep at daily times that are incompatible with the current phase of one's circadian rhythms as well as the possibility of internal desynchronization among components of the circadian system. What is worse about shift work (besides not getting to go to Fiji or Rome) is that environmental cues are largely unchanged for those who switch abruptly from a day shift to a night shift. Family members and friends maintain their usual routines of work, school, meals, socializing, and sleeping and the external lighting cycle does not change (although the shift worker's exposure to it likely would).

Thus, the local environmental cues that gradually resynchronize jet-lagged travelers to a new time zone remain at least partially unchanged for the shift worker. In addition, many shift-work schedules rotate too rapidly for the circadian system to fully resynchronize. There is physiological evidence that those switching rapidly between different work shifts show little or no adaptation of circadian rhythms to an altered work schedule (Costa et al., 1997; Touitou et al., 1990). In other words, despite working for 2 or 3 days during what would be daytime in New Delhi or Tokyo, the shift worker's circadian system remains anchored to Halifax nighttime. Even most "permanent" night-shift workers show little sign of circadian synchronization to their nocturnal work hours, although a few people with extreme delayed chronotypes may show physiological adaptation to nocturnal work (Dumont et al., 2001; Roden et al., 1993). Not surprisingly, rotating shift workers can suffer many of the same symptoms as the jet traveler who has crossed eight or 12 time zones.

Not only are external cues incompatible with resynchronizing their rhythms but also many workers are not motivated to do so. Shifting all of their daily rhythms while working at night would conflict with their interest in being with family and friends or doing chores during the day. Adapting to a nocturnal rhythm is also discouraged because most workers know that they will return to a different schedule after a few days on the night shift. A typical strategy is to tolerate reduced daytime sleep length and quality while on the night shift, trying to catch up with naps, and changing other aspects of their daily routines as little as possible. Inevitably, however, they will wind up eating during the night and trying to sleep during the day. During this period of disruption, workers and their families would also be at risk of experiencing some of the mood and interpersonal problems associated with inadequate sleep (see Section 13.8.2) in addition to their physiological symptoms.

13.10.3 Health consequences of shift work

Shift work leads to immediate personal discomfort and increases the risks of poor performance and safety problems during night shifts. But those who work rotating shifts for many years also experience increased personal health risks over the long term (Boivin & Boudreau, 2014). Evidence is available for several different professions, but the largest body of evidence that links adverse work schedules to the development of chronic diseases relates to nurses.

A history of engaging in rotating shifts or working at night was associated with higher rates of heart disease, diabetes, reproductive disorders, dementia, and cancer in nurses (and in other professions) (Bokenberger et al., 2018; Jørgensen et al., 2020; Schernhammer et al., 2001; Vetter et al., 2015; Vetter et al., 2016). More years of shift work were linked to more weight gain, increased abdominal obesity (van Amelsvoort et al., 1999), and increased risk of heart disease (Vetter et al., 2016). A mismatch between work schedules and individual chronotypes (e.g., people with morning chronotypes working at night) further increased the risk of shift-work related illnesses (Vetter et al., 2015).

A study of a large cohort of female nurses in the United States starting in 1988 assessed the chances of healthy aging as a function of years of rotating shift work. Healthy aging was defined as surviving to at least age 70 with no major chronic illness, with intact physical and cognitive functions, and no impairment in mental health. The initial cohort included >46,000 nurses aged 46–68 years and free of major health conditions in 1988. Their development of chronic illnesses, of declining physical and cognitive health, and of mental health issues was followed for 24 years (until 2012) and was related to their history of different lengths of rotating shift work.

There was a consistent trend of decreasing chances of healthy aging in general as the history of shift work lengthened from 1 to >10 years, with a clear increase in risk among those working rotating shifts for 6–9 and >10 years. This pattern of a declining probability of global healthy aging as the duration of shift work lengthened also applied to each of the major domains of health studied (Shi et al., 2022).

Starting shift work early in life (before age 20) may be particularly harmful. There is evidence, for example, that it further increased the risk of developing multiple sclerosis, above the already elevated risk among shift workers in general (Hedstrom et al., 2011). Younger (<40 years old) textile factory shift workers on rapidly rotating shifts (every 2 days) had higher chronic cortisol levels and increased body mass indices relative to control day workers. But among older workers in this environment, differences between workers on these shifts and controls did not reach significance. One interpretation is that there may be a selection bias in some work environments, such that only those who were able to adapt successfully to rapidly rotating shifts continued on those schedules beyond age 40 (Manenschijn et al., 2011).

A review of population-based findings that linked long-term shift work to increased reproductive risks in women (reduced fertility, disrupted menstrual cycles, increases in miscarriages) evaluated these results as being of mixed quality, with the strongest evidence related to increased miscarriages (Fernandez et al., 2016). More recent studies reported that shift-working nurses with more insomnia symptoms (possibly reflecting poor adaptation to their work schedules) had an increased risk of developing irregular menstrual cycles (Kang et al., 2019) and that a recent history of shift work accelerated onset of menopause (Stock et al., 2019).

A prospective cohort study found a large increased risk of developing gestational diabetes in pregnant women working evening shifts, which was mediated in part by variability in sleep schedules (Wallace et al., 2022). A recent meta-analysis identified increased pregnancy-related risks among women who worked long hours, had rotating shifts, or worked nights. Across these work conditions, there were variably increased risks of miscarriage, premature birth, hypertension of pregnancy, small birthweight infants, and preeclampsia, a dangerous form of hypertension during pregnancy that can harm both the mother and the fetus (Cai et al., 2019).

Studies have also identified an increased risk of cancer in shift workers. A meta-analysis of studies from several countries involving >3.5 million people concluded that a history of shift work increased the risk of a diagnosis of melanoma, the most dangerous form of skin cancer. The risk of melanoma increased as a function of years of shift work; a dose response analysis concluded that each additional year of shift work increased the risk by ~2% (Yousef et al., 2020).

There have been many studies examining the links between night or shift work and the risk of developing breast cancer. Meta-analyses conducted in different ways have concluded that the evidence for this association ranged from robust to nonexistent (Jia et al., 2013; Kamdar et al., 2013; Megdal et al., 2005; Travis et al., 2016). Despite methodological differences and inconsistencies among studies (Haus & Smolensky, 2013), the associations were seen as strong enough for the International Agency for Cancer Research (World Health Organization) to conclude that shift work involving circadian disruption is "probably carcinogenic in humans" (report summarized in Straif et al., 2007). One variable contributing to inconsistencies across these reviews is the difference between retrospective and prospective studies of shift-work participation, with the latter showing no significant impact on risk of breast cancer, regardless of length of shift work (Travis et al., 2016). Given the mixed evidence depending on methods used, it is possible that increased risk relates to a combination of shift work with other factors that remain to be identified (see next section).

13.10.4 Mechanisms that may contribute to increased risks

The mechanisms responsible for reported links between night/shift work and serious illnesses are not clear, but it is likely that multiple factors contribute to increased risk. Identifying these risks depends on the population being studied, the particular patterns and histories of shift work involved, and the kinds of potentially confounding factors that are controlled for in the analysis. Potential contributing factors include chronic disruption of circadian organization; disturbed sleep patterns and physiology; blunting of nocturnal melatonin secretion by light at night; increased DNA damage; behavioral changes (e.g., diet quality, drug use); increased inflammation; and impaired immune system function (Davis & Mirick, 2006; Haus & Smolensky, 2013; Puttonen et al., 2010; Schernhammer et al., 2001; Straif et al., 2007).

The reproductive effects that have been linked to night/shift work may reflect changes in rhythms of female reproductive hormones. Daily rhythms of release of luteinizing hormone and follicle-stimulating hormone from the pituitary gland are lost under constant routine conditions, indicating that these are not endogenously generated rhythms in people. The observed rhythms of these hormones depend on other daily cycles, such as light–dark exposure, sleep–wake rhythms, and/or meal patterns (Klingman et al., 2011). Reversal or disruption of these cues as a result of working at night and trying to sleep during the day could disturb these hormonal rhythms and affect reproductive functions.

Disruption of melatonin rhythms, which are very sensitive to light exposure at night (Lewy et al., 1980), is another mechanism that could contribute to disease risk. Melatonin has been proposed, but not proven, to help protect against various diseases. This idea is based in part on evidence that it is an effective scavenger of free oxygen radicals and has protective effects against agents that can damage DNA and cellular physiology (Galano et al., 2018; Tan et al., 1993). In a study that monitored a marker of melatonin production in nurses working variable numbers of night shifts, those with more than eight night shifts per month produced less melatonin (Peplonska et al., 2012). A systematic review and meta-analysis concluded that workers on night shifts showed a significant decrease in melatonin production (Wei et al., 2020).

Night work inevitably involves increased exposure to light at night (LAN), which reduces melatonin production. Given the sensitivity of melatonin production to light exposure and the suggestive evidence that melatonin plays a protective role against developing cancer, countries with more light exposure at night would be predicted to have higher cancer rates. A study compared the incidence of five common cancers in women across 164 nations and correlated the risks of these cancers with average levels of LAN. There was no relationship between the incidence of four cancers and LAN, but there was a significant correlation between breast cancer incidence and LAN. After controlling for many other potential factors, there was a 30–50% higher risk of breast cancer in women in countries with the highest, as compared to the lowest, levels of LAN (Kloog et al., 2010).

A similar study concluded that LAN is associated with increased risk of prostate cancer in men (Kloog et al., 2009). Higher levels of nocturnal light exposure in older people were also correlated with higher rates of components of the metabolic syndrome: obesity, diabetes, and hypertension (Kim et al., 2022); see Chapter 14. It is, therefore, likely that work schedules that increase exposure to LAN would increase the risk of developing some types of cancer and metabolic abnormalities.

Studies using animal models provide indirect support for a role for melatonin disruption in the development of breast cancer. In rats implanted with human breast cancer tissue, treatment with exogenous melatonin reduced markers of tumor cell proliferation (Blask et al., 2005). In rats bearing a breast tumor that is estrogen-sensitive (i.e., estrogen increases growth of the tumor), nocturnal light exposure promoted tumor growth and increased resistance to anti-estrogen therapy. These effects of light in promoting tumor growth were mediated by suppression of endogenous melatonin production, as was shown by reversing these effects by treatment with exogenous melatonin (Dauchy et al., 2014).

These findings demonstrate a role for melatonin and for the effects of light exposure at night (at least in nocturnal animals) on tumor proliferation, which could contribute to increased risk of women developing breast cancer. Nevertheless, the extent of the cancer risk associated with LAN for people, and how it interacts with other factors, remain uncertain (Haus & Smolensky, 2013; Travis et al., 2016).

Cancers can result from DNA damage that is not adequately repaired. A study of physicians whose blood was collected in the morning after nights of adequate sleep and after overnight work shifts found that they had increased levels of DNA damage and reduced levels of DNA repair molecules after overnight work (Cheung et al., 2019). Reductions in molecules that repair DNA damage were also demonstrated in sleep-deprived zebra fish (Zada et al., 2021). In mice, there was increased expression of DNA repair molecules and accelerated DNA repair during sleep relative to waking (Bellesi et al., 2016). The impact of sleep loss on DNA repair mechanisms may interact with reduced melatonin levels resulting from nocturnal light exposure to prevent adequate repair of damaged DNA, leading to increased risk of developing cancers.

Another potential effect of both chronic shift work and jet lag is disruption of the internal organization of the circadian system by exposure to abnormal lighting patterns and repeatedly shifting daily rhythms. As previously reviewed in Section 13.9.1, even a single abrupt shift of external lighting cycles can transiently disrupt the internal organization of the circadian pacemaker and its coordination of peripheral circadian rhythms. People experiencing repeated episodes of jet lag or shifting work schedules likely experience similarly disrupted phase relations among internal circadian rhythms. In animal models, chronic disruption of circadian rhythm organization has been shown to increase the risk of developing serious illnesses, including cardiovascular disease (Martino et al., 2008) and cancer (Van Dycke et al., 2015).

This effect may be especially relevant to older shift workers. In a study in mice, lighting phase shifts caused changes in the phase relations between gene expression rhythms in different organs, and these differences were larger in older than in younger mice. These results suggest that resynchronization of rhythms to shifted cycles was slower or less complete in older mice (Leise et al., 2013). If similar disruption of circadian organization occurs in people working rotating shifts, it could contribute to making adaptation to shift work more difficult for older workers (Reilly et al., 1997).

Repeated shift work cycles are associated with periodic reductions in the amount of sleep and disruptions of its structure and timing. Differences in sleep patterns have been associated with increased risks of several different diseases, as reviewed in Chapters 14 and 15. One example links sleep changes related to work schedules to a well characterized health risk factor. Bus drivers working rotating shift-work schedules that involved early morning starts had more variable sleep–wake schedules over the week than those not working shifts. This difference was associated with a dramatic increase in the proportion of drivers showing a non-dipping blood pressure pattern during sleep (McHill et al., 2022). This lack of substantial reductions in blood pressure during the sleep phase has been linked to increased risk of developing vascular diseases (Fagard et al., 2008; Verdecchia, 2000), as discussed in detail in Section 14.8.

Working at night can also contribute to developing chronic diseases because of its impact on behavior. Hospital staff working night shifts, for example, likely eat less healthy diets. Cafeterias are often closed at night, while typically low-quality food in vending machines is available at all hours. Eating at night is also associated with making unhealthy food choices and with altered physiological responses to food intake. These changes in meal timing and composition promote metabolic disorders, including weight gain and the many negative health impacts of excess weight, which include increased risk of cancer and vascular disease (see Section 14.7). In a retrospective analysis, the number of years of previous shift work was positively correlated with higher waist-to-hip ratios and increased abdominal obesity in both men and women (van Amelsvoort et al., 1999). It is not known to what extent these effects relate to the altered timing and type of food intake or to metabolic changes resulting from circadian rhythm disruption.

Those who work extended, night, or rotating shifts also tend to consume more drugs than day workers, which could have long-term negative health consequences. Drugs used included sedatives, alcohol, and tobacco, which were sometimes used in attempts to regulate their sleep (Niedhammer et al., 1995; Trinkoff & Storr, 1998). Reduced supervision of hospital staff at night could also allow opportunities for unauthorized use of restricted medications, including stimulants and sedatives that are available in hospitals.

A meta-analysis of studies of alcohol use in numerous countries found increased cross-sectional risk of alcohol use, and increased prospective risk of developing risky alcohol use, in those working more hours weekly than is typically recommended (>40 h) (Virtanen et al., 2015). An American study using insurance claims records found that people working >56 h weekly had increased use of prescription sedatives and drugs with sedative properties than those working shorter hours. This effect of long work hours was greater among women and professionals but also among those using food stamps, probably reflecting lower incomes (Ezekekwu et al., 2023).

Another risk factor associated with shift work is likely to be the general life stress and social disruption that occurs in relation to scheduling family functions and meeting personal needs. Along with the physiological effects of shift work, these additional stressors could contribute to the increased rates of health problems that have been identified among long-term shift workers.

13.10.5 Addressing shift work-related problems

Some health risks associated with long-term shift work are clearly established and others are uncertain, with conflicting population-based findings. What remains clear are the immediate impacts of working overnight on human performance. Except for a few extreme "night-owls" who may prefer to work permanent night shifts, most people who periodically work at night have difficulty remaining alert and performing optimally during that time. Even those who work "permanent" night shifts may revert to more typical sleep–wake patterns on days off, so their rhythms must be adjusted again when they return to work. The many documented and suspected impacts on performance during night work, rotating shift work, and extended work periods raise questions about how performance could be enhanced during these challenging schedules. These questions include the following:

- What helps people adapt quickly to a shifted work schedule?
- How long should people stay on any one shifted work schedule?
- How should people rotate from one work schedule to another?
- How long a break should there be between different work shifts?
- Are short or long shifts better overnight (e.g., 8 h vs. 12 h)?

The answers to these questions are often very complex. They are related not only to the function of physiological mechanisms that regulate sleep and circadian rhythms (and individual differences in these mechanisms) but also to the influence of social and environmental pressures and personal preferences (Knauth, 2009). A recent review summarized many of these issues and offered a set of guiding principles for instituting and evaluating methods for reducing the health and safety risks associated with shift work (Gurubhagavatula et al., 2021). This section cannot address the full scope of these issues, but it will focus on a few selected topics.

Manipulating light exposure and taking melatonin are the most consistently effective circadian phase-shifting methods that have been applied to help people adapt to shifting work schedules and to jet lag. To produce optimal phase shifts, these methods require careful timing of bright light exposure at particular circadian phases, avoidance of light at other phases (including wearing strongly tinted goggles when exposed to sunlight), and precise timing of melatonin treatments (Eastman & Burgess, 2009).

Even using ideal treatments under controlled laboratory conditions, the amount of phase shift produced in one day is relatively small (~0.5–3 h). At least several days of treatments would be needed to shift the circadian system to match a work schedule that is shifted by 8–12 h. No known manipulation can produce immediate physiological synchronization after a large shift in an individual's work schedule. The result is that most people working night shifts are not physiologically adapted to working at that phase (Costa et al., 1997; Touitou et al., 1990). Complete physiological adaptation to nocturnal work during rotating schedules would also not be desirable for those workers who stay on one shift for only a few days and would need subsequently to resynchronize quickly to a different schedule.

An alternative approach was proposed to try to achieve a compromise phase for night workers that reduces sleepiness during work at night and confines most of the phase of maximal sleepiness (the hours around the body temperature minimum) to a sleep period. This approach uses the known phase-shifting tools (timed light exposures, melatonin, tinted goggles), along with planned shifts in sleep–wake schedules, to achieve reasonably good performance at night, while preserving nightly melatonin secretion and allowing adaptation to more normal schedules during days off (Eastman, 2016; Smith & Eastman, 2012; Smith et al., 2009).

This approach may facilitate adaptation to night work for both permanent night workers and rotating shift workers, but it would require careful adherence to schedules of sleep, melatonin treatments, and light exposure. In addition, aspects of these approaches can conflict with workers' desire to schedule some of their daily activities to match those of family and friends. Another recently studied approach used a shift work-adapted version of Cognitive Behavioral Therapy (CBT) that was able to improve daytime sleep during rotating shifts and reduce symptoms of depression and anxiety in health care shift workers (Vallières et al., 2024).

The direction of shift rotation could theoretically influence adaptation to new shifts because most people find delaying their circadian schedules (= westward flights) easier than advancing them (= eastward flights). Although this might suggest that delaying work schedules would be easier, most workers don't delay their entire circadian cycle as they switch shifts, unlike the shifts that occur when people fly to a different time zone. Someone on a day shift will typically sleep during the night immediately *before* going to work in the morning; but when working on a night shift, they may sleep immediately *after* coming back from work (Åkerstedt, 2003).

Workers rearrange their daily schedules to suit a combination of the demands of work, family, social interactions, and lifestyle preferences, making it unclear which rotation direction would be optimal (Turek, 1986). Nevertheless, some large-scale empirical studies have reported that backward-rotating shifts are more disruptive of sleep quality and family life and are associated with poorer health outcomes (van Amelsvoort et al., 2004; Wangsan et al., 2022).

With respect to the patterns and timing of night work and of rotation between shifts, these vary among professions, institutions, and individual workers, resulting in differential effects on the health of workers. One study in South Korea involved polysomnography technologists who worked nights conducting sleep studies but also worked days scoring these studies and conducting daytime nap studies. Night work occurred on a variety of schedules: permanent night shift; slow rotation between working nights and days (at 3–12 month intervals); fast rotations between night and day work within a week; and permanent day work (with only rare night work). Those who worked on any of the schedules involving regular nighttime work reported more anxiety and insomnia than "day-only" workers, and those working on fast rotations and permanent night shifts generally rated their physical and mental health worse than those on slow rotations (Lee et al., 2020).

An example of the social complexities that interact with physiological constraints relates to the preferred duration of shifts. Given the difficulty of performing well at night and the fatigue caused by lengthy work periods (especially at night), it would seem sensible to institute relatively short overnight work shifts. Instead, 8, 10, or 12 h shifts may be standard in different jurisdictions and work settings.

A review of the available literature highlighted the fact that workers' and employers' attitudes toward different shift lengths depended on which variables were the focus of a decision about work schedules: worker productivity, workplace accidents, worker health and safety, quality of personal and family life, etc. (Ferguson & Dawson, 2012). One factor that is important to some workers is that working three 12 h shifts usually comprises a week's work, giving them four days off work every week. They may see the advantages of this schedule for organizing parental and other responsibilities as outweighing the disadvantages of difficult overnight work periods.

An interesting example of how different factors influence attitudes toward shift-work durations is a study involving members of the Phoenix, Arizona police department. The study compared the impacts of their standard 40 h workweek (4 consecutive 10 h shifts) in a control precinct and a 6-month trial of an experimental schedule involving 3 consecutive 13.33 h shifts weekly in another precinct. Compared to the control precinct, officers on the longer work shifts got less sleep: <6 h between shifts, so they were awake for >18 h on workdays. They also reported worse sleep, had more daytime sleepiness, slower reaction times, more lapses on the PVT, and rated themselves as having a worse overall quality of life. The long-shift precinct also recorded an increase in citizens' serious complaints about police conduct relative to the previous year (when they were on the standard shift), while the control precinct recorded a decrease in this category of complaints.

Before the trial began, only a minority of officers in the experimental and control precincts indicated a preference for the 13.33 h shift (28% in the experimental group). Over the course of the trial, the proportion preferring the longer shift fell even further in the experimental precinct and also in the control precinct (perhaps as a result of communication among officers). This increase in negative attitudes toward the new schedule is consistent with the poorer sleep quality and amount, reduced daytime alertness, and worse reported quality of life while working the longer shifts.

Two months after their return to the traditional 10 h shifts, this preference was further strengthened, with only 17% of the experimental group still preferring the longer shift schedule. However, among spouses/partners of officers in the long-shift precinct, the proportion preferring the longer shift schedule near the end of the trial had *increased* from ~7% before the trial to >33%. This change among officers' family members presumably reflected the perceived benefits for the family of the officers' extra days off (Bell et al., 2015).

A potentially related finding is from a study of law-enforcement officers in the United Kingdom. It found a high incidence of sleep problems among officers but a difference between measures of long-term sleep difficulties and short-term problems. Actigraphic studies showed that participants who worked 12 h rotating shifts had the worst sleep efficiency, compared to participants who worked only day shifts and those on 8 h rotating shifts, and significantly shorter total sleep time than those on day shifts. Consistent with these objective findings, subjective evaluations of sleep that were obtained concurrently with each sleep episode also showed that those on the 12 h shifts reported more awakenings and less optimal behavior after waking. Nevertheless, when asked about their sleep over the last month, those on 12 h rotating shifts self-reported better sleep than those on 8 h rotating shifts (Sharma et al., 2023). Although this difference between short-term and long-term attitudes is difficult to interpret, it may indicate a general sense that 12 h shifts provided significant benefits, despite the immediate objective and subjective evidence that 12 h shifts disrupted sleep and waking performance.

13.10.6 Summary

In addition to effects on job performance and risks to individual safety, a lifetime history of adverse work schedules is also associated with an increased incidence of negative health outcomes. Although there is conflicting evidence related to some conditions, the outcomes identified include increased risk of being overweight, developing heart disease and several cancers, experiencing changes in menstrual cycles, and having adverse pregnancy outcomes. These effects may be related to a complex of factors including disrupted circadian rhythms, sleep loss, suppression of melatonin secretion, DNA damage and its inadequate repair, increased drug and alcohol use, and environmental and social stressors related to the complexity of accommodating shift-work scheduling.

Jet lag is a model of some of the effects of shift work because both involve trying to function and sleep at times that conflict with the dictates of circadian rhythms and sleep needs. Shift workers also have the disadvantage of not being exposed to environmental cues consistent with their work timing, not usually having the time to adapt physiologically to their shifted schedule, and not being motivated to do so, given the short time they may spend on a new shift and conflicting personal demands. In fact, there is little evidence of significant physiological adaptation to short-term shifted work schedules. Workers on night shifts are therefore working with suboptimal alertness at night and inadequate sleep during the day.

Manipulations of light exposure and treatments with melatonin can achieve a compromise phase of adaptation to a shifted schedule to partially reduce worktime sleepiness and sleep loss and improve the ability to return to normal schedules on days off. But these interventions require several days of planned, carefully timed manipulations to achieve these outcomes, which may not be practical for many workers.

Studies in animal models involving abrupt, large shifts of lighting cycles found that components of the distributed circadian system shifted at different rates and that even two parts of the SCN pacemaker become desynchronized from each other. These changes led to transient internal desynchrony among circadian system components, which may contribute further to the malaise and health risks associated with both jet lag and rotating shift work schedules.

Addressing problems related to adverse work schedules is complicated because of the many conflicting motivations and requirements involved. The issues for individual workers in a health care setting, for example, might include risks to personal safety (on the job or during commutes to and from work); long-term health risks that are poorly understood; disruption of family and personal life; impacts on the quality of their job performance and (in the case of health care staff) their patients' health; and the quality of their training.

For patients in a hospital, the relevant variables include the quality of performance of the staff treating them at night, and, over the longer term, the quality of training that staff receive, which may affect their future care. For administrators running health care systems, the issues include not only the liabilities (and insurance costs) associated with health and safety risks for both staff and patients but also the cost of implementing systems and hiring additional staff to reduce these risks. The general public may be interested in reducing the costs associated with health care, but they will have conflicting priorities, depending on their own and their families' current and future needs for health care.

Similar conflicting pressures would influence attempts to increase the time allowed for shift workers to get more sleep and to recover from the effects of sleep loss and rhythm disruptions, with similar implications for costs and liabilities. How much risk should society tolerate in each of these situations? How much would we be willing to pay to reduce that risk? One study involving a test of longer shift durations and more days off for police officers illustrated both the negative health and personal effects of extended work shifts and the conflicting motivations between the officers involved and their spouses/partners with respect to the costs and benefits of different schedules.

Issues related to shift work have no easy answers. The reality is that we are a diurnal species, with relatively inelastic circadian systems and sleep needs that evolved in relation to environments and lifestyles that are very different from those most people experience today. No single solution can address all of the challenges posed by the perceived need for around-the-clock services; each situation requires a series of difficult compromises that try to balance the many factors and motivations involved (Gurubhagavatula et al., 2021). One study that is currently planned will attempt to combine the best available information about shift-work scheduling with targeted education and training programs for both workers and shift planners in a randomized, controlled trial (Declercq et al., 2022). Its outcomes may help inform future approaches to dealing with the inherent complexities of shift-work scheduling.

Literature cited

Aeschbach, D., Postolache, T. T., Sher, L., Matthews, J. R., Jackson, M. A., & Wehr, T. A. (2001). Evidence from the waking electroencephalogram that short sleepers live under higher homeostatic sleep pressure than long sleepers. *Neuroscience, 102*(2), 493–502.

Åkerstedt, T. (2003). Shift work and disturbed sleep/wakefulness. *Occup Med, 53*(2), 89–94. doi: 10.1093/occmed/kqg046

Åkerstedt, T., & Wright Jr., K. P. (2009). Sleep loss and fatigue in shift work and shift work disorder. *Sleep Med Clin, 4*(2), 257–271. doi: 10.1016/j.jsmc.2009.03.001

Anderson, C., & Platten, C. R. (2011). Sleep deprivation lowers inhibition and enhances impulsivity to negative stimuli. *Behav Brain Res, 217*(2), 463–466. doi: 10.1016/j.bbr.2010.09.020

Anderson, C., Sullivan, J. P., Flynn-Evans, E. E., Cade, B. E., Czeisler, C. A., & Lockley, S. W. (2012). Deterioration of neurobehavioral performance in resident physicians during repeated exposure to extended duration work shifts. *Sleep, 35*(8), 1137–1146. doi: 10.5665/sleep.2004

Armstrong, J. M., Ruttle, P. L., Klein, M. H., Essex, M. J., & Benca, R. M. (2014). Associations of child insomnia, sleep movement, and their persistence with mental health symptoms in childhood and adolescence. *Sleep, 37*(5), 901–909. doi: 10.5665/sleep.3656

Arnal, P. J., Sauvet, F., Leger, D., van Beers, P., Bayon, V., Bougard, C., … Chennaoui, M. (2015). Benefits of sleep extension on sustained attention and sleep pressure before and during total sleep deprivation and recovery. *Sleep, 38*(12), 1935–1943. doi: 10.5665/sleep.5244

Arnedt, J. T., Owens, J., Crouch, M., Stahl, J., & Carskadon, M. A. (2005). Neurobehavioral performance of residents after heavy night call vs after alcohol ingestion. *JAMA, 294*, 1025–1033.

Astill, R. G., Van der Heijden, K. B., Van Ijzendoorn, M. H., & Van Someren, E. J. (2012). Sleep, cognition, and behavioral problems in school-age children: a century of research meta-analyzed. *Psychol Bull, 138*(6), 1109–1138. doi: 10.1037/a0028204

Baddeley, A. (1998). The central executive: a concept and some misconceptions. *J Int Neuropsych Soc, 4*, 523–526.

Banks, S., & Dinges, D. F. (2007). Behavioral and physiological consequences of sleep restriction. *J Clin Sleep Med, 3*(5), 519–528.

Banks, S., Jones, C. W., McCauley, M. E., Dorrian, J., Basner, M., Maislin, G., … Dinges, D. F. (2023). Long-term influence of sleep/wake history on the dynamic neurobehavioural response to sustained sleep restriction. *J Sleep Res*, e14117. doi: 10.1111/jsr.14117

Banks, S., Van Dongen, H. P. A., Maislin, G., & Dinges, D. F. (2010). Neurobehavioral dynamics following chronic sleep restriction: dose-response effects of one night for recovery. *Sleep, 33*(8), 1013–1026.

Barger, L. K., Cade, B. E., Ayas, N., Cronin, J. W., Rosner, B., Speizer, F. E., … Harvard Work Hours, Health, and Safety Group. (2005). Extended work shifts and the risk of motor vehicle crashes among interns. *New Engl J Med, 352*(2), 125–134.

Basner, M., Hermosillo, E., Nasrini, J., McGuire, S., Saxena, S., Moore, T. M., … Dinges, D. F. (2018). Repeated administration effects on Psychomotor Vigilance Test performance. *Sleep, 41*(1). doi: 10.1093/sleep/zsx187

Baum, K. T., Desai, A., Field, J., Miller, L. E., Rausch, J., & Beebe, D. W. (2014). Sleep restriction worsens mood and emotion regulation in adolescents. *J Child Psychol Psychiatry, 55*(2), 180–190. doi: 10.1111/jcpp.12125

Becker, S. P., Epstein, J. N., Tamm, L., Tilford, A. A., Tischner, C. M., Isaacson, P. A., … Beebe, D. W. (2019). Shortened sleep duration causes sleepiness, inattention, and oppositionality in adolescents with attention-deficit/hyperactivity disorder: findings from a crossover sleep restriction/extension study. *J Am Acad Child Adolesc Psychiatry, 58*(4), 433–442. doi: 10.1016/j.jaac.2018.09.439

Bédard, M.-A., Montplaisir, J., Malo, J., Richer, F., & Rouleau, I. (1993). Persistent neuropsychological deficits and vigilance impairment in sleep apnea syndrome after treatment with continuous positive airway pressure (CPAP). *J Clin Exp Neuropsyc, 15*(2), 330–341. doi: 10.1080/01688639308402567

Beebe, D. W. (2011). Cognitive, behavioral, and functional consequences of inadequate sleep in children and adolescents. *Pediatr Clin N Am, 58*(3), 649–665. doi: 10.1016/j.pcl.2011.03.002

Beebe, D. W., & Gozal, D. (2002). Obstructive sleep apnea and the prefrontal cortex: towards a comprehensive model linking nocturnal upper airway obstruction to daytime cognitive and behavioral deficits. *J Sleep Res, 11*, 1–16.

Beebe, D. W., Groesz, L., Wells, C., Nichols, A., & McGee, K. (2003). The neuropsychological effects of obstructive sleep apnea: a meta-analysis of norm-referenced and case-controlled data. *Sleep, 26*(3), 298–307.

Belenky, G., Wesensten, N. J., Thorne, D. R., Thomas, M. L., Sing, H. C., Redmond, D. . . . Balkin, T. J. (2003). Patterns of performance degradation and restoration during sleep restriction and subsequent recovery: a sleep dose-response study. *J Sleep Res, 12*, 1–12.

Bell, L. B., Virden, T. B., Lewis, D. J., & Cassidy, B. A. (2015). Effects of 13-hour 20-minute work shifts on law enforcement officers' sleep, cognitive abilities, health, quality of life, and work performance: the Phoenix study. *Police Q, 18*(3), 293–337. doi: 10.1177/1098611115584910

Bellesi, M., Bushey, D., Chini, M., Tononi, G., & Cirelli, C. (2016). Contribution of sleep to the repair of neuronal DNA double-strand breaks: evidence from flies and mice. *Sci Rep, 6*, 36804. doi: 10.1038/srep36804

Ben Simon, E., Oren, N., Sharon, H., Kirschner, A., Goldway, N., Okon-Singer, H., . . . Hendler, T. (2015). Losing neutrality: the neural basis of impaired emotional control without sleep. *J Neurosci, 35*(38), 13194–13205. doi: 10.1523/JNEUROSCI.1314-15.2015

Ben Simon, E., Vallat, R., Rossi, A., & Walker, M. P. (2022). Sleep loss leads to the withdrawal of human helping across individuals, groups, and large-scale societies. *PLoS Biol, 20*(8), e3001733. doi:10.1371/journal.pbio.3001733

Bernier, A., Beauchamp, M. H., Bouvette-Turcot, A. A., Carlson, S. M., & Carrier, J. (2013). Sleep and cognition in preschool years: specific links to executive functioning. *Child Dev, 84*(5), 1542–1553. doi: 10.1111/cdev.12063

Bernier, A., Carlson, S. M., Bordeleau, S., & Carrier, J. (2010). Relations between physiological and cognitive regulatory systems: infant sleep regulation and subsequent executive functioning. *Child Dev, 81*(6), 1739–1752. doi: 10.1111/j.1467-8624.2010.01507.x

Blask, D. E., Brainard, G. C., Dauchy, R. T., Hanifin, J. P., Davidson, L. K., Krause, J. A., . . . Zalatan, F. (2005). Melatonin-depleted blood from premenopausal women exposed to light at night stimulates growth of human breast cancer xenografts in nude rats. *Cancer Res, 65*(23), 11174–11184. doi: 10.1158/0008-5472.can-05-1945

Bodenmann, S., Hohoff, C., Freitag, C., Deckert, J., Rétey, J. V., Bachmann, V., & Landolt, H. P. (2012). Polymorphisms of ADORA2A modulate psychomotor vigilance and the effects of caffeine on neurobehavioural performance and sleep EEG after sleep deprivation. *Br J Pharmacol, 165*(6), 1904–1913. doi: 10.1111/j.1476-5381.2011.01689.x

Boivin, D. B., & Boudreau, P. (2014). Impacts of shift work on sleep and circadian rhythms. *Pathol Biol (Paris), 62*(5), 292–301. doi: 10.1016/j.patbio.2014.08.001

Bokenberger, K., Sjolander, A., Dahl Aslan, A. K., Karlsson, I. K., Akerstedt, T., & Pedersen, N. L. (2018). Shift work and risk of incident dementia: a study of two population-based cohorts. *Eur J Epidemiol, 33*(10), 977–987. doi: 10.1007/s10654-018-0430-8

Bonuck, K., Freeman, K., Chervin, R. D., & Xu, L. (2012). Sleep-disordered breathing in a population-based cohort: behavioral outcomes at 4 and 7 years. *Pediatrics, 129*(4), e857–e865. doi: 10.1542/peds.2011-1402

Braun, A. R., Balkin, T. J., Wesenten, N. J., Carson, R. E., Varga, M., Baldwin, P., . . . Herscovitch, P. (1997). Regional cerebral blood flow throughout the sleep-wake cycle. An $H_2{}^{15}O$ PET study. *Brain, 120*, 1173–1197.

Brunner, D. P., Dijk, D. J., Tobler, I., & Borbély, A. A. (1990). Effect of partial sleep deprivation on sleep stages and EEG power spectra: evidence for non-REM and REM sleep homeostasis. *Electroencephalogr Clin Neurophysiol, 75*, 492–499.

Cai, C., Vandermeer, B., Khurana, R., Nerenberg, K., Featherstone, R., Sebastianski, M., & Davenport, M. H. (2019). The impact of occupational shift work and working hours during pregnancy on health outcomes: a systematic review and meta-analysis. *Am J Obstet Gynecol, 221*(6), 563–576. doi: 10.1016/j.ajog.2019.06.051

Cai, Y., Mai, Z., Li, M., Zhou, X., & Ma, N. (2021). Altered frontal connectivity after sleep deprivation predicts sustained attentional impairment: a resting-state functional magnetic resonance imaging study. *J Sleep Res*, **e13329**. doi: 10.1111/jsr.13329

Cajochen, C., Brunner, D. P., Kräuchi, K., Graw, P., & Wirz-Justice, A. (1995). Power density in theta/alpha frequencies of the waking EEG progressively increases during sustained wakefulness. *Sleep, 18*(10), 890–894.

Cajochen, C., Foy, R., & Dijk, D.-J. (1999). Frontal predominance of a relative increase in sleep delta and theta EEG activity after sleep loss in humans. *Sleep Res Online, 2*(3), 65–69.

Carskadon, M. A., & Dement, W. C. (1981). Cumulative effects of sleep restriction on daytime sleepiness. *Psychophysiology, 18*(2), 107–113.

Carskadon, M. A., & Dement, W. C. (1982). Nocturnal determinants of daytime sleepiness. *Sleep, 5*(Suppl. 2), S73–S81.

Carskadon, M. A., & Dement, W. C. (1987). Daytime sleepiness: quantification of a behavioral state. *Neurosci Biobehav Rev, 11*, 307–317.

Carskadon, M. A., Dement, W. C., Mitler, M. M., Roth, T., Westbrook, P. R., & Keenan, S. (1986). Guidelines for the Multiple Sleep Latency Test (MSLT): a standard measure of sleepiness. *Sleep, 9*(4), 519–524.

Carskadon, M. A., Harvey, K., & Dement, W. C. (1981). Sleep loss in young adolescents. *Sleep, 4*(3), 299–312.

CDC. (2011). Unhealthy sleep-related behaviors-12 states, 2009. *Morb Mort Wkly Rep, 60*(8), 233–266.

CDC. (2014). Short sleep duration (<7 hours) among adults, by congressional district: US, 2014. Retrieved from http://www.sleepresearchsociety.org/PDFs/SAE_CD113_2014_Sleep.pdf

Chee, M. W. L., & Choo, W. C. (2004). Functional imaging of working memory after 24 hr of total sleep deprivation. *J Neurosci, 24*(19), 4560–4567. doi: 10.1523/jneurosci.0007-04.2004

Chee, M. W. L., Tan, J. C., Zheng, H., Parimal, S., Weissman, D. H., Zagorodnov, V., & Dinges, D. F. (2008). Lapsing during sleep deprivation is associated with distributed changes in brain activation. *J Neurosci, 28*(21), 5519–5528. doi: 10.1523/jneurosci.0733-08.2008

Chervin, R. D., Dillon, J. E., Bassetti, C., Ganoczy, D. A., & Pituch, K. J. (1997). Symptoms of sleep disorders, inattention, and hyperactivity in children. *Sleep, 20*(12), 1185–1192.

Chervin, R. D., Ruzicka, D. L., Giordani, B. J., Weatherly, R. A., Dillon, J. E., Hodges, E. K., . . . Guire, K. E. (2006). Sleep-disordered breathing, behavior, and cognition in children before and after adenotonsillectomy. *Pediatrics, 117*(4), e769–e778.

Cheung, V., Yuen, V. M., Wong, G. T. C., & Choi, S. W. (2019). The effect of sleep deprivation and disruption on DNA damage and health of doctors. *Anaesthesia, 74*(4), 434–440. doi: 10.1111/anae.14533

Christie, M. A., Bolortuya, Y., Chen, L. C., McKenna, J. T., McCarley, R. W., & Strecker, R., E. (2008). Microdialysis elevation of adenosine in the basal forebrain produces vigilance impairments in the rat psychomotor vigilance task. *Sleep, 31*(10), 1393–1398.

Christie, M. A., McKenna, J. T., Connolly, N. P., McCarley, R. W., & Strecker, R. E. (2008). 24 hours of sleep deprivation in the rat increases sleepiness and decreases vigilance: introduction of the rat-psychomotor vigilance task. *J Sleep Res, 17*(4), 376–384. doi: 10.1111/j.1365-2869.2008.00698.x

Chua, E. C., Yeo, S. C., Lee, I. T., Tan, L. C., Lau, P., Cai, S., . . . Gooley, J. J. (2014). Sustained attention performance during sleep deprivation associates with instability in behavior and physiologic measures at baseline. *Sleep, 37*(1), 27–39. doi: 10.5665/sleep.3302

Clasadonte, J., McIver, S. R., Schmitt, L. I., Halassa, M. M., & Haydon, P. G. (2014). Chronic sleep restriction disrupts sleep homeostasis and behavioral sensitivity to alcohol by reducing the extracellular accumulation of adenosine. *J Neurosci, 34*(5), 1879–1891. doi: 10.1523/JNEUROSCI.2870-12.2014

Cohen, D. A., Wang, W., Wyatt, J. K., Kronauer, R. E., Dijk, D.-J., Czeisler, C. A., & Klerman, E. B. (2010). Uncovering residual effects of chronic sleep loss on human performance. *Sci Transl Med, 2*, 14ra3. doi:10.1126/scitranslmed.3000458

Costa, G., Bertoldi, A., Kovacic, M., Ghirlanda, G., Minors, D. S., & Waterhouse, J. M. (1997). Hormonal secretion of nurses engaged in fast-rotating shift systems. *Int J Occup Env Health, 3*(Supplement 2), S35–S39.

Cote, K. A., Mondloch, C. J., Sergeeva, V., Taylor, M., & Semplonius, T. (2014). Impact of total sleep deprivation on behavioural neural processing of emotionally expressive faces. *Exp Brain Res, 232*(5), 1429–1442. doi: 10.1007/s00221-013-3780-1

Cremone, A., McDermott, J. M., & Spencer, R. M. C. (2017). Naps enhance executive attention in preschool-aged children. *J Pediatr Psychol, 42*(8), 837–845. doi: 10.1093/jpepsy/jsx048

Cunningham, J. E. A., Jones, S. A. H., Eskes, G. A., & Rusak, B. (2018). Acute sleep restriction has differential effects on components of attention. *Front Psychiatry, 9*, 499. doi: 10.3389/fpsyt.2018.00499

Curtis, B. J., McKinney, T. L., Euler, M., Anderson, J. S., Baron, K. G., Smith, T. W., & Williams, P. G. (2024). Sleepy without stimulation: subjective and objective sleepiness in actigraphy-verified natural short sleepers. *J Sleep Res*, e14170. doi:10.1111/jsr.14170

Curtis, B. J., Williams, P. G., & Anderson, J. S. (2018). Objective cognitive functioning in self-reported habitual short sleepers not reporting daytime dysfunction: examination of impulsivity via delay discounting. *Sleep, 41*(9), zsy115. doi:10.1093/sleep/zsy115

Dagys, N., McGlinchey, E. L., Talbot, L. S., Kaplan, K. A., Dahl, R. E., & Harvey, A. G. (2012). Double trouble? The effects of sleep deprivation and chronotype on adolescent affect. *J Child Psychol Psychiatry, 53*(6), 660–667. doi: 10.1111/j.1469-7610.2011.02502.x

Dauchy, R. T., Xiang, S., Mao, L., Brimer, S., Wren, M. A., Yuan, L., … Hill, S. M. (2014). Circadian and melatonin disruption by exposure to light at night drives intrinsic resistance to tamoxifen therapy in breast cancer. *Cancer Res, 74*(15), 4099–4110. doi: 10.1158/0008-5472.CAN-13-3156

Davidson, A. J., Castanon-Cervantes, O., Leise, T. L., Molyneux, P. C., & Harrington, M. E. (2009). Visualizing jet lag in the mouse suprachiasmatic nucleus and peripheral circadian timing system. *Eur J Neurosci, 29*(1), 171–180. doi: 10.1111/j.1460-9568.2008.06534.x

Davidson, F., Rusak, B., Chambers, C., & Corkum, P. (2019). The impact of sleep restriction on daytime functioning in school-age children with and without ADHD: a narrative review of the literature. *Can J School Psychol, 34*(3), 188–214.

Davis, S., & Mirick, D. K. (2006). Circadian disruption, shift work and the risk of cancer: a summary of the evidence and studies in Seattle. *Cancer Cause Control, 17*(4), 539–545. doi: 10.1007/s10552-005-9010-9

Dawson, D., & Reid, K. (1997). Fatigue, alcohol and performance impairment. *Nature, 388*(6639), 236.

de Bruin, E. J., van Run, C., Staaks, J., & Meijer, A. M. (2017). Effects of sleep manipulation on cognitive functioning of adolescents: A systematic review. *Sleep Med Rev, 32*, 45–57. doi: 10.1016/j.smrv.2016.02.006

Declercq, I., Van Den Eede, F., Roelant, E., & Verbraecken, J. (2022). SHIFTPLAN: a randomized controlled trial investigating the effects of a multimodal shift-work intervention on drivers' fatigue, sleep, health, and performance parameters. *Trials, 23*(1), 662. doi: 10.1186/s13063-022-06573-6

Demichelis, O. P., Grainger, S. A., Burr, L., & Henry, J. D. (2022). Emotion regulation mediates the effects of sleep on stress and aggression. *J Sleep Res*, e13787. doi: 10.1111/jsr.13787

Deurveilher, S., Bush, J. E., Rusak, B., Eskes, G. A., & Semba, K. (2015). Psychomotor vigilance task performance during and following chronic sleep restriction in rats. *Sleep, 38*(4), 515–528. doi: 10.5665/sleep.4562

Dijk, D.-J., & Archer, S. N. (2010). PERIOD3, circadian phenotypes, and sleep homeostasis. *Sleep Med Rev, 14*(3), 151–160. doi: 10.1016/j.smrv.2009.07.002

Dinges, D. F., Pack, F., Williams, K., Gillen, K. A., Powell, J. W., Ott, G. E., … Pack, A. I. (1997). Cumulative sleepiness, mood disturbance, and psychomotor vigilance performance decrements during a week of sleep restricted to 4–5 hours per night. *Sleep, 20*(4), 267–277.

Doran, S. M., Van Dongen, H. P. A., & Dinges, D. F. (2001). Sustained attention performance during sleep deprivation: evidence of state instability. *Arch Ital Biol, 139*, 253–267.

Drummond, S. P., Anderson, D. E., Straus, L. D., Vogel, E. K., & Perez, V. B. (2012). The effects of two types of sleep deprivation on visual working memory capacity and filtering efficiency. *PLoS One, 7*(4), e35653. doi: 10.1371/journal.pone.0035653

Drummond, S. P., Brown, G. G., Salamat, J. S., & Gillin, J. C. (2004). Increasing task difficulty facilitates the cerebral compensatory response to total sleep deprivation. *Sleep, 27*(3), 445–451.

Drummond, S. P. A., Bischoff-Grethe, A., Dinges, D. F., Ayalon, L., Mednick, S. C., & Meloy, M. J. (2005). The neural basis of the psychomotor vigilance task. *Sleep, 28*(9), 1059–1068.

Dumont, M., Benhaberou-Brun, D., & Paquet, J. (2001). Profile of 24-h light exposure and circadian phase of melatonin secretion in night workers. *J Biol Rhythms, 16*(5), 502–511.

Eastman, C. I. (2016). How to reduce circadian misalignment in rotating shift workers. *ChronoPhysiol Ther, 6*, 41–46. doi: 10.2147/CPT.S111424

Eastman, C. I., & Burgess, H. J. (2009). How to travel the world without jet lag. *Sleep Med Clin, 4*(2), 241–255. doi: 10.1016/j.jsmc.2009.02.006

Ezekekwu, E., Johnson, C., Karimi, S., Antimisiaris, D., & Lorenz, D. (2023). Examining the relationship between long working hours and the use of prescription sedatives among U.S. workers. *Sleep Med, 109*, 226–239. doi: 10.1016/j.sleep.2023.06.026

Fagard, R. H., Celis, H., Thijs, L., Staessen, J. A., Clement, D. L., De Buyzere, M. L., & De Bacquer, D. A. (2008). Daytime and nighttime blood pressure as predictors of death and cause-specific cardiovascular events in hypertension. *Hypertension, 51*(1), 55–61. doi: 10.1161/HYPERTENSIONAHA.107.100727

Fallone, G., Acebo, C., Arnedt, J. T., Seifer, R., & Carskadon, M. A. (2001). Effects of acute sleep restriction on behavior, sustained attention, and response inhibition in children. *Percept Mot Skills, 93*, 213–229.

Fallone, G., Acebo, C., Seifer, R., & Carskadon, M. A. (2005). Experimental restriction of sleep opportunity in children: effects on teacher ratings. *Sleep, 28*(12), 1561–1567.

Ferguson, S. A., & Dawson, D. (2012). 12-h or 8-h shifts? It depends. *Sleep Med Rev, 16*(6), 519–528. doi: 10.1016/j.smrv.2011.11.001

Fernandez, R. C., Marino, J. L., Varcoe, T. J., Davis, S., Moran, L. J., Rumbold, A. R., … Moore, V. M. (2016). Fixed or rotating night shift work undertaken by women: implications for fertility and miscarriage. *Semin Reprod Med, 34*(2), 74–82. doi: 10.1055/s-0036-1571354

Filtness, A. J., Anund, A., Fors, C., Ahlström, C., Åkerstedt, T., & Kecklund, G. (2014). Sleep-related eye symptoms and their potential for identifying driver sleepiness. *J Sleep Res, 23*, 568–575. doi: 0.1111/jsr.12163

Finan, P. H., Quartana, P. J., Remeniuk, B., Garland, E. L., Rhudy, J. L., Hand, M., … Smith, M. T. (2017). Partial sleep deprivation attenuates the positive affective system: effects across multiple measurement modalities. *Sleep, 40*(1). doi: 10.1093/sleep/zsw017

Finan, P. H., Quartana, P. J., & Smith, M. T. (2015). The effects of sleep continuity disruption on positive mood and sleep architecture in healthy adults. *Sleep, 38*(11), 1735–1742. doi: 10.5665/sleep.5154

Finelli, L. A., Baumann, H., Borbély, A. A., & Achermann, P. (2000). Dual electroencephalogram markers of human sleep homeostasis: correlation between theta activity in waking and slow-wave activity in sleep. *Neuroscience, 101*(3), 523–529.

Fischman, S., Kuffler, D. P., & Bloch, C. (2015). Disordered sleep as a cause of attention deficit/hyperactivity disorder: recognition and management. *Clin Pediatr, 54*(8), 713–722. doi: 10.1177/0009922814548673

Flo, E., Pallesen, S., Moen, B. E., Waage, S., & Bjorvatn, B. (2014). Short rest periods between work shifts predict sleep and health problems in nurses at 1-year follow-up. *Occup Environ Med, 71*(8), 555–561. doi: 10.1136/oemed-2013-102007

Foley, J. E., & Weinraub, M. (2017). Sleep, affect, and social competence from preschool to preadolescence: distinct pathways to emotional and social adjustment for boys and for girls. *Front Psychol, 8*, 711. doi: 10.3389/fpsyg.2017.00711

Franken, P., & Dijk, D.-J. (2009). Circadian clock genes and sleep homeostasis. *Eur J Neurosci, 29*(9), 1820–1829. doi: 10.1111/j.1460-9568.2009.06723.x

Friedman, B.-C., Hendeles-Amitai, A., Kozminsky, E., Leiberman, A., Friger, M., Tarasiuk, A., & Tal, A. (2003). Adenotonsillectomy improves neurocognitive function in children with obstructive sleep apnea syndrome. *Sleep, 26*(8), 999–1005.

Friedman, N. P., Corley, R. P., Hewitt, J. K., & Wright Jr, K. P. (2009). Individual differences in childhood sleep problems predict later cognitive executive control. *Sleep, 32*(3), 323–333.

Friedman, N. P., & Robbins, T. W. (2022). The role of prefrontal cortex in cognitive control and executive function. *Neuropsychopharmacology, 47*(1), 72–89. doi: 10.1038/s41386-021-01132-0

Galano, A., Tan, D. X., & Reiter, R. J. (2018). Melatonin: a versatile protector against oxidative DNA damage. *Molecules, 23*(3), 530. doi:10.3390/molecules23030530

Galli, O., Jones, C. W., Larson, O., Basner, M., & Dinges, D. F. (2022). Predictors of interindividual differences in vulnerability to neurobehavioral consequences of chronic partial sleep restriction. *Sleep, 45*(1), zsab278. doi: 10.1093/sleep/zsab278

George, C. F. P., & Smiley, A. (1999). Sleep apnea and automobile crashes. *Sleep, 22*(6), 790–795.

Gillberg, M., Kecklund, G., & Åkerstedt, T. (1994). Relations between performance and subjective ratings of sleepiness during a night awake. *Sleep, 17*(3), 236–241.

Goel, N., Banks, S., Mignot, E., & Dinges, D. F. (2010). *DQB1*0602* predicts interindividual differences in physiologic sleep, sleepiness, and fatigue. *Neurology, 75*, 1509–1519.

Goitein, L., Shanafelt, T., Wipf, J., Slatore, C., & Back, A. (2005). The effects of work-hour limitations on resident well-being, patient care, and education in an internal medicine residency program. *Arch Intern Med, 165*(22), 2601–2606. doi: 10.1001/archinte.165.22.2601

Goldstein-Piekarski, A. N., Greer, S. M., Saletin, J. M., & Walker, M. P. (2015). Sleep deprivation impairs the human central and peripheral nervous system discrimination of social threat. *J Neurosci, 35*(28), 10135–10145. doi: 10.1523/JNEUROSCI.5254-14.2015

Gopal, R., Glasheen, J. J., Miyoshi, T. J., & Prochazka, A. V. (2005). Burnout and internal medicine resident work-hour restrictions. *Arch Intern Med, 165*(22), 2595–2600. doi: 10.1001/archinte.165.22.2595

Gordon, A. M., & Chen, S. (2014). The role of sleep in interpersonal conflict: do sleepless nights mean worse fights? *Soc Psychol Pers Sci, 5*(2), 168–175. doi: 10.1177/1948550613488952

Grant, D. A., & Van Dongen, H. P. A. (2013). Individual differences in sleep duration and responses to sleep loss. In P. Shaw, M. Tafti, & M. J. Thorpy (Eds.),

The Genetic Basis of Sleep and Sleep Disorders (pp. 189–196). Cambridge: Cambridge University Press.

Gregory, A. M., & O'Connor, T. G. (2002). Sleep problems in childhood: a longitudinal study of developmental change and association with behavioral problems. *J Am Acad Child Adolesc Psychiatry, 41*(8), 964–971.

Gregory, A. M., & Sadeh, A. (2016). Annual research review: sleep problems in childhood psychiatric disorders--a review of the latest science. *J Child Psychol Psychiatry, 57*(3), 296–317. doi: 10.1111/jcpp.12469

Gruber, R., Cassoff, J., Frenette, S., Wiebe, S., & Carrier, J. (2012). Impact of sleep extension and restriction on children's emotional lability and impulsivity. *Pediatrics, 130*(5), e1155–1161. doi: 10.1542/peds.2012-0564

Gruber, R., Sommerville, G., Panaitescu, A., & Saha, S. (2023). Sleep duration, but not insomnia symptoms, is associated with poor executive functions in adolescents. *Sleep Med, 101*, 36–39. doi: 10.1016/j.sleep.2022.10.009

Gruber, R., Wiebe, S., Montecalvo, L., Brunetti, B., Amsel, R., & Carrier, J. (2011). Impact of sleep restriction on neurobehavioral functioning of children with attention deficit hyperactivity disorder. *Sleep, 34*(3), 315–323.

Gujar, N., McDonald, S. A., Nishida, M., & Walker, M. P. (2011). A role for REM sleep in recalibrating the sensitivity of the human brain to specific emotions. *Cereb Cortex, 21*(1), 115–123. doi: 10.1093/cercor/bhq064

Gujar, N., Yoo, S. S., Hu, P., & Walker, M. P. (2011). Sleep deprivation amplifies reactivity of brain reward networks, biasing the appraisal of positive emotional experiences. *J Neurosci, 31*(12), 4466–4474. doi: 10.1523/JNEUROSCI.3220-10.2011

Gurubhagavatula, I., Barger, L. K., Barnes, C. M., Basner, M., Boivin, D. B., Dawson, D., ... Van Dongen, H. P. A. (2021). Guiding principles for determining work shift duration and addressing the effects of work shift duration on performance, safety, and health: guidance from the American Academy of Sleep Medicine and the Sleep Research Society. *J Clin Sleep Med, 17*(11), 2283–2306. doi: 10.5664/jcsm.9512

Hare, T. A., Camerer, C. F., Knoepfle, D. T., & Rangel, A. (2010). Value computations in ventral medial prefrontal cortex during charitable decision making incorporate input from regions involved in social cognition. *J Neurosci, 30*(2), 583–590. doi: 10.1523/JNEUROSCI.4089-09.2010

Harrison, Y., Horne, J. A., & Rothwell, A. (2000). Prefrontal neuropsychological effects of sleep deprivation in young adults - a model for healthy aging? *Sleep, 23*(8), 1067–1073.

Haus, E. L., & Smolensky, M. H. (2013). Shift work and cancer risk: potential mechanistic roles of circadian disruption, light at night, and sleep deprivation. *Sleep Med Rev, 17*(4), 273–284. doi: 10.1016/j.smrv.2012.08.003

He, Y., Jones, C. R., Fujiki, N., Xu, Y., Guo, B., Holder, J. L., ... Fu, Y. H. (2009). The transcriptional repressor DEC2 regulates sleep length in mammals. *Science, 325*(5942), 866–870. doi: 10.1126/science.1174443

Hedstrom, A. K., Åkerstedt, T., Hillert, J., Olsson, T., & Alfredsson, L. (2011). Shift work at young age is associated with increased risk for multiple sclerosis. *Ann Neurol, 70*(5), 733–741. doi: 10.1002/ana.22597

Hirsch Allen, A. J., Park, J. E., Adhami, N., Sirounis, D., Tholin, H., Dodek, P., ... Ayas, N. (2014). Impact of work schedules on sleep duration of critical care nurses. *Am J Crit Care, 23*(4), 290–295. doi: 10.4037/ajcc2014876

Holding, B. C., Lauka, P., Fischer, H., Bänziger, T., Axelsson, J., & Sundelin, T. (2017). Multimodal emotion recognition is resilient to insufficient sleep: results from cross-sectional and experimental studies. *Sleep, 40*(11), zsx145. doi: 10.1093/sleep/zsx145.

Horne, J. (2011). The end of sleep: "sleep debt" versus biological adaptation of human sleep to waking needs. *Biol Psychol, 87*(1), 1–14. doi: 10.1016/j.biopsycho.2010.10.004

Horne, J. A. (1993). Human sleep, sleep loss and behaviour. Implications for the prefrontal cortex and psychiatric disorder. *Br J Psychiatry, 162*, 413–419. doi: 10.1192/bjp.162.3.413

Horne, J. A., & Burley, C. V. (2010). We know when we are sleepy: subjective versus objective measurements of moderate sleepiness in healthy adults. *Biol Psychol, 83*(3), 266–268. doi: 10.1016/j.biopsycho.2009.12.011

Horne, J. A., Reyner, L. A., & Barrett, P. R. (2003). Driving impairment due to sleepiness is exacerbated by low alcohol intake. *Occup Environ Med, 60*, 689–692.

Huang, Z. L., Qu, W. M., Eguchi, N., Chen, J. F., Schwarzschild, M. A., Fredholm, B. B., ... Hayaishi, O. (2005). Adenosine A2A, but not A1, receptors mediate the arousal effect of caffeine. *Nat Neurosci, 8*(7), 858–859. doi: 10.1038/nn1491

Jackson, M. L., Gunzelmann, G., Whitney, P., Hinson, J. M., Belenky, G., Rabat, A., & Van Dongen, H. P. (2013). Deconstructing and reconstructing cognitive performance in sleep deprivation. *Sleep Med Rev, 17*(3), 215–225. doi: 10.1016/j.smrv.2012.06.007

Jia, Y., Lu, Y., Wu, K., Lin, Q., Shen, W., Zhu, M., ... Chen, J. (2013). Does night work increase the risk of breast cancer? A systematic review and meta-analysis of epidemiological studies. *Cancer Epidemiol, 37*(3), 197–206. doi: 10.1016/j.canep.2013.01.005

Jones, K., & Harrison, Y. (2001). Frontal lobe function, sleep loss and fragmented sleep. *Sleep Med Rev, 5*(6), 463–475. doi: 10.1053/smrv.2001.0203

Jørgensen, J. T., Hansen, J., Westendorp, R. G. J., Nabe-Nielsen, K., Stayner, L. T., Simonsen, M. K., & Andersen, Z. J. (2020). Shift work and incidence of dementia: a Danish nurse cohort study. *Alzheimers Dement, 16*(9), 1268–1279. doi: 10.1002/alz.12126

Kahn-Greene, E. T., Killgore, D. B., Kamimori, G. H., Balkin, T. J., & Killgore, W. D. S. (2007). The effects of sleep deprivation on symptoms of psychopathology in healthy adults. *Sleep Med, 8*, 215–221. doi: 0.1016/j.sleep.2006.08.007

Kamdar, B. B., Tergas, A. I., Mateen, F. J., Bhayani, N. H., & Oh, J. (2013). Night-shift work and risk of breast cancer: a systematic review and meta-analysis. *Breast Cancer Res Treat, 138*, 291–301. doi: 10.1007/s10549-013-2433-1)

Kamphuis, J., Dijk, D. J., Spreen, M., & Lancel, M. (2014). The relation between poor sleep, impulsivity and aggression in forensic psychiatric patients. *Physiol Behav, 123*, 168–173. doi: 10.1016/j.physbeh.2013.10.015

Kang, W., Jang, K. H., Lim, H. M., Ahn, J. S., & Park, W. J. (2019). The menstrual cycle associated with insomnia in newly employed nurses performing shift work: a 12-month follow-up study. *Int Arch Occup Environ Health, 92*(2), 227–235. doi: 10.1007/s00420-018-1371-y

Killgore, W. D. S., Balkin, T. J., & Wesensten, N. J. (2006). Impaired decision making following 49 h of sleep deprivation. *J Sleep Res, 15*, 7–13.

Kim, M., Vu, T. H., Maas, M. B., Braun, R. I., Wolf, M. S., Roenneberg, T., ... Zee, P. C. (2022). Light at night in older age is associated with obesity, diabetes, and hypertension. *Sleep, 46*(3), zsac130. doi:10.1093/sleep/zsac130

Kim, Y., Bolortuya, Y., Chen, L., Basheer, R., McCarley, R. W., & Strecker, R. E. (2012). Decoupling of sleepiness from sleep time and intensity during chronic sleep restriction: evidence for a role of the adenosine system. *Sleep, 35*(6), 861–869. doi: 10.5665/sleep.1890

Kim, Y., Elmenhorst, D., Weisshaupt, A., Wedekind, F., Kroll, T., McCarley, R. W., ... Bauer, A. (2015). Chronic sleep restriction induces long-lasting changes in adenosine and noradrenaline receptor density in the rat brain. *J Sleep Res, 24*(5), 549–558. doi: 10.1111/jsr.12300

Klerman, E. B., & Dijk, D. J. (2005). Interindividual variation in sleep duration and its association with sleep debt in young adults. *Sleep, 28*(10), 1253–1259.

Klingman, K. M., Marsh, E. E., Klerman, E. B., Anderson, E. J., & Hall, J. E. (2011). Absence of circadian rhythms of gonadotropin secretion in women. *J Clin Endocr Metab, 96*(5), 1456–1461. doi: 10.1210/jc.2010-2739

Kloog, I., Haim, A., Stevens, R. G., & Portnov, B. A. (2009). Global co-distribution of light at night (LAN) and cancers of prostate, colon, and lung in men. *Chronobiol Int, 26*(1), 108–125. doi: 10.1080/07420520802694020

Kloog, I., Stevens, R. G., Haim, A., & Portnov, B. A. (2010). Nighttime light level co-distributes with breast cancer incidence worldwide. *Cancer Cause Control, 21*(12), 2059–2068. doi: 10.1007/s10552-010-9624-4

Knauth, P. (2009). Changing schedules: shiftwork. *Chronobiol Int, 14*(2), 159–171. doi: 10.3109/07420529709001153

Krause, A. J., Ben Simon, E., Mander, B. A., Greer, S. M., Saletin, J. M., Goldstein-Piekarski, A. N., & Walker, M. P. (2017). The sleep-deprived human brain. *Nat Rev Neurosci, 18*, 404–418. doi: 0.1038/nrn.2017.55

Kuna, S. T., Maislin, G., Pack, F. M., Staley, B., Hachadoorian, R., Coccaro, E. F., & Pack, A. I. (2012). Heritability of performance deficit accumulation during acute sleep deprivation in twins. *Sleep, 35*(9), 1223–1233. doi: 10.5665/sleep.2074

Lam, J. C., Mahone, E. M., Mason, T., & Scharf, S. M. (2011). The effects of napping on cognitive function in preschoolers. *J Dev Behav Pediatr, 32*(2), 90–97. doi: 10.1097/DBP.0b013e318207ecc7

Lamond, N., & Dawson, D. (1999). Quantifying the performance impairment associated with fatigue. *J Sleep Res, 8*, 255–262.

Landrigan, C. P., Rothschild, J. M., Cronin, J. W., Kaushal, R., Burdick, E., Katz, J. T., ... Czeisler, C. A. (2004). Effect of reducing interns' work hours on serious medical errors in intensive care units. *N Engl J Med, 351*(18), 1838–1848. doi: 10.1056/NEJMoa041406

Lau, E. Y. Y., Eskes, G. A., Morrison, D. L., Rajda, M., & Spurr, K. F. (2010). Executive function in patients with obstructive sleep apnea treated with continuous positive airway pressure. *J Int Neuropsych Soc, 16*(06), 1077–1088. doi: 10.1017/s1355617710000901

Lau, E. Y. Y., Wong, M. L., Rusak, B., Lam, Y. C., Wing, Y. K., Tseng, C. H., & Lee, T. M. C. (2019). The coupling of short sleep duration and high sleep need predicts riskier decision making. *Psychol Health, 34*(10), 1196–1213. doi: 10.1080/08870446.2019.1594807

Lee, S. Y., Song, P., Choi, S. J., Suh, S., Kwon, S. O., & Joo, E. Y. (2020). The impact of the shift system on health and quality of life of sleep technicians. *Sleep Med, 76*, 72–79. doi: 10.1016/j.sleep.2020.09.026

Leise, T., Harrington, M., Molyneux, P., Song, I., Queenan, H., Zimmerman, E., Lall, G., & Biello, S. (2013). Voluntary exercise can strengthen the circadian system in aged mice. *Age, 35*, 2137–2152. doi: 10.1007/s11357-012-9502-y)

Leise, T. L., Goldberg, A., Michael, J., Montoya, G., Solow, S., Molyneux, P., ... Harrington, M. E. (2020). Recurring circadian disruption alters circadian clock sensitivity to resetting. *Eur J Neurosci, 51*(12), 2343–2354. doi: 10.1111/ejn.14179

Lenzer, J. (2015). Doctors underwent "extreme sleep deprivation" in studies of effect on patient deaths. *Br Med J, 351*, h6295. doi: 10.1136/bmj.h6295

Leproult, R., Colecchia, E. F., Berardi, M., Stickgold, R., Kosslyn, S. M., & Van Cauter, E. (2003). Individual differences in subjective and objective alertness during sleep deprivation are stable and unrelated. *Am J Physiol, 284*, R280-R290.

Lewy, A. J., Wehr, T. A., Goodwin, F. K., Newsome, D. A., & Markey, S. P. (1980). Light suppresses melatonin secretion in humans. *Science, 210*, 1267–1269.

Libedinsky, C., Smith, D. V., Teng, C. S., Namburi, P., Chen, V. W., Huettel, S. A., & Chee, M. W. (2011). Sleep deprivation alters valuation signals in the ventromedial prefrontal cortex. *Front Behav Neurosci, 5*. doi:10.3389/fnbeh.2011.00070

Lim, J., & Dinges, D. F. (2008). Sleep deprivation and vigilant attention. *Ann NY Acad Sci, 1129*(1), 305–322. doi: 10.1196/annals.1417.002

Lim, J., & Dinges, D. F. (2010). A meta-analysis of the impact of short-term sleep deprivation on cognitive variables. *Psychol Bull, 136*(3), 375–389. doi: 10.1037/a0018883

Liu, S. Y., Perez, M. A., & Lau, N. (2018). The impact of sleep disorders on driving safety-findings from the Second Strategic Highway Research Program naturalistic driving study. *Sleep, 41*(4), zsy023. doi: 10.1093/sleep/zsy023

Liu, Z., Wang, Y., Cai, L., Li, Y., Chen, B., Dong, Y., & Huang, Y. H. (2016). Prefrontal cortex to accumbens projections in sleep regulation of reward. *J Neurosci, 36*(30), 7897–7910. doi: 10.1523/JNEUROSCI.0347-16.2016

Lo, J. C., Groeger, J. A., Santhi, N., Arbon, E. L., Lazar, A. S., Hasan, S., ... Dijk, D.-J. (2012). Effects of partial and acute total sleep deprivation on performance across cognitive domains, individuals and circadian phase. *PLoS One, 7*(9), e45987. doi: 10.1371/journal.pone.0045987

Lollies, F., Schnatschmidt, M., Bihlmeier, I., Genuneit, J., In-Albnon, T., Holtmann, M., ... Schlarb, A. A. (2022). Associations of sleep and emotion regulation processes in childhood and adolescence - a systematic review, report of methodological challenges and future directions. *Sleep Sci, 15*(4), 490–514. doi: 10.5935/1984-0063.20220082

Louca, M., & Short, M. A. (2014). The effect of one night's sleep deprivation on adolescent neurobehavioral performance. *Sleep, 37*(11), 1799–1807. doi: 10.5665/sleep.4174

Lundahl, A., Kidwell, K. M., Van Dyk, T. R., & Nelson, T. D. (2015). A meta-analysis of the effect of experimental sleep restriction on youth's attention and hyperactivity. *Dev Neuropsychol, 40*(3), 104–121. doi: 10.1080/87565641.2014.939183

Ma, N., Dinges, D. F., Basner, M., & Rao, H. (2015). How acute total sleep loss affects the attending brain: a meta-analysis of neuroimaging studies. *Sleep, 38*(2), 233–240. doi: 10.5665/sleep.4404

Manenschijn, L., van Kruysbergen, R. G., de Jong, F. H., Koper, J. W., & van Rossum, E. F. (2011). Shift work at young age is associated with elevated long-term cortisol levels and body mass index. *J Clin Endocrinol Metab, 96*(11), E1862–E1865. doi: 10.1210/jc.2011-1551

Martino, T. A., Oudit, G. Y., Herzenberg, A. M., Tata, N., Koletar, M. M., Kabir, G. M., ... Sole, M. J. (2008). Circadian rhythm disorganization produces profound cardiovascular and renal disease in hamsters. *Am J Physiol Regul Integr Comp Physiol, 294*(5), R1675–R1683. doi: 10.1152/ajpregu.00829.2007

Maski, K. P., & Kothare, S. V. (2013). Sleep deprivation and neurobehavioral functioning in children. *Int J Psychophysiol, 89*(2), 259–264. doi: 10.1016/j.ijpsycho.2013.06.019

McCann, M., Bayliss, D. M., Pestell, C., Hill, C. M., & Bucks, R. S. (2018). The relationship between sleep and working memory in children with neurological conditions. *Child Neuropsychol, 24*(3), 304–321. doi: 10.1080/09297049.2016.1231298

McClure, D. J., Zuckerman, S. L., Kutscher, S. J., Gregory, A. J., & Solomon, G. S. (2014). Baseline neurocognitive testing in sports-related concussions: the importance of a prior night's sleep. *Am J Sports Med, 42*(2), 472–478. doi: 10.1177/0363546513510389

McHill, A. W., Czeisler, C. A., & Shea, S. A. (2018). Resident physician extended work hours and burnout. *Sleep, 41*(8), zsy112. doi: 10.1093/sleep/zsy112

McHill, A. W., Hull, J. T., Cohen, D. A., Wang, W., Czeisler, C. A., & Klerman, E. B. (2019). Chronic sleep restriction greatly magnifies performance decrements immediately after awakening. *Sleep, 42*(5), zsz032. doi: 10.1093/sleep/zsz032

McHill, A. W., Hull, J. T., Wang, W., Czeisler, C. A., & Klerman, E. B. (2018). Chronic sleep curtailment, even without extended (>16-h) wakefulness, degrades human vigilance performance. *Proc Natl Acad Sci U S A, 115*(23), 6070–6075. doi: 10.1073/pnas.1706694115

McHill, A. W., Velasco, J., Bodner, T., Shea, S. A., & Olson, R. (2022). Rapid changes in overnight blood pressure after transitioning to early-morning shiftwork. *Sleep, 45*(3), zsab203. doi: 10.1093/sleep/zsab203

McMakin, D. L., Dahl, R. E., Buysse, D. J., Cousins, J. C., Forbes, E. E., Silk, J. S., ... Franzen, P. L. (2016). The impact of experimental sleep restriction on affective functioning in social and nonsocial contexts among adolescents. *J Child Psychol Psychiatry, 57*(9), 1027–1037. doi: 10.1111/jcpp.12568

Megdal, S. P., Kroenke, C. H., Laden, F., Pukkala, E., & Schernhammer, E. S. (2005). Night work and breast cancer risk: a systematic review and meta-analysis. *Eur J Cancer, 41*(13), 2023–2032. doi: 10.1016/j.ejca.2005.05.010

Mu, Q., Mishory, A., Johnson, K. A., Nahas, Z., Kozel, F. A., Yamanaka, K., ... George, M. S. (2005). Decreased brain activation during a working memory task at rested baseline is associated with vulnerability to sleep deprivation. *Sleep, 28*(4), 433–446.

Mulhall, M. D., Sletten, T. L., Magee, M., Stone, J. E., Ganesan, S., Collins, A., ... Rajaratnam, S. M. W. (2019). Sleepiness and driving events in shift workers: the impact of circadian and homeostatic factors. *Sleep, 42*(6), zsz074. doi:10.1093/sleep/zsz074

Munkhjargal, O., Oka, Y., Tanno, S., Shimizu, H., Fujino, Y., Kira, T., ... Higaki, T. (2022). Discrepancy between subjective and objective sleepiness in adolescents. *Sleep Med, 96*, 1–7. doi: 10.1016/j.sleep.2022.04.025

Nagano, M., Adachi, A., Nakahama, K., Nakamura, T., Tamada, M., Meyer-Bernstein, E., ... Shigeyoshi, Y. (2003). An abrupt shift in the day/night cycle causes desynchrony in the mammalian circadian center. *J Neurosci, 23*(14), 6141–6151.

National-Sleep-Foundation. (2003). Sleep in America poll 2003. Retrieved from https://www.thensf.org/wp-content/uploads/2021/03/2003-SleepPollExecSumm.pdf

Nicholls, S. K., Casiraghi, L. P., Wang, W., Weber, E. T., & Harrington, M. E. (2019). Evidence for internal desynchrony caused by circadian clock resetting. *Yale J Biol Med, 92*, 259–270.

Niedhammer, I., Lert, F., & Marne, M. J. (1995). Psychotropic drug use and shift work among French nurses (1980-1990). *Psychol Med, 25*, 329–338.

Nigro, S. E., Peugh, J., Yolton, K., Chen, A., Lanphear, B. P., & Beebe, D. (2023). Early childhood sleep quantity, but not caregiver-reported sleep problems, predicts impulse control in children at age 8 years. *Child Neuropsychol, 30*(4), 602–614. doi: 10.1080/09297049.2023.2247602

Ojio, Y., Nishida, A., Shimodera, S., Togo, F., & Sasaki, T. (2016). Sleep duration associated with the lowest risk of depression/anxiety in adolescents. *Sleep, 39*(8), 1555–1562. doi: 10.5665/sleep.6020

Oonk, M., Davis, C. J., Krueger, J. M., Wisor, J. P., & Van Dongen, H. P. (2015). Sleep deprivation and time-on-task performance decrement in the rat psychomotor vigilance task. *Sleep, 38*(3), 445–451. doi: 10.5665/sleep.4506

Pace-Schott, E. F., Hutcherson, C. A., Bemporad, B., Morgan, A., Kumar, A., Hobson, J. A., & Stickgold, R. (2009). Failure to find executive function deficits following one night's total sleep deprivation in university students under naturalistic conditions. *Behav Sleep Med, 7*(3), 136–163. doi: 10.1080/15402000902976671

Palmer, C. A., Bower, J. L., Cho, K. W., Clementi, M. A., Lau, S., Oosterhoff, B., & Alfano, C. A. (2023). Sleep loss and emotion: A systematic review and meta-analysis of over 50 years of experimental research. *Psychol Bull, 150*(4), 440–463. doi: 10.1037/bul0000410

Patrick, G. T. W., & Gilbert, J. A. (1896). On the effects of loss of sleep. *Psych Rev, 3*(5), 469–483.

Pellegrino, R., Kavakli, I. H., Goel, N., Cardinale, C. J., Dinges, D. F., Kuna, S. T., ... Pack, A. I. (2014). A novel BHLHE41 variant is associated with short sleep and resistance to sleep deprivation in humans. *Sleep, 37*(8), 1327–1336. doi: 10.5665/sleep.3924

Peplonska, B., Bukowska, A., Gromadzinska, J., Sobala, W., Reszka, E., Lie, J. A., ... Wasowicz, W. (2012). Night shift work characteristics and 6-sulfatoxymelatonin (MT6s) in rotating night shift nurses and midwives. *Occup Environ Med, 69*(5), 339–346. doi: 10.1136/oemed-2011-100273

Peters, J. D., Biggs, S. N., Bauer, K. M., Lushington, K., Kennedy, D., Martin, J., & Dorrian, J. (2009). The sensitivity of a PDA-based psychomotor vigilance task to sleep restriction in 10-year-old girls. *J Sleep Res, 18*(2), 173–177. doi: 10.1111/j.1365-2869.2008.00716.x

Petit, D., Touchette, E., Pennestri, M. H., Paquet, J., Cote, S., Tremblay, R. E., ... Montplaisir, J. Y. (2023). Nocturnal sleep duration trajectories in early childhood and school performance at age 10 years. *J Sleep Res*, *32*(5), e13893. doi:10.1111/jsr.13893

Philibert, I. (2005). Sleep loss and performance in residents and nonphysicians: a meta-analytic examination. *Sleep*, *28*(11), 1392–1402.

Philip, P., Sagaspe, P., Prague, M., Tassi, P., Capelli, A., Bioulac, B., ... Taillard, J. (2012). Acute versus chronic partial sleep deprivation in middle-aged people: differential effect on performance and sleepiness. *Sleep*, *35*(7), 997–1002. doi: 10.5665/sleep.1968

Porkka-Heiskanen, T., & Kalinchuk, A. V. (2011). Adenosine, energy metabolism and sleep homeostasis. *Sleep Med Rev*, *15*(2), 123–135. doi: 10.1016/j.smrv.2010.06.005

Porkka-Heiskanen, T., Strecker, R. E., & McCarley, R. W. (2000). Brain site-specificity of extracellular adenosine concentration changes during sleep deprivation and spontaneous sleep: an in vivo microdialysis study. *Neuroscience*, *99*(3), 507–517.

Posner, M. I., & Rothbart, M. K. (1998). Attention, self-regulation and consciousness. *Phil Trans R Soc Lond B*, *353*, 1915–1927.

Poudel, G. R., Innes, C. R., & Jones, R. D. (2012). Cerebral perfusion differences between drowsy and nondrowsy individuals after acute sleep restriction. *Sleep*, *35*(8), 1085–1096. doi: 10.5665/sleep.1994

Powell, N. B., Schechtman, K. B., Riley, R. W., Li, K., Troell, R., & Guilleminault, C. (2001). The road to danger: the comparative risks of driving while sleepy. *Laryngoscope*, *111*(5), 887–893.

Puttonen, S., Harma, M., & Hublin, C. (2010). Shift work and cardiovascular disease - pathways from circadian stress to morbidity. *Scand J Work Environ Health*, *36*(2), 96–108. doi: 10.5271/sjweh.2894

RAND. (2016). Why sleep matters-the economic costs of insufficient sleep: a cross-country comparative analysis. Retrieved from http://www.rand.org/randeurope/research/projects/the-value-of-the-sleep-economy.html

Randazzo, A. C., Muehlbach, M. J., Schweitzer, P. K., & Walsh, J. K. (1998). Cognitive function following acute sleep restriction in children ages 10-14. *Sleep*, *21*(8), 861–868.

Reilly, T., Waterhouse, J., & Atkinson, G. (1997). Aging, rhythms of physical performance, and adjustment to changes in the sleep-activity cycle. *Occup Environ Med*, *54*, 812–816.

Rétey, J. V., Adam, M., Gottselig, J. M., Khatami, R., Durr, R., Achermann, P., & Landolt, H. P. (2006). Adenosinergic mechanisms contribute to individual differences in sleep deprivation-induced changes in neurobehavioral function and brain rhythmic activity. *J Neurosci*, *26*(41), 10472–10479. doi: 10.1523/jneurosci.1538-06.2006

Rétey, J. V., Adam, M., Khatami, R., Luhmann, U. F., Jung, H. H., Berger, W., & Landolt, H. P. (2007). A genetic variation in the adenosine A2A receptor gene (ADORA2A) contributes to individual sensitivity to caffeine effects on sleep. *Clin Pharmacol Ther*, *81*(5), 692–698. doi: 10.1038/sj.clpt.6100102

Reynaud, E., Vecchierini, M. F., Heude, B., Charles, M. A., & Plancoulaine, S. (2018). Sleep and its relation to cognition and behaviour in preschool-aged children of the general population: a systematic review. *J Sleep Res*, *27*(3), 1–18. doi:10.1111/jsr.12636

Riggins, T., & Spencer, R. M. C. (2020). Habitual sleep is associated with both source memory and hippocampal subfield volume during early childhood. *Sci Rep*, *10*(1), 15304. doi:10.1038/s41598-020-72231-z

Roca, J., Fuentes, L. J., Marotta, A., López-Ramón, M.-F., Castro, C., Lupiáñez, J., & Martella, D. (2012). The effects of sleep deprivation on the attentional functions and vigilance. *Acta Psycholog*, *140*, 164–176. doi: 0.1016/j.actpsy.2012.03.007

Roden, M., Koller, M., Pirich, K., Vierhapper, H., & Waldhauser, F. (1993). The circadian melatonin and cortisol secretion pattern in permanent night shift workers. *Am J Physiol Regul Integr Comp Physiol*, *265*(1, Part 2), R261–R267.

Roehrs, T., & Roth, T. (1992). Multiple Sleep Latency Test: technical aspects and normal values. *J Clin Neurophysiol*, *9*(1), 63–67.

Roehrs, T., Timms, V., Zwyghuizen-Doorenbos, A., & Roth, T. (1989). Sleep extension in sleepy and alert normals. *Sleep*, *12*(5), 449–457.

Rollinson, D. C., Rathlev, N. K., Moss, M., Killiany, R., Sassower, K. C., Auerbach, S., & Fish, S. S. (2003). The effects of consecutive night shifts on neuropsychological performance of interns in the emergency department: a pilot study. *Ann Emerg Med*, *41*(3), 400–406. doi: 10.1067/mem.2003.77

Rupp, T. L., Wesensten, N. J., & Balkin, T. J. (2009). Sleep history affects task acquisition during subsequent sleep restriction and recovery. *J Sleep Res*, *19*(2), 289–297. doi: 10.1111/j.1365-2869.2009.00800.x

Rupp, T. L., Wesensten, N. J., & Balkin, T. J. (2012). Trait-like vulnerability to total and partial sleep loss. *Sleep*, *35*(8), 1163–1172. doi: 10.5665/sleep.2010

Sadeh, A., Gruber, R., & Raviv, A. (2003). The effects of sleep restriction and extension on school-age children: what a difference an hour makes. *Child Dev*, *74*(2), 444–455.

Salthouse, T. A. (2005). Relations between cognitive abilities and measures of executive functioning. *Neuropsychology*, *19*(4), 532–545. doi: 10.1037/0894-4105.19.4.532

Schernhammer, E. S., Laden, F., Speizer, F. E., Willett, W. C., Hunter, D. J., Kawachi, I., & Colditz, G. A. (2001). Rotating night shifts and risk of breast cancer in women participating in the nurses' health study. *J Natl Cancer Inst*, *93*(20), 1563–1568.

Sharma, L., Pedlar, C. R., Burgess, P. W., Kanagasabai, S., & Ronca, F. (2023). Acute and long-term sleep measurements produce opposing results on sleep quality in 8 and 12 hour shift patterns in law enforcement officers. *J Sleep Res*, *32*(5), e13862. doi:10.1111/jsr.13862

Sharpe, R., Koval, V., Ronco, J. J., Qayumi, K., Dodek, P., Wong, H., ... Ayas, N. T. (2010). The impact of prolonged continuous wakefulness on resident clinical performance in the intensive care unit: a patient simulator study. *Crit Care Med*, *38*(3), 766–770. doi: 10.1097/CCM.0b013e3181cd122a

Sheehan, C. M., Frochen, S. E., Walsemann, K. M., & Ailshire, J. A. (2019). Are U.S. adults reporting less sleep?: findings from sleep duration trends in the National Health Interview Survey, 2004–2017. *Sleep*, *42*(2), zsy221. doi:10.1093/sleep/zsy221

Shen, L., van Schie, J., Ditchburn, G., Brook, L., & Bei, B. (2018). Positive and negative emotions: differential associations with sleep duration and quality in adolescents. *J Youth Adolesc*, *47*(12), 2584–2595. doi: 10.1007/s10964-018-0899-1

Shi, H., Huang, T., Schernhammer, E. S., Sun, Q., & Wang, M. (2022). Rotating night shift work and healthy aging after 24 years of follow-up in the Nurses' Health Study. *JAMA Netw Open*, *5*(5), e2210450. doi:10.1001/jamanetworkopen.2022.10450

Skorucak, J., Arbon, E. L., Dijk, D. J., & Achermann, P. (2018). Response to chronic sleep restriction, extension, and subsequent total sleep deprivation in humans: adaptation or preserved sleep homeostasis? *Sleep*, *41*(7), zsy078. doi:10.1093/sleep/zsy078

Smith, M. G., Wusk, G. C., Nasrini, J., Baskin, P., Dinges, D. F., Roma, P. G., & Basner, M. (2021). Effects of six weeks of chronic sleep restriction with weekend recovery on cognitive performance and wellbeing in high-performing adults. *Sleep*, *44*(8), zsab051. doi:10.1093/sleep/zsab051

Smith, M. R., & Eastman, C. I. (2012). Shift work: health, performance and safety problems, traditional countermeasures, and innovative management strategies to reduce circadian misalignment. *Nat Sci Sleep*, *4*, 111–132. doi: 10.2147/NSS.S10372

Smith, M. R., Fogg, L. F., & Eastman, C. I. (2009). A compromise circadian phase position for permanent night work improves mood, fatigue and performance. *Sleep*, *32*(11), 1481–1489.

Smithson, L., Baird, T., Tamana, S. K., Lau, A., Mariasine, J., Chikuma, J., ... Mandhane, P. J. (2018). Shorter sleep duration is associated with reduced cognitive development at two years of age. *Sleep Med*, *48*, 131–139. doi: 10.1016/j.sleep.2018.04.005

Stenuit, P., & Kerkhofs, M. (2005). Age modulates the effects of sleep restriction in women. *Sleep*, *28*(10), 1283–1286.

Stock, D., Knight, J. A., Raboud, J., Cotterchio, M., Strohmaier, S., Willett, W., ... Schernhammer, E. (2019). Rotating night shift work and menopausal age. *Hum Reprod*, *34*(3), 539–548. doi: 10.1093/humrep/dey390

Straif, K., Baan, R., Grosse, Y., Secretan, B., Ghissassi, F. E., Bouvard, V., ... Cogliano, V. (2007). Carcinogenicity of shift-work, painting, and fire-fighting. *Lancet Oncol*, *8*(12), 1065–1066. doi: 10.1016/s1470-2045(07)70373-x

Studler, M., Gianotti, L. R. R., Lobmaier, J., Maric, A., & Knoch, D. (2024). Human prosocial preferences are related to slow-wave activity in sleep. *J Neurosci*, *44*(15). doi:10.1523/jneurosci.0885-23.2024

Talbot, L. S., McGlinchey, E. L., Kaplan, K. A., Dahl, R. E., & Harvey, A. G. (2010). Sleep deprivation in adolescents and adults: changes in affect. *Emotion*, *10*(6), 831–841. doi: 10.1037/a0020138

Tan, D. X., Chen, L. D., Poeggeler, B., Manchester, L. C., & Reiter, R. J. (1993). Melatonin: a potent, endogenous hydroxyl radical scavenger. *Endocr J*, *1*, 57–60.

Tomaso, C. C., Johnson, A. B., & Nelson, T. D. (2021). The effect of sleep deprivation and restriction on mood, emotion, and emotion regulation: three meta-analyses in one. *Sleep*, *44*(6), zsaa289. doi:10.1093/sleep/zsaa289

Torsvall, L., & Åkerstedt, T. (1987). Sleepiness on the job: continuously measured EEG changes in train drivers. *Electroencephalogr Clin Neurophysiol*, *66*(6), 502–511. doi: 10.1016/0013-4694(87)90096-4

Touitou, Y., Motohashi, Y., Reinberg, A., Touitou, C., Bourdeleau, P., Bogdan, A., & Auzéby, A. (1990). Effect of shift work on the night-time secretory patterns of melatonin, prolactin, cortisol and testosterone. *Eur J Appl Physiol, 60*, 288–292.

Travis, R. C., Balkwill, A., Fensom, G. K., Appleby, P. N., Reeves, G. K., Wang, X. S., … Beral, V. (2016). Night shift work and breast cancer incidence: three prospective studies and meta-analysis of published studies. *J Natl Cancer Inst, 108*(12), djw169. doi: 10.1093/jnci/djw169

Trinkoff, A. M., & Storr, C. L. (1998). Work schedule characteristics and substance use in nurses. *Am J Ind Med, 34*(3), 266–271. doi: 10.1002/(sici)1097-0274(199809)34:3<266::Aid-ajim9>3.0.Co;2-t

Tucker, A. M., Whitney, P., Belenky, G., Hinson, J. M., & Van Dongen, H. P. A. (2010). Effects of sleep deprivation on dissociated components of attention. *Sleep, 33*(1), 47–57.

Turek, F. W. (1986). Circadian principles and design of rotating shift work schedules. *Am J Physiol, 251*(3, part 2), R636–R638.

Vallières, A., Pappathomas, A., Garnier, S. B., Mérette, C., Carrier, J., Paquette, T., & Bastien, C. H. (2024). Behavioural therapy for shift work disorder improves shift workers' sleep, sleepiness and mental health: a pilot randomised control trial. *J Sleep Res*, e14162. doi:10.1111/jsr.14162

van Amelsvoort, L. G., Jansen, N. W., Swaen, G. M., van den Brandt, P. A., & Kant, I. (2004). Direction of shift rotation among three-shift workers in relation to psychological health and work-family conflict. *Scand J Work Environ Health, 30*(2), 149–156. doi: 10.5271/sjweh.772

van Amelsvoort, L. G. P. M., Schouten, E. G., & Kok, F. J. (1999). Duration of shift work related to body mass index and waist to hip ratio. *Int J Obesity, 23*, 973–978.

van der Helm, E., Gujar, N., & Walker, M. P. (2010). Sleep deprivation impairs the accurate recognition of human emotions. *Sleep, 33*(3), 335–342.

Van Dongen, H. P., Vitellaro, K. M., & Dinges, D. F. (2005). Individual differences in adult human sleep and wakefulness: leitmotif for a research agenda. *Sleep, 28*(4), 479–496.

Van Dongen, H. P. A., Baynard, M. D., Maislin, G., & Dinges, D. F. (2004). Systematic individual differences in neurobehavioral impairment from sleep loss: evidence of trait-like differential vulnerability. *Sleep, 27*(3), 423–433.

Van Dongen, H. P. A., Maislin, G., Mullington, J. M., & Dinges, D. F. (2003). The cumulative cost of additional wakefulness: dose-response effects on neurobehavioral functions and sleep physiology from chronic sleep restriction and total sleep deprivation. *Sleep, 26*(2), 117–126.

Van Dycke, K. C., Rodenburg, W., van Oostrom, C. T., van Kerkhof, L. W., Pennings, J. L., Roenneberg, T., … van der Horst, G. T. (2015). Chronically alternating light cycles increase breast cancer risk in mice. *Curr Biol, 25*(14), 1932–1937. doi: 10.1016/j.cub.2015.06.012

Van Dyk, T. R., Zhang, N., Catlin, P. A., Cornist, K., McAlister, S., Whitacre, C., & Beebe, D. W. (2017). Feasibility and emotional impact of experimentally extending sleep in short-sleeping adolescents. *Sleep, 40*(9), zsx123. doi: 10.1093/sleep/zsx123

Verdecchia, P. (2000). Prognostic value of ambulatory blood pressure: current evidence and clinical implications. *Hypertension, 35*(3), 844–851. doi: 10.1161/01.hyp.35.3.844

Vetter, C., Devore, E. E., Ramin, C. A., Speizer, F. E., Willett, W. C., & Schernhammer, E. S. (2015). Mismatch of sleep and work timing and risk of type 2 diabetes. *Diabetes Care, 38*, 1707–1713. doi: 10.2337/dc15-0302/-/DC1

Vetter, C., Devore, E. E., Wegrzyn, L. R., Massa, J., Speizer, F. E., Kawachi, I., Rosner, B., Stampfer, M. J., & Schernhammer, E. S. (2016). Association between rotating night shift work and risk of coronary heart disease among women. *J Am Med Assoc, 315*(16), 1726–1734. doi: 10.1001/jama.2016.4454

Virtanen, M., Jokela, M., Nyberg, S. T., Madsen, I. E., Lallukka, T., Ahola, K., … Kivimaki, M. (2015). Long working hours and alcohol use: systematic review and meta-analysis of published studies and unpublished individual participant data. *Br Med J, 350*, g7772. doi: 10.1136/bmj.g7772

Vriend, J. L., Davidson, F. D., Corkum, P. V., Rusak, B., Chambers, C. T., & McLaughlin, E. N. (2013). Manipulating sleep duration alters emotional functioning and cognitive performance in children. *J Pediatr Psychol, 38*(10), 1058–1069. doi: 10.1093/jpepsy/jst033

Vriend, J. L., Davidson, F. D., Corkum, P. V., Rusak, B., McLaughlin, E. N., & Chambers, C. T. (2012). Sleep quantity and quality in relation to daytime functioning in children. *Child Health Care, 41*(3), 204–222. doi: 10.1080/02739615.2012.685039

Vyazovskiy, V. V., & Tobler, I. (2005). Theta activity in the waking EEG is a marker of sleep propensity in the rat. *Brain Res, 1050*((1-2)), 64–71. doi: 0.1016/j.brainres.2005.05.022

Wallace, D. A., Reid, K., Grobman, W. A., Facco, F. L., Silver, R. M., Pien, G. W., … Sofer, T. (2022). Associations between evening shift work, irregular sleep timing, and gestational diabetes in the Nulliparous Pregnancy Outcomes Study: Monitoring Mothers-to-be (nuMoM2b). *Sleep, 46*(4), zsac297. doi:10.1093/sleep/zsac297

Wangsan, K., Chaiear, N., Sawanyawisuth, K., Klainin-Yobas, P., Simajareuk, K., & Boonsawat, W. (2022). Which shiftwork pattern Is the strongest predictor for poor sleep quality in nurses? *Int J Environ Res Public Health, 19*(21). doi: 10.3390/ijerph192113986

Waters, F., & Bucks, R. S. (2011). Neuropsychological effects of sleep loss: implication for neuropsychologists. *J Int Neuropsychol Soc, 17*(4), 571–586. doi: 10.1017/S1355617711000610

Watson, N. F., Badr, M. S., Belenky, G., Bliwise, D. L., Buxton, O. M., Buysse, D., … Tasali, E. (2015). Joint consensus statement of the American Academy of Sleep Medicine and Sleep Research Society on the recommended amount of sleep for a healthy adult: methodology and discussion. *Sleep, 38*(8), 1161–1183. doi: 10.5665/sleep.4886

Webb, W. B., & Agnew, H. W. (1965). Sleep: effects of a restricted regime. *Science, 150*(3704), 1745–1747.

Wei, T., Li, C., Heng, Y., Gao, X., Zhang, G., Wang, H., … Hou, H. (2020). Association between night-shift work and level of melatonin: systematic review and meta-analysis. *Sleep Med, 75*, 502–509. doi: 10.1016/j.sleep.2020.09.018

Werth, E., Achermann, P., & Borbély, A. (1997). Fronto-occipital power gradients in human sleep. *J Sleep Res, 6*, 102–112.

Williamson, A. M., & Feyer, A., -M. (2000). Moderate sleep deprivation produces impairments in cognitive and motor performance equivalent to legally prescribed levels of alcohol intoxication. *Occup Environ Med, 57*, 649–655.

Womack, S. D., Hook, J. N., Reyna, S. H., & Ramos, M. (2013). Sleep loss and risk-taking behavior: a review of the literature. *Behav Sleep Med, 11*(5), 343–359. doi: 10.1080/15402002.2012.703628

Yamaguchi, Y., Suzuki, T., Mizoro, Y., Kori, H., Okada, K., Chen, Y., … Okamura, H. (2013). Mice genetically deficient in vasopressin V1a and V1b receptors are resistant to jet lag. *Science, 342*(6154), 85–90.

Yamazaki, E. M., Antler, C. A., Lasek, C. R., & Goel, N. (2021). Residual, differential neurobehavioral deficits linger after multiple recovery nights following chronic sleep restriction or acute total sleep deprivation. *Sleep, 44*(4), zsaa224. doi:10.1093/sleep/zsaa224

Yamazaki, E. M., & Goel, N. (2020). Robust stability of trait-like vulnerability or resilience to common types of sleep deprivation in a large sample of adults. *Sleep, 43*(6), zsz292. doi:10.1093/sleep/zsz292

Yamazaki, S., Numan, R., Abe, M., Hida, A., Takahashi, R.-I., Ueda, M., … Tei, H. (2000). Resetting central and peripheral circadian oscillators in transgenic rats. *Science, 288*(5466), 682–685. doi: 10.1126/science.288.5466.682

Yang, C.-M., Lin, F.-W., & Spielman, A. J. (2004). A standard procedure enhances the correlation between subjective and objective measures of sleepiness. *Sleep, 27*(2), 329–332.

Yoo, S. S., Gujar, N., Hu, P., Jolesz, F. A., & Walker, M. P. (2007). The human emotional brain without sleep--a prefrontal amygdala disconnect. *Curr Biol, 17*(20), R877–878. doi: 10.1016/j.cub.2007.08.007

Yousef, E., Mitwally, N., Noufal, N., & Tahir, M. R. (2020). Shift work and risk of skin cancer: a systematic review and meta-analysis. *Sci Rep, 10*(1), 2012. doi: 10.1038/s41598-020-59035-x

Yu, Y., Chen, Y. X., Liu, L., Yu, Z. Y., & Luo, X. (2017). Neuropsychological functioning after adenotonsillectomy in children with obstructive sleep apnea: a meta-analysis. *J Huazhong Univ Sci Technol Med Sci, 37*(3), 453–461. doi: 10.1007/s11596-017-1756-2

Zada, D., Sela, Y., Matosevich, N., Monsonego, A., Lerer-Goldshtein, T., Nir, Y., & Appelbaum, L. (2021). Parp1 promotes sleep, which enhances DNA repair in neurons. *Mol Cell, 81*(24), 4979–4993.e4977. doi: 10.1016/j.molcel.2021.10.026

CHAPTER 14

Sleep and Human Health, Part A

14.1 OVERVIEW

This chapter reviews how sleep duration is manipulated in research studies, including methods that produce partial sleep restriction or total sleep deprivation, and reviews the challenges and complexities involved in interpreting the results obtained. It also reviews the reported effects of extreme sleep loss on health.

The chapter then reviews evidence from population-based, observational studies that differences in sleep duration and quality are associated with increased risk of illness. It includes discussion of the relations between sleep and conditions such as elements of the metabolic syndrome (insulin resistance, hypertension, lipid dysregulation, and excess body weight/abdominal fat), Type 2 diabetes, obesity, and vascular disease. It also reviews how sleep duration influences immune system function and susceptibility to infection.

The chapter then reviews the results of experimental studies of the metabolic effects of sleep restriction. These acute effects on physiological measures suggest how chronic short sleep can contribute to development of the diseases that are associated with short sleep in population-based studies.

14.2 Studying sleep deprivation

Our society is ambivalent about sleep. Many people behave as if they believe that sleep is a waste of precious time that should be limited as much as possible. But there are also frequent stories in print and electronic media about the harmful health effects of inadequate sleep; indeed, concerns that children were not getting enough sleep were expressed at least a century ago (see Chapter 6). The idea of a physiological need for sleep, similar to that for motivated behaviors linked to other basic drives, is supported by the fact that lack of sleep leads to a progressively stronger, ultimately irresistible, drive to sleep as well as to rebound increases in sleep once it is allowed (see Chapter 5).

The usual approach to studying the effects of not satisfying basic drives like hunger or thirst is to prevent access to the relevant external resources—food or water—and to study the physiological consequences. Sleep, however, is different because it is an internal process that does not rely on external resources. Depriving an animal or person of sleep does not involve removing access to something; instead, it requires sustained interventions to maintain waking. This fact complicates interpretation of the results of sleep deprivation studies. Are changes in the physiology of an animal or person after sleep deprivation the result *only* of the loss of sleep, or are they also related to other effects of the interventions that must be used to prevent sleep? (See **Box 14.1**.)

Various methods have been used to study the effects of sleep deprivation. In human research studies, voluntary cooperation is the starting point; but that must be supplemented by a researcher's interventions to keep a person awake when the drive to sleep eventually becomes overwhelming. In animal studies, voluntary cooperation is not possible, so three main approaches are used:

- Passive methods in which the environment is designed so that sleep onset triggers an event that rapidly wakes the animal;
- Active methods that force the animal to do something that is incompatible with sustaining sleep, such as walking continuously;
- Gentle methods that provide a stimulating environment and frequent, novel distractions so that an animal stays awake to explore these stimuli.

Some of these methods are only suitable for producing short-term sleep loss within a 24 h period, while others may be applied over longer periods to produce either continuous or repeated sleep loss over many days. As discussed briefly in Section 5.4, the physiological mechanisms that respond to acute and sustained sleep loss may be quite different.

BOX 14.1 Sleep Deprivation and Stress

One issue in interpreting the health effects of sleep deprivation is that the interventions used to prevent sleep may also evoke stress responses. Sustained stress is itself a cause of illness and physiological damage. To attribute any effects to sleep loss itself, we need to be able to distinguish them from the effects of nonspecific situational stressors.

Hans Selye first introduced the concept of stress in the 1920s. He described a "general adaptation syndrome" consisting of common patterns of physiological damage resulting from prolonged exposure to various kinds of stress (initially different illnesses) (Selye, 1946). The responses to stress included activation of the hypothalamic-pituitary-adrenal (HPA) axis and the sympathetic nervous system as well as other physiological changes, some of which could be adaptive and others harmful. The meaning of "stress" and "stressor," however, as they are used today, is not always clear. The terms are sometimes used imprecisely to refer to a variety of environmental events, to the perception of these events, or to the physiological responses they evoke.

A critical review of the concept of stress concluded that neuroendocrine changes alone do not define an event as a stressor. This is because neuroendocrine responses to rewarding stimuli or to voluntary intense activity (presumably not stressors) can be similar to those evoked by threatening or painful stimuli (presumably stressors). The authors advocated that stressors should be considered environmental events that "exceed an animal's natural regulatory capacity," and especially events that are unpredictable and evoke physiological changes that are uncontrollable (Koolhaas et al., 2011). Based on these criteria, some methods of sleep restriction in animals would qualify as stressors.

Stressors can also be discussed in relation to the concept of allostasis, which also refers to events that exceed an animal's regulatory abilities (see Chapter 5). Allostasis can be defined as adaptive physiological adjustments that occur in response to the inability to satisfy a need using the usual homeostatic mechanisms, but which also impose a physiological cost on the organism (McEwen, 2006). Given these definitions, the physiological effects of extreme sleep deprivation likely reflect a combination of specific changes related to lost sleep (or excess waking) and more general effects shared with other stressors that provoke allostatic responses and their physiological costs.

One passive method is called a platform or flowerpot method. It originally involved housing an animal (rat, mouse, or cat) on an upside-down flowerpot set in a shallow pool of water (Mendelson et al., 1974). An appropriately sized flowerpot (or a manufactured platform) has a small surface on which the animal can sit or stand as long as it is awake. Onset of sleep, especially REM sleep, causes reduced postural muscle tone that makes the animal fall partially or completely off the small surface and contact the water. Falling and contacting the water awaken the animal, so it is forced to stay awake to avoid the results of falling asleep.

This method is most effective for chronic REM sleep deprivation, although there may also be an initial reduction in NREM sleep (Mendelson et al., 1974). To control for the reduced mobility involved, several small platforms can be placed close enough to each other to allow an animal to move between them, but not close enough to support it if it falls asleep. A standard control for the general housing situation is to have an animal live on a similar, but larger, platform that allows it to sleep without falling off.

A related approach was developed in the University of Chicago laboratory of Allan Rechtschaffen in the 1980s. This disk-over-water (DOW) method (introduced in Chapter 5; see **Figure 5.7**) controlled for some of the confounds in previous studies and permitted long-term sleep deprivation. Sleep deprivation was the passive result of disk rotation that was triggered automatically when a computer detected sleep features in the EEG of a rat; but there was also an active component because the awakened rat had to walk briefly to avoid contacting the water beneath the rotating disk.

A control rat lived in the same environment and had some of the same physical experiences as the experimental rat, but it could sleep freely without triggering disk rotation, as long as the experimental rat did not also fall asleep. As a result, it got most of its usual sleep: for example, a 28% reduction in total sleep time in one study, while the experimental rat was severely sleep deprived by a 91% reduction (Rechtschaffen & Bergmann, 1995). An advantage of this method is that it is automated and allows very long-term deprivation studies over periods of weeks, rather than hours or days, and can be made relatively selective by using a specific sleep stage as the trigger for disk rotation.

Active methods of deprivation involve forcing animals to walk slowly and continuously on a motorized treadmill or rotating wheel, which is incompatible with producing more than very brief sleep episodes. To control for the effects of exercise, researchers often compare sleep-deprived animals to others that engage voluntarily in similar, or higher, activity levels during their daily active phase, but sleep freely. Many rodents will run for miles daily in a wheel that they can rotate voluntarily. However, the timing, intensity, and voluntary nature of spontaneous wheel running distinguish it from the features of enforced slow walking. Applying the criteria of predictability and control (Koolhaas et al., 2011), enforced activity would be seen as having a stress component, but voluntary activity would not, even if it were more intense.

The final category of methods is intended to reduce the potentially stressful effects of other sleep deprivation approaches by using so-called gentle handling (which now usually includes very little, if any, direct handling of animals) (see, e.g., Franken et al., 1991). This method involves an experimenter responding immediately to EEG and/or postural signs of sleep onset in an animal by introducing novel objects into its environment, moving bedding or other objects near the animal, or gently blowing on it or stroking it with a brush to attract its attention and keep it from sleeping. This method is effective in preventing sleep for relatively short periods, but it is unclear whether it would lose its effectiveness over longer durations (see the summary in **Table 14.1**).

One indicator of a stress response is an increased release of adrenal corticosteroid hormones (primarily corticosterone in rats and cortisol in people). Unambiguous stressors, like acute pain, cause very large increases in adrenal steroid secretion, but other forms of strong arousal can also increase levels (Koolhaas et al., 2011). Increased release of adrenal steroids might be an initial indication of whether a method of sleep deprivation like gentle handling can avoid generating stress responses. However, the effects of sleep loss on adrenal hormone measurements have been inconsistent across studies.

For example, sleep deprivation for 3–6 h by gentle handling caused increases in corticosterone levels that ranged from small to very large in rats and mice (Gip et al., 2004; Mongrain et al., 2010; Zant et al., 2011). This variability may be related in part to a lack of standardization across laboratories of the procedures and components used to keep animals from sleeping. However, even using the same method in a single study produced increases in corticosterone levels ranging from 2- to nearly 8-fold over baseline in different inbred mouse strains, indicating genetic differences in responsiveness (Mongrain et al., 2010). These increases were still lower, however, than would be caused by a stressor like pain, so they may reflect mostly increased arousal rather than stress. Gentle handling appears therefore to minimize, if not eliminate, nonspecific stress responses, but not to the same extent in all species or strains of animals. It is most useful for short-term deprivation (e.g., 3–6 h), but it is unlikely to be effective over very long durations.

14.2.1 Summary

Depriving animals or people of sleep requires some form of intervention to keep them awake since sleep is an internally generated activity. People can engage in voluntary sleep deprivation, but experimenters' interventions are often necessary to maintain waking during extended sleep loss. For animal studies, there are passive and active methods of sleep deprivation that are effective to different degrees, each of which has strengths and limitations. Different methods may be most useful for producing either acute or sustained sleep loss, and these may have different physiological effects.

Automated systems, such as the DOW procedure, have the advantage of allowing very long-term sleep deprivation without direct intervention from experimenters as well as including a control animal that shares both the environment and many aspects of the experience. All methods carry the risk of combining specific effects of sleep loss with those of nonspecific stress resulting from the interventions. Gentle handling methods reduce stress responses to a large extent, but not identically across species and strains of rodents, and they are most useful for short-term sleep deprivation.

Discussions about the effects of increased stress versus lost sleep in these studies may be partially circular since the sustained loss of sleep itself may induce physiological stress

Table 14.1 Methods of Sleep Deprivation

Method	Type of Deprivation	Approach/Method	Controls
• Voluntary (people only)	• "Total" or stage-selective; short or long-term (days)	• Social, auditory, or physical stimulation to supplement cooperation	• Free sleep
• Small platform or flowerpot (animals)	• Principally of REM sleep; short- or long-term	• Passive; risk of falling into shallow water after (REM) sleep onset	• Multiple small platforms permitting movement but not sleep, and/or large platforms permitting sleep
• Disk over water (animals)	• "Total" or stage- selective; short or very long-term (weeks)	• Passive (and active); sleep onset triggers disk rotation, causing waking and walking briefly to avoid contacting shallow water	• Control animal in the same environment has similar experiences but loses much less sleep
• Motorized wheel/ treadmill (animals)	• "Total"; short- or long-term	• Active; continuous forced locomotion	• Voluntary locomotion or free sleep
• Gentle handling (animals)	• "Total"; short-term	• Distraction, alerting	• Free sleep

responses (Meerlo et al., 2008). Nevertheless, it is possible to distinguish the physiological patterns of responses to severe sleep loss from those to classical stressors, as discussed in the following section.

14.3 Effects of "total" sleep deprivation

14.3.1 Total sleep deprivation in animals

Early reports indicated that animals of several species died after prolonged sleep deprivation induced by forced continuous activity (see discussion of the term "total sleep deprivation" in Section 5.5.2). These studies typically did not include controls for the effects of continuous activity, and most were done before EEG recordings were available (see, e.g., Leake et al., 1927; see Ross, 1965 for other references). Studies using the DOW procedure were later conducted on rats monitored with EEG recordings and with yoked control animals in the same environment. After periods of days or weeks of severe sleep loss, experimental rats, but not controls, developed many physiological abnormalities. These included skin and other lesions, changes in the digestive system, severe disruption of body temperature regulation, increased metabolic rates, and very large increases in food intake that were paradoxically accompanied by weight loss.

This unique symptom profile reflected seriously disturbed physiological functions that were unlikely to reflect stress responses alone. These symptoms did not, for example, resemble those seen in rats that were stressed by frequent foot shocks over a period of weeks (Paré, 1964), nor were they similar to the features of stress syndromes in general (Rechtschaffen & Bergmann, 2002). Some symptoms (weight loss and dysregulated body temperature) resembled those seen in rabbits that were sleep deprived by forced continuous walking (Leake et al., 1927). But rats in the DOW studies did not have to walk continuously, so these symptoms in both species were more likely related to sleep loss than to the effects of continuous walking. After 11 days, the first sleep-deprived experimental rat in a DOW study died, and none survived the procedure for more than 32 days,[1] while all control rats survived (Rechtschaffen & Bergmann, 1995).

It has been difficult to identify the mechanisms by which long-term sleep loss results in the unusual cluster of metabolic symptoms seen in rats (Bergmann et al., 1989). Some studies suggested that bacterial infections resulting from failure of the immune system played an important role (Everson, 1993; Everson & Toth, 2000). Others concluded that infections were secondary consequences of primary metabolic changes (Benca & Quintans, 1997). However, a role for immune system involvement at some stage of sleep deprivation is supported by evidence that more modest sleep loss alters several aspects of immune system function (see Section 14.9).

The effects observed in DOW studies did not depend specifically on loss of NREM sleep since similar results were seen after selective REM sleep deprivation, although the symptoms appeared more slowly (Rechtschaffen & Bergmann, 2002). It is not clear what the minimum degree and pattern of sleep loss is that would produce these symptoms. A sleep deprivation procedure that mimicked the pattern of sleep loss typical of DOW studies produced severe disruptions of sleep continuity and amounts. This procedure was applied for 10-day periods to experimental rats, followed by 2 recovery days with essentially free sleep opportunities. Despite the recovery opportunities, repetitions of these 10 + 2 day cycles resulted in the gradual emergence of a pattern of symptoms similar to those of DOW studies. Rats in the experimental group showed increased food and water intake, body weight loss, and severe metabolic and anatomical abnormalities, leading to a moribund condition for two of the animals (Everson & Szabo, 2009). Thus, neither continuous sleep loss without interruption, nor loss of NREM sleep, appear to be essential to inducing features of this syndrome.

There have been few recent, long-term sleep deprivation studies in other species. Pigeons (*Columba livia*) and rats were studied using DOW and a modified version of this method. Sleep-deprived rats showed the expected metabolic changes within 7 days of starting sleep deprivation, but pigeons did not show systematic changes in body weight, food intake, or body temperature over 24 days, despite comparable degrees of sleep loss in experimental animals of both species (Newman et al., 2009; Newman et al., 2008) (**Figure 14.1**). It is not clear how to account for these differences. It is possible that these species can tolerate extreme sleep interruption and loss to different degrees or for different lengths of time (see Section 14.3.3). Alternatively, it is possible that rats are more vulnerable to other features of the experimental situation.

There have also been studies of the effects of long-term sleep deprivation in the fruit fly *Drosophila melanogaster*. As reviewed in Section 7.3, several laboratories have shown that fruit flies meet the formal behavioral criteria usually applied to determine whether animals sleep. A study using wild-type fruit flies found that they began to die after 60–70 h of continuous sleep deprivation (Shaw et al., 2002). A later study, however, used abrupt rotation of the tubes in which flies lived to arouse them if they were inactive for >20 s over their entire lifespan (~40–50 days) in order to cause a >95% reduction in

[1] In later studies, rats that showed a similar syndrome and would eventually have died were euthanized before they reached that stage.

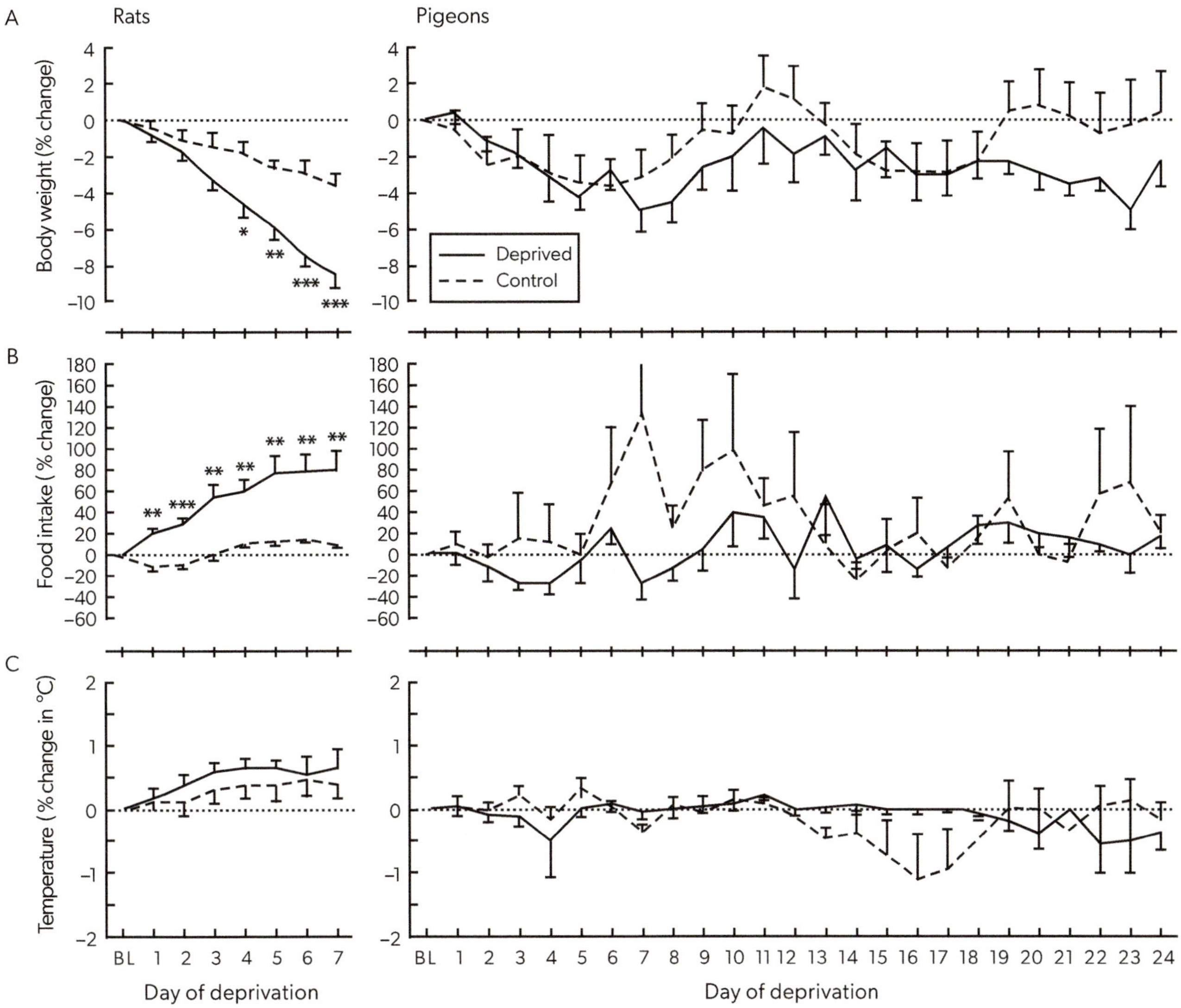

Figure 14.1 Body weights (**A**), food intake (**B**), and body temperature change (**C**) in rats (left panel) and pigeons (right panel) undergoing sleep deprivation under similar conditions (disk-over-water method) for 7 days (rats) or 24 days (pigeons). Experimental rats undergoing sleep deprivation (Deprived; solid lines) showed steep declines in body weight (**A**), despite significantly increased food intake (**B**), and with small temperature increases (**C**), relative to their yoked controls (Control; dashed lines). Despite fluctuations in these measures, neither experimental nor control pigeons showed systematic, sustained changes in body weight, food intake, or body temperature over a 24-day period with similar levels of sleep loss as the rats in the Deprived group. * $p < .05$, ** $p < .01$, *** $p < .001$ relative to controls. Reprinted with permission of Oxford University Press from Newman, S.M. et al. (2009) Sleep deprivation in pigeons and rats using motion detection. *Sleep* 32:1299–1312. © Sleep Research Society (2009). doi: 10.1093/sleep/32.10.1299.

sleep. There was no effect on survival of male flies, and females showed an average reduction in lifespan of only ~9% relative to controls (Geissmann et al., 2019).

Another study deprived fruit flies of sleep using a different approach. A genetic mutation was introduced into flies that caused specific ion channels to open at high ambient temperatures. These mutations were targeted to neurons that are known to suppress sleep in flies. Exposure to high temperatures opened the channels and activated the sleep-suppressing neurons. Applying this method resulted in flies losing ~90% of their sleep and starting to die after about 10 days; the entire group had died after ~20 days (versus ~40 days for controls without the mutation housed at the same temperature) (Vaccaro et al., 2020).

Sleep-deprived (mutant) flies accumulated large amounts of highly reactive oxygen species (ROS) in their guts, which led to oxidative stress. Treatment with a variety of drugs that reduce oxidative stress (including melatonin, which is a scavenger of free oxygen radicals; see Section 9.5.1) was able to prevent early death, despite continuing sleep loss (Vaccaro et al., 2020). These results are discussed further in Section 14.3.3.

14.3.2 Total sleep loss in people

A previous chapter reviewed the case of Randy Gardner, a 17-year-old high school student in San Diego, California, who voluntarily stayed awake in early 1964 for a total of 264 h (11 days) as part of a science fair project (Ross, 1965); see Section 5.3.1. There have been reports of others breaking this record (with over 18 days of sleep loss), but there is little documentation to support these claims.

Despite the lack of continuous EEG recordings or a controlled laboratory environment, there was a degree of supervision and monitoring of Gardner's condition. The distinguished sleep researcher, William Dement, came from Stanford University to observe the latter part of the deprivation period, and a neurologist serving in the US Navy, John Ross, conducted neurological and EEG tests on Gardner both during and after his sleepless ordeal (Ross, 1965). One result noted in EEG recordings obtained late in the period of sleep loss was that there were increases in theta- and delta-band activity while awake, as is typical of people who have experienced much shorter periods of sleep loss (Cajochen et al., 1995). Nevertheless, without continuous EEG recordings, and despite the efforts of collaborators to keep him awake, we cannot be certain how much he might have slept unintentionally. As is typical of animal studies attempting to produce total sleep deprivation, it is likely that he was deprived of nearly all sleep but experienced some short sleep bouts before being awakened.

Gardner showed only a small increase in sleep duration immediately after his lengthy time awake and seemed to recover with no obvious ill effects. As a result, this event is sometimes cited as evidence that prolonged sleep loss in people has no significant physiological consequences. Ross's published medical evaluation of Gardner, however, indicated that the experience of sleep loss was not entirely benign. He reported that Gardner showed abnormal eye movements, an inability to show convergence (moving eyes inward to focus on an object in the near field), nausea, abnormal sensory and reflex thresholds, growth of lymphoid tissue in the throat, the presence of a cardiac murmur that disappeared two days after the end of sleep deprivation, and other physical symptoms.

There were also reports of marked effects on behavior and cognition, including motor dysfunctions, memory lapses, irritability, visual illusions, loss of ability to identify familiar objects by touch, slurred speech, and fragmented thoughts (Ross, 1965). Some aspects of Gardner's deficits appear to be exaggerated forms of the symptoms seen during shorter periods of sleep deprivation: difficulty focusing attention or sustaining cognitive activities, and extreme sleepiness leading to brief sleep episodes (microsleeps) intruding into waking activities. Microsleeps accompanied by hypnogogic (sleep-onset) hallucinations could account for some of his reported misperceptions of the environment (imagining fog around a streetlight, mistaking a street sign for a person, "seeing" forest or garden scenes). Why sleep loss led to other physiological signs (e.g., a heart murmur, growth of lymphoid tissue, motor problems) is unknown.

Other than these features, Gardner's metabolic and physiological measures were generally normal, and he seemed to recover rapidly and fully. An interview published in an online magazine in 2006 revealed that Gardner, 60 years old at the time, had recently retired from his job with an interior landscaping business, and remained in good health (http://tinyurl.com/2a6mw3c). Four years later, a New York Times columnist met him and reported that he then had symptoms of insomnia (http://tinyurl.com/zymhqgh), which is not an unusual development for someone in his 60s.

14.3.3 Species comparisons

Why did roughly similar durations of sleep loss have more severe effects on rats than on pigeons and on this one human? It is difficult to compare species that are separated by wide taxonomic gaps and have very different physiologies, but there are some possibilities to consider. One possibility is that the voluntary nature of Gardner's sleep loss was important. If unpredictability and lack of control are key features of stressors, then rats and pigeons would have suffered more stress than Gardner, in addition to the effects of sleep loss. But the pattern of symptoms shown by rats in DOW studies did not match those triggered by chronic, severe stress, nor can this interpretation explain the differences between pigeons and rats who were exposed to similar involuntary experiences.

Another consideration is that some birds can sleep unihemispherically while keeping the eye connected to the waking hemisphere open, probably to reduce predation risk (e.g., as in ducks; see Section 7.5.3), or allow continuous flight (see **Figure 7.13**). However, pigeons do not show completely unihemispheric sleep similar to that of ducks. They do often sleep with only one eye closed and the contralateral hemisphere showing more power in the low-frequency SWS range than the hemisphere linked to the open eye. Thus, they have the ability to show independent expression of slower EEG frequencies in the two hemispheres (Rattenborg et al., 2001). Although there was no clear evidence of unihemispheric sleep among the pigeons in the long-term deprivation studies, it is possible that they reduced the impact of sleep deprivation to some degree by generating slower EEG frequencies unihemispherically while remaining awake (Newman et al., 2008).

Another possibility is that the physiological consequences of sleep loss are related to metabolic rate and to lifespan, which are closely linked. Smaller organisms within a taxonomic group tend to live shorter lives and to have higher metabolic rates; that is, they appear to live faster (= age more quickly). Rats in captivity typically live less than 3 years (https://tinyurl.com/yj7tf555) and humans can live 80–85 years or longer (http://tinyurl.com/5kt4p9), giving a ratio of ~28:1. If sleep is important because it reverses some of the metabolic costs of being awake, the impact of losing sleep could be related to an organism's "rate of living." From this perspective, rats losing most of their sleep over 11–30 days may suffer metabolic damage equivalent to that of a person not sleeping for 10–28 months. No human has been kept awake for a duration even approaching 10 months, and this explanation is unlikely to ever be tested in people.

The idea of a role for lifespan also applies to the pigeons who were minimally affected by extended sleep loss. Pigeons are relatively long-lived and can survive for 15 years in captivity; there is a record lifespan of 35 years claimed for one pigeon. This hypothesis, however, does not address results from other species that were studied in the past. Rabbits are typically longer-lived than rats, but when forced to walk continuously, died within a similar time frame (8–31 days) (Leake et al., 1927). This similarity might be coincidental since the method used with rabbits was very different from the DOW procedure.

If we add to the species comparisons the study of fruit flies who died sooner when they were continuously sleep deprived, the phylogenetic gap increases, yet there are suggestive connections between the findings in fruit flies and rats. Flies apparently died as a result of the accumulation of reactive oxygen species in their guts, which caused visible damage to their digestive systems (Vaccaro et al., 2020). This result echoes the severe metabolic dysregulation seen in rats in the DOW studies. The rats ate very large amounts of food, yet lost weight and had notable changes in the structure of their digestive systems (Everson et al., 1989). Rats that underwent 10 days of sleep loss also showed increased DNA oxidative damage, and cell death in their liver, lungs, and intestines, which could have interfered with nutrient utilization, among other harmful consequences (Everson et al., 2014).

Thus, in both rats and fruit flies, sustained sleep loss caused severe oxidative damage in several organs including the digestive system, which could have contributed to inadequate nutrition and ultimately to debilitation and death. The idea that nutritional deficits mediate some of the effects of sleep loss is supported by the results of another DOW study in which rats were given either a high-calorie diet or standard laboratory food. The sleep-deprived rats ate large amounts of food, as in previous studies, but those on the high-calorie diet maintained their weights more successfully and survived longer than those on the control diet before becoming seriously ill (Everson & Wehr, 1993).

Despite the intriguing parallels between these rat and fruit fly studies, it is also the case that two studies using very different methods to sleep-deprive fruit flies reached different conclusions about whether sleep loss shortens lifespan (Geissmann et al., 2019; Vaccaro et al., 2020). In the absence of more studies using the same methods across species, it remains a challenge to explain either the differences or similarities that were observed, or to speculate about which findings would generalize to other species, including people.

The possibility that oxidative stress plays a role in mediating the health effects of sleep loss in rats and fruit flies raises the question of whether its involvement can also explain the lack of physiological damage in sleep-deprived pigeons. A study of the relation of oxidative stress to lifespan in 78 bird species reported a negative correlation between longevity and levels of a marker of oxidative stress, and a corresponding positive correlation of longevity with markers of antioxidant activity. Pigeons were the longest lived species included (at 35 years) and had the fourth lowest level of a marker of oxidative damage, malondialdehyde, which reacts with DNA and has been linked to aging. Their levels of antioxidants were low or mid-range (Xia & Møller, 2018). The potential link between pigeons' resistance to the effects of sleep loss and their spontaneous low levels of oxidative damage is intriguing. Future studies will have to determine whether the levels of markers of DNA oxidative damage and repair systems in different species predict the degree to which they would be physiologically affected by severe sleep loss.

14.3.4 People who "never" sleep

Another potential source of information about the physiological effects of a complete lack of sleep are people who claim never to sleep at all, or to survive indefinitely on remarkably little sleep. The existence of such individuals would argue that the negative effects of sleep loss seen in most people are not inevitable, and that others could perhaps train themselves to sleep very little without affecting their health.

Most accounts of such short sleep are anecdotal and not accompanied by objective evidence. There are reports, however, of a handful of people who claimed to sleep very little, were in good health, and were studied in a laboratory using polysomnography (PSG). They slept ~1–3 h nightly over several nights and claimed that these durations were normal for them (Jones & Oswald, 1968; Meddis, 1977; Meddis et al., 1973). Although these findings were interpreted as showing that sleep serves no essential recuperative function (Meddis, 1977), an alternative interpretation is that some very rare individuals achieve the benefits of sleep over extremely short durations. Other physiological parameters also show a range of values across a population.

One study investigated the genetic makeup of two related individuals with unusually short habitual sleep durations for their family: ~6.25 h vs. ~8.0 h for other family members. It found that the short sleepers differed from other family members in having a mutation in a regulatory gene called *DEC2* (He et al., 2009). Introducing this mutation into a mouse genome also shortened sleep and was associated with increased brain levels of the wake-promoting peptide hypocretin (Hirano et al., 2018); see Section 11.3.4.

Although people with *DEC2* mutations slept much longer than the rare cases of those who slept 1–3 h nightly, these results and related findings (Jones et al., 2019) demonstrated that sleep duration in people is genetically influenced. Other genetic features might be responsible for some of the more extreme cases of short sleep without negative health effects. Similarly, many genetic loci have been identified in populations of fruit flies that are associated with the expression of a broad range of sleep durations (Harbison et al., 2013).

If genetic features regulate sleep duration in people, what does this imply about the degree to which baseline sleep durations can be modified? An attempt by a few people in their 20s to reduce their sleep gradually over a period of months from a baseline of ~8 h was successful to the extent that they reached durations of 4.5–5.5 h, and when allowed to sleep freely over the next year, rebounded to only 5.5–7.0 h. At the shortest durations achieved, however, participants complained of overwhelming fatigue, reduced efficiency, falling asleep in inappropriate situations, and being at risk of sleeping while driving (Friedmann et al., 1977). This is a very different condition from that of the few healthy ultra-short sleepers that have been identified. People who spontaneously sleep 7–8 h seem unable to function effectively on much less sleep over the long term, indicating limited elasticity in sleep need. Extreme short sleep in otherwise healthy people does not appear to represent a conscious choice, but rather a rare, genetically determined phenotype.

In contrast to the handful of documented short sleepers, more typical PSG findings from people who claimed to sleep very little were reported in a study of two self-described, extreme short sleepers. One was a 28 year-old man who claimed to have slept 0–1 h nightly for 4.5 years, and the other was a 39 year-old woman who reported that she had not slept at all for 13 years. Neither showed any signs of psychiatric abnormalities or ill health. During an overnight laboratory study, the man slept for 7.2 h and the woman for 6.9 h. Most remarkably, when interviewed the next morning, both denied having slept at all during their night in the laboratory (McCall & Edinger, 1992).

This phenomenon appears to be an extreme example of sleep state misperception, a condition in which people perceive some or all of their sleep periods as waking and may therefore report that they were awake for long periods when they were objectively asleep. A possible explanation for this condition comes from studies of people complaining of insomnia (note the definition of insomnia in Box 4.3, Section 4.4.5). Chronic insomnia patients were studied overnight using PSG; when asked later about their sleep, they underestimated their total sleep time and overestimated their latency to fall asleep (Carskadon et al., 1976). Insomnia patients also had more short arousals during the night (13–25, depending on age) than is typical for those without insomnia, were inaccurate in estimating how many arousals they experienced, and misperceived PSG-defined sleep periods as being wake periods (Carskadon et al., 1976; Harvey & Tang, 2012).

A meta-analysis of studies that compared PSG findings from patients with primary insomnia to those of good sleepers reported that insomnia patients slept 23 min less on average, had 20 min less SWS, and 10 min less REM sleep, were awake for 20 min more, and had six more awakenings during the night (WASO). Insomnia patients, however, self-reported worse sleep parameters than the objective data. They reported ~50 min less total sleep and 50 min more WASO than the PSG data indicated (Baglioni et al., 2014). A recent study also found that insomnia patients underestimated, but healthy sleepers overestimated, their PSG-determined sleep durations (Benz et al., 2023). Thus, sleep state misperception is common among primary insomnia patients, as it is in those with other sleep disorders (Valko et al., 2021), although it is usually less extreme than among those who claim (incorrectly) that they never sleep.

Another study reported that underestimation of sleep amounts was especially characteristic of the subset of people with insomnia who have normal sleep durations. People with chronic insomnia and normal sleep durations (≥6 h) underestimated their sleep durations, but those with objectively short sleep (<6 h) were actually accurate in estimating their sleep durations. On personality tests, those showing sleep state misperception also had increased scores for anxious rumination, depression, and poor coping skills (Fernandez-Mendoza et al., 2011).

People showing extreme forms of sleep state misperception may be especially good at detecting and remembering being awake during the night and poor at detecting the intervening sleep periods. As a result, they may interpret their memories of repeated, brief wake episodes as part of extended wake periods. This interpretation can account for their failure to report repeatedly awakening from sleep as well as for their perception of having been awake most of the night, leading to the most extreme claims of never sleeping.

Discrepancies between subjective and objective assessments of sleep quality are relevant not only to insomnia but also to other clinical conditions. For example, in people with chronic fatigue syndrome, subjective ratings of sleep quality predicted next-day fatigue levels, but sleep duration measured by actigraphy did not. Thus, the degree of fatigue reported was related to patients' experience of the quality of their recent sleep, not to their objective sleep amounts (Russell et al., 2016). Objective evidence and subjective reports of sleep quality have also been reported to be poorly correlated in other populations, such as among older people (Unruh et al., 2008).

14.3.5 Summary

Experimental (near-)total sleep deprivation over many days has harmful effects on physiology and behavior, ultimately leading to death, at least in some species. These include animals in older studies that involved intense, continuous exercise, but also rats deprived of sleep using the DOW method that does not involve continuous activity. Randy Gardner also developed unusual physiological abnormalities during his extended sleep loss, but these did not resemble those seen in rats, and he recovered rapidly and remained in good health. Although contributions of nonspecific stress cannot be ruled out, the pattern of physiological abnormalities observed in rats after extreme sleep loss did not match those generated by traditional stressors.

The effects seen in rats were not observed in studies of similarly treated pigeons. It is unclear whether the ability of pigeons to show more asymmetric (but not unihemispheric) sleep in their two hemispheres could have helped protect them from the debilitating effects seen in rats. With few species studied, it is difficult to speculate about why some were less affected than others. One possibility relates to differences in lifespans of species and the proportion of the expected lifespan during which sleep was eliminated. The rate of accumulation of physiological damage from being awake may differ among species with different lifespans.

Fruit flies that were continuously sleep-deprived died sooner than controls in some studies, but not others. There is evidence that oxidative damage, especially in the digestive systems of both rats and fruit flies, contributed to poor absorption or utilization of nutrients and ultimately to debilitation and early death. This suggestion is supported by evidence that rats fed a diet with a high caloric density were partially protected against the effects of sleep loss. There is indirect support for the idea that differences in oxidative stress responses to sleep loss may contribute to species differences in physiological damage suffered. The net oxidative stress (i.e., levels of markers of oxidative stress minus levels of antioxidant agents) of bird species, for example, correlates with their lifespans. Pigeons, who appeared largely unaffected by degrees of sleep loss that severely damaged the physiology of rats, are very long-lived relative to other birds and have very low spontaneous levels of oxidative damage.

A very small number of people appear to do well on very little sleep, perhaps reflecting their unusual genetic makeup, rather than a conscious decision to sleep less. Gene mutations have been linked to more modest shortening of habitual sleep durations in people and in other species. Most claims by people of very short or no sleep over long periods, however, are probably the result of sleep state misperception. This is also a common characteristic of many patients with primary insomnia and other sleep disorders.

Although modest, voluntary reductions in habitual sleep durations may be possible, most people cannot choose to substantially reduce their sleep over the long term without developing extreme daytime sleepiness and increasing deficits in performance.

14.4 Studying effects of sleep duration

Few people undergo long-term, complete sleep loss, but many people in industrial societies experience more modest, but chronic, sleep restriction or disruption. The following sections review how the effects of differences in sleep duration and quality are studied through observational and experimental research and what the results of these studies indicate about the consequences for human health of short or disrupted sleep.

14.4.1 Observational and experimental approaches

Among people responding to surveys, there are large individual differences in reported sleep durations. The impact of these differences on human health have been studied using two approaches: experimental studies and observational (population-based) studies.

Experimental studies involve manipulation of a single variable—typically the length of sleep allowed—and measurement of the resulting physiological effects. These studies are usually conducted in a laboratory in which all environmental variables are held constant, and experimenters control the participants' activity level, diet, and sleep choices (e.g., timing, lighting conditions, etc.). Participants are assigned randomly to treatment and control conditions (or are matched between conditions), so their individual characteristics are balanced across groups. With all other variables held constant, the main advantage of this approach is that it allows conclusions about whether the manipulated variable (imposed sleep length) caused an observed physiological effect.

Experimental studies also have disadvantages. They are expensive to run and therefore only a relatively small number of people can be studied for limited durations (days or weeks at most). The resulting small sample sizes cannot represent all of the variability (environmental, cultural, socioeconomic,

Table 14.2 Features of Human Population-Based and Experimental Approaches

Method	Strengths	Limitations	Controls

Experimental (sleep restriction; typically laboratory-based)	• Controlled:
	  • Environment
	  • Time in bed
	  • Diet
	  • Activity, etc.
	• Manipulation of only one variable: sleep length
	• Allows causal inferences
		• Expensive, thus usually small numbers
		• Short duration
		• Few endpoints
		• Not representative of entire population
		• Studies surrogate health markers, not illnesses
		• Cannot observe long-term outcomes
			• Randomly assigned or matched control & treatment groups
			• Control group gets adequate sleep

Observational (population-based studies; often based on survey data)	• Representative of diverse population(s) • Large number of potential endpoints • Time frame of years/decades allows studies of the development of illnesses • Natural settings	• No control of behavior or environment • Sleep duration is often self-reported in response to limited questions, or a single measure • "Hidden" confounders • Correlational results	• Statistical control of potential confounding variables, but only for those known or suspected ahead of time

ethnic, etc.) present in the general population from which participants were recruited. In addition, those willing and able to participate in laboratory research studies are often healthier and more fit than the majority of that population. Together, these factors limit the extent to which findings can be generalized to the wider population.

Another critical limitation is that the duration of experimental studies does not allow the observation of long-term health consequences. The health effects of differences in sleep duration (e.g., a serious illness or early death) may take years or decades to emerge in people. These health outcomes cannot be studied directly with experimental approaches, which instead focus on immediate changes in physiology that serve as surrogate (substitute) markers for longer-term effects on health.

In contrast, observational studies do not involve manipulating sleep amounts. They document the relations that occur spontaneously between sleep duration or quality and physiological functions or health outcomes within a population. They can involve collecting data from very large groups of participants, who can represent a range of fitness and health, because they can be sampled randomly from the general population. They can also include people from a broader range of ages, ethnicities, and socioeconomic conditions than might typically get recruited to participate in laboratory studies. These features improve generalizability of results to the population of interest, which varies along all of these dimensions. People can also be studied repeatedly over long periods of time (years or decades) in naturalistic settings, so that correlations between sleep features and long-term health outcomes can be observed.

Observational studies, however, also have limitations. Participants choose their own sleep durations; what determines these choices is generally not known. There is also no control over participants' environments and behavior. These studies usually rely on surveys to get self-reports about both sleep and health variables, which are less reliable than data obtained by direct measurement, as in laboratory studies. Surveys aimed principally at other health issues may include only one or a few questions about sleep, typically addressing only average durations, and these questions may be ambiguous (e.g., whether naps are included or not) (Kurina et al., 2013). Surveys also typically rely on retrospective self-reports of sleep duration (e.g., "over the last week") in contrast to time-use or daily-diary studies, which are completed in real time (see Section 14.4.2), or objective measurements of sleep. A few studies have, however, combined objective sleep measurements with survey data to reduce some of these concerns.

Because of these features, observational studies can detect correlations between variables related to sleep and health, but they do not allow strong conclusions about whether these represent causal relations.[2] Thus, experimental and observational studies have complementary strengths and weaknesses that should be considered when evaluating their results, as outlined in **Table 14.2**.

[2] For an amusing look at spurious correlations (i.e., those that clearly do *not* represent a causal relation), see http://www.tylervigen.com/spurious-correlations, which demonstrates some very robust and meaningless correlations between changes in variables measured over a period of years. These include a robust correlation between changes in the divorce rate in Maine and the per capita consumption of margarine, and between changes in the number of Apple iPhones sold and the number of people who died by falling down stairs. (On second thought, the latter correlation may turn out not to be spurious, given the effects of smartphones on attention.)

Observational studies can be either cross-sectional or longitudinal. Cross-sectional studies compare the health of groups (e.g., short, long, and "normal" sleepers)[3] at a single time point to establish correlations with current health status. In longitudinal (prospective) studies, a cohort of participants is studied at baseline and then over many years (often repeatedly at long intervals) to measure changes over time. Participants who are similarly healthy at the beginning of the study, but report sleeping more or less, may develop health problems to different extents. Although such results do not establish a causal relation, the gradual development of a health issue in parallel to differences in sleep behavior strengthens the association between these variables.

When sleep duration or quality correlates with the development of a health problem, other variables may also correlate with that outcome (confounding variables); these must be controlled for using statistical methods. Examining longitudinal trends, controlling for confounding variables, along with several other methods, are usually considered necessary to meet what are called the "Bradford Hill criteria." These criteria were summarized by the British medical statistician Sir Austin Bradford Hill (Bradford Hill, 1965). The goal of applying these criteria is to identify highly likely (not proven) causal relations between variables for situations in which experimental approaches are not possible and/or not ethical, but the health risks of ignoring observational evidence are very high.

In addition to controlling statistically for confounders, these criteria include, e.g., demonstrating consistent dose-response effects, or showing that onset of an illness (or recovery from it) regularly follows a change in behavior or environmental exposure. The most famous example to which these criteria were applied was establishing the link between smoking tobacco and developing lung cancer in a series of studies investigating the causes of death among British physicians during the 1950s (see, e.g., Doll & Bradford Hill, 1954).[4] The hypothesis that smoking tobacco causes lung cancer was supported by a range of evidence that was overwhelming and convincing,[5] even if not proven by a controlled experimental study in people, which would be impossible and unethical to perform.

Assessing possible confounding variables is critical. Reported sleep duration in a population may be correlated with development of a health problem, but so may age, body weight, or alcohol consumption, which may also be correlated with sleep duration. If sleep duration remains a predictor of the target health outcome when other potentially relevant variables are controlled for, it strengthens the argument that there is a unique association between sleep duration and that outcome.

There remains a risk, however, that other variables that are correlated with sleep duration were not measured because of the limitations of survey methods, or because they were not suspected ahead of time to be relevant. Not controlling for variables that turn out to be relevant can result in misleading conclusions about the role of sleep.[6] The selection of variables to control for and the interpretation of the resulting correlations are not automatic; they require a sophisticated understanding of both the range of possibly relevant variables and the statistical issues involved (Rohrer, 2018). See **Box 14.2** for a brief introduction to a different approach to using population-based data.

14.4.2 Measuring sleep duration

Sleep duration is the independent variable in most studies reviewed in the following sections and in Chapter 15. In population-based studies, it is often assessed by self-report, which can take different forms: responding to a question about habitual sleep durations; keeping daily sleep logs; answering well-validated sleep quality questionnaires; or recording diaries that detail all activities within a day ("time-use" studies).

[3] These terms are not used identically in all studies, but normal sleep durations are typically considered to be in the 6–9 h range for adults (with an average of ~7–7.5 h according to surveys), so short and long sleepers are often considered to be those falling outside that range. A 2018 analysis of the results of 6 billion sleep nights obtained from Fitbit activity monitors in the United States, however, reported somewhat lower averages: ~6.5 h for men and 6.8 h for women (https://tinyurl.com/y9h823jd). As for other accelerometer-based devices, there are differences between Fitbit and PSG in estimating some sleep features (de Zambotti et al., 2018), and results from objective measurements using any device may differ from those obtained in surveys.

[4] Some, however, recognized the harms associated with smoking tobacco much earlier. King James 1 of England published an otherwise repulsive, racist essay in 1604, which included a description of tobacco smoking as *"[a] custome lothsome to the eye, hatefull to the Nose, harmefull to the braine, dangerous to the Lungs ...* " (https://www.exclassics.com/blasts/tob.htm). The US Centers for Disease Control and Prevention estimate cigarette smoking to be responsible for one third of all cancer deaths and 90% of all lung cancer deaths annually in the United States https://www.cdc.gov/tobacco/about/cigarettes-and-cancer.html.

[5] Convincing to most people, but not to one of the most important statisticians of the 20th century, Ronald A. Fisher (a devoted pipe smoker), who objected to people drawing any form of causal inference from correlational data, however strong the correlations, and however potentially dangerous the consequences of not inferring causality (http://tinyurl.com/heu7fwo).

[6] Results of observational studies are often reported in news media and are frequently misunderstood as demonstrating causal relations. Thus, eating fish or jogging might be reported to be *correlated*, respectively, with lower risks of heart disease or needing a hip replacement. These are correlations, so one cannot conclude that jogging leads to a reduced need for hip replacement surgery. People with healthy, pain-free hip joints will certainly not get hip replacements, and pain-free hip joints may also make jogging more likely. Thus, rather than jogging reducing the need for hip replacements, having healthy hip joints is a confounding variable that leads to both more jogging and fewer hip surgeries. Without accounting for confounding variables and establishing causality, adopting the behavior involved (jogging) will not necessarily produce the desired result (no hip replacement needed).

BOX 14.2 Mendelian Randomization

A different approach to using population-based data is to analyze disease risk in a large observational database using genetic data (Mendelian randomization or MR). The impact of genetic variations is evaluated as if the presence of these variations were treatments in a clinical trial involving very large, diverse populations. In these analyses, associations are examined between genes that, for example, promote production of either "good" (HDL) or "bad" (LDL) cholesterol and the risk of cardiovascular disease, while behaviors that could affect cholesterol levels (e.g., diet, exercise, etc.) are controlled for. Note that the levels of different kinds of cholesterol are not manipulated by the experimenter; rather, peoples' genes provide the hypothetical "manipulation."

Another example is correlating genes that are known to be related to chronotype and sleep timing to the risk of developing major depression (Daghlas et al., 2021). This method mimics conducting an experiment on a large population to determine whether chronotype/sleep timing affects the probability of major depression, without actually experimentally manipulating chronotype or sleep timing. Although there are controversies about the assumptions underlying MR and how the results should be reported and interpreted, MR is a promising approach to making population-based studies more "experiment-like" (see https://tinyurl.com/yba55mag).

Objective measures of sleep include PSG, video observation, and actigraphy (see Sections 2.2.1 and 2.7). PSG is typically used in laboratory studies but has also been used in home studies and in some population-based research. Actigraphy has also been used in some population-based studies. Results from actigraphy studies can differ from those using PSG or video recordings, especially in specific populations (de Zambotti et al., 2018; Pollak et al., 2001; Sitnick et al., 2008; Waldon et al., 2016). Nevertheless, estimates of several sleep parameters derived from actigraphy are highly correlated with PSG results in many studies (Ancoli-Israel et al., 2003; Marino et al., 2013; Meltzer et al., 2012).

Using different methods can produce systematically different results (e.g., subjective estimates of sleep duration may be shorter than those obtained using actigraphy). In a study of older people (57–97 years old), women reported getting ~15 min less sleep than men in their sleep diaries, but averaged ~15 min more sleep than men according to actigraphy (Van Den Berg et al., 2008), consistent with the data from Fitbit studies mentioned earlier: https://tinyurl.com/y9h823jd. Time diaries that require detailed reporting of each activity and its duration during a 24 h period yielded longer estimates of sleep duration among 10–18 year-olds than did simply asking participants how long they "usually" slept. Surprisingly, the time-diary and self-report measures were statistically independent and differed in how well they correlated with measures of body weight (Knutson & Lauderdale, 2007); see Section 14.7.

Understanding how best to interpret self-reported sleep durations remains a challenge. One characteristic of sleep is limited awareness of the passage of time, so it is not surprising that subjective estimates of sleep duration can be unreliable. Responses to questions about habitual sleep patterns may also be affected by memory distortion, participants' expectations of normal sleep, and social desirability (providing answers that participants believe are most socially acceptable).

Participants' feelings about their sleep quality are also likely to affect responses about sleep duration. The principal factors determining self-reports of sleep quality were reported to be sleep efficiency (i.e., sleep-onset latency and continuity of sleep), total sleep duration, and amount of SWS (Keklund & Åkerstedt, 1997; Åkerstedt et al., 1994). Those who experience their sleep as inadequate or of low quality for any reason are unlikely to endorse having what they consider a "normal" sleep duration, regardless of its actual length (Bliwise & Young, 2007; Knutson & Lauderdale, 2007). As previously discussed, people diagnosed with insomnia tended to report shorter sleep durations than PSG recordings showed, while many good sleepers tended to overestimate their sleep durations (Benz et al., 2023; Carskadon et al., 1976); see Section 14.3.4.

Thus, survey results based solely on self-reports of sleep duration (or quality) should be interpreted cautiously and, when possible, in relation to results from studies that included objective sleep measures. It is also worth noting that regardless of how self-evaluations of sleep quality and duration differ from objective measures, it is these subjective judgments that affect peoples' motivation to change their sleep patterns, to self-medicate, or to seek treatment for perceived sleep problems.

Most surveys include a small number of responses indicating extreme habitual sleep durations (e.g., 3 or 11 h nightly), which may be accurate for a small subset of people, but may more commonly reflect personal characteristics that influence self-reports. These characteristics include age, racial self-identification, income level, education, and self-reported health quality (Jackson et al., 2018; Lauderdale et al., 2008). Americans with lower socioeconomic status or income, members of minority ethnic/racial groups, and those who were never married reported short sleep (and for some groups also long sleep) more often than others, after controlling for many potential confounding variables (Whinnery et al., 2014). It is unclear whether these findings indicate that extreme sleep durations are more common in these groups, or whether they reflect an influence of personal variables and feelings about sleep quality on subjective estimates of sleep duration.

14.4.3 Summary

As summarized in **Table 14.2**, observational and experimental approaches to identifying the effects of sleep duration on health have different strengths and weaknesses. Well-controlled experimental studies can establish causality, but they are limited by cost and time to relatively small groups, who may not represent the full range of personal characteristics in the general population. They also cannot be conducted long enough to evaluate whether experimental sleep restriction causes health consequences that take years to develop. These studies can instead examine sleep effects on surrogate measures that are linked to the health consequences of interest.

Although they cannot theoretically prove causality, properly controlled observational studies make critical contributions to understanding how sleep duration is related to health. They permit collecting data from large, diverse populations, and longitudinal versions can be conducted over the years or decades it takes for diseases to emerge. It is important in these studies to control for potential confounding variables, but some of these may not be recognized ahead of time.

The strongest case for a causal role for sleep duration in determining health outcomes can be made when the results of observational and experimental studies are combined and point to the same conclusion. Some examples discussed in the following sections involve observational studies showing correlations between sleep duration and the development of specific illnesses, and experimental studies that showed parallel effects of sleep manipulations on surrogate markers linked to the same illnesses.

14.5 Sleep-disordered breathing

A text focused on clinical sleep disorders would have a large section devoted to sleep-disordered breathing (SDB). The several conditions that cause SDB are major contributors to the enormous financial costs and personal suffering related to inadequate sleep. They are also the most frequently evaluated and treated disorders in clinical sleep laboratories (AlGhanim et al., 2008; Hillman et al., 2018).

Obstructive sleep apnea (OSA), the most common of these disorders, involves cycles of stopping breathing for seconds or even minutes at a time, along with reductions in oxygen levels in the blood (oxygen desaturation), followed by a gasping intake of breath and arousal. These events may be repeated dozens or hundreds of times a night.

OSA is a major contributor to shortened sleep and disruption of sleep continuity. Repeated episodes of reduced oxygen supply to the brain at night also lead to changes in brain function. OSA results in increased daytime sleepiness, increased risk of transportation accidents, cognitive problems, and vascular disease. Because OSA is a common condition and closely linked to metabolic and vascular disorders, it is often included as a potential confounding variable in analyses of sleep duration effects on human health, such as those discussed in the following sections. This is not always possible, however, because OSA and related conditions are often not diagnosed or are diagnosed only after years of illness. As a result, some affected participants in survey studies would not be aware that they have these conditions and would not report them.

A summary of basic information about some aspects of OSA is presented in Appendix B.

14.6 Sleep, metabolic syndrome, and glucose regulation

14.6.1 Observational studies

Population-based studies have examined how sleep duration relates to the risk of developing abnormalities that are part of the metabolic syndrome. This syndrome includes several linked conditions: obesity (especially abdominal obesity); hyperlipidemia (elevated blood cholesterol and/or triglyceride levels); hypertension (high blood pressure); and disturbed glucose regulation. Abnormal glucose regulation can result from inadequate responses to the effects of the hormone insulin (increased insulin resistance, or stated differently, decreased insulin sensitivity). Increased insulin resistance can lead to hyperglycemia (elevated circulating glucose levels), hyperinsulinemia (elevated blood insulin levels), and Type 2 diabetes mellitus (T2D) (Kyrou et al., 2006); see **Box 14.3**.

The metabolic syndrome is very common in many countries and its prevalence is increasing. At the time of the studies cited, it affected ~32% of the population in the United States (Ford et al., 2004; Hall et al., 2012), and 16.5%-23.3% of the population in a Chinese survey (Yang et al., 2007). The presence of this syndrome greatly increases the risk of developing serious illnesses like heart disease, stroke, and T2D, all of which have major impacts on quality of life, health care costs, and the risk of premature death.

Both cross-sectional and prospective population-based studies have reported increased risks of having or developing elevated glucose levels or T2D among men and women who self-reported short sleep, long sleep, or sleep maintenance difficulties. These associations were observed after adjusting for many potential confounds: age, gender, alcohol consumption, obesity, hypertension, depression, and physical activity, among others (Ayas et al., 2003; Beihl et al., 2009; Cappuccio et

BOX 14.3 Diabetes

Type 2 diabetes (T2D) is an acquired resistance to the physiological effects of the pancreatic hormone insulin. It is different from Type 1 diabetes (T1D), which is an autoimmune disease that destroys the insulin-secreting pancreatic islet cells. Insulin is normally released into the bloodstream in response to the rise in blood glucose levels that follows food intake. It causes some cells (e.g., muscle cells) to take up glucose from the circulation and thereby limits meal-related spikes in blood glucose levels. Mild insulin resistance (i.e., reduced uptake of glucose in response to insulin) causes compensatory increases in insulin release (hyperinsulinemia) to try to maintain blood glucose in the normal range. Increased insulin levels may allow people with mild insulin resistance to keep levels within this range, but they are still at increased risk of developing vascular disease and other health problems (Einhorn, 2003).

When insulin resistance is severe, even increased insulin release no longer controls blood glucose levels, which rise into the diabetic range. The excess circulating glucose is taken up by other cells, including those lining blood vessels, resulting in damage to these vessels throughout the body. The vascular damage caused by uncontrolled increases in glucose levels impairs blood flow, causing tissue damage in many organs, and ultimately increases the risk of blindness from diabetic retinopathy (loss of retinal cells), kidney failure, heart attack, stroke, lower limb amputation, and several types of cancer (Bhandari et al., 2014; Fowler, 2008; Rose et al., 2007).

al., 2010; Chaput et al., 2007; Gangwisch et al., 2007; Gottlieb et al., 2005; Mallon et al., 2005; Matthews et al., 2012; Yaggi et al., 2006).

In a UK population sample, the risk of having T2D increased progressively with shorter sleep durations. Eating healthy diets (low consumption of processed and red meat, and increased fruits, vegetables, and fish) was protective against developing T2D in the entire sample. However, the increased risks of T2D among those sleeping <6 h nightly did not differ between those with healthy and unhealthy diets. Thus, healthy diets alone did not alter the risk associated with short sleep (Nôga et al., 2024).

Other metabolic syndrome features (obesity, hypertension, hyperlipidemia) were also found to be associated with self-reported short sleep durations (Cappuccio et al., 2007; Gangwisch et al., 2005; Grandner et al., 2014; Park, 2013). Among those who already had T2D, both short and long sleep durations were associated with the presence of all features of the metabolic syndrome and with insulin resistance, after controlling for many variables, including ongoing treatments for diabetes (Ohkuma et al., 2014).

Other studies used the Pittsburgh Sleep Quality Index (PSQI), a well-validated questionnaire (Buysse et al., 1989), to evaluate sleep efficiency, complaints about sleep quality, and impaired daytime alertness. Poor sleep quality, assessed using the PSQI, was associated with several of the components of the metabolic syndrome (increased body weight, elevated blood glucose and insulin levels, and reduced levels of high-density lipoprotein (HDL) cholesterol, which is protective against vascular disease (Hung et al., 2013; Jennings et al., 2007).

A combined actigraphic/questionnaire study of people with T2D found that variability in sleep durations, short and long average sleep amounts, and poor subjective sleep quality were important predictors of long-term impaired glucose regulation (Brouwer et al., 2020). Similarly, an actigraphic study of adult patients with T1D found that those with irregular sleep schedules (short weekday sleep with catch-up sleep on weekends) had the poorest long-term regulation of blood glucose levels (Larcher et al., 2016).

A delayed chronotype, assessed by self-reported sleep timing on weekends and weekdays, and corrected for apparent sleep debt, was associated with poorer control of blood glucose levels in people already diagnosed with T2D (Reutrakul et al., 2013). Social jet lag (usually defined as the reported difference in midsleep timing between "free" and work/school days) was assessed in T2D patients using the Munich ChronoType Questionnaire. Increased social jet lag was associated with poorer long-term regulation of blood glucose (Kelly et al., 2020). This association was not observed in a study involving only a single question about chronotype preference, perhaps because this measure lacked sufficient sensitivity (Xie et al., 2021).

Delayed chronotype, short sleep durations, irregular sleep schedules, and social jet lag often overlap, especially in young adults, so it can be difficult to use questionnaires to disentangle their respective contributions to metabolic symptoms. Studies using objective measures like actigraphy or PSG can help to clarify these associations. A study using actigraphy in children (4–10 years old) found that those who were overweight or obese (see Section 14.7) had shorter sleep durations and more variable sleep patterns (typically involving increased catch-up sleep on weekends). Short and variable sleep were also associated with metabolic abnormalities, including increased levels of insulin, triglycerides, LDL cholesterol, and C-reactive protein (CRP)[7] (Spruyt et al., 2011). A study of adolescents using actigraphy

[7] CRP is a product of the liver that is regulated by immune system components. Elevated CRP levels are considered a marker of persistent, low-grade inflammation, which has been linked to increased risk of many serious diseases; see Section 14.9.

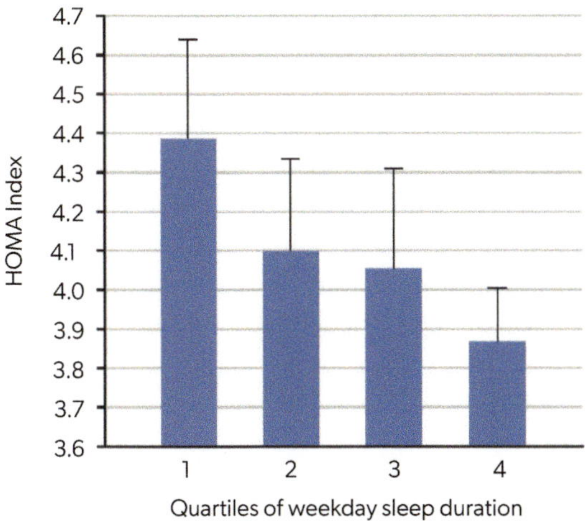

Figure 14.2 Insulin resistance (shown as a HOMA (Homeostasis Model Assessment) Index (Y axis) on a weekday morning in male and female adolescents in relation to their weekday sleep durations, measured using actigraphy. Sleep durations were divided into four equal-sized groups (quartiles), shown on the X axis, with sleep duration increasing from group 1 to 4. Those with the shortest average sleep durations (quartile 1) had the highest levels of insulin resistance (the opposite of insulin sensitivity). Elevated insulin resistance is associated with an increased risk of developing T2D and/or vascular disease. Reprinted with permission of Oxford University Press from Matthews, K.A. et al. (2012) Sleep duration and insulin resistance in healthy black and white adolescents. *Sleep* 35:1353–1358. © Sleep Research Society (2012). doi: 10.5665/sleep.2112.

found that those with the shortest spontaneous sleep durations (especially during weekdays) had the greatest degree of insulin resistance (Matthews et al., 2012) (**Figure 14.2**).[8]

A possible confounding factor in studies based on questionnaire data is the presence of sleep-disordered breathing (SDB), which may not be reported by participants, in part because sleep-related respiratory symptoms may be present but undiagnosed for many years. PSG studies can identify these symptoms, but these are not usually included in population-based studies. When PSG studies were available, the conclusions reached were somewhat inconsistent. One study found that symptoms of the metabolic syndrome were associated with sleep features in middle-aged women (sleep apnea symptoms, lighter NREM sleep, and low sleep efficiency). After controlling for confounders, including sleep apnea symptoms, only low sleep efficiency was significantly associated with the metabolic syndrome (Hall et al., 2012). A larger cohort of both men and women that used home PSG studies found that after controlling for confounders, including SDB symptoms and activity levels, no sleep features were associated with metabolic syndrome symptoms (Haba-Rubio et al., 2015).

Another study obtained PSG recordings at two time points separated by 12–30 years (average: ~19 years). SDB symptoms were associated with features of the metabolic syndrome both cross-sectionally and prospectively. Other objective sleep features at baseline did not predict the presence of metabolic symptoms at the second time point. However, self-reported long sleep latencies (over the last month) predicted elevated glucose and other metabolic symptoms at the second time point, after adjustment for multiple confounders including SDB symptoms (Bowman et al., 2019). One potential interpretation is that self-reports of sleep problems during a recent month may be a better reflection of habitual sleep patterns than a single PSG study.

These studies confirmed that SDB has important impacts on metabolic symptoms. Differences among their results may be related to the participants' gender, ethnicity, or the baseline prevalence of SDB among the study participants as well as on the specific confounders included in the analyses.

Despite the advantages of obtaining PSG data, they are usually available at only a single timepoint. It is unknown to what extent these results represent habitual sleep patterns during the years over which metabolic symptoms may develop. A few studies have examined stability of PSG features over multiple nights. In one study, PSG recordings were obtained from insomnia patients and controls over three successive nights. The percentage of N3 sleep and EEG characteristics derived from power-spectral analyses of NREM sleep were stable over these nights. However, other objective sleep features (total sleep duration, sleep continuity, and sleep onset latency) were poorly correlated over the recording nights (Israel et al., 2012). These are features that are sometimes linked to metabolic symptoms when obtained by self-report.

A study that obtained 5 nights of at-home recordings using a novel headband that can distinguish sleep features (Dreem^{TM} headband) reported different degrees of variability over these nights depending on sleep measures. For example, variability was reported to be low for total sleep time and sleep efficiency, but high for sleep-onset latency, WASO, and N3 percentage (Chouraki et al., 2023).

An analysis of eight previous studies that used actigraphy, self-reports, or EEG measurement over multiple nights (at least 3) reported variability over nights in sleep duration and efficiency. The most common self-reported measure in survey studies (total sleep time) was similarly variable using all three methods, with coefficients of variation of ~19%, but EEG measures had somewhat lower variability than the other measures,

[8] High values of the measure of insulin resistance used in this and other studies (HOMA) are strongly associated with disturbed glucose regulation, but there is no agreement on the cut-off HOMA values that identify increased clinical risk for developing T2D (Gayosa-Diz et al., 2013). The impacts of high insulin resistance interact with variables like the composition of the population being studied and levels of obesity in a sample, so there is no single threshold value that reliably predicts who is highly likely to develop T2D.

at least using some criteria (Messman et al., 2022).[9] These results raise the question of how stable either self-reported or objective measures (using a variety of devices) would be over years or decades, rather than days.

PSG studies are clearly valuable for identifying the presence of SDB and other potentially confounding conditions, of which participants are often unaware. However, it is not clear that a single objective study using PSG or actigraphy will provide a reliable estimate of participants' habitual sleep patterns over decades. It remains to be established whether a single self-report asking about "habitual sleep" provides a better or worse estimate of long-term sleep patterns than single actigraphy, PSG, or time-use studies. The financial and logistical constraints inherent in large, population-based studies also raise the question of whether multiple assessments over many years using any of these methods would provide more useful information than single studies, and whether the benefits would outweigh the costs involved.

14.6.2 Experimental studies

Experimental sleep restriction has been used to help clarify whether the associations documented in observational studies are likely to reflect causal relations between short or disrupted sleep and metabolic symptoms. In these studies, acute metabolic changes in response to short-term sleep restriction serve as surrogate markers for the risk of developing clinical conditions that have been identified in observational studies.

Reduced sleep for as little as one or a few nights caused increased insulin levels and/or increased insulin resistance (i.e., reduced insulin sensitivity) in both people and rats (Buxton et al., 2010; Donga et al., 2010; Jha et al., 2016; Reynolds et al., 2012); for reviews, see Reutrakul & Van Cauter, 2018; Rogers et al., 2024; Zhu et al., 2019. The dynamics of glucose regulation under sleep restriction are illustrated in a study of healthy, young men (average age, 27 years) who had 2 nights of 10 h time in bed (TIB) followed by 5 nights of 4 h TIB (**Figure 14.3**). Despite controlled, weight-appropriate caloric intake during each day and no overnight snacks, those with restricted sleep showed sustained increases in circulating glucose and insulin levels after meals and throughout the night (Reynolds et al., 2012).

These effects can be modified by altered energy balance. When men and women (age 30-45 years) were allowed 4 h TIB for 4 nights, but food intake was restricted to the extent of causing small losses in body weight, sleep loss did not cause increased insulin resistance (St-Onge et al., 2012). It is likely that endocrine responses to reduced food intake and/or decreasing body weight obscured effects of sleep loss on glucose metabolism that were seen in studies that did not involve participant weight loss.

There is evidence that SWS is particularly important for regulating glucose metabolism. Disrupting SWS with noise over 3 nights caused increased insulin resistance that was proportional to the amount of SWS lost, despite normal total sleep durations (Tasali et al., 2008). Even a single night with a large reduction in SWS (~80% decrease) in young-adult men increased insulin resistance, but REM sleep reductions did not (Herzog et al., 2013). A decrease of ~40% in SWS for one night among young adolescents (11–14 years) had less impact on glucose regulation (Shaw et al., 2016). It is unclear whether the difference between these results was related to the age of the participants or to the more modest reduction in SWS for the adolescents.

Not only does reduced sleep disrupt glucose regulation, but increasing sleep has the opposite effect. People with relatively short habitual sleep durations on weeknights (6.5 h) and at least 1 h more on weekends (in response to their cumulative sleep debt) attempted to increase their weeknight sleep for a 6-week period. There were large individual differences in how successful these attempts were, but the entire group averaged increases of ~50 min sleep nightly. Those with the largest increases showed the most improvement in insulin sensitivity (Leproult et al., 2015). Similarly, in people with experimentally restricted sleep (5 h nightly) that resulted in reduced insulin sensitivity, 3–5 subsequent nights with an extended sleep opportunity (9 h) partially restored insulin sensitivity (Eckel et al., 2015).

Although recovery sleep after sleep loss can improve glucose regulation, these benefits may be rapidly reversible. People who had been restricted to 5 h TIB for 5 nights showed improved insulin sensitivity during 2 nights of recovery sleep (simulating a weekend of extended sleep). However, the improvement was rapidly reversed and resulted in decreased muscle and liver insulin sensitivity when they were again restricted to 5 h sleep for 2 nights (Depner et al., 2019). Despite its immediate benefits, extending sleep over the "weekend" did not prevent an immediate impact of subsequent short sleep on insulin sensitivity.

In contrast to these results, an observational study of Korean adults evaluated the effects of real weekend catch-up sleep among those who self-reported similarly short sleep durations on weekdays (<6 h). The study found that those who had more weekend catch-up sleep (at least 40 min more, but averaging ~2 h more on each weekend night) showed reduced prevalence of symptoms of the metabolic syndrome (levels of blood glucose, triglycerides, and amount of abdominal obesity) compared to those who did not increase their sleep on weekends. Although the two groups differed along other

[9] An actigraphic study conducted over 6 months identified four categories of rest-activity patterns. About 23% of participants shifted between categories at least once during this period, but almost all those classified as "short sleepers" stayed in that category (Crosley-Lyons et al., 2025).

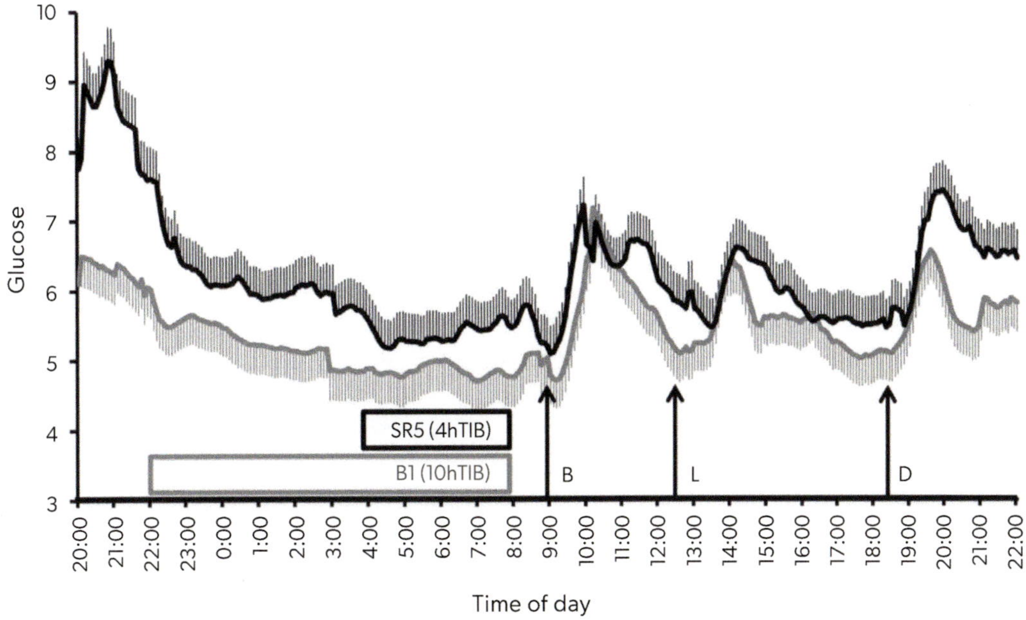

Figure 14.3 Daily pattern of circulating glucose levels at baseline (gray line) following a night with 10 h time in bed (TIB) and after 5 nights of sleep restriction (SR5) to 4 h TIB nightly (black line); vertical lines indicate standard errors. The actual TIB at baseline (10 h; B1) and during restriction (4 h; SR5) are shown as horizontal bars above the X axis. Blood glucose levels rose in response to each meal (breakfast [B], lunch [L] and dinner [D]) but showed more sustained increases after each meal in the 4 h TIB condition. In addition, glucose levels were strongly increased throughout the evening and night after sleep restriction, despite strict control of food consumption with no snacking allowed after meals. Reprinted with permission from Reynolds, A.C. et al. (2012) Impact of five nights of sleep restriction on glucose metabolism, leptin and testosterone in young adult men. *PLoS ONE* 7:e41218. © Reynolds et al. (2012). Licensed under a Creative Commons Attribution License (CC-BY). doi:10.1371/journal.pone.0041218.

dimensions (type of employment, alcohol use, and others), the results were similar when these variables were controlled for in the analysis (Kim et al., 2020).

These two studies reached different conclusions about the benefits of weekend catch-up sleep but based their conclusions on different approaches. The experimental restriction study observed the acute effects of sleep restriction and the immediate reversal of the benefits of extra "weekend" sleep when sleep was again restricted (Depner et al., 2019). The observational study instead compared the metabolic consequences of self-reported, habitual short sleep in those who either voluntarily increased sleep on weekends or did not, presumably over a period of years (Kim et al., 2020).

The participants in these studies also differed in several ways. The experimental study used a within-participant design and imposed controlled sleep amounts in a Boston laboratory. Participants were men and women with an average age of 25 years; most were identified as White, with smaller numbers of Asian, Latino/Hispanic and a few with other ethnic backgrounds. The observational study included results from a database of adult Koreans with an average age of 47 years. It examined the effects on a different set of features of the metabolic syndrome, based on self-reported sleep patterns (Kim et al., 2020). Two other population-based studies that used an earlier version of the same Korean national database found that weekend catch-up sleep reduced the probability of having high levels of CRP, although this effect was limited in one study to those who slept <6 h on weekdays and were non-obese (Han et al., 2020; Jung et al., 2019).

It is unclear whether the age or ethnic/racial characteristics of the participants in these studies, or the structural differences in the studies' designs, contributed to these contrasting conclusions. One possible interpretation is that the benefits for metabolic functions of long-term, habitual increases in total sleep amounts, averaging 4 h each weekend (Kim et al., 2020), may have outweighed the negative effects of short-term fluctuations in glucose metabolism resulting from alternating reductions and increases in sleep amounts, as in Depner et al., 2019. The results of these studies indicate the need for more long-term experimental and observational studies to address the factors that determine whether weekend recovery sleep has only acute, or also long-term, benefits in reducing metabolic health risks.

The effects of both reduced and extended sleep durations in experimental studies are consistent with a role for sleep duration, especially the amount of SWS, in regulating glucose metabolism. Experimental results demonstrated a mechanism that likely underlies the population-based evidence linking habitual short sleep to impaired glucose metabolism, obesity (see Section 14.7), and other features of the metabolic syndrome as well as the many health problems that result secondarily from these conditions (WHO, 2020).

14.6.3 Summary

Self-reported and objectively observed short sleep were associated with many of the features of the metabolic syndrome: hypertension, insulin resistance, diabetes, and hyperlipidemia. This cluster of abnormal features predicts increased risk of developing serious illnesses, including diabetes, heart disease, and stroke. This association was sometimes stronger in women than in men. Controlling for the presence of SDB symptoms (which themselves disrupt and shorten sleep) reduced the apparent connection between sleep duration and metabolic abnormalities in some studies, but not in others.

Experimental studies of acute reductions in sleep duration strengthened the interpretation from observational studies that chronic short sleep can cause these conditions; even a single night of SWS restriction decreased insulin sensitivity. The conclusion that short sleep impairs glucose regulation was further strengthened by evidence that insulin sensitivity was improved in chronic short sleepers to the extent that they increased their sleep amounts over several weeks. Food restriction sufficient to reduce body weight may, however, alter metabolism sufficiently to obscure the effects of short sleep on insulin sensitivity.

Both survey responses and PSG recordings are typically obtained at one or two time points, and it is uncertain whether they reflect sleep characteristics over the longer term. Asking about "habitual" sleep characteristics is intended to overcome this problem, but such self-reports may be affected by memory distortions and several kinds of reporting biases. Thus, in attempting to predict the future risk of developing T2D, it is not clear whether single measures using PSG recordings, actigraphy, current sleep diaries, or retrospective self-reports are most useful. Repeated objective measurements over time may partially address these issues, but these are often not feasible.

Irregular sleep schedules, including high levels of social jet lag, in children, adolescents, and adults were also associated with disturbed regulation of glucose and cholesterol. However, population-based studies found that among chronic short sleepers, habitual weekend catch-up sleep improved several of the features of the metabolic syndrome and markers of inflammation. A laboratory-based study of the effects of catch-up sleep instead found that the benefits for insulin sensitivity were immediately reversed by a return to short sleep. Extra sleep on weekends may be beneficial for chronic short sleepers over the long term, despite the potential disruptive effects of changing sleep patterns during the week, relative to those with stable, adequate sleep amounts. Future studies that assess the impact of the many differences between these studies will be needed to better understand whether or not weekend catch-up sleep has long-term health benefits or costs.

Taken together, these results imply that chronic short sleep is causally related to impaired metabolic regulation, which can lead over the long term to major metabolic illnesses and their many serious health consequences. The question of why reported long sleep is also often associated with metabolic disorders and other health problems will be discussed in the next chapter (Section 15.6.2).

14.7 Sleep and body weight regulation

14.7.1 Relations between sleep duration and body weight

It is widely recognized that there is an ongoing epidemic of increased body weights. A 2020 report indicated that 1.9 billion adults worldwide were considered overweight (body-mass index (BMI) >25) and about 650 million were considered obese (BMI >30) as of 2016 (WHO, 2020).[10] A more recent international review found a continuing increase in obesity, with accelerating increases in childhood obesity, so that the estimate for 2022 was that about 1 billion people worldwide now meet criteria for being obese (NCD-RisC, 2024). Excess weight is associated with many serious health consequences, including increased risk of developing vascular disease, insulin resistance, diabetes, arthritis, and cancer. For example, of all cancer deaths in the United States, 14% in men and 20% in women were attributed to being overweight or obese (Calle et al., 2003).[11] A recent review found that elevated BMI was the third leading cause of all risk-attributable cancer deaths worldwide, trailing only smoking and alcohol use (Tran et al., 2022).[12]

---

[10] BMI is defined as body mass (in kilograms) divided by the square of a person's height (in meters).

[11] Being overweight or moderately obese on its own is not a perfect predictor of the extent and immediacy of the risk of serious health problems (e.g., cardiovascular disease). The distribution of body fat, waist circumference, and several metabolic markers modify the health risks associated with these conditions. Severe obesity, however, indicates a very high risk of cardiovascular and other diseases (Després et al., 2021).

[12] The health risks of being overweight do not apply equally to all ages. Older people (~65–85 years old) with recommended, "normal" BMIs had fewer functional disabilities than those who were overweight or obese, but also had increased mortality rates (Lang et al., 2008; Stessman et al., 2009). A meta-analysis of 20 studies of mortality in nursing-home residents (average age, ~84 years) showed increased mortality for those who were underweight, but reduced mortality for those overweight or obese, relative to those with normal BMIs (Veronese et al., 2015). These results may reflect the fact that many older people lose muscle mass and have poor nutrition, resulting in reduced body weights, but also reducing their metabolic reserve and their capacity to survive serious infections and injuries.

Increased calorie intake combined with decreased energy expenditure from more sedentary lifestyles are usually considered the principal contributors to increasing rates of obesity. But other factors have also been proposed to play a role, for example, consumption of high-sugar soft drinks that provide calories in liquid form (Hu, 2013); personality characteristics (Chaput et al., 2009); increased exposure to environmental toxins; and increased use of medications that have the side effect of causing weight gain (McAllister et al., 2009; Nicol et al., 2018). Another contributing factor that is supported by increasingly strong evidence is sleep duration. Observational studies have consistently found that adults sleeping 7–8 h nightly have the lowest BMIs; short sleepers (and less consistently, long sleepers) have higher BMIs (Kripke et al., 2002; Taheri et al., 2004).

Many studies and meta-analyses have reported strong links between short sleep and higher body weights in children, both cross-sectionally and prospectively (Chaput et al., 2006; Chaput et al., 2016; Felsö et al., 2017; Magee & Hale, 2012; Miller et al., 2018; Nielsen et al., 2011; Spaeth et al., 2019; Spruyt et al., 2011; Taveras et al., 2014). A study of children 8.8–13.5 years old, for example, found that short sleep, poor sleep quality, delayed bedtime, and increased sleep-onset latency were all significantly associated with being overweight or obese (Morrissey et al., 2022).

Short sleep at a young age seems to be a particularly strong predictor of later weight gain during both childhood (Bell & Zimmerman, 2010; Magee & Hale, 2012) and young adulthood, even after controlling for current sleep durations as adults (Landhuis et al., 2008). Adolescents (age ~15 years) with sleep difficulties that persisted to age 20 had increased risk of overweight/obesity, as did those who reported short sleep only at age 20 (Wang et al., 2023). Factors associated with short sleep that could mediate its effects on body weight in adolescents include increased food reward properties, decreased insulin sensitivity, disrupted meal patterns, and increased sedentary behavior/screen time (DiFrancesco et al., 2023; Duraccio et al., 2019). The temporal direction of many of these associations—early short sleep or sleep difficulties followed by later weight gain—is consistent with, but does not prove, a causal interpretation.

Associations observed in children and young adults between short sleep and body weight become less consistent in older adults (Grandner et al., 2015; Hasler et al., 2004; Magee & Hale, 2012; Nielsen et al., 2011). Among studies that found a cross-sectional association of short sleep with higher BMIs in older adults, some found that it also predicted future increases in weight or BMI (Chaput et al., 2008; Patel et al., 2006; Xiao et al., 2013) (**Figure 14.4**), but others did not (Gangwisch et al., 2005; Stranges et al., 2008).

A prospective study of people in China across adulthood observed more weight gain over 8 years in those sleeping <6 h compared to those sleeping 7 h at baseline (Ning et al., 2020). A study including data from American survey participants ranging in age from mid-adolescence to >65 years found that shorter sleep was linearly related to increased BMI in the adolescent and young adult groups. However, higher BMI was associated with both short and long sleep in older middle-aged

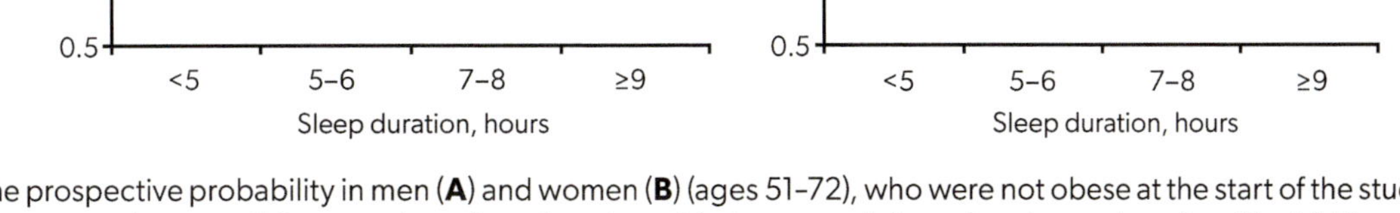

Figure 14.4 The prospective probability in men (**A**) and women (**B**) (ages 51-72), who were not obese at the start of the study), of developing obesity over the next ~7.5 years, plotted as a function of their reported sleep durations at baseline (X axis). Those with stroke, heart disease, or cancer at baseline, or who developed these conditions during the study, were excluded, leaving a sample of >83,000 people. In each case, risk among those showing 7–8 h of sleep is the reference value (Referent; red line), and probabilities are expressed relative to these reference values. For both sexes, those with shortest sleep (<5 h) had the greatest increase in risk of developing obesity (45% and 37% higher for men and women, respectively), while the 5–6 h sleep group among women also had a significantly increased risk (15% higher). Error bars are 95% confidence intervals, so means with error bars that do not cross the red line are statistically significantly different from the reference value. Adapted with permission from Xiao, Q. et al. (2013) A large prospective investigation of sleep duration, weight change, and obesity in the NIH-AARP Diet and Health Study cohort. *Am J Epidemiol* 178 (11):1600–1610. Published by Oxford University Press on behalf of the Johns Hopkins Bloomberg School of Public Health © (2013). doi: 10.1093/aje/kwt180.

adults, and the relationship between sleep and BMI was weak in the oldest group (Grandner et al., 2015).

Some studies also reported gender differences in links between short sleep and obesity, but these have not been consistent. There are reports of a significant association of short sleep with risk of obesity in women but not men (Mercy et al., 2022), and of short sleep with later development of overweight/obesity in young women but less so in young men (Wang et al., 2023). While both genders with very short sleep had increased risk of developing obesity, moderately short sleep increased obesity risk in women but not in men (Xiao et al., 2013), and short sleep in another study was associated with abdominal obesity only in men (Zhou et al., 2020).

Several factors might contribute to different results in these population-based studies: the definitions of short sleepers and their comparison groups; the range of confounders included; and the nationality, ethnicity, and other demographic characteristics of the study population. Differences among studies in the inclusion/exclusion criteria that are used may also be important. For example, serious, chronic illnesses increase in frequency with age, and participants who had or developed such illnesses were excluded in some studies but not in others (Xiao et al., 2013).

Weaker effects of sleep duration on body weight in older people may be related to the fact that most middle-aged and older adults gain weight over the years, develop more medical conditions, and experience endocrine changes (including menopause) that can affect body weight regulation. These changes may make it more difficult to detect any additional impact of sleep duration on weight (Grandner et al., 2015; Xiao et al., 2013). The effects of short sleep later in life may also differ among individuals. In some people, short sleep early in development may contribute to increased weight, but short sleep as adults may contribute only to maintaining the excess weight gained earlier. In others, short sleep may contribute to weight gain both as children and as adults.

Behavioral habits probably also interact with sleep duration to influence weight regulation. These include, for example, activity levels, tobacco smoking, dieting habits, and personality variables, such as the tendency to show disinhibited food intake (increased intake in response to emotional states or to the palatability of food) (Chaput et al., 2011; Chaput et al., 2009; Ning et al., 2020; Xiao et al., 2013). Conclusions about the impact of sleep may be affected by the extent to which these behavioral factors are incorporated into the analysis.

Among adults, both successfully losing weight with dieting and exercise and subsequently regaining weight are also associated with sleep quality or duration. A Danish study involving participants in a weight loss and maintenance program reported on effects of both sleep quality (assessed using the PSQI) and sleep duration (assessed using actigraphy). It found that those with poor sleep quality lost less weight and body fat than those with better sleep quality. In addition, among the subset of participants (average age ~44 years) who managed to achieve a target weight reduction, those classified as short sleepers (<6 h nightly) regained more weight and body fat over the following year than those sleeping ≥6 h nightly (Bogh et al., 2023).

When short sleep and excess weight are found to be associated in young adults, there is also the possibility of reverse causation or a mutually reinforcing effect. One study observed cross-sectional associations between short sleep and obesity as well as a prospective association between short sleep at one age and later development of obesity. However, the study also detected the opposite association: obesity at one age (without short sleep) predicted the appearance of short sleep at a later age (Hasler et al., 2004). Another study also reported that persistent overweight/obesity from adolescence to young adulthood predicted emergence of sleep difficulties and short sleep in young adults (Wang et al., 2023).

The mechanisms involved in these "reverse" associations are not known. Suggested possibilities include a common causal factor contributing to the development of both short sleep and weight gain (e.g., chronic inflammation); a lifetime history of overweight contributing to sleep difficulties (e.g., because of emergence of SDB or reduced likelihood of regular exercise); or bidirectional influences involving unidentified mechanisms (Nielsen et al., 2011).

14.7.2 Sleep duration and energy balance

Although behavioral mechanisms have been suggested as mediators that contribute to the links between short sleep and weight gain (Duraccio et al., 2019), most experimental studies have focused on physiological mechanisms; for reviews, see Reutrakul & Van Cauter, 2018; St-Onge, 2017. Body weight reflects the long-term balance between total energy intake and total energy expenditure, so studies have investigated whether sleep affects mechanisms involved in both processes. Hormones involved in appetite regulation are one of these mechanisms.

Early studies of fit young men found that sleep restriction over several nights reduced levels of the hormone leptin (a product of fat cells), increased levels of ghrelin (a gut peptide), altered how insulin and glucose responded to food intake, and modified the daily cortisol rhythm (**Figure 14.5**) (Spiegel, Leproult, et al., 2004; Spiegel, Tasali, et al., 2004). Ghrelin levels rise in anticipation of meals and stimulate hunger and food intake, but leptin inhibits appetite. Thus, the opposite changes in these hormones during sleep restriction would be predicted to promote increased food consumption and weight gain

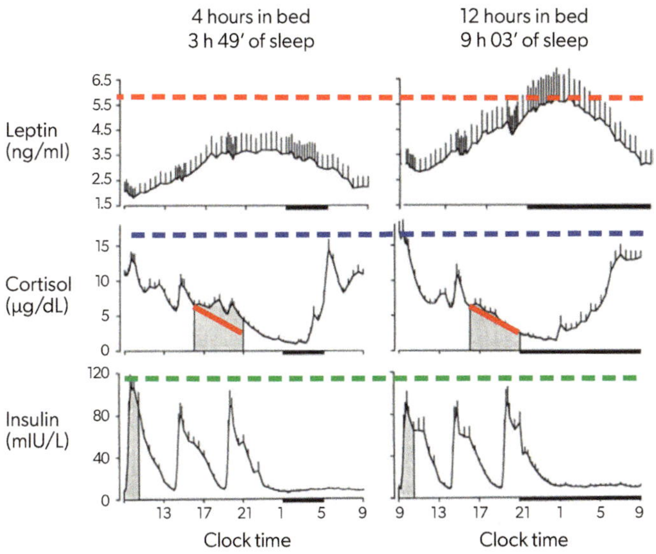

Figure 14.5 Effects on endocrine variables of 7 nights of 12 h time in bed (TIB) (right) or 6 nights of 4 h TIB (left) in healthy young men (corresponding respectively to ~9 h and <4 h of actual sleep nightly). The black box on the X axis of each graph represents the TIB, and endocrine values (Y axes) are plotted against clock time (X axis). The top panels show a decrease in levels of the hormone leptin, which is involved in promoting satiety, among participants restricted to 4 h TIB. The horizontal red line indicates the peak average leptin level in the 12 h sleep group, which is higher than any average value in the 4 h sleep group (left). The middle panels show the patterns of blood cortisol levels across the day. The red line in the right panel illustrates the steep decline in cortisol during the late afternoon/early evening in those with 12 h TIB. A similarly positioned red line in the left panel shows that cortisol levels were elevated for longer during the evening in those with 4 h TIB, resulting in higher cortisol levels at that time. The dashed blue line shows the peak cortisol level after waking in the morning (09:00) in the 12 h condition, which is higher than the value at the same clock time after 4 h TIB, and higher than the peak value immediately after waking in that condition (05:00). The bottom panels show insulin responses to meals. Those with short sleep (left) showed an increased spike of insulin secretion in response to the morning meal, relative to the value for the 12 h sleep group (dashed green line). Adapted with permission of Oxford University Press from Spiegel, K. et al. (2004) Leptin levels are dependent on sleep duration: relationships with sympathovagal balance, carbohydrate regulation, cortisol, and thyrotropin. *J Clin Endocrinol Metab* 89(11): 5762–5771. © The Endocrine Society (2004). doi: 10.1210/jc.2004-1003.

(Cummings et al., 2001; Ferrario et al., 2016; Spiegel et al., 2011; Wren et al., 2001).

These hormonal changes during sleep restriction have not, however, been seen consistently across studies of men, women, and adolescents. In addition to the original reports of decreased leptin levels, sleep loss has also been found to not affect levels (Calvin et al., 2013; Klingenberg et al., 2013; Nedeltcheva et al., 2009; Schmid et al., 2009; St-Onge et al., 2012), or to increase them (Bosy-Westphal et al., 2008; Hayes et al., 2011; Markwald et al., 2013; Omisade et al., 2010; Reynolds et al., 2012; Simpson et al., 2010). Increased ghrelin levels during sleep restriction were seen in men, but not in women, when no snacking was allowed (St-Onge et al., 2012); but studies with free access to food during sleep restriction reported decreased ghrelin (Markwald et al., 2013) or no change (Bosy-Westphal et al., 2008).

Total overnight sleep loss may have different effects from those of partial sleep restriction. Plasma and salivary ghrelin levels normally rise overnight, but total sleep deprivation in young adult men and adolescent boys and girls blunted the rise (Dzaja et al., 2004; Felsö et al., 2022). Among adolescents, there was a particularly strong attenuation of the nocturnal rise among those considered overweight/obese (average BMI of 25.8), compared to participants with normal weights (average BMI of 19.5) (Felsö et al., 2022).

The timing of sampling is important for measuring both leptin and ghrelin. Leptin levels show a daily rhythm, the form of which is modified by sleep loss (Mullington et al., 2003), and leptin levels change across the menstrual cycle (Gröschl et al., 2002; Wunder et al., 2006). Ghrelin levels rise before meals and fall afterwards, show a daily rhythm, and are affected by calorie restriction (Cummings et al., 2001; Spiegel et al., 2011).

One meta-analysis of a subset of published studies that met inclusion criteria (Lin et al., 2020) concluded that the evidence indicates that ghrelin levels are elevated in both spontaneous short sleepers and in those with experimentally restricted sleep lengths (although this effect may be limited to men when food is not freely available) (St-Onge et al., 2012). This conclusion is consistent with the idea that short sleep increases ghrelin, which promotes food intake and results in increased weights. The meta-analysis also found that experimental sleep restriction in many studies also increased leptin levels, which is proposed to function as a satiety agent. These results suggest that short sleep increased levels of hormones that both decrease and increase hunger, which would not account for the apparent effects of short sleep on body weight. A limitation that was noted was that there was insufficient information to assess potential interactions with diet, food intake, and activity levels (Lin et al., 2020), so the possible influence of these factors, and others discussed above, could not be evaluated.

Many factors likely contributed to different findings among studies of how sleep restriction affects ghrelin and leptin levels. These include the severity of sleep restriction imposed; differences in access to food and the resulting metabolic consequences; the gender and age of participants; the level of activity permitted; the sampling method and its timing; unreported lighting conditions during overnight sleep deprivation; and body weights of participants (Felsö et al., 2022; Schmid et al., 2008; Spiegel, Leproult, et al., 2004; St-Onge et al., 2012;

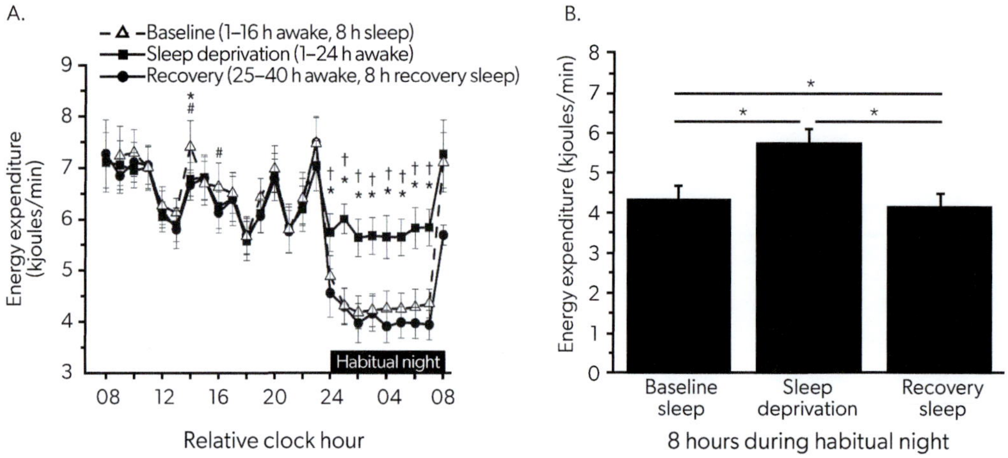

Figure 14.6 **A.** Energy expenditure across the day and habitual night (usual sleep phase) in participants studied under modified constant routine conditions. There was a large increase in energy expenditure when kept awake at night (black squares) compared to when sleeping at night (white triangles), even though motor activity was severely restricted. When allowed recovery sleep for 8 h at the same daily phase after sleep deprivation (black circles), there was a small *decrease* in energy expenditure during the sleep period, probably reflecting more consolidated sleep and more rebound SWS compared to baseline conditions (see panel B). * Significant difference between Baseline and Sleep deprivation days. † Significant difference between Sleep deprivation and Recovery days. # Significant difference between Baseline and Recovery days. **B.** Average energy expenditure per minute (Y axis) during the 8 h habitual sleep phase, under three different conditions, as shown in panel **A**: during the Baseline day with 16 h awake and 8 h of sleep; during the next day with 24 h awake (Sleep deprivation); and during the following Recovery day with 16 h awake followed by an 8 h sleep period. * Statistically significant comparison. Reprinted with permission of John Wiley and Sons from Jung, C.M. et al. (2011) Energy expenditure during sleep, sleep deprivation and sleep following sleep deprivation in adult humans. *J Physiol* 589: 235–244. © The Authors (2010). Journal compilation © The Physiological Society and John Wiley and Sons (2010). doi: 10.1113/jphysiol.2010.197517. Permission conveyed through Copyright Clearance Center Inc.

St-Onge, 2013); for reviews, see Rogers et al., 2024; St-Onge, 2013; Zhu et al., 2019.

Despite uncertainty about the hormonal mechanisms that may be involved, there is consistent evidence that experimental sleep restriction over just a few nights produces measurable weight gains (Markwald et al., 2013; Nedeltcheva et al., 2009; Spaeth et al., 2013). These gains tended to be larger in men than in women and in those who identified as African-American (Spaeth et al., 2013; 2014).

These effects of sleep restriction over short periods are counterintuitive because people who stay awake longer necessarily increase their energy expenditure relative to when they sleep (i.e., they burn more calories while awake). This increased energy expenditure is not only the obvious result of people being more active while awake than while asleep. It occurs even in a constant routine procedure during which people stay awake but are kept completely inactive for ≥24 h (see Section 3.5.2). Energy expenditure during a 24 h constant routine with no sleep allowed was increased overall by ~7% compared to during a baseline day that included an 8 h sleep opportunity. This change resulted from a >30% increase in energy expenditure during the usual 8 h sleep period while participants were awake and immobile, as compared to the same 8 h interval while asleep and immobile (Jung et al., 2011); sleeping itself reduces energy expenditure. Participants also showed a small decrease in energy expenditure while sleeping during a recovery period compared to sleeping during the same 8 h interval at baseline, probably reflecting increased amounts of SWS and more sustained sleep following a night with no sleep (**Figure 14.6**).

In another study, more moderate sleep restriction of adults (5 h TIB for 5 nights, with no enforced immobility) increased total 24 h energy expenditure by 9% relative to a baseline condition with 9 h TIB. Despite burning more calories when they were awake for longer, participants in the 5 h TIB condition still gained 0.82 kg (1.8 lb) over 5 days (Markwald et al., 2013), principally because of an increase in energy intake from snacks during the extended wake time (**Figure 14.7**).[13]

Several mechanisms contributed to body weight increases during sleep restriction, even in the face of higher energy

[13] This average increase combines results for men and women. Both men and women gained weight in the 5 h TIB condition, but men gained more (1.11 vs. 0.52 kg). In the 9 h TIB condition, women lost a nonsignificant amount of weight while men actually gained weight (0.78 kg). The availability of snacks appears to have motivated more calorie intake in men than women even in the 9 h TIB condition, but more strongly when allowed only 5 h TIB.

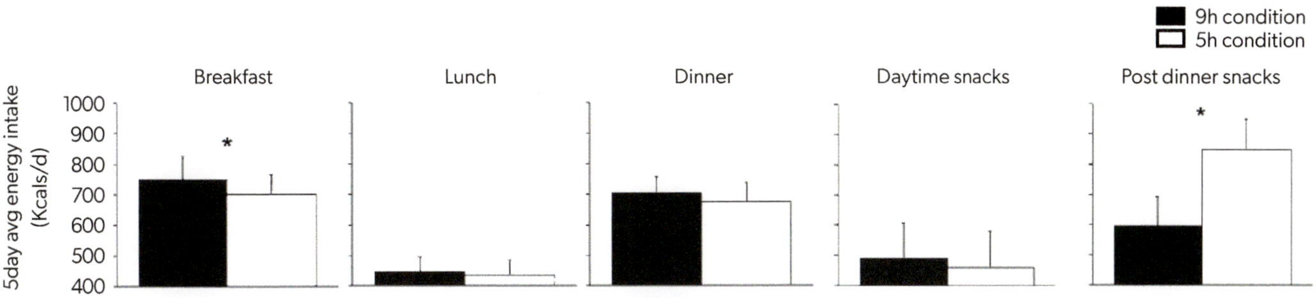

Figure 14.7 Calorie intake (kilocalories per day averaged over 5 days: Kcals/d) from breakfast, lunch, dinner, daytime snacks, and post-dinner snacks among men and women allowed 9 h time in bed (TIB) nightly (black columns), compared to when allowed 5 h TIB nightly for 5 nights (white columns). There was a large increase in calorie intake from snacks consumed during the evening hours (Post dinner snacks) in the 5 h TIB condition. The additional calories consumed overcompensated for the larger amount of energy expended as a result of being awake longer, resulting in a net weight gain over the 5 days of the study. The significant decrease in calorie intake at breakfast in the 5 h TIB condition may reflect the fact that these young adults were awakened 2 h earlier than in the 9 h TIB condition and were eating breakfast at a non-preferred circadian phase. Alternatively, this small reduction could have been the result of their increased calorie intake from snacks during the previous evening. * $p < 0.05$. Reprinted with permission from Markwald, R.R. et al. (2013) Impact of insufficient sleep on total daily energy expenditure, food intake, and weight gain. *Proc Natl Acad Sci (USA)* 110:5695–5700. doi: 10.1073/pnas.1216951110.

expenditure from being awake longer. Sleep restriction increased self-reported hunger during the following day in both men (Brondel et al., 2010; Spiegel, Tasali, et al., 2004) and women (LeRoux et al., 2014); for a meta-analysis of the effects of total and partial sleep deprivation on subjective hunger, see Zhu et al., 2019. Sleep reductions also increased total food intake as well as preferences for high-calorie foods (when participants were allowed food choices). In particular, there was increased intake of high-calorie snacks during extended waking at night (Bosy-Westphal et al., 2008; Calvin et al., 2013; Hogenkamp et al., 2013; Markwald et al., 2013; Nedeltcheva et al., 2009; Schmid et al., 2008; Spaeth et al., 2013; Spiegel et al., 2005; Spiegel et al., 1999; Spiegel, Tasali, et al., 2004; Zhu et al., 2019). Total overnight sleep loss was also reported to increase subjective valuation of food items and brain activation in the amygdala and hypothalamus in response to food images. These results are consistent with sleep loss increasing the anticipated reward value of food (Rihm et al., 2019).

Similar effects on food intake were seen in children of both genders (8–11 years old) who were required to increase or decrease their usual sleep durations for a week each, in random order. This procedure produced a 2.3 h difference in average sleep durations between the two conditions. During sleep restriction, children reported consuming more calories daily than during sleep extension, mostly during the extra hours awake. The children weighed an average of 0.22 kg (~0.5 lb) more after the sleep-restriction week than after the sleep-extension week (Hart et al., 2013). Although the weight increases observed during a few days of reduced sleep in both adults and children sound relatively small, consistent short sleep over months or years could result in significant cumulative increases in body weights.

Studies have reached different conclusions about whether increased intake of fat or carbohydrates was most important for weight gain during sleep restriction. A meta-analysis concluded that sleep-restricted adults increased 24 h energy intake in large part by increasing fat intake at the expense of protein (Al Khatib et al., 2017).

The critical role of voluntary increases in food intake during short sleep was reinforced by the results of the study discussed earlier in which participants ate a consistent, rigid diet that did not permit additional nighttime snacks. As a result, participants were in a state of negative energy balance during 4 days of either 9 h TIB or 4 h TIB. They lost 1.0 kg (2.2 lb) during 9 h TIB days and 0.8 kg (1.7 lb) during the 4 h TIB days (St-Onge et al., 2012). Thus, weight gain during sleep restriction did not occur in the absence of free access to food. However, the slightly reduced weight *loss* during sleep restriction might suggest that short sleep promoted weight gain (or prevented weight loss) by a mechanism other than increasing food intake.[14]

[14] Women in this study did not show increased ghrelin levels but instead showed *decreased* levels of the gut hormone glucagon-like peptide-1 (GLP-1) (St-Onge et al., 2012). GLP-1 promotes insulin release and reduces appetite, so decreased GLP-1 levels might have acted as an appetite-promoting response to inadequate food availability or to weight loss. Agonists acting on GLP-1 receptors (e.g., semaglutide, sold as Ozempic™ or Wegovy™ are increasingly used to treat diabetes and to promote weight loss (Nauck et al., 2021).

14.7.3 Effects of meal timing on metabolism

Staying awake longer allows more time for late-night snacking that contributes to measurable weight gain within a few days (Markwald et al., 2013; Nedeltcheva et al., 2009; Spaeth et al., 2013) (see **Figure 14.7**). These effects may be related not only to increased calorie consumption, but also to the time at which sleep-restricted participants eat. Delayed bedtimes and reduced sleep amounts result in more food consumption during the circadian night phase if free food intake is allowed.

Studies in mice found that the daily phase at which calories were consumed affected how energy was utilized. Mice that were allowed to eat a high-fat diet for six weeks only during the 12 h light phase (when they normally eat very little) gained significantly more weight than those fed similarly during their 12 h dark phase, despite comparable calorie consumption and activity levels (Arble et al., 2009). Mice given free access to a very attractive, high-fat diet ate small amounts at all times of day and developed obesity, fatty deposits in their livers and elevated insulin levels. When mice had access to the same diet for 8 h only in the daily dark phase, they ate similar total amounts but did not develop these metabolic symptoms. Preventing mice from eating the attractive, high-fat diet during the light phase (their "wrong" time of day) protected them from its negative metabolic effects (Hatori et al., 2012).

The results of studies in people are consistent with the idea that the timing of food intake affects weight regulation. One example is a Spanish observational study of overweight people taking part in a structured weight-loss program over a 20-week period. In Spain, the largest daily meal is typically eaten in the afternoon, not in the evening (see Chapter 6). Participants who usually ate their principal daily meal (~40% of daily calorie intake) before 15:00 lost more weight than those who ate their largest meal after 15:00, despite a similar level of total energy intake (Garaulet et al., 2013) (**Figure 14.8**).

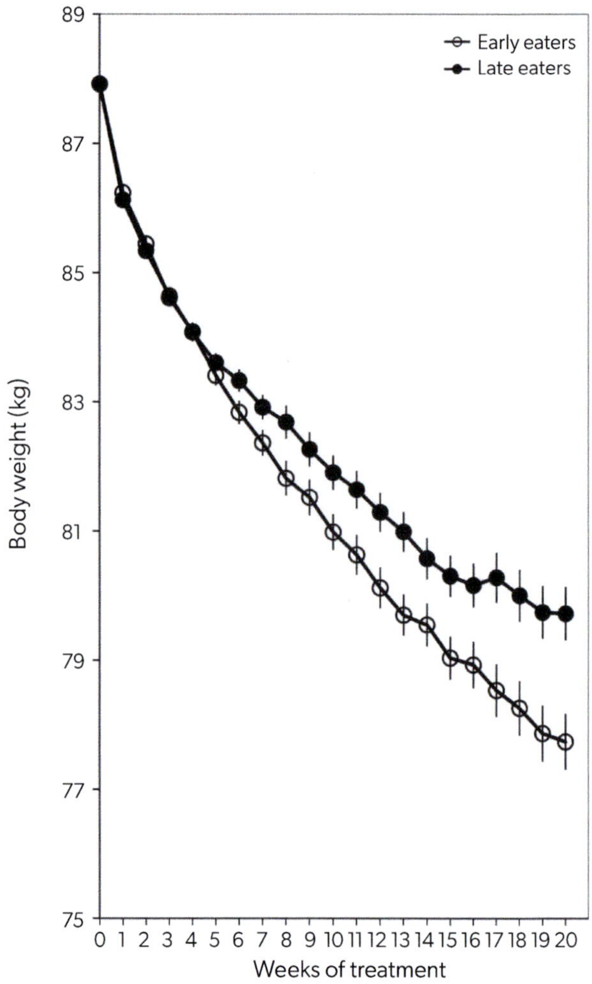

Figure 14.8 Participants who were overweight (starting at an average weight of ~88 kg or 204 lb) participated in a structured weight-loss program. Those with later meal timing, defined as eating their principal daily meal after 15:00 (Late eaters, black symbols) lost body weight (Y axis) more slowly than those eating their principal meal before 15:00 (Early eaters, white symbols) during 20 weeks of the program (X axis). Reprinted with permission of Springer: Nature from Garaulet, M. et al. (2013) Timing of food intake predicts weight loss effectiveness. *Int J Obes (Lond)* 37:604–611. © Macmillan Publishers Ltd (2013). doi:10.1038/ijo.2012.229.

Consistent with these findings, people with a strongly delayed chronotype, including later preferred mealtimes, had higher BMIs than those with an advanced chronotype. They also tended to have shorter sleep durations, later sleep timing, and poorer quality diets. However, the number of calories consumed after 20:00 remained a significant, independent predictor of increased BMI after controlling for sleep duration and timing (Baron et al., 2011). In another observational study, adults who ate larger meals earlier in the day, had substantial breakfasts, consumed fewer snacks, and went for longer durations overnight without food gained less weight than those who ate larger meals later in the day (Kahleova et al., 2017).

Meal timing is also associated with greater body weights in children, independently of differences in sleep duration. Children in Australia with later bedtimes and wake times had higher BMIs than those with an early chronotype, even though both groups had similar sleep durations (Olds et al., 2011). This finding may be related to evidence in another study that later bedtimes in children were associated with later mealtimes and higher daily fat intake (Spaeth et al., 2019). In a Spanish study, school-age children with typically later evening meal timing (after ~21:00) had higher rates of overweight/obesity as well as higher levels of markers of inflammation, including CRP levels, than those with earlier mealtimes (Martínez-Lozano et al., 2020). A study of American preschoolers (3–5 years old) found that a later sleep midpoint (measured using actigraphy) was associated with later morning and evening meal timing and cross-sectionally with higher levels of body fat. Shorter sleep durations and later meal timing also predicted higher body fat levels a year later (Goetz et al., 2022).

A delayed circadian chronotype in people with T2D was associated with less adequate control of blood glucose levels and a lack of blood pressure dipping at night (Reutrakul et al., 2013); see Section 14.8. Similarly, women with longer "fasting" periods overnight (i.e., those who consumed fewer late-night snacks) had better regulation of blood glucose after a morning glucose challenge test (probably reflecting improved insulin sensitivity), and lower values of hemoglobin A1c, an indicator of improved long-term glucose regulation (Marinac et al., 2015).

Experimental research supports the conclusions from these observational studies. An experimental study of people with T2D found that those assigned to eat only during the window of 12:00 to 20:00, with no enforced calorie restrictions, lost more weight than controls, while a group assigned to reduce calorie intake, with no time restriction, did not lose significantly more weight than controls. Both intervention groups had similar reductions in a marker of blood glucose regulation. The temporal restriction group also had a larger spontaneous reduction in calorie intake than the other groups, so it is unclear to what extent the benefits can be attributed to changes in the timing of meals or to the associated reduction in calorie intake (Pavlou et al., 2023).

A laboratory study of overweight/obese, middle-aged participants involved a cross-over design in which they switched from early to late eating, or the opposite, for several days, while metabolic responses were assessed. Early eating involved meals at 1 h, 5 h:10 min, and 9 h:20 min after waking, while late eating involved meals 5 h:10 min, 9 h:20 min, and 13 h:30 min after waking. Late eating resulted in several metabolic and behavioral effects, all of which would favor weight gain. Late eaters rated themselves as hungrier, had reduced 24 h levels of leptin (a satiety signal), reduced 24 h core body temperature, reduced energy expenditure, and changes in gene expression in fat cells that are consistent with increased fat production and storage (Vujovic et al., 2022).

Taken together, these observational and experimental results indicate that reducing the length of time during which people can eat may affect body weight regulation by reducing snacking opportunities and overall calorie intake, regardless of the timing of meals. But it is clear in both animal and human studies that eating at the "wrong" circadian phase (i.e., nighttime for people) can disrupt glucose regulation, alter hormonal signals, increase hunger, increase calorie capture, reduce energy expenditure, and, ultimately, promote weight gain.

Short sleep can therefore affect weight regulation through at least five mechanisms: allowing extra time for food intake; increasing hunger; shifting food preferences toward high-calorie snack foods (when permitted); modifying patterns of hormone release that affect metabolism; and facilitating food consumption during the circadian night phase.

14.7.4 Summary

In most observational studies, current short sleep was associated with higher body weights. The effects of short sleep on future weight gains, however, were most robust in younger populations and observed less consistently in older people, especially in the very old. Short sleep during adulthood may help maintain overweight developed in childhood in some people, rather than further increasing weight gain. The tendency to gain weight in general during aging may obscure some sleep duration effects. Long sleep was also sometimes associated with increased cross-sectional and prospective risks of being overweight or obese, and this effect appeared most clearly in late middle age.

In experimental studies, sleep restriction over a few days resulted in increases in body weight in both adults and children. These effects were primarily related to the extra time available to eat, and especially to an increase in snacking during the hours between dinner and the delayed sleep opportunity. These effects were more robust in men than in women in some studies. When food access was strongly restricted in one study (no snacking), so that participants were in a state of negative energy balance, they lost weight even when allowed 9 h TIB but lost slightly less when they had 4 h TIB. Whether this small difference was related to an opposing effect of short sleep in promoting weight gain is unknown.

Changes in hormones that affect food intake and metabolism may contribute to the effects of short sleep on body weight, but these hormonal changes differed among studies of experimental sleep restriction. These differences may be related to whether food was freely available or restricted, the timing of sampling, and the mixture of men and women in the studies.

Experimental sleep restriction increased the apparent reward properties of food and increased food intake during the extra waking hours when participants were allowed free access to food. The additional calorie intake during the night resulted in measurable weight gain in just a few days, despite increased energy expenditure as a result of being awake longer. Studies differed as to whether nocturnal snacking involved mostly foods higher in carbohydrate, protein, or fat content, but a meta-analysis emphasized the role of an increased preference for high-fat foods at night in promoting weight gain. If sustained over years of chronic short sleep, the resulting cumulative weight increases could account for the association between habitual short sleep and higher body weights that was reported in many observational studies.

Shorter sleep durations can influence body weight both because the resulting longer time spent awake allows for more calorie consumption and because more food intake can occur during the physiological night phase. Animal studies showed severe metabolic effects of food consumption during their circadian rest phase. Similarly, adults and children who ate more at later circadian phases, even without enforced sleep restriction, tended to have increased weights, higher body fat levels, and worse blood glucose regulation.

Overweight people studied with both early and late meal patterns showed behavioral, metabolic, and gene expression changes that are likely to promote more energy intake, lower energy expenditure, and more fat deposition when eating later in the circadian day. Human physiology appears to be adapted to deal metabolically with food eaten primarily during the day. Delayed sleep–wake timing and associated delays in meal timing would tend to promote increased food intake and negative metabolic consequences related to the circadian phase of consumption.

Some of the metabolic effects of short sleep can be modified by factors that have received less experimental attention: attitudes toward perceived sleep problems; a tendency toward disinhibited eating; and a sedentary lifestyle. The interactions among personality characteristics, lifestyle variables, and sleep length in influencing metabolism and weight regulation are important targets for future research.

14.8 **Sleep and vascular disease**

Hypertension is a component of the metabolic syndrome that does not usually cause obvious symptoms, but increases the risk of cardiovascular disease, stroke, and other end-organ damage (e.g., kidney failure, retinal damage). There are several proposed links between the risk of hypertension and sleep characteristics.

A meta-analysis of 11 prospective cohort studies concluded that the risk of developing hypertension was increased by self-reported short sleep and by insomnia complaints (disrupted sleep continuity and early-morning waking) (Meng et al., 2013). Sleep disruption was also proposed to mediate the impact of environmental conditions that elevate blood pressure, such as high levels of noise at night (Akinseye et al., 2015; Chang et al., 2009). A population-based study of Korean adults found an increased risk of reporting hypertension among those sleeping <6 h nightly. This risk was reduced for short-sleepers who also reported an additional 1 h of catch-up sleep on weekend nights. Respondents' judgments about their sleep quality were also important. The increased risk of hypertension among those reporting short sleep and the benefits of catch-up sleep were both more robust among those who complained that their sleep was inadequate, compared to those who did not (Hwangbo et al., 2013).

SWS amounts may be especially important in relation to hypertension. Reduced SWS strongly predicted development of hypertension, independently of total sleep duration or other potential confounders (Fung et al., 2011; Javaheri et al., 2017). This result echoes the finding that reduced SWS was specifically associated with disruption of glucose metabolism (Herzog et al., 2013; Tasali et al., 2008); see Section 14.6.2.

Several sleep disorders could contribute to the reported association between short sleep and hypertension. OSA, the most common form of SDB, is well-documented to both shorten sleep and increase blood pressure (see Appendix B). High numbers of periodic limb movements (PLMs) during sleep, which are often accompanied by blood pressure surges, apneas, or brief arousals, also increase the risk of hypertension (Srivali et al., 2023). Participants in survey studies can be asked whether they have OSA or other sleep-related disorders, but people who have these conditions may not be diagnosed for years (or decades), so participants might not be aware of their condition. PSG studies are therefore needed to address their potential role as confounders.

Some PSG studies reported that associations between sleep duration and hypertension were lost after controlling for the presence of SDB (Fung et al., 2013; Haba-Rubio et al., 2015). However, even after controlling for SDB symptoms, the presence of insomnia symptoms along with objective short sleep (<6 h nightly)[15] predicted increased risk of hypertension and other vascular conditions (Bertisch et al., 2018; Fernandez-Mendoza et al., 2012; Vgontzas et al., 2013; Vgontzas et al., 2009). Thus, in some cases, SDB may be responsible for the link between short sleep and vascular diseases, but the combination of short sleep and insomnia symptoms is an independent risk factor for these conditions.

One model proposed that insomnia with objective short sleep is a severe form of insomnia involving stress system activation, which increases the risk of developing hypertension and chronically elevated cortisol levels.[16] Insomnia patients with objectively normal sleep durations were instead proposed

[15] "Insomnia with objective short sleep" is proposed to differ from typical insomnia, which can be diagnosed without objective evidence of short sleep, as defined in Section 4.4.5. This distinction assumes that short sleep is a stable feature of individuals. A recent study, however, found that some insomnia patients with <6 h sleep during a first night of recording did not show short sleep during a second night (Cox et al., 2024), so appropriate classification may depend on more than a single PSG study. For a recent review discussing the role of PSG in assessing insomnia complaints, see Frase et al., 2023.

[16] Cortisol is an important regulatory hormone secreted by the adrenal glands that influences glucose metabolism and mediates stress responses. It is secreted with a strong daily rhythm, peaking after waking and falling to low levels at night.

to be at increased risk of developing other features of the metabolic syndrome, such as obesity. The risk of developing obesity was reported to be more closely linked to subjective reports of sleep disturbance and to emotional distress than to objective sleep duration (Vgontzas et al., 2013; Vgontzas et al., 2014). This conclusion is consistent with other evidence that personality and behavioral variables interact with sleep duration to affect weight regulation (see Section 14.7.1).

The daily rhythm of blood pressure has important impacts on the magnitude of the health risk associated with hypertension in people. Blood pressure usually rises during the day and falls ("dips")[17] at night during sleep, but some people do not show nocturnal dipping. Regardless of whether people show elevated blood pressure during a daytime assessment, they may be either nighttime "dippers" or "non-dippers." Blood pressure must be monitored across 24 h to determine the daily pattern (Sherwood et al., 2002) (**Figure 14.9**).

There are many chronic health conditions that are associated with the non-dipping pattern: sleep apnea, insomnia, cardiac arrhythmias, neurodegenerative diseases, and kidney disease, among others. In a meta-analysis of patients with OSA, ~60% showed the non-dipping pattern (Cuspidi et al., 2019). Non-dipping may also be an acute response to disruptions in sleep patterns. Bus drivers who started a split shift work schedule (including early morning start times) showed a rapid increase in the proportion with a non-dipping pattern, which was linked to higher variability in their sleep timing over a week (McHill et al., 2022).

The mechanism responsible for blood pressure dipping has been controversial. One constant-routine study (see Chapter 3) found that dipping at night was a response to sleep rather than an endogenous circadian rhythm (Kerkhof et al., 1998), a finding that is consistent with evidence that blood pressure also drops during daytime naps (Bursztyn et al., 1994). More recent studies using constant-routine and forced-desynchronization protocols, however, provided clear evidence that there is endogenous circadian modulation of blood pressure that is independent of sleep (Scheer et al., 2010; Shea et al., 2011). Thus, blood pressure dipping at night is under circadian control but it is further reinforced by sleep. The presence of a non-dipping pattern may be related to sustained sympathetic nervous system activation during the night (Sherwood et al., 2002).

Although increased 24 h average blood pressure raises the risk of vascular disease and vascular death, non-dipping is an additional risk factor that remains significant even when corrected for the daily average pressure (Ben-Dov et al., 2007; Metoki et al., 2006; Routledge et al., 2007; Salles et al., 2016). Similarly, patients with kidney disease who showed nocturnal hypertension were at increased risk of developing kidney failure and cardiac damage compared to patients without nocturnal hypertension (Fu et al., 2022).

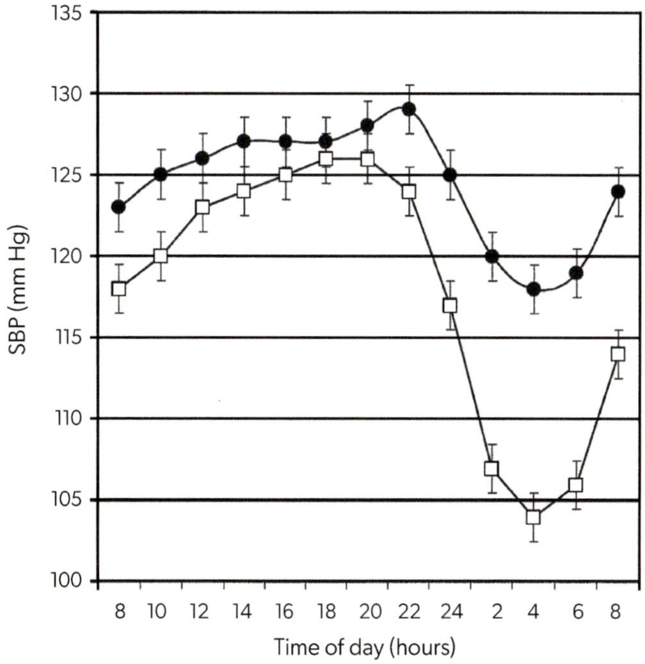

Figure 14.9 Twenty-four-hour patterns of systolic blood pressure (SBP in mm of mercury, Y axis) in people with a dipping pattern (white symbols) or a non-dipping pattern (black symbols) plotted against time of day (X axis). A minimal decline of 10% is the usual definition of a dipping pattern. Reprinted with permission from Sherwood, A. et al. (2002) Nighttime blood pressure dipping: role of the sympathetic nervous system. *Am J Hypertens* 15:111–118. © Oxford University Press (2002). doi: 10.1016/s0895-7061(01)02251-8.

Elevated nighttime blood pressure alone is a stronger predictor of vascular risk than daytime blood pressure, which on its own does not predict cardiovascular disease when nocturnal pressure is controlled for (Fagard et al., 2008; Verdecchia, 2000) (**Figure 14.10**). The highest risk for developing vascular disease and death from vascular causes is observed in people with elevated average daily pressure combined with a non-dipping pattern at night (Hermida et al., 2013; Staplin et al., 2023; Verdecchia, 2000; Yang et al., 2019) (**Figure 14.11**).

OSA disrupts sleep, dampens blood pressure dipping, and is associated with increased risk of vascular disease (Hla et al., 2008; Seif et al., 2014). Among those with OSA, successful treatment with continuous positive airway pressure (CPAP) to open obstructed air passages restored a nocturnal fall in blood pressure (Phillips & O'Driscoll, 2013), probably in part by reducing sleep disruption. Although OSA can be a

[17] "Dipping" is typically defined as showing ≥10% decline in systolic and diastolic blood pressure. "Systolic" refers to the pressure exerted by blood flowing in arteries while it is being pumped during contractions of the heart's ventricles, and "diastolic" refers to the arterial pressure between ventricular contractions.

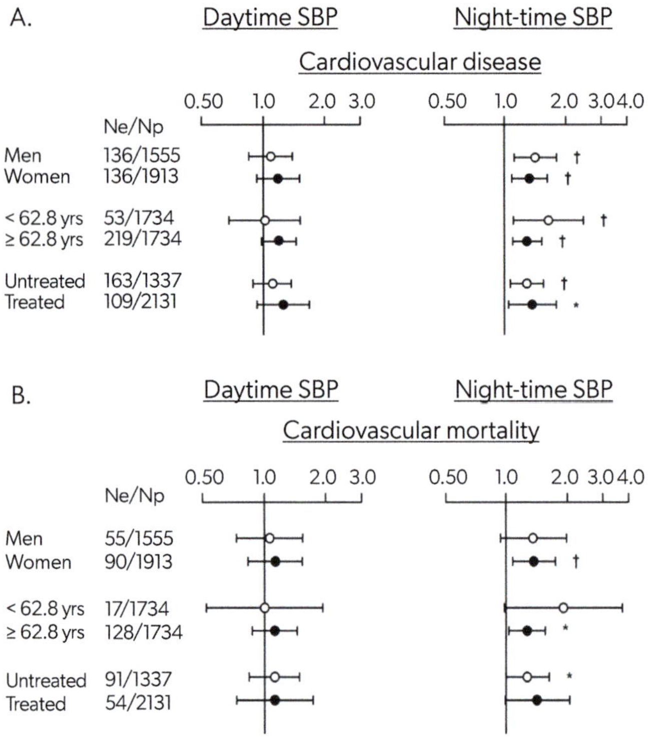

Figure 14.10 Results of a meta-analysis of the hazard ratio for **A.** cardiovascular disease and **B.** cardiovascular mortality associated with systolic blood pressure (SBP) recorded during the daytime (Daytime SBP, left column) or night-time (Night-time SBP, right column) in patients with hypertension. The hazard ratio is the risk of occurrence of the target event over time for those with elevated as compared to normal SBP during the day or night. Plots show the hazard ratio as a mean value (symbol) with horizontal error bars indicating the 95% confidence intervals. These values are presented separately by gender (Men, Women), age (<62.8 years, ≥62.8 years) and whether they were receiving treatment for hypertension (Treated, Untreated). A significant increase in the hazard ratio associated with elevated SBP is indicated by error bars that do not cross the vertical line (1.0, indicating equal risk for those with and without elevated SBP at those phases, and by a symbol (*p <0.05; † p<0.01). After controlling for daytime SBP, nighttime SBP predicted increased risk of cardiovascular disease and cardiovascular mortality in most subgroups. After controlling for nighttime SBP, daytime SBP was not a significant predictor for any subgroup. These results indicate that elevated nocturnal blood pressure is a robust predictor of cardiovascular risk after controlling for elevated daytime blood pressure, but the reverse is not the case. Ne/Np indicates the number of observed events (cardiovascular disease or death) over the number of patients in that group. Reprinted with permission of Wolters Kluwer Health Inc. from Fagard, R.H. et al. (2008) Daytime and nighttime blood pressure as predictors of death and cause-specific cardiovascular events in hypertension. *Hypertension* 51 (1): 55–61. © American Heart Association (2008). doi: 10.1161/HYPERTENSIONAHA.107.100727.

confounding factor in evaluating the interaction among sleep disruption, dipping, and hypertension, even in those without OSA, nocturnal non-dipping was an independent risk factor for vascular disease (Hermida et al., 2013).

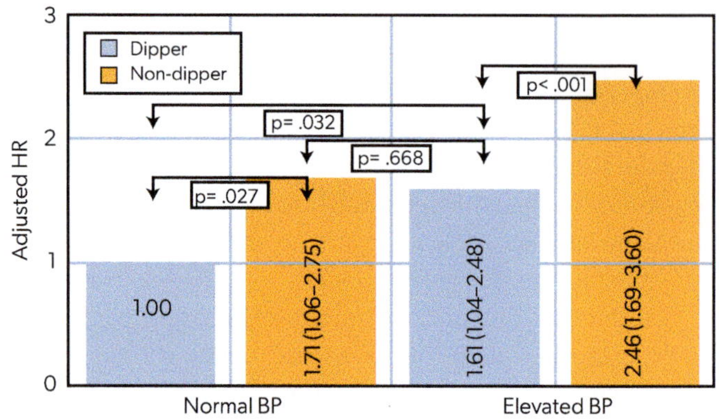

Figure 14.11 Risk of all subsequent cardiovascular events in a population sample presented as a hazard ratio (HR), after adjustment for confounding variables (Y axis). Risk for those with normal blood pressure at baseline (before the ~5.5 year observation period) (left side: Normal BP) and a nocturnal dipping pattern (Dipper; blue) is set at 1.0. Risks were similarly elevated for those with normal BP and a non-dipping pattern (left side, orange; ~1.7-fold increase; values shown are the mean and 95% confidence interval) and those with elevated blood pressure and a dipping pattern (right side, blue, ~1.6-fold increase). Risk was highest for those with both elevated blood pressure and a non-dipping pattern (right side, orange; ~2.5-fold increase. This value corresponds to a nearly 150% increase in risk of cardiovascular events over time relative to dippers with normal blood pressure. Comparisons and their associated statistical probabilities are indicated by the arrows. Reprinted with permission of Taylor & Francis Ltd and Dr. Ramón Hermida from Hermida, R.C. et al. (2013) Blunted sleep-time relative blood pressure decline increases cardiovascular risk independent of blood pressure level--the "normotensive non-dipper" paradox. *Chronobiol Int* 30:87–98. © Taylor & Francis, Ltd. (2013) (www.tandfonline.com). doi: 10.3109/07420528.2012.701127.

Drug treatments to lower blood pressure can also restore the dipping pattern (Uzu & Kimura, 1999) (**Figure 14.12**). Studies of the time of day at which antihypertensive medications were taken found that taking medications at bedtime improved blood pressure control and restored dipping better than morning treatments (Kaur et al., 2016; Sun et al., 2016). Whether these differences led to different outcomes (risk of heart attack, stroke, or death from vascular disease) is less clear.

Evening timing of antihypertensive medications was reported to reduce these risks more than morning treatments in some studies (Hermida et al., 2007; Hermida et al., 2010), but another trial found no benefit of evening treatments over morning treatments (Mackenzie et al., 2022). There were criticisms raised about the positive studies (Turgeon et al., 2021), but there were also concerns about the reliability of the negative study (Salah & Mehta, 2022). A general problem with the design of these studies is uncertainty about the extent and consistency with which patients adhere to their assigned daily timing of drug treatments over many months

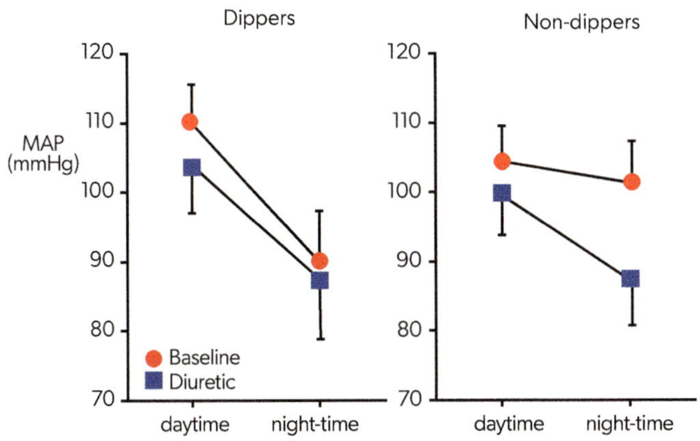

Figure 14.12 Effects of treatment with a diuretic agent on patterns of mean arterial blood pressure (MAP, measured in mm of mercury, mmHg; Y axis) in both dippers (left panel) and non-dippers (right panel). MAP combines measures of systolic and diastolic blood pressure. Results are shown before treatment (red symbols) and after diuretic treatment (blue symbols). Diuretic treatment had no effect on the daily pattern in dippers but restored the dipping pattern in non-dippers. Adapted with permission from Uzu, T. & Kimura, G. (1999) Diuretics shift circadian rhythm of blood pressure from nondipper to dipper in essential hypertension. *Circulation* 100:1635–1638. © Wolters Kluwer Health (P&E) Limited (1999). doi: 10.1161/01.cir.100.15.1635.

or years. This concern makes it difficult to interpret either positive or negative outcomes. The issue of whether timing of antihypertensive treatments affects mortality risk remains to be addressed with more rigorously controlled, large-scale studies that monitor times of treatments, which are reportedly under way.

Another potential cause of elevated nocturnal blood pressure is reduced production of melatonin. Endogenous melatonin is released at night from the pineal gland under the control of the suprachiasmatic nucleus, and its rise promotes the transition to sleep (see Chapter 9). Melatonin reduces blood pressure by dilating peripheral blood vessels as well as by promoting sleep, which itself also reduces blood pressure (Cagnacci et al., 2005; Cagnacci et al., 1992; Kräuchi et al., 2000). Nocturnal production of melatonin can be reduced by aging and by light exposure at night, whether from ordinary home/workplace illumination (Phillips et al., 2019), or from the screens of electronic devices (Cajochen et al., 2011; Carter et al., 2016; Chang et al., 2015; Gooley et al., 2011; Wood et al., 2013); see Section 9.2.2.

Treating healthy men with exogenous melatonin acutely during the day (Arangino et al., 1999) or treating both healthy and hypertensive women with a sustained-release formulation at night (Cagnacci et al., 2005) reduced blood pressure (**Figure 14.13**). The effects of immediate-release melatonin in reducing blood pressure are, however, limited by its very short half-life, which is often less than an hour for an oral dose (Harpsøe et al., 2015). Controlled-release formulations that sustain melatonin levels for more of the night were most effective in reducing blood pressure in hypertensive patients (Cagnacci et al., 2005; Grossman et al., 2011).

Melatonin's effects extend beyond its immediate pharmacological action on blood vessels. A single dose of

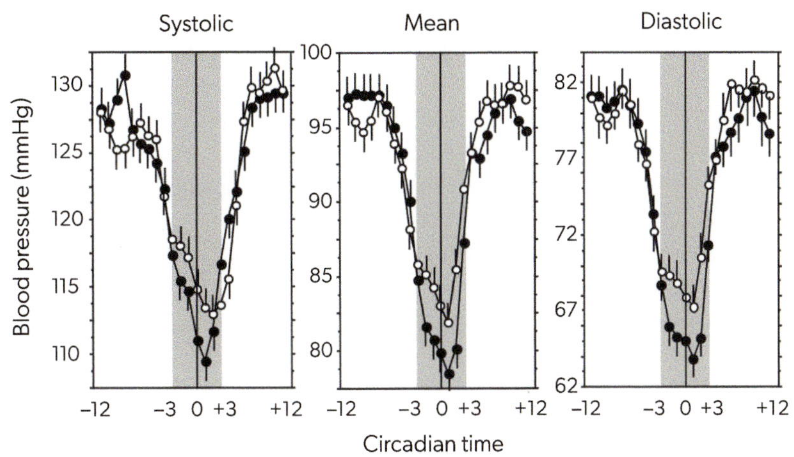

Figure 14.13 Effects of 3 weeks of nightly controlled-release melatonin (3 mg, given 1 h before bedtime) (black symbols) or placebo (white symbols) on systolic (left), diastolic (right), and mean (center) blood pressure (Y axis) in a group of 18 women, including those with normal and elevated blood pressure, aged 47–63 years. Women were studied twice in a cross-over design with either melatonin or placebo treatment first. Data are plotted relative to the time of the minimum values of blood pressure/heart rate, which is set as circadian time 0 (X axis). This phase would correspond to the late night (~04:00–05:00) for most people. The shaded areas represent the 6 h surrounding circadian time 0. The largest decreases in blood pressure attributable to melatonin treatment occurred shortly after circadian time 0. Reprinted with permission from Cagnacci, A. et al. (2005) Prolonged melatonin administration decreases nocturnal blood pressure in women. Am J Hypertens 18:1614–1618. © Oxford University Press (2005). doi:10.1016/j.amjhyper.2005.05.008.

controlled-release melatonin at bedtime was ineffective in hypertensive men during the first night, but repeated doses for 3 weeks reduced nocturnal blood pressure, advanced sleep onset, and increased sleep duration and efficiency (Scheer et al., 2004). These beneficial effects of melatonin may be related in part to an indirect effect on the amplitude of daily rhythms, including the sleep–wake rhythm, presumably as a result of its action on the suprachiasmatic nucleus; see Section 9.7. Despite these potential benefits, there are also reasons to be cautious in using melatonin as an over-the-counter medication, as discussed in Section 9.8.

14.8.1 Summary

Short sleep (especially in those with insomnia symptoms) and reduced amounts of SWS are associated with an increased risk of developing hypertension and the associated risk of heart disease, stroke, or other vascular diseases. The impact of hypertension on the risk of vascular disease depends in part on the daily rhythm of blood pressure; specifically, the lack of a dipping pattern during the night is associated with increased vascular risk, independently of daytime levels. Daytime blood pressure is not a robust predictor of cardiovascular disease or cardiac death after controlling for nighttime blood pressure. These results indicate the importance of 24 h monitoring of blood pressure to assess vascular risk.

Several factors can contribute to inadequate nocturnal dipping, including disrupted sleep, reduced melatonin levels, and a variety of illnesses. OSA is one condition that disrupts and shortens sleep and is associated with vascular disease, but non-dippers who do not have OSA are also at increased risk. Treatment with antihypertensive drugs or melatonin can reduce blood pressure. The effects of melatonin on blood pressure appear to be mediated by a combination of dilating blood vessels and reinforcing the rhythm amplitude of the circadian pacemaker. In patients taking multiple drugs for hypertension, there is evidence that taking at least one at bedtime enhances nocturnal dipping of blood pressure, but there are conflicting findings about whether this change improves health outcomes. Clinical trials that are currently being conducted may help to clarify this issue.

14.9 Sleep and the immune system

Many people suspect that they are more likely to develop a viral infection (specifically, cold or flu symptoms) if they are "run-down," working too hard, and not getting enough sleep, presumably because these conditions impair the function of their immune systems. Is there evidence to support the idea that sleep loss contributes to susceptibility to infection? One early observation was that 2 of 5 healthy participants in a study involving 64 h of sustained waking developed cold symptoms a few days later (Dickstein & Moldofsky, 1999), suggesting that sleep loss disrupted immune system function.

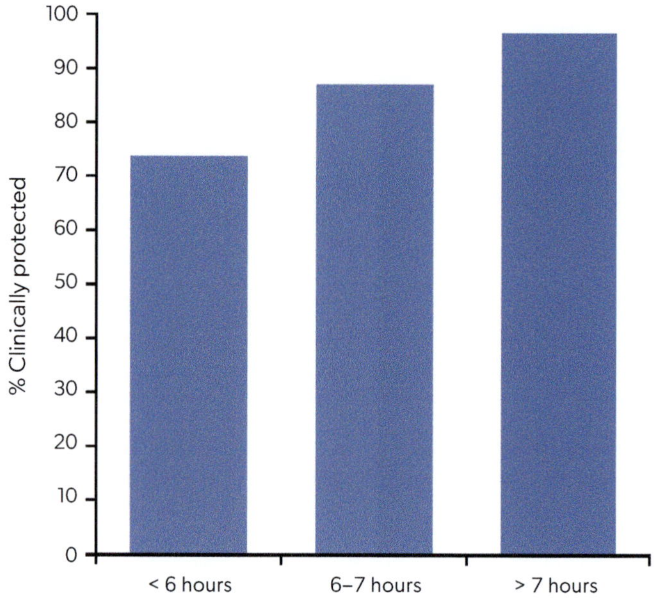

Figure 14.14 Percentage of participants who produced adequate protective levels of antibodies to hepatitis B 6 months after their final (third) immunization (Y axis), as a function of their self-reported typical sleep durations at the time of immunization (X axis). Shorter self-reported sleep (<6 h) was associated with a smaller percentage of people developing adequate clinical protection, suggesting a reduced immune system response to the antigens contained in the hepatitis B vaccine. Reprinted with permission of Oxford University Press from Prather, A.A. et al. (2012) Sleep and antibody response to hepatitis B vaccination. *Sleep* 35(8):1063–1069. © Sleep Research Society (2012). doi: 10.5665/sleep.1990.

Later observational studies supported the interpretation that short sleep or poor quality sleep affects immune system responses. Among people being vaccinated against hepatitis B, those who reported sleeping <6 h spontaneously had an inadequate immune response compared to those who slept >7 h. Among normal or long sleepers, ~95% developed adequate clinical protection after vaccination, as compared to only ~70% of short sleepers (Prather et al., 2012) (**Figure 14.14**). Similarly, more self-reported insomnia symptoms were associated with weaker antibody responses after inoculation against the COVID-19 virus (Athanasiou et al., 2023).

Development of viral infections was also linked to sleep amounts. The risk of a diagnosis of pneumonia over a 4-year period in women was elevated among those who habitually slept ≤5 h and ≥9 h or reported inadequate sleep (Patel et al., 2012). Participants who were exposed to a rhinovirus (common cold virus) and reported sleeping <7 h nightly for

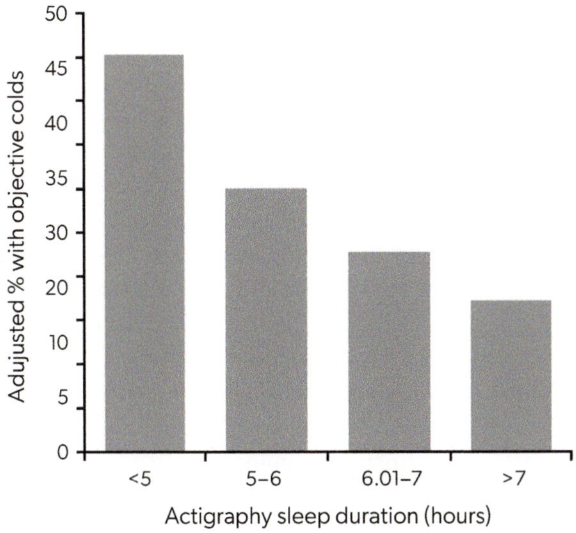

Figure 14.15 Percentage of people who developed cold symptoms during a 5-day period of quarantine after controlled exposure to a cold virus (Y axis), plotted against their sleep durations during the preceding week, measured using actigraphy (X axis). Those with the shortest sleep durations (< 5 h) were ~2.5 times more likely to develop cold symptoms than those averaging more than 7 h sleep nightly. Reprinted with permission of Oxford University Press from Prather, A.A. et al. (2015) Behaviorally assessed sleep and susceptibility to the common cold. *Sleep* 38(9):1353–1359. © Sleep Research Society (2015). doi: 10.5665/sleep.4968.

the previous 2 weeks were nearly three times more likely to develop cold symptoms than those who slept >8 h (Cohen et al., 2009). Very short sleepers (<5 h, as measured by actigraphy) had a nearly 3-fold increase in the risk of developing cold symptoms after experimental exposure to a rhinovirus, relative to those sleeping >7 h (Prather et al., 2015) (**Figure 14.15**).

Results from studies involving experimental manipulations of sleep are consistent with the findings from these observational studies. Participants who were immunized against influenza after the 4th of 6 nights with sleep restricted to 4 h nightly showed less increase in antibody levels than those who maintained their usual sleep durations around the time of immunization (Spiegel et al., 2002). People who were kept awake overnight after immunization against hepatitis A showed a blunted antibody response compared to those who slept freely (Lange et al., 2003). Thus, both observational and experimental studies support the conclusion that chronically or acutely reduced sleep impairs the immune system's ability to respond effectively to viruses or to viral components in a vaccine.

Despite the consistent evidence that immune system function is impaired by sleep loss, the mechanisms involved are less clear. The reported effects of both sleep and sleep loss on immune system components are complex and sometimes inconsistent across studies (Axelsson et al., 2013; Dickstein & Moldofsky, 1999; Dinges et al., 1995). This variability limits the conclusions that can be reached about the mechanisms by which sleep affects the immune system (Benca & Quintans, 1997; Grandner, Sands-Lincoln, et al., 2013).

The immune system includes many interacting components that are regulated by both endocrine and neural inputs and are responsive to infections and illnesses. Among the components that respond to infection are several kinds of leucocytes (white blood cells) that are produced in bone marrow and circulate in the bloodstream and lymphatic system. Leucocytes produce small regulatory proteins called cytokines, which serve as important signals in the immune system. Some cytokines are usually classified as pro-inflammatory and are important for fighting infections and disease (e.g., interleukin (IL)-1, IL-6, IL-12, and tumor-necrosis factor (TNF)-α). Others are considered anti-inflammatory, inhibiting inflammatory responses and promoting tissue healing (e.g., IL-4, IL-10, IL-13) (Irwin, 2015). However, some cytokines (e.g., IL-6) can play either pro- or anti-inflammatory roles depending on conditions (Xing et al., 1998). This finding is consistent with evidence that adrenal glucocorticoids (e.g., cortisol in people), which are classically considered anti-inflammatory agents that are used chronically to treat inflammatory conditions, including rheumatoid arthritis, asthma, and colitis, also have an immediate pro-inflammatory effect (e.g., in response to an acute stress; see Cruz-Topete & Cidlowski, 2015).

Acute, short-term sleep loss has usually been reported to suppress pro-inflammatory cytokines (e.g., IL-6), decreasing the number of natural killer cells (leucocytes that respond to infections and tumors) and increasing levels of anti-inflammatory cytokines (Irwin, 2015; Lange et al., 2010; Moldofsky et al., 1989; Redwine, 2000). These results are consistent with evidence that acute sleep loss reduces the capacity to respond effectively to infection or immunization (see **Figures 14.14 and 14.15**).

There are, however, conflicting findings about the responses of specific cytokines, with both pro- and anti-inflammatory cytokines being increased in different studies in response to acute sleep loss and differences being observed between genders. In response to very modest sleep restriction for a week, both IL-6 and TNF-α increased in men, while only IL-6 increased in women (Vgontzas et al., 2004). Gender differences were also observed in how these cytokines responded across the day after acute overnight sleep restriction (Irwin et al., 2010).

The differences in immune system responses across studies are probably related in part to the methods used and to the timing of measurements of immune system components, which are regulated dynamically (Chennaoui et al., 2011; Frey et al., 2007; Haack et al., 2002; Haack et al., 2007;

Meier-Ewert et al., 2004; Vgontzas et al., 2004). Some studies measured spontaneous levels of immune system activity (e.g., circulating cytokine levels). Others extracted immune cells from blood and studied their responses in vitro to chemical agents that provoke cytokine production. In some cases, mixtures of immune system cell types that have different functions were studied together, making interpretation of results difficult; for reviews, see Benca & Quintans, 1997; Born et al., 1997.

A commonly used method involves sampling blood repeatedly from chronically implanted venous catheters, but this approach may have unintended effects. One study used this method to assess the effects of overnight sleep deprivation on IL-6 levels measured over 24 h, including a period of either overnight sleep or total sleep deprivation. There were apparently larger increases in IL-6 levels during sleep relative to sleep deprivation. However, the results obtained from blood draws through a catheter that had been in place for over 24 h were also compared to those from samples obtained by needle sticks (venipuncture), once at the start and once at the end of the 24 h study.

There were increased IL-6 levels in the samples from the implanted catheter, especially in the sleep condition, but there was no similar increase in levels in the venipuncture group, regardless of sleep condition. Increases were attributed to greater difficulties in blood sampling by suction using catheters from sleeping participants, which apparently resulted in local IL-6 production. Thus, increases in IL-6 levels were largely the result of a local immune response to the implanted catheter or to manipulations needed to sample during sleep, rather than to a system-wide change in IL-6 levels related to sleep (Haack et al., 2002).

The timing of sampling in studies is also important because the release of some cytokines triggers activation of other cellular and humoral immune components. These interactions result in a cascade of changes over time, so when samples are taken after an intervention can determine the response observed. For example, in a 40 h constant routine study, pro- and anti-inflammatory cytokines increased at different times during the sustained waking period (Frey et al., 2007).

There are also strong daily rhythms in the expression of immune system components, which are influenced by both circadian and sleep-related mechanisms. Adrenal stress hormones (cortisol and epinephrine), for example, modulate immune system activity (Irwin, 2015; Lange et al., 2010). Partial sleep restriction alters the daily rhythm of cortisol levels in men, women, and children, and does so differently in women depending on menstrual cycle phase (Gribbin et al., 2012; LeRoux et al., 2014; Omisade et al., 2010; Spiegel, Leproult, et al., 2004). Specifically, some of the effects of sleep restriction on cortisol rhythms were present during the follicular phase, but not during the luteal phase (LeRoux et al., 2014).[18]

The morning rise of cortisol presumably prepares people physiologically for increased activity, while the afternoon decline prepares them for the nightly rest phase. Both of these functions of the daily cortisol rhythm are disrupted by sleep loss. Sleep restriction increases late-day cortisol levels by slowing the afternoon decline, but also reduces the amplitude of the morning peak (Gribbin et al., 2012; LeRoux et al., 2014; Omisade et al., 2010; Spiegel, Leproult, et al., 2004). Thus, sampling immune system components that are affected by cortisol levels at different times of day (and during different menstrual cycle phases in women) could affect the results obtained, especially when only a single time point is studied (Axelsson et al., 2013; Born et al., 1997; Dinges et al., 1995; Irwin, 2015; Irwin et al., 2010).

In contrast to the effects of acute sleep restriction, *chronic* self-selected short sleep, lengthy periods of sleep restriction, and delayed sleep phases have most often been associated with *increases* in pro-inflammatory cytokines and other markers of inflammation, for example, higher levels of CRP (Grandner, Sands-Lincoln, et al., 2013; Meier-Ewert et al., 2004; Mullington et al., 2010; Nowakowski et al., 2018; Zhang et al., 2022). Chronic inflammation has been linked to the development of serious illnesses, including obesity and cancer (Fair & Montgomery, 2009), dementia (Darweesh et al., 2018), diabetes and vascular disease (Grandner, Sands-Lincoln, et al., 2013; Wilson et al., 2006), and depression (Dantzer et al., 2008). A further complication is that in some populations, indicators of inflammation were elevated among short sleepers (or long sleepers) of one gender, but not the other (Bakour et al., 2017; Grandner, Buxton, et al., 2013; Miller et al., 2009), and these effects were also modified by race/ethnicity and age (Blair et al., 2015; Grandner, Buxton, et al., 2013; Irwin, 2015; Zhang et al., 2022).

Thus, probes of immune system function can produce different results depending on the methods used; the cytokines studied; the degree, duration, and pattern of sleep loss; the timing and methods of sampling; the ethnic/racial composition of the groups studied; and their age, gender, and hormonal status.

Obesity and chronic inflammation interact to promote the development and progression of many cancers (Coussens & Werb, 2002; Iyengar et al., 2016). Since chronic inadequate sleep is associated with both weight gain and inflammation, studies have examined whether short or inadequate sleep are associated with later development of cancer. Although some meta-analyses concluded that sleep duration did not affect the

[18] Women studied during constant routines were also relatively protected during the luteal phase against the effects of sleep loss on vigilance performance that were seen during the follicular phase (Vidafar et al., 2018).

risk of developing specific cancers (e.g., Liu et al., 2020), recent, high-quality studies using large databases found that sleep duration and poor sleep quality are linked to increased risk of developing cancer.

For example, a study of the incidence of cancer in a longitudinal database from the UK showed that worse reported sleep quality at baseline (also associated with shorter sleep) predicted a higher risk of developing any cancer over an 8 year period in people over 50 years old at baseline (Song et al., 2021). Another recent study examined whether sleep duration, chronotype, and insomnia symptoms predicted the occurrence over a ~7 year period of new-onset lung cancer in a UK sample of nearly half a million people. There was an increased risk of developing lung cancer in short and long sleepers and in those with an evening chronotype, but not in those with insomnia symptoms, after controlling for many other potential risk factors (Xie et al., 2021).

14.9.1 Summary

Observational and experimental studies found that acute sleep deprivation and habitual short sleep reduced resistance to infections and impaired the development of immunity in response to vaccines. These effects were presumably related to reductions in pro-inflammatory immune responses, but there is less consensus about the specific molecular pathways involved.

Conflicting findings about which cytokines and other immune system components are affected by chronic short or long sleep, and by acute changes in sleep amounts, are probably influenced by several factors. These include different methods of measuring immune system function; sampling at different times after an intervention; differences in the circadian (and menstrual, and perhaps seasonal) timing of sampling; and the gender, age, and ethnic/racial composition of groups being studied. The inherent complexity of the immune system and the dynamic interactions that occur over time among its components complicate analyses of responses to sleep duration.

Over the longer term, chronic short (and sometimes long) sleep in people and in animal models was associated with several markers of increased inflammation, including increased CRP levels. Chronic inflammation and high CRP levels have in turn been linked to many serious diseases, including vascular disease and cancer. The risk of cancer is influenced by both chronic inflammation and obesity, both of which are affected by short sleep. Recent longitudinal, population-based studies demonstrated increased risks of developing cancers in those who reported poor sleep quality and either short or long habitual sleep at baseline.

Literature cited

Åkerstedt, T., Hume, K., Minors, D., & Waterhouse, J. (1994). The meaning of good sleep: a longitudinal study of polysomnography and subjective sleep quality. *J Sleep Res*, *3*(3), 152–158. doi: 10.1111/j.1365-2869.1994.tb00122.x

Akinseye, O. A., Williams, S. K., Seixas, A., Pandi-Perumal, S. R., Vallon, J., Zizi, F., & Jean-Louis, G. (**2015**). Sleep as a mediator in the pathway linking environmental factors to hypertension: a review of the literature. *Int J Hypertens*, *2015*, 926414. doi: 10.1155/2015/926414

AlGhanim, N., Comondore, V. R., Fleetham, J., Marra, C. A., & Ayas, N. T. (2008). The economic impact of obstructive sleep apnea. *Lung*, *186*, 7–12. doi: 10.1007/s00408-007-9055-5

Al Khatib, H. K., Harding, S. V., Darzi, J., & Pot, G. K. (2017). The effects of partial sleep deprivation on energy balance: a systematic review and meta-analysis. *Eur J Clin Nutr*, *71*(5), 614–624. doi: 10.1038/ejcn.2016.201

Ancoli-Israel, S., Cole, R., Alessi, C., Chambers, M., Moorcroft, W., & Pollak, C. P. (2003). The role of actigraphy in the study of sleep and circadian rhythms. *Sleep*, *26*(3), 342–392.

Arangino, S., Cagnacci, A., Angiolucci, M., Vacca, A. M. B., Longu, G., Volpe, A., & Melis, G. B. (1999). Effects of melatonin on vascular reactivity, catecholamine levels, and blood pressure in healthy men. *Am J Cardiol*, *83*, 1417–1419.

Arble, D. M., Bass, J., Laposky, A. D., Vitaterna, M. H., & Turek, F. W. (2009). Circadian timing of food intake contributes to weight gain. *Obesity*, *17*, 2100–2102. doi: 0.1038/oby.2009.264

Athanasiou, N., Baou, K., Papandreou, E., Varsou, G., Amfilochiou, A., Kontou, E., … Vagiakis, E. (2023). Association of sleep duration and quality with immunological response after vaccination against severe acute respiratory syndrome coronavirus-2 infection. *J Sleep Res*, *32*(1), e13656. doi:10.1111/jsr.13656

Axelsson, J., Rehman, J., Åkerstedt, T., Ekman, R., Miller, G. E., Höglund, C. O., & Lekander, M. (2013). Effects of sustained sleep restriction on mitogen-stimulated cytokines, chemokines and T helper 1/ T helper 2 balance in humans. *PLoS One*, *8*(12), e82291. doi:10.1371/journal.pone.0082291

Ayas, N. T., White, D. P., Al-Delaimy, W. K., Manson, J. E., Stampfer, M. J., Speizer, F. E., … Hu, F. B. (2003). A prospective study of self-reported sleep duration and incident diabetes in women. *Diabetes Care*, *26*, 380–384.

Baglioni, C., Regen, W., Teghen, A., Spiegelhalder, K., Feige, B., Nissen, C., & Riemann, D. (2014). Sleep changes in the disorder of insomnia: a meta-analysis of polysomnographic studies. *Sleep Med Rev*, *18*(3), 195–213. doi: 10.1016/j.smrv.2013.04.001

Bakour, C., Schwartz, S., O'Rourke, K., Wang, W., Sappenfield, W., Couluris, M., & Chen, H. (2017). Sleep trajectories and systemic inflammation in young adults: results from the National Longitudinal Study of Adolescent to Adult Health (Add Health). *Sleep*, *40*(11), zsz156. doi: 10.1093/sleep/zsx156

Baron, K. G., Reid, K. J., Kern, A. S., & Zee, P. C. (2011). Role of sleep timing in caloric intake and BMI. *Obesity*, *19*, 1374–1381. doi: 0.1038/oby.2011.100

Beihl, D. A., Liese, A. D., & Haffner, S. M. (2009). Sleep duration as a risk factor for incident type 2 diabetes in a multiethnic cohort. *Ann Epidemiol*, *19*(5), 351–357. doi: 10.1016/j.annepidem.2008.12.001

Bell, J. F., & Zimmerman, F. J. (2010). Shortened nighttime sleep duration in early life and subsequent childhood obesity. *Arch Pediatr Adolesc Med*, *164*(9), 8440–8845.

Benca, R. M., & Quintans, J. (1997). Sleep and host defenses: a review. *Sleep*, *20*(11), 1027–1037.

Ben-Dov, I. Z., Kark, J. D., Ben-Ishay, D., Mekler, J., Ben-Arie, L., & Bursztyn, M. (2007). Blunted heart rate dip during sleep and all-cause mortality. *Arch Intern Med*, *167*(19), 2116–2121.

Benz, F., Riemann, D., Domschke, K., Spiegelhalder, K., Johann, A. F., Marshall, N. S., & Feige, B. (2023). How many hours do you sleep? A comparison of subjective and objective sleep duration measures in a sample of insomnia patients and good sleepers. *J Sleep Res*, *32*(2), e13802. doi:10.1111/jsr.13802

Bergmann, B. M., Everson, C. A., Kushida, C. A., Fang, V. S., Leitch, C. A., Schoeller, D. A., … Rechtschaffen, A. (1989). Sleep deprivation in the rat: V. energy use and mediation. *Sleep*, *12*(1), 31–41.

Bertisch, S. M., Pollock, B. D., Mittleman, M. A., Buysse, D. J., Bazzano, L. A., Gottlieb, D. J., & Redline, S. (2018). Insomnia with objective short sleep duration and risk of incident cardiovascular disease and all-cause mortality: Sleep Heart Health Study. *Sleep, 41*(6), zsy047. doi: 10.1093/sleep/zsy047

Bhandari, R., Kelley, G. A., Hartley, T. A., & Rockett, I. R. H. (2014). Metabolic syndrome is associated with increased breast cancer risk: a systematic review and meta-analysis. *Int J Breast Cancer, 2014*, 189384. doi: 0.1155/2014/189384

Blair, L. M., Porter, K., Leblebicioglu, B., & Christian, L. M. (2015). Poor sleep quality and associated inflammation predict preterm birth: heightened risk among African Americans. *Sleep, 38*(8), 1259–1267. doi: 10.5665/sleep.4904

Bliwise, D. L., & Young, T. B. (2007). The parable of parabola: what the U-shaped curve can and cannot tell us about sleep. *Sleep, 30*(12), 1614–1615.

Bogh, A. F., Jensen, S. B. K., Juhl, C. R., Janus, C., Sandsdal, R. M., Lundgren, J. R., ... Torekov, S. S. (2023). Insufficient sleep predicts poor weight loss maintenance after one year. *Sleep, 26*(5), zsac295. doi:10.1093/sleep/zsac295

Born, J., Lange, T., Hansen, K., Mölle, M., & Fehm, H. L. (1997). Effects of sleep and circadian rhythm on human circulating immune cells. *J Immunol, 158*, 4454–4464.

Bosy-Westphal, A., Hinrichs, S., Jauch-Chara, K., Hitze, B., Later, W., Wilms, B., ... Muller, M. J. (2008). Influence of partial sleep deprivation on energy balance and insulin sensitivity in healthy women. *Obes Facts, 1*(5), 266–273. doi: 10.1159/000158874

Bowman, M. A., Duggan, K. A., Brindle, R. C., Kline, C. E., Krafty, R. T., Thayer, J. F., & Hall, M. H. (2019). Prospective associations among objectively and subjectively assessed sleep and the metabolic syndrome. *Sleep Med, 58*, 1–6. doi: 10.1016/j.sleep.2019.02.005

Bradford Hill, A. (1965). The environment and disease: association or causation? *Proc Roy Soc Med, 58*, 295–300.

Brondel, L., Romer, M. A., Nougues, P. M., Touyarou, P., & Davenne, D. (2010). Acute partial sleep deprivation increases food intake in healthy men. *Am J Clin Nutr, 91*(6), 1550–1559. doi: 10.3945/ajcn.2009.28523

Brouwer, A., van Raalte, D. H., Rutters, F., Elders, P. J. M., Snoek, F. J., Beekman, A. T. F., & Bremmer, M. A. (2020). Sleep and HbA1c in patients with type 2 diabetes: which sleep characteristics matter most? *Diabetes Care, 43*(1), 235–243. doi: 10.2337/dc19-0550

Bursztyn, M., Mekler, J., Wachtel, N., & Ben-Ishay, D. (1994). Siesta and ambulatory blood pressure monitoring: comparability of the afternoon nap and night sleep. *Am J Hypertens, 7*, 217–221.

Buxton, O. M., Pavlova, M., Reid, E. W., Wang, W., Simonson, D. C., & Adler, G. K. (2010). Sleep restriction for 1 week reduces insulin sensitivity in healthy men. *Diabetes, 59*(9), 2126–2133. doi: 10.2337/db09-0699

Buysse, D., Reynolds Iii, C. F., Monk, T., Berman, S., & Kupfer, D. (1989). The Pittsburgh Sleep Quality Index: a new instrument for psychiatric practice and research. *Psychiatry Res, 28*, 193–213.

Cagnacci, A., Cannoletta, M., Renzi, A., Baldassari, F., Arangino, S., & Volpe, A. (2005). Prolonged melatonin administration decreases nocturnal blood pressure in women. *Am J Hypertens, 18*(12 Pt 1), 1614–1618. doi: 10.1016/j.amjhyper.2005.05.008

Cagnacci, A., Elliott, J. A., & Yen, S. S. C. (1992). Melatonin: a major regulator of the circadian rhythm of core temperature in humans. *J Clin Endocr Metab, 75* (2), 447–452.

Cajochen, C., Brunner, D. P., Kräuchi, K., Graw, P., & Wirz-Justice, A. (1995). Power density in theta/alpha frequencies of the waking EEG progressively increases during sustained wakefulness. *Sleep, 18*(10), 890–894.

Cajochen, C., Frey, S., Anders, D., Spati, J., Bues, M., Pross, A., ... Stefani, O. (2011). Evening exposure to a light emitting diodes (LED)-backlit computer screen affects circadian physiology and cognitive performance. *J Appl Physiol, 110*(5), 1432–1438. doi: 10.1152/japplphysiol.00165.2011

Calle, E. E., Rodriguez, C., Walker-Thurmond, K., & Thun, M. J. (2003). Overweight, obesity and mortality from cancer in a prospectively studied cohort of U.S. adults. *New Engl J Med, 348*(17), 1625–1638.

Calvin, A. D., Carter, R. E., Adachi, T., Macedo, P. G., Albuquerque, F. N., van der Walt, C., ... Somers, V. K. (2013). Effects of experimental sleep restriction on caloric intake and activity energy expenditure. *Chest, 144*(1), 79–86. doi: 10.1378/chest.12-2829

Cappuccio, F. P., D'Elia, L., Strazzullo, P., & Miller, M. A. (2010). Quantity and quality of sleep and incidence of type 2 diabetes: a systematic review and meta-analysis. *Diabetes Care, 33*(2), 414–420. doi: 10.2337/dc09-1124

Cappuccio, F. P., Stranges, S., Kandala, N. B., Miller, M. A., Taggart, F. M., Kumari, M., ... Marmot, M. G. (2007). Gender specific associations of short sleep duration with prevalent and incident hypertension: the Whitehall II study. *Hypertension, 50*(4), 693–700. doi: 10.1161/hypertensionaha.107.095471

Carskadon, M. A., Dement, W. C., Mitler, M. M., Guilleminault, C., Zarcone, V. P., & Spiegel, R. (1976). Self-reports versus sleep laboratory findings in 122 drug-free subjects with complaints of chronic insomnia. *Am J Psychiatry, 133*, 1382–1388.

Carter, B., Rees, P., Hale, L., Bhattacharjee, D., & Paradkar, M. S. (2016). Association between portable screen-based media device access or use and sleep outcomes: a systematic review and meta-analysis. *JAMA Pediatr, 170*(12), 1202–1208. doi: 10.1001/jamapediatrics.2016.2341

Chang, A. M., Aeschbach, D., Duffy, J. F., & Czeisler, C. A. (2015). Evening use of light-emitting eReaders negatively affects sleep, circadian timing, and next-morning alertness. *Proc Natl Acad Sci U S A, 112*(4), 1232–1237. doi: 10.1073/pnas.1418490112

Chang, T. Y., Lai, Y. A., Hsieh, H. H., Lai, J. S., & Liu, C. S. (2009). Effects of environmental noise exposure on ambulatory blood pressure in young adults. *Environ Res, 109*(7), 900–905. doi: 10.1016/j.envres.2009.05.008

Chaput, J.-P., Després, J.-P., Bouchard, C., & Tremblay, A. (2011). The association between short sleep duration and weight gain is dependent on disinhibited eating behavior in adults. *Sleep, 34*(10), 1291–1297.

Chaput, J.-P., Leblanc, C., Pérusse, L., Després, J.-P., Bouchard, C., & Tremblay, A. (2009). Risk factors for adult overweight and obesity in the Quebec Family Study: have we been barking up the wrong tree? *Obesity, 17*(10), 1964–1970. doi: 10.1038/oby.2009.116

Chaput, J. P., Brunet, M., & Tremblay, A. (2006). Relationship between short sleeping hours and childhood overweight/obesity: results from the "Quebec en Forme" Project. *Int J Obes (Lond), 30*(7), 1080–1085. doi: 10.1038/sj.ijo.0803291

Chaput, J. P., Després, J. P., Bouchard, C., & Tremblay, A. (2007). Association of sleep duration with type 2 diabetes and impaired glucose tolerance. *Diabetologia, 50*(11), 2298–2304. doi: 10.1007/s00125-007-0786-x

Chaput, J. P., Després, J. P., Bouchard, C., & Tremblay, A. (2008). The association between sleep duration and weight gain in adults: a 6-year prospective study from the Quebec Family Study. *Sleep, 31*(4), 517–523.

Chaput, J. P., Gray, C. E., Poitras, V. J., Carson, V., Gruber, R., Olds, T., ... Tremblay, M. S. (2016). Systematic review of the relationships between sleep duration and health indicators in school-aged children and youth. *Appl Physiol Nutr Metab, 41*(6 Suppl 3), S266–282. doi: 10.1139/apnm-2015-0627

Chennaoui, M., Sauvet, F., Drogou, C., Van Beers, P., Langrume, C., Guillard, M., ... Gomez-Merino, D. (2011). Effect of one night of sleep loss on changes in tumor necrosis factor alpha (TNF-alpha) levels in healthy men. *Cytokine, 56*(2), 318–324. doi: 10.1016/j.cyto.2011.06.002

Chouraki, A., Tournant, J., Arnal, P., Pepin, J. L., & Bailly, S. (2023). Objective multi-night sleep monitoring at home: variability of sleep parameters between nights and implications for the reliability of sleep assessment in clinical trials. *Sleep, 46*(5), zsac319. doi:10.1093/sleep/zsac319

Cohen, S., Doyle, W. J., Alper, C. M., Janicki-Deverts, D., & Turner, R. B. (2009). Sleep habits and susceptibility to the common cold. *Arch Intern Med, 169*(1), 62–67. doi: 10.1001/archinternmed.2008.505

NCD-RisC. (2024). Worldwide trends in underweight and obesity from 1990 to 2022: a pooled analysis of 3663 population-representative studies with 222 million children, adolescents, and adults. *Lancet, 403*(10431), 1027–1050. doi: 10.1016/S0140-6736(23)02750-2

Coussens, L. M., & Werb, Z. (2002). Inflammation and cancer. *Nature, 420*(6917), 860–867. doi: 10.1038/nature01322

Cox, R., Rosler, L., Weber, F. D., Blanken, T. F., Wassing, R., Ramautar, J. R., & Van Someren, E. J. W. (2024). The first-night effect and the consistency of short sleep in insomnia disorder. *J Sleep Res, 33*(1), e13897. doi:10.1111/jsr.13897

Crosley-Lyons, R., Li, J., Wang, W. L., Wang, S. D., Huh, J., Bae, D., Intille, S. S., & Dunton, G. F. (2025). Exploring person-centred sleep and rest-activity cycle dynamics over 6 months. *J Sleep Res*, Feb. 5, e144471. doi:10.1111/jsr.14471

Cruz-Topete, D., & Cidlowski, J. A. (2015). One hormone, two actions: anti- and pro-inflammatory effects of glucocorticoids. *Neuroimmunomodulation, 22*(1–2), 20–32. doi: 10.1159/000362724

Cummings, D. E., Purnell, J. Q., Frayo, R. S., Schmidova, K., Wisse, B. E., & Weigle, D. S. (2001). A preprandial rise in plasma ghrelin levels suggests a role in meal initiation in humans. *Diabetes, 50*, 1714–1719.

Cuspidi, C., Tadic, M., Sala, C., Gherbesi, E., Grassi, G., & Mancia, G. (2019). Blood pressure non-dipping and obstructive sleep apnea syndrome: a meta-analysis. *J Clin Med, 8*(9), 1367. doi:10.3390/jcm8091367

Daghlas, I., Lane, J. M., Saxena, R., & Vetter, C. (2021). Genetically proxied diurnal preference, sleep timing, and risk of major depressive disorder. *JAMA Psychiatry, 78*(8), 903–910. doi:10.1001/jamapsychiatry.2021.0959

Dantzer, R., O'Connor, J. C., Freund, G. G., Johnson, R. W., & Kelley, K. W. (2008). From inflammation to sickness and depression: when the immune system subjugates the brain. *Nat Rev Neurosci, 9*(1), 46–56. doi: 10.1038/nrn2297

Darweesh, S. K. L., Wolters, F. J., Ikram, M. A., de Wolf, F., Bos, D., & Hofman, A. (2018). Inflammatory markers and the risk of dementia and Alzheimer's disease: A meta-analysis. *Alzheimers Dement, 14*(11), 1450–1459. doi: 10.1016/j.jalz.2018.02.014

Depner, C. M., Melanson, E. L., Eckel, R. H., Snell-Bergeon, J. K., Perreault, L., Bergman, B. C., … Wright, K. P., Jr. (2019). Ad libitum weekend recovery sleep fails to prevent metabolic dysregulation during a repeating pattern of insufficient sleep and weekend recovery sleep. *Curr Biol, 29*(6), 957–967 e954. doi: 10.1016/j.cub.2019.01.069

Després, J. P., Carpentier, A. C., Tchernof, A., Neeland, I. J., & Poirier, P. (2021). Management of obesity in cardiovascular practice: JACC focus seminar. *J Am Coll Cardiol, 78*(5), 513–531. doi: 10.1016/j.jacc.2021.05.035

de Zambotti, M., Goldstone, A., Claudatos, S., Colrain, I. M., & Baker, F. C. (2018). A validation study of Fitbit Charge 2 compared with polysomnography in adults. *Chronobiol Int, 35*(4), 465–476. doi: 10.1080/07420528.2017.1413578

Dickstein, J. B., & Moldofsky, H. (1999). Sleep, cytokines and immune function. *Sleep Med Rev, 3*(3), 219–228.

DiFrancesco, M. W., Alsameen, M., St-Onge, M. P., Duraccio, K. M., & Beebe, D. W. (2023). Altered neuronal response to visual food stimuli in adolescents undergoing chronic sleep restriction. *Sleep, 47*(4), zsad036. doi:10.1093/sleep/zsad036

Dinges, D. F., Douglas, S. D., Hamarman, S., Zaugg, L., & Kapoor, S. (1995). Sleep deprivation and human immune function. *Adv Neuroimmunol, 5*, 97–110.

Doll, R., & Bradford Hill, A. (1954). The mortality of doctors in relation to their smoking habits: a preliminary report. *Br Med J, 328*(7455), 1529–1533.

Donga, E., van Dijk, M., van Dijk, J. G., Biermasz, N. R., Lammers, G. J., van Kralingen, K. W., … Romijn, J. A. (2010). A single night of partial sleep deprivation induces insulin resistance in multiple metabolic pathways in healthy subjects. *J Clin Endocr Metab, 95*(6), 2963–2968. doi: 10.1210/jc.2009-2430

Duraccio, K. M., Krietsch, K. N., Chardon, M. L., Van Dyk, T. R., & Beebe, D. W. (2019). Poor sleep and adolescent obesity risk: a narrative review of potential mechanisms. *Adolesc Health Med Ther, 10*, 117–130. doi: 10.2147/AHMT.S219594

Dzaja, A., Dalal, M. A., Himmerich, H., Uhr, M., Pollmächer, T., & Schuld, A. (2004). Sleep enhances nocturnal plasma ghrelin levels in healthy subjects. *Am J Endocrinol Metab, 286*, E963–E967. doi: 10.1152/ajpendo.00527.2003

Eckel, R. H., Depner, C. M., Perreault, L., Markwald, R. R., Smith, M. R., McHill, A. W., … Wright, K. P., Jr. (2015). Morning circadian misalignment during short sleep duration impacts insulin sensitivity. *Curr Biol, 25*(22), 3004–3010. doi: 10.1016/j.cub.2015.10.011

Einhorn, D. (2003). American College of Endocrinology position statement on the insulin resistance syndrome. *Endocr Prac, 9*(3), 236–252.

Everson, C. A. (1993). Sustained sleep deprivation impairs host defense. *Am J Physiol, 265*, R1148–R1154.

Everson, C. A., Bergmann, B. M., & Rechtschaffen, A. (1989). Sleep deprivation in the rat: III. Total sleep deprivation. *Sleep, 12*(1), 13–21.

Everson, C. A., Henchen, C. J., Szabo, A., & Hogg, N. (2014). Cell injury and repair resulting from sleep loss and sleep recovery in laboratory rats. *Sleep, 37*(12), 1929–1940. doi: 10.5665/sleep.4244

Everson, C. A., & Szabo, A. (2009). Recurrent restriction of sleep and inadequate recuperation induce both adaptive changes and pathological outcomes. *Am J Physiol, 297*(5), R1430–R1440. doi: 10.1152/ajpregu.00230.2009

Everson, C. A., & Toth, L. A. (2000). Systemic bacterial invasion induced by sleep deprivation. *Am J Physiol, 278*, R905–R916.

Everson, C. A., & Wehr, T. A. (1993). Nutritional and metabolic adaptations to prolonged sleep deprivation in the rat. *Am J Physiol, 264*(2), R376–R387.

Fagard, R. H., Celis, H., Thijs, L., Staessen, J. A., Clement, D. L., De Buyzere, M. L., & De Bacquer, D. A. (2008). Daytime and nighttime blood pressure as predictors of death and cause-specific cardiovascular events in hypertension. *Hypertension, 51*(1), 55–61. doi: 10.1161/HYPERTENSIONAHA.107.100727

Fair, A. M., & Montgomery, K. (2009). Energy balance, physical activity, and cancer risk. In M. Verma (Ed.), *Cancer Epidemiology. Volume 2, Modifiable Factors* (Vol. 472, pp. 57–88). New York: Humana Press.

Felsö, R., Lányi, E., Erhardt, E., Laufer, Z., Kardos, D., Herczeg, R., … Molnár, D. (2022). Total sleep deprivation decreases saliva ghrelin levels in adolescents. *J Sleep Res*, e13746. doi: 10.1111/jsr.13746

Felsö, R., Lohner, S., Hollódy, K., Erhardt, É., & Molnár, D. (2017). Relationship between sleep duration and childhood obesity: systematic review including the potential underlying mechanisms. *Nutr Metab Cardiovasc Dis, 27*(9), 751–761. doi: 10.1016/j.numecd.2017.07.008

Fernandez-Mendoza, J., Calhoun, S. L., Bixler, E. O., Karataraki, M., Liao, D., Vela-Bueno, A., … Vgontzas, A. N. (2011). Sleep misperception and chronic insomnia in the general population: role of objective sleep duration and psychological profiles. *Psychosom Med, 73*(1), 88–97. doi: 10.1097/PSY.0b013e3181fe365a

Fernandez-Mendoza, J., Vgontzas, A. N., Liao, D., Shaffer, M. L., Vela-Bueno, A., Basta, M., & Bixler, E. O. (2012). Insomnia with objective short sleep duration and incident hypertension: the Penn State Cohort. *Hypertension, 60*(4), 929–935. doi: 10.1161/HYPERTENSIONAHA.112.193268

Ferrario, C. R., Labouebe, G., Liu, S., Nieh, E. H., Routh, V. H., Xu, S., & O'Connor, E. C. (2016). Homeostasis meets motivation in the battle to control food intake. *J Neurosci, 36*(45), 11469–11481. doi: 10.1523/JNEUROSCI.2338-16.2016

Ford, E. S., Giles, W. H., & Mokdad, A. H. (2004). Increasing prevalence of the metabolic syndrome among U. S. adults. *Diabetes Care, 27*, 2444–2449.

Fowler, M. J. (2008). Microvascular and macrovascular complications of diabetes. *Clin Diabet, 26*(2), 77–82.

Franken, P., Dijk, D. J., Tobler, I., & Borbély, A. A. (1991). Sleep deprivation in rats: effects on EEG power spectra, vigilance states, and cortical temperature. *Am J Physiol, 261*, R198–R208.

Frase, L., Nissen, C., Spiegelhalder, K., & Feige, B. (2023). The importance and limitations of polysomnography in insomnia disorder-a critical appraisal. *J Sleep Res, 32*(6), e14036. doi: 10.1111/jsr.14036

Frey, D. J., Fleshner, M., & Wright, K. P. (2007). The effects of 40 hours of total sleep deprivation on inflammatory markers in healthy young adults. *Brain Behav Immun, 21*(8), 1050–1057. doi: 10.1016/j.bbi.2007.04.003

Friedmann, J., Globus, G., Huntley, A., Mullaney, D., Naitoh, P., & Johnson, L. (1977). Performance and mood during and after gradual sleep reduction. *Psychophysiology, 14*(3), 245–250.

Fu, X., Ren, H., Xie, J., Wang, W., Li, Y., Gao, P., & Chen, N. (2022). Association of nighttime masked uncontrolled hypertension with left ventricular hypertrophy and kidney function among patients with chronic kidney disease not receiving dialysis. *JAMA Netw Open, 5*(5), e2214460. doi:10.1001/jamanetworkopen.2022.14460

Fung, M. M., Peters, K., Ancoli-Israel, S., Redline, S., Stone, K. L., Barrett-Connor, E., & MrOS Research Group. (2013). Total sleep time and other sleep characteristics measured by actigraphy do not predict incident hypertension in a cohort of community-dwelling older men. *J Clin Sleep Med, 9*(6), 585–591. doi: 10.5664/jcsm.2756

Fung, M. M., Peters, K., Redline, S., Ziegler, M. G., Ancoli-Israel, S., Barrett-Connor, E., Stone, K. L., & MrOS Research Group. (2011). Decreased slow wave sleep increases risk of developing hypertension in elderly men. *Hypertension, 58*(4), 596–603. doi: 0.1161/HYPERTENSIONAHA.111.174409

Gangwisch, J., Malaspina, D., Boden-Albala, B., & Heymsfield, S. (2005). Inadequate sleep as a risk factor for obesity: analyses of the NHANES I. *Sleep, 28*(10), 1289–1296.

Gangwisch, J. E., Heymsfield, S. B., Boden-Albala, B., Buijs, R. M., Kreier, F., Pickering, T. G., … Malaspina, D. (2007). Sleep duration as a risk factor for diabetes incidence in a large US sample. *Sleep, 30*(12), 1667–1673.

Garaulet, M., Gomez-Abellan, P., Alburquerque-Bejar, J. J., Lee, Y. C., Ordovas, J. M., & Scheer, F. A. (2013). Timing of food intake predicts weight loss effectiveness. *Int J Obes (Lond), 37*(4), 604–611. doi: 10.1038/ijo.2012.229

Gayosa-Diz, P., Otero-González, A., Rodriguez-Alvarez, M. X., Gude, F., Garciá, F., De Francisco, A., & Quintela, A. G. (2013). Insulin-resistance (HOMA-IR) cut-off values and the metabolic syndrome in general adult populations: effect of gender and age: EPIRCE cross-sectional study. *BMC Endocr Disord, 13*(47). doi:10.1186/1472-6823-13-47

Geissmann, Q., Beckwith, E. J., & Gilestro, G. F. (2019). Most sleep does not serve a vital function: evidence from *Drosophila melanogaster*. *Sci Adv, 5*(2), eaau9253. doi:10.1126/sciadv.aau9253

Gip, P., Hagiwara, G., Sapolsky, R. M., Cao, V. H., Heller, H. C., & Ruby, N. F. (2004). Glucocorticoids influence brain glycogen levels during sleep deprivation. *Am J Physiol Regul Integr Comp Physiol, 286*, R1057–R1062.

Goetz, A. R., Jindal, I., Moreno, J. P., Puyau, M. R., Adolph, A. L., Musaad, S., … Bacha, F. (2022). The role of sleep and eating patterns in adiposity gain among preschool-aged children. *Am J Clin Nutr, 116*(5), 1334–1342. doi: 10.1093/ajcn/nqac197

Gooley, J. J., Chamberlain, K., Smith, K. A., Khalsa, S. B. S., Rajaratnam, S. M. W., Van Reen, E., … Lockley, S. W. (2011). Exposure to room light before bedtime suppresses melatonin onset and shortens melatonin duration in humans. *J Clin Endocr Metab, 96*, E463–E472. doi: 10.1210/jc.2010-2098

Gottlieb, D. J., Punjabi, N. M., Newman, A. B., Resnick, H. E., Redline, S., Baldwin, C. M., & Nieto, F. J. (2005). Association of sleep time with diabetes mellitus and impaired glucose tolerance. *Arch Intern Med, 165*, 863–868.

Grandner, M. A., Buxton, O. M., Jackson, N., Sands-Lincoln, M., Pandey, A., & Jean-Louis, G. (2013). Extreme sleep durations and increased C-reactive protein: effects of sex and ethnoracial group. *Sleep, 36*(5), 769–779E. doi: 10.5665/sleep.2646

Grandner, M. A., Chakravorty, S., Perlis, M. L., Oliver, L., & Gurubhagavatula, I. (2014). Habitual sleep duration associated with self-reported and objectively determined cardiometabolic risk factors. *Sleep Med, 15*(1), 42–50. doi: 10.1016/j.sleep.2013.09.012

Grandner, M. A., Sands-Lincoln, M. R., Pak, V. M., & Garland, S. N. (2013). Sleep duration, cardiovascular disease, and proinflammatory biomarkers. *Nat Sci Sleep, 5*, 93–107. doi: 10.2147/NSS.S31063

Grandner, M. A., Schopfer, E. A., Sands-Lincoln, M., Jackson, N., & Malhotra, A. (2015). Relationship between sleep duration and body mass index depends on age. *Obesity (Silver Spring), 23*(12), 2491–2498. doi: 10.1002/oby.21247

Gribbin, C. E., Watamura, S. E., Cairns, A., Harsh, J. R., & Lebourgeois, M. K. (2012). The cortisol awakening response (CAR) in 2- to 4-year-old children: effects of acute nighttime sleep restriction, wake time, and daytime napping. *Dev Psychobiol, 54*(4), 412–422. doi: 10.1002/dev.20599

Gröschl, M., Rauh, M., Dörr, H. G., Blum, W. F., Rascher, W., & Dötsch, J. (2002). Salivary leptin levels during the menstrual cycle and their relation to progesterone. *Fertil Steril, 77*(6), 1306–1307.

Grossman, E., Laudon, M., & Zisapel, N. (2011). Effect of melatonin on nocturnal blood pressure: meta-analysis of randomized controlled trials. *Vasc Health Risk Manag, 7*, 577–584. doi: 10.2147/VHRM.S24603

Haack, M., Kraus, T., Schuld, A., Dalal, M., Koethe, D., & Pollmächer, T. (2002). Diurnal variations of interleukin-6 plasma levels are confounded by blood drawing procedures. *Psychoneuroendocrinology, 27*, 921–931.

Haack, M., Sanchez, E., & Mullington, J. M. (2007). Elevated inflammatory markers in response to prolonged sleep restriction are associated with increased pain experience in healthy volunteers. *Sleep, 30*(9), 1145–1152.

Haba-Rubio, J., Marques-Vidal, P., Andries, D., Tobback, N., Preisig, M., Vollenweider, P., … Heinzer, R. (2015). Objective sleep structure and cardiovascular risk factors in the general population: the HypnoLaus Study. *Sleep, 38*(3), 391–400. doi: 10.5665/sleep.4496

Hall, M. H., Okun, M. L., Sowers, M., Matthews, K. A., Kravitz, H. M., Hardin, K., … Sanders, M. H. (2012). Sleep is associated with the metabolic syndrome in a multi-ethnic cohort of midlife women: the SWAN Sleep Study. *Sleep, 35*(6), 783–790. doi: 10.5665/sleep.1874

Han, K. M., Lee, H. J., Kim, L., & Yoon, H. K. (2020). Association between weekend catch-up sleep and high-sensitivity C-reactive protein levels in adults: a population-based study. *Sleep, 43*(8), zsaa010. doi:10.1093/sleep/zsaa010

Harbison, S. T., McCoy, L. J., & Mackay, T. F. C. (2013). Genome-wide association study of sleep in *Drosophila melanogaster. BMC Genomics, 14*, 281. doi:10.1186/1471-2164-14-281

Harpsøe, N. G., Andersen, L. P., Gögenur, I., & Rosenberg, J. (2015). Clinical pharmacokinetics of melatonin: a systematic review. *Eur J Clin Pharmacol, 71*(8), 901–909. doi: 10.1007/s00228-015-1873-4

Hart, C. N., Carskadon, M. A., Considine, R. V., Fava, J. L., Lawton, J., Raynor, H. A., … Owens, J. (2013). Changes in children's sleep duration on food intake, weight, and leptin. *Pediatrics, 132*, e1473-e1480.

Harvey, A. G., & Tang, N. K. (2012). (Mis)perception of sleep in insomnia: a puzzle and a resolution. *Psychol Bull, 138*(1), 77–101. doi: 10.1037/a0025730

Hasler, G., Buysse, D. J., Klaghofer, R., Gamma, A., Ajdacic, V., Eich, D., … Angst, J. (2004). The association between short sleep duration and obesity in young adults: a 13-year prospective study. *Sleep, 27*(4), 661–666.

Hatori, M., Vollmers, C., Zarrinpar, A., DiTacchio, L., Bushong, E. A., Gill, S., … Panda, S. (2012). Time-restricted feeding without reducing caloric intake prevents metabolic diseases in mice fed a high-fat diet. *Cell Metab, 15*, 848–860. doi: 10.1016/j.cmet.2012.04.019

Hayes, A. L., Xu, F., Babineau, D., & Patel, S. R. (2011). Sleep duration and circulating adipokine levels. *Sleep, 34*(2), 147–152.

He, Y., Jones, C. R., Fujiki, N., Xu, Y., Guo, B., Holder, J. L., Rossner, M. J., Nishino, S., & Fu, Y. H. (2009). The transcriptional repressor DEC2 regulates sleep length in mammals. *Science, 325*(5942), 866–870. doi: 10.1126/science.1174443

Hermida, R. C., Ayala, D. E., Fernandez, J. R., & Calvo, C. (2007). Chronotherapy improves blood pressure control and reverts the nondipper pattern in patients with resistant hypertension. *Hypertension, 51*(1), 69–76. doi: 10.1161/HYPERTENSIONAHA.107.096933

Hermida, R. C., Ayala, D. E., Mojon, A., & Fernandez, J. R. (2013). Blunted sleep-time relative blood pressure decline increases cardiovascular risk independent of blood pressure level--the "normotensive non-dipper" paradox. *Chronobiol Int, 30*(1-2), 87–98. doi: 10.3109/07420528.2012.701127

Hermida, R. C., Ayala, D. E., Mojón, A., & Fernández, J. R. (2010). Influence of circadian time of hypertension treatment on cardiovascular risk: results of the MAPEC study. *Chronobiol Int, 27*(8), 1629–1651. doi: 10.3109/07420528.2010.510230

Herzog, N., Jauch-Chara, K., Hyzy, F., Richter, A., Friedrich, A., Benedict, C., & Oltmanns, K. M. (2013). Selective slow wave sleep but not rapid eye movement sleep suppression impairs morning glucose tolerance in healthy men. *Psychoneuroendocrinology, 38*(10), 2075–2082. doi: 10.1016/j.psyneuen.2013.03.018

Hillman, D., Mitchell, S., Streatfeild, J., Burns, C., Bruck, D., & Pezzullo, L. (2018). The economic cost of inadequate sleep. *Sleep, 41*(8), zsy083. doi:10.1093/sleep/zsy083

Hirano, A., Hsu, P. K., Zhang, L., Xing, L., McMahon, T., Yamazaki, M., Ptacek, L. J., & Fu, Y. H. (2018). DEC2 modulates orexin expression and regulates sleep. *Proc Natl Acad Sci USA, 115*(13), 3434–3439. doi: 10.1073/pnas.1801693115

Hla, K. M., Young, T., Finn, L., Peppard, P. E., Szklo-Coxe, M., & Stubbs, M. (2008). Longitudinal association of sleep-disordered breathing and nondipping in nocturnal blood pressure In the Wisconsin Sleep Cohort study. *Sleep, 31*(6), 795–800.

Hogenkamp, P. S., Nilsson, E., Nilsson, V. C., Chapman, C. D., Vogel, H., Lundberg, L. S., … Schiöth, H. B. (2013). Acute sleep deprivation increases portion size and affects food choice in young men. *Psychoneuroendocrinology, 38*(9), 1668–1674. doi: 0.1016/j.psyneuen.2013.01.012

Hu, F. B. (2013). Resolved: there is sufficient scientific evidence that decreasing sugar-sweetened beverage consumption will reduce the prevalence of obesity and obesity-related diseases. *Obes Rev, 14*(8), 606–619. doi: 10.1111/obr.12040

Hung, H. C., Yang, Y. C., Ou, H. Y., Wu, J. S., Lu, F. H., & Chang, C. J. (2013). The association between self-reported sleep quality and metabolic syndrome. *PLoS One, 8*(1), e54304. doi: 10.1371/journal.pone.0054304

Hwangbo, Y., Kim, W. J., Chu, M. K., Yun, C. H., & Yang, K. I. (2013). Association between weekend catch-up sleep duration and hypertension in Korean adults. *Sleep Med, 14*(6), 549–554. doi: 10.1016/j.sleep.2013.02.009

Irwin, M. R. (2015). Why sleep is important for health: a psychoneuroimmunology perspective. *Annu Rev Psychol, 66*, 143–172. doi: 10.1146/annurev-psych-010213-115205

Irwin, M. R., Carrillo, C., & Olmstead, R. (2010). Sleep loss activates cellular markers of inflammation: sex differences. *Brain Behav Immun, 24*(1), 54–57. doi: 10.1016/j.bbi.2009.06.001

Israel, B., Buysse, D. J., Krafty, R. T., Begley, A., Miewald, J., & Hall, M. (2012). Short-term stability of sleep and heart rate variability in good sleepers and patients with insomnia: for some measures, one night is enough. *Sleep, 35*(9), 1285–1291. doi: 10.5665/sleep.2088

Iyengar, N. M., Gucalp, A., Dannenberg, A. J., & Hudis, C. A. (2016). Obesity and cancer mechanisms: tumor microenvironment and inflammation. *J Clin Oncol, 34*(35), 4270–4276. doi: 10.1200/JCO.2016.67.4283

Jackson, C. L., Patel, S. R., Jackson, W. B., 2nd, Lutsey, P. L., & Redline, S. (2018). Agreement between self-reported and objectively measured sleep duration among white, black, Hispanic, and Chinese adults in the United States: Multi-Ethnic Study of Atherosclerosis. *Sleep, 41*(6), zsy057. doi: 10.1093/sleep/zsy057

Javaheri, S., Zhao, Y. Y., Punjabi, N. M., Quan, S. F., Gottlieb, D. J., & Redline, S. (2017). Slow wave sleep is associated with incident hypertension: the Sleep Heart Health Study. *Sleep, 41*(1), zsx179. doi: 10.1093/sleep/zsx179

Jennings, J. R., Muldoon, M. F., Hall, M., Buysse, D. J., & Manuck, S. B. (2007). Self-reported sleep quality is associated with the metabolic syndrome. *Sleep, 30*(2), 219–223.

Jha, P. K., Foppen, E., Kalsbeek, A., & Challet, E. (2016). Sleep restriction acutely impairs glucose tolerance in rats. *Physiol Rep, 4*(12), e12839. doi:10.14814/phy2.12839

Jones, H. S., & Oswald, I. (1968). Two cases of healthy insomnia. *Electroencephalogr Clin Neurophysiol, 24*(4), 378–380.

Jones, S. E., van Hees, V. T., Mazzotti, D. R., Marques-Vidal, P., Sabia, S., van der Spek, A., … Wood, A. R. (2019). Genetic studies of accelerometer-based sleep measures in 85,670 individuals yield new insights into human sleep behaviour. *Nat Commun, 10*(1), 1585. doi: 10.1038/s41467-019-09576-1

Jung, C. M., Melanson, E. L., Frydendall, E. J., Perreault, L., Eckel, R. H., & Wright, K. P. (2011). Energy expenditure during sleep, sleep deprivation and sleep following sleep deprivation in adult humans. *J Physiol, 589*(1), 235–244. doi: 10.1113/jphysiol.2010.197517

Jung, S. W., Lee, K. J., & Lee, J. H. (2019). Does weekend catch-up sleep affect high-sensitivity C-reactive protein levels among Korean workers?: a cross-sectional study using KNHANES. *J Occup Environ Med, 61*(9), e367–e373. doi: 10.1097/JOM.0000000000001657

Kahleova, H., Lloren, J. I., Mashchak, A., Hill, M., & Fraser, G. E. (2017). Meal frequency and timing are associated with changes in body mass index in Adventist Health Study 2. *J Nutrition, 147*(9), 1722–1728. doi: 10.3945/jn.116.244749

Kaur, G., Phillips, C. L., Wong, K., McLachlan, A. J., & Saini, B. (2016). Timing of administration: for commonly-prescribed medicines in Australia. *Pharmaceutics, 8*(2), 13. doi:10.3390/pharmaceutics8020013
Keklund, G., & Åkerstedt, T. (1997). Objective components of individual differences in subjective sleep quality. *J Sleep Res, 6*(4), 217–220. doi: 10.1111/j.1365-2869.1997.00217.x
Kelly, R. M., Finn, J., Healy, U., Gallen, D., Sreenan, S., McDermott, J. H., & Coogan, A. N. (2020). Greater social jetlag associates with higher HbA1c in adults with type 2 diabetes: a cross sectional study. *Sleep Med, 66*, 1–9. doi: 10.1016/j.sleep.2019.07.023
Kerkhof, G. A., Van Dongen, H. P. A., & Bobbert, A. C. (1998). Absence of circadian rhythmicity in blood pressure? *Am J Hypertens, 11*, 373–377.
Kim, D. J., Mun, S. J., Choi, J. S., Kim, J., Lee, G.-h., Kim, H.-w., … Cho, J. W. (2020). Beneficial effects of weekend catch-up sleep on metabolic syndrome in chronic short sleepers. *Sleep Med, 76*, 26–32. doi: 10.1016/j.sleep.2020.09.025
Klingenberg, L., Chaput, J. P., Holmback, U., Visby, T., Jennum, P., Nikolic, M., Astrup, A., & Sjodin, A. (2013). Acute sleep restriction reduces insulin sensitivity in adolescent boys. *Sleep, 36*(7), 1085–1090. doi: 10.5665/sleep.2816
Knutson, K. L., & Lauderdale, D. S. (2007). Sleep duration and overweight in adolescents: self-reported sleep hours versus time diaries. *Pediatrics, 119*(5), e1056–e1062. doi: 10.1542/peds.2006-2597
Koolhaas, J. M., Bartolomucci, A., Buwalda, B., de Boer, S. F., Flugge, G., Korte, S. M., … Fuchs, E. (2011). Stress revisited: a critical evaluation of the stress concept. *Neurosci Biobehav Rev, 35*(5), 1291–1301. doi: 10.1016/j.neubiorev.2011.02.003
Kräuchi, K., Cajochen, C., Werth, E., & Wirz-Justice, A. (2000). Functional link between distal vasodilation and sleep-onset latency? *Am J Physiol Regul Integr Comp Physiol, 278*(3), R741–748.
Kripke, D. F., Garfinkel, L., Wingard, D. L., Klauber, M. R., & Marler, M. R. (2002). Mortality associated with sleep duration and insomnia. *Arch Gen Psychiatr, 59*, 131–136.
Kurina, L. M., McClintock, M. K., Chen, J. H., Waite, L. J., Thisted, R. A., & Lauderdale, D. S. (2013). Sleep duration and all-cause mortality: a critical review of measurement and associations. *Ann Epidemiol, 23*(6), 361–370. doi: 10.1016/j.annepidem.2013.03.015
Kyrou, I., Chrousos, G. P., & Tsigos, C. (2006). Stress, visceral obesity, and metabolic complications. *Ann N Y Acad Sci, 1083*, 77–110. doi: 10.1196/annals.1367.008
Landhuis, C. E., Poulton, R., Welch, D., & Hancox, R. J. (2008). Childhood sleep time and long-term risk for obesity: a 32-year prospective birth cohort study. *Pediatrics, 122*(5), 955–960. doi: 10.1542/peds.2007-3521
Lang, I. A., Llewellyn, D. J., Alexander, K., & Melzer, D. (2008). Obesity, physical function, and mortality in older adults. *J Am Geriatr Soc, 56*(8), 1474–1478. doi: 10.1111/j.1532-5415.2008.01813.x
Lange, T., Dimitrov, S., & Born, J. (2010). Effects of sleep and circadian rhythm on the human immune system. *Ann N Y Acad Sci, 1193*, 48–59. doi: 10.1111/j.1749-6632.2009.05300.x
Lange, T., Perras, B., Fehm, H. L., & Born, J. (2003). Sleep enhances the human antibody response to hepatitis A vaccination. *Psychosom Med, 65*, 831–835. doi: 0.1097/01.PSY.0000091382.61178.F1
Larcher, S., Gauchez, A. S., Lablanche, S., Pepin, J. L., Benhamou, P. Y., & Borel, A. L. (2016). Impact of sleep behavior on glycemic control in type 1 diabetes: the role of social jetlag. *Eur J Endocrinol, 175*(5), 411–419. doi: 10.1530/EJE-16-0188
Lauderdale, D. S., Knutson, K. L., Yan, L. L., Liu, K., & Rathouz, P. J. (2008). Self-reported and measured sleep duration: how similar are they? *Epidemiology, 19*(6), 838–845. doi: 10.1097/EDE.0b013e318187a7b0
Leake, C., Grab, J. A., & Senn, M. J. (1927). Studies in exhaustion due to lack of sleep. II. Symptomatology in rabbits. *Am J Physiol, 82*(1), 127–130.
Leproult, R., Deliens, G., Gilson, M., & Peigneux, P. (2015). Beneficial impact of sleep extension on fasting insulin sensitivity in adults with habitual sleep restriction. *Sleep, 38*(5), 707–715. doi: 10.5665/sleep.4660
LeRoux, A., Wright, L., Perrot, T., & Rusak, B. (2014). Impact of menstrual cycle phase on endocrine effects of partial sleep restriction in healthy women. *Psychoneuroendocrinology, 49*, 34–46. doi: 10.1016/j.psyneuen.2014.06.002
Lin, J., Jiang, Y., Wang, G., Meng, M., Zhu, Q., Mei, H., Liu, S., & Jiang, F. (2020). Associations of short sleep duration with appetite-regulating hormones and adipokines: A systematic review and meta-analysis. *Obes Rev, 21*(11), e13051. doi: 10.1111/obr.13051
Liu, R., Wu, S., Zhang, B., Guo, M., & Zhang, Y. (2020). The association between sleep duration and prostate cancer: a systematic review and meta-analysis. *Medicine (Baltimore), 99*(28), e21180. doi:10.1097/MD.0000000000021180
Mackenzie, I. S., Rogers, A., Poulter, N. R., Williams, B., Brown, M. J., Webb, D. J., … MacDonald, T. M. (2022). Cardiovascular outcomes in adults with hypertension with evening versus morning dosing of usual antihypertensives in the UK (TIME study): a prospective, randomised, open-label, blinded-endpoint clinical trial. *Lancet, 400*(10361), 1417–1425. doi: 10.1016/s0140-6736(22)01786-x
Magee, L., & Hale, L. (2012). Longitudinal associations between sleep duration and subsequent weight gain: a systematic review. *Sleep Med Rev, 16*(3), 231–241. doi: 10.1016/j.smrv.2011.05.005
Mallon, L., Broman, J.-E., & Hetta, J. (2005). High incidence of diabetes in men with sleep complaints or short sleep duration. *Diabetes Care, 27*, 2762–2767.
Marinac, C. R., Natarajan, L., Sears, D. D., Gallo, L. C., Hartman, S. J., Arredondo, E., & Patterson, R. E. (2015). Prolonged nightly fasting and breast cancer risk: findings from NHANES (2009-2010). *Cancer Epidemiol Biomarkers Prev, 24*(5), 783–789. doi: 10.1158/1055-9965.EPI-14-1292
Marino, M., Li, Y., Rueschman, M. N., Winkelman, J. W., Ellenbogen, J. M., Solet, J. M., … Buxton, O. M. (2013). Measuring sleep: accuracy, sensitivity, and specificity of wrist actigraphy compared to polysomnography. *Sleep, 36*(11), 1747–1755. doi: 10.5665/sleep.3142
Markwald, R. R., Melanson, E. L., Smith, M. R., Higgins, J., Perreault, L., Eckel, R. H., & Wright Jr, K. P. (2013). Impact of insufficient sleep on total daily energy expenditure, food intake, and weight gain. *Proc Natl Acad Sci USA, 110*(14), 5695–5700.
Martínez-Lozano, N., Tvarijonaviciute, A., Ríos, R., Barón, I., Scheer, F., & Garaulet, M. (2020). Late eating Is associated with obesity, inflammatory markers and circadian-related disturbances in school-aged children. *Nutrients, 12*, 1–12. doi: 10.3390/nu12092881
Matthews, K. A., Dahl, R. E., Owens, J. F., Lee, L., & Hall, M. (2012). Sleep duration and insulin resistance in healthy black and white adolescents. *Sleep, 35*(10), 1353–1358. doi: 10.5665/sleep.2112
McAllister, E. J., Dhurandhar, N. V., Keith, S. W., Aronne, L. J., Barger, J., Baskin, M., … Allison, D. B. (2009). Ten putative contributors to the obesity epidemic. *Crit Rev Food Sci Nutr, 49*(10), 868–913. doi: 10.1080/10408390903372599
McCall, W. V., & Edinger, J. D. (1992). Subjective total insomnia: An example of sleep state misperception. *Sleep, 15*, 71–73.
McEwen, B. S. (2006). Sleep deprivation as a neurobiologic and physiologic stressor: allostasis and allostatic load. *Metabolism Clin Exp, 55*(Supplenment 2), S20–S23. doi: 0.1016/j.metabol.2006.07.008
McHill, A. W., Velasco, J., Bodner, T., Shea, S. A., & Olson, R. (2022). Rapid changes in overnight blood pressure after transitioning to early-morning shiftwork. *Sleep, 45*(3), zsab203. doi: 10.1093/sleep/zsab203
Meddis, R. (1977). *The sleep instinct*. London: Routledge & Kegan Paul.
Meddis, R., Pearson, A. J. D., & Langford, G. (1973). An extreme case of healthy insomnia. *Electroencephalogr Clin Neurophysiol, 35*, 213–214.
Meerlo, P., Sgoifo, A., & Suchecki, D. (2008). Restricted and disrupted sleep: effects on autonomic function, neuroendocrine stress systems and stress responsivity. *Sleep Med Rev, 12*(3), 197–210. doi: 10.1016/j.smrv.2007.07.007
Meier-Ewert, H. K., Ridker, P. M., Rifai, N., Regan, M. M., Price, N. J., Dinges, D. F., & Mullington, J. M. (2004). Effect of sleep loss on C-reactive protein, an inflammatory marker of cardiovascular risk. *J Am Coll Cardiol, 43*(4), 678–683. doi: 10.1016/j.jacc.2003.07.050
Meltzer, L. J., Montgomery-Downs, H. E., Insana, S. P., & Walsh, C. M. (2012). Use of actigraphy for assessment in pediatric sleep research. *Sleep Med Rev, 16*(5), 463–475. doi: 10.1016/j.smrv.2011.10.002
Mendelson, W., Guthrie, R. D., Guynn, R., Harris, R. L., & Wyatt, R. J. (1974). Rapid eye movement (REM) sleep deprivation, stress and intermediary metabolism. *J Neurochem, 22*, 1157–1159.
Meng, L., Zheng, Y., & Hui, R. (2013). The relationship of sleep duration and insomnia to risk of hypertension incidence: a meta-analysis of prospective cohort studies. *Hypertens Res, 36*(11), 985–995. doi: 10.1038/hr.2013.70
Mercy, U. C., Elenwa, F., Ogunsola, A. S., Eniola, O. A., Yunusa, I., & Karaye, I. M. (2022). Sex differences in the association between short sleep duration and obesity among US adults: findings from NHANES, 2015-2020. *Sleep Med, 92*, 59–63. doi: 10.1016/j.sleep.2022.03.004
Messman, B. A., Wiley, J. F., Yap, Y., Tung, Y. C., Almeida, I. M., Dietch, J. R., … Slavish, D. C. (2022). How much does sleep vary from night-to-night? A quantitative summary of intraindividual variability in sleep by age, gender, and racial/ethnic identity across eight-pooled datasets. *J Sleep Res, 31*(6), e13680. doi:10.1111/jsr.13680
Metoki, H., Ohkubo, T., Kikuya, M., Asayama, K., Obara, T., Hashimoto, J., … Imai, Y. (2006). Prognostic significance for stroke of a morning pressor surge and a nocturnal blood pressure decline: the Ohasama study. *Hypertension, 47*(2), 149–154. doi: 10.1161/01.HYP.0000198541.12640.0f
Miller, M. A., Kandala, N. B., Kivimaki, M., Kumari, M., Brunner, E. J., Lowe, G. D., … Cappuccio, F. P. (2009). Gender differences in the cross-sectional

relationships between sleep duration and markers of inflammation: Whitehall II study. *Sleep, 32*(7), 857–864.

Miller, M. A., Kruisbrink, M., Wallace, J., Ji, C., & Cappuccio, F. P. (2018). Sleep duration and incidence of obesity in infants, children, and adolescents: a systematic review and meta-analysis of prospective studies. *Sleep, 41*(4). doi: 10.1093/sleep/zsy018

Moldofsky, H., Lue, F. A., Davidson, J. R., & Gorczynski, R. (1989). Effects of sleep deprivation on human immune functions. *FASEB J, 3*, 1972–1977.

Mongrain, V., Hernandez, S. A., Pradervand, S., Dorsaz, S., Curie, T., Hagiwara, G., … Franken, P. (2010). Separating the contribution of glucocorticoids and wakefulness to the molecular and electrophysiological correlates of sleep homeostasis. *Sleep, 33*(9), 1147–1157.

Morrissey, B., Orellana, L., Allender, S., & Strugnell, C. (2022). The sleep-obesity nexus: assessment of multiple sleep dimensions and weight status among Victorian primary school children. *Nat Sci Sleep, 14*, 581–591. doi: 10.2147/nss.S352357

Mullington, J. M., Chan, J. L., Van Dongen, H., Szuba, M. P., Samaras, J., Price, N. J., … Mantzoros, C. S. (2003). Sleep loss reduces diurnal rhythm amplitude of leptin in healthy men. *J Neuroendocrinol, 15*(9), 851–854.

Mullington, J. M., Simpson, N. S., Meier-Ewert, H. K., & Haack, M. (2010). Sleep loss and inflammation. *Best Pract Res Clin Endocrinol Metab, 24*(5), 775–784. doi: 10.1016/j.beem.2010.08.014

Nauck, M. A., Quast, D. R., Wefers, J., & Meier, J. J. (2021). GLP-1 receptor agonists in the treatment of type 2 diabetes - state-of-the-art. *Mol Metab, 46*, 101102. doi:10.1016/j.molmet.2020.101102

Nedeltcheva, A. V., Kilkus, J. M., Imperial, J., Kasza, K., Schoeller, D. A., & Penev, P. D. (2009). Sleep curtailment is accompanied by increased intake of calories from snacks. *Am J Clin Nutr, 89*(1), 126–133. doi: 10.3945/ajcn.2008.26574

Newman, S. M., Paletz, E. M., Obermeyer, W. H., & Benca, R. M. (2009). Sleep deprivation in pigeons and rats using motion detection. *Sleep, 32*(10), 1299–1312.

Newman, S. M., Paletz, E. M., Rattenborg, N. C., Obermeyer, W. H., & Benca, R. M. (2008). Sleep deprivation in the pigeon using the disk-over-water method. *Physiol Behav, 93*(1–2), 50–58. doi: 10.1016/j.physbeh.2007.07.012

Nicol, G. E., Yingling, M. D., Flavin, K. S., Schweiger, J. A., Patterson, B. W., Schechtman, K. B., & Newcomer, J. W. (2018). Metabolic effects of antipsychotics on adiposity and insulin sensitivity in youths: a randomized clinical trial. *JAMA Psychiatry, 75*(8), 788–796. doi: 10.1001/jamapsychiatry.2018.1088

Nielsen, L. S., Danielsen, K. V., & Sorensen, T. I. (2011). Short sleep duration as a possible cause of obesity: critical analysis of the epidemiological evidence. *Obes Rev, 12*(2), 78–92. doi: 10.1111/j.1467-789X.2010.00724.x

Ning, X., Lv, J., Guo, Y., Bian, Z., Tan, Y., Pei, P., … China Kadoorie Biobank Collaborative, G. (2020). Association of sleep duration with weight gain and general and central obesity risk in Chinese adults: a prospective study. *Obesity (Silver Spring), 28*(2), 468–474. doi: 10.1002/oby.22713

Nôga, D. A., Meth, E., Pacheco, A. P., Tan, X., Cedernaes, J., van Egmond, L. T., … Benedict, C. (2024). Habitual short sleep duration, diet, and development of type 2 diabetes in adults. *JAMA Netw Open, 7*(3), e241147. doi:10.1001/jamanetworkopen.2024.1147

Nowakowski, S., Matthews, K. A., von Kanel, R., Hall, M. H., & Thurston, R. C. (2018). Sleep characteristics and inflammatory biomarkers among midlife women. *Sleep, 41*(5), zsy049. doi: 10.1093/sleep/zsy049

Ohkuma, T., Fujii, H., Iwase, M., Ogata-Kaizu, S., Ide, H., Kikuchi, Y., … Kitazono, T. (2014). U-shaped association of sleep duration with metabolic syndrome and insulin resistance in patients with type 2 diabetes: the Fukuoka Diabetes Registry. *Metabolism, 63*(4), 484–491. doi: 10.1016/j.metabol.2013.12.001

Olds, T. S., Maher, C. A., & Matricciani, L. A. (2011). Sleep duration or bedtime? Exploring the relationship between sleep habits and weight status and activity patterns. *Sleep, 34*(10), 1299–1307.

Omisade, A., Buxton, O. M., & Rusak, B. (2010). Impact of acute sleep restriction on cortisol and leptin levels in young women. *Physiol Behav, 99*(5), 651–656. doi: 10.1016/j.physbeh.2010.01.028

Paré, W. P. (1964). The effect of chronic environmental stress on stomach ulceration, adrenal function, and consummatory behavior in the rat. *J Psychol, 57*, 143–151.

Park, S. (2013). The association between short sleep duration and body mass index among South Korean children and adolescents. *J Sch Nurs, 29*(2), 142–150. doi: 10.1177/1059840512450582

Patel, S. R., Malhotra, A., Gao, X., Hu, F. B., Neuman, M. I., & Fawzi, W. W. (2012). A prospective study of sleep duration and pneumonia risk in women. *Sleep, 35*(1), 97–101. doi: 10.5665/sleep.1594

Patel, S. R., Malhotra, A., White, D. P., Gottlieb, D. J., & Hu, F. B. (2006). Association between reduced sleep and weight gain in women. *Am J Epidemiol, 164*(10), 947–954. doi: 10.1093/aje/kwj280

Pavlou, V., Cienfuegos, S., Lin, S., Ezpeleta, M., Ready, K., Corapi, S., … Varady, K. A. (2023). Effect of time-restricted eating on weight loss in adults with type 2 diabetes: a randomized clinical trial. *JAMA Netw Open, 6*(10), e2339337. doi:10.1001/jamanetworkopen.2023.39337

Phillips, A. J. K., Vidafar, P., Burns, A. C., McGlashan, E. M., Anderson, C., Rajaratnam, S. M. W., … Cain, S. W. (2019). High sensitivity and interindividual variability in the response of the human circadian system to evening light. *Proc Natl Acad Sci U S A, 116*(24), 12019–12024. doi: 10.1073/pnas.1901824116

Phillips, C. L., & O'Driscoll, D. M. (2013). Hypertension and obstructive sleep apnea. *Nat Sci Sleep, 5*, 43–52. doi: 10.2147/NSS.S34841

Pollak, C. P., Tryon, W. W., Nagaraja, H., & Dzwonczyk, R. (2001). How accurately does wrist actigraphy identify the states of sleep and wakefulness? *Sleep, 24*(8), 957–965.

Prather, A. A., Hall, M., Fury, J. M., Ross, D. C., Muldoon, M. F., Cohen, S., & Marsland, A. L. (2012). Sleep and antibody response to hepatitis B vaccination. *Sleep, 35*(8), 1063–1069. doi: 10.5665/sleep.1990

Prather, A. A., Janicki-Deverts, D., Hall, M. H., & Cohen, S. (2015). Behaviorally assessed sleep and susceptibility to the common cold. *Sleep, 38*(9), 1353–1359. doi: 10.5665/sleep.4968

Rattenborg, N. C., Amlaner, C. J., & Lima, S. L. (2001). Unilateral eye closure and interhemispheric EEG asymmetry during sleep in the pigeon (*Columba livia*). *Brain Behav Evol, 58*, 323–332.

Rechtschaffen, A., & Bergmann, B. M. (1995). Sleep deprivation in the rat by the disk-over-water method. *Behav Brain Res, 69*(1–2), 55–63.

Rechtschaffen, A., & Bergmann, B. M. (2002). Sleep deprivation in the rat: an update of the 1989 paper. *Sleep, 25*(1), 18–24.

Redwine, L. (2000). Effects of sleep and sleep deprivation on interleukin-6, growth hormone, cortisol, and melatonin levels in humans. *J Clin Endocr Metab, 85*(10), 3597–3603. doi: 10.1210/jc.85.10.3597

Reutrakul, S., Hood, M. M., Crowley, S. J., Morgan, M. K., Teodori, M., Knutson, K., & Van Cauter, E. (2013). Chronotype is independently associated with glycemic control in type 2 diabetes. *Diabetes Care, 36*(9), 2523–2529. doi: 10.2337/dc12-2697

Reutrakul, S., & Van Cauter, E. (2018). Sleep influences on obesity, insulin resistance, and risk of type 2 diabetes. *Metabolism, 84*, 56–66. doi: 10.1016/j.metabol.2018.02.010

Reynolds, A. C., Dorrian, J., Liu, P. Y., Van Dongen, H. P., Wittert, G. A., Harmer, L. J., & Banks, S. (2012). Impact of five nights of sleep restriction on glucose metabolism, leptin and testosterone in young adult men. *PLoS One, 7*(7), e41218. doi: 10.1371/journal.pone.0041218

Rihm, J. S., Menz, M. M., Schultz, H., Bruder, L., Schilbach, L., Schmid, S. M., & Peters, J. (2019). Sleep deprivation selectively upregulates an amygdala-hypothalamic circuit involved in food reward. *J Neurosci, 39*(5), 888–899. doi: 10.1523/JNEUROSCI.0250-18.2018

Rogers, E. M., Banks, N. F., & Jenkins, N. D. M. (2024). The effects of sleep disruption on metabolism, hunger, and satiety, and the influence of psychosocial stress and exercise: a narrative review. *Diabetes Metab Res Rev, 40*(2), e3667. doi:10.1002/dmrr.3667

Rohrer, J. M. (2018). Thinking clearly about correlations and causation: graphical causal models for observational data. *Adv Meth Prac Psychol Sci, 1*(1), 27–42.

Rose, D. P., Haffner, S. M., & Baillargeon, J. (2007). Adiposity, the metabolic syndrome, and breast cancer in African-American and white American women. *Endocr Rev, 28*(7), 763–777. doi: 10.1210/er.2006-0019

Ross, J. J. (1965). Neurological findings after prolonged sleep deprivation. *Arch Neurol, 12*, 399–403.

Routledge, F. S., McFetridge-Durdle, J. A., & Dean, C. R. (2007). Night-time blood pressure patterns and target organ damage: a review. *Can J Cardiol, 23*(2), 132–138.

Russell, C., Wearden, A. J., Fairclough, G., Emsley, R. A., & Kyle, S. D. (2016). Subjective but not actigraphy-defined sleep predicts next-day fatigue in chronic fatigue syndrome: a prospective daily diary study. *Sleep, 39*(4), 937–944. doi: 10.5665/sleep.5658

Salah, H. M., & Mehta, J. L. (2022). Best time for administration of antihypertensive medications: morning or evening? *Lancet, 400*(10361), 1383–1385. doi: 10.1016/s0140-6736(22)01900-6

Salles, G. F., Reboldi, G., Fagard, R. H., Cardoso, C. R., Pierdomenico, S. D., Verdecchia, P., … Investigators, A.-H. (2016). Prognostic effect of the nocturnal blood pressure fall in hypertensive patients: the ambulatory blood pressure collaboration in patients with hypertension (ABC-H) meta analysis. *Hypertension, 67*(4), 693–700. doi: 10.1161/HYPERTENSIONAHA.115.06981

Scheer, F. A. J. L., Hu, K., Evoniuk, H., Kelly, E. E., Malhotra, A., Hilton, M. F., & Shea, S. A. (2010). Impact of the human circadian system, exercise, and their interaction on cardiovascular function. *Proc Natl Acad Sci USA*, *107*(47), 20541–20546. doi: 10.1073/pnas.1006749107

Scheer, F. A. J. L., Van Montfrans, G. A., van Someren, E. J. W., Mairuhu, G., & Buijs, R. M. (2004). Daily nighttime melatonin reduces blood pressure in male patients with essential hypertension. *Hypertension*, *43*(2), 192–197. doi: 10.1161/01.HYP.0000113293.15186.3b

Schmid, S. M., Hallschmid, M., Jauch-Chara, K., Born, J., & Schultes, B. (2008). A single night of sleep deprivation increases ghrelin levels and feelings of hunger in normal-weight healthy men. *J Sleep Res*, *17*(3), 331–334. doi: 10.1111/j.1365-2869.2008.00662.x

Schmid, S. M., Hallschmid, M., Jauch-Chara, K., Wilms, B., Benedict, C., Lehnert, H., ... Schultes, B. (2009). Short-term sleep loss decreases physical activity under free-living conditions but does not increase food intake under time-deprived laboratory conditions in healthy men. *Am J Clin Nutr*, *90*(6), 1476–1482. doi: 10.3945/ajcn.2009.27984

Seif, F., Patel, S. R., Walia, H. K., Rueschman, M., Bhatt, D. L., Blumenthal, R. S., ... Mehra, R. (2014). Obstructive sleep apnea and diurnal nondipping hemodynamic indices in patients at increased cardiovascular risk. *J Hypertens*, *32*(2), 267–275. doi: 10.1097/HJH.0000000000000011

Selye, H. (1946). The general adaptation syndrome and the diseases of adaptation. *J Clin Endocrinol*, *6*(2), 117–230.

Shaw, N. D., McHill, A. W., Schiavon, M., Kangarloo, T., Mankowski, P. W., Cobelli, C., ... Hall, J. E. (2016). Effect of slow wave sleep disruption on metabolic parameters in adolescents. *Sleep*, *39*(8), 1591–1599. doi: 10.5665/sleep.6028

Shaw, P. J., Tononi, G., Greenspan, R. J., & Robinson, D. F. (2002). Stress response genes protect against lethal effects of sleep deprivation in *Drosophila*. *Nature*, *417*(6886), 287–291.

Shea, S. A., Hilton, M. F., Hu, K., & Scheer, F. A. (2011). Existence of an endogenous circadian blood pressure rhythm in humans that peaks in the evening. *Circ Res*, *108*(8), 980–984. doi: 10.1161/CIRCRESAHA.110.233668

Sherwood, A., Steffen, P. R., Blumenthal, J. A., Kuhn, C., & Hinderliter, A. L. (2002). Nighttime blood pressure dipping: role of the sympathetic nervous system. *Am J Hypertens*, *15*, 111–118.

Simpson, N. S., Banks, S., & Dinges, D. F. (2010). Sleep restriction Is associated with increased morning plasma leptin concentrations, especially in women. *Biological Research For Nursing*, *12*(1), 47–53. doi: 10.1177/1099800410366301

Sitnick, S. L., Goodlin-Jones, B. L., & Anders, T. F. (2008). The use of actigraphy to study sleep disorders in preschoolers: some concerns about detection of nighttime awakenings. *Sleep 31*(3), 395–401.

Song, C., Zhang, R., Wang, C., Fu, R., Song, W., Dou, K., & Wang, S. (2021). Sleep quality and risk of cancer: findings from the English longitudinal study of aging. *Sleep*, *44*(3), zsaa192. doi: 10.1093/sleep/zsaa192

Spaeth, A. M., Dinges, D. F., & Goel, N. (2013). Effects of experimental sleep restriction on weight gain, caloric intake, and meal timing in healthy adults. *Sleep*, *36*(7), 981–990. doi: 0.5665/sleep.2792

Spaeth, A. M., Dinges, D. F., & Goel, N. (2014). Sex and race differences in caloric intake during sleep restriction in healthy adults. *Am J Clin Nutr*, *100*(2), 559–566. doi: 10.3945/ajcn.114.086579

Spaeth, A. M., Hawley, N. L., Raynor, H. A., Jelalian, E., Greer, A., Crouter, S. E., ... Hart, C. N. (2019). Sleep, energy balance, and meal timing in school-aged children. *Sleep Med*, *60*, 139–144. doi:10.1016/j.sleep.2019.02.003

Spiegel, K., Knutson, K., Leproult, R., Tasali, E., & Van Cauter, E. (2005). Sleep loss: a novel risk factor for insulin resistance and Type 2 diabetes. *J Appl Physiol*, *99*(5), 2008–2019. doi: 10.1152/japplphysiol.00660.2005

Spiegel, K., Leproult, R., L'Hermite-Balériaux, M., Copinschi, G., Penev, P. D., & Van Cauter, E. (2004). Leptin levels are dependent on sleep duration: relationships with sympathovagal balance, carbohydrate regulation, cortisol, and thyrotropin. *J Clin Endocr Metab*, *89*(11), 5762–5771. doi: 10.1210/jc.2004-1003

Spiegel, K., Leproult, R., & Vancauter, E. (1999). Impact of sleep debt on metabolic and endocrine function. *Lancet*, *354*(9188), 1435–1439. doi: 10.1016/s0140-6736(99)01376-8

Spiegel, K., Sheridan, J. F., & Van Cauter, E. (2002). Effect of sleep deprivation on response to immunization. *JAMA*, *288*(12), 1471–1472.

Spiegel, K., Tasali, E., Leproult, R., Scherberg, N., & Van Cauter, E. (2011). Twenty-four-hour profiles of acylated and total ghrelin: relationship with glucose levels and impact of time of day and sleep. *J Clin Endocrinol Metab*, *96*(2), 486–493. doi: 10.1210/jc.2010-1978

Spiegel, K., Tasali, E., Penev, P., & Van Cauter, E. (2004). Brief communication: Sleep curtailment in healthy young men is associated with decreased leptin levels, elevated ghrelin levels, and increased hunger and appetite. *Ann Intern Med*, *141*(11), 846–850.

Spruyt, K., Molfese, D. L., & Gozal, D. (2011). Sleep duration, sleep regularity, body weight, and metabolic homeostasis in school-aged children. *Pediatrics*, *127*(2), e345–352. doi: 10.1542/peds.2010-0497

Srivali, N., Thongprayoon, C., Tangpanithandee, S., Krisanapan, P., Mao, M. A., Zinchuk, A., ... Cheungpasitporn, W. (2023). Periodic limb movements during sleep and risk of hypertension: a systematic review. *Sleep Med*, *102*, 173–179. doi: 10.1016/j.sleep.2023.01.008

St-Onge, M. P. (2013). The role of sleep duration in the regulation of energy balance: effects on energy intakes and expenditure. *J Clin Sleep Med*, *9*(1), 73–80. doi: 10.5664/jcsm.2348

St-Onge, M. P. (2017). Sleep-obesity relation: underlying mechanisms and consequences for treatment. *Obes Rev*, *18 Suppl 1*, 34–39. doi: 10.1111/obr.12499

St-Onge, M.-P., O'Keeffe, M., Roberts, A. L., RoyChoudhury, A., & Laferrère, B. (2012). Short sleep duration, glucose dysregulation and hormonal regulation of appetite in men and women. *Sleep*, *35*(11), 1503–1510. doi: 10.5665/sleep.2198

Staplin, N., de la Sierra, A., Ruilope, L. M., Emberson, J. R., Vinyoles, E., Gorostidi, M., ... Williams, B. (2023). Relationship between clinic and ambulatory blood pressure and mortality: an observational cohort study in 59 124 patients. *Lancet*, *401*, 2041–2050. doi: 10.1016/S0140-6736(23)00733-X

Stessman, J., Jacobs, J. M., Ein-Mor, E., & Bursztyn, M. (2009). Normal body mass index rather than obesity predicts greater mortality in elderly people: the Jerusalem longitudinal study. *J Am Geriatr Soc*, *57*(12), 2232–2238. doi: 10.1111/j.1532-5415.2009.02567.x

Stranges, S., Cappuccio, F. P., Kandala, N. B., Miller, M. A., Taggart, F. M., Kumari, M., ... Marmot, M. G. (2008). Cross-sectional versus prospective associations of sleep duration with changes in relative weight and body fat distribution: the Whitehall II Study. *Am J Epidemiol*, *167*(3), 321–329. doi: 10.1093/aje/kwm302

Sun, Y., Yu, X., Liu, J., Zhou, N., Chen, L., Zhao, Y., ... Cui, L. (2016). Effect of bedtime administration of blood-pressure lowering agents on ambulatory blood pressure monitoring results: a meta-analysis. *Cardiol J*, *23*(4), 473–481. doi: 10.5603/CJ.a2016.0027

Taheri, S., Lin, L., Austin, D., Young, T., & Mignot, E. (2004). Short sleep duration is associated with reduced leptin, elevated ghrelin, and increased body mass index. *PLoS Med*, *1*(3), e62. doi: 10.1371/journal.pmed.0010062

Tasali, E., Leproult, R., Ehrmann, D. A., & Van Cauter, E. (2008). Slow-wave sleep and the risk of type 2 diabetes in humans. *Proc Natl Acad Sci USA*, *105*(3), 1044–1049. doi: 10.1073/pnas.0706446105

Taveras, E. M., Gillman, M. W., Pena, M. M., Redline, S., & Rifas-Shiman, S. L. (2014). Chronic sleep curtailment and adiposity. *Pediatrics*, *133*(6), 1013–1022. doi: 10.1542/peds.2013-3065

Tran, K. B., Lang, J. J., Compton, K., Xu, R., Acheson, A. R., Henrikson, H. J., ... Murray, C. J. L. (2022). The global burden of cancer attributable to risk factors, 2010–19: a systematic analysis for the Global Burden of Disease Study 2019. *Lancet*, *400*(10352), 563–591. doi: 10.1016/s0140-6736(22)01438-6

Turgeon, R. D., Althouse, A. D., Cohen, J. B., Enache, B., Hogenesch, J. B., Johansen, M. E., ... Hiremath, S. (2021). Lowering nighttime blood pressure with bedtime dosing of antihypertensive medications: controversies in hypertension - con side of the argument. *Hypertension*, *78*(3), 871–878. doi: 10.1161/HYPERTENSIONAHA.121.16501

Unruh, M. L., Redline, S., An, M. W., Buysse, D. J., Nieto, F. J., Yeh, J. L., & Newman, A. B. (2008). Subjective and objective sleep quality and aging in the Sleep Heart Health Study. *J Am Geriatr Soc*, *56*(7), 1218–1227. doi: 10.1111/j.1532-5415.2008.01755.x

Uzu, T., & Kimura, G. (1999). Diuretics shift circadian rhythm of blood pressure from nondipper to dipper in essential hypertension. *Circulation*, *100*(15), 1635–1638.

Vaccaro, A., Kaplan Dor, Y., Nambara, K., Pollina, E. A., Lin, C., Greenberg, M. E., & Rogulja, D. (2020). Sleep loss can cause death through accumulation of reactive oxygen species in the gut. *Cell*, *181*(6), 1307–1328. doi: 10.1016/j.cell.2020.04.049

Valko, P. O., Hunziker, S., Graf, K., Werth, E., & Baumann, C. R. (2021). Sleep-wake misperception: a comprehensive analysis of a large sleep lab cohort. *Sleep Med*, *88*, 96–103. doi: 10.1016/j.sleep.2021.10.023

Van Den Berg, J. F., Van Rooij, F. J., Vos, H., Tulen, J. H., Hofman, A., Miedema, H. M., ... Tiemeier, H. (2008). Disagreement between subjective and actigraphic measures of sleep duration in a population-based study of elderly persons. *J Sleep Res*, *17*(3), 295–302. doi: 10.1111/j.1365-2869.2008.00638.x

Verdecchia, P. (2000). Prognostic value of ambulatory blood pressure: current evidence and clinical implications. *Hypertension*, *35*(3), 844–851. doi: 10.1161/01.hyp.35.3.844

Veronese, N., Cereda, E., Solmi, M., Fowler, S. A., Manzato, E., Maggi, S., ... Correll, C. U. (2015). Inverse relationship between body mass index and mortality in older nursing home residents: a meta-analysis of 19,538 elderly subjects. *Obes Rev, 16*(11), 1001–1015. doi: 10.1111/obr.12309

Vgontzas, A. N., Fernandez-Mendoza, J., Liao, D., & Bixler, E. O. (2013). Insomnia with objective short sleep duration: the most biologically severe phenotype of the disorder. *Sleep Med Rev, 17*(4), 241–254. doi: 10.1016/j.smrv.2012.09.005

Vgontzas, A. N., Fernandez-Mendoza, J., Miksiewicz, T., Kritikou, I., Shaffer, M. L., Liao, D., ... Bixler, E. O. (2014). Unveiling the longitudinal association between short sleep duration and the incidence of obesity: the Penn State Cohort. *Int J Obes (Lond), 38*(6), 825–832. doi: 10.1038/ijo.2013.172

Vgontzas, A. N., Liao, D., Bixler, E. O., Chrousos, G. P., & Vela-Bueno, A. (2009). Insomnia with objective short sleep duration is associated with a high risk of hypertension. *Sleep, 32*(4), 491–497.

Vgontzas, A. N., Zoumakis, E., Bixler, E. O., Lin, H. M., Follett, H., Kales, A., & Chrousos, G. P. (2004). Adverse effects of modest sleep restriction on sleepiness, performance, and inflammatory cytokines. *J Clin Endocrinol Metab, 89*(5), 2119–2126. doi: 10.1210/jc.2003-031562

Vidafar, P., Gooley, J. J., Burns, A. C., Rajaratnam, S. M. W., Rueger, M., Van Reen, E., ... Cain, S. W. (2018). Increased vulnerability to attentional failure during acute sleep deprivation in women depends on menstrual phase. *Sleep, 41*(8), zsy098. doi:10.1093/sleep/zsy098

Vujovic, N., Piron, M. J., Qian, J., Chellappa, S. L., Nedeltcheva, A., Barr, D., ... Scheer, F. A. J. L. (2022). Late isocaloric eating increases hunger, decreases energy expenditure, and modifies metabolic pathways in adults with overweight and obesity. *Cell Metab, 34*(10), 1486–1498 e1487. doi: 10.1016/j.cmet.2022.09.007

Waldon, J., Begum, E., Gendron, M., Rusak, B., Andreou, P., Rajda, M., & Corkum, P. (2016). Concordance of actigraphy with polysomnography in children with and without attention-deficit/hyperactivity disorder. *J Sleep Res, 25*(5), 524–533. doi: 10.1111/jsr.12402

Wang, M., Flexeder, C., Kilanowski, A., Kress, S., Herberth, G., Schikowski, T., ... Standl, M. (2023). Changes in sleep duration and sleep difficulties from adolescence to young adulthood and the risk of obesity: bidirectional evidence in the GINIplus and LISA studies. *Sleep Med, 101*, 401–410. doi: 10.1016/j.sleep.2022.11.031

Whinnery, J., Jackson, N., Rattanaumpawan, P., & Grandner, M. A. (2014). Short and long sleep duration associated with race/ethnicity, sociodemographics, and socioeconomic position. *Sleep, 37*(3), 601–611. doi: 10.5665/sleep.3508

WHO. (2020). Obesity and overweight. Retrieved July 15, 2020, from https://www.who.int/news-room/fact-sheets/detail/obesity-and-overweight

Wilson, A. M., Ryan, M. C., & Boyle, A. J. (2006). The novel role of C-reactive protein in cardiovascular disease: risk marker or pathogen. *Int J Cardiol, 106*(3), 291–297. doi: 10.1016/j.ijcard.2005.01.068

Wood, B., Rea, M. S., Plitnick, B., & Figueiro, M. G. (2013). Light level and duration of exposure determine the impact of self-luminous tablets on melatonin suppression. *Appl Ergon, 44*(2), 237–240. doi: 10.1016/j.apergo.2012.07.008

Wren, A. M., Seal, L. J., Cohen, M. A., Brynes, A. E., Frost, G. S., Murphy, K. G., ... Bloom, S. R. (2001). Ghrelin enhances appetite and increases food intake in humans. *J Clin Endocr Metab, 86*(12), 5992–5995.

Wunder, D. M., Yared, M., Bersinger, N. A., Widmer, D., Kretschmer, R., & Birkhauser, M. H. (2006). Serum leptin and C-reactive protein levels in the physiological spontaneous menstrual cycle in reproductive age women. *Eur J Endocrinol, 155*(1), 137–142. doi: 10.1530/eje.1.02178

Xia, C., & Møller, A. P. (2018). Long-lived birds suffer less from oxidative stress. *Avian Res, 9*, 41. doi:10.1186/s40657-018-0133-6

Xiao, Q., Arem, H., Moore, S. C., Hollenbeck, A. R., & Matthews, C. E. (2013). A large prospective investigation of sleep duration, weight change, and obesity in the NIH-AARP Diet and Health Study cohort. *Am J Epidemiol, 178*(11), 1600–1610. doi: 10.1093/aje/kwt180

Xie, J., Zhu, M., Ji, M., Fan, J., Huang, Y., Wei, X., ... Shen, H. (2021). Relationships between sleep traits and lung cancer risk: a prospective cohort study in UK Biobank. *Sleep, 44*(9), zsab089. doi:10.1093/sleep/zsab089

Xing, Z., Gauldie, J., Cox, G., Baumann, H., Jordana, M., Lei, X.-F., & Achong, M. K. (1998). IL-6 is an antiinflammatory cytokine required for controlling local or systemic acute inflammatory responses. *J Clin Invest, 101*, 301–320.

Yaggi, H. K., Araujo, A. B., & McKinlay, J. B. (2006). Sleep duration as a risk factor for the development of type 2 diabetes. *Diabetes Care, 29*(3), 657–661.

Yang, W., Reynolds, K., Gu, D., Chen, J., & He, J. (2007). A comparison of two proposed definitions for metabolic syndrome in the Chinese adult population. *Am J Med Sci, 334*(3), 184–189.

Yang, W. Y., Melgarejo, J. D., Thijs, L., Zhang, Z. Y., Boggia, J., Wei, F. F., ... International Database on Ambulatory Blood Pressure in Relation to Cardiovascular Outcomes, I. (2019). Association of office and ambulatory blood pressure with mortality and cardiovascular outcomes. *JAMA, 322*(5), 409–420. doi: 10.1001/jama.2019.9811

Zant, J. C., Leenaars, C. H., Kostin, A., Van Someren, E. J., & Porkka-Heiskanen, T. (2011). Increases in extracellular serotonin and dopamine metabolite levels in the basal forebrain during sleep deprivation. *Brain Res, 1399*, 40–48. doi: 10.1016/j.brainres.2011.05.008

Zhang, K. P., Buxton, M., Rodriguez-Carmona, Y., Peterson, K. E., Liu, Y., Burgess, H. J., ... Jansen, E. C. (2022). Duration, timing, and consistency of sleep in relation to inflammatory cytokines in Mexican adolescents. *Sleep Med, 100*, 103–111. doi: 10.1016/j.sleep.2022.08.007

Zhou, Q., Wu, X., Zhang, D., Liu, L., Wang, J., Cheng, R., ... Hu, F. (2020). Age and sex differences in the association between sleep duration and general and abdominal obesity at 6-year follow-up: the rural Chinese cohort study. *Sleep Med, 69*, 71–77. doi: 10.1016/j.sleep.2019.12.025

Zhu, B., Shi, C., Park, C. G., Zhao, X., & Reutrakul, S. (2019). Effects of sleep restriction on metabolism-related parameters in healthy adults: a comprehensive review and meta-analysis of randomized controlled trials. *Sleep Med Rev, 45*, 18–30. doi: 10.1016/j.smrv.2019.02.002

CHAPTER 15

Sleep and Human Health, Part B

15.1 OVERVIEW

This chapter continues the discussion of how sleep duration and quality are related to human health, with a focus on conditions with major behavioral, emotional, and cognitive features. It addresses how sleep is related to the experience of pain and of several major psychiatric conditions, including anxiety disorders, depression, bipolar disorder, and schizophrenia. It discusses whether changes in sleep are only symptoms of these illnesses or also contribute to their development and maintenance. It reviews the relations between sleep and the risk of development of neurodegenerative conditions, especially Alzheimer's disease, and of early death. It discusses how the results of experimental research related to these topics can be linked to findings from population-based observational research. Finally, this chapter considers how we can interpret evidence from some studies that both short and long sleep are related to increased disease and mortality risk.

15.2 Sleep and pain

Pain is a complex physiological/behavioral phenomenon. It is usually caused by tissue damage from injury or disease, but people also experience pain in the absence of such damage. Examples include tension headaches, intense pain in response to light touch in patients with shingles,[1] and phantom limb pain that is perceived as coming from a missing limb. People may also not report experiencing pain despite serious injury under extreme, stressful conditions, such as during a battle or following a serious accident. Similarly, acute exposure to a stressor can reduce pain sensitivity in animals (Sorge et al., 2014) and people (Le Bars, 2002). These variations in the experience of pain are the result of processes occurring in peripheral sensory nerves, the spinal cord, and the brain that can moderate, intensify, or even create the experience of pain, often independently of the extent of tissue damage (Mendell, 2014).

Chronic pain is closely linked to disturbed sleep. One estimate is that 67–88% of patients with chronic pain disorders also have sleep complaints; conversely, at least 50% of insomnia patients also experience chronic pain (Finan et al., 2013). An obvious interpretation would be that chronic pain is the driver of this relationship because it prevents people from sleeping well. But there is also evidence from observational and experimental studies for the opposite effect: that sleep loss contributes to pain sensitivity.

For example, patients with fibromyalgia[2] or burn injuries reported that days with more pain were followed by more disrupted sleep, and that nights of poor sleep were followed by days with more severe pain (Affleck et al., 1996; Raymond et al., 2001). High variability in total sleep amounts reported in 2 weeks of daily diaries were associated with more reports of pain, depression, and other conditions (Slavish et al., 2019). Other correlational studies also found that sleep quality and/or duration at night predicted next-day pain experience in people with various painful conditions (Edwards et al., 2008; Lewandowski et al., 2010; Tang et al., 2012). In some of these studies, there was surprisingly little evidence supporting the intuitively more obvious correlation: between daytime pain levels and the quality of sleep during the following night.

[1] Shingles is a skin rash that results from previous infection by the *Varicella zoster* virus. This virus causes chicken pox in childhood and then remains in nerves innervating the skin for the rest of one's life. After decades of being dormant, the virus can be reactivated in adulthood and produce the symptoms of shingles. These include the experience of sometimes extreme pain in response to light contact with the affected skin areas.

[2] Fibromyalgia is a fairly common condition characterized by widespread musculoskeletal pain persisting for many months, painful responses to gentle touch on certain trigger points, unrefreshing sleep, fatigue, and disturbances of mood and memory (Boissevain & McCain, 1991). These symptoms partially overlap those of depression (depressed mood, lack of energy, and memory and sleep problems). As a result, there have been arguments about whether this syndrome is a form of depression that includes body pain symptoms, or whether the mood, memory, and sleep complaints are instead a predictable consequence of suffering chronically from debilitating pain and fatigue that lack an identified cause or effective treatment.

Studies that included polysomnogram (PSG) recordings suggested that the amount and/or quality of slow-wave sleep (SWS) was an important predictor of next-day pain. Older people who had shorter total sleep times reported more moderate to severe pain over the preceding weeks, and less SWS in male participants was significantly correlated with more reported pain (Weingarten et al., 2016). This finding is consistent with findings in an early study that bursts of alpha EEG activity that intruded on SWS ("alpha-delta sleep") were associated with increased pain reports by patients with fibromyalgia (Moldofsky et al., 1975). However, alpha-delta sleep does not appear to be specific to this condition, and not all fibromyalgia patients show this EEG pattern; see discussion in Older et al., 1998. It is unclear whether these EEG features are partial arousals or mixed states caused by episodes of pain, or whether they contribute to pain by disrupting SWS, thereby reducing its benefits.

The effects of experimental manipulations of sleep support the proposal based on observational studies that sleep loss alters pain sensitivity. An early study in Nathaniel Kleitman's laboratory demonstrated that 60 h of sleep deprivation caused increased sensitivity (hyperalgesia) in people to experimental application of painful stimuli, without an increase in sensitivity to light touch. These results indicated that sleep loss had a specific effect on the experience of pain rather than on general skin sensitivity (Cooperman et al., 1934). Other studies confirmed that sensitivity to pain evoked by pressure, electrical, or thermal stimulation increased after acute partial or complete sleep deprivation (Matre et al., 2015; Onen et al., 2001; Ødegard et al., 2015) or chronic restriction to 4 h time in bed (TIB) for 8 days (Haack et al., 2007).

Based on the observation of abnormal EEG patterns during SWS in patients with fibromyalgia (Moldofsky et al., 1975), healthy control participants were selectively deprived of either SWS or REM sleep overnight. Deprivation of SWS, but not of REM sleep, resulted in next-day hyperalgesia (Moldofsky & Scarisbrick, 1976). Similarly, 3 successive nights of selective SWS deprivation resulted in lower pain thresholds in middle-aged women (Lentz et al., 1999). In another study, the degree of analgesia (reduced pain sensitivity) for mechanical pain was significantly correlated with how much SWS was regained during recovery sleep after combined total and selective SWS deprivation (Onen et al., 2001).

Another study compared the effects of two methods of reducing sleep amounts by 50% over 3 nights. One group was allowed to sleep for half their usual duration in a single block of time, which preserved total SWS amounts at the expense of N2 and REM sleep (see Section 5.4.2). The other group was exposed to repeated forced awakenings to reduce their total sleep duration by similar amounts; they showed a significant reduction in SWS on the first night and increases in N1 sleep over the 3 nights. Pain reports and induced analgesia were unaffected by reducing sleep by 50% in a single block with preserved N3 sleep amounts. However, repeated sleep disruption caused increases in pain reports and impaired analgesia[3] (Smith et al., 2007). These effects appeared to result from acute reductions in SWS and chronic increases in N1 sleep. Repeated cycles of 3 nights of sleep disruption over a 2-week period also impaired induced analgesia in healthy, young women participants but not significantly in men (Haack et al., 2023).

Sleep stages other than SWS have also been implicated in regulating pain sensitivity. In one study, reducing total sleep amounts in people increased thermal pain sensitivity, as did selective reductions of REM sleep, but not of NREM (mostly N2) sleep (Roehrs et al., 2006). Similarly, most studies of selective sleep deprivation in animal models have concluded that loss of REM sleep is responsible for inducing hyperalgesia (Lautenbacher et al., 2006).

Differences between the results of most human and animal studies may be related to the fact that most human studies involve pain that is produced by mechanical pressure. Many animal studies, however, and the selective REM sleep reduction study in people (Roehrs et al., 2006), produced pain using heat. The pain modulatory outputs from the brain to the spinal cord generally have a greater impact on mechanical than thermal pain sensitivity. It is these descending signals from the brain to the spinal cord, and therefore sensitivity to mechanically induced pain, that appear to be most affected by reductions in SWS (Lautenbacher et al., 2006).

The conclusion that sleep duration/quality regulates pain sensitivity is strengthened by evidence that increasing sleep can reduce pain. A study of healthy young adults selected those with unusually short sleep-onset latencies during Multiple Sleep Latency Tests (MSLTs; see Section 2.7). This increased daytime sleepiness likely reflects a chronic sleep debt. After baseline pain sensitivity testing, some participants were allowed extended TIB (10 h) for 4 nights, while others slept their usual amounts, and both were then retested. The more participants increased their sleep durations during the nights between tests, the less sleepy they were during the day, and the less sensitive they were to painful stimuli. Thus, reducing an apparent, chronic sleep debt also reduced pain sensitivity (Roehrs et al., 2012) (**Figure 15.1**). Sleep extension in healthy young people by ~2 h nightly for 5 nights also produced analgesia, in this case by increasing maximum pain tolerance without altering pain thresholds (Simonelli et al., 2019).

[3] The analgesia-inducing procedure used in this study involved immersing one hand in ice-cold water, thereby triggering activity in descending inhibitory projections to pain-responsive neurons in the spinal cord. This procedure results in a 20–30% reduction in acute sensitivity to a painful pressure stimulus applied to the contralateral limb (Le Bars, 2002).

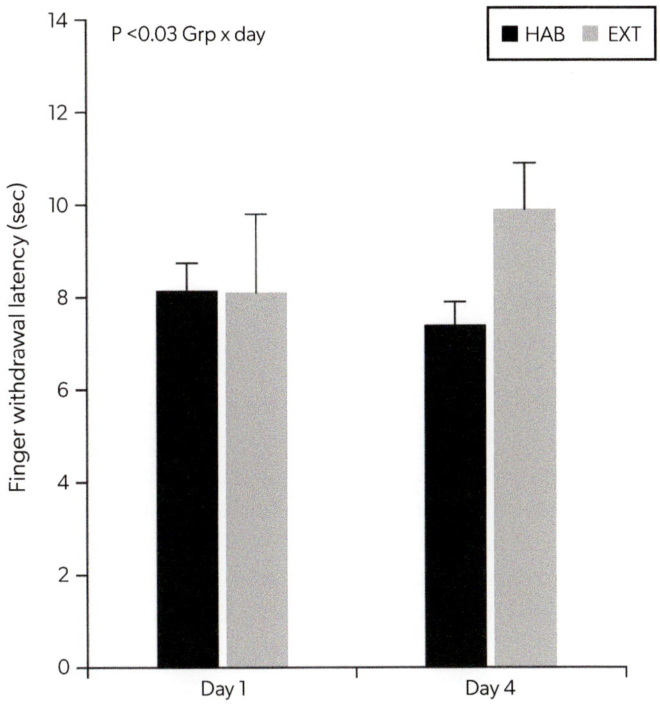

Figure 15.1 Effects of several nights of sleep extension on participants who had short sleep-onset latencies during MSLTs at baseline (implying unsatisfied sleep need). Both groups showed similar latencies to withdraw a finger from a hot stimulus (Finger Withdrawal Latency, Y axis) at baseline (Day 1). But unlike the control group with habitual sleep durations (HAB, black columns), those allowed extended time in bed (10 h) over 4 nights (EXT, gray columns) showed a significantly longer finger-withdrawal latency (Day 4). The resulting significant ($p < 0.03$) group X day interaction indicated that the extra sleep significantly reduced pain sensitivity. The extended sleep group increased average nightly sleep durations by ~1.8 h. Reprinted with permission of Oxford University Press from Roehrs, T.A. et al. (2012) Pain sensitivity and recovery from mild chronic sleep loss. *Sleep* 35:1667–1672. © Sleep Research Society (2012). doi: 10.5665/sleep.2240.

Other approaches to enhancing sleep quality or duration have included both non-drug treatments for insomnia (e.g., CBT-I)[4] and drug treatments. A meta-analysis of how non-drug treatments for sleep problems affect patients with various chronic pain conditions concluded that these treatments produced substantial improvements in sleep, moderate reductions in fatigue, and small reductions in self-reported pain (Tang et al., 2015).

A pharmacological approach was used to enhance sleep in women with fibromyalgia. They were treated with sodium oxybate, a commercial form of γ-hydroxybutyrate (GHB).[5] Compared to placebo controls, treated patients had increased SWS amounts at night; during the next day, they experienced less pain sensitivity at typical fibromyalgia pressure points. They also self-reported significantly less spontaneous pain and fatigue (Scharf et al., 2003). It is unlikely that effects on next-day pain of GHB at night represented a direct drug effect on pain sensitivity because GHB has a very short half-life. Thus, the effects of treatments on pain sensitivity were likely mediated by improved sleep, especially increased SWS.

The mechanisms linking poor sleep to increased pain are uncertain, but one possibility is the involvement of inflammatory responses (McMahon et al., 2015). As discussed in Section 14.9, chronic short sleep is associated with increases in markers of chronic inflammation (Mullington et al., 2010). In a study of the effects of chronic sleep restriction on young men and women, increases in subjective pain reports were strongly correlated with higher levels of the pro-inflammatory cytokine IL-6 (Haack et al., 2007) (**Figure 15.2**). In a study involving recurring disrupted and shortened sleep over a 2-week period, the cyclooxygenase system that produces inflammatory prostaglandins was activated in healthy young men, but not in women (Haack et al., 2023). These findings provide preliminary evidence suggesting that changes in immune system activity may mediate some effects of inadequate sleep on pain sensitivity, at least in men.

15.2.1 Summary

Sleep disruption and short sleep (less commonly, long sleep) are associated with increased sensitivity to experimentally generated pain and increased general complaints of pain. Poor quality sleep and the experience of pain are reciprocally related, so that sleep disturbance often predicts increased pain the following day.

A role for SWS in modulating pain was implied by evidence for abnormal alpha-delta patterns during SWS in some fibromyalgia patients. It was also supported by evidence for increased pain sensitivity after selective deprivation of SWS, but not REM sleep, and the opposite effect on pain sensitivity of the robust recovery of SWS after deprivation. But some human and many animal studies also found that REM sleep loss increased pain sensitivity. These different conclusions may in some cases be related to the species being studied but may also be influenced by the kind of pain stimulus used. Most

[4] Cognitive Behavioral Therapy for Insomnia (CBT-I) involves several psychological treatment approaches aimed at reducing the behavioral, cognitive, and environmental factors that sustain chronic insomnia symptoms (Edinger & Means, 2005; Morin, 1993).

[5] GHB can be prescribed to treat narcolepsy symptoms, especially daytime sleepiness; see Section 11.3.4. It is taken at night to improve sleep consolidation, increase N3 sleep, and reduce daytime sleepiness (Black et al., 2009; Dauvilliers et al., 2017); the mechanism underlying its effectiveness in treating narcolepsy remains uncertain (Kilduff, 2023).

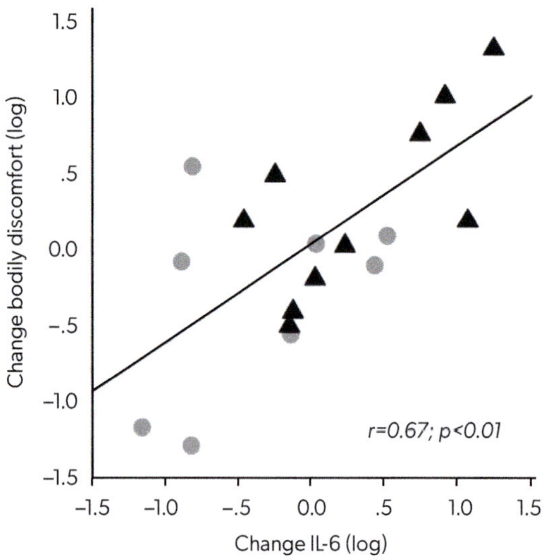

Figure 15.2 One group of women were allowed 4 h time in bed (TIB) for 10 nights (triangles; ~50% reduction in sleep) and another were maintained on 8 h TIB for the same duration (circles). There was a robust positive correlation between changes in blood levels of the cytokine interleukin (IL)-6 (X axis) and changes in bodily discomfort (Y axis). Those with 4 h TIB tended to show increased IL-6 levels, while those with 8 h TIB mostly showed decreases, probably as a result of their stable sleep durations and adherence to other aspects of the study protocol. Although sleep restriction was also associated with increased fatigue/tiredness ratings, the correlation between higher IL-6 levels and increased bodily discomfort remained significant after controlling for fatigue ratings. Reprinted with permission of Oxford University Press from Haack, M. et al. Elevated inflammatory markers in response to prolonged sleep restriction are associated with increased pain experience in healthy volunteers. *Sleep* 30(9):1145–1152, 2007. © Sleep Research Society (2012). doi: 10.1093/sleep/30.9.1145.

human studies used mechanical pain, but thermal pain was used in most animal studies. Studies in both animals and people that used thermal pain found effects of REM sleep deprivation. SWS appeared to be more involved in regulating mechanical pain, which may be more influenced by cortical modulation than other kinds of pain.

Increasing sleep amounts in those with inadequate sleep can improve pain symptoms. Improving or lengthening sleep with non-drug treatments or extending TIB in those with evidence of a habitual sleep debt, reduced pain sensitivity. Treatment with GHB, which increased SWS amounts and helped maintain sleep, also reduced pain in fibromyalgia patients.

How sleep loss increases pain sensitivity is not well understood, but correlational evidence and some experimental results suggest a role for chronic activation of inflammatory immune system components as a result of inadequate sleep. Other evidence supports a role for sleep in supporting neural modulation of acquired analgesia. Some preliminary results suggest possible gender differences in the degree to which immune system activity or cortical modulation mediate sleep effects on pain.

15.3 Sleep, anxiety, and mood disorders

The links between sleep and many psychiatric disorders were recognized because disrupted or unusually short or long sleep are often obvious features of these conditions, and for some disorders are recognized as core symptoms of the condition (Boivin, 2000). These observations led to studies that investigated whether sleep problems are not only symptoms but also perpetuate, or predict, the emergence of psychiatric disorders. Although the discussion of these linkages is organized around psychiatric diagnoses, it should be recognized that sleep disturbance is a transdiagnostic symptom and that many patients have complex diagnoses, for example, comorbid depression and anxiety or psychosis with depression/mania (schizoaffective disorder).

15.3.1 Anxiety disorders

Among the most common psychiatric conditions globally are anxiety disorders (Baxter et al., 2013). There are many recognized subtypes of anxiety disorders, but the most common include generalized anxiety disorder (GAD), panic disorder (PD), and post-traumatic stress disorder (PTSD) (which is not currently classified as an anxiety disorder but has strong anxiety components). In addition, anxiety is often a prominent feature of other psychiatric disorders, especially major depression. For GAD, PTSD, and depression, sleep disturbance is common enough to be included among their diagnostic criteria (Breslau et al., 1996).

One review identified three key sleep features that characterize anxiety disorders: decreased total sleep time, increased sleep-onset latency, and more wake episodes interrupting sleep, which together result in reduced sleep efficiency (Benca et al., 1992). In addition to these objective features, anxiety is associated with subjective insomnia symptoms, including self-reports of poor sleep quality, unrefreshing sleep, and daytime sleepiness. These features are also often seen in patients with depression, but their occurrence in anxiety disorders is independent of the presence of comorbid depression (Cox & Olatunji, 2020).

Extended periods of waking before sleep onset and during sleep interruptions are often filled with rumination (repetitive thoughts about negative past or current events), worry about future events, hopelessness, and distress. Persistent rumination may be linked to evidence supporting the idea that cortical hyperarousal contributes to both nighttime sleep disturbances and daytime anxiety symptoms (Richards et al., 2020).

Distressing thoughts and the cortical arousal associated with them are likely to disturb sleep, but decreased and disrupted sleep may also contribute to the development and maintenance of anxiety disorders. For example, the presence of insomnia symptoms predicted an elevated lifetime risk of developing an anxiety disorder (Breslau et al., 1996). A study of Australian adults with no diagnosis at baseline also found increased risk for a diagnosis of GAD or PD within 4 years among those who reported sleep disturbances. The presence of rumination and specific personality features partially mediated the link between disturbed sleep and development of an anxiety disorder, but the link with sleep disturbances remained significant after accounting for these variables (Batterham et al., 2012). In PTSD patients, waking from frightening nightmares may increase anxiety. This anxiety can then become associated with sleep itself, further promoting insomnia symptoms and reducing sleep quality (Richards et al., 2020). Thus, sleep disturbances and anxiety are often reciprocally causally related.

Treatment studies further reinforce this conclusion. One study involved CBT that was focused on treatment of anxiety symptoms in patients with GAD. It found that the anxiety treatment reduced self-reported insomnia symptoms, even though treatments were not directed specifically at sleep problems (Bélanger et al., 2004). Conversely, internet-based CBT for insomnia (CBT-I) in patients with GAD reduced insomnia symptoms as intended, but also reduced anxiety symptoms as effectively as a treatment aimed specifically at anxiety (Mason et al., 2023). A meta-analysis of studies in which CBT-I was given to patients who also had coexisting anxiety confirmed that specific treatment of insomnia symptoms produced significant reductions in levels of anxiety (Belleville et al., 2011).

15.3.2 Depression

Major (unipolar) depressive disorder involves sustained negative mood, reduced energy, rumination, sleep problems, and loss of enjoyment of previously pleasurable activities, among other symptoms (Kaplan & Harvey, 2009; Lorenzo-Luaces et al., 2021). Those diagnosed with major depression typically report insomnia symptoms, such as difficulty falling asleep, frequent arousals, and inability to return to sleep after early morning waking, resulting in reduced sleep amounts. Among seven commonly used scales for measuring depression, all include insomnia features as diagnostic symptoms, and three also include excessive sleep (hypersomnia) (Fried et al., 2022). In some studies, sleep symptoms similar to those associated with depression persisted even after remission from a depressive episode (Harvey, 2011).

In comparison to those with only depression or anxiety, those with comorbid anxiety and depression had the highest insomnia scores and shortest reported sleep durations, although a proportion of patients also reported very long sleep durations (van Mill et al., 2010). The latter group included, but were not limited to, those diagnosed with seasonal affective disorder (SAD), who often report hypersomnia during winter (Rosenthal et al., 1984). Self-reports of long sleep in depression (and other conditions) should be interpreted cautiously. An actigraphic study reported small increases in sleep duration in winter compared to summer among patients with SAD, but not as large as indicated by self-report, and total sleep time did not differ significantly from that of controls (Wescott et al., 2023). Some self-reports of long sleep may include hours spent in bed trying to sleep but with less actual sleep time because of long sleep-onset latencies, frequent arousals, and difficulty returning to sleep.

Many clinicians, however, recognize a subtype of depression that includes "atypical" features such as hypersomnia, lethargy, overeating, and a chronic course of illness with early onset (Kaplan & Harvey, 2009; Stewart et al., 2009). Although hypersomnia is usually identified by self-report, one PSG study of sleep in depressed patients with self-reported hypersomnia found significantly longer sleep durations with no increase in the number of arousals during sleep, relative to age- and gender-matched healthy controls (Plante et al., 2017). Thus, self-reports of hypersomnia in some patients do reflect increased sleep amounts. Some estimates suggest that about a quarter of depressed patients meet the criteria for atypical depression, but there is continuing controversy about whether it is a physiologically and clinically distinct subtype; see reviews by Łojko & Rybakowski, 2017; Lorenzo-Luaces et al., 2021.

PSG studies of most patients with typical major depression find substantial changes in sleep. These include earlier onsets of REM sleep during the sleep period, shorter total sleep durations, increased amounts of REM sleep as a proportion of the shortened time asleep, and reduced SWS amounts (**Figure 15.3**) (Benca et al., 1992; Kupfer, 1976; Nutt et al., 2008).

Some of these sleep symptoms are likely related to the role of serotonin (5-HT) and/or norepinephrine (NE) in regulation of REM sleep. As discussed in Section 10.7.2, onset of REM sleep is triggered by acetylcholine (ACh) and opposed by both 5-HT and NE. Early onset of REM sleep during the sleep period and increased total amounts are both consistent with reduced 5-HT and NE activity, implying functional deficits in these neurotransmitter systems. Consistent with this interpretation, many drugs that are used to treat depression increase 5-HT and/or NE neurotransmission by inhibiting their synaptic reuptake (Wilson & Argyropoulos, 2005). Many antidepressants suppress REM sleep production, especially early in treatment, which is also consistent with the expected effects of increasing 5-HT and

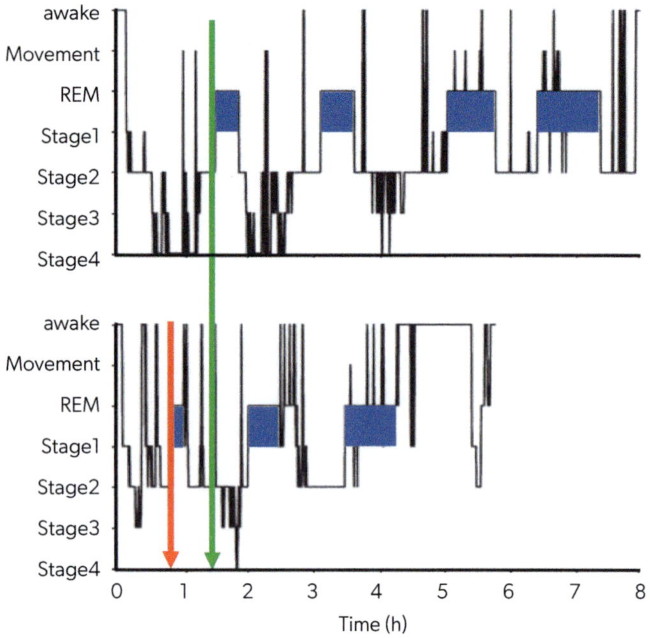

Figure 15.3 Overnight sleep patterns of a healthy control participant (top) and of a patient with major depression (bottom). REM sleep episodes are shown in blue. The onset of the first REM sleep episode in the patient with depression is indicated by the red arrow and the onset of REM sleep in the control participant is indicated by the green arrow. The characteristic features in the depressed patient include early onset of the first REM sleep episode, a higher percentage of REM sleep relative to a reduced total sleep time, more arousals (including a lengthy wake episode after hour 4), a large reduction in the amount of SWS (Stages 3 & 4), and an early morning final arousal ending a shortened sleep period. Adapted with permission of Taylor & Francis Ltd. and Dr. David Nutt from Nutt, D. et al. (2008) Sleep disorders as core symptoms of depression. *Dialogues Clin Neurosci* 10:329–336. © Taylor & Francis Ltd. (2008) (www.tandfonline.com). doi: 10.31887/DCNS.2008.10.3/dnutt.

NE activity; see discussion of the effects of antidepressants in Section 10.5.1.

There is evidence that sleep problems are not only a common symptom of depression but may also contribute causally to the expression of other symptoms. For example, in healthy controls, mimicking the typical pattern of sleep in patients with depression by disrupting sleep continuity resulted in reduced SWS amounts, decreases in positive mood, and increases in negative mood, although not into the clinical range. These effects on mood were greater than those caused by simply reducing the total time available for sleep by an equal amount, and they were mediated by the resulting reduction in the amount of SWS (Finan et al., 2015).

Links between sleep quality and depression also appear in clinical populations. Having insomnia strongly increased the lifetime risk of developing depression (Breslau et al., 1996), and insomnia symptoms or disturbed sleep predicted an increased risk of developing depression over the next four years (Batterham et al., 2012; Szklo-Coxe et al., 2010). In another study, one insomnia symptom (difficulty initiating sleep) predicted increased risk of onset of major depression (Blanken et al., 2020).

Persistent insomnia symptoms *after* successful treatment for depression also predicted worse functional outcomes in the long-term (Li et al., 2012) and an increased risk of relapse into depression (Dombrovski et al., 2008). Among adolescents (12–16 years old), rumination was found to be a significant mediator of the correlation between insomnia and depression symptoms (Li et al., 2023). For adults, both rumination and personality characteristics mediated the link between sleep disturbances and the risk of depression (Batterham et al., 2012).

Another approach to assessing whether disturbed sleep contributes to symptoms of depression is to assess whether reducing sleep problems improves depression. Adding CBT-I to treat insomnia symptoms in depressed patients along with their usual treatments had very potent effects in reducing both insomnia and depression symptoms, even in patients with drug treatment-resistant depression (Manber et al., 2008; Wagley et al., 2013; Watanabe et al., 2011) (**Figure 15.4**). CBT-I

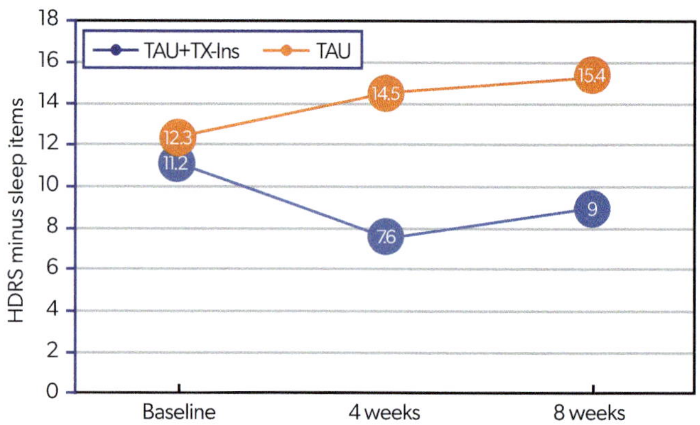

Figure 15.4 GRID-Hamilton Depression Rating Scale (HDRS) scores for two groups of treatment-resistant patients with major depression at baseline, and after 4 weeks and 8 weeks of treatments; higher scores (Y axis) indicate worse depression. Patients either continued to receive their anti-depressant medications as usual (TAU; orange) or also received a brief behavioral intervention (CBT-I) to treat insomnia symptoms (TAU + TX-Ins; blue) between baseline and 8 weeks (X axis). Values shown are group means of HDRS scores with all sleep-related items removed. Depression symptoms in those undergoing only TAU either stayed the same or got worse, while adding the treatment for insomnia symptoms not only improved sleep, but also reduced symptoms of depression, outside of sleep symptoms. In the TAU group, only 6% reached a level indicating remission of depression, while 50% achieved remission in the TAU + TX-Ins group. This figure is based on data published in Watanabe, N. et al. (2011) Brief behavioral therapy for refractory insomnia in residual depression: an assessor-blind, randomized control trial. *J Clin Psychiatry* 72:1651–1658, 2011. doi: 10.4088/JCP.10m06130gry.

given alone to treat insomnia in patients with both insomnia and depression improved their sleep quality and also reduced their depressive symptoms as effectively as an antidepressant (Carney et al., 2017).

In another study, CBT-I alone reduced depressive symptoms in those with depression at baseline and reduced the risk of new onset of depression by ~50% over the following year in those without depression at baseline (Cheng et al., 2019). In adolescents with insomnia symptoms, CBT-I reduced depressive symptoms, and the effect was significantly mediated by reductions in rumination (Li et al., 2023). In older patients with insomnia (average age of ~70), CBT-I was similarly effective in reducing the risk of developing or having a recurrence of depression over a 3-year follow-up period (Irwin et al., 2021).

A meta-analysis of studies in which patients with PTSD were given CBT-I found the anticipated improvement in sleep but also observed improvements in self-reported and clinician-evaluated PTSD symptoms and a more modest reduction in associated depressive symptoms (Ho et al., 2016).

Improvements in depression severity as a result of CBT-I treatment may involve both a direct benefit of cognitive and behavioral changes linked to the treatment components in improving depression symptoms, as well as an indirect effect mediated by reductions in the consequences of sleep-related symptoms (Irwin & Olmstead, 2022; Lin et al., 2022). For example, among patients with insomnia, but without depression, who were treated with CBT-I, the degree of improvement in scores on the Insomnia Severity Index (ISI) was related in part to the extent of reduction in fatigue and generalized anxiety. These are common symptoms shown by patients with insomnia, but also by those with anxiety and depressive disorders (Marway et al., 2023); reductions in fatigue and anxiety symptoms would reduce scores on depression rating scalse.

An analysis of the effects of the dissociative anesthetic ketamine in patients with treatment-resistant depression also points to an important therapeutic role for changes in sleep. Unlike most commonly used antidepressant drugs, which act by increasing 5-HT and/or NE neurotransmission, ketamine blocks a subtype of glutamate receptors, N-methyl-D-aspartate (NMDA) receptors. Intravenous infusions of ketamine have rapid antidepressant and mood-elevating effects (within hours) in many depressed patients (Berman et al., 2000). These benefits may not last beyond a few days, and repeated treatments are often needed to maintain the antidepressant response (Duncan & Zarate, 2013; aan het Rot et al., 2012).

Human clinical and animal model studies both indicated that the effects of ketamine on depression involve an immediate change in glutamatergic neurotransmission, but there are a variety of proposed routes by which these changes might affect mood. One proposed mechanism is that ketamine acts by increasing SWS/SWA and thereby promotes neural plasticity mechanisms that are active during sleep (Alitalo et al., 2021; Duncan & Zarate, 2013; Duncan et al., 2013). In a study using rats, ketamine caused an immediate increase in activity, a delay in onset of REM sleep, and increased SWA during NREM sleep (Wang et al., 2023). These changes are the opposite of the sleep features seen in depression: earlier onset of REM sleep and decreased SWS; see **Figure 15.3**. A study of the mediators of treatment effects of ketamine in patients with treatment-resistant depression found that benefits for depression symptoms and suicidality were mediated in part by improvements in self-reported sleep symptoms, which included insomnia symptoms, reduced total sleep amounts, nighttime restlessness, and early morning awakening (Rodrigues et al., 2022).

Another mechanism by which improvements in sleep can potentially affect depression is through indirect effects on immune system function. Symptoms triggered by pro-inflammatory cytokines in response to infection (Benca et al., 1992; Gresham et al., 1965; Nutt et al., 2008; Rumble et al., 2015) overlap those seen in depression: lack of energy, reduced activity, negative mood state, and disrupted sleep (Felger & Lotrich, 2013; Wohleb et al., 2016). A meta-analysis concluded that depressed patients are 50% more likely to have significantly elevated CRP levels (a marker of inflammation) than matched healthy controls (Osimo et al., 2019).

The overlap between symptoms of depression and responses to infection prompted the hypothesis that increases in pro-inflammatory cytokines and CRP as a result of sleep loss contribute to the symptoms of depression (Dantzer et al., 2008; Hayley, 2011; Raison & Miller, 2013). That hypothesis suggests that by improving sleep amounts and quality, ketamine can reduce the inflammatory responses that help maintain depression symptoms. Similarly, improved sleep after treatment with CBT-I may reduce inflammatory responses and thereby improve mood and reduce the risk of relapse into depression.

15.3.3 Bipolar disorder

Bipolar disorder (formerly "manic-depression") is a major psychiatric condition characterized by repeated bouts of depression and low energy, alternating at variable intervals with periods of high energy, irritability, euphoria, grandiosity, and behavioral disinhibition. The activated phase of the illness may involve either milder, shorter-lasting versions of these symptoms (hypomania) or extreme and more sustained versions (mania). Bipolar disorder has high heritability (~70%), shares genetic liability with other illnesses, including schizophrenia, major depression, and attention deficit disorder, and presents a higher lifetime risk of suicide than any other mental illness (Gordovez & McMahon, 2020; McIntyre et al., 2020).

Sleep in patients with bipolar disorder changes with the stage of the illness. During depressive episodes, sleep is disrupted by wake episodes, SWS is reduced, and REM sleep is modified, with an earlier onset during sleep and an increase in REM density (measured as rapid eye movements per unit time). These sleep symptoms are generally similar to those seen in unipolar major depression, but depressed bipolar patients matched for age, gender, and depression severity to those with unipolar depression showed more extreme sleep changes (Riemann et al., 2002). During (hypo) manic episodes, sleep amounts are reduced, sometimes to an extreme extent, while activity levels and arousal are strongly increased. PSG studies are difficult to conduct in this population, but a study of stable, manic inpatients who had been removed from drug treatments for a week showed features that overlapped some symptoms seen in depression: reduced sleep durations, increased density of eye movements during REM sleep, reduced sleep efficiency, and more N1 sleep (Hudson et al., 2002).

The most common treatment used to stabilize mood in bipolar patients is lithium (in the form of lithium carbonate), which is effective in reducing mania and can also reduce depression symptoms, but perhaps less effectively. Lithium treatment also reverses some bipolar sleep features by increasing SWS and decreasing REM sleep amounts (Roux & Kryger, 2010). Other mood stabilizers (e.g., valproate, lamotrigine) are also used, in part because lithium is effective in only some bipolar patients. Its use may be limited by side effects in a subset of patients. Depressive episodes are difficult to treat and may require both a mood stabilizer and another treatment, either an antipsychotic medication or an antidepressant. However, the use of antidepressants, alone or in combination with a mood stabilizer, is controversial because there is little evidence of benefit and some increased risk of triggering a manic episode. This risks associated with using an antidepressant appear to be highest for drugs that increase NE neurotransmission and in patients with rapid cycling between depression and mania (Post, 2016).

Even bipolar patients receiving drug treatments to maintain a stable mood state (euthymia), may still show disrupted sleep based on actigraphy, with frequent interruptions of sleep during the night (Ortiz et al., 2016). Self-reported short or highly variable sleep patterns in bipolar patients undergoing their usual treatments predicted more severe episodes of mania and depression over the next year (Gruber et al., 2011). Spontaneous, acute reductions in sleep amounts are also an important signal, and likely a trigger, for an impending transition from depression to (hypo)mania in most patients (Leibenluft et al., 1996; Wehr et al., 1987).

The inherent alternation of states that characterizes bipolar illness and the presence of circadian rhythm disruptions in many bipolar patients suggest that abnormalities in circadian organization are involved in generating some of its symptoms (Wehr et al., 1983). A case-study of a patient with longstanding bipolar illness showed that early daily timing of increased activity (and therefore reduced sleep) was associated with transitions out of depression into a (hypo)manic phase. This shift in activity onset resembled the effects of a phase-advance of the circadian activity rhythm. Mimicking this effect by deliberately phase-advancing the patient's sleep–wake cycles by 6 h during a depressive episode similarly reduced depressive symptoms, an effect which lasted for several days (Wehr et al., 1979). This patient also showed mood improvement in response to sleep deprivation, as discussed further in Section 15.3.4.

The evidence suggesting involvement of sleep disruption in the expression of bipolar symptoms extends to the pattern of emergence of bipolar disorder during development. Children of one or both parents with bipolar disorder are at higher risk for developing the illness. They have been studied to determine whether there are precursors that predict the subsequent onset of bipolar disorder. Among children who went on to develop bipolar disorder, usually in late adolescence, earlier symptoms appeared in childhood in the following general order: sleep difficulties, anxiety, minor mood and adjustment disorders, one or more major depressive episodes, and a first bipolar episode (Duffy et al., 2010; Duffy et al., 2018). Other studies confirmed the appearance of sleep symptoms in childhood or around puberty as a predictor of later onset of bipolar disorder, depression, or emotional problems in adolescence (Quach et al., 2018; Ritter et al., 2011).

Most patients with bipolar disorder have a habitual delayed chronotype, even between periods of illness (Takaesu, 2018), and irregular sleep timing is associated with more disease severity (Gruber et al., 2011), but these features are not necessarily specific to bipolar disorder. One study showed that young people with a variety of psychiatric conditions (including bipolar disorder) had more delayed, interrupted, and irregular sleep patterns than controls, which could not be accounted for by the effects of any current drug treatments (Robillard et al., 2015).

Irregular sleep patterns are also characteristic of those who are not currently ill but are at elevated risk of developing a bipolar disorder, based on their scores on psychological tests of hypomanic tendencies. University students who had high scores on these tests also had shorter and more variable sleep durations, and more fragmented and interrupted sleep than controls, as assessed using actigraphy (Ankers & Jones, 2009). In another actigraphy study, children at high genetic risk of developing a mood disorder (one parent with bipolar disorder and one with major depression) had the most irregular weekly sleep schedules, showing both less sleep during weeknights and more sleep on weekends than controls (Wescott et al., 2019).

15.3.4 Sleep deprivation effects on depression

One of the most surprising connections between sleep and psychiatric disorders is the well-established finding that sleep deprivation can improve mood and reduce other symptoms of depression in unipolar and bipolar depressed patients. This phenomenon has been recognized for more than half a century (Pflug & Tölle, 1971). Reviews of the published literature have concluded that overnight complete or partial sleep deprivation (usually during the second half of the night) alleviates depressive symptoms acutely in ~50% of depressed patients (Boland et al., 2017; Wu & Bunney, 1990). These findings may be related to the evidence discussed in the preceding section that spontaneously shortened sleep (i.e., early waking) often precedes a switch from depression to euthymia or (hypo)mania, and deliberately waking patients for the second half of the night mimics this pattern and its effects (Boland et al., 2017; Leibenluft et al., 1996; Wehr et al., 1987; Wehr et al., 1979).

These findings seem counterintuitive for several reasons. First, most people without depression respond to sleep deprivation with reduced vigor and negative moods, not mood improvement and increased energy (Dinges et al., 1997). Second, reduced sleep amounts that result from extended sleep-onset latencies, disrupted sleep continuity, and early waking often precede the onset of a depressive episode, rather than improving mood. These symptoms may also persist during a depressive episode, and even continue after treatments successfully reduce other symptoms of depression. Third, the rapid antidepressant effects of ketamine treatments have been attributed in part to improved sleep and increased SWS after treatment (Duncan & Zarate, 2013; Duncan et al., 2013; Rodrigues et al., 2022). Finally, there is substantial evidence that cognitive treatments aimed specifically at improving sleep quality can reduce depressive symptoms and the risk of relapse after successful treatment (Carney et al., 2017; Cheng et al., 2019; Irwin et al., 2021); see Section 15.3.2. These findings do not suggest that deliberately reducing sleep amounts would result in mood improvement in patients with depression.

Nevertheless, there is a wealth of evidence that deliberate sleep restriction consistently improves mood and activation levels in a subset of depressed patients. These effects are also surprisingly rapid. Treatment with most antidepressant drugs (except ketamine; see Section 15.3.2) typically takes days or weeks to begin to improve symptoms. During sleep deprivation in depressed unipolar or bipolar patients, mood and energy improvements occur very rapidly—literally overnight (Wehr et al., 1979).

For adult humans, staying awake continuously for 16 h is generally considered normal (see Section 13.3.2); cognitive deficits and increased sleepiness associated with overnight sleep deprivation start to develop when people are awake for longer than 16 h; see, for example, **Figures 13.7** and **13.10**. Consistent with this interpretation that sleep deprivation involves being awake for more than 16 h, for one unipolar depressed patient, repeated tests during depressive episodes showed that about 16–18 h of continuous waking triggered rapid mood improvement (Knowles et al., 1979). Equally remarkable is that mood improvements in this patient and others were completely or partially reversed just as quickly by sleep the next night or even, in some cases, by a very brief (e.g., 15 min) nap during the day (Bunney & Bunney, 2013; Gillin et al., 1989; Knowles et al., 1979) (**Figure 15.5**).

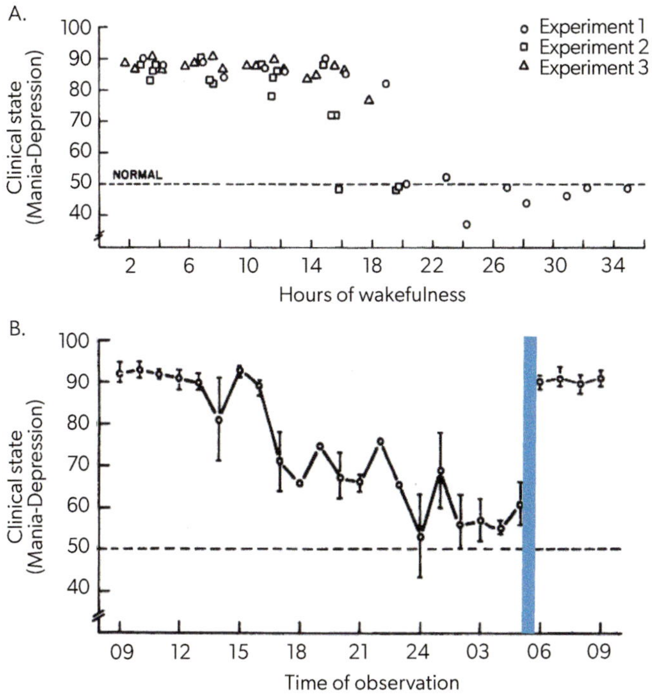

Figure 15.5 A. Depression ratings (Y axis) of a female patient plotted as a function of the length of time she had been awake (X axis) during three different studies (Experiments 1-3). A state of severe clinical depression (ratings of 80-90 on the Y axis) was maintained from waking until about 16-18 h later, when mood began to improve, leading rapidly to a normal mood or slight hypomania (~50 on the Y axis) by about 19-20 h awake, which was maintained as long as she remained awake (up to ~35 h in one study). **B.** The clinical state of the same woman during an overnight trial of sleep deprivation. She started with severe depression (90; Y axis) and showed a gradual improvement in mood starting after ~16 h awake, leading to a near-normal mood state (55-60) in the late night. She took a 15 min nap just before 06:00 (blue line), which was followed by an immediate relapse to severe depression (90). Reprinted with permission from Knowles, J.B. et al. (1979) Five variations of sleep deprivation in a depressed woman. *Brit J Psychiatry* 135:403-410. © Cambridge University Press (1979). doi: 10.1192/bjp.135.5.403.

It is surprising how consistently similar proportions of depressed patients respond, despite large differences in the composition of the groups being studied and the assessment methods used. Sleep deprivation was similarly effective (i.e., 40–60% showed improvement) in very different groups: in patients who were either recently diagnosed or had experienced years of recurrent depressive episodes; in men and women; regardless of the severity of baseline symptoms; regardless of the use of different criteria for mood improvement;[6] regardless of ongoing (ineffective) antidepressant treatment or lack of treatment; whether patients were exposed to bright light or darkness during the deprivation period; and in those with unipolar major depression or those who were in the depressive phase of a bipolar disorder (Boland et al., 2017; Gottlieb et al., 2021; Wehr et al., 1985). The effectiveness of sleep deprivation appears to be related to the state of being depressed, regardless of the specific diagnosis, psychiatric history, ongoing treatment, or personal characteristics of patients.

Many hypotheses have been proposed for why sleep loss can have antidepressant effects and what distinguishes the ~50% of patients who respond from those who do not. These include effects of sleep loss on circadian rhythms and circadian clock gene expression; differences in the rate of increase of the drive for SWA (represented by the rate of increase in Process S; see Section 5.3.3); effects on arousal levels; the impact of lost REM sleep; neurochemical changes in brain regions involved in sleep and/or mood regulation; and altered synaptic plasticity or strength (Bernier et al., 2009; Borbély & Wirz-Justice, 1982; Bunney & Bunney, 2013; Duncan & Zarate, 2013; Van den Hoofdakker et al., 1989; Vogel et al., 1980; Wehr, 1990; Wirz-Justice & Van den Hoofdakker, 1999). There remains, however, no consensus about why sleep loss has the observed effects on mood in a consistent subset of patients with depression.

Although there is no agreement about the mechanisms involved, there is evidence supporting the clinical use of sleep deprivation as an adjunct to the treatment of depression, despite the significant risk of a switch into mania in patients with bipolar depression (Ioannou et al., 2021). When used along with other treatments (e.g., antidepressant drugs, bright light exposure, or phase advances of circadian rhythms), single or multiple trials of sleep deprivation resulted in enhanced, more rapid, or more sustained improvements in symptoms (Benedetti et al., 2005; D'Agostino et al., 2020; Ramirez-Mahaluf et al., 2020; Riemann et al., 2002; Wu et al., 2009).

[6] Different criteria have been used to define "responders" and "non-responders" to treatments (e.g., 30, 40, or 50% reduction in depression rating scores). Despite applying these different criteria, similar proportions of patients were classified as responders (Boland et al., 2017). It appears that the specific threshold used to define a positive response had little impact on the results because patients responded either strongly (e.g., **Figure 15.5**) or not at all to sleep deprivation.

A meta-analysis of seven studies, using one or several nights of total sleep deprivation in combination with ongoing treatments, found a significant improvement in depression rating scores 1 week after treatment, relative to usual treatment alone, but no sustained benefit when assessed 2 weeks later. However, this significant benefit across studies was present only if a single study of older, late-onset depressed patients was excluded (Ioannou et al., 2021). The basis for the exclusion was not clear, but older patients are more likely to have cognitive problems, multiple illnesses, and multiple ongoing pharmacological treatments (Kok & Reynolds, 2017). Given the small number of studies reviewed and the uncertainty of benefits, further research is needed to determine whether sleep deprivation has a sustained benefit as an add-on to other treatments.

There is also a need to determine the basis for the differences between patients who do and do not respond to sleep deprivation, which could provide more insight into the mechanisms involved. It remains unclear whether there is a single best form of deprivation (early- or late-night partial deprivation, complete overnight deprivation, focused on one sleep stage or not), whether the number of treatments affects long-term results, and whether there is additional benefit from combining sleep deprivation with other treatments.

15.3.5 Summary

Major psychiatric disorders are typically accompanied by changes in sleep and/or circadian rhythms. In anxiety disorders, these changes include longer latencies to fall asleep, decreased sleep amounts, and more interrupted sleep, as well as subjective symptoms of insomnia. These sleep features contribute to further increasing anxiety, especially about sleep, which, in turn, further disturbs sleep. These reciprocal influences were illustrated by the results of treatment studies. Cognitive-behavioral treatments aimed at sleep symptoms also reduced some of the symptoms of PTSD, and, similarly, psychological treatments aimed at GAD improved sleep quality.

People with major depression show similarly disturbed sleep, in part because depression is often comorbid with an anxiety disorder or anxiety symptoms. Another characteristic of sleep in patients with depression is the early appearance of REM sleep during the night and an overall increase in REM sleep density and amounts. These features are consistent with the idea of a deficit in monoamine activity in depression, since the monoamines 5-HT and NE oppose the onset of REM sleep. Similarly, most antidepressant drugs promote increased activity of 5-HT and NE, and also reduce REM sleep amounts, at least initially during treatment. The benefits of the novel antidepressant ketamine are also mediated in part by effects on sleep quality.

Sleep disturbances are not only symptoms of depression but may contribute to the onset of depressive episodes and increase the probability of relapse after successful treatment. Treating sleep problems in depression with CBT-I reduced the risk of relapse into another depressive episode.

Depressed patients have increased rates of chronic inflammation, suggesting that some of the symptoms of the illness may be related to overactivity of pro-inflammatory cytokines. Chronic sleep disruption also increases markers of inflammation, leading to the hypothesis that inflammation may mediate some of the influence of sleep disturbances on the risk of developing depression.

Sleep during depressive episodes in patients with bipolar disorder resembles sleep in unipolar depression, but the changes may be more extreme. During (hypo)manic episodes, sleep is instead dramatically shortened and patients are tonically activated and aroused. Advances of sleep–wake cycles and loss of sleep often herald a spontaneous transition from depression to a (hypo)manic phase, and instituting these changes deliberately can improve depression symptoms, at least transiently.

Irregular and disrupted sleep and a delayed chronotype are seen in children and adolescents at high risk of later developing bipolar disorder. However, these symptoms are not specific to bipolar disorder and are also antecedents of other developing psychiatric conditions. This finding is consistent with evidence that children of parents with bipolar disorder are at increased risk of developing either that illness or another major psychiatric disorder.

Although sleep disruption characterizes depression, overnight complete or partial sleep deprivation has the surprising effect of immediately reducing depressive symptoms in ~50% of patients. These mood improvements are rapidly reversed in most patients by even brief sleep episodes during the next day. Similar proportions of depressed patients respond to sleep loss with improved mood, regardless of their other characteristics or ongoing treatments. Although the mechanisms involved remain unknown, the effects of sleep deprivation have been tested for the capacity to accelerate mood improvement in patients in combination with other antidepressant treatments. Despite some positive results, more research is needed to identify which treatment procedures involving sleep deprivation could produce more sustained improvements in depressive symptoms.

15.4 Sleep and schizophrenia

15.4.1 Sleep changes and underlying mechanisms

Schizophrenia is another serious mental illness with very high heritability (~80%) (Legge et al., 2021). It is characterized by "positive" psychotic symptoms (e.g., hallucinations, delusions) and "negative" symptoms (e.g., cognitive and attentional deficits, flat affect, social withdrawal). Many studies of sleep in people with schizophrenia have involved those who are currently being medicated or had been withdrawn from prior antipsychotic medication; the latter are usually referred to as "drug-free." Because some physiological effects may persist long after medications have been withdrawn, sleep features may continue to be influenced by a prior history of drug treatments. A few studies of sleep in people with schizophrenia, however, involved first-episode patients who had not begun antipsychotic treatments and were therefore referred to as "drug-naïve."

The typical sleep features seen in people with schizophrenia resemble those in other psychiatric conditions: disrupted sleep continuity, delayed sleep onset, and reduced total sleep duration (Chouinard et al., 2004; Lauer et al., 1997; Van Cauter et al., 1991). Features observed less consistently across studies include reduced amounts of REM sleep, N2 sleep, or SWS (Boivin, 2000; Chan et al., 2017; Chouinard et al., 2004; Cohrs, 2008; Lauer et al., 1997; Poulin et al., 2003; Van Cauter et al., 1991).

A meta-analysis confirmed that, relative to controls, sleep quality was worse and sleep disturbance more frequent in those at clinical high risk for developing psychosis, as well as in those with either early-stage or chronic schizophrenia. Features of sleep architecture, including sleep-onset latency, sleep efficiency, total sleep amount, and REM density were variably affected in either early-stage or chronic schizophrenia but not in those at high risk (Bagautdinova et al., 2023). However, another study found that the single most frequently reported symptom during the prodromal phase preceding an initial diagnosis of a psychotic disorder (including schizophrenia) was sleep disturbance (Yung & McGorry, 1996).

Antipsychotic medications generally increase total sleep amounts and reduce sleep disruptions, often in parallel to the degree to which they reduce psychotic symptoms, although some treated patients continue to show unstable and disrupted sleep–wake rhythms (Wulff et al., 2011). Most antipsychotics reduce the actions of neurotransmitters that have activating effects, including dopamine, serotonin, and histamine, which would likely result in some degree of sedation (Aringhieri et al., 2018).

Sleep improvements during antipsychotic treatments might result from either direct effects on sleep regulatory systems or from the effects of reduced stress and arousal as a result of reductions in psychotic symptoms. Because antipsychotic drugs have sleep-promoting effects on healthy controls as well as on patients, it is likely that specific pharmacological effects on sleep mechanisms are involved (Cohrs, 2008). Countering this benefit for sleep, however, is the risk among at least 10% of treated patients, depending on the specific drug and dosage used, of developing a side-effect called akathisia (Bratti et al., 2007). This condition involves motor restlessness (especially in the legs), agitation, and a subjective need to move, which can interfere with initiating and maintaining sleep.

Transgenic mouse models of schizophrenia have been produced by introducing genetic changes that are linked to human schizophrenia into the mouse genome. Among these mouse models, several have shown effects on sleep or circadian rhythms. One mouse model involves the *Bdr* mutation that affects the *SNAP-25* gene, which has been implicated in abnormal synaptic transmission and hippocampal function in people with schizophrenia (Johnson et al., 2008). Transgenic mice with this mutation showed phase-advanced circadian rhythms in a light–dark cycle so that the main bout of "nocturnal" activity actually started in the light phase. The rhythms affected included activity, adrenal corticosterone, and suprachiasmatic nucleus vasopressin, resulting in severely fragmented and unstable daily rest-activity cycles.[7] The mechanism responsible for the advanced circadian phase is unknown, but under free-running conditions, circadian organization appeared normal and rhythm periods were unchanged relative to wild-type mice. These results suggest that the mutation affected entrainment processes rather than rhythm generation (Oliver et al., 2012).

Another gene that is linked to schizophrenia is the *STOP* gene (also called *MAP6*), which regulates stability of microtubules, synaptic function, and synaptic plasticity (Andrieux et al., 2002). In mice with a knockout of this gene, sleep was strongly disrupted. There was an overall decrease in NREM sleep and increase in waking, both in lighting cycles and in free-running conditions. These mice also showed many more transitions in both directions between waking and NREM sleep, without similar changes in REM sleep regulation. During NREM sleep in the daily light phase, mice showed a decrease in EEG activity in the sigma-band range (the frequency range of sleep spindles; see Section 15.4.2), but showed increased delta-band activity. Despite these sleep abnormalities, they showed normal circadian organization, except for an increase in free-running period in constant conditions (Deurveilher et al., 2021; Profitt et al., 2016).

These results indicate that changes in some genes linked to schizophrenia in people affected aspects of sleep regulation in mice, including the stability of sleep, amounts of NREM sleep, and the expression of EEG activity in the spindle-frequency range. The effects on the circadian system were more subtle, but changes observed under entrained conditions could contribute to instability of sleep–wake patterns. Thus, these mutations in mice recapitulate some of the abnormalities in regulation of sleep seen in people with schizophrenia.

15.4.2 Reductions in sleep spindles

Studies of medicated patients with chronic schizophrenia reported decreased numbers, density, and coherence of sleep spindles across all NREM sleep stages, despite no change in amounts of N2 sleep, during which spindles are most prominent (Ferrarelli et al., 2007; Wamsley et al., 2012).[8] To assess whether current medications contributed to these differences, a later study compared sleep spindle numbers in treated schizophrenia patients to those of healthy controls given similar medications (presumably acutely). It still found a decrease in spindle numbers in those with schizophrenia compared to these partial controls (Ferrarelli et al., 2010).

To avoid any potential influence of medications or length of prior illness, another study recorded sleep in early-stage, unmedicated people with psychosis, including a subset with a diagnosis of schizophrenia and others with mood or other disorders that included psychotic features. It found a decrease in spindle density and amplitude during N2 sleep in the full group of people with psychosis compared to controls, but this difference was driven entirely by those who had been diagnosed with schizophrenia. Other people with psychotic symptoms did not differ from controls (Manoach et al., 2014) (**Figure 15.6**).

High-density (64-channel) EEG recordings were made from another group of people experiencing a first-episode of schizophrenia. The group included a majority who were drug-naïve and some with limited prior exposure to antipsychotic medications. There were decreases relative to controls in spindle density and duration, but not amplitude, in recordings from a cluster of electrodes above the frontal cortical region. These changes were not correlated with antipsychotic doses in the previously treated subset of patients, suggesting that they were unrelated to drug effects in that subgroup (Kaskie et al., 2019). A meta-analysis confirmed that spindle density, duration, and amplitude were significantly reduced relative to controls in people during both early-stage and chronic schizophrenia (Bagautdinova et al., 2023).

Because of the high heritability of schizophrenia, another study examined sleep in first-degree relatives of people diagnosed with schizophrenia. This group included children with a variety of other conditions (ADHD, anxiety, depression, etc.)

[7] An advanced phase of entrainment would result in the early part of the daily active phase overlapping the light phase of the lighting cycle. The conflicting effects of the circadian active phase (promoting activity) and of bright light (inhibiting activity) could be responsible for producing irregular, fragmented activity.

[8] An earlier study of drug-naïve patients with schizophrenia reported a significant reduction in absolute amounts of N2 sleep, but expressed as a percentage of total sleep time, there was no difference between patients and controls (Lauer et al., 1997).

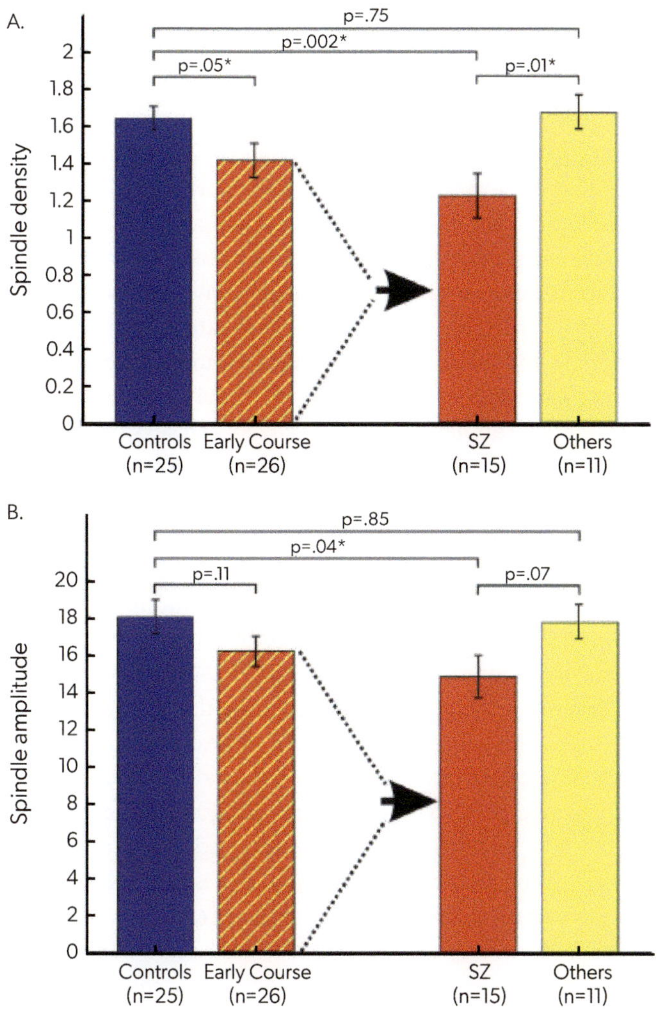

Figure 15.6 Left side: **A.** Spindle density and **B.** spindle amplitude of Controls (blue columns) and of patients with psychosis studied before any drug treatment (Early Course; hatched columns), showing trends toward reduced spindle parameters in all psychotic patients relative to controls. Right side: The patient group's results were broken down into those with a diagnosis of schizophrenia (SZ, red columns) and those with psychosis for other reasons (Others, yellow columns). Patients with schizophrenia showed a large, significant reduction in both spindle measures relative to controls and, for density, to other patients with psychosis. Patients with schizophrenia accounted for the marginal differences between controls and patients with psychosis in general. Patients with psychosis who were not diagnosed with schizophrenia did not differ significantly from controls on either measure. Probabilities associated with different comparisons between groups are shown at the top of each panel. Reprinted with permission from Manoach D.S. et al. (2014) Sleep spindle deficits in antipsychotic-naive early course schizophrenia and in non-psychotic first-degree relatives. *Front Hum Neurosci* 0.3389/fnhum.2014.00762, 2014. © 2014 Manoach, Demanuele, Wamsley, Vangel, Montrose, Miewald, Kupfer, Buysse, Stickgold and Keshavan. This is an open-access article distributed under the terms of a Creative Commons Attribution License (CC-BY). doi: 10.3389/fnhum.2014.00762.

but no psychotic disorders. The first-degree relatives showed significantly reduced spindle amplitudes and a nonsignificant trend toward reduced spindle density relative to controls (Manoach et al., 2014). This partial replication of the changes seen in those with schizophrenia among close relatives without psychosis suggests that the underlying changes leading to altered spindle characteristics are linked to the degree of familial (presumably genetic) risk of developing schizophrenia.

The frequent observation of reduced number, density, and/or amplitude of sleep spindles in drug-naïve and minimally antipsychotic-exposed patients leads to two important conclusions. First, these changes are not a product of medication effects, and second, they are characteristic of early as well as chronic phases of schizophrenia. Thus, they are not the result of deterioration of brain function from a history of chronic illness. The finding that some changes were only observed in a limited frontal region of the brain (Kaskie et al., 2019) suggests that some earlier electrophysiological studies that did not assess differences among cortical regions could have missed these region-specific changes.

15.4.3 Effects of sleep spindle reductions

Reduced sleep spindle numbers may be related to the intellectual decline seen in many people with chronic schizophrenia. There are claims that some features of sleep spindles are positively correlated with measures of general intelligence (see Section 18.9). In addition, sleep spindles and their interaction with cortical slow waves are implicated in the "offline" strengthening of memories through consolidation during sleep (see Section 18.6.2). Deficits in memory consolidation that are maintained over time could contribute cumulatively to impaired performance on tests of intellectual abilities.

When tested for overnight improvement of a newly learned motor sequence task, people with schizophrenia showed deficits relative to controls that were correlated with the degree of reduction in number and density of sleep spindles (Wamsley et al., 2012). Both reduced density of sleep spindles and altered timing of spindles relative to slow waves also predicted deficits in overnight improvement on a motor sequence task among patients with schizophrenia (Demanuele et al., 2017).

Individuals at clinical high risk for potentially developing schizophrenia (based on the presence of sub-syndromal symptoms) showed reduced spindle durations relative to controls, especially in a prefrontal region. Spindle duration changes in the high-risk individuals were correlated with reductions in performance on a working memory task, which is also often impaired in patients with schizophrenia (Mayeli et al., 2022). A study of children (8–15 years old) with depression or high familial risk of depression also found both the depressed and high-risk groups had lower frontal spindle densities in N2 sleep than controls (Lopez et al., 2010).

Sleep spindles are the product of interactions among the thalamic reticular nucleus (TRN), the cortex, and thalamic relay nuclei (see Section 12.2.4). The TRN is also involved in regulating sensory filtering and attention while awake (Halassa et al., 2014; Wimmer et al., 2015; Yu et al., 2009). Tests of prepulse inhibition (PPI) of startle responses showed performance deficits in several groups: patients with chronic schizophrenia who were medicated; first-episode, antipsychotic-naïve schizophrenia patients; and siblings of people with schizophrenia (Braff et al., 1992; Kumari et al., 2005; Kumari et al., 2007). PPI involves a reduction in the strength of a startle response to a strong stimulus when it is preceded with short latency by a weaker stimulus. Altered PPI performance appears to reflect changes in sensorimotor filtering and habituation. This interpretation is consistent with other evidence for changes in low-level filtering and processing of sensory inputs in people with schizophrenia (Freedman et al., 1991).

Total sleep deprivation can mimic some of the characteristics of people with schizophrenia. For example, total overnight sleep loss in healthy people resulted in deficits in PPI responses, perceptual distortions, cognitive disorganization, and anhedonia, all of which are seen in stronger form in those with schizophrenia (Petrovsky et al., 2014). Sleep deprivation (1–3 days) can also produce PPI deficits in a rat model, which can be prevented by giving antipsychotic drugs (Frau et al., 2008). As discussed in Section 14.3.2, very long-term sleep deprivation also caused perceptual distortions and fragmented thinking in Randy Gardner (Ross, 1965). People with schizophrenia do not stop sleeping, but it is possible that their often disrupted and shortened sleep, along with changes like reductions in the number and timing of sleep spindles in prefrontal cortical regions, could contribute to some of their perceptual and cognitive symptoms.

Given the reported role of the TRN in sensory filtering and in sleep spindle production, deficits in the function of the TRN in people with schizophrenia could contribute to altered PPI and to reduced overnight memory consolidation that depends on the number and timing of sleep spindles. Altered sensory filtering may also contribute to people with schizophrenia being overwhelmed by complex sound environments and unable to focus attention on relevant inputs and exclude distracting sounds (Freedman et al., 1991). Deficits in sensory filtering may also contribute to altered attributions and interpretation of sensory inputs, which may, in turn, contribute to misperceptions and hallucinations.

Although most people with schizophrenia show general intellectual decline, some have well-preserved intellectual functions. Regardless of their extent of general intellectual decline or stability, however, they show impairments in executive and attention tasks that are linked to frontal lobe activity (Shallice et al., 1991; Weickert et al., 2000). The observation that sleep spindles were selectively modified over frontal cortical regions in people with schizophrenia (Kaskie et al., 2019), combined with the role of spindles in sensory filtering and attention, suggests that some of their cognitive deficits are related to altered thalamic interactions with the frontal lobes.

Altered production and function of sleep spindles have also been reported in children, adolescents, and adults with autism spectrum disorder (ASD). Some studies of adults and children with autism reported either a reduced number or density of sleep spindles in N2 sleep (Farmer et al., 2018; Limoges et al., 2005). Another study observed reduced N3 spindle numbers and altered timing of spindles relative to slow oscillations, compared to controls. Although both controls and people with ASD showed sleep-dependent memory consolidation, controls with more sleep spindles showed better memory consolidation, while the opposite correlation was found in those with ASD (Mylonas et al., 2022). The basis for this surprising difference is unknown.

Taken together, these results indicate that abnormal spindle production may be characteristic of several kinds of major psychiatric conditions. An analysis of overlap in genetic variation among psychiatric disorders found that genetic markers in those with schizophrenia overlapped significantly with markers from individuals with major depression and ASD. The genetic variation overlap with schizophrenia was moderate for depression and low for ASD (Lee et al., 2013). These findings hint that there may be a common genetic contribution to the decreases in sleep spindle activity seen in these disorders, which may reflect altered interactions between the TRN and frontal cortical regions.

15.4.4 Summary

Sleep and daily rhythms are disrupted in people with schizophrenia. There is consistent evidence for shortened and disturbed sleep, as well as increased sleep-onset latencies. Disrupted sleep is improved by treatment with antipsychotic drugs, which reduce the activity of several neurotransmitter systems linked to arousal. Animal models that incorporate genetic abnormalities seen in many people with schizophrenia also show abnormal sleep and circadian rhythm characteristics. This evidence suggests that some aspects of sleep/circadian disruptions seen in those with schizophrenia may be related to genetic changes characteristic of their disorder.

Alterations in sleep spindles have been observed in people with schizophrenia, including both those with a history of longstanding illness and prior drug treatments and those who are newly diagnosed and drug-naïve. There is some evidence indicating that these changes are most prominent in frontal cortical regions. Depending on the study and the recording methods used, the number, density, amplitude, or duration of spindles have been reported to be reduced. The fact that first-degree relatives of people with schizophrenia also show altered sleep spindle features suggests that some of these changes are heritable and linked to the degree of genetic risk of developing schizophrenia. Frontal cortical reductions in spindle numbers have also been reported in children with depression or who are at high risk of developing depression, which may reflect overlap of genetic features that are associated with increased risk of developing schizophrenia, depression, and other major psychiatric disorders.

Sleep spindles, which are generated by the TRN, are known to interact with slow cortical oscillations during sleep to strengthen consolidation of new learning. The timing of spindles relative to slow oscillations was also altered in people with schizophrenia. Reduced overnight improvements following new learning in those with schizophrenia are consistent with the observed differences in sleep spindle numbers, characteristics, and timing.

People with schizophrenia show altered low-level sensory functions (e.g., on tests of PPI) and deficits in higher level cognitive functions, such as working memory. These altered functions may reflect changes in the interaction between the TRN and the frontal cortex. Modified sensory functions, in particular reduced filtering and inadequate attentional selection, may contribute to perceptual changes that are linked to the development of hallucinations and other cognitive abnormalities.

Studies of children and adults with ASD also found reduced spindle density/numbers in N2 and N3 sleep, altered spindle timing relative to slow oscillations, and functional relations opposite to those seen in controls between spindle numbers and memory consolidation. Schizophrenia, depression, and ASD share significant overlap in genetic marker variations. This overlap and similar changes in sleep spindle features suggest a possible common genetic basis in several psychiatric conditions for changes in TRN-cortical functional interactions.

15.5 Sleep and Alzheimer's disease

15.5.1 Sleep quality/duration and risk of AD

Disturbed sleep and daily rhythms are characteristic of several neurodegenerative diseases, including Alzheimer's disease (AD), which is the most common cause of dementia (loss of cognitive abilities, including memory) (Bliwise, 1993; McCurry et al., 1999). Disruption of sleep and rhythms is important not only because of its effects on patients, but also because of the increased burden it places on families and the health system. Family caregivers of patients with dementia frequently cite sleep disruption, along with associated agitation and wandering at night, as major problems that contribute to institutionalization earlier than might otherwise be required (Pollak & Perlick, 1991; Pollak & Stokes, 1997; Sanford, 1975).

AD patients show reduced SWS amounts, reduced number of spindles, and increasing disruption of both sleep and daily rhythms as the disease progresses from mild to severe forms, even compared to older insomnia patients (Tao et al., 2023; Vitiello & Prinz, 1989). Some sleep-related symptoms may reflect loss of normal suprachiasmatic nucleus function in AD (Hofman & Swaab, 1994; Wang et al., 2015) (see Sections 8.4.3 and 8.4.4); others may be related to degeneration in other brain regions involved in sleep regulation. Sleep disruption in AD patients (reported by a family member or other close informant) was associated with more severe brain changes, including increases in ventricular size and brain volume losses, especially of gray matter, in the hippocampus, frontal and temporal cortical regions (Burke et al., 2022).

Disturbed sleep, assessed by self-report or actigraphy in older people, often appears before cognitive symptoms and is associated with an increased risk within a few years of being diagnosed with dementia, AD, or cognitive decline (Lim et al., 2013; Lo et al., 2014; Luojus et al., 2017; Shi et al., 2018; Sterniczuk et al., 2013; Tranah et al., 2011). Among older people studied with actigraphy, those with the most disrupted sleep patterns had a 50% increased risk of developing AD within the next few years, relative to those with the least disrupted patterns (Lim et al., 2013) (**Figure 15.7**). A longitudinal study obtained five self-reports of sleep duration at 3–5 year intervals over a period of 19 years. It identified habitual short sleep (<7 h) and inconsistent sleep durations over time as being significantly associated with cognitive decline in an older population (Keil et al., 2023).

A recent study reported that among patients referred for evaluation to a sleep clinic, those with PSG-determined reductions in sleep efficiency, N3 sleep, and REM sleep had an increased likelihood of a subsequent diagnosis of a neurodegenerative disease over a median follow-up period of ~13 years. Neurodegenerative diseases included AD, Parkinson's disease, vascular dementia, and others, but associations of sleep features to specific diseases could not be determined (Ibrahim et al., 2024). Female nurses who engaged in sustained night-shift work over a period of years, which is likely to have disrupted their sleep patterns, also had an elevated risk of developing dementia (Jørgensen et al., 2020).

A related observation linking sleep disturbance and AD is that objectively determined (actigraphy or PSG) disrupted sleep was more common among healthy older people (mean

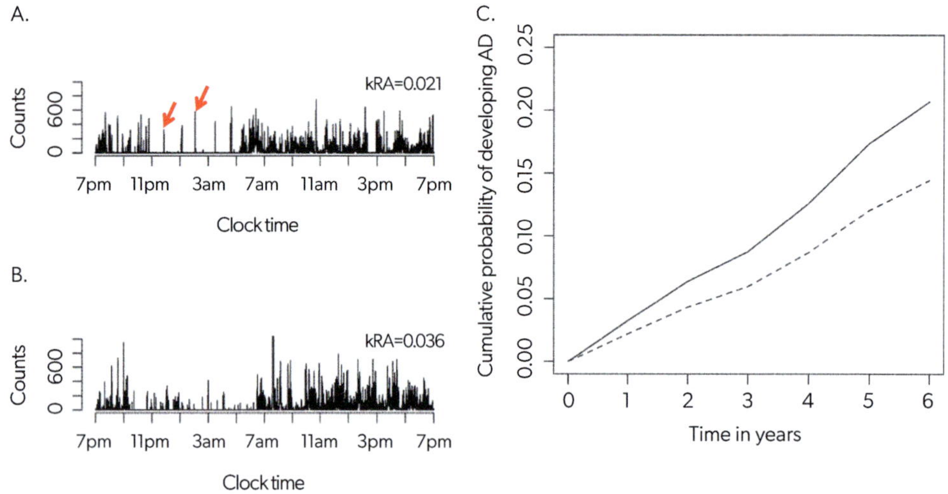

Figure 15.7 Actigraphic records of 24 h periods (X axis) illustrating examples of (**A**) the least disrupted sleep (lowest 10%) and (**B**) most disrupted sleep (highest 10%) among a group of older people (average age, ~82 years). **C**. Based on longitudinal studies of ~750 participants, these curves represent the cumulative probability of a diagnosis of Alzheimer's disease in later years among those with the most disrupted sleep patterns at baseline (kRA = 0.036, solid line) and those with the least disrupted sleep (kRA = 0.021, dashed line). "kRA" is a measure that reflects the probability of a transition from rest to activity during sleep; higher values, as in (**B**) indicate more disrupted sleep. The record in **A** shows several discrete, brief episodes of what likely were arousals to wakefulness (arrows indicate two of these), with sustained sleep between arousals. The record in **B** shows nearly continuous low levels of activity during most of the night, reflecting many transitions from rest to activity. Adapted with permission of Oxford University Press from Lim, A.S.P. et al. (2013) Sleep fragmentation and the risk of incident Alzheimer's disease and cognitive decline in older persons. *Sleep* 36:1027–1032. © Sleep Research Society (2013). doi: 10.5665/sleep.2802.

age ~65 years) who carry the epsilon (ε) 4 variant allele of the APOE gene than among those without it. Those with the allele showed more WASO and shorter total sleep times, but did not have significantly increased subjective complaints about sleep quality. The presence of this allele does not determine that AD will develop, but it greatly increases the risk, especially if both copies of the gene are the APOE ε4 variant (Drogos et al., 2016).

A meta-analysis of 27 studies concluded that sleep problems (including short and long sleep, sleep-related breathing disorders, sleep fragmentation, and insomnia) were significantly associated with an increased risk of developing cognitive impairment and AD (Bubu et al., 2017). However, this conclusion may be too general, since it encompassed a variety of ways of assessing sleep problems, which may not carry equivalent risk. Some subjective measures may not show this association; for example, subjectively reported "poor sleep quality" alone was not linked to increased risk of developing dementia or AD (Lysen et al., 2018).

15.5.2 Sleep features and markers of risk of AD

There are several lines of physiological evidence that may account for the observed association of disrupted sleep with an increased risk of developing cognitive decline and a diagnosis of AD. Many studies have suggested that accumulation in the brain of neuronal plaques containing forms of the peptide amyloid beta (Aβ), especially the $A\beta_{42}$ form, is a key step in the development of AD and its cognitive symptoms (Blennow et al., 2015; Selkoe & Hardy, 2016). Retention of high levels of $A\beta_{42}$ in brain tissue is seen as an initial step in the development of Aβ plaques and associated neuronal damage. Older people with normal cognition who had elevated levels of $A\beta_{42}$ in the brain were found to be at higher risk of showing cognitive decline within a few years than those with normal levels (Donohue et al., 2017).

The level of $A\beta_{42}$ in CSF sampled from a spinal tap follows a different course. It is normal in individuals who do not develop AD, even among those with mild cognitive impairment (MCI), which increases the risk of later developing AD. MCI patients who still had only MCI for up to 10 years after initial assessment, or developed another neurodegenerative condition, also had normal CSF $A\beta_{42}$ levels. However, those MCI patients without dementia at the time of sampling, but who were diagnosed with AD over the next 0–10 years, already had low levels of CSF $A\beta_{42}$, presumably reflecting retention of $A\beta_{42}$ in brain tissue (Buchhave et al., 2012).

Low CSF levels of $A\beta_{42}$ remain characteristic of patients who have been diagnosed with AD, because sequestering $A\beta_{42}$ in neuronal plaques in the brain reduces circulating levels in the CSF (Andreasen & Blennow, 2002). Among older patients with Aβ plaques in the brain, as determined by positron emission tomography (PET) imaging, CSF Aβ_{42} levels were low compared to both healthy young and healthy older individuals with no Aβ plaques. CSF levels also varied on an hourly basis over 36 h in healthy participants of both ages but remained low and stable in those with established amyloid plaques in the brain (Huang et al., 2012).

Another molecular change involved in human neurodegenerative diseases is the intracellular aggregation of tangles containing hyperphosphorylated forms of the microtubule-associated protein tau (P-tau), the presence of which correlates with neuronal damage in several conditions, including AD (Williams, 2006). There are different views on the roles of Aβ and tau in the development of AD. Some focus on the role of Aβ accumulation and plaque formation in the brain as the trigger for aggregation of tau protein in tangles and accompanying neural damage (Hardy & Higgins, 1992; Jack et al., 2010). This model is supported, for example, by evidence that low CSF Aβ levels were present in MCI patients (presumably reflecting sequestering in the brain) at least as early as 10 years before a diagnosis of AD, while CSF levels of tau and P-tau (which are increased in diagnosed AD patients) were only elevated in those who converted to AD within 5 years or less (Buchhave et al., 2012).

Others emphasize the very early appearance of tau-related pathology in the brain before detectable Aβ pathology, and the independence of these markers. They do not support the hypothesis that Aβ accumulation initiates the cascade of events leading to AD neuropathology (Armstrong, 2014; Herrup, 2015; Stratmann et al., 2016). One example of the apparent independence of the presence of Aβ accumulation and P-tau was reported in a postmortem study of somatostatin neurons in the hypothalamus of AD patients and controls. A marker of abnormal tau protein was observed mainly in the brains of older AD patients while Aβ-related plaques were present mostly in the brains of younger AD patients (van de Nes et al., 2006).

A recent study provided indirect support for a primary role for tau pathology in cognitive decline. It demonstrated preserved cognitive function at an older age in an individual with a gene that usually triggers very early-onset, familial AD. The preservation of cognitive functions was apparently related to the presence of a rare variant of another gene. This individual had low levels of tau-related pathology in the brain along with preserved cognitive function, despite the presence of widespread Aβ plaques (Lopera et al., 2023).

Tau pathology is detectable in neuronal projections from several subcortical nuclei at very early stages of AD, before the appearance of Aβ-related pathology in the cortex (Stratmann et al., 2016). The form of tau protein that is measured appears to determine when it appears in the sequence of AD development. A form of P-tau that is phosphorylated at residue 231 increased in the CSF in association with the earliest PET markers of abnormal Aβ physiology in the brain and earlier than other P-tau forms that were studied (Ashton et al., 2022).

There is also evidence that the brain regions associated with different patterns of functional deficits in AD match the anatomical distribution of tau protein aggregation better than the distribution of Aβ plaques (Ossenkoppele et al., 2016). The anatomical distribution of tau protein is also linked to the amount of gray matter loss across different brain regions in patients with dementia, and to functional deficits related to those regions. For example, increased tau levels in the medial temporal lobe were linked to episodic memory deficits, and tau in bilateral frontoparietal regions was related to executive function deficits (Bejanin et al., 2017). However, this evidence is not inconsistent with the interpretation that disrupted Aβ processing triggers the spread of tau pathology that becomes closely associated with late-stage neurodegenerative changes (Jack et al., 2010).

Whichever hypothesis one accepts, there is evidence that sleep patterns are related to the risk of developing AD and that they influence the regulation of both Aβ and tau. One review concluded that sleep disruption is associated with abnormal regulation of both Aβ and tau protein as well as with signs of neurodegeneration (Van Egroo et al., 2019). In genetically engineered mice that develop tau pathologies during aging, chronic sleep restriction or sleep disruption in young adulthood accelerated the appearance of these pathological changes and the associated neuronal loss later in life. Neuronal damage was especially enhanced in structures related to sleep–wake regulation, such as the locus coeruleus (Zhu et al., 2018).

Many human studies found that sleep quality or amount correlated with levels of brain or CSF markers related to increased AD risk. Cognitively intact older people were studied at baseline and either 7 or 16 years later. Aβ levels were measured using PET imaging, and sleep quality was measured using questionnaires, actigraphy, or EEG recordings. Participants who reported excessive daytime sleepiness at baseline showed increased brain Aβ levels during the second imaging studies compared to those without daytime sleepiness at baseline (Carvalho et al., 2018; Spira et al., 2018). Self-reported short sleep or low-quality sleep were also associated cross-sectionally with increased brain Aβ levels (Spira et al., 2013), and objectively increased sleep disturbances were associated with an increased burden of tau protein (Winer et al., 2021).

A study that assessed sleep using >2 weeks of actigraphy in people without signs of cognitive decline (mean age, 59 years) found an inverted-U shaped function for Aβ_{42} in the CSF. Highest CSF levels were seen in those with a median sleep duration of 7.2 h, and lowest levels (presumably reflecting sequestering of Aβ in the brain) were seen in those with a median sleep duration of 5.8 h; levels were also decreased for those sleeping 7–9 h. There were no sleep duration-related differences in CSF levels of tau protein. These results may imply a bimodal increased risk of formation of Aβ plaques in those sleeping less and more than ~7 h nightly (Gibson et al., 2023).

Nevertheless, the dynamics of CSF Aβ levels over the many years during which AD may develop are complex and not well characterized. High CSF Aβ levels at an early stage may reflect higher circulating levels, including in the brain, and therefore increased risk of later plaque formation and AD. But as Aβ becomes sequestered in neural plaques, CSF levels fall so that they are low in those with established AD, as described previously (Huang et al., 2012). As a result, it can be difficult to interpret cross-sectional information about CSF levels of Aβ without simultaneous measurement of brain levels of Aβ or of plaques. In addition, the ratio between different forms of Aβ and of tau protein circulating in plasma may be more relevant to the later accumulation of amyloid plaques in the brain, and presumably increased risk of AD, than overall levels of all forms of Aβ and tau (Janelidze et al., 2024).

SWS was reported to be important for the regulation of CSF Aβ levels in cognitively normal older people. Those with the most SWS, especially SWA in frontal regions, had the lowest levels of Aβ in the CSF, which was interpreted as reflecting a lower risk of later development of AD (Varga et al., 2016). In a study of participants without cognitive symptoms, those with the highest amounts of SWA (especially in the 1-2 Hz range) had the lowest levels of both Aβ and tau protein in the brain and CSF. These associations were strongest between high SWA amounts and a low level of PET-imaged tau, which predicts a low risk of developing AD symptoms (Lucey et al., 2019). Participants with the greatest reduction of SWA as a result of experimental noise disruption overnight had increased CSF Aβ levels the next morning, consistent with a role for SWA in reducing circulating Aβ levels (Ju et al., 2017).

The implied neuroprotective role of SWS was supported by evidence from young adults who underwent several nights of partial sleep restriction, during which they lost other sleep stages but produced normal amounts of SWS (see **Figures 5.11, 13.6**, and Section 5.4.2). They did not show changes in Aβ levels or other markers suggestive of increased risk of AD (Olsson et al., 2018; Olsson et al., 2019). Evidence from a rat model of traumatic brain injury also supported a neuroprotective role for SWS. Brain injury resulted in diffuse damage to axonal pathways, increased levels of the precursor protein from which Aβ is formed, and measurable cognitive deficits. Treating rats with sodium oxybate (GHB) to increase SWS after traumatic brain injury reduced both axonal damage and its associated cognitive deficits (Morawska et al., 2016).

Cognitively normal older people were studied at baseline and 2 years later using anatomical MRI to measure changes in brain regional volumes. Those who had poor sleep quality at baseline relative to those with good sleep quality (assessed using the Pittsburgh Sleep Quality Index) showed much greater loss of neural volume during the second scan in two key brain regions: the right hippocampus and right posterior cingulate cortex. These structures play important roles in the control of attention, memory, and emotions, all of which are often disrupted in patients with AD (Liu et al., 2022).

Taken together, these results demonstrate that measures of sleep quality and of SWA amounts in older people are correlated with levels of tau and Aβ, with damage to brain mechanisms linked to AD symptoms, and with an increased risk of a subsequent diagnosis of AD. Sleep changes are also linked, but in different ways, to other neurodegenerative conditions, as discussed in **Box 15.1**.

15.5.3 Mechanisms of sleep effects on AD risk

Several approaches have been taken to assess why measures of sleep quality are correlated with markers of AD risk. In mouse models, Aβ levels in the brain were reduced after normal sleep and were increased by interventions that reduced sleep. These included either acute sleep disruption or treatment with the wake-promoting peptide, hypocretin (also called orexin; see Chapter 11). In mice that were genetically engineered to produce high amounts of Aβ, chronic sleep restriction further increased Aβ plaque formation; these effects were prevented by treating mice with antagonists that blocked hypocretin receptors (Kang et al., 2009).

Consistent with the conclusion that waking promotes Aβ accumulation, mice showed a daily rhythm of Aβ levels in the brain's interstitial fluid (found in the spaces surrounding brain cells), with high levels at night when they were most often awake (Kang et al., 2009). Healthy young people also showed a robust daily rhythm with increasing levels of $Aβ_{42}$ and $Aβ_{40}$ in the CSF during daytime waking and lowest levels after a night's sleep. The amplitude of this daily rhythm was attenuated in people older than 60 years and virtually abolished for $Aβ_{42}$ in participants with established amyloid plaques (Huang et al., 2012). Overnight sleep deprivation in people prevented the usual morning decline of Aβ levels in the CSF (Ooms et al., 2014) and increased Aβ levels in the brain, primarily in the right hippocampus and thalamus, as assessed using PET imaging (Shokri-Kojori et al., 2018).

A mechanism that could account for how sleep and waking affect Aβ levels was described in a study showing that the rate of clearance of Aβ from mouse brains via the "glymphatic"[9] (or

[9] This term, derived from "glia" and "lymphatic," refers to a role for glial cells in maintaining a flow of fluids through the brain's interstitial (i.e., extracellular) space, thereby helping to clear out metabolic waste products, similarly to the function of the lymphatic system elsewhere in the body. Although the nervous system was generally considered to lack a classic lymphatic system, recent evidence suggests that it exists and can serve as the route by which waste collected through the glymphatic system leaves the brain (Ahn et al., 2019; Louveau et al., 2015).

BOX 15.1 Sleep Disturbances in Other Diseases

Sleep disruption has been linked to other neurodegenerative conditions, in addition to AD. The presence of REM Sleep Behavior Disorder (REMBD) predicts a subsequent diagnosis of Parkinson's disease (PD) or another tau-related neurodegenerative condition (see Section 10.8). The sleep symptoms of REMBD appear to be related to damage to pontine mechanisms regulating REM sleep atonia. These symptoms occur before the development of motor symptoms of PD that result from degeneration of dopamine neurons in the midbrain substantia nigra. There is also evidence that among patients who already have a diagnosis of PD, the presence of REMBD predicts the later emergence of dementia symptoms. These findings imply a close link between REMBD and the later development of both motor and cognitive symptoms of PD (Nomura et al., 2013).

A very rare genetic condition called Fatal Familial Insomnia (FFI) is a neurodegenerative disease involving severe reductions in sleep amounts and quality. This condition has sometimes been cited as evidence that lack of sleep can be fatal in humans. FFI is characterized by a lack of N3 sleep and sleep spindles, preserved N1 sleep, daytime sleepiness, dysregulation of body temperature, flattened circadian rhythms, and a broad array of severe autonomic, intellectual, and motor symptoms, leading ultimately to death (Montagna, 2005).

The name of the condition reflects the fact that disturbed sleep regulation is often an early sign of developing FFI, but the disease affects many physiological systems. It is known to involve misfolding of a prion protein in the brain, as seen in "mad cow" disease in cattle or Creutzfeldt-Jakob disease in humans. It results in widespread pathological changes in cortical and brainstem areas, and especially profound degeneration in thalamic nuclei that are involved in the production of delta waves and sleep spindles (Montagna, 2005). It is possible that sustained sleep loss contributes to progression of other features of FFI, but it is the prion disease and resulting broad neurodegeneration that is the root cause of these symptoms and ultimately of death. Thus, sleep loss in FFI is best considered a symptom of this disorder rather than a principal cause, as might be suggested by its name.

Similarly, an exceedingly rare condition called Morvan syndrome includes a sustained loss of deep sleep, an abnormal REM sleep-like state with enacted dreams, and serious autonomic and motor abnormalities. Although the cause is unknown, there are hints that this syndrome may result from an autoimmune condition, and that the loss of sleep features, such as slow waves and sleep spindles, is the result of functional disruption of thalamocortical communication (Fischer-Perroudon et al., 1974; Josephs et al., 2004; Montagna & Lugaresi, 2002).

A retrospective review of a national database in Taiwan of all diagnoses of neurodegenerative diseases between 2000 and 2015 found that some conditions were associated with diagnoses of sleep disorders, including sleep apnea and insomnia. Given the nature of the study, these associations could reflect co-morbidities or sleep symptoms secondary to the diseases. However, longer durations of sleep disorders were associated with higher probabilities of developing a neurodegenerative disease, suggesting that the sleep disorder was either, or both, an early symptom of the disease or a contributor to its development (Lin et al., 2023).

proto-lymphatic) system (Iliff et al., 2012) was faster during sleep or anesthesia than during waking. These differences were the result of sleep/anesthesia enhancing the flow of CSF through the depth of the cortex by expanding the volume of the interstitial space surrounding cells (Xie et al., 2013) (**Figure 15.8**).

The reported strong correlations between SWS and lower Aβ levels (Ju et al., 2017; Varga et al., 2016) could be explained by evidence that SWA is associated with an increased flow of blood and CSF into the human brain. During SWS, high amounts of SWA were followed by waves of increased blood flow into the cortex that were not seen during waking, followed by inflow of CSF into the ventricles (Fultz et al., 2019; Helakari et al., 2022) (**Figure 15.9**).

These findings suggest that sleep (especially SWS) plays an important role in facilitating removal of potentially toxic products of cellular metabolism throughout the depth of cortical tissue, which during waking occurs mainly near the cortical surface.[10] One implication of these results is that the reduced amounts of SWS in older people (especially in men) (see Chapter 4), may allow faster buildup of neurotoxic agents like Aβ and tau protein in the brain.

However, both theoretical arguments and experimental findings have raised questions about whether an active transport system based on glial activity is involved in removing molecules from the brain; for contrasting reviews, see Beschorner & Nedergaard, 2024; Smith & Verkman, 2018. In some studies, movement of molecules through brain tissue has been ascribed to passive mechanisms, such as diffusion, with no evidence of active transport via the glymphatic system. Most relevant to the present discussion, one study concluded that the clearance

[10] This evidence led to development of a hypothesis to explain differences among species in sleep amounts, which is discussed in Section 16.3.1 (Herculano-Houzel, 2015).

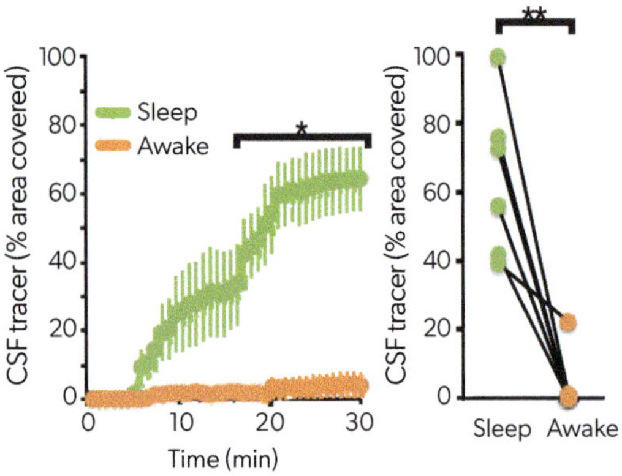

Figure 15.8 **A.** Two-photon imaging was used to observe regions of the cortex of living mice while awake and asleep. A tracer was injected into the cerebrospinal fluid of mice, and the area of the cortical region in which the tracer appeared (Y axis) was observed over a 30 min period (X axis). During sleep (green) the tracer penetrated a much larger volume of the cortex than while the mice were awake (orange). **B.** The final area of cortex labeled by the injected tracer at the end of 30 min of sleep (green) or wake (orange) is shown for individual mice. **p <0.01. Adapted with permission of the AAAS and Dr. Maiken Nedergaard (University of Copenhagen) from Xie L. et al. (2013) Sleep drives metabolite clearance from the adult brain. *Science* 342:373–377. © American Association for the Advancement of Science (2013); permission conveyed through Copyright Clearance Center, Inc. doi: 10.1126/science.1241224.

of molecules from brain tissue was actually slower, rather than faster, during sleep or anesthesia (Miao et al., 2024). These contradictory conclusions came from studies with many technical and procedural differences, so this issue remains to be resolved by future research.

Regardless of the mechanism(s) involved, animal studies consistently showed that sleep loss increased levels of Aβ in the brain. Human studies, however, present a less consistent picture. One review concluded that there remains uncertainty about the degree to which sleep loss or disruption produces a pattern of brain changes that is consistent with the characteristic changes seen in AD. It also indicated that correlations between reduced sleep/SWA and markers of brain pathology may appear either because sleep loss affects brain health or because brain pathology alters sleep. For example, loss of gray matter volume, which accompanies increases in Aβ plaques and tau protein during the progression of AD, may reduce the capacity to generate large-amplitude slow waves (André et al., 2021).

A systematic review of the literature related to how sleep parameters affect levels of neurochemical markers related to risk of AD and other diseases in people also concluded that the available evidence is weak and often conflicting. A major concern was the variety of methods used to assess sleep parameters, making it difficult to compare results among studies. The review also stressed that studies with small numbers of participants increased the risk of reaching conclusions that are not supported by larger studies (Sangalli & Boggero, 2023).

One apparently consistent finding was that studies that included participants younger than 65 years showed a

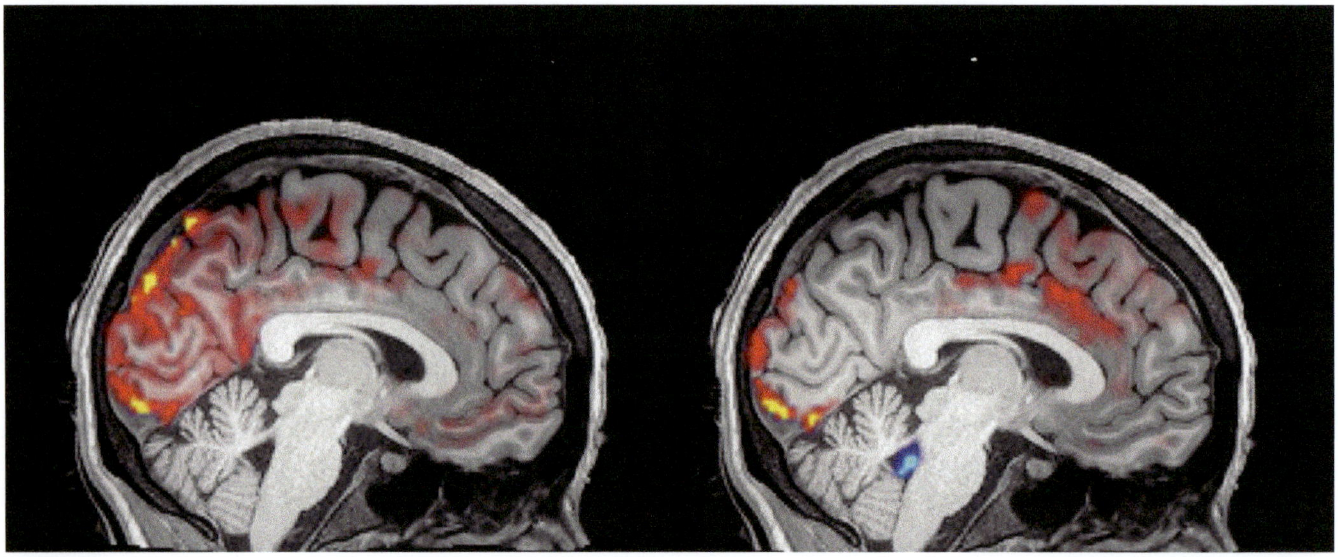

Figure 15.9 Functional magnetic resonance imaging was combined with EEG recordings to assess patterns of flow of blood and cerebrospinal fluid in the brain associated with sleep. Regions of pulsatile increases (at ~20 sec intervals) in blood flow into the brain (red/yellow; left panel), followed high levels of slow-wave activity during slow-wave sleep, and were followed in turn by an influx of cerebrospinal fluid (blue; right panel). The images were extracted from a video recording and were provided courtesy of Dr. Laura Lewis, Massachusetts Institute of Technology. For more details, see Fultz N.E. et al. (2019) Coupled electrophysiological, hemodynamic, and cerebrospinal fluid oscillations in human sleep. *Science* 366:628–631. doi: 10.1126/science.aax5440.

correlation between shorter total sleep time and higher Aβ levels, while studies with older participants showed mixed or contradictory results. One possibility is that aging-related increases in brain pathology (in the absence of AD) could obscure the effects of sleep deficits on Aβ levels in older populations (Sangalli & Boggero, 2023). An example is that the size of the basal forebrain cholinergic system decreases with age in the absence of dementia but decreases further in those with AD (Grothe et al., 2012).

The issue is further complicated by evidence that sleep disruption and AD are reciprocally related. Evidence supporting a role for sleep loss in promoting Aβ plaques came from studies showing that mice that were genetically engineered to spontaneously develop amyloid plaques showed even greater plaque numbers if they also underwent experimental sleep deprivation (Kang et al., 2009). Other AD model mice developed disrupted circadian rhythms and disrupted sleep patterns after Aβ plaques had appeared (Roh et al., 2012; Sterniczuk et al., 2010). The degree of sleep disruption observed in these mice was positively correlated with the extent of Aβ plaque development, which is ambiguous as to the direction of causality. But, critically, immunization against Aβ prevented the deterioration of sleep quality, suggesting that increased Aβ levels disrupted sleep (Roh et al., 2012). Studies using zebrafish have also shown that genetic manipulations that produced a variety of changes in amyloid physiology also affect sleep duration and activity levels (Özcan et al., 2024).

Factors contributing to the development of AD may influence sleep mechanisms at very early stages of the development of the disease, long before cognitive deficits and cortical changes are seen. Evidence supporting this idea came from a postmortem study of the brains of people who died at the earliest stages of potentially developing AD. These people were considered to be at Braak Stage I (Braak & Braak, 1991), based on the presence of tau pathology in the medial temporal lobe (MTL) or at Braak Stage 0 (those with no evident MTL pathology). Tau-related pathology appeared in an array of subcortical nuclei that are involved in sleep–wake regulation (among other subcortical structures). These included the cholinergic basal forebrain, perifornical and lateral hypothalamus, substantia nigra, ventral tegmental area, periaqueductal gray, dorsal raphe, and locus coeruleus; see Chapters 10 & 11. Three individuals considered to be at Braak Stage 0 at death showed the earliest signs of tau pathology in these subcortical structures; they had died at an average age of 29 years (Stratmann et al., 2016).

Postmortem studies of patients who had been diagnosed with AD showed that a key sleep regulatory structure in the ventrolateral preoptic area (VLPO) had a reduced number of galanin-immunoreactive neurons (involved in promoting sleep continuity; see Section 11.4), relative to controls without AD (Lim et al., 2014). This reduction in sleep-regulatory neurons may have been the result of neurodegeneration caused by AD, and it could also have contributed to additional cell loss because the resulting disruption of sleep further increased Aβ levels.

Sleep loss may also act indirectly to increase the risk of developing AD. Sleep loss in mice and rats increased the risk of having a leaky blood-brain barrier (BBB) (Gómez-González et al., 2013; He et al., 2014; Hurtado-Alvarado et al., 2017), possibly as a result of chronic inflammation (Hurtado-Alvarado et al., 2016).[11] The BBB is the lining of blood vessels in the brain that both protects brain tissue from circulating pathogens and regulates the exchange of molecules between brain tissue and the circulatory system. People with early stage AD also showed broadly distributed increases in BBB leakage (van den Haar et al., 2016). Whether BBB leakage and inflammation contribute to the development of AD or are consequences of the sleep disruption seen in patients with AD, is not clear; both may be true.

The evidence that SWS protects against the accumulation of Aβ can be linked to the findings reviewed in earlier sections that reductions in sleep, and especially loss of SWS, are associated with disturbed glucose regulation and development of diabetes (Section 14.6), hypertension (Section 14.8), and inflammation (Section 14.9), all of which also contribute to neural damage and increase the risk of dementia or AD (Abell et al., 2018; Darweesh et al., 2018; Kloppenborg et al., 2008; McGrath et al., 2018). Thus, loss of sleep (especially SWS) may have direct effects on the risk of AD by reducing brain clearance of toxins. But sleep loss may also act indirectly by increasing the risk of developing these metabolic and regulatory disorders, which themselves increase the risk of AD.

Similarly, self-reported difficulty initiating sleep (one symptom of insomnia) was associated 14 years later with poorer cognitive functioning in several domains. These associations were mediated in part through the presence of depressive symptoms and vascular disease (Zaheed et al., 2023). Depression is associated with hippocampal tissue loss, and vascular disease can lead to microvascular damage in the brain, both of which contribute to cognitive decline and increased risk of developing dementia.

The path to developing AD may be best understood as involving multiple interacting processes and several feedback loops. Sleep disruption and loss, like other component processes, may both contribute to the development of AD and be further intensified by the consequences of the disease. **Figure 15.10** illustrates a web of functional, reciprocal connections that likely link inadequate sleep and AD.

[11] A later study did not find evidence for leakage of the BBB after chronic sleep restriction in rats (Hall et al., 2020) possibly because of the use of less severe patterns and durations of sleep loss.

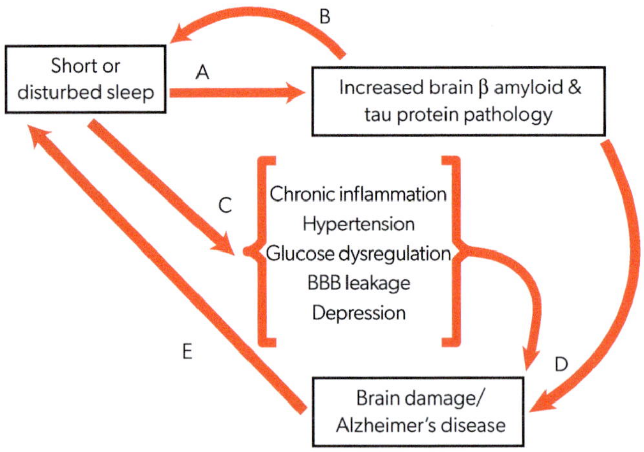

Figure 15.10 This flow diagram summarizes some of the proposed connections between chronically short and/or disturbed sleep and an increased risk of developing Alzheimer's disease. **A.** Short or disturbed sleep increases brain levels of beta (β) amyloid by reducing its clearance from the brain as well as the clearance of tau protein. **B.** Increased beta amyloid levels also disturb sleep further, leading to a positive feedback loop. **C.** Short/disturbed sleep is also linked to increased risk of chronic inflammation, hypertension, glucose dysregulation, blood-brain barrier (BBB) leakage, and depression. **D.** High levels of beta amyloid and tau protein, chronic inflammation, hypertension, glucose dysregulation, BBB leakage, and depression, which are related to short and disturbed sleep, have all been proposed to contribute to neurodegeneration, and ultimately to increase the risk of developing Alzheimer's disease or other dementias. **E.** The associated brain damage (e.g., to the ventrolateral preoptic area, suprachiasmatic nuclei, and other sleep-regulatory systems) may in turn disrupt sleep and disturb daily rhythms, which further accelerates the processes leading to neural degeneration.

In addition to effects of short sleep, prospective cohort studies have also reported that long (≥9 h) sleep is associated with increased risk of developing dementia or AD. Progressive lengthening of sleep duration, in particular, has been associated with an increased risk of AD and with decreased cerebral volumes, possibly reflecting neural degeneration (Benito-León et al., 2009; Lu et al., 2018; Westwood et al., 2017). The connection between long sleep durations and dementia is surprising, given other evidence that sleep promotes removal of potentially toxic waste products from the brain and is neuroprotective. The basis for this linkage is discussed in Section 15.7.

15.5.4 Summary

Sleep and rhythm disturbances are common symptoms of AD and can serve as early markers of the disease before core cognitive symptoms appear. Sleep disruption (especially reduced SWS) is associated with high levels of Aβ in the brain in animal studies and increased risk of a subsequent diagnosis of AD or dementia in some human research. Other research indicates that tau-related pathology precedes the development of Aβ plaques and that its distribution best matches the patterns of cognitive dysfunction that occur. The relative roles of Aβ and tau protein in triggering neurodegeneration and dementia are the subject of continuing debate, but it appears that sleep disruption is associated with abnormal regulation of both Aβ and tau protein.

The evidence in humans, however, is inconsistent, probably as a result of the use of varying measures of sleep duration and quality across studies. The effects of short sleep on neurodegeneration may be clearer in younger populations because aging-related neural damage can make it more difficult to detect additional degenerative changes attributable to sleep characteristics.

The processes linking sleep problems and increased risk of developing AD are not firmly established, but there are several identified mechanisms in animal and human studies that could contribute to this association. Waking increases levels of Aβ in the brain, presumably as a by-product of brain metabolic activity. There is evidence that sleep is associated with increases in the volume of interstitial space in the cortex, which promotes faster clearance of Aβ, and presumably other toxins, from the brain. SWA is also specifically associated with increased flow of blood and CSF into the brain. These sleep-related changes may play an important role in removing toxic waste products from the brain and reducing the buildup of proteins linked to neuropathology. However, contradictory results obtained using different methods have raised questions about these proposed mechanisms and about whether sleep increases the rates of clearance of molecules from the brain.

Animal research has indicated that the interactions between sleep and AD may be reciprocal. Increased Aβ plaque levels in mice were associated with increased sleep disruption, which can be prevented by reducing Aβ plaque formation. Thus, sleep loss appears to increase levels of Aβ, and these increased levels can further disrupt sleep, leading to a positive feedback loop that promotes the development of brain damage and AD symptoms. Chronic short sleep also increases the probability of developing other conditions (e.g., Type 2 diabetes, hypertension, inflammation) that are, in turn, associated with an increased risk of brain damage and the development of AD. Therefore, chronic sleep reduction may act both directly and indirectly to promote physiological changes that increase the risk of brain damage and the development of AD.

15.6 Sleep and mortality risk

15.6.1 Association of mortality risk with both short and long sleep

A variety of population-based, observational studies found that short sleep, long sleep, or both were associated with increased mortality risk (i.e., the risk of dying within the multiyear period of a study), resulting in many reports of U-shaped relations between sleep duration and risk. Cut-off values defining short and long sleep differed among studies, but several studies reported the lowest mortality risk for those sleeping ~7 h or 7–8 h, and increasing risk for those sleeping either <7 h or ≥8 h (Kripke et al., 2002; Patel et al., 2004; Shen et al., 2016; Yin et al., 2017). Studies that applied more extreme cut-off values, such as ≤5 for short sleep and ≥9 h for long sleep, often found higher relative risk estimates linked to these definitions: 1.25–1.27 and 1.3–1.47 (or averages of ~26% and ~39% increases in risk, respectively), relative to the reference group (Gangwisch et al., 2008; Soh et al., 2018; Tao et al., 2021).

Some of the complexities inherent in trying to compare results among studies are illustrated by comparing the conclusions reached about how the age and gender of participants influenced the apparent risk associated with sleep duration differences in a selection of these studies. A Swedish study (~34,000 participants) used the ≤5 and ≥9 h cut-offs and a reference value of 6 h of sleep. Self-reported sleep was assessed at the start of the study based on a question about usual sleep on "weekday nights." Participants averaged ~50 years old at baseline and the follow-up period for assessing mortality risk was up to 20.5 years.

This study reported similar relative risks for short and long sleep for the entire sample (1.28 and 1.29, respectively), after full adjustment for confounding variables. Separate analyses of mortality risk for men and women found that risk was significantly elevated among women for both short and long sleep (1.54 and 1.30). But for men, only long sleep was significantly associated with increased mortality risk (1.28); men with short sleep did not have increased risk relative to the reference group (Åkerstedt et al., 2024).

Another large-scale study using a United Kingdom database (>400,000 participants) asked participants to estimate their sleep over 24 h periods, including naps. It compared short (≤5 h) and long (≥9 h) sleepers to a reference group reporting 7 h of sleep. During up to a 10-year follow-up period, the study found increased all-cause mortality risk in the entire sample for both short and long sleepers (1.25 and 1.30, respectively). Separated by gender, there was significantly increased mortality risk for long sleepers among both men (1.34) and women (1.21). Among short sleepers, men also showed a significantly increased risk (1.33), but the result for women was ambiguous, with a relative risk of 1.12 and a 95% confidence interval of 1.00–12.6 (Tao et al., 2021).

An American population-based study (n ≈9,800) asked about usual hours of sleep at night or when participants usually slept, without reference to weekdays, weekends, or naps. It used ≤5 and ≥9 h as cut-offs and 7 h as a reference value, with an 8–10 year follow-up. It found that both short and long sleep increased risk in men and women in an unadjusted model, but in a fully adjusted model,[12] long sleep remained a significant risk for both men and women, as did short sleep for men, but it was no longer significantly associated with increased risk in women (Gangwisch et al., 2008). Thus, this study and the (Tao et al., 2021) study agreed that short sleep in men, but not in women, was significantly associated with mortality risk, while the (Åkerstedt et al., 2024) study found that short sleep increased risk in women but not in men.

Another American study, that included only female nurses and used 7.0 h as the reference value and cut-offs of <5 and 8 h or more, found that both short and long sleep were associated with increased risk over 14 years of follow-up in an unadjusted model. In a fully adjusted model, however, the impact of short sleep was no longer significant, but long sleep remained a significant risk factor (Patel et al., 2004). This result is consistent with those for women in (Gangwisch et al., 2008) and (Tao et al., 2021) but not with the increased risk for women with short sleep in (Åkerstedt et al., 2024).

Earlier studies cited in these reports had a variety of results, but the largest study of sleep effects on mortality risk (using a reference value of 7 h and a 6 year follow-up) found that both short and long sleep were associated with significantly increased mortality risk in both men and women and that the effects were most robust for long sleep (Kripke et al., 2002).

It is not clear why these large studies conducted on populations in relatively wealthy, industrialized societies reached different conclusions about the effects of short sleep on risk in men and women. One potential contributing factor is that the elevated mortality risk for women with short sleep increased progressively with the length of follow-up in the (Åkerstedt et al., 2024) study, while it was stable for men. Mortality rates for women increased especially between 10 and 20 years of the follow-up period. This study had the longest follow-up (~20 years), compared to ~10–14 years for the other studies (Gangwisch et al., 2008; Patel et al., 2004; Tao et al., 2021). Studies with shorter follow-up periods might have missed the interval of greatest increase in mortality risk for older women who were short sleepers. Another important difference is that the reference value used in the (Åkerstedt et al., 2024) study was 6 h, but the other studies used 7 h.

The questions asked about sleep also differed among studies. Participants in the Swedish survey were asked about their usual sleep on weekday nights. Those in the two American

[12] To illustrate the range of potentially confounding variables applied in fully adjusted models, in the (Gangwisch et al., 2008) study these included age, physical activity, smoking, depression, gender (for the full cohort), education, living alone, low income, daytime sleepiness, nighttime awakening, ethnicity, sleeping pill use, body weight, diabetes, hypertension, general health, and cancer. For a listing of confounders used across 27 studies, see the meta-analysis by (da Silva et al., 2016).

studies were asked about the number of hours of sleep participants "usually get a night (or when you usually sleep)" (Gangwisch et al., 2008), and the "total hours of actual sleep in a 24-hour period" (Patel et al., 2004). The UK-based study asked, "About how many hours sleep do you get in every 24 hours?" and added a request to please include naps.

Thus, the implication of the key question asked in three of these studies is that weekend and weekday nights might (or might not) be included, while one study explicitly excluded weekend sleep. One study asked about sleep over 24 h and explicitly included naps. Another asked about sleep over 24 h without explicitly including or excluding naps. A third asked about sleep only at night (presumably excluding naps), and the fourth study was ambiguous because it asked about sleep at night "or when you usually sleep", which may have been especially relevant to habitual shift workers. Whether participants chose to include weekend sleep or not in their estimates could be important. There is evidence that the metabolic health of chronic short sleepers may benefit from weekend catch-up sleep (at least in a Korean population) (Kim et al., 2020), but there are also conflicting findings about the consequences of irregular weekly sleep schedules, as discussed in Section 14.6.2.

There are also cultural, ethnic, and environmental differences among the countries in which these studies were conducted. One American study (Gangwisch et al., 2008), for example, included ~14.5% of participants listed as "non-Caucasian," with the highest proportions of this population appearing in the most extreme short and long sleep groups. The Swedish report did not comment on racial or ethnic background but may have included a more homogeneous sample. The UK study used a Biobank that included ethnic information, but the publication did not include discussion of this feature of the sample. Several studies have reported that Black Americans are more likely to report both short and long sleep than White Americans, after adjusting for many social and demographic factors (Nunes et al., 2008; Seixas et al., 2017).

Another factor that was considered in some studies was whether the effect of sleep duration on mortality risk was related to the age of participants at baseline. An American study (Gangwisch et al., 2008) found that sleep duration affected mortality risk over 8–10 years in those who were 60–86 years old but not in those who were 32–59 years old at baseline. The overall lower probability of dying in middle age may have reduced the chances of detecting a significant effect of sleep duration in the younger cohort. However, another report based on a Swedish cohort (Åkerstedt et al., 2017) that included participants with an average age of ~50 years at baseline and a longer follow-up period (~18.3 years), concluded that sleep duration affected mortality risk for those up to 65 years old at baseline but not for those older than 65.

Although these results seem to point to different conclusions about whether effects of sleep duration on mortality risk are most evident in older or younger participants, the effect of the starting age of participants in a study may interact with the length of follow-up to determine the outcome. A short follow-up period may favor detecting an effect on older participants, because younger participants are at lower risk of dying. A longer follow-up may instead favor detecting effects on younger participants, since variability in mortality risk is likely reduced in very old participants.

Although several studies used 7 h as the reference sleep duration, they had different lengths of follow-up and used different questions to ask about sleep duration (the same questions mentioned previously in the discussion of gender differences). It is unclear whether differences in methods, follow-up duration, or in racial/ethnic composition of the samples studied contributed to the different conclusions reached. Ambiguity in some studies' instructions with respect to inclusion of naps may also be important. A British study involving >1,700 men aged 71–92 at baseline, with a 9-year follow-up period asked about both nighttime sleep and daytime naps. It reported no association of nighttime short or long sleep with mortality risk in a fully adjusted model, but observed a significantly increased risk of dying among those reporting daytime naps >1 h (Chen et al., 2023).

There have also been several meta-analyses summarizing results across studies of sleep duration and mortality risk. Because many of these studies were based on extracting information about sleep from large population surveys, the researchers interested in the effects of sleep typically had no control over the nature of the questions asked or the categories participants used to report on their sleep. For example, participants might be given a choice among ≤5, 6, 7, 8 and ≥9 h or be asked to provide a whole number as their estimate.

As a result, reviews and meta-analyses necessarily included studies that used different questions about sleep and different forms of data. The studies also used several different cut-off values for short and long sleep and, less frequently, different reference values, although these were most often ~7 h. A sample of several meta-analyses reported relative mortality risks among studies for short and long sleep (variously defined in the contributing studies) of 1.06 to 1.12 and 1.23 to 1.36 (or ~10% and ~30% increases), respectively (Cappuccio et al., 2010; da Silva et al., 2016; Gallicchio & Kalesan, 2009).

15.6.2 Other factors affecting studies of mortality risk

The fact that both short and long sleep were identified in many studies as being associated with increased mortality risk does not imply that the effects of short and long sleep are equivalent.

In most studies, as indicated by the size of the risk ratios mentioned above, long sleep was a stronger predictor than short sleep of increased risk. Despite this difference, one meta-analysis concluded that the association with short sleep was consistent regardless of starting age, gender, definition of short sleep, length of follow-up, geographic location, or adjustment for socioeconomic status. The association with long sleep, however, varied depending on the definition of long sleep, the age of the cohort, the length of follow-up, and the geographic location of studies (Cappuccio et al., 2010). One meta-analysis suggested that short sleep was associated with increased mortality risk primarily in American studies (da Silva et al., 2016), but another analysis did not support this interpretation (Cappuccio et al., 2010).

Despite some consistent findings related to short and long self-reported sleep in most studies, there are limitations in the available data that suggest caution in interpreting some of the results. First, with few exceptions, most studies relied on participants responding to one or a few survey questions about sleep length. This approach raises the issue of the accuracy of participants' responses and the degree to which other factors influenced them. As discussed in Section 14.4.2, responses to questions about sleep duration can be affected by memory distortion, wanting to provide socially acceptable responses, cultural influences, feelings about their sleep quality (rather than duration), and sleep-state misperception, among other factors.

Responses will also be affected by the terminology used in survey questions and how participants interpret them. Thus, questions in different surveys about sleep length that include terms such as "last week," "last month," "typical/usual/average," "weeknights," "including weekend nights," "in 24 h," "including naps," or not referring to naps or to weeknight-weekend differences, can influence how participants respond and make it difficult to compare results across studies.

Second, although different studies control for a variety of potential confounders, it is possible that unsuspected ("hidden") confounders exist that are not controlled for in most studies (Kurina et al., 2013). Finally, whether subjective or objective measures are used, only one or a very few assessments were obtained in most studies. It is not clear how stable sleep durations are over the decades during which health conditions emerge that may affect mortality risk (see discussion in Section 14.6.1).

A few studies obtained two self-reports separated by a few years. Mortality risk was reported to be higher for people who reported substantial changes in nightly sleep durations or daily napping behavior during aging (Cheng et al., 2018; Ferrie et al., 2007; Hublin et al., 2007; Soh et al., 2018). In a Finnish study that involved two surveys 6 years apart, only about 2/3 of respondents stayed in the same category (short, average, or long sleep) in both surveys; both stable short and stable long sleep were associated with increased risk. About equal proportions of participants shifted to the short and long categories, and these changes were also associated with increased risk in most cases (Hublin et al., 2007).

In a British study, two surveys were completed 4–5 years apart, for followup periods of 17 and 12 years, relative to the first and second surveys. Reported short (≤5 h) and long (≥9 h) sleep on the second survey were both associated with increased mortality risk, regardless of responses on the first survey. In addition, shortening sleep on the second survey from 6, 7, or 8 h on the first survey, or lengthening from 7 or 8 h were associated with increased mortality risk. (Ferrie et al., 2007). A study in Scotland that surveyed people 4–7 years apart found that those who reported short sleep (<7 h) on both surveys had increased mortality risk relative to those reporting average sleep (7 to 8 h) on both surveys (Heslop et al., 2002).

A study in China of people with a starting median age of 82 years reported that increasing sleep duration by >1 h per year over the next ~4 years increased the risk of all-cause mortality by 29% relative to a group with stable sleep; shortening sleep did not affect relative mortality rates (Ruan et al., 2023).

In addition to confirming the increased risks of self-reported short and long sleep, these studies with repeated measurements indicated that a substantial proportion of individuals change sleep duration categories over a period of a few years. Although not formally tested in these studies, there is suggestive evidence that responses closer to the time of death may better predict mortality risk.

A meta-analysis of studies that examined the relation of insomnia symptoms, rather than sleep duration, to mortality risk found no significant difference in risk between those who did or did not report insomnia symptoms (Lovato & Lack, 2019), confirming a similar conclusion from the largest single study of sleep duration effects on mortality (>1.1 million participants) (Kripke et al., 2002).

Other factors that may not be detected in studies involving questionnaires can also affect the outcome. A study that measured sleep using PSG also asked whether participants had at least a 1-year history of insomnia (see the definition of insomnia in Box 4.3, Chapter 4). Mortality risk in men over a 14-year period was highly elevated among those who had objective short sleep and reported insomnia symptoms[13] but not among those with only one of these characteristics (Vgontzas et al., 2010). This result is consistent with the previously cited studies

[13] The apparent distinctiveness of this subgroup was supported by a report that Cognitive Behavioral Therapy for Insomnia (CBT-I) was less successful for insomnia patients with objective short sleep (Bathgate et al., 2017). More recent studies, however, reported that CBT-I had similar benefits for insomnia patients regardless of their objectively measured sleep duration before treatment (Crönlein et al., 2020; Galbiati et al., 2021; Rochefort et al., 2019).

that the presence of insomnia symptoms alone did not affect mortality risk (Kripke et al., 2002; Lovato & Lack, 2019).

Partially consistent with these studies were the results of a study of ethnic Chinese participants in Taiwan. It found that long sleep (≥9 h) was associated with increased mortality risk, but short sleep, occasional insomnia, and frequent insomnia were not. However, insomnia "nearly every day" significantly increased mortality risk after full adjustment for confounders. The highest mortality risk was found among those reporting both ≥9 h sleep and insomnia symptoms nearly every day (Chien et al., 2010). Long sleep combined with frequent insomnia symptoms and daytime sleepiness were also associated with increased mortality risk in a Swedish cohort, while long sleep without insomnia symptoms was not, nor was the presence of insomnia in those sleeping 8 h or less (Hedström et al., 2019).

A PSG study included data from two American cohorts over a 15-year period. It found that there was increased mortality risk related to a cluster of PSG-based sleep measures, but not for self-reported short sleep, after controlling for many other variables. The strongest predictors derived from PSG were low sleep efficiency and longer periods of blood oxygen saturation below 90%. Oxygen saturation would likely be affected by sleep-disordered breathing (SDB; e.g., sleep apnea) and other respiratory conditions. Reduced sleep efficiency could be the result of sleep disruptions from SDB, restless legs syndrome (RLS), or insomnia (Wallace et al., 2021). SDB and RLS were detected during PSG studies, but they might not emerge as potential confounders from studies relying on self-reports, because many people are unaware that they have these conditions.

A study that collected a week of actigraphic data from >1800 people (average age ~63 years) assessed mortality risk over the next >6 years. It reported that sleep duration was linked to mortality risk, but that there was a stronger association with more irregular sleep patterns. The measure used to assess sleep regularity captured variability in timing of not only sleep onset and end but also the pattern of sleep and wake throughout 24 h periods, which would include sleep disruption and napping patterns. Higher degrees of sleep irregularity were associated with increased risk of cardiovascular and all-cause mortality after controlling for many variables, including sleep duration (Windred et al., 2023).

Sleep duration and sleep irregularity were not independent of each other. Sleep durations up to ~7.8 h were associated with increasing regularity, but regularity then decreased for those with longer sleep durations (Windred et al., 2023). These results suggest that long sleep may be associated with more disrupted and less consistent sleep patterns. The finding that irregularity in sleep patterns predicts higher mortality risk is consistent with other evidence for increased risk of AD in those with more disrupted daily rest-activity patterns (Lim et al., 2013); see Section 15.5.1.

15.6.3 Summary

Studies that found an association of sleep duration with mortality risk often reported that both short and long sleep were associated with increased mortality risk relative to those sleeping ~7–8 h nightly. Long sleep predicted increased mortality risk across most studies, and usually more robustly than short sleep, even when short sleep was a significant predictor. In addition, increasing sleep durations over years among older people also predicted increased mortality risk. Studies that involved two surveys several years apart indicated that consistent short or long sleep increased risk, but those who increased or decreased sleep from near the reference value on a second survey were also at increased mortality risk. The finding that a significant proportion of respondents moved between sleep duration categories within a few years raises questions about the stability of self-reported sleep durations and therefore about the reliability of classifying survey respondents into one sleep duration category based on a single self-report.

Even studies that did not find significant effects of specific short sleep durations on mortality risk often reported U-shaped functions for risk in relation to sleep duration, with lowest risk around 7 h. The lack of significant effects of short sleep in some studies may reflect a lack of sufficient statistical power to measure these effects in smaller studies, since the effects of short sleep were generally weaker than those of long sleep. However, the largest single study of mortality risk found statistically significant increases in relative risk for both short and long sleep.

The results in individual studies, however, appeared to be affected by several factors: the gender of participants; the presence of comorbidities, including insomnia, SDB, or other sleep disorders; the baseline age composition of the groups; the length of follow-up; the cut-off and reference values used for sleep durations; the wording of questions in self-report questionnaires; the ethnic/racial/national composition of the study samples; and the types of potential confounders that were considered. The variety of questions about sleep duration used in different studies (e.g., weekday, usual, 24 h, including naps or not) and how these forms of question affect participants' responses deserves careful analysis. One meta-analysis reported that several factors affected the strength of the reported association with long sleep, but the association of mortality risk with short sleep was largely independent of demographic and study design factors.

Disruption of daily sleep rhythms, assessed using actigraphy, also predicted increased cardiovascular and all-cause mortality risk, even when controlling for the effects of sleep duration. The linked factors of shorter sleep durations and more irregular rhythms each predicted increased mortality risk.

15.7 Why long and short sleep are related to illness and mortality risk

The often observed association of short or disrupted sleep with increased mortality risk can reasonably be attributed to the increased risk of serious health problems that observational studies find are also correlated with short sleep. These include diabetes, obesity, vascular disease, chronic inflammation, psychiatric illnesses, and the accumulation of neural markers related to development of AD/dementia (Itani et al., 2017; Knapik et al., 2023). In addition, experimental studies have shown that acute sleep restriction affects surrogate markers for these conditions in ways that would likely produce poor health outcomes if short sleep were a chronic condition. These experimental results strengthen the interpretation from observational studies that chronic short sleep over decades could contribute to developing these illnesses, and ultimately to increasing mortality risk.

Nevertheless, it remains a challenge to decide whether these associations indicate that particular illnesses are consequences or causes of short sleep (Kurina et al., 2013). Longitudinal studies showing that short sleep at one age in the absence of illness is followed by a later increased risk of emergence of the illness can partially address this issue. For example, a meta-analysis of studies in adults concluded that there was a cross-sectional association of both short and long sleep with the presence of the metabolic syndrome. Prospective cohort studies, however, showed that only short sleep predicted later development of the metabolic syndrome (Hua et al., 2021).

These results support the interpretation that short sleep is a risk factor for the future development of conditions that could lead to early death. Long sleep in the studies reviewed, however, occurred at the same time as symptoms of the metabolic syndrome, rather than preceding its appearance (Hua et al., 2021). This result could be consistent with alternative interpretations: that long sleep is a consequence of metabolic abnormalities, or that both are attributable to an unidentified common cause.

It is uncertain why long sleep (defined in different studies as >8, 9, or 10 h nightly) should be linked to several of the clinical conditions discussed in Chapters 14 and 15 (diabetes, vascular disease, obesity, some forms of depression) and to increased relative mortality risk (Grandner & Drummond, 2007; Jike et al., 2018); see Section 15.6.1. Experimental tests of whether long sleep causes physiological effects that might reasonably contribute to these risks would involve laboratory studies that lengthen sleep beyond, for example, 8 or 9 h. These studies would be designed to observe effects on surrogate markers of disease as a parallel to experimental studies that restrict sleep to <6 or 7 h. Conducting such studies by lengthening the sleep of otherwise healthy, average sleepers is, however, a difficult challenge. It is easy in a laboratory to get willing, 7–8 h sleepers to sleep less by keeping them out of bed beyond a target duration, monitoring them continuously, and alerting them as needed. But participants cannot be compelled by experimenters to sleep more than they choose to.

A few studies have, however, tried to assess the effects of extending sleep on health markers. It is important, however, to consider baseline sleep durations in such studies. Among habitual short sleepers, increasing sleep durations toward the recommended range would be predicted to have health benefits, rather than being harmful. These benefits of extending sleep for short sleepers have been shown, in fact, for symptoms of the metabolic syndrome (Eckel et al., 2015; Kim et al., 2020; Leproult et al., 2015; Tasali et al., 2022) (see Section 14.6.2); for pain sensitivity (Roehrs et al., 2012; Simonelli et al., 2019) (see Section 15.2); and for mood, negative emotions, and daytime sleepiness (Casement et al., 2020; Dewald-Kaufmann et al., 2014; Parsons & Young, 2022; Van Dyk et al., 2017). A meta-analysis of studies involving sleep extension among those starting with habitual short sleep found that the approaches used can be very effective, and it confirmed these benefits and others (Baron et al., 2021).

One study that was planned to increase sleep duration among short sleepers (<6.5 h), who were also obese and had symptoms of the metabolic syndrome, found that participants "spontaneously" increased sleep by an average of ~30 min during a ~3-month period intended to establish baseline sleep and metabolic features. This increase occurred *before* participants were assigned to either a treatment or control condition. Increased sleep was accompanied by reduced sleepiness and significant improvements in metabolic syndrome features (Cizza et al., 2014). It is unclear what caused the increase in sleep duration. One possibility is that participants were sensitized to issues related to their sleep and diet habits by the careful, daily record-keeping required during the baseline period. Whatever the explanation, these self-generated increases in sleep amounts among habitual short sleepers improved several aspects of their health.

Increasing sleep durations among those who usually sleep 7–8 h nightly is more difficult. Although unable to compel increased sleep, a few studies have successfully encouraged people with normal baseline durations to lengthen sleep in different ways: keeping them for 14 h nightly in a darkened laboratory for up to 28 nights (Wehr et al., 1993); scheduling extended sleep times at home (Harrison & Horne, 1996); or scheduling longer sleep opportunities in a laboratory (Taub et al., 1971). The effects of sleep extension were neutral or mildly beneficial in these studies, except that increasing sleep (from 7–8 to ~9 h for 2 nights) reduced performance on some cognitive tests (Taub et al., 1971).[14] There were reports of reduced fatigue and improved mood among those who spent 14 h nightly in the dark for several weeks and increased their sleep time, except for one individual who became depressed soon after the transfer to 14 h nights and was removed from the study[15] (Wehr et al., 1993). No mood improvements or declines were reported in those sleeping up to 10 h nightly at home (Harrison & Horne, 1996).

These studies included few physiological measures that could serve as surrogate markers for the clinical conditions associated with long sleep in observational studies. The few hormonal changes observed in one study were unlikely to be harmful (Wehr et al., 1993). This evidence is very limited, but it does not suggest that long sleep itself alters physiological parameters acutely in ways that, if sustained, are likely to contribute over the longer term to illness or shorter lifespans. Other explanations are needed for the observed association between long (or lengthening) sleep and increased risk of illness or mortality.

It is likely that reverse causality accounts for some of these associations; that is, self-reported long sleep is the result, not the cause, of illnesses that lead to early death. Conditions that reduce activity and increase fatigue and insomnia symptoms may result in frequent napping, disrupted sleep, and lengthy times in bed; for example, excess body weight, undetected depression or sleep apnea, disrupted daily rhythms, or early stages of diabetes or neurodegenerative conditions. Lengthy periods spent in bed may then be self-reported as long sleep durations, even though actual time asleep may not be increased (Grandner & Drummond, 2007).

In a 2001 poll in the United States, both short and long sleepers reported more sleep complaints than those who slept 8 h. Complaints included difficulty falling asleep, waking during the night, daytime sleepiness, waking too early, and unrefreshing sleep. Short sleep is logically linked to these complaints, but they are unlikely consequences of long sleep. The fact that these complaints accompanied self-reports of long sleep suggests that many such reports reflect poor quality, disrupted sleep during extended times in bed, which result from physical or mental health conditions (Grandner & Kripke, 2004).

[14] Extended time in bed for people with normally adequate sleep may disrupt daily rhythms or encourage sleep fragmentation, which could affect cognitive test performance by, paradoxically, increasing next-day sleepiness; for a review, see Grandner & Drummond, 2007.

[15] This individual had second-degree relatives with a history of depression, which could suggest an undetected genetic predisposition to depression; he recovered quickly when returned to normal lighting conditions.

An example of how self-reports of long sleep can be influenced by psychological state is the finding that depressed patients with bipolar illness self-reported excessive sleep but showed normal sleep durations according to PSG studies (Nofzinger et al., 1991). Self-reported increased sleep durations and napping were characteristic of some patients diagnosed with a variety of mood disorders, but objective studies indicated that only a minority showed unusually long sleep or increased daytime sleepiness (Kaplan & Harvey, 2009).

The trajectories by which a condition like depression could contribute to self-reported long sleep and ultimately to increased mortality risk are not known, but a plausible sequence might include the following. Depression is often characterized by insomnia symptoms along with reduced levels of energy, motivation, and sense of self-worth. These symptoms could lead to, or reinforce, behavioral changes, including more time spent in bed (but not necessarily asleep), limited social interactions, inadequate self-care or diet, and a more sedentary lifestyle. These outcomes could act together to promote poor physical health (e.g., metabolic or vascular diseases) and ultimately to increased mortality risk, which would be statistically associated with self-reported long sleep.

Depression may be related to an increase in specific causes of death. A population-based study showed that people with a significantly depressed mood at baseline (in the early 1970s) had higher rates of dying from vascular diseases in the following decades compared to those without depressed mood. For example, among women who died in the last decade of the 40-year follow-up period, 50% of those who had reported a depressed mood decades earlier died of a vascular disease, compared to only 13.6% of those without depression at baseline (Wyman et al., 2012).

Population-based studies found that long sleep is often associated with poor general physical health, low physical activity levels, depression, and disrupted daily rhythms (Bellavia et al., 2014; Patel et al., 2006; Stranges et al., 2008; Zuurbier et al., 2015). One study that reported a U-shaped function for sleep duration in relation to mortality risk also found that long sleepers were at increased risk only if they also reported daytime sleepiness or difficulty initiating sleep; risk increased as the frequency of these insomnia-related symptoms increased. These features most likely reflect undetected physical or mental health problems that influence sleep (Hedström et al., 2019). Another study found that self-reported ≥9 h sleep increased the risk of cardiovascular death or all-cause mortality primarily in those with insomnia symptoms (Chien et al., 2010).

There is also evidence supporting the interpretation that neural damage resulting from aging and neurodegenerative diseases could promote longer sleep durations. Because of the length of time over which neurodegeneration develops (decades for some forms of AD), people at very early stages of disease have few or no obvious symptoms and are unlikely to be examined for neural changes. But reductions in the size and function of neural mechanisms that promote waking have been detected and might contribute to increased sleep durations in older people and in those at early stages of (undetected) neurodegenerative conditions.

A study of the brains of people who had died of unrelated conditions at young ages found signs of tau pathology in several subcortical nuclei that contribute to maintaining arousal and waking (Stratmann et al., 2016). The basal forebrain cholinergic system, which plays an important role in maintaining arousal, waking, and cognitive functions, was found to decrease in size during aging, and these reductions were more extreme in even the early stages of AD (Grothe et al., 2012).

A postmortem study of the brains of patients with established AD who had undergone PSG studies an average of ~5 years before death found that those with the fewest surviving neurons in the lateral hypothalamus and tuberomammillary nucleus (see Sections 11.2 and 11.3) had shown longer sleep during the PSG studies (Oh et al., 2022). These results can be restated as showing that AD patients with more neuronal loss in wake-promoting hypothalamic structures at the time of death had shown longer sleep durations earlier in the development of the disease.

The impact of a sedentary lifestyle may also be an important factor. A study that found a U-shaped function for mortality risk over a 15-year period asked participants to report their activity levels. Long sleepers who were the most sedentary, but not those with average or high activity levels, had increased mortality risk. Thus, a sedentary lifestyle was a confounding factor that contributed to the apparent link between self-reported long sleep and mortality risk. In contrast, the increased mortality risk associated with short sleep was similar regardless of habitual activity levels (Bellavia et al., 2014).

In a study that used actigraphy, disruption of circadian rest-activity cycles was associated with increased mortality risk, but sleep duration was not. However, those with the most circadian disruption also showed reduced total activity levels (Zuurbier et al., 2015). Later analyses indicated that differences in the degree to which people led a sedentary lifestyle accounted for part of the increased risk that was attributed to disruption of circadian rest-activity cycles.[16]

15.7.1 Summary

Population-based, observational research found that short and long sleep were associated with many medical conditions and with increased mortality risk but inconsistently across studies. In some studies, short sleep predicted later emergence of metabolic syndrome features, but long sleep was associated with these symptoms only cross-sectionally. These results suggest that short sleep may be causally involved in producing these conditions, while long sleep may be the consequence of metabolic or other conditions; alternatively, both long sleep and metabolic disorders may be caused by a different, common factor.

Sleep restriction studies demonstrated acute physiological changes that are consistent with the hypothesis that chronic short sleep can contribute causally to serious medical conditions, which, in turn, could contribute to increased mortality risk. See **Table 15.1** for a summary of how physiological observations (e.g., lack of nocturnal blood pressure dipping) and physiological effects of experimental sleep restriction (e.g., increased insulin resistance) could be related to increased disease and mortality risk in population-based studies.

Experimental sleep extension in people with short sleep at baseline conferred health benefits rather than harms, which provides no hint as to why long sleep should be associated with increased illness or mortality risk. In people with normal sleep amounts, conducting sleep extension studies is difficult because experimenters cannot enforce additional sleep as they can enforce reduced sleep. In the few studies that have successfully encouraged additional sleep in participants with apparently adequate baseline sleep, there has been little or no indication of harmful consequences.

Table 15.1 Effects of Short Sleep in Experimental and Observational Studies

Physiological Effects of Experimentally Reduced Sleep	Population-Based Outcomes Associated with Short Sleep
Increased insulin resistance	Type 2 diabetes
Altered metabolic hormones; short-term weight gain & increased calorie intake	Overweight/obesity; increased risk of vascular disease & cancer
Suppressed immune responses to antigens	Increased risk of viral infections
Complex immune system changes	Chronic inflammation
Acute increases in pain sensitivity	Chronic pain syndromes
Increased amyloid β levels and tau protein abnormalities in the brain	Increased risk of Alzheimer's disease/dementia
Changes in multiple surrogate markers	Increased mortality risk

Table 15.1 The left-hand column lists observed effects of experimental sleep restriction in laboratory studies. The right-hand column shows diseases and chronic conditions in population-based studies that could result from the cumulative effects over years of the corresponding conditions in the left-hand column. Note that many of these chronic conditions interact (e.g., chronic inflammation, type 2 diabetes, and vascular disease have also been linked to increased risk of dementia).

[16] I am grateful to Dr. H. Tiemeier for this information; personal communication (November 2016).

Long sleep (>9 h) does not appear to contribute directly to health risks. Instead, self-reports of long sleep probably reflect misreporting of time in bed as sleep, reverse causality, or the presence of uncontrolled confounders, such as undetected depression, a sedentary lifestyle, or undetected diseases that affect sleep (or at least time in bed) and daytime alertness. In some studies, long sleep, after adjustments for many confounders, was only significantly linked to increased mortality risk when it was accompanied by symptoms of insomnia. These symptoms may be signs of chronic mental or physical health problems or of early stages of developing neurological or other illnesses.

Among short sleepers, mortality risk was similar across all habitual activity levels, but only the most sedentary long-sleepers showed increased mortality risk. Sustained lengthening of sleep durations over years in old age, however, does predict increased mortality. The causes of progressive increases in self-reported sleep duration are unknown, but it is possible that they result from undetected early stages of neurodegenerative conditions, high rates of cell loss in wake-promoting systems, poor general health, or a sedentary or socially restricted lifestyle.

The available evidence supports the conclusion that adults who report sleeping an average of 7–8 h nightly have the lowest risk of developing several serious diseases and the lowest mortality risk. Acutely shortened sleep produces physiological changes that are consistent with the conclusion that habitual short sleep contributes to several chronic health conditions and, ultimately, to increased mortality risk.

Literature cited

Aan Het Rot, M., Zarate, C. A., Jr., Charney, D. S., & Mathew, S. J. (2012). Ketamine for depression: where do we go from here? *Biol Psychiatry, 72*(7), 537–547. doi: 10.1016/j.biopsych.2012.05.003

Abell, J. G., Kivimaki, M., Dugravot, A., Tabak, A. G., Fayosse, A., Shipley, M., ... Singh-Manoux, A. (2018). Association between systolic blood pressure and dementia in the Whitehall II cohort study: role of age, duration, and threshold used to define hypertension. *Eur Heart J, 39*(33), 3119–3125. doi: 10.1093/eurheartj/ehy288

Affleck, G., Urrows, S., Tennen, H., Higgins, P., & Abeles, M. (1996). Sequential daily relations of sleep, pain intensity, and attention to pain among women with fibromyalgia. *Pain, 68*, 363–368.

Ahn, J. H., Cho, H., Kim, J. H., Kim, S. H., Ham, J. S., Park, I., ... Koh, G. Y. (2019). Meningeal lymphatic vessels at the skull base drain cerebrospinal fluid. *Nature, 572*(7767), 62–66. doi: 10.1038/s41586-019-1419-5

Åkerstedt, T., Bellocco, R., Widman, L., Eriksson, J., Ye, W., Adami, H. O., & Trolle Lagerros, Y. (2024). The association of short and long sleep with mortality in men and women. *J Sleep Res, 33*(2), e13931. doi:10.1111/jsr.13931

Åkerstedt, T., Ghilotti, F., Grotta, A., Bellavia, A., Lagerros, Y. T., & Bellocco, R. (2017). Sleep duration, mortality and the influence of age. *Eur J Epidemiol, 32*(10), 881–891. doi10.1007/s10654-017-0297-0

Alitalo, O., Saarreharju, R., Henter, I. D., Zarate, C. A., Jr., Kohtala, S., & Rantamaki, T. (2021). A wake-up call: sleep physiology and related translational discrepancies in studies of rapid-acting antidepressants. *Prog Neurobiol, 206*, 102140. doi:10.1016/j.pneurobio.2021.102140

André, C., Laniepce, A., Chételat, G., & Rauchs, G. (2021). Brain changes associated with sleep disruption in cognitively unimpaired older adults: a short review of neuroimaging studies. *Ageing Res Rev, 66*, 101252. doi: 10.1016/j.arr.2020.101252

Andreasen, N., & Blennow, K. (2002). β-Amyloid (Aβ) protein in cerebrospinal fluid as a biomarker for Alzheimer's disease. *Peptides, 23*, 1205–1214.

Andrieux, A., Salin, P. A., Vernet, M., Kujala, P., Baratier, J., Gory-Faure, S., ... Job, D. (2002). The suppression of brain cold-stable microtubules in mice induces synaptic defects associated with neuroleptic-sensitive behavioral disorders. *Gene Dev, 16*(18), 2350–2364. doi: 10.1101/gad.223302

Ankers, D., & Jones, S. H. (2009). Objective assessment of circadian activity and sleep patterns in individuals at behavioural risk of hypomania. *J Clin Psychol, 65*(10), 1071–1086. doi: 10.1002/jclp.20608

Aringhieri, S., Carli, M., Kolachalam, S., Verdesca, V., Cini, E., Rossi, M., ... Scarselli, M. (2018). Molecular targets of atypical antipsychotics: from mechanism of action to clinical differences. *Pharmacol Therapeut, 192*, 20–41. doi: 10.1016/j.pharmthera.2018.06.012

Armstrong, R. A. (2014). A critical analysis of the "amyloid cascade hypothesis." *Folia Neuropathol, 3*, 211–225. doi: 10.5114/fn.2014.45562

Ashton, N. J., Benedet, A. L., Pascoal, T. A., Karikari, T. K., Lantero-Rodriguez, J., Brum, W. S., ... Rosa-Neto, P. (2022). Cerebrospinal fluid p-tau231 as an early indicator of emerging pathology in Alzheimer's disease. *EBioMedicine, 76*, 103836. doi:10.1016/j.ebiom.2022.103836

Bagautdinova, J., Mayeli, A., Wilson, J. D., Donati, F. L., Colacot, R. M., Meyer, N., ... Ferrarelli, F. (2023). Sleep abnormalities in different clinical stages of psychosis: a systematic review and meta-analysis. *JAMA Psychiatry, 80*(3), 202–210. doi:10.1001/jamapsychiatry.2022.4599

Baron, K. G., Duffecy, J., Reutrakul, S., Levenson, J. C., McFarland, M. M., Lee, S., & Qeadan, F. (2021). Behavioral interventions to extend sleep duration: a systematic review and meta-analysis. *Sleep Med Rev, 60*, 101532. doi:10.1016/j.smrv.2021.101532

Bathgate, C. J., Edinger, J. D., & Krystal, A. D. (2017). Insomnia patients with objective short sleep duration have a blunted response to cognitive behavioral therapy for insomnia. *Sleep, 40*(1), zsw012. doi: 10.1093/sleep/zsw012

Batterham, P. J., Glozier, N., & Christensen, H. (2012). Sleep disturbance, personality and the onset of depression and anxiety: prospective cohort study. *Aust NZ J Psychiatry, 46*(11), 1089–1098. doi: 10.1177/0004867412457997

Baxter, A. J., Scott, K. M., Vos, T., & Whiteford, H. A. (2013). Global prevalence of anxiety disorders: a systematic review and meta-regression. *Psychol Med, 43*(5), 897–910. doi: 10.1017/S003329171200147X

Bejanin, A., Schonhaut, D. R., La Joie, R., Kramer, J. H., Baker, S. L., Sosa, N., ... Rabinovici, G. D. (2017). Tau pathology and neurodegeneration contribute to cognitive impairment in Alzheimer's disease. *Brain, 140*(12), 3286–3300. doi: 10.1093/brain/awx243

Bélanger, L., Morin, C. M., Langlois, F., & Ladouceur, R. (2004). Insomnia and generalized anxiety disorder. *J Anxiety Disord, 18*(4), 561–571. doi: 10.1016/s0887-6185(03)00031-8

Bellavia, A., Åkerstedt, T., Bottai, M., Wolk, A., & Orsini, N. (2014). Sleep duration and survival percentiles across categories of physical activity. *Am J Epidemiol, 179*(4), 484–491. doi: 10.1093/aje/kwt280

Belleville, G., Cousineau, H., Levrier, K., & St-Pierre-Delorme, M. E. (2011). Meta-analytic review of the impact of cognitive-behavior therapy for insomnia on concomitant anxiety. *Clin Psychol Rev, 31*(4), 638–652. doi: 10.1016/j.cpr.2011.02.004

Benca, R. M., Obermeyer, W. H., Thisted, R. A., & Gillin, J. C. (1992). Sleep and psychiatric disorders, a meta-analysis. *Arch Gen Psychiatr, 49*, 651–668.

Benedetti, F., Barbini, B., Fulgosi, M. C., Colombo, C., Dallaspezia, S., Pontiggia, A., & Smeraldi, E. (2005). Combined total sleep deprivation and light therapy in the treatment of drug-resistant bipolar depression: acute response. *J Clin Psychiatry, 66*(12), 1535–1540.

Benito-Léon, J., Bermejo-Pareja, F., Vega, S., & Louis, E. D. (2009). Total daily sleep duration and the risk of dementia: a prospective population-based study. *Eur J Neurol, 16*(9), 990–997. doi: 10.1111/j.1468-1331.2009.02618.x

Berman, R. M., Cappiello, A., Anand, A., Oren, D. A., Heninger, G. R., Charney, D. S., & Krystal, J. H. (2000). Antidepressant effects of ketamine in depressed patients. *Biol Psychiatry, 47*, 351–354.

Bernier, D., Bartha, R., Devarajan, S., MacMaster, F. P., Schmidt, M., & Rusak, B. (2009). Effects of overnight sleep restriction on brain chemistry and mood in women with unipolar depression and healthy controls. *J Psychiatr Neurosci, 34*(5), 352–360.

Beschorner, N., & Nedergaard, M. (2024). Glymphatic system dysfunction in neurodegenerative diseases. *Curr Opin Neurol, 37*(2), 182–188. doi: 10.1097/WCO.0000000000001252

Black, J., Pardi, D., Hornfeldt, C. S., & Inhaber, N. (2009). The nightly administration of sodium oxybate results in significant reduction in the nocturnal sleep disruption of patients with narcolepsy. *Sleep Med, 10*(8), 829–835. doi: 10.1016/j.sleep.2009.05.004

Blanken, T. F., Borsboom, D., Penninx, B. W. J. H., & Van Someren, E. J. W. (2020). Network outcome analysis identifies difficulty initiating sleep as a primary target for prevention of depression: a 6-year prospective study. *Sleep, 43*(5). doi: 10.1093/sleep/zsz288

Blennow, K., Mattsson, N., Scholl, M., Hansson, O., & Zetterberg, H. (2015). Amyloid biomarkers in Alzheimer's disease. *Trends Pharacol Sci, 36*(5), 297–309. doi: 10.1016/j.tips.2015.03.002

Bliwise, D. L. (1993). Sleep in normal aging and dementia. *Sleep, 16*, 40–81.

Boissevain, M. D., & McCain, G. A. (1991). Toward an integrated understanding of fibromyalgia syndrome. I. Medical and pathophysiological aspects. *Pain, 45*, 227–238.

Boivin, D. (2000). Influence of sleep-wake and circadian rhythm disturbances in psychiatric disorders. *J Psychiatry Neurosci, 25*(5), 446–458.

Boland, E. M., Rao, H., Dinges, D. F., Smith, R. V., Goel, N., Detre, J. A., ... Gehrman, P. R. (2017). Meta-analysis of the antidepressant effects of acute sleep deprivation. *J Clin Psychiatry, 78*(8), e1020–e1034. doi: 10.4088/JCP.16r11332

Borbély, A. A., & Wirz-Justice, A. (1982). Sleep, sleep deprivation and depression. A hypothesis derived from a model of sleep regulation. *Hum Neurobiol, 1*(3), 2015–2210.

Braak, H., & Braak, E. (1991). Neuropathological stageing of Alzheimer-related changes. *Acta Neuropathologica, 82*, 239–259.

Braff, D. L., Grillon, C., & Geyer, M. A. (1992). Gating and habituation of the startle reflex in schizophrenic patients. *Arch Gen Psychiatr, 49*, 206–215.

Bratti, I. M., Kane, J. M., & Marder, S. R. (2007). Chronic restlessness with antipsychotics. *Am J Psychiatry, 164*(11), 1648–1654.

Breslau, N., Roth, T., Rosenthal, L., & Andreski, P. (1996). Sleep disturbance and psychiatric disorders: a longitudinal epidemiological study of young adults *Biol Psychiatry, 39*, 411–418.

Bubu, O. M., Brannick, M., Mortimer, J., Umasabor-Bubu, O., Sebastiao, Y. V., Wen, Y., ... Anderson, W. M. (2017). Sleep, cognitive impairment, and Alzheimer's disease: a systematic review and meta-analysis. *Sleep, 40*(1), 1–18. doi: 0.1093/sleep/zsw032

Buchhave, P., Minthon, L., Zetterberg, H., Wallin, A. K., Blennow, K., & Hansson, O. (2012). Cerebrospinal fluid levels of β-amyloid 1–42, but not tau, are fully changed already 5 to 10 years before the onset of Alzheimer dementia. *Arch Gen Psychiatr, 69*(1), 98–106.

Bunney, B. G., & Bunney, W. E. (2013). Mechanisms of rapid antidepressant effects of sleep deprivation therapy: clock genes and circadian rhythms. *Biol Psychiatry, 73*(12), 1164–1171. doi: 10.1016/j.biopsych.2012.07.020

Burke, S., Grudzien, A., Li, T., Abril, M., Spadola, C., Barnes, C., ... DeKosky, S. (2022). Correlations between sleep disturbance and brain structures associated with neurodegeneration in the National Alzheimer's Coordinating Center Uniform Data Set. *J Clin Neurosci, 106*, 204–212. doi: 10.1016/j.jocn.2022.07.012

Cappuccio, F. P., D'Elia, L., Strazzullo, P., & Miller, M. A. (2010). Sleep duration and all-cause mortality: a systematic review and meta-analysis of prospective studies. *Sleep, 33*(5), 585–592.

Carney, C. E., Edinger, J. D., Kuchibhatla, M., Lachowski, A. M., Bogouslavsky, O., Krystal, A. D., & Shapiro, C. M. (2017). Cognitive behavioral insomnia therapy for those with insomnia and depression: a randomized controlled clinical trial. *Sleep, 40*(4), zsx019. doi: 10.1093/sleep/zsx019

Carvalho, D. Z., St Louis, E. K., Knopman, D. S., Boeve, B. F., Lowe, V. J., Roberts, R. O., ... Vemuri, P. (2018). Association of excessive daytime sleepiness with longitudinal β-amyloid accumulation in elderly persons without dementia. *JAMA Neurol, 75*(6), 672–680. doi: 10.1001/jamaneurol.2018.0049

Casement, M. D., Livingston, N. R., Allen, N. B., & Forbes, E. E. (2020). Feasibility, acceptability and affective consequences of at-home sleep extension in young women with depressive symptoms: A pilot study. *J Sleep Res, 30*(2), e13045. doi:10.1111/jsr.13045

Chan, M. S., Chung, K. F., Yung, K. P., & Yeung, W. F. (2017). Sleep in schizophrenia: A systematic review and meta-analysis of polysomnographic findings in case-control studies. *Sleep Med Rev, 32*, 69–84. doi: 10.1016/j.smrv.2016.03.001

Chen, A., Lennon, L., Pappacosta, O., & Wannamethee, S. G. (2023). Association of night-time sleep duration and daytime napping with all-cause and cause-specific mortality in older British men: findings from the British Regional Heart Study. *Sleep Med, 109*, 32–39. doi: 10.1016/j.sleep.2023.06.020

Cheng, G. H., Malhotra, R., Ostbye, T., Chan, A., Ma, S., & Lo, J. C. (2018). Changes in nocturnal sleep and daytime nap durations predict all-cause mortality among older adults: the Panel on Health and Ageing of Singaporean Elderly. *Sleep, 41*(7). doi: 10.1093/sleep/zsy087

Cheng, P., Kalmbach, D. A., Tallent, G., Joseph, C. L., Espie, C. A., & Drake, C. L. (2019). Depression prevention via digital cognitive behavioral therapy for insomnia: a randomized controlled trial. *Sleep, 42*(10), zsz150. doi: 10.1093/sleep/zsz150

Chien, K.-L., Chen, P.-C., Hsu, H.-C., Su, T.-C., Sung, F.-C., Chen, M.-F., & Lee, Y.-T. (2010). Habitual sleep duration and insomnia and the risk of cardiovascular events and all-cause death: report from a community-based cohort. *Sleep, 33*(2), 177–184.

Chouinard, S., Poulin, J., Stip, E., & Godbout, R. (2004). Sleep in untreated patients with schizophrenia: a meta-analysis *Schizophrenia Bull, 30*(4), 957–967.

Cizza, G., Piaggi, P., Rother, K. I., Csako, G., & Sleep Extension Study Group. (2014). Hawthorne effect with transient behavioral and biochemical changes in a randomized controlled sleep extension trial of chronically short-sleeping obese adults: implications for the design and interpretation of clinical studies. *PLoS One, 9*(8), e104176. doi: 10.1371/journal.pone.0104176

Cohrs, S. (2008). Sleep disturbances in patients with schizophrenia: impact and effect of antipsychotics. *CNS Drugs, 22*(11), 939–962.

Cooperman, N. R., Mullin, F. J., & Kleitman, N. (1934). Studies on the physiology of sleep. XI. Further observations on the effects of prolonged sleeplessness. *Am J Physiol, 107*(3), 589–593.

Cox, R. C., & Olatunji, B. O. (2020). Sleep in the anxiety-related disorders: A meta-analysis of subjective and objective research. *Sleep Med Rev, 51*, 101282. doi: 10.1016/j.smrv.2020.101282

Crönlein, T., Wetter, T. C., Rupprecht, R., & Spiegelhalder, K. (2020). Cognitive behavioral treatment for insomnia is equally effective in insomnia patients with objective short and normal sleep duration. *Sleep Med, 66*, 271–275. doi: 10.1016/j.sleep.2018.10.038

D'Agostino, A., Ferrara, P., Terzoni, S., Ostinelli, E. G., Carrara, C., Prunas, C., ... Destrebecq, A. (2020). Efficacy of triple chronotherapy in unipolar and bipolar depression: A systematic review of the available evidence. *J Affect Disord, 276*, 297–304. doi: 10.1016/j.jad.2020.07.026

da Silva, A. A., de Mello, R. G., Schaan, C. W., Fuchs, F. D., Redline, S., & Fuchs, S. C. (2016). Sleep duration and mortality in the elderly: a systematic review with meta-analysis. *Br Med J Open, 6*(2), 1–13. doi:10.1136/bmjopen-2015-008119

Dantzer, R., O'Connor, J. C., Freund, G. G., Johnson, R. W., & Kelley, K. W. (2008). From inflammation to sickness and depression: when the immune system subjugates the brain. *Nat Rev Neurosci, 9*(1), 46–56. doi: 10.1038/nrn2297

Darweesh, S. K. L., Wolters, F. J., Ikram, M. A., de Wolf, F., Bos, D., & Hofman, A. (2018). Inflammatory markers and the risk of dementia and Alzheimer's disease: a meta-analysis. *Alzheimers Dement, 14*(11), 1450–1459. doi: 10.1016/j.jalz.2018.02.014

Dauvilliers, Y., Roth, T., Guinta, D., Alvarez-Horine, S., Dynin, E., & Black, J. (2017). Effect of sodium oxybate, modafinil, and their combination on disrupted nighttime sleep in narcolepsy. *Sleep Med, 40*, 53–57. doi: 10.1016/j.sleep.2017.07.030

Demanuele, C., Bartsch, U., Baran, B., Khan, S., Vangel, M. G., Cox, R., ... Manoach, D. S. (2017). Coordination of slow waves with sleep spindles predicts sleep-dependent memory consolidation in schizophrenia. *Sleep, 40*(1), 1–10. doi: 10.1093/sleep/zsw013

Deurveilher, S., Ko, K. R., Saumure, B. S. C., Robertson, G. S., Rusak, B., & Semba, K. (2021). Altered circadian activity and sleep/wake rhythms in the stable tubule only polypeptide (STOP) null mouse model of schizophrenia. *Sleep, 44*(4), 1–15. doi:10.1093/sleep/zsaa237

Dewald-Kaufmann, J. F., Oort, F. J., & Meijer, A. M. (2014). The effects of sleep extension and sleep hygiene advice on sleep and depressive symptoms in adolescents: a randomized controlled trial. *J Child Psychol Psychiatry, 55*(3), 273–283. doi: 10.1111/jcpp.12157

Dinges, D. F., Pack, F., Williams, K., Gillen, K. A., Powell, J. W., Ott, G. E., ... Pack, A. I. (1997). Cumulative sleepiness, mood disturbance, and psychomotor vigilance performance decrements during a week of sleep restricted to 4–5 hours per night. *Sleep, 20*(4), 267–277.

Dombrovski, A. Y., Cyranowski, J. M., Mulsant, B. H., Houck, P. R., Buysse, D. J., Andreescu, C., ... Frank, E. (2008). Which symptoms predict recurrence of depression in women treated with maintenance interpersonal psychotherapy? *Depress Anxiety, 25*(12), 1060–1066. doi: 10.1002/da.20467

Donohue, M. C., Sperling, R. A., Petersen, R., Sun, C. K., Weiner, M. W., Aisen, P. S., & Initiative, A. s. D. N. (2017). Association between elevated brain amyloid and subsequent cognitive decline among cognitively normal persons. *JAMA, 317*(22), 2305–2316. doi: 10.1001/jama.2017.6669

Drogos, L. L., Gill, S. J., Tyndall, A. V., Raneri, J. K., Parboosingh, J. S., Naef, A., … Poulin, M. J. (2016). Evidence of association between sleep quality and *APOE ε4* in healthy older adults. *Neurology, 87*, 1836–1842.

Duffy, A., Alda, M., Hajek, T., Sherry, S. B., & Grof, P. (2010). Early stages in the development of bipolar disorder. *J Affect Disorders, 121*(1-2), 127–135. doi: 10.1016/j.jad.2009.05.022

Duffy, A., Goodday, S., Keown-Stoneman, C., & Grof, P. (2018). The emergent course of bipolar disorder: observations over two decades from the Canadian High-Risk Offspring Cohort. *Am J Psychiatry, 176*(9), 720–729. doi: 10.1176/appi.ajp.2018.18040461

Duncan, W. C., Sarasso, S., Ferrarelli, F., Selter, J., Riedner, B. A., Hejazi, N. S., … Zarate, C. A. (2013). Concomitant BDNF and sleep slow wave changes indicate ketamine-induced plasticity in major depressive disorder. *Int J Neuropsychopharmacol, 16*(2), 301–311. doi: 10.1017/S1461145712000545

Duncan, W. C., Jr., & Zarate, C. A., Jr. (2013). Ketamine, sleep, and depression: current status and new questions. *Curr Psychiatry Rep, 15*(9), 1–7. doi:10.1007/s11920-013-0394-z

Eckel, R. H., Depner, C. M., Perreault, L., Markwald, R. R., Smith, M. R., McHill, A. W., … Wright, K. P., Jr. (2015). Morning circadian misalignment during short sleep duration impacts insulin sensitivity. *Curr Biol, 25*(22), 3004–3010. doi: 10.1016/j.cub.2015.10.011

Edinger, J. D., & Means, M. K. (2005). Cognitive-behavioral therapy for primary insomnia. *Clin Psychol Rev, 25*(5), 539–558. doi: 10.1016/j.cpr.2005.04.003

Edwards, R. R., Almeida, D. M., Klick, B., Haythornthwaite, J. A., & Smith, M. T. (2008). Duration of sleep contributes to next-day pain report in the general population. *Pain, 137*(1), 202–207. doi: 10.1016/j.pain.2008.01.025

Farmer, C. A., Chilakamarri, P., Thurm, A. E., Swedo, S. E., Holmes, G. L., & Buckley, A. W. (2018). Spindle activity in young children with autism, developmental delay, or typical development. *Neurology, 91*(2), e112–e122. doi: 10.1212/WNL.0000000000005759

Felger, J. C., & Lotrich, F. E. (2013). Inflammatory cytokines in depression: neurobiological mechanisms and therapeutic implications. *Neuroscience, 246*, 199–229. doi: 10.1016/j.neuroscience.2013.04.060

Ferrarelli, F., Huber, R., Peterson, M. J., Massimini, M., Murphy, M., Riedner, B. A., … Tononi, G. (2007). Reduced sleep spindle activity in schizophrenia patients. *Am J Psychiatry, 164*, 483–492.

Ferrarelli, F., Peterson, M. J., Sarasso, S., Riedner, B. A., Murphy, M. J., Benca, R. M., … Tononi, G. (2010). Thalamic dysfunction in schizophrenia suggested by whole-night deficits in slow and fast spindles. *Am J Psychiatry, 167*(11), 1339–1348. doi: 10.1176/appi.ajp.2010.09121731

Ferrie, J. E., Shipley, M. J., & Cappuccio, F. P. (2007). A prospective study of change in sleep duration: associations with mortality in the Whitehall II cohort. *Sleep, 30*(12), 1659–1666.

Finan, P. H., Goodin, B. R., & Smith, M. T. (2013). The association of sleep and pain: an update and a path forward. *J Pain, 14*(12), 1539–1552. doi: 10.1016/j.jpain.2013.08.007

Finan, P. H., Quartana, P. J., & Smith, M. T. (2015). The effects of sleep continuity disruption on positive mood and sleep architecture in healthy adults. *Sleep, 38*(11), 1735–1742. doi: 0.5665/sleep.5154

Fischer-Perroudon, C., Trillet, M., Mouret, J., Tommasi, M., Jouvet, M., Schott, B., & Girard, P. F. (1974). Polygraphic and metabolic studies of persistent insomnia with hallucinations. [In French] *Rev Neurol (Paris), 130*(3-4), 111–125.

Frau, R., Orru, M., Puligheddu, M., Gessa, G. L., Mereu, G., Marrosu, F., & Bortolato, M. (2008). Sleep deprivation disrupts prepulse inhibition of the startle reflex: reversal by antipsychotic drugs. *Int J Neuropsychopharmacol, 11*(7), 947–955. doi: 10.1017/S1461145708008900

Freedman, R., Waldo, M., Bickford-Wimer, P., & Nagamoto, H. (1991). Elementary neuronal dysfunctions in schizophrenia. *Schizophrenia Res, 4*, 233–243.

Fried, E. I., Flake, J. K., & Robinaugh, D. J. (2022). Revisiting the theoretical and methodological foundations of depression measurement. *Nat Rev Psychol, 1*, 358–368. doi: 10.1038/s44159-022-00050-2

Fultz, N. E., Bonmassar, G., Setsompop, K., Stickgold, R. A., Rosen, B. R., Polimeni, J. R., & Lewis, L. D. (2019). Coupled electrophysiological, hemodynamic, and cerebrospinal fluid oscillations in human sleep. *Science, 366*, 628–631.

Galbiati, A., Sforza, M., Leitner, C., Castelnovo, A., D'Este, G., Ferini-Strambi, L., … Castronovo, V. (2021). The reliability of objective total sleep time in predicting the effectiveness of cognitive-behavioral therapy for insomnia. *Sleep Med, 82*, 43–46. doi: 10.1016/j.sleep.2021.03.021

Gallicchio, L., & Kalesan, B. (2009). Sleep duration and mortality: a systematic review and meta-analysis. *J Sleep Res, 18*(2), 148–158. doi: 10.1111/j.1365-2869.2008.00732.x

Gangwisch, J. E., Heymsfield, S. B., Boden-Albala, B., Buijs, R. M., Kreier, F., Opler, M. G., … Malaspina, D. (2008). Sleep duration associated with mortality in elderly, but not middle-aged, adults in a large US sample. *Sleep, 31*(8), 1087–1096.

Gibson, M., Nicolazzo, J., Cavuoto, M., Rowsthorn, E., Cribb, L., Bransby, L., … Pase, M. P. (2023). Short sleep duration is associated with lower cerebrospinal fluid amyloid beta 42 levels in midlife: a preliminary report. *Sleep, 46*(4), zsac307. doi:10.1093/sleep/zsac307

Gillin, J. C., Kripke, D. F., Janowsky, D. S., & Risch, S. C. (1989). Effects of brief naps on mood and sleep in sleep-deprived depressed patients. *Psychiatry Res, 27*(3), 253–265.

Gómez-González, B., Hurtado-Alvarado, G., Esqueda-Leon, E., Santana-Miranda, R., Rohas-Zamorano, J. A., & Velazquez-Moctezuma, J. (2013). REM sleep loss and recovery regulates blood-brain barrier function. *Curr Neurovasc Res, 10*, 197–207.

Gordovez, F. J. A., & McMahon, F. J. (2020). The genetics of bipolar disorder. *Mol Psychiatry, 25*(3), 544–559. doi: 10.1038/s41380-019-0634-7

Gottlieb, J. F., Goel, N., Chen, S., & Young, M. A. (2021). Meta-analysis of sleep deprivation in the acute treatment of bipolar depression. *Acta Psychiatr Scand, 143*(4), 319–327. doi: 10.1111/acps.13255

Grandner, M. A., & Drummond, S. P. (2007). Who are the long sleepers? Towards an understanding of the mortality relationship. *Sleep Med Rev, 11*(5), 341–360. doi: 10.1016/j.smrv.2007.03.010

Grandner, M. A., & Kripke, D. F. (2004). Self-reported sleep complaints with long and short sleep: a nationally representative sample. *Psychosom Med, 66*(2), 239–241.

Gresham, S. C., Agnew Jr., H. W., & Williams, R. L. (1965). The sleep of depressed patients. *Arch Gen Psychiatr, 13*, 503–507.

Grothe, M., Heinsen, H., & Teipel, S. J. (2012). Atrophy of the cholinergic Basal forebrain over the adult age range and in early stages of Alzheimer's disease. *Biol Psychiatry, 71*(9), 805–813. doi: 10.1016/j.biopsych.2011.06.019

Gruber, J., Miklowitz, D. J., Harvey, A. G., Frank, E., Kupfer, D., Thase, M. E., … Ketter, T. A. (2011). Sleep matters: sleep functioning and course of illness in bipolar disorder. *J Affect Disord, 134*(1-3), 416–420. doi: 10.1016/j.jad.2011.05.016

Haack, M., Engert, L. C., Besedovsky, L., Goldstein, M. R., Devine, J. K., Dang, R., … Simpson, N. (2023). Alterations of pain pathways by experimental sleep disturbances in humans: central pain-inhibitory, cyclooxygenase, and endocannabinoid pathways. *Sleep, 46*(6), zsad061. doi:10.1093/sleep/zsad061

Haack, M., Sanchez, E., & Mullington, J. M. (2007). Elevated inflammatory markers in response to prolonged sleep restriction are associated with increased pain experience in healthy volunteers. *Sleep, 30*(9), 1145–1152.

Halassa, M. M., Chen, Z., Wimmer, R. D., Brunetti, P. M., Zhao, S., Zikopoulos, B., W… Wilson, M. A. (2014). State-dependent architecture of thalamic reticular subnetworks. *Cell, 158*(4), 808–821. doi: 10.1016/j.cell.2014.06.025

Hall, S., Deurveilher, S., Robertson, G. S., & Semba, K. (2020). Homeostatic state of microglia in a rat model of chronic sleep restriction. *Sleep, 43*(11), zsaa108. doi:10.1093/sleep/zsaa108

Hardy, J. A., & Higgins, G. A. (1992). Alzheimer's disease: the amyloid cascade hypothesis. *Science, 256*(5054), 184–185.

Harrison, Y., & Horne, J. A. (1996). Long-term extension to sleep – are we really chronically sleep deprived? *Psychophysiology, 33*, 22–30.

Harvey, A. G. (2011). Sleep and circadian functioning: critical mechanisms in the mood disorders? *Annu Rev Clin Psychol, 7*, 297–319. doi: 10.1146/annurev-clinpsy-032210-104550

Hayley, S. (2011). Toward an anti-inflammatory strategy for depression. *Front Behav Neurosci, 5*. doi: 10.3389/fnbeh.2011.00019

He, J., Hsuchou, H., He, Y., Kastin, A. J., Wang, Y., & Pan, W. (2014). Sleep restriction impairs blood-brain barrier function. *J Neurosci, 34*(44), 14697–14706. doi: 10.1523/JNEUROSCI.2111-14.2014

Hedström, A. K., Bellocco, R., Ye, W., Trolle Lagerros, Y., & Åkerstedt, T. (2019). Association between insomnia and mortality is only evident among long sleepers. *Nat Sci Sleep, 11*, 333–342. doi: 10.2147/nss.S222049

Helakari, H., Korhonen, V., Holst, S. C., Piispala, J., Kallio, M., Väyrynen, T., … Kiviniemi, V. (2022). Human NREM sleep promotes brain-wide vasomotor and respiratory pulsations. *J Neurosci, 42*(12), 2503–2515. doi: 10.1523/JNEUROSCI.0934-21.2022

Herculano-Houzel, S. (2015). Decreasing sleep requirement with increasing numbers of neurons as a driver for bigger brains and bodies in mammalian evolution. *Proc Biol Sci, 282*(1816), 20151853. doi:10.1098/rspb.2015.1853

Herrup, K. (2015). The case for rejecting the amyloid cascade hypothesis. *Nat Neurosci, 18*(6), 794–799. doi: 10.1038/nn.4017

Heslop, P., Smith, G. D., Metcalfe, C., Macleod, J., & Hart, C. (2002). Sleep duration and mortality: the effect of short or long sleep duration on cardiovascular and all-cause mortality in working men and women. *Sleep Med, 3*, 305–314.

Ho, F. Y., Chan, C. S., & Tang, K. N. (2016). Cognitive-behavioral therapy for sleep disturbances in treating posttraumatic stress disorder symptoms: A meta-analysis of randomized controlled trials. *Clin Psychol Rev, 43*, 90–102. doi: 10.1016/j.cpr.2015.09.005

Hofman, M. A., & Swaab, D. F. (1994). Alterations in circadian rhythmicity of the vasopressin-producing neurons of the human suprachiasmatic nucleus (SCN) with aging. *Brain Res, 651*, 134–142.

Hua, J., Jiang, H., Wang, H., & Fang, Q. (2021). Sleep duration and the risk of metabolic syndrome in adults: a systematic review and meta-analysis. *Front Neurol, 12*, 635564. doi:10.3389/fneur.2021.635564

Huang, Y., Potter, R., Sigurdson, W., Santacruz, A., Shih, S., Ju, Y. E., ... Bateman, R. J. (2012). Effects of age and amyloid deposition on Aβ dynamics in the human central nervous system. *Arch Neurol, 69*(1), 51–58. doi: 10.1001/archneurol.2011.235

Hublin, C., Partinen, M., Koskenvuo, M., & Kaprio, J. (2007). Sleep and mortality: a population-based 22-year follow-up study. *Sleep, 30*(10), 1245–1253.

Hudson, J. I., Lipinski, J. F., Keck Jr, P. E., Aizley, H. G., Lukas, S. E., Rothschild, A. J., . . . Kupfer, D. J. (2002). Polysomnographic characteristics of young manic patients. Comparison with unipolar depressed and normal control subjects. *Arch Gen Psychiatr, 49*, 378–383.

Hurtado-Alvarado, G., Dominguez-Salazar, E., Pavon, L., Velazquez-Moctezuma, J., & Gomez-Gonzalez, B. (2016). Blood-brain barrier disruption induced by chronic sleep loss: low-grade inflammation may be the link. *J Immunol Res, 2016*, 4576012. doi: 10.1155/2016/4576012

Hurtado-Alvarado, G., Velazquez-Moctezuma, J., & Gomez-Gonzalez, B. (2017). Chronic sleep restriction disrupts interendothelial junctions in the hippocampus and increases blood-brain barrier permeability. *J Microsc, 268*(1), 28–38. doi: 10.1111/jmi.12583

Ibrahim, A., Cesari, M., Heidbreder, A., Defrancesco, M., Brandauer, E., Seppi, K., ... Stefani, A. (2024). Sleep features and long-term incident neurodegeneration: a polysomnographic study. *Sleep, 47*(3), zsad304. doi:10.1093/sleep/zsad304

Iliff, J. J., Wang, M., Liao, Y., Plogg, B. A., Peng, W., Gundersen, G. A., ... Nedergaard, M. (2012). A paravascular pathway facilitates CSF flow through the brain parenchyma and the clearance of interstitial solutes, including amyloid beta. *Sci Transl Med, 4*(147), 147ra111. doi: 10.1126/scitranslmed.3003748

Ioannou, M., Wartenberg, C., Greenbrook, J. T. V., Larson, T., Magnusson, K., Schmitz, L., ... Steingrimsson, S. (2021). Sleep deprivation as treatment for depression: systematic review and meta-analysis. *Acta Psychiatr Scand, 143*(1), 22–35. doi: 10.1111/acps.13253

Irwin, M. R., Carrillo, C., Sadeghi, N., Bjurstrom, M. F., Breen, E. C., & Olmstead, R. (2021). Prevention of incident and recurrent major depression in older adults with insomnia: a randomized clinical trial. *JAMA Psychiatry, 79*(1), 33–41. doi: 10.1001/jamapsychiatry.2021.3422

Irwin, M. R., & Olmstead, R. (2022). Suicide risk and lithium-reply. *JAMA Psychiatry, 79*(5), 515. doi: 10.1001/jamapsychiatry.2022.0084

Itani, O., Jike, M., Watanabe, N., & Kaneita, Y. (2017). Short sleep duration and health outcomes: a systematic review, meta-analysis, and meta-regression. *Sleep Med, 32*, 246–256. doi: 10.1016/j.sleep.2016.08.006

Jack, C. R., Jr., Knopman, D. S., Jagust, W. J., Shaw, L. M., Aisen, P. S., Weiner, M. W., ... Trojanowski, J. Q. (2010). Hypothetical model of dynamic biomarkers of the Alzheimer's pathological cascade. *Lancet Neurol, 9*(1), 119–128. doi: 10.1016/S1474-4422(09)70299-6

Janelidze, S., Barthelemy, N. R., Salvado, G., Schindler, S. E., Palmqvist, S., Mattsson-Carlgren, N., ... Hansson, O. (2024). Plasma phosphorylated Tau 217 and Aβ42/40 to predict early brain Aβ accumulation in people without cognitive impairment. *JAMA Neurol, 81*(9), 947–957. doi: 10.1001/jamaneurol.2024.2619

Jike, M., Itani, O., Watanabe, N., Buysse, D. J., & Kaneita, Y. (2018). Long sleep duration and health outcomes: a systematic review, meta-analysis and meta-regression. *Sleep Med Rev, 39*, 25–36. doi: 10.1016/j.smrv.2017.06.011

Johnson, R. D., Oliver, P. L., & Davies, K. E. (2008). SNARE proteins and schizophrenia: linking synaptic and neurodevelopmental hypotheses. *Acta Biochimica Polonica, 55*(4), 619–628.

Jørgensen, J. T., Hansen, J., Westendorp, R. G. J., Nabe-Nielsen, K., Stayner, L. T., Simonsen, M. K., & Andersen, Z. J. (2020). Shift work and incidence of dementia: a Danish Nurse Cohort study. *Alzheimers Dement, 16*(9), 1268–1279. doi: 10.1002/alz.12126

Josephs, K. A., Silber, M. H., Fealey, R. D., Nippoldt, T. B., Auger, R. G., & Vernino, S. (2004). Neurophysiologic studies in Morvan syndrome *J Clin Neurophysiol, 21*, 440–445.

Ju, Y. S., Ooms, S. J., Sutphen, C., Macauley, S. L., Zangrilli, M. A., Jerome, G., ... Holtzman, D. M. (2017). Slow wave sleep disruption increases cerebrospinal fluid amyloid-beta levels. *Brain, 140*(8), 2104–2111. doi: 10.1093/brain/awx148

Kang, J. E., Lim, M. M., Bateman, R. J., Lee, J. J., Smyth, L. P., Cirrito, J. R., ... Holtzman, D. M. (2009). Amyloid-β dynamics are regulated by orexin and the sleep-wake cycle. *Science, 326*(5955), 1005–1007. doi: 10.1126/science.1180962

Kaplan, K. A., & Harvey, A. G. (2009). Hypersomnia across mood disorders: a review and synthesis. *Sleep Med Rev, 13*(4), 275–285. doi: 10.1016/j.smrv.2008.09.001

Kaskie, R. E., Graziano, B., & Ferrarelli, F. (2019). Topographic deficits in sleep spindle density and duration point to frontal thalamo-cortical dysfunctions in first-episode psychosis. *J Psychiatr Res, 113*, 39–44. doi: 10.1016/j.jpsychires.2019.03.009

Keil, S. A., Schindler, A. G., Wang, M. X., Piantino, J., Silbert, L. C., Elliott, J. E., ... Iliff, J. J. (2023). Longitudinal sleep patterns and cognitive impairment in older adults. *JAMA Netw Open, 6*(12), e2346006. doi:10.1001/jamanetworkopen.2023.46006

Kilduff, T. S. (2023). The mystery of gamma-hydoxybutyrate efficacy in narcolepsy type 1. *Sleep, 46*(9), zsad156. doi:10.1093/sleep/zsad156

Kim, D. J., Mun, S. J., Choi, J. S., Kim, J., Lee, G.-H., Kim, H.-W., ... Cho, J. W. (2020). Beneficial effects of weekend catch-up sleep on metabolic syndrome in chronic short sleepers. *Sleep Med, 76*, 26–32. doi: 10.1016/j.sleep.2020.09.025

Kloppenborg, R. P., van den Berg, E., Kappelle, L. J., & Biessels, G. J. (2008). Diabetes and other vascular risk factors for dementia: which factor matters most? A systematic review. *Eur J Pharmacol, 585*(1), 97–108. doi: 10.1016/j.ejphar.2008.02.049

Knapik, J. J., Caldwell, J., Steelman, R. A., Trone, D. W., Farina, E. K., & Lieberman, H. R. (2023). Short sleep duration is associated with a wide variety of medical conditions among United States military service members. *Sleep Med, 101*, 283–295. doi: 10.1016/j.sleep.2022.11.015

Knowles, J. B., Southmayd, S. E., Delva, N., MacLean, A. W., Cairns, J., & Letemendia, F. J. (1979). Five variations of sleep deprivation in a depressed woman. *Br J Psychiatry, 135*, 403–410.

Kok, R. M., & Reynolds, C. F., 3rd. (2017). Management of depression in older adults: a review. *JAMA, 317*(20), 2114–2122. doi: 10.1001/jama.2017.5706

Kripke, D. F., Garfinkel, L., Wingard, D. L., Klauber, M. R., & Marler, M. R. (2002). Mortality associated with sleep duration and insomnia. *Arch Gen Psychiatr, 59*, 131–136.

Kumari, V., Das, M., Zachariah, E., Ettinger, U., & Sharma, T. (2005). Reduced prepulse inhibition in unaffected siblings of schizophrenia patients. *Psychophysiology, 42*(5), 588–594. doi: 10.1111/j.1469-8986.2005.00346.x

Kumari, V., Fannon, D., Sumich, A. L., & Sharma, T. (2007). Startle gating in antipsychotic-naive first episode schizophrenia patients: one ear is better than two. *Psychiatry Res, 151*(1-2), 21–28. doi: 10.1016/j.psychres.2006.09.013

Kupfer, D. J. (1976). REM latency: a psychobiologic marker for primary depressive disease. *Biol Psychiatry, 11*(2), 159–174.

Kurina, L. M., McClintock, M. K., Chen, J. H., Waite, L. J., Thisted, R. A., & Lauderdale, D. S. (2013). Sleep duration and all-cause mortality: a critical review of measurement and associations. *Ann Epidemiol, 23*(6), 361–370. doi: 10.1016/j.annepidem.2013.03.015

Lauer, C. J., Schreiber, W., Pollmächer, T., Holsboer, F., & Krieg, J.-C. (1997). Sleep in schizophrenia: a polysomnographic study on drug-naive patients. *Neuropsychopharmacology, 16*, 51–60.

Lautenbacher, S., Kundermann, B., & Krieg, J. (2006). Sleep deprivation and pain perception. *Sleep Med Rev, 10*(5), 357–369. doi: 10.1016/j.smrv.2005.08.001

Le Bars, D. (2002). The whole body receptive field of dorsal horn multireceptive neurones. *Brain Res Rev, 40*, 29–44.

Lee, S. H., Ripke, S., Neale, B. M., Faraone, S. V., Purcell, S. M., Perlis, R. H., ... Wray, N. R. (2013). Genetic relationship between five psychiatric disorders estimated from genome-wide SNPs. *Nat Genet, 45*(9), 984–994. doi: 10.1038/ng.2711

Legge, S. E., Santoro, M. L., Periyasamy, S., Okewole, A., Arsalan, A., & Kowalec, K. (2021). Genetic architecture of schizophrenia: a review of major advancements. *Psychol Med, 51*(13), 2168–2177. doi:10.1017/S0033291720005334

Leibenluft, E., Albert, P. S., Rosenthal, N. E., & Wehr, T. A. (1996). Relationship between sleep and mood in patients with rapid-cycling bipolar disorder. *Psychiatry Res, 63*, 161–168.

Lentz, M. J., Landis, C. A., Rothermel, J., & Shaver, J. L. F. (1999). Effects of selective slow wave sleep disruption on musculoskeletal pain and fatigue in middle aged women. *J Rheumatol, 26*, 1586–1592.

Leproult, R., Deliens, G., Gilson, M., & Peigneux, P. (2015). Beneficial impact of sleep extension on fasting insulin sensitivity in adults with habitual sleep restriction. *Sleep, 38*(5), 707–715. doi: 10.5665/sleep.4660

Lewandowski, A. S., Palermo, T. M., De la Motte, S., & Fu, R. (2010). Temporal daily associations between pain and sleep in adolescents with chronic pain versus healthy adolescents. *Pain, 151*(1), 220–225. doi: 10.1016/j.pain.2010.07.016

Li, S. H., Corkish, B., Richardson, C., Christensen, H., & Werner-Seidler, A. (2023). The role of rumination in the relationship between symptoms of insomnia and depression in adolescents. *J Sleep Res, 33*(2), e13932. doi:10.1111/jsr.13932

Li, S. X., Lam, S. P., Chan, J. W., Yu, M. W., & Wing, Y. K. (2012). Residual sleep disturbances in patients remitted from major depressive disorder: a 4-year naturalistic follow-up study. *Sleep, 35*(8), 1153–1161. doi: 10.5665/sleep.2008

Lim, A. S., Ellison, B. A., Wang, J. L., Yu, L., Schneider, J. A., Buchman, A. S., Bennett, D. A., & Saper, C. B. (2014). Sleep is related to neuron numbers in the ventrolateral preoptic/intermediate nucleus in older adults with and without Alzheimer's disease. *Brain, 137*(Pt 10), 2847–2861. doi: 10.1093/brain/awu222

Lim, A. S., Kowgier, M., Yu, L., Buchman, A. S., & Bennett, D. A. (2013). Sleep fragmentation and the risk of incident Alzheimer's disease and cognitive decline in older persons. *Sleep, 36*(7), 1027–1032. doi: 10.5665/sleep.2802

Limoges, E., Mottron, L., Bolduc, C., Berthiaume, C., & Godbout, R. (2005). Atypical sleep architecture and the autism phenotype. *Brain, 128*(Pt 5), 1049–1061. doi: 10.1093/brain/awh425

Lin, W., Lin, Y.-K., Yang, F.-C., Chung, C.-H., Hu, J.-M., Tsao, C.-H., … Chien, W.-C. (2023). Risk of neurodegenerative diseases in patients with sleep disorders: A nationwide population-based case-control study. *Sleep Med, 107*, 289–299. doi: 10.1016/j.sleep.2023.05.014

Lin, Y.-H., Lin, S.-H., & Chen, I.-M. (2022). The direct effect of cognitive behavioral rherapy for insomnia on depression prevention and the mediation effect via insomnia remission. *JAMA Psychiatry, 79*(5), 514–515. doi: 10.1001/jamapsychiatry.2022.0084

Liu, C., Lee, S. H., Loewenstein, D. A., Galvin, J. E., Camargo, C. J., & Alperin, N. (2022). Poor sleep accelerates hippocampal and posterior cingulate volume loss in cognitively normal healthy older adults. *J Sleep Res, 31*(4), e13538. doi:10.1111/jsr.13538

Lo, J. C., Loh, K. K., Zheng, H., Sim, S. K., & Chee, M. W. (2014). Sleep duration and age-related changes in brain structure and cognitive performance. *Sleep, 37*(7), 1171–1178. doi: 10.5665/sleep.3832

Łojko, D., & Rybakowski, J. K. (2017). Atypical depression: current perspectives. *Neuropsychiatr Dis Treat, 13*, 2447–2456. doi: 10.2147/NDT.S147317

Lopera, F., Marino, C., Chandrahas, A. S., O'Hare, M., Villalba-Moreno, N. D., Aguillon, D., … Quiroz, Y. T. (2023). Resilience to autosomal dominant Alzheimer's disease in a Reelin-COLBOS heterozygous man. *Nat Med, 29*(5), 1243–1252. doi:10.1038/s41591-023-02318-3

Lopez, J., Hoffmann, R., & Armitage, R. (2010). Reduced sleep spindle activity in early-onset and elevated risk for depression. *J Am Acad Child Adolesc Psychiatry, 49*(9), 934–943. doi: 10.1016/j.jaac.2010.05.014

Lorenzo-Luaces, L., Buss, J. F., & Fried, E. I. (2021). Heterogeneity in major depression and its melancholic and atypical specifiers: a secondary analysis of STAR*D. *BMC Psychiatry, 21*(1), 454. doi:10.1186/s12888-021-03444-3

Louveau, A., Smirnov, I., Keyes, T. J., Eccles, J. D., Rouhani, S. J., Peske, J. D., … Kipnis, J. (2015). Structural and functional features of central nervous system lymphatic vessels. *Nature, 523*(7560), 337–341. doi: 10.1038/nature14432

Lovato, N., & Lack, L. (2019). Insomnia and mortality: a meta-analysis. *Sleep Med Rev, 43*, 71–83. doi: 10.1016/j.smrv.2018.10.004

Lu, Y., Sugawara, Y., Zhang, S., Tomata, Y., & Tsuji, I. (2018). Changes in sleep duration and the risk of incident dementia in the elderly Japanese: the Ohsaki Cohort 2006 Study. *Sleep, 41*(10), 1–8. doi: 10.1093/sleep/zsy143

Lucey, B. P., McCullough, A., Landsness, E. C., Toedebusch, C. D., McLeland, J. S., Zaza, A. M., … Holtzman, D. M. (2019). Reduced non-rapid eye movement sleep is associated with tau pathology in early Alzheimer's disease. *Sci Transl Med, 11*(474), eaau6550. doi:10.1126/scitranslmed.aau6550

Luojus, M. K., Lehto, S. M., Tolmunen, T., Brem, A. K., Lonnroos, E., & Kauhanen, J. (2017). Self-reported sleep disturbance and incidence of dementia in ageing men. *J Epidemiol Commun Health, 71*(4), 329–335. doi: 10.1136/jech-2016-207764

Lysen, T. S., Wolters, F. J., Luik, A., Kamran, M., Tiemeier, H., & Ikram, M. A. (2018). Subjective sleep quality is not associated with incident dementia: the Rotterdam study. *J Alzheimer Dis, 64*(1), 239–247.

Manber, R., Edinger, J. D., Gress, J. L., San Pedro-Salcedo, M. G., Kuo, T. F., & Kalista, T. (2008). Cognitive behavioral therapy for insomnia enhances depression outcome in patients with comorbid depressive disorder and insomnia. *Sleep, 31*(4), 489–495.

Manoach, D. S., Demanuele, C., Wamsley, E. J., Vangel, M., Montrose, D. M., Miewald, J., … Keshavan, M. S. (2014). Sleep spindle deficits in antipsychotic-naive early course schizophrenia and in non-psychotic first-degree relatives. *Front Hum Neurosci, 8*, 762. doi: 10.3389/fnhum.2014.00762

Marway, O. S., Lau, P. H., Carmona, N. E., & Carney, C. E. (2023). What are patients completing Cognitive Behavioral Insomnia Therapy telling us with their post-treatment Insomnia Severity Index scores? *Sleep Med, 103*, 187–194. doi: 10.1016/j.sleep.2023.02.008

Mason, E. C., Grierson, A. B., Sie, A., Sharrock, M. J., Li, I., Chen, A. Z., & Newby, J. M. (2023). Co-occurring insomnia and anxiety: A randomized controlled trial of internet CBT for insomnia vs. internet CBT for anxiety. *Sleep, 46*(2), zsac205. doi: 10.1093/sleep/zsac205

Matre, D., Hu, L., Viken, L. A., Hjelle, I. B., Wigemyr, M., Knardahl, S., … Nilsen, K. B. (2015). Experimental sleep restriction facilitates pain and electrically induced cortical responses. *Sleep, 38*(10), 1607–1617. doi: 10.5665/sleep.5058

Mayeli, A., Wilson, J. D., Donati, F. L., LaGoy, A. D., & Ferrarelli, F. (2022). Sleep spindle alterations relate to working memory deficits in individuals at clinical high-risk for psychosis. *Sleep, 45*(11), 1–9. doi:10.1093/sleep/zsac193

McCurry, S. M., Logsdon, R. G., Teri, L., Gibbons, L. E., Kukull, W. A., Bowen, J. D., … Larson, E. B. (1999). Characteristics of sleep disturbance in community-dwelling Alzheimer's disease patients. *J Geriatr Psych Neurol, 12*, 53–59.

McGrath, E. R., Beiser, A. S., DeCarli, C., Plourde, K. L., Vasan, R. S., Greenberg, S. M., & Seshadri, S. (2018). Blood pressure from mid- to late life and risk of incident dementia. *Neurology, 89*, 2447–2454.

McIntyre, R. S., Berk, M., Brietzke, E., Goldstein, B. I., López-Jaramillo, C., Kessing, L. V., … Mansur, R. B. (2020). Bipolar disorders. *Lancet, 396*(10265), 1841–1856. doi: 10.1016/s0140-6736(20)31544-0

McMahon, S. B., La Russa, F., & Bennett, D. L. (2015). Crosstalk between the nociceptive and immune systems in host defence and disease. *Nat Rev Neurosci, 16*(7), 389–402. doi: 10.1038/nrn3946

Mendell, L. M. (2014). Constructing and deconstructing the gate theory of pain. *Pain, 155*(2), 210–216. doi: 10.1016/j.pain.2013.12.010

Miao, A., Luo, T., Hsieh, B., Edge, C. J., Gridley, M., Wong, R. T. C., Constandinou, T. G., Wisden, W., & Franks, N. P. (2024). Brain clearance is reduced during sleep and anesthesia. *Nat Neurosci*. doi: 10.1038/s41593-024-01638-y

Moldofsky, H., & Scarisbrick, P. (1976). Induction of neurasthenic musculoskeletal pain syndrome by selective sleep stage deprivation. *Psychosom Med, 38*(1), 35–44.

Moldofsky, H., Scarisbrick, P., England, R., & Smythe, H. (1975). Musculoskeletal symptoms and non-REM sleep disturbance in patients with "fibrositis syndrome" and healthy subjects. *Psychosom Med, 37*(4), 341–351.

Montagna, P. (2005). Fatal familial insomnia: a model disease in sleep physiopathology. *Sleep Med Rev, 9*(5), 339–353. doi: 10.1016/j.smrv.2005.02.001

Montagna, P., & Lugaresi, E. (2002). Agrypnia Excitata: a generalized overactivity syndrome and a useful concept in the neurophysiopathology of sleep. *Clin Neurophysiol, 113*, 552.560.

Morawska, M. M., Buchele, F., Moreira, C. G., Imbach, L. L., Noain, D., & Baumann, C. R. (2016). Sleep modulation alleviates axonal damage and cognitive decline after rodent traumatic brain injury. *J Neurosci, 36*(12), 3422–3429. doi: 10.1523/JNEUROSCI.3274-15.2016

Morin, C. M. (1993). *Insomnia: Psychological Assessment and Management*. New York: Guilford Press.

Mullington, J. M., Simpson, N. S., Meier-Ewert, H. K., & Haack, M. (2010). Sleep loss and inflammation. *Best Pract Res Clin Endocrinol Metab, 24*(5), 775–784. doi: 10.1016/j.beem.2010.08.014

Mylonas, D., Machado, S., Larson, O., Patel, R., Cox, R., Vangel, M., … Manoach, D. S. (2022). Dyscoordination of non-rapid eye movement sleep oscillations in autism spectrum disorder. *Sleep, 45*(3), 1–15. doi: 10.1093/sleep/zsac010

Nofzinger, E. A., Thase, M. E., Reynolds Iii, C. F., Himmelhoch, J. M., Mallinger, A., Houck, P., & Kupfer, D. J. (1991). Hypersomnia in bipolar depression: a comparison with narcolepsy using the multiple sleep latency test. *Am J Psychiatry, 148*, 1177–1181.

Nomura, T., Inoue, Y., Kagimura, T., & Nakashima, K. (2013). Clinical significance of REM sleep behavior disorder in Parkinson's disease. *Sleep Med, 14*(2), 131–135. doi: 10.1016/j.sleep.2012.10.011

Nunes, J., Jean-Louis, G., Zizi, F., Casimir, G. J., von Gizycki, H., Brown, C. D., & McFarlane, S. I. (2008). Sleep duration among black and white Americans: results of the National Health Interview Survey. *J Natl Med Assoc, 100*(3), 317–322.

Nutt, D., Wilson, S., & Paterson, L. (2008). Sleep disorders as core symptoms of depression *Dialogues Clin Neurosci, 10*(3), 329–336.

Ødegard, S. S., Omland, P. M., Nilsen, K. B., Stjern, M., Gravdahl, G. B., & Sand, T. (2015). The effect of sleep restriction on laser evoked potentials, thermal sensory and pain thresholds and suprathreshold pain in healthy subjects. *Clin Neurophysiol, 126*(10), 1979–1987. doi: 10.1016/j.clinph.2014.12.011

Oh, J. Y., Walsh, C. M., Ranasinghe, K., Mladinov, M., Pereira, F. L., Petersen, C., … Grinberg, L. T. (2022). Subcortical neuronal correlates of sleep in neurodegenerative diseases. *JAMA Neurol, 79*(5), 498–508. doi: 10.1001/jamaneurol.2022.0429

Older, S. A., Battafarano, D. F., Danning, C. L., Ward, J. A., Grady, E. P., Derman, S., & Russell, I. J. (1998). The effects of delta wave sleep interruption on pain thresholds and fibromyalgia-like symptoms in healthy subjects; correlations with insulin-like growth factor I. *J Rheumatol, 25*, 1180–1186.

Oliver, P. L., Sobczyk, M. V., Maywood, E. S., Edwards, B., Lee, S., Livieratos, A., ... Foster, R. G. (2012). Disrupted circadian rhythms in a mouse model of schizophrenia. *Curr Biol, 22*(4), 314–319. doi: 10.1016/j.cub.2011.12.051

Olsson, M., Arlig, J., Hedner, J., Blennow, K., & Zetterberg, H. (2018). Sleep deprivation and cerebrospinal fluid biomarkers for Alzheimer's disease. *Sleep, 41*(5), zsy025. doi: 10.1093/sleep/zsy025

Olsson, M., Arlig, J., Hedner, J., Blennow, K., & Zetterberg, H. (2019). Sleep deprivation and plasma biomarkers for Alzheimer's disease. *Sleep Med, 57*, 92–93. doi: 10.1016/j.sleep.2018.12.029

Onen, S. H., Alloui, A., Gross, A., Eschallier, A., & Dubray, C. (2001). The effects of total sleep deprivation, selective sleep interruption and sleep recovery on pain tolerance thresholds in healthy subjects. *J Sleep Res, 10*, 35–42.

Ooms, S., Overeem, S., Besse, K., Rikkert, M. O., Verbeek, M., & Claassen, J. A. (2014). Effect of 1 night of total sleep deprivation on cerebrospinal fluid β-amyloid 42 in healthy middle-aged men: a randomized clinical trial. *JAMA Neurol, 71*(8), 971–977. doi: 10.1001/jamaneurol.2014.1173

Ortiz, A., Bradler, K., Radu, L., Alda, M., & Rusak, B. (2016). Exponential state transition dynamics in the rest-activity architecture of patients with bipolar disorder. *Bipolar Disord, 18*(2), 116–123. doi: 10.1111/bdi.12372

Osimo, E. F., Baxter, L. J., Lewis, G., Jones, P. B., & Khandaker, G. M. (2019). Prevalence of low-grade inflammation in depression: a systematic review and meta-analysis of CRP levels. *Psychol Med, 49*(12), 1958–1970. doi: 10.1017/S0033291719001454

Ossenkoppele, R., Schonhaut, D. R., Scholl, M., Lockhart, S. N., Ayakta, N., Baker, S. L., ... Rabinovici, G. D. (2016). Tau PET patterns mirror clinical and neuroanatomical variability in Alzheimer's disease. *Brain, 139*(Pt 5), 1551–1567. doi: 10.1093/brain/aww027

Özcan, G. G., Lim, S., Canning, T., Tirathdas, L., Donnelly, J., Kundu, T., & Rihel, J. (2024). Genetic and chemical disruption of amyloid precursor protein processing impairs zebrafish sleep maintenance. *iScience, 27*(2), 108870. doi:10.1016/j.isci.2024.108870

Parsons, C. E., & Young, K. S. (2022). Beneficial effects of sleep extension on daily emotion in short-sleeping young adults: an experience sampling study. *Sleep Health, 8*(5), 505–513. doi: 10.1016/j.sleh.2022.05.008

Patel, S. R., Ayas, N. T., Malhotra, M. R., White, D. P., Schernhammer, E. S., Speizer, F. E., ... Hu, F. B. (2004). A prospective study of sleep duration and mortality risk in women. *Sleep, 27*(3), 440–444.

Patel, S. R., Malhotra, A., Gottlieb, D. J., White, D. P., & Hu, F. B. (2006). Correlates of long sleep duration. *Sleep, 29*(7), 881–889.

Petrovsky, N., Ettinger, U., Hill, A., Frenzel, L., Meyhofer, I., Wagner, M., ... Kumari, V. (2014). Sleep deprivation disrupts prepulse inhibition and induces psychosis-like symptoms in healthy humans. *J Neurosci, 34*(27), 9134–9140. doi: 10.1523/JNEUROSCI.0904-14.2014

Pflug, B., & Tölle, R. (1971). Disturbance of the 24-hour rhythm in endogenous depression and the treatment of endogenous depression by sleep deprivation. *Int Pharmacopsychiatry*, 6, 187–196.

Plante, D. T., Cook, J. D., & Goldstein, M. R. (2017). Objective measures of sleep duration and continuity in major depressive disorder with comorbid hypersomnolence: a primary investigation with contiguous systematic review and meta-analysis. *J Sleep Res, 26*(3), 255–265. doi: 10.1111/jsr.12498

Pollak, C. P., & Perlick, D. (1991). Sleep problems and institutionalization of the elderly. *J Geriatri Psychiatry Neurology, 4*, 204–210.

Pollak, C. P., & Stokes, P. E. (1997). Circadian rest-activity rhythms in demented and nondemented older community residents and their caregivers. *J Am Geriatr Soc, 45*, 446–452.

Post, R. M. (2016). Treatment of bipolar depression: evolving recommendation *Psychiatr Clin N Am, 39*(1), 11–33.

Poulin, J., Daoust, A.-M., Forest, G., Stip, E., & Godbout, R. (2003). Sleep architecture and its clinical correlates in first episode and neuroleptic-naive patients with schizophrenia. *Schizophrenia Res, 62*(1-2), 147–153. doi: 10.1016/s0920-9964(02)00346-8

Profitt, M. F., Deurveilher, S., Robertson, G. S., Rusak, B., & Semba, K. (2016). Disruptions of sleep/wake patterns in the stable tubule only polypeptide (STOP) null mouse model of schizophrenia. *Schizophrenia Bull, 42*(5), 1207–1215. doi: 10.1093/schbul/sbw017

Quach, J. L., Nguyen, C. D., Williams, K. E., & Sciberras, E. (2018). Bidirectional associations between child sleep problems and internalizing and externalizing difficulties from preschool to early adolescence. *JAMA Pediatr, 172*(2), 1–8. doi: 10.1001/jamapediatrics.2017.4363

Raison, C. L., & Miller, A. H. (2013). Malaise, melancholia and madness: the evolutionary legacy of an inflammatory bias. *Brain Behav Immun, 31*, 1–8. doi: 10.1016/j.bbi.2013.04.009

Ramirez-Mahaluf, J. P., Rozas-Serri, E., Ivanovic-Zuvic, F., Risco, L., & Vohringer, P. A. (2020). Effectiveness of sleep deprivation in treating acute bipolar depression as augmentation strategy: a systematic review and meta-analysis. *Front Psychiatry, 11*(70), 1–9. doi: 10.3389/fpsyt.2020.00070

Raymond, I., Nielsen, T. A., Lavigne, G., Manzini, C., & Choinière, M. (2001). Quality of sleep and its daily relationship to pain intensity in hospitalized adult burn patients. *Pain, 92*, 381–388.

Richards, A., Kanady, J. C., & Neylan, T. C. (2020). Sleep disturbance in PTSD and other anxiety-related disorders: an updated review of clinical features, physiological characteristics, and psychological and neurobiological mechanisms. *Neuropsychopharmacology, 45*(1), 55–73. doi: 10.1038/s41386-019-0486-5

Riemann, D., Voderholzer, U., & Berger, M. (2002). Sleep and sleep-wake manipulations in bipolar depression. *Neuropsychobiology, 45*, 7–12.

Ritter, P. S., Marx, C., Bauer, M., Leopold, K., & Pfennig, A. (2011). The role of disturbed sleep in the early recognition of bipolar disorder: a systematic review. *Bipolar Disord, 13*(3), 227–237. doi: 10.1111/j.1399-5618.2011.00917.x

Robillard, R., Hermens, D. F., Naismith, S. L., White, D., Rogers, N. L., Ip, T. K., ... Hickie, I. B. (2015). Ambulatory sleep-wake patterns and variability in young people with emerging mental disorders. *J Psychiatry Neurosci, 40*(1), 28–37.

Rochefort, A., Jarrin, D. C., Belanger, L., Ivers, H., & Morin, C. M. (2019). Insomnia treatment response as a function of objectively measured sleep duration. *Sleep Med*. doi: 10.1016/j.sleep.2019.01.016

Rodrigues, N. B., McIntyre, R. S., Lipsitz, O., Cha, D. S., Cao, B., Lee, Y., ... Rosenblat, J. D. (2022). Do sleep changes mediate the anti-depressive and anti-suicidal response of intravenous ketamine in treatment-resistant depression? *J Sleep Res, 31*(1), e13400. doi: 10.1111/jsr.13400

Roehrs, T., Hyde, M., Blaisdell, B., Greenwald, M., & Roth, T. (2006). Sleep loss and REM sleep loss are hyperalgesic. *Sleep, 29*(2), 145–151.

Roehrs, T. A., Harris, E., Randall, S., & Roth, T. (2012). Pain sensitivity and recovery from mild chronic sleep loss. *Sleep, 35*(12), 1667–1672. doi: 10.5665/sleep.2240

Roh, J. H., Huang, Y., Bero, A. W., Kasten, T., Stewart, F. R., Bateman, R. J., & Holtzman, D. M. (2012). Disruption of the sleep-wake cycle and diurnal fluctuation of beta-amyloid in mice with Alzheimer's disease pathology. *Sci Transl Med, 4*(150), 150ra122. doi: 10.1126/scitranslmed.3004291

Rosenthal, N. E., Sack, D. A., Gillin, J. C., Lewy, A. J., Goodwin, F. K., Davenport, Y., ... Wehr, T. A. (1984). Seasonal affective disorder: a description of the syndrome and preliminary findings with light therapy. *Arch Gen Psychiatr, 41*, 72–80.

Ross, J. J. (1965). Neurological findings after prolonged sleep deprivation. *Arch Neurol, 12*, 399–403.

Roux, F. J., & Kryger, M. H. (2010). Medication effects on sleep. *Clin Chest Med, 31*(2), 397–405. doi: 10.1016/j.ccm.2010.02.008

Ruan, H., Zheng, Y., Yang, J., Li, L., Zhang, M., Wang, Z., & He, S. (2023). Changes in daily sleep duration and subsequent risk of mortality among older people. *Sleep Med, 101*, 252–259. doi:10.1016/j.sleep.2022.11.016

Rumble, M. E., White, K. H., & Benca, R. M. (2015). Sleep disturbances in mood disorders. *Psychiatr Clin N Am, 38*(4), 743–759. doi: 10.1016/j.psc.2015.07.006

Sanford, J. R. A. (1975). Tolerance of debility in elderly dependants by supporters at home: its significance for hospital practice. *Br Med J, 3*(471–473).

Sangalli, L., & Boggero, I. A. (2023). The impact of sleep components, quality and patterns on glymphatic system functioning in healthy adults: a systematic review. *Sleep Med, 101*, 322–349. doi: 10.1016/j.sleep.2022.11.012

Scharf, M. B., Baumann, M., & Berkowitz, D. V. (2003). The effects of sodium oxybate on clinical symptoms and sleep patterns in patients with fibromyalgia. *J Rheumatol, 30*, 1070–1074.

Seixas, A. A., Auguste, E., Butler, M., James, C., Newsome, V., Auguste, E., ... Jean-Louis, G. (2017). Differences in short and long sleep durations between blacks and whites attributed to emotional distress: analysis of the National Health Interview Survey in the United States. *Sleep Health, 3*(1), 28–34. doi: 10.1016/j.sleh.2016.11.003

Selkoe, D. J., & Hardy, J. (2016). The amyloid hypothesis of Alzheimer's disease at 25 years. *EMBO Mol Med, 8*(6), 595–608. doi: 10.15252/emmm.201606210

Shallice, T., Burgess, P. W., & Frith, C. D. (1991). Can the neuropsychological case-study approach be applied to schizophrenia? *Psychol Med, 21*(3), 661–673. doi: 10.1017/s0033291700022303

Shen, X., Wu, Y., & Zhang, D. (2016). Nighttime sleep duration, 24-hour sleep duration and risk of all-cause mortality among adults: a meta-analysis of prospective cohort studies. *Sci Rep, 6*, 21480. doi: 10.1038/srep21480

Shi, L., Chen, S. J., Ma, M. Y., Bao, Y. P., Han, Y., Wang, Y. M., … Lu, L. (2018). Sleep disturbances increase the risk of dementia: A systematic review and meta-analysis. *Sleep Med Rev*, *40*, 4–16. doi: 10.1016/j.smrv.2017.06.010

Shokri-Kojori, E., Wang, G. J., Wiers, C. E., Demiral, S. B., Guo, M., Kim, S. W., … Volkow, N. D. (2018). β-Amyloid accumulation in the human brain after one night of sleep deprivation. *Proc Natl Acad Sci U S A*, *115*(17), 4483–4488. doi: 10.1073/pnas.1721694115

Simonelli, G., Mantua, J., Gad, M., St Pierre, M., Moore, L., Yarnell, A. M., … Capaldi, V. F. (2019). Sleep extension reduces pain sensitivity. *Sleep Med*, *54*, 172–176. doi: 10.1016/j.sleep.2018.10.023

Slavish, D. C., Taylor, D. J., & Lichstein, K. L. (2019). Intraindividual variability in sleep and comorbid medical and mental health conditions. *Sleep*, *42*(6), zsz052. doi:10.1093/sleep/zsz052

Smith, A. J., & Verkman, A. S. (2018). The "glymphatic" mechanism for solute clearance in Alzheimer's disease: game changer or unproven speculation? *FASEB J*, *32*(2), 543–551. doi: 10.1096/fj.201700999

Smith, M. T., Edwards, R. R., McCann, U. D., & Haythornthwaite, J. A. (2007). The effects of sleep deprivation on pain inhibition and spontaneous pain in women. *Sleep*, *30*(4), 494–505.

Soh, A. Z., Chee, M. W. L., Yuan, J. M., & Koh, W. P. (2018). Sleep lengthening in late adulthood signals increased risk of mortality. *Sleep*, *41*(3). doi: 10.1093/sleep/zsy005

Sorge, R. E., Martin, L. J., Isbester, K. A., Sotocinal, S. G., Rosen, S., Tuttle, A. H., … Mogil, J. S. (2014). Olfactory exposure to males, including men, causes stress and related analgesia in rodents. *Nat Methods*, *11*(6), 629–632. doi: 10.1038/nmeth.2935

Spira, A. P., An, Y., Wu, M. N., Owusu, J. T., Simonsick, E. M., Bilgel, M., … Resnick, S. M. (2018). Excessive daytime sleepiness and napping in cognitively normal adults: associations with subsequent amyloid deposition measured by PiB PET. *Sleep*, *41*(10), zsy152. doi: 10.1093/sleep/zsy152

Spira, A. P., Gamaldo, A. A., An, Y., Wu, M. N., Simonsick, E. M., Bilgel, M., … Resnick, S. M. (2013). Self-reported sleep and beta-amyloid deposition in community-dwelling older adults. *JAMA Neurol*, *70*(12), 1537–1543. doi: 10.1001/jamaneurol.2013.4258

Sterniczuk, R., Dyck, R. H., LaFerla, F. M., & Antle, M. C. (2010). Characterization of the 3xTg-AD mouse model of Alzheimer's disease: part 1. circadian changes. *Brain Res*, *1348*, 139–148. doi: 10.1016/j.brainres.2010.05.013

Sterniczuk, R., Theo, O., Rusak, B., & Rockwood, K. (2013). Sleep disturbance is associated with incident dementia and mortality. *Curr Alzheimer Res*, *10*(7), 767–775. doi: 10.2174/15672050113109990134

Stewart, J. W., McGrath, P. J., Quitkin, F. M., & Klein, D. F. (2009). DSM-IV depression with atypical features: is it valid? *Neuropsychopharmacology*, *34*(13), 2625–2632. doi: 10.1038/npp.2009.99

Stranges, S., Dorn, J. M., Shipley, M. J., Kandala, N. B., Trevisan, M., Miller, M. A., … Cappuccio, F. P. (2008). Correlates of short and long sleep duration: a cross-cultural comparison between the United Kingdom and the United States: the Whitehall II Study and the Western New York Health Study. *Am J Epidemiol*, *168*(12), 1353–1364. doi: 10.1093/aje/kwn337

Stratmann, K., Heinsen, H., Korf, H. W., Del Turco, D., Ghebremedhin, E., Seidel, K., … Rüb, U. (2016). Precortical phase of Alzheimer's disease (AD)-related tau cytoskeletal pathology. *Brain Pathol*, *26*(3), 371–386. doi: 10.1111/bpa.12289

Szklo-Coxe, M., Young, T., Peppard, P. E., Finn, L. A., & Benca, R. M. (2010). Prospective associations of insomnia markers and symptoms with depression. *Am J Epidemiol*, *171*(6), 709–720. doi: 10.1093/aje/kwp454

Takaesu, Y. (2018). Circadian rhythm in bipolar disorder: a review of the literature. *Psychiatr Clin Neurosci*, *72*(9), 673–682. doi: 10.1111/pcn.12688

Tang, N. K., Goodchild, C. E., Sanborn, A. N., Howard, J., & Salkovskis, P. M. (2012). Deciphering the temporal link between pain and sleep in a heterogeneous chronic pain patient sample: a multilevel daily process study. *Sleep*, *35*(5), 675–687A. doi: 10.5665/sleep.1830

Tang, N. K., Lereya, S. T., Boulton, H., Miller, M. A., Wolke, D., & Cappuccio, F. P. (2015). Nonpharmacological treatments of insomnia for long-term painful conditions: a systematic review and meta-analysis of patient-reported outcomes in randomized controlled trials. *Sleep*, *38*(11), 1751–1764. doi: 10.5665/sleep.5158

Tao, F., Cao, Z., Jiang, Y., Fan, N., Xu, F., Yang, H., … Wang, Y. (2021). Associations of sleep duration and quality with incident cardiovascular disease, cancer, and mortality: a prospective cohort study of 407,500 UK biobank participants. *Sleep Med*, *81*, 401–409. doi: 10.1016/j.sleep.2021.03.015

Tao, P., Svetnik, V., Bliwise, D. L., Zammit, G., Lines, C., & Herring, W. J. (2023). Comparison of polysomnography in people with Alzheimer's disease and insomnia versus non-demented elderly people with insomnia. *Sleep Med*, *101*, 515–521. doi: 10.1016/j.sleep.2022.11.027

Tasali, E., Wroblewski, K., Kahn, E., Kilkus, J., & Schoeller, D. A. (2022). Effect of sleep extension on objectively assessed energy intake among adults with overweight in real-life settings: a randomized clinical trial. *JAMA Intern Med*, *182*(4), 365–374. doi:10.1001/jamainternmed.2021.8098

Taub, J. M., Globus, G. G., Phoebus, E., & Drury, R. (1971). Extended sleep and performance. *Nature*, *233*, 142–143.

Tranah, G. J., Blackwell, T., Stone, K. L., Ancoli-Israel, S., Paudel, M. L., Ensrud, K. E., … Group, S. O. F. R. (2011). Circadian activity rhythms and risk of incident dementia and mild cognitive impairment in older women. *Ann Neurol*, *70*(5), 722–732. doi: 10.1002/ana.22468

Van Cauter, E., Linkowski, P., Kerkhofs, M., Hubain, P., L'Hermite-Balériaux, M., Leclerq, R., … Mendlewicz, J. (1991). Circadian and sleep-related endocrine rhythms in schizophrenia. *Arch Gen Psychiatr*, *48*, 348–356.

van de Nes, J. A., Konermann, S., Nafe, R., & Swaab, D. F. (2006). Beta-protein/A4 deposits are not associated with hyperphosphorylated tau in somatostatin neurons in the hypothalamus of Alzheimer's disease patients. *Acta Neuropathologica*, *111*(2), 126–138. doi: 10.1007/s00401-005-0018-8

van den Haar, H., Burgmans, S., Jansen, J. F. A., van Osch, M. J. P., van Buchem, M. A., Muller, M., … Backes, W. H. (2016). Blood-brain barrier leakage in patients with early Alzheimer disease. *Radiology*, *281*(2), 527–535.

Van den Hoofdakker, R. H., Bouhuys, A. L., & Beersma, D. G. M. (1989). The effects of sleep deprivation and sleep on depressive mood and subjective arousal. *Biol Psychiatry*, *26*, 733–736.

Van Dyk, T. R., Zhang, N., Catlin, P. A., Cornist, K., McAlister, S., Whitacre, C., & Beebe, D. W. (2017). Feasibility and emotional impact of experimentally extending sleep in short-sleeping adolescents. *Sleep*, *40*(9), zsx123. doi: 10.1093/sleep/zsx123

Van Egroo, M., Narbutas, J., Chylinski, D., Villar González, P., Maquet, P., Salmon, E., … Vandewalle, G. (2019). Sleep-wake regulation and the hallmarks of the pathogenesis of Alzheimer's disease. *Sleep*, *42*(4), zsz017. doi: 10.1093/sleep/zsz017

van Mill, J. G., Hoogendijk, W. J., Vogelzangs, N., van Dyck, R., & Penninx, B. W. (2010). Insomnia and sleep duration in a large cohort of patients with major depressive disorder and anxiety disorders. *J Clin Psychiatry*, *71*(3), 239–246. doi: 10.4088/JCP.09m05218gry

Varga, A. W., Wohlleber, M. E., Giménez, S., Romero, S., Alonso, J. F., Ducca, E. L., … Osorio, R. S. (2016). Reduced slow-wave sleep is associated with high cerebrospinal fluid Aβ42 levels in cognitively normal elderly. *Sleep*, *39*(11), 2041–2048. doi: 0.5665/sleep.6240

Vgontzas, A. N., Liao, D., Pejovic, S., Calhoun, S., Karataraki, M., Basta, M., … Bixler, E. O. (2010). Insomnia with short sleep duration and mortality: the Penn State Cohort. *Sleep*, *33*(9), 1159–1164.

Vitiello, M., & Prinz, P. N. (1989). Alzheimer's disease: sleep and sleep/wake patterns. *Clin Geriatr Med*, *5*(2), 289–299.

Vogel, G. W., Vogel, F., McAbee, R., & Thurmond, A. J. (1980). Improvement of depression by REM sleep deprivation. New findings and a theory. *Arch Gen Psychiatr*, *37*, 247–253.

Wagley, J. N., Rybarczyk, B., Nay, W. T., Danish, S., & Lund, H. G. (2013). Effectiveness of abbreviated CBT for insomnia in psychiatric outpatients: sleep and depression outcomes. *J Clin Psychol*, *69*(10), 1043–1055. doi: 10.1002/jclp.21927

Wallace, M. L., Coleman, T. S., Mentch, L. K., Buysse, D. J., Graves, J. L., Hagen, E. W., … Peppard, P. E. (2021). Physiological sleep measures predict time to 15-year mortality in community adults: application of a novel machine learning framework. *J Sleep Res*, *30*(6), e13386. doi:10.1111/jsr.13386

Wamsley, E. J., Tucker, M. A., Shinn, A. K., Ono, K. E., McKinley, S. K., Ely, A. V., … Manoach, D. S. (2012). Reduced sleep spindles and spindle coherence in schizophrenia: mechanisms of impaired memory consolidation? *Biol Psychiatry*, *71*(2), 154–161. doi: 10.1016/j.biopsych.2011.08.008

Wang, J. L., Lim, A. S., Chiang, W. Y., Hsieh, W. H., Lo, M. T., Schneider, J. A., … Saper, C. B. (2015). Suprachiasmatic neuron numbers and rest-activity circadian rhythms in older humans. *Ann Neurol*, *78*(2), 317–322. doi: 10.1002/ana.24432

Wang, Y., Melgers, M., Meijer, J. H., & Deboer, T. (2023). Comparison of sleep deprivation and a low dose of ketamine on sleep and the electroencephalogram in Brown Norway rats. *J Sleep Res*, *32*(5), e13863. doi:10.1111/jsr.13863

Watanabe, N., Furukawa, T., Shimodera, S., Morokuma, I., Katsuki, F., Fujita, H., … Perlis, M. (2011). Brief behavioral therapy for refractory insomnia in residual depression: an assessor-blind, randomized control trial. *J Clin Psychiatry*, *72*(12), 1651–1658. doi: 10.4088/JCP.10m06130gry

Wehr, T. A. (1990). Effects of wakefulness and sleep on depression and mania. In J. Montplaisir & R. Godbout (Eds.), *Sleep and Biological Rhythms: Basic Mechanisms and Applications to Psychiatry* (pp. 42–86). Oxford: Oxford University Press.

Wehr, T. A., Moul, D. E., Barbato, G., Giesen, H. A., Seidel, J. A., Barker, C., & Bender, C. (1993). Conservation of photoperiod-responsive mechanisms in humans. *Am J Physiol, 265*(4 Pt 2), R846–R857.

Wehr, T. A., Rosenthal, N. E., Sack, D. A., & Gillin, J. C. (1985). Antidepressant effects of sleep deprivation in bright and dim light. *Acta Psychiatr Scan, 72*, 161–165.

Wehr, T. A., Sack, D., Rosenthal, N., Duncan, W., & Gillin, J. C. (1983). Circadian rhythm disturbances in manic-depressive illness. *Fed Proc, 42*, 2809–2814.

Wehr, T. A., Sack, D. A., & Rosenthal, N. E. (1987). Sleep reduction as a final common pathway in the genesis of mania *Am J Psychiatry, 144*, 201–204.

Wehr, T. A., Wirz-Justice, A., Goodwin, F. K., Duncan, W., & Gillin, J. C. (1979). Phase advance of the circadian sleep-wake cycle as an antidepressant. *Science, 206*(4419), 710–713.

Weickert, T. W., Goldberg, T. E., Gold, J. M., Bigelow, L. B., Egan, M. F., & Weinberger, D. R. (2000). Cognitive impairments in patients with schizophrenia displaying preserved or compromised intellect. *Arch Gen Psychiatr, 57*, 907–913.

Weingarten, J. A., Dubrovsky, B., Basner, R. C., Redline, S., George, L., & Lederer, D. J. (2016). Polysomnographic measurement of sleep duration and bodily pain perception in the Sleep Heart Health Study. *Sleep, 39*(8), 1583–1589. doi: 0.5665/sleep.6026

Wescott, D. L., Franzen, P. L., Hasler, B. P., Miller, M. A., Soehner, A. M., Smagula, S. F., … Roecklein, K. A. (2023). Elusive hypersomnolence in seasonal affective disorder: actigraphic and self-reported sleep in and out of depressive episodes. *Psychol Med, 53*(4), 1313–1322. doi: 10.1017/S003329172100283X

Wescott, D. L., Morash-Conway, J., Zwicker, A., Cumby, J., Uher, R., & Rusak, B. (2019). Sleep in offspring of parents with mood disorders. *Front Psychiatry, 10*, 225. doi: 10.3389/fpsyt.2019.00225

Westwood, A. J., Jain, N., Himali, J. J., DeCarli, C., Auerbach, S. H., Pase, M. P., & Seshadri, S. (2017). Prolonged sleep duration as a marker of early neurodegeneration predicting incident dementia. *Neurology, 88*, 1–8.

Williams, D. R. (2006). Tauopathies: classification and clinical update on neurodegenerative diseases associated with microtubule-associated protein tau. *Intern Med J, 36*(10), 652–660. doi: 10.1111/j.1445-5994.2006.01153.x

Wilson, S., & Argyropoulos, S. (2005). Antidepressants and sleep: a qualitative review of the literature. *Drugs, 65*(7), 927–947.

Wimmer, R. D., Schmitt, L. I., Davidson, T. J., Nakajima, M., Deisseroth, K., & Halassa, M. M. (2015). Thalamic control of sensory selection in divided attention. *Nature, 526*(7575), 705–709. doi: 10.1038/nature15398

Windred, D. P., Burns, A. C., Lane, J. M., Saxena, R., Rutter, M. K., Cain, S. W., & Phillips, A. J. K. (2023). Sleep regularity is a stronger predictor of mortality risk than sleep duration: a prospective cohort study. *Sleep, 47*(1), zsad253. doi: 10.1093/sleep/zsad253

Winer, J. R., Morehouse, A., Fenton, L., Harrison, T. M., Ayangma, L., Reed, M., … Walker, M. P. (2021). Tau and beta-amyloid burden predict actigraphy-measured and self-reported impairment and misperception of human sleep. *J Neurosci, 41*(36), 7687–7696. doi: 10.1523/JNEUROSCI.0353-21.2021

Wirz-Justice, A., & Van den Hoofdakker, R. H. (1999). Sleep deprivation in depression: what do we know, where do we go? *Biol Psychiatry, 46*, 445–453.

Wohleb, E. S., Franklin, T., Iwata, M., & Duman, R. S. (2016). Integrating neuro-immune systems in the neurobiology of depression. *Nat Rev Neurosci, 17*(8), 497–511. doi: 10.1038/nrn.2016.69

Wu, J. C., & Bunney, W. E. (1990). The biological basis of an antidepressant response to sleep deprivation and relapse: review and hypothesis. *Am J Psychiatry, 147*, 14–21.

Wu, J. C., Kelsoe, J. R., Schachat, C., Bunney, B. G., DeModena, A., Golshan, S., … Bunney, W. E. (2009). Rapid and sustained antidepressant response with sleep deprivation and chronotherapy in bipolar disorder. *Biol Psychiatry, 66*(3), 298–301. doi: 10.1016/j.biopsych.2009.02.018

Wulff, K., Dijk, D. J., Middleton, B., Foster, R. G., & Joyce, E. M. (2011). Sleep and circadian rhythm disruption in schizophrenia. *Brit J Psychiatry, 200*(4), 308–316. doi: 10.1192/bjp.bp.111.096321

Wyman, L., Crum, R. M., & Celentano, D. (2012). Depressed mood and cause-specific mortality: a 40-year general community assessment. *Ann Epidemiol, 22*(9), 638–643. doi: 10.1016/j.annepidem.2012.06.102

Xie, L., Kang, H., Xu, Q., Chen, M. J., Liao, Y., Thiyagarajan, M., … Nedergaard, M. (2013). Sleep drives metabolite clearance from the adult brain. *Science, 342*(6156), 373–377. doi: 10.1126/science.1241224

Yin, J., Jin, X., Shan, Z., Li, S., Huang, H., Li, P., Peng, X., Peng, Z., … Liu, L. (2017). Relationship of sleep duration with all-cause mortality and cardiovascular events: a systematic review and dose-response meta-analysis of prospective cohort studies. *J Am Heart Assoc, 6*(9), 1–15. doi: 10.1161/JAHA.117.005947

Yu, X.-J., Xu, X.-X., He, S., & He, J. (2009). Change detection by thalamic reticular neurons. *Nat Neurosci, 12*(9), 1165–1170. doi: 10.1038/nn.2373

Yung, A. R., & McGorry, P. D. (1996). The initial prodrome in psychosis: descriptive and qualitative aspects. *Aust NZ J Psychiatry, 30*(5), 587–599.

Zaheed, A. B., Chervin, R. D., Spira, A. P., & Zahodne, L. B. (2023). Mental and physical health pathways linking insomnia symptoms to cognitive performance 14 years later. *Sleep, 46*(3), zsac262. doi: 10.1093/sleep/zsac262

Zhu, Y., Zhan, G., Fenik, P., Brandes, M., Bell, P., Francois, N., Shulman, K., & Veasey, S. (2018). Chronic sleep disruption advances the temporal progression of tauopathy in P301S mutant mice. *J Neurosci, 38*(48), 10255–10270. doi: 10.1523/JNEUROSCI.0275-18.2018

Zuurbier, L. A., Luik, A. I., Hofman, A., Franco, O. H., Van Someren, E. J., & Tiemeier, H. (2015). Fragmentation and stability of circadian activity rhythms predict mortality: the Rotterdam study. *Am J Epidemiol, 181*(1), 54–63. doi: 10.1093/aje/kwu245

E.

Functions of Sleep

CHAPTER 16

Models of the Functions of Sleep

16.1 OVERVIEW

The central mystery of sleep is why we spend about a third of our lives in a state of unconsciousness, rather than spending that time awake, fulfilling biological needs, earning income, studying for exams, or making music. What benefits do we obtain from the investment of time asleep that are more valuable than we might get from other, more "productive," activities? Despite the vast amount of information that we have acquired about the mechanisms that regulate sleep, there is little agreement about the answer to this central question about sleep: *Why* do humans and other animals sleep?

Early answers to this question were based on introspection and on observation of other animals. These led to ideas such as the need for the central perceiving organ of animals to rest (Aristotle, 350 BCE) (see Section 1.2), or for recovery from the general rigors of waking (knitting up "the ravell'd sleeve of care," as in Shakespeare's *Macbeth*). In the scientific era, researchers have also addressed this issue, but it is not surprising that their efforts have not resulted in agreement on an answer. Questions about function are inherently more difficult to answer than questions about mechanism. In addition, since sleep occurs universally among vertebrates, and perhaps among all animals, any answer to the question will also have to account for why this function is served by such radically different durations of total sleep time and of individual sleep stages among species; see Chapter 7.

There is no shortage of ideas about the function of sleep or why sleep takes different form in different species, and new hypotheses continue to be proposed. Among the many explanations for why we sleep, some focus on the role of each species' ecological niche in the external environment in shaping differences among species in sleep-wake patterns. Others focus instead on the idea that sleep satisfies one or more internal physiological needs, especially needs related to brain health or neurobehavioral functions (for a recent discussion of these issues, see Krueger et al., 2016). This chapter reviews some of these ideas and the arguments and evidence that have been marshaled for and against them. The following chapters address one specific function of sleep which is the focus of considerable current research—the process of consolidating memories.

16.2 Ecological/circadian models

Explanations for why animals sleep that focus on the role of environmental factors have been called ecological/circadian models (Meddis, 1977; Siegel, 2009). These models emphasize that sleep is a feature of the rest phase of the circadian cycle that organizes an animal's physiology and behavior to suit the particular ecological niche it occupies. In this view, sleep functions as a form of "adaptive inactivity" (Siegel, 2009), implying that it adapts an organism to its ecological niche by restricting its periods of being active and interacting with its environment. Differences in life habits and environmental pressures are invoked to explain observed differences among species in the duration and pattern of their sleep.

The view that these differences among species are related to ecological pressures is reinforced by the interpretation that large variations in sleep parameters are incompatible with the idea that sleep satisfies an essential physiological need. If animals sleep to satisfy a universal physiological need, how can they do so with such diverse amounts and patterns of sleep? Skepticism that there is a core physiological need for sleep is also provoked by reports of very short, habitual sleep durations in a few people who appeared to be healthy, energetic, and otherwise normal (Meddis, 1977; Meddis et al., 1973); see Section 14.3.4.

An evolutionary example is the divergence of sleep patterns among related species of Mexican cave fish. Surface-dwelling species, which have eyes, show sleep-like inactivity for over 13 h daily, while their blind relatives, which live in darkness in deep underwater caves, sleep for as little as 1.8–4 h daily (Duboue et al., 2011). Presumably, neither set of these related species has a physiological need to sleep for 13 h daily; rather, this sleep duration accompanied adaptation to a specific ecological niche. Species that adapted to a different niche co-evolved a different sleep pattern.

There is also evidence that species that sleep for substantial durations at some life stages may sleep very little, if any, at other times. Examples of species that show periods of near-continuous activity across the day and night include swimming marine mammals, migrating birds, polar species during constant daylight, and continuously active "nurse" bees that care for the young in a hive (Bloch et al., 2013; Siegel, 2009); see Chapter 7.

The argument that sleep is sometimes dispensable is weakened by the fact that sleep has not actually been measured directly in many of these species. In fact, "near-continuous" activity need not indicate a complete lack of sleep. In one species (the great frigate bird, *Fregata minor*), sleep is not absent during multiday flights over water, but it is greatly reduced relative to their sleep on land. The sleep that is expressed is unihemispheric or strongly asymmetric (Rattenborg et al., 2016); see **Figure 7.13**. Similarly, marine mammals and some amphibious species that have been studied using EEG show sleep alternately in their two cerebral hemispheres during period of continuous swimming (see Chapter 7). Thus, sleep can coexist with near-continuous activity, even if its amount is significantly reduced or its pattern drastically altered. In fact, the evidence that selection pressures have driven the evolution of adaptations to permit alternating sleep between hemispheres may be considered a potent argument in favor of the physiological importance of sleep for these species.

A core idea about the function of circadian rest-activity rhythms is that they restrict an animal's engagement with its environment and its energy expenditure to its daily active phase, when its activities are likely to be most effective, while exposing it to the least potential danger (see Section 7.4.2). In this view, sleep during the daily rest phase is useful because sleep is especially effective at preventing activity during the "wrong" circadian phase. This phase is defined as the period when external risks are high and potential benefits are minimal (e.g., because of the presence of predators, the absence of prey, or lighting conditions that do not match that species' sensory abilities). At the same time, sleep/rest helps to conserve valuable energy that can be used more profitably at other times, and does so more effectively than simply resting while awake (see Section 14.7.2).

Conserving metabolic energy may not seem like a very important issue to people living in wealthy, industrialized nations in the 21st century. In these countries, up to ~50% of the population are classified as overweight or obese. People in these societies are often more concerned with finding ways to expend excess energy than to conserve it, including purchasing exercise equipment for themselves (or for their overweight pets). However, conserving energy is a critical issue for other animals in their natural environments (see **Box 16.1**), as it was for most humans throughout our evolutionary history. Even today, getting sufficient energy remains a vital concern for people in many countries, especially when armed conflict, drought, or flooding threaten access to adequate food.

There is support for the idea that sleep conserves more energy than resting. Energy expenditure was ~32% lower in people during an 8 h sleep opportunity than during an equivalent period spent awake, but completely inactive, during a constant-routine protocol (Jung et al., 2011). One argument against the idea that sleep is primarily an energy conservation strategy is that some species that normally sleep are capable of more effective methods of energy conservation. Some mammals and many small birds can reduce their body temperatures and metabolic rates profoundly when they are under thermal or nutritional stress (Ruf & Geiser, 2015). These bouts of daily torpor (similar to brief periods of hibernation) greatly reduce energy expenditure (Heldmaier et al., 2004). If energy conservation were

BOX 16.1 Energy Balance in Hibernating Bats

One example of the delicate metabolic balance other species face relates to the steep decline over the last few years in the number of bats in parts of eastern North America. This catastrophic loss of bat populations has been linked to the spread of a fungus (*Geomyces destructans*) that causes "white-nose disease" in hibernating bats, particularly in the common little brown bat (*Myotis lucifugus*). Temperate zone bats usually hibernate throughout the winter in order to conserve energy at a time of year when their food resources are almost completely absent. Like many hibernators, they rely on stored fat and low metabolic rates to survive the winter, much of which they spend dormant at low body temperatures in protected roosting sites, such as caves.

Bats appear to be dying because the painful "white-nose" infections cause them to rewarm to high body temperatures more frequently and for longer than usual during their winter hibernation period. The resulting increase in energy expenditure causes them to fly out of their hibernation sites in search of food, but their insect prey are not available in winter. This behavior further magnifies their energy losses. For large numbers of infected bats, the excess energy expenditure is enough to tip the balance from survival to death before spring arrives, resulting in overwintering losses of up to 90% of some local populations (Reeder et al., 2012; Warnecke et al., 2012).

the main reason for sleeping, it is not clear why these species would sleep under most circumstances and resort to a more effective method like torpor only under conditions of energy stress.

As discussed in Chapter 7, the role played by each species in the ecosystem can be seen as shaping its pattern of sleep and waking. Top predators (e.g., lions and other large cats), which have little risk of being the target of predation, sleep for many hours daily, presumably to conserve energy for when it is needed and is most likely to be spent effectively. Prey species, especially those living in open environments that offer little or no secure shelter (e.g., antelopes, horses), sleep briefly and in short bouts to maintain vigilance (individually or as a herd) and to reduce the risk of attack by potential predators. However, other species that are regularly preyed on, like rats and mice, sleep about 12 h or more daily, although typically in sheltered places to reduce risk. Thus, aspects of life history, predation risk, metabolism, food quality, and environment all have to be considered in order to generate coherent accounts of how ecological/circadian models can explain sleep patterns.

These models can identify life-history factors and ecological pressures that account for the daily timing and duration of sleep and wake in some species (Bloch et al., 2013; Siegel, 2009), but not in others. For example, adult African elephants (*Loxodonta africana*), who are at little or no predation risk, sleep very briefly. During an actigraphic study conducted in the field, they slept only ~2 h daily, and during some days appeared not to sleep at all (Gravett et al., 2017).

Another challenge to these models is the need to explain why sleep in vulnerable prey species involves loss of awareness of their potentially dangerous external environment. From a safety perspective, it seems counter-productive to become unconscious for ~12 h every day, albeit intermittently, rather than remaining conscious and resting quietly in a safe retreat. The thalamocortical filtering mechanisms discussed in Chapter 12 can facilitate early detection of some potential dangers, but these mechanisms cannot be as effective as remaining awake and alert during the daily rest phase. The fact that a form of sleep occurs across much or all of the animal kingdom, despite the inherent increase in predation risk, suggests that sleep serves fundamental physiological needs, as well as ecological adaptations.[1]

Ecological accounts also do not address other features of sleep and its regulation. Among these are the key observation of homeostatic regulation of total sleep durations, of specific stages of sleep, and, especially, of slow-wave activity (SWA) (see Chapter 5). Sleep homeostasis is difficult to explain based on the idea that the function of sleep is to keep an animal from engaging with the environment at the wrong time of day. If environmental disturbances prevented an animal from sleeping for a period of time, what ecological purpose would be served by later making up for the lost sleep time, for particular sleep stages, or for the missing cortical SWA?

Although these objections might also be countered by further arguments, there remain key features of sleep and its regulation that are difficult to account for on the basis of ecological/circadian models. Among these are the internal rhythmic structure of sleep and its complex electrophysiological architecture (Chapters 2 and 10); the elaborate neural systems that are involved in regulating sleep features and their timing relations (Chapters 8–12); the behavioral deficits and health damage resulting from insufficient sleep (Chapters 13–15); and the remarkable changes in brain physiology and anatomy that occur during sleep (Section 15.5.3).

16.2.1 Summary

Several different approaches have been taken to developing hypotheses about the function of sleep. The large differences among species in total sleep amounts and types of sleep suggested that these are shaped by ecological and life-history factors through evolution, and are regulated proximally by the circadian system. These ecological/circadian models hypothesize that sleep is a form of adaptive inactivity that prevents dangerous and costly expenditure of energy when it would be least effective—and most risky. Sleep is therefore regulated by the circadian system in each species in order to prevent active engagement with the environment at times of day when waking activities would reduce, rather than enhance, chances for survival and reproductive success.

Evidence that some animals sleep very little, if at all, for at least part of their lives is often used to support this class of models and to refute the idea that sleep serves a core physiological function. A related argument is that it is improbable that any mechanism that serves a core physiological function could vary as widely in its expression as sleep does.

Ecological/circadian models can account for some specific examples of sleep patterns, but there are also counter-examples that do not readily fit these models. In addition, the idea that sleep is a mechanism to restrict activity to the right circadian phase and to conserve energy expenditure does not explain other features of sleep. These include the homeostatic regulation of sleep and of its stages, especially of SWA; the complex neural mechanisms underlying its regulation and internal structure; and the development of mechanisms to permit

[1] A potential counter-argument is that it could be advantageous to be unaware of stimuli (e.g., from potential mates or competitors) that could disrupt rest and provoke risky behaviors. In addition, increased energy costs of quiet wakefulness compared to those of sleep may be important, especially for small mammals with high metabolic rates. It is not clear how to calculate the net costs and benefits of vigilant rest (risk of being provoked into activity along with increased energy expenditure vs. reduced predation risk) against the risks and benefits of sleep (increased risk of predation vs. reduced energy expenditure and isolation from arousing stimuli).

alternating unihemispheric sleep in situations where bihemispheric sleep would not be feasible. Nor does it account for the damaging effects of acute sleep loss on cognitive functions and the many health consequences of chronic sleep loss.

16.3 Physiological models

In contrast to ecological models, most hypotheses about the function of sleep relate to the internal physiology of animals, especially the physiology of the brain.[2] Different hypotheses focus on different aspects of physiology, for example, regulating energy homeostasis; reversing the effects of waking activities on the brain and body; rehearsing instinctive behavioral patterns; storing, discarding, or integrating newly acquired information; and evaluating alternative solutions to problems. This section reviews some arguments for and against this general class of models.

16.3.1 Addressing species differences

As discussed above, one argument against sleep serving one or more essential physiological functions relates to the large differences in lengths and patterns of sleep shown by different species. Why do some mammals sleep for 3 h and others for 20 h daily? If sleep, for example, serves the function of consolidating newly acquired information, how do we account for the very long sleep durations of sloths (~16 h in a laboratory study, but reportedly <10 h in the wild) (Rattenborg et al., 2008) and of opossums (19 h) (Van Twyver & Allison, 1970)? Without getting into difficult arguments about how to compare intelligence across species, most people would not consider sloths and opossums to be the most intellectually active among mammalian species. What rich set of new information and skills do they acquire during the few hours that they are awake every day, and why does consolidating that information require a sleep period that is significantly longer than that of the average human?

One way of responding to this general criticism is to consider the evidence for differences in the way species fulfill other drives that are clearly related to physiological needs, such as those for food and water.[3] There are, for example, large differences in the amount of water consumed by different species. Many birds drink water, but some do so rarely: raptors (e.g., hawks, falcons) typically satisfy their fluid needs from the bodies of the prey they consume. With respect to food intake, shrews are tiny mammals with very high metabolic rates that must eat almost continuously to survive, while lions can gorge on a large meal and not eat for many days. Snakes can go months between meals, and hibernating mammals may also not eat for months at a time.

The fact that different species eat and drink in very different ways and with different temporal constraints does not contradict the conclusion that there is a universal physiological need for animals to have sufficient food and fluids, and to actively regulate energy and fluid balance. Similarly, evidence that sleep patterns and durations vary widely among species, and even to some extent among people, does not rule out the idea that it serves a core physiological need. As is the case for food or water intake, sleep may satisfy a universal physiological need in different ways for different species. Ecological and life history factors can account for differences among species in how they regulate sleep, energy, and water balance, but they do not rule out the idea that each of these functions serves a universal, physiological need in species-specific ways.

One proposed model can be used to illustrate why different species might need different sleep durations to satisfy a proposed need, namely, the need for mammals to eliminate metabolic toxins from their brains. The model is based on evidence that structural changes that occur in the brain during sleep facilitate removing metabolic toxins from the cortex (Iliff et al., 2012; Xie et al., 2013); see Section 15.5.3. In this model, sleep duration differences among species are the result of balancing the time needed to detoxify the full depth of the cortex during sleep with the time needed to find sufficient food to meet each species' energy requirements. The factors proposed to determine each species' sleep duration include the size of the brain and the body, the animal's energy requirements (and the sources of this energy), and a critical anatomical feature—the ratio of neuronal density to the brain's cortical surface area (Herculano-Houzel, 2015).

Regardless of the generality of this model, it illustrates in principle how anatomy, physiology, and ecology can interact to produce quite different sleep patterns that still serve a single physiological need that is common to all mammals, that is, detoxifying the cortex during sleep.

16.3.2 Generating physiological hypotheses

Another approach to thinking about why we sleep is to examine the large number of physiological functions that change during sleep relative to waking. For example, the hypothesis that an important function of sleep is to regulate energy

[2] "Sleep is of the brain, by the brain and for the brain," according to the title of one review (Hobson, 2005). However, a recent publication demonstrated that genetic changes to endoplasmic reticulum function in peripheral tissues in the nematode *Caenorhabditis elegans* and in mice can regulate the amount of sleep shown, suggesting that sleep amounts are also related to the function of peripheral tissues (Kawano et al., 2023).

[3] I am indebted to my late colleague Serge Daan, a leader in the fields of animal ecology and circadian biology, for this discussion about species differences in the performance of essential physiological functions.

utilization in either the brain or the entire body stems from evidence of sleep-related changes in brain metabolism and energy balance (Benington & Heller, 1995; Kong et al., 2002; Nofzinger et al., 2002; Schmidt, 2014). This idea is further supported for mammals by evidence of physiological overlap between mechanisms that regulate sleep and body temperature. Individual neurons in the medial preoptic area, for example, are involved in both the promotion of NREM sleep and the regulation of body temperature (Harding et al., 2018).

A second potential source of ideas about the physiological functions of sleep is the evidence for increased risks of illness and disturbed behavioral functions as a result of sleep loss or disruption. These risks include increases in conditions such as hypertension, obesity, chronic pain, insulin resistance, type 2 diabetes, vascular disease, and Alzheimer's disease (AD) (see Chapters 14 and 15). Behavioral consequences of sleep loss include impaired ability to sustain attention, to regulate emotions, and to consolidate new learning (see Chapters 13 and 17). These findings do not, however, suggest a direct answer to the question of what the core function of sleep is. It is unlikely that sleep evolved primarily to regulate body weight, blood pressure, or emotional balance—or to prevent AD.

The increased health risks associated with inadequate sleep are more likely to be indirect results of disruptions in critical regulatory and repair mechanisms that are compromised by sleep loss. Tracing the specific physiological mechanisms by which sleep, or sleep loss, influences other regulatory systems can potentially provide insights into the general functions sleep serves. One example is the discovery of a mechanism linking sleep duration to a protein, amyloid beta (Aβ), involved in the development of AD. The specific observation is that sleep facilitates clearance of Aβ by increasing the volume of extracellular space in the brain, while extended waking impairs this process (Iliff et al., 2012; Xie et al., 2013); see Section 15.5.3. As discussed in the preceding section, this finding contributed to a model that attempts to account for the daily sleep requirements of different species based on the rate at which toxic products of neural metabolism can be removed from the brain, as modulated by other critical needs (Herculano-Houzel, 2015). This example can be generalized to suggest that one function of sleep is the elimination of toxins from the brain that accumulate as a result of its waking activities. Increased risk of developing AD may be a downstream consequence of disrupting this physiological regulatory function of sleep.

Identifying specific mechanisms by which sleep or sleep loss influence the risk of developing other illnesses (e.g., vascular disease, type 2 diabetes) may also provide insights into more general functions of sleep. For example, people show a circadian variation in blood pressure, reaching a low point during the night (dipping), probably as a result of parasympathetic dominance during the circadian rest phase (Scheer et al., 2010; Shea et al., 2011); see Section 14.8. The lack of nocturnal dipping in blood pressure is the vascular marker that most strongly predicts increased risk of vascular disease or death (Fagard et al., 2008; Staplin et al., 2023; Verdecchia, 2000). Sleep facilitates nocturnal dipping, and conditions that disturb sleep (e.g., obstructive sleep apnea) disrupt this pattern and increase vascular risk.

Why a lack of nocturnal dipping is the most potent risk factor for developing vascular disease is less clear. It may reflect a need for repair of vascular tissue to recover from cellular stresses and damage that are produced by tonically higher blood pressure while awake, as well as acute increases in blood pressure in response to ordinary waking activities. Adequate sleep has been linked to DNA repair mechanisms that restore damaged tissues in both the brain and peripheral organs (Cheung et al., 2019; Everson et al., 2014; Zada et al., 2021). Based on this evidence, we might propose that one function of sleep is to facilitate repair of molecular/cellular damage to vascular tissues, which in the absence of adequate sleep accumulates and increases the risk of developing cardiovascular and cerebrovascular disease.

The immediate and downstream consequences of these and other disruptions of physiological organization that result from lost sleep, including, for example, disruption of the circadian cortisol rhythm (Omisade et al., 2010; Spiegel et al., 2004) and loss of insulin sensitivity (Reutrakul & Van Cauter, 2018; Reynolds et al., 2012), contribute ultimately to increased risk of developing the diseases discussed in Chapters 14 and 15. These mechanisms imply a general function for sleep in repairing and restoring physiological systems that are stressed in different ways by the impacts of waking. More detailed analysis of the causal chains that link sleep loss (and often associated circadian disruption) to development of specific illnesses remains to be done. But currently available evidence provides empirical support for the view expressed by philosophers and poets that we cannot sustain waking activity continuously, and that one function of sleep is to permit the repair and restoration of our bodies to health and optimal function.

A third source of ideas about the physiological function of sleep is the extensive literature demonstrating that sleep plays a role in neural plasticity and, more specifically, in the consolidation of memory. Research on this topic has led to broad acceptance of the idea that one function of sleep is stabilizing and strengthening plastic changes in the nervous system that occur during waking, or "rewiring" the brain based on waking experience (Horner, 2014; Krueger et al., 2016; Spencer et al., 2017; Vorster & Born, 2015). The following two chapters review evidence for the role of sleep in brain plasticity and in the consolidation of new learning (Chapter 17) as well as evidence related to the neural mechanisms involved in these processes (Chapter 18).

16.3.3 Summary

The variability of sleep patterns among species, and in some cases in a single species at different life stages, seems to challenge the idea that sleep serves one or more universal physiological functions. But it is important to note that other core physiological functions, like regulation of energy and water balance, are, in fact, expressed in highly variable forms across species. Thus, some animals eat almost continuously while others may not eat for months, and some may not normally drink water to maintain fluid balance. It is possible to model how a combination of physiological, anatomical, and ecological constraints could result in a universal physiological need being met with very different amounts of sleep.

Several lines of evidence have led to the view that sleep does, in fact, serve important physiological functions. One source of ideas for the nature of these functions derives from evidence for major differences in key physiological functions between wake and sleep. One example is energy utilization and restoration, especially in the brain. This evidence led to the hypothesis that energy resources for the brain are depleted during waking and are restored selectively during sleep.

Other ideas about the physiological function of sleep derive from evidence of functional deficits and illnesses that are associated with insufficient sleep. These include the inadequate removal from the brain of toxic waste products generated by waking activity. One model proposed a specific account of how different patterns and durations of sleep would be required to satisfy the universal need to remove toxins from the brain in relation to each species' unique anatomical and physiological features and in the context of its ecological constraints.

Other functions of sleep are also implied by the kinds of physiological damage that accumulate when sleep is lost or disrupted, such as when daily blood pressure rhythms are disrupted and lead to increased risk of vascular damage. The implied repair functions that occur during sleep can be related to processes of DNA and tissue repair, which appear to be best performed during sleep and during its linked circadian phase.

Another key physiological function that has been proposed for sleep is facilitating plastic changes in the brain that result from waking experiences, including specific learning episodes. The following chapters review some of the large body of evidence related to this idea.

Sleep may serve several common, core physiological functions but still be expressed differently in different species in response to their unique ecological constraints, metabolic requirements, and anatomical features. Large species differences in sleep amounts and patterns do not prove that sleep does not serve common, core physiological function; they invite exploration of how physiological and ecological mechanisms have been adapted to allow satisfaction of sleep-related functions in different ways.

Literature cited

Aristotle. (350 BCE). *On Sleep and Sleeplessness* (J. I. Beare, Trans.). Retrieved from http://tinyurl.com/yxqw5qda

Benington, J. H., & Heller, H. C. (1995). Restoration of brain energy metabolism as the function of sleep. *Prog Neurobiol, 45*, 347–360.

Bloch, G., Barnes, B. M., Gerkema, M. P., & Helm, B. (2013). Animal activity around the clock with no overt circadian rhythms: patterns, mechanisms and adaptive value. *Proc Roy Soc Lon B, 280*(1765), 20130019. doi: 10.1098/rspb.2013.0019

Cheung, V., Yuen, V. M., Wong, G. T. C., & Choi, S. W. (2019). The effect of sleep deprivation and disruption on DNA damage and health of doctors. *Anaesthesia, 74*(4), 434–440. doi: 10.1111/anae.14533

Duboue, E. R., Keene, A. C., & Borowsky, R. L. (2011). Evolutionary convergence on sleep loss in cavefish populations. *Curr Biol, 21*(8), 671–676. doi: 10.1016/j.cub.2011.03.020

Everson, C. A., Henchen, C. J., Szabo, A., & Hogg, N. (2014). Cell injury and repair resulting from sleep loss and sleep recovery in laboratory rats. *Sleep, 37*(12), 1929–1940. doi: 10.5665/sleep.4244

Fagard, R. H., Celis, H., Thijs, L., Staessen, J. A., Clement, D. L., De Buyzere, M. L., & De Bacquer, D. A. (2008). Daytime and nighttime blood pressure as predictors of death and cause-specific cardiovascular events in hypertension. *Hypertension, 51*(1), 55–61. doi: 10.1161/HYPERTENSIONAHA.107.100727

Gravett, N., Bhagwandin, A., Sutcliffe, R., Landen, K., Chase, M. J., Lyamin, O. I., ... Manger, P. R. (2017). Inactivity/sleep in two wild free-roaming African elephant matriarchs - Does large body size make elephants the shortest mammalian sleepers? *PLoS One, 12*(3), e0171903. doi: 10.1371/journal.pone.0171903

Harding, E. C., Yu, X., Miao, A., Andrews, N., Ma, Y., Ye, Z., ... Franks, N. P. (2018). A neuronal hub binding sleep initiation and body cooling in response to a warm external stimulus. *Curr Biol, 28*(14), 2263–2273 e2264. doi: 10.1016/j.cub.2018.05.054

Heldmaier, G., Ortmann, S., & Elvert, R. (2004). Natural hypometabolism during hibernation and daily torpor in mammals. *Respir Physiol Neurobiol, 141*(3), 317–329. doi: 10.1016/j.resp.2004.03.014

Herculano-Houzel, S. (2015). Decreasing sleep requirement with increasing numbers of neurons as a driver for bigger brains and bodies in mammalian evolution. *Proc Biol Sci, 282*(1816), 20151853. doi:10.1098/rspb.2015.1853

Hobson, J. A. (2005). Sleep is of the brain, by the brain and for the brain. *Nature, 437*(7063), 1254–1256. doi: 10.1038/nature04283

Horner, R. L. (2014). *The Universal Pastime: Sleep and Rest Explained* Retrieved from https://store.bookbaby.com/book/the-universal-pastime-sleep-and-rest-explained

Iliff, J. J., Wang, M., Liao, Y., Plogg, B. A., Peng, W., Gundersen, G. A., ... Nedergaard, M. (2012). A paravascular pathway facilitates CSF flow through the brain parenchyma and the clearance of interstitial solutes, including amyloid beta. *Sci Transl Med, 4*(147), 147ra111. doi: 10.1126/scitranslmed.3003748

Jung, C. M., Melanson, E. L., Frydendall, E. J., Perreault, L., Eckel, R. H., & Wright, K. P. (2011). Energy expenditure during sleep, sleep deprivation and sleep following sleep deprivation in adult humans. *J Physiol, 589*(1), 235–244. doi: 10.1113/jphysiol.2010.197517

Kawano, T., Kashiwagi, M., Kanuka, M., Chen, C. K., Yasugaki, S., Hatori, S., ... Hayashi, Y. (2023). ER proteostasis regulators cell-non-autonomously control sleep. *Cell Rep, 42*(3), 112267. doi:10.1016/j.celrep.2023.112267

Kong, J., Shepel, P., Holden, C., Mackiewicz, M., Pack, A., & Geiger, J. (2002). Brain glycogen decreases with increased periods of wakefulness: implications for homeostatic drive to sleep. *J Neurosci, 22*(13), 5581–5587.

Krueger, J. M., Frank, M. G., Wisor, J. P., & Roy, S. (2016). Sleep function: toward elucidating an enigma. *Sleep Med Rev, 28*, 46–54. doi: 10.1016/j.smrv.2015.08.005

Meddis, R. (1977). *The sleep instinct*. London: Routledge & Kegan Paul.

Meddis, R., Pearson, A. J. D., & Langford, G. (1973). An extreme case of healthy insomnia. *Electroencephalogr Clin Neurophysiol, 35*, 213–214.

Nofzinger, E., Buysse, D., Miewald, J. M., Meltzer, C., Price, J., Sembrat, R., … Moore, R. (2002). Human regional cerebral glucose metabolism during non-rapid eye movement sleep in relation to waking. *Brain, 125*, 1105–1115.

Omisade, A., Buxton, O. M., & Rusak, B. (2010). Impact of acute sleep restriction on cortisol and leptin levels in young women. *Physiol Behav, 99*(5), 651–656. doi: 10.1016/j.physbeh.2010.01.028

Rattenborg, N. C., Voirin, B., Cruz, S. M., Tisdale, R., Dell'Omo, G., Lipp, H. P., … Vyssotski, A. L. (2016). Evidence that birds sleep in mid-flight. *Nat Commun, 7*, 12468. doi: 10.1038/ncomms12468

Rattenborg, N. C., Wikelski, M., Heidrich, W., Kuemmeth, F., Spoelstra, K., Kays, R. W., … Voirin, B. (2008). Sleeping outside the box: electroencephalographic measures of sleep in sloths inhabiting a rainforest. *Biol Lett, 4*(4), 402–405. doi: 10.1098/rsbl.2008.0203

Reeder, D. M., Frank, C. L., Turner, G. G., Meteyer, C. U., Kurta, A., Britzke, E. R., … Blehert, D. S. (2012). Frequent arousal from hibernation linked to severity of infection and mortality in bats with white-nose syndrome. *PLoS One, 7*(6), e38920. doi: 10.1371/journal.pone.0038920

Reutrakul, S., & Van Cauter, E. (2018). Sleep influences on obesity, insulin resistance, and risk of type 2 diabetes. *Metabolism, 84*, 56–66. doi: 10.1016/j.metabol.2018.02.010

Reynolds, A. C., Dorrian, J., Liu, P. Y., Van Dongen, H. P., Wittert, G. A., Harmer, L. J., & Banks, S. (2012). Impact of five nights of sleep restriction on glucose metabolism, leptin and testosterone in young adult men. *PLoS One, 7*(7), e41218. doi: 10.1371/journal.pone.0041218

Ruf, T., & Geiser, F. (2015). Daily torpor and hibernation in birds and mammals. *Biol Rev Camb Philos Soc, 90*(3), 891–926. doi: 10.1111/brv.12137

Scheer, F. A. J. L., Hu, K., Evoniuk, H., Kelly, E. E., Malhotra, A., Hilton, M. F., & Shea, S. A. (2010). Impact of the human circadian system, exercise, and their interaction on cardiovascular function. *Proc Natl Acad Sci USA, 107*(47), 20541–20546. doi: 10.1073/pnas.1006749107

Schmidt, M. H. (2014). The energy allocation function of sleep: a unifying theory of sleep, torpor, and continuous wakefulness. *Neurosci Biobehav Rev, 47*, 122–153. doi: 0.1016/j.neubiorev.2014.08.001

Shea, S. A., Hilton, M. F., Hu, K., & Scheer, F. A. (2011). Existence of an endogenous circadian blood pressure rhythm in humans that peaks in the evening. *Circ Res, 108*(8), 980–984. doi: 10.1161/CIRCRESAHA.110.233668

Siegel, J. M. (2009). Sleep viewed as a state of adaptive inactivity. *Nat Rev Neurosci, 10*, 747–753. doi: 0.1038/nrn2697

Spencer, R. M. C., Walker, M. P., & Stickgold, R. (2017). Sleep and memory consolidation. In M. H. Kryger, A. Roth, & W. C. Dement (Eds.), *Sleep Disorders Medicine* (pp. 205–223). St. Louis: Elsevier.

Spiegel, K., Leproult, R., L'Hermite-Balériaux, M., Copinschi, G., Penev, P. D., & Van Cauter, E. (2004). Leptin levels are dependent on sleep duration: relationships with sympathovagal balance, carbohydrate regulation, cortisol, and thyrotropin. *J Clin Endocr Metab, 89*(11), 5762–5771. doi: 10.1210/jc.2004-1003

Staplin, N., de la Sierra, A., Ruilope, L. M., Emberson, J. R., Vinyoles, E., Gorostidi, M., … Williams, B. (2023). Relationship between clinic and ambulatory blood pressure and mortality: an observational cohort study in 59 124 patients. *Lancet, 401*, 2041–2050. doi: 10.1016/S0140-6736(23)00733-X

Van Twyver, H., & Allison, T. (1970). Sleep in the opossum *Didelphis marsupialis*. *Electroencephalogr Clin Neurophysiol, 29*(2), 181–189.

Verdecchia, P. (2000). Prognostic value of ambulatory blood pressure: current evidence and clinical implications. *Hypertension, 35*(3), 844–851. doi: 10.1161/01.hyp.35.3.844

Vorster, A. P., & Born, J. (2015). Sleep and memory in mammals, birds and invertebrates. *Neurosci Biobehav Rev, 50*, 103–119. doi: 10.1016/j.neubiorev.2014.09.020

Warnecke, L., Turner, J. M., Bollinger, T. K., Lorch, J. M., Misra, V., Cryan, P. M., … Willis, C. K. (2012). Inoculation of bats with European Geomyces destructans supports the novel pathogen hypothesis for the origin of white-nose syndrome. *Proc Natl Acad Sci U S A, 109*(18), 6999–7003. doi: 10.1073/pnas.1200374109

Xie, L., Kang, H., Xu, Q., Chen, M. J., Liao, Y., Thiyagarajan, M., … Nedergaard, M. (2013). Sleep drives metabolite clearance from the adult brain. *Science, 342*(6156), 373–377. doi: 10.1126/science.1241224

Zada, D., Sela, Y., Matosevich, N., Monsonego, A., Lerer-Goldshtein, T., Nir, Y., & Appelbaum, L. (2021). Parp1 promotes sleep, which enhances DNA repair in neurons. *Mol Cell, 81*(24), 4979–4993.e4977. doi: 10.1016/j.molcel.2021.10.026

CHAPTER 17

The Role of Sleep in Memory

17.1 OVERVIEW

This chapter reviews a function of sleep that has been the focus of extensive research over recent decades—its role in memory.[1] It first describes how memory for new learning is affected by interference and by the process of consolidation. It reviews some of the methods commonly used to assess the involvement of sleep and of different sleep stages in memory consolidation. It discusses the effects of sleep, and of sleep loss, on consolidation of several types of learning: explicit/declarative, sensory/perceptual, motor/procedural, and emotional, and the involvement of NREM and REM sleep in these effects.

The chapter then discusses other factors that influence whether and how sleep affects memory, including participants' motivation, expectations, and age. Finally, it reviews the role of sleep in developing insights and solving problems. The next chapter (Chapter 18) reviews the physiological mechanisms in different sleep stages that underlie the involvement of sleep in memory.

17.2 Introduction to sleep and memory

17.2.1 Interference and consolidation

It is not surprising that being deprived of sleep *before* trying to learn something can interfere with later performance. Sleepy brains have difficulty maintaining attention, encoding and storing new information, and retrieving it (Cousins et al., 2018; Drummond et al., 2000; Kurinec et al., 2021; Walker & Stickgold, 2006; Yoo et al., 2007), and restoring alertness with a daytime nap can facilitate later learning (Ong et al., 2020).

What is more surprising is the idea that sleep *after* learning can improve retention of the learned information. The first English-language publication describing such "backward" effects of sleep on memory was (Jenkins & Dallenbach, 1924).[2] They reported that people who had learned a list of nonsense syllables remembered more of them when they were tested after periods of sleep (1–8 h long) than after the same durations spent awake (**Figure 17.1**).

Memory performance at the end of each training session was equal, so differences in recall were not the result of differences in initial learning. Instead, memory performance depended on something that occurred after learning, while participants were either asleep or awake. Jenkins & Dallenbach concluded that the rate of forgetting ("obliviscence," as they called it) after learning was higher while awake than during sleep because interference from waking experiences disrupted the newly formed memory traces in the brain. Thus, they saw sleep as playing a passive role in preserving new memories by shielding them from interfering input that occurs while awake.

This interpretation relates to the idea that new, short-term memories are the product of changes in neural circuits that are initially relatively unstable. As a result, they are subject to interference from later inputs that can prevent them from being stabilized into a long-term memory. For example, memory for a newly learned phone number can be disrupted and lost if a person were immediately exposed to related information (e.g., hearing a list of other numbers).

How well memories are retained depends on processes that occur during learning, for example, while rehearsing new information or practicing a new skill (online effects), and also on processes that occur later without active practice (offline effects). Offline effects can occur while either awake or asleep, and can include interference from new inputs that disrupt memory, as well as processes of memory consolidation, which produce a more stable form of memory[3] (**Figure 17.2**). Similar

[1] The association of sleep with memory was a theme in the 1967 novel (translated in 1970) *One Hundred Years of Solitude*, by Gabriel García Márquez. The novel described an epidemic of insomnia (in this case, literally not sleeping) that led to hardly any fatigue, but rather to a loss of memory (Márquez, 1970).

[2] See reference 528 in (Rasch & Born, 2013) for an earlier publication in German by Rosa Heine as well as their discussion of earlier work related to this issue by Hermann Ebbinghaus.

[3] The "more stable" form should not be considered permanent, however, because even established memories can be forgotten. In addition, each act of recalling long-term memories makes them more labile and susceptible to modification, a process referred to as reconsolidation (Lewis, 1979; Roediger & Abel, 2022; Sara, 2010).

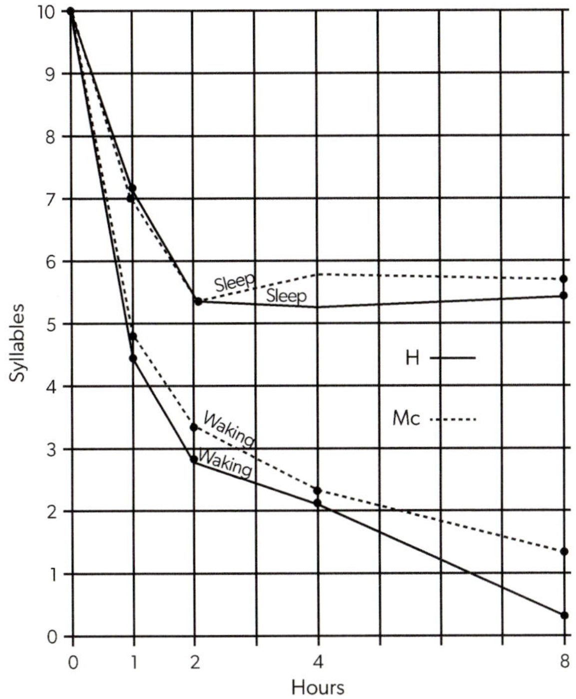

Figure 17.1 The two participants whose data are shown (H and Mc) were tested for their memory of newly learned nonsense syllables during different sessions spent either waking (two lower curves) or asleep (two upper curves) after learning. The figure shows the number of syllables successfully recalled during testing (Y axis) plotted against the number of hours of waking or sleep following training: 1, 2, 4, or 8 h (X axis). Because they matched the participants' performance at the end of each learning session, the authors concluded that the effect of sleep was to slow the rate of forgetting that occurred during waking. (The values plotted after 4 h Waking were reversed for the two participants in a data table in the publication relative to what is shown in the published figure (as noted by Rasch & Born [Physiological Reviews 93: 681–766, 2013]. There is no independent way to determine which of these values is correct, but they have no impact on the interpretation of the results.) Reprinted with permission of the University of Illinois Press from Jenkins J.G. & Dallenbach K.M. (1924) Obliviscence during sleep and waking. *Am J Psychol* 35:605–612. © by the Board of Trustees of the University of Illinois (1924). doi: 10.2307/1414040.

or different consolidation mechanisms may be active during waking and sleep, but their effectiveness in stabilizing memory will also depend on the degree to which the post-learning interval includes interfering experiences, which typically occur while awake (Dastgheib et al., 2022; Mednick et al., 2009).

In the Jenkins and Dallenbach study, sleep during the 1–8 h after learning could have improved memory relative to waking either by reducing interference, as they proposed, or by better strengthening consolidation of the recent learning, or both. There is, in fact, experimental evidence that sleep can benefit some kinds of memory by protecting it from interfering new input and that undisturbed, quiet waking can sometimes have similar protective effects (Ellenbogen et al., 2006; Gottselig et al., 2004; Korman et al., 2007; Mednick et al., 2009), although the extent of this protective effect has also been questioned (Pöhlchen et al., 2020).

There is also a large body of behavioral and physiological evidence showing that mechanisms operating during sleep play an active role in stabilizing or strengthening new memories and integrating the acquired information into existing knowledge (Diekelmann et al., 2009; Hoedlmoser et al., 2022; Rasch & Born, 2013; Spencer et al., 2017; Vorster & Born, 2015; Walker & Stickgold, 2006). See **Box 17.1** for some practical applications, especially applicable to students, related to the role of sleep in memory consolidation.

17.2.2 Types of learning and sleep effects

A standard way of classifying learning is to distinguish explicit from implicit learning (**Table 17.1**). Explicit (or declarative) learning refers to situations in which an individual is aware of a learning task (e.g., learning a list of word-pairs or nonsense syllables, as in the Jenkins and Dallenbach study), memorizing a sequence of numbers, or learning new facts (semantic learning). Explicit learning also includes the process of acquiring autobiographical memories, for example, memories of a

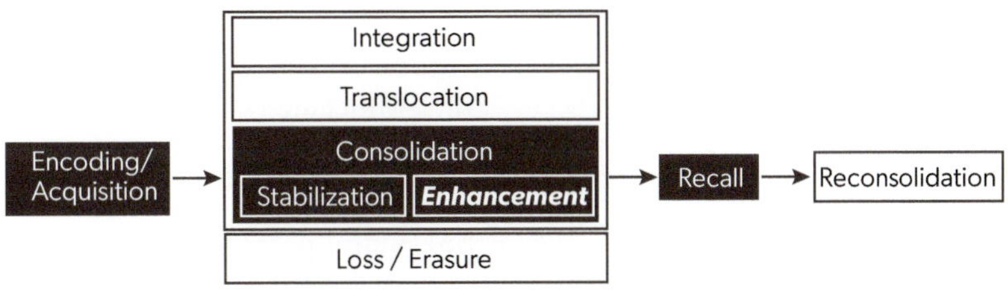

Figure 17.2 Memory is modeled here as involving several steps. Initial acquisition of memory involves encoding neural traces reflecting the new information. That information can then undergo consolidation, leading to either stabilization of the memory as encoded or its further offline enhancement (i.e., strengthening the memory). The neural traces forming the memory can also be translocated (moved) to other parts of the nervous system and integrated with existing stored memories. The initial memory trace can also be lost or erased, so it can no longer be retrieved. If the memory is preserved and then recalled, it is also reconsolidated and stored again. A reconsolidated memory may differ in some ways from the originally encoded and stored memory. Reprinted with permission from Walker, M.P. (2008) Sleep-dependent memory processing. *Harv Rev Psychiatry* 16:287–298. © President and Fellows of Harvard College (2008). doi: 10.1080/10673220802432517.

BOX 17.1 Effects of Naps and Sleep Loss on Student Performance

Students faced with a fast-approaching examination have to decide whether to stay up late to cram for it over one or several nights or to study until roughly their usual bedtime and then get adequate sleep. How should they choose to spend their nights—studying or sleeping?

There are two related risks of inadequate sleep before an examination. One is that those who are partially or completely sleep-deprived overnight perform poorly on some cognitive tasks (see Chapter 13), so overnight sleep loss is likely to impair next-day performance. The second issue is that not allowing sufficient time for sleep to help consolidate newly acquired information could impair its later retrieval.

One study suggested that the answer might depend on the timing of the exam and the pattern of studying. It compared the effects of extra cramming to those of a nap for students who had been studying novel biological information about different species of crabs and ants. Students either took a ~60 min nap after the initial study period or spent that time cramming.

Both taking a nap and cramming improved retention 30 min after the end of the study period, as compared to staying awake and watching an unrelated movie. However, 8 days later, those who had napped showed better retention than those who either crammed or stayed awake without studying. Thus, both additional studying and naps after learning improved immediate retention of new information, but only naps after learning improved retention over the longer term (Cousins et al., 2019). As a result, cramming could produce different results depending on whether it is for an immediately following test or for a cumulative final exam at the end of a course.

Another study compared memory performance of students who were restricted to 5 or 9 h time in bed (TIB) over 7 nights. Students learned the definitions of words either by studying them eight times in a single session (massed learning) or by studying them twice per session over four daily sessions (spaced learning). Students who had 9 h TIB performed well regardless of which studying method they used. Those who had 5 h TIB also performed well on items that were studied with spaced learning but performed poorly on items studied using massed learning (Huang et al., 2016).

When students used an efficient (spaced) learning method, chronic sleep restriction for a week had little effect on later performance. But using a less effective strategy (massed learning or cramming) combined with repeated sleep restriction resulted in significantly poorer performance. Taken together, these studies indicate that the timing of a test, the pattern of sleep loss (acute vs. chronic), and the method of studying interact in complex ways to determine how sleep or sleep loss will affect memory and performance.

Table 17.1 Principal Types of Learning

Explicit/Declarative		Implicit/Non-Declarative		
Semantic	Episodic	Sensory/ Perceptual	Motor/ Procedural/Skill	Incidental/ Insight

childhood trip, or the first time you met a particular person (episodic learning). Explicit learning produces memories that include facts, events, or experiences that an individual can state verbally or declare (hence, "declarative" memory); see Section 17.4.

Implicit (or non-declarative) learning relates to acquisition of knowledge/skills, or to a change in performance as a result of experience, that occurs without conscious awareness and is not readily verbalized. This category groups together several different types of learning: perceptual/sensory learning (e.g., learning to rapidly identify a specific visual feature in a complex array) (Section 17.6), motor/procedural/skill learning (learning to play a piano or ride a bicycle) (Section 17.7), incidental learning (e.g., acquiring information about a text or image without conscious awareness of doing so), and insight (recognizing the solution to a problem, often abruptly) (Section 17.11). The broad categories of explicit and implicit learning can be further modified by the degree to which the learning tasks involve novelty, contextual information, emotional arousal, and other characteristics.

Beyond agreement that sleep after learning improves memory in many studies, there is also evidence that different sleep stages and features are involved in consolidating different types of learning. There are, however, different views about which sleep stages and which sleep features affect different kinds of memory (Ackermann et al., 2015; Fogel et al., 2007; Mantua, 2018; Pesonen et al., 2019; Rasch & Born, 2013; Smith, 1995; Ujma et al., 2014); see Section 17.8.

Several factors contribute to these different views. Performance in human learning studies is very sensitive to the overall experimental design used (see Section 17.3), the exact instructions given, and the details of the procedures used. These characteristics vary across studies. In addition, a single type of learning can be studied using many different tests. One review included a list of the tests that were used to assess sleep effects on memory consolidation in human studies. It listed 19 different tests for episodic/declarative memory and eight for procedural/perceptual memory, among a total of 40 different tests that had been used (Scullin & Bliwise, 2015). Studies of parallel memory systems in nonhuman species necessarily used other methods.

One advantage of using a variety of tests and procedures is that it allows researchers to determine the limits to which specific models of memory consolidation apply. In addition, analysis of the factors contributing to different outcomes can provide insights into the underlying mechanisms involved, as illustrated in several of the following sections. A disadvantage, however, is that differences between tests and procedures can influence the results obtained, leading to inconsistent conclusions, for example, about which sleep stages affect consolidation of different types of memories. Many studies have also involved relatively small numbers of participants, which can increase the risk of false positive results that are not replicated consistently in later studies (Ackermann et al., 2015; Davidson et al., 2021).

17.2.3 Summary

Memory depends on forming and strengthening neural connections during the learning process (online processes). These network connections are initially unstable and susceptible to interference; they become more stable through a later process of consolidation without additional learning (offline processes). Sleep after learning may sometimes help preserve memories passively by reducing interfering input, but there is extensive evidence that sleep in many cases also actively improves memory by strengthening offline consolidation.

There are two principal categories of learning, explicit/declarative and implicit/non-declarative, and several types of learning in each category. Studies have reached different conclusions about which sleep stages or features are involved in strengthening memories related to these different kinds of memory. The experimental strategies, number of participants, specific procedures, instructions to participants, and statistical analyses used in different studies probably contribute to these differences. But the variety of testing conditions used also has value in setting the limits of generality for models of consolidation processes and in helping to identify the mechanisms involved.

17.3 Studying how sleep affects memory

To orient readers to the methods used to study the involvement of sleep in memory, this section reviews the principal experimental approaches used and some of their respective strengths and weaknesses, although this is not an exhaustive list of methods that have been used. Many studies using these methods also involved variations, including manipulations of the stimuli used (e.g., their context, meaning, salience, emotional valence); various ways of measuring memory (e.g., recognition, retrieval, ratings of emotional valence, and susceptibility to interference); and the timing of sleep and of memory testing after learning.

17.3.1 Types of studies

> ***Method 1. Daytime vs. nighttime retention:*** In this method, participants are trained either in the morning or evening and are then retested after equivalent periods of time, including either a daytime wake period or a nighttime period including sleep. The length of the retention interval can therefore be identical for the groups.

A potential confounding factor in this design is that training and testing both occur at different circadian phases in the two groups. Differences in outcomes between treatments could be related in part to circadian effects on either learning (during training) or performance (during testing) rather than to effects attributable to what happened between training and testing. A partial control is to ensure that immediate performance after learning is equivalent between treatment groups. Another issue is that the daytime period could include potentially interfering experiences or could allow opportunities for explicit rehearsal of learned material, both of which would be less likely during the sleep period.

> ***Method 2. AM-PM-AM design:*** This is a variation on the daytime/nighttime method that controls for some nonspecific factors. It involves training one group in the morning and testing them in the evening; participants then sleep overnight and are retested in the morning (AM-PM-AM). A second group (PM-AM-PM) is trained in the evening, allowed to sleep overnight, and tested in the morning, followed by a retest in the evening after being awake all day. Neither group is sleep-deprived and each is tested in both the morning and evening. Both groups experience their usual sleep and wake periods before one of their two tests, but in different orders (**Figure 17.3**).

This approach assesses at which time point memory improves, either after a sleep period or after a wake period, in the absence of sleep deprivation and without differences between groups in the circadian times of testing. There are, however, group differences in the circadian phase of initial learning, in the length of time between learning and the sleep opportunity, and in the order of the sleep and wake periods after training.

> ***Method 3. Overnight sleep deprivation:*** The simplest approach to assessing whether sleep is important for consolidation is to have participants learn a task in the evening, either allow them to sleep overnight or keep them awake, and then test them in the morning.

The obvious potential confound is that effects on performance in the morning could result either from differences in consolidation overnight or from morning sleepiness after having been awake for ~24 h.

A control procedure that has been used is to allow one or more recovery nights for both groups before assessing memory, in an attempt to eliminate differences in current sleepiness during testing. This procedure then allows a test

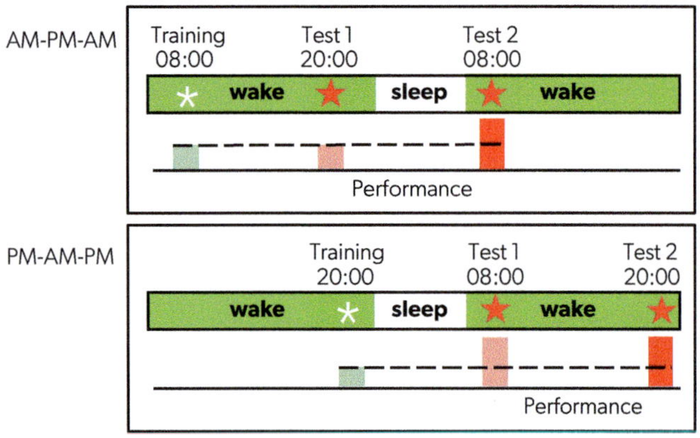

Figure 17.3 The top part of each panel shows the timeline of an experimental procedure, and the bottom part shows the performance effects that might be seen in a study using an AM-PM-AM design. Participants in two groups (AM-PM-AM and PM-AM-PM) are given baseline performance tests immediately after learning a task, which occurs either early or late in the wake period (white ✻). Both groups are also tested twice afterwards at 12 h intervals (red stars). The total sleep (white) and wake (green) durations after training are identical for both groups by the time of Test 2. The effects of sleep versus wake on consolidation can be measured by comparing performance on Test 1 (pink) in the AM-PM-AM condition (wake period) to performance on Test 1 in the PM-AM-PM condition (sleep period), and by determining whether performance improves after Test 1 or after Test 2 for each group. Note, however, that the groups differ in the circadian phase of training and whether the sleep period follows immediately after training or occurs after a period of wake following training. In the hypothetical bar graphs showing memory performance below each schedule, baseline performance after training is shown as a green column. For the AM-PM-AM group (Top), there was no improvement at Test 1 (pink) relative to baseline performance (black dashed line), when they were tested after 12 h awake. But there was immediate improvement in the PM-AM-PM group (Bottom) after the same interval that included sleep before Test 1 (pink). When the AM-PM-AM group (Top) was then allowed to sleep, they showed improvement on Test 2 (red). But in the PM-AM-PM group (Bottom) after the same interval spent awake there was no further improvement on Test 2 (red).

of whether sleep immediately after learning contributed to the strength of consolidation, assuming that any possible additional effects of sleep during recovery nights would be common to both groups.

A related, but opposite, approach is to attempt to improve memory consolidation by increasing sleep amounts after learning. This approach could involve either prior sleep deprivation to promote more sleep during recovery after training, or pharmacological methods, such as blocking arousal-promoting hypocretin receptors in order to enhance sleep (Pittaras et al., 2022); see Section 11.3.1.

Method 4. Selective sleep deprivation: Another approach addresses whether specific sleep features/stages are related to memory consolidation. In these studies, participants are selectively deprived of one sleep stage or of specific sleep features (e.g., slow waves). Memory performance of deprived participants is compared to that of participants who slept freely or were deprived of a different sleep stage. Thus, selective REM sleep deprivation may impair consolidation of only one type of learning while selective N3 deprivation may impair consolidation only of another type. The results are interpreted as showing that these different sleep stages are involved in consolidation of different kinds of learning.

Some studies have used forced awakenings selectively from N3 or REM sleep to reduce these stages. A challenge in these studies is that sleep stages are linked. For example, NREM sleep (including mostly N3) typically precedes the first REM sleep episode in adults at sleep onset. Depriving participants of N3 could also affect REM sleep expression. To address this issue, some studies have used relatively subtle sound stimuli that do not usually cause waking but can disrupt production of features like slow waves. This method can produce very substantial reductions in the targeted sleep stage or features, but they do not eliminate them completely, and total sleep time may also be reduced (Casey et al., 2016).

Method 5. Split-night studies: Split-night studies depend on the fact that sleep in adult humans at night includes large amounts of N3 during the first half of the night and of REM sleep during the second half of the night. The role of N3-enriched sleep is assessed by giving participants a learning experience before sleep onset and testing memory after a half-night of sleep. The role of REM-enriched sleep is assessed in one of two ways. Participants stay awake for the first part of the night and are then trained; or they can be allowed to sleep and are then woken halfway through the night to have the learning experience. In each case, after training, they are allowed to experience REM-enriched sleep and are then tested (Plihal & Born, 1997).

Studies may also include control participants who are treated similarly but stay awake between learning and testing during corresponding first or second halves of the night (Barrett & Ekstrand, 1972; Rauchs et al., 2004). This design can allow the training, the retention interval, and the testing to occur at relatively similar circadian phases in control and experimental groups, but with different amounts of N3 or REM sleep occurring during the post-training retention intervals.

A limitation of this design is that participants will have different amounts of sleep before their learning experience as well as after it. When all participants are trained in the middle of the night, some are kept awake until that point so they have their "early sleep" afterwards, while others sleep for ~4 h before training so they have "late sleep" afterwards (Barrett & Ekstrand, 1972). It is very challenging to control simultaneously for sleep amounts before training, degree of alertness, circadian phases of training and testing, and lengths of delays between training and testing; for a discussion, see (Diekelmann et al., 2013).

Another limitation of this approach is that sleep stages are not confined completely to half of the sleep period, so the sleep stage differences between treatment groups are relative rather than absolute. Some REM sleep and N2 occur along with N3 early in the sleep period, and both N2 and REM sleep occur during the second half. Different effects of early vs. late sleep on different types of learning can therefore only be tentatively attributed to the involvement of specific sleep stages.

Method 6. Correlational studies: A commonly used method is to measure sleep using PSG during a baseline night and during the next night after an intervening learning experience. *Changes* in sleep stages or features during the night after learning (relative to the baseline night) are then correlated with *differences* in memory performance among participants. For example, the amount of REM sleep or the density of N2 sleep spindles can be measured on a baseline night and then again after a specific learning experience. A positive correlation between the degree of improvement in memory performance and the extent of increase in a sleep feature or stage after learning indicates its potential involvement in consolidation.

A variation on this approach is to use brain-imaging methods to measure neural activity patterns during sleep on nights preceding and after learning (e.g., the strength of functional connectivity between particular brain structures), and to correlate changes in these measures with differences in later memory performance.

Because these methods are correlational, they cannot determine causality. However, they can strongly imply a specific role for a sleep stage in relation to one kind of learning if there is a "double dissociation." As a hypothetical example, this could refer to finding that increased N3 after learning is correlated with better consolidation of explicit, but not implicit, learning, while the reverse is true for increases in REM sleep.

Method 7. Nap studies: In nap studies, participants first have a learning experience and are then allowed a short, daytime sleep opportunity, typically lasting 60–90 min (although as little as 10–30 min in a few studies). Participants sleep for as long as they can within this nap opportunity window. They are then tested for their memory of what they learned before the nap, and performance is compared to that of control participants who stayed awake. To reduce the risk of uncontrolled rehearsal of the learned material, participants who stay awake may be kept busy performing an unrelated, distracting task.

These studies have the advantage that learning and testing occur at the same circadian phases in both the sleep and wake groups, and these times fall within a very limited part of the circadian cycle. Because people differ in how long they sleep and in the sleep stages and features they produce during a nap, it is possible to correlate differences in later memory performance with the amount of total sleep or of a particular sleep stage or feature produced during the nap.

One possible concern is that any built up homeostatic sleep drive would be reduced by the nap but not by continued waking, and that could benefit performance in the nap group. The significance of this factor is reduced by timing the learning and nap to occur relatively early in the day, when there would be minimal homeostatic sleep drive rather than in the late afternoon or evening. Another issue might be the presence of sleep inertia in the nap condition, but that can be addressed by allowing a sufficient period after waking before testing.

One limitation to nap studies is uncertainty as to whether the effects of short daytime naps generalize to overnight sleep, because there are many differences in neuroendocrine and other physiological functions between day and night, some of which can influence memory (Born & Wagner, 2004). In addition, some models of how sleep affects memory consolidation propose a combined role for SWS and REM sleep and for their alternation during NREM–REM sleep cycles. The timing and length of naps may not allow for production of such cycles. Nevertheless, the effectiveness of naps in some studies indicates that NREM–REM cycles may not be essential for sleep to benefit consolidation of at least some memories.

Method 8. Manipulations during sleep: Another approach is to test the effects on memory of manipulations during sleep that are designed to either reinforce or interfere with consolidation processes. One method involves presenting stimuli associated with the learning event (e.g., one of two words in a paired-associate word list) during specific sleep stages to try to trigger the neural activity that is linked to those stimuli. This approach to reinforcing the consolidation process is usually called targeted memory reactivation; it is discussed in Section 18.11).

A variation involves enhancing neural activity associated with only a subset of cues from the learning experience. This method allows comparison of memory for associations linked to cues that were presented during sleep with memory linked to cues that were not targeted during sleep. An alternative method involves presenting a stimulus that was globally present during training (e.g., a distinctive odor) to try to reactivate neural activity associated with the overall learning experience.

Another approach is altering specific sleep features (e.g., slow oscillations, sleep spindles, or hippocampal theta waves) during sleep after participants have learned something and measuring the effects on later memory performance. Studies have used sounds, electrical stimulation, drugs, or (in animal studies) optogenetic methods to trigger or suppress specific sleep features. These methods have the important advantage that controlled manipulations allow stronger inferences about causality than correlational studies (i.e., an experimentally induced change in targeted neural features can be shown to produce a change in memory consolidation; see Section 18.12).

Method 9. Interference: This modification is applicable to many kinds of experimental designs. Rather than assessing only how well newly learned information/skills are retained, researchers can assess how resistant memories are to interference from new, related information. For example, after learning a paired-associate list, participants either sleep or stay awake. They then learn a second list that includes a subset of words from the original list that are now paired with new words, before being tested for their memory of the original pairings (Ellenbogen et al., 2006). Similarly, participants may learn to perform a finger-tapping sequence at high speed and accuracy followed by either sleeping or staying awake. They then learn to finger-tap a new sequence, after which performance on the original sequence is reassessed.

The logic of this design is that more effectively consolidated memories are more resistant to interference effects, while weakly consolidated memories remain labile and subject to disruption by new input. Therefore, the degree to which retention of the original learning is better after sleep than after waking reflects how effectively sleep strengthened consolidation.

17.3.2 A case study of an experiment

Given this overview of the variety of methods that have been used and some of their strengths and weaknesses, it is useful to consider one study as an example of the complexity that can arise in designing and executing these studies. This study was the largest investigation (up to that time, 929 participants) that assessed which differences in sleep features/stages among participants after learning were correlated with the benefits of sleep for memory consolidation. The test involved incidental learning about pictures which participants were instructed simply to rate for their emotional valence; there was no instruction to memorize the pictures.

The memory test used in the main experiment (free recall of pictures) had been shown previously in a smaller pilot study to benefit from overnight sleep during the retention interval, as compared to a daytime retention interval spent awake (see Method #1 in the preceding section). Participants in the main study were tested for their memory of a set of pictures immediately after an exposure session (short-delay recall) and the next day after a night of sleep (long-delay recall). The results indicated no statistically significant correlations between differences in sleep features among participants and differences in overnight changes in memory (long-delay test scores minus short-delay test scores) (Ackermann et al., 2015).[4]

Before concluding from this result that there is no point in reading more about studies addressing how sleep stages and EEG features relate to memory consolidation, there are several points to consider. These issues illustrate some of the complexities involved in comparing results across studies. First, participants in the main study observed a set of pictures but were not told that they would be tested for their memory of the pictures immediately after training, nor that they would be retested the next day on their memory for the same pictures. The fact that participants were not aware that they would be retested on the original set of pictures may be relevant because participants' expectations of the future need for newly learned information has been shown in some studies to affect whether memory is enhanced by later sleep (see Section 17.9.3). However, this kind of "incidental" learning, without instructions about later testing, was found to be influenced by sleep in other studies.

Second, when participants returned the next day, they viewed a second set of pictures and were then retested for their memories of both the first and second sets. As a result, this was a study of the possible effects of interference from new learning on overnight retention of old learning (see Method #9 in the preceding section). The choice of an interference paradigm was based on previous findings that this approach was especially useful for demonstrating the benefits of sleep for consolidation of memory. A third point noted by the authors is that there was a ~6 h delay from exposure to the pictures before sleep; some other studies involved sleep immediately after a learning experience. Finally, participants also completed a working

[4] The one exception was a very small *negative* correlation between % REM sleep and amount of retention from the short-delay to the long-delay test, accounting for roughly 1% of the variance in memory performance. The direction of this minimal effect had not been predicted based on previous research.

memory task and a motor-sequence learning task on both days of the main experiment. The pilot study that showed that sleep affected memory for pictures did not include an interfering picture-learning experience nor working memory and motor learning tasks.

There was also no wake control group in the main study, so it is not known whether sleep in general would have benefited memory retention relative to an awake control group (as in the pilot study), given the context of the participants' lack of expectations of retesting, their participation in other tests, and the use of an interference paradigm. Without evidence that sleep affects performance on this memory task under these conditions, it is difficult to interpret the finding that there were no significant correlations between differences among participants in specific sleep features and differences in memory performance.

Despite these issues, this study had many strengths that others often lack. The experimenters tested a few planned, primary hypotheses, rather than only exploring their data for significant correlations afterwards. The very large number of participants also ensured that there was more than sufficient power in the study to test these hypotheses. The pilot study also showed that performance on the free recall of pictures task was improved by overnight sleep and that this improvement was not an artefact of the time of day of learning. In addition, the experimenters used a stringent correction (Bonferroni correction) for multiple statistical comparisons, which is not always done, especially in studies that are considered "exploratory." Other types of corrections for multiple comparisons could have resulted in different conclusions.

The fact that the largest study intended to assess which features of sleep are associated with better consolidation of memories did not identify any such features should not be interpreted as evidence that no aspect of sleep affects memory. That is clearly not the case, as discussed in the following sections. Rather, this experiment could be considered an informative case study demonstrating that specific combinations of experimental design and analysis features and procedural differences can have large, and not readily predictable, impacts on the conclusions reached. It remains to be determined which of these factors were most relevant to the outcomes of this study.

17.3.3 Summary

Several methods have been developed to assess the role of sleep and its features in stabilizing or strengthening memories, including correlational, deprivation, enhancement, and manipulation methods. Attempts to interfere with previous learning can also be used as a tool to assess the strength of memory consolidation after sleep. Each experimental approach has both strengths and weaknesses.

Correlational studies assess how sleep stages or features change after different types of learning experiences and correlate these results with memory performance. Deprivation studies assess memory after attempting to selectively deprive participants of specific sleep stages, of sleep features, or of sleep in general, using behavioral or pharmacological approaches. Manipulation studies attempt to increase or decrease expression of sleep stages or features, or to provoke increased neural activity related to a subset of learned associations while participants sleep. Compared to correlational research, studies using experimental manipulations of sleep features allow stronger causal inferences about the involvement of these features in memory consolidation.

In designing overnight correlational and deprivation studies, it is difficult to simultaneously control for all of the potentially relevant variables: the circadian phases of training, testing, and sleep; the length of time between training and testing; and participants' alertness at each stage of the study. Variations on the AM-PM-AM design can avoid some of these potential confounds but not others.

Nap studies overcome most of these challenges by using short daytime sleep periods and having identical training and testing times for control and experimental groups within a constrained circadian time window. The timing of naps is important in order to reduce the chance that they could improve performance by overcoming built up homeostatic sleep drive rather than enhancing consolidation. It is possible, however, that the many differences in physiological functions during brief daytime and lengthy nighttime sleep (e.g., levels of hormones; cycling of sleep stages) could limit generalization from the effects on memory observed after naps to those following overnight sleep.

A very large study did not identify any inter-individual differences in sleep features that correlated significantly with overnight memory retention, although the same test that was used previously showed a significant benefit of sleep for memory retention relative to a control daytime waking period. It is unclear whether these results indicate that only within-participant changes in sleep features (which were not studied) are predictably related to memory enhancement by sleep or whether other procedural and analytic features of this study affected the ability to detect statistically significant effects.

17.4 Explicit (declarative) learning

A comprehensive review of research related to sleep and memory is beyond the scope of this volume. The following sections focus on studies of the involvement of sleep in consolidation of memories related to a few types of learning. They also review evidence that the apparent involvement of sleep is modified by factors such as study procedures, experimental instructions, and participants' age. Chapter 18 reviews the neural mechanisms that have been proposed to underlie the effects of sleep on memory consolidation.

Explicit learning has probably been the most common target of research related to sleep and memory. Explicit learning studies have involved verbal material, spatial information, and episodic memory in people as well as a variety of tasks in laboratory animals, using methods of correlation, deprivation, and manipulation. The majority of these studies have found that NREM sleep (N2 and/or N3) is involved in consolidation of explicit learning.

Most explicit memory results have been linked to the role of the hippocampus in memory. It is involved in acquisition and short-term retention of explicit information and, through interactions with the cortex, in consolidation of new information into long-term memory traces.[5] The hippocampal role in consolidation during sleep is hypothesized to involve reactivation and replay of neural activity patterns corresponding to recently acquired information, followed by the storage of this information in the cortex. The neural mechanisms involved in hippocampal-cortical consolidation of memories are reviewed in detail in Section 18.6, with a focus on EEG features that occur during N2/N3 sleep: hippocampal sharp-wave ripples, cortical slow waves, and sleep spindles.

In contrast, there is evidence that REM sleep reinforces memory for several forms of implicit learning that are preserved after hippocampal damage (e.g., motor or sensory learning; see following sections). Together, these findings led to the hypothesis that hippocampal-dependent (explicit) and hippocampal-independent (implicit) memories are consolidated during different sleep stages: NREM sleep for explicit memories and REM sleep for implicit memories (Alger et al., 2012; Born et al., 2006; Gais & Born, 2004; Plihal & Born, 1997; Plihal & Born, 1999; Ravassard et al., 2016; Smith, 1995). Some versions of this model emphasize a specific role for N3 sleep in explicit memory consolidation, but there is also evidence supporting an important role for sleep spindles, which are most prominent in N2 but also occur in N3 sleep (Purcell et al., 2017); see Section 18.6.2.

Studies that supported the different roles of NREM and REM sleep included split-night designs that assessed effects of sleep on memory for both explicit and implicit learning tasks. For example, split-night studies showed more explicit memory benefits from SWS-enriched early sleep than REM-enriched late sleep (e.g., Barrett & Ekstrand, 1972; Plihal & Born, 1997; Plihal & Born, 1999). (See **Figure 17.4**) Another split-night study found that spatial memory (explicit) was strengthened by early-night (SWS-enriched) sleep, while performance on an implicit, verbal learning task (word-stem priming) was strengthened by late-night (REM-enriched) sleep (Plihal & Born, 1999). One split-night study, however, also supported REM sleep involvement in spatial aspects of episodic memory (Rauchs et al., 2004). Involvement of NREM sleep in explicit memory has also been inferred from observation of post-learning changes in NREM EEG features and their timing in both people and rats (Mölle et al., 2009).

This model was also supported by evidence that naps including only NREM sleep improved memory for an explicit task (paired-associate words) but not for an implicit visuomotor skill (Tucker et al., 2006). Similarly, memories of word-pairs were protected from potentially interfering input of other words after naps that included N3 sleep but not those that included REM sleep (Deliens et al., 2013).

Consistent with these findings, studies that are reviewed in Chapter 18 showed that explicit (but not implicit) memories can be strengthened in people and rats by manipulating hippocampal and cortical EEG features of NREM sleep that are hypothesized to be involved in consolidation (e.g., Barham et al., 2016; Maingret et al., 2016). Together with evidence from studies using correlation and deprivation methods, the results of these manipulation studies support the idea that NREM sleep features are selectively involved in offline consolidation of explicit memories.

In contrast to these results linking explicit memory consolidation to NREM sleep and implicit memories to REM sleep, there is also a line of research that emphasized the role of REM sleep in *explicit* memory consolidation. Studies in both rats and people reported increases in REM sleep amounts either immediately after an explicit learning experience or following a short delay period. Preventing REM sleep during these post-training "REM windows" (but not later) impaired memory for the new information (Hennevin & Leconte, 1977; Pearlman & Becker, 1973; Smith et al., 2004). Overnight deprivation of REM sleep in people also reduced recall of learned narratives more than loss of Stage 4 sleep (Tilley & Empson, 1978). In this study, participants deprived of REM sleep also got less N2 sleep, so memory impairment might also be interpreted as being related to loss of N2 sleep. Arguing against this interpretation was evidence that the degree of memory impairment was correlated with the degree of reduction of REM sleep and not with the degree of reduction of N2 sleep.

[5] The classic human examples demonstrating the essential role of the hippocampus in explicit memory are those of HM and similar patients, who had undergone surgical ablation of the temporal lobe (including the hippocampus) to control epileptic seizures. They were subsequently unable to retain short-term, explicit memories without continuous verbal rehearsal, nor form new long-term memories of events, people's names, or their own activities. They were nevertheless able to learn and retain new motor skills based on implicit memory (Milner, 2005; Scoville & Milner, 1957).

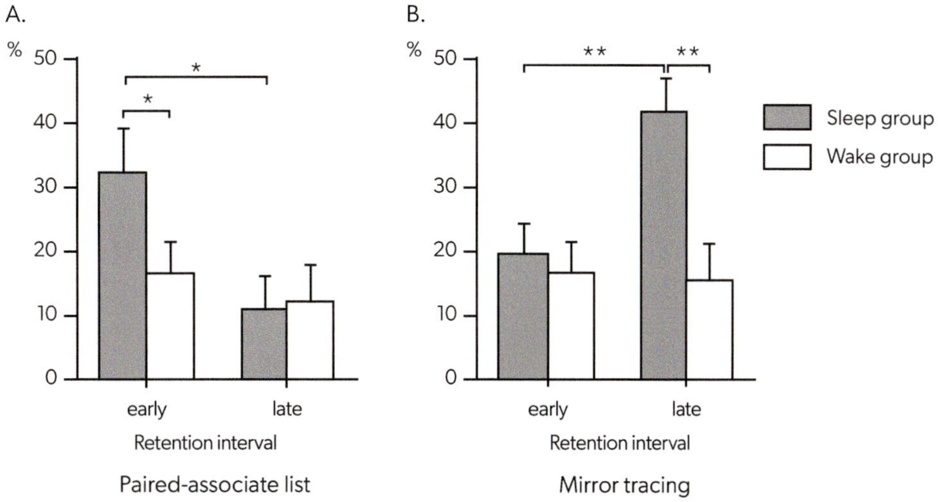

Figure 17.4 **A.** Percentage of paired-associate words that were retained (Y axis) from lists learned before the usual sleep phase. The 3 h retention interval after learning was spent either awake (white) or asleep (gray) early in the sleep phase (~23:00–02:00) or late in the sleep phase (~03:00–06:00). Retention was improved by sleep relative to wake only during the early part of the night. **B:** An identical design tested the effects of the same sleep or wake intervals on the degree to which participants retained skill at tracing complex figures seen through a mirror (i.e., left-right reversed). They performed the mirror-tracing task before and then after early or late retention intervals spent either asleep or awake. Only the late sleep group showed a significant benefit of sleep for retention of skill at mirror-tracing. *: $p < 0.05$; **$p < 0.01$. Adapted with permission of Dr. Jan Born from Plihal, W. & Born, J. (1997) Effects of early and late nocturnal sleep on declarative and procedural memory. *J Cogn Neurosci* 9(4): 534–547. © Massachusetts Institute of Technology (1997). doi: 10.1162/jocn.1997.9.4.534.

A link between REM sleep and explicit memory was also supported by evidence in people of increased cortical theta- and sigma-band activity during overnight REM sleep after paired-associate learning (explicit) but not after training on two motor-skill tasks (implicit) (Fogel et al., 2007). Both explicit and procedural learning have been linked to the expression of electrical patterns during REM sleep, namely, hippocampal theta rhythms and ponto-geniculo-occipital (PGO) waves (which are recorded sequentially in the pons, the lateral geniculate nuclei, and the occipital cortex)[6] (Datta, 2000; Peigneux & Smith, 2017; Sakai & Cespuglio, 1974).

Another link between REM sleep and explicit memories is the effect of REM sleep deprivation on an important neurophysiological model of hippocampal-dependent memory, namely, long-term potentiation (LTP) (Ishikawa et al., 2006). The mechanism underlying LTP is thought to play a key role in explicit memory formation, as discussed in Section 18.2.

The hypothesis that REM sleep is important for memory consolidation was criticized on several grounds (Vertes & Eastman, 2000). In addition to pointing out inconsistencies in this literature, critics noted that the methods used to prevent REM sleep in rodent studies could have contributed to memory disruption, because these are potentially stressful (see Section 14.2) and may have other physiological consequences that could affect memory (Siegel, 2001; Vertes & Eastman, 2000); for a review, see Boyce et al., 2017. These are significant issues, but more recent studies have used non-stressful deprivation methods and physiological manipulations other than deprivation to implicate REM sleep in explicit memory consolidation (Boyce et al., 2016; Ravassard et al., 2016).

Another criticism of the REM sleep/memory hypothesis was that the durations of REM sleep observed across different species do not seem related to these species' abilities to form memories. Some species that are clearly very capable of learning show little REM sleep (horse, rhesus monkey, elephant) or none (dolphin). Species with large amounts of REM sleep (e.g., armadillos and opossums) are not noted for having sophisticated learning abilities (Siegel, 2001). The same point could, however, also be made in relation to total sleep durations and learning. Despite the apparent lack of correlation between amounts of REM sleep (or sleep in general) and memory abilities across species, our earlier discussion about the function of sleep (Section 16.3.1) also applies here. Different species may accomplish the same physiological goal using different mechanisms or may use the same mechanism (e.g., REM sleep) for different functions.

[6] PGO waves were originally described in cats and some other mammals (Callaway et al., 1987), and their putative analog has also been recorded in humans (Lim et al., 2007). They are linked (to different extents) to the timing of rapid eye movements in REM sleep. In rats, these waves are usually recorded only in the pons, and their propagation pattern is less certain (Farber et al., 1980); they are often referred to as P-waves in both rat and human studies since their degree of homology to feline PGO waves is uncertain; see Section 12.2.6.

Finally, involvement of REM sleep in memory was questioned because people who chronically use drugs that suppress REM sleep (e.g., benzodiazepines, cannabis, alcohol, and some antidepressants)[7] (Naiman, 2017) do not show obvious memory deficits and may be successful in demanding professional careers (Siegel, 2001; Vertes & Eastman, 2000). To be clear, these arguments appear to be aimed at the idea that REM sleep is essential for explicit memory formation. Most laboratory studies, however, observed *quantitative* differences in some forms of memory consolidation as a function of REM sleep amounts rather than a complete inability to form new memories without REM sleep. It would be difficult to guess how such quantitative differences would, or would not, impact the professional success of individuals with different habits and intellectual abilities in the uncontrolled world outside the laboratory.

These critiques of the idea that REM sleep is the principal mechanism for consolidating explicit memories raised important issues and highlighted inconsistencies and gaps in this literature. More recent research has, however, provided new lines of evidence supporting the involvement of REM sleep in memory consolidation, including some forms of explicit memory (see next section). What has not been supported is the idea that REM sleep is the principal or only mechanism responsible for explicit memory consolidation; there is also considerable support for the involvement of NREM sleep.

17.4.1 Summary

There is extensive evidence based on ablation studies indicating that the hippocampus plays a critical role in acquiring and temporarily storing explicit memories in both people and animals. This conclusion is also supported by other physiological evidence that is reviewed in Chapter 18. There is also evidence indicating that NREM sleep (N2 and/or N3) is involved in consolidating explicit memories. This form of consolidation depends on reactivation of recent memory traces by the hippocampus, followed by hippocampal-cortical communication involving sharp-wave ripples, cortical slow waves, and sleep spindles (see Chapter 18). REM sleep was instead proposed to be involved in consolidating implicit learning, although other studies also demonstrated its involvement in some forms of explicit learning in both animals and people.

Early proposals that REM sleep is of central importance for memory consolidation in general were criticized on several grounds; these criticisms were partly justified and raised important issues. More modest claims for the involvement of REM sleep in consolidation of several kinds of learning, including some types of explicit learning, have been supported by more recent research, as discussed in the following sections.

17.5 REM sleep, emotional content, and memory

The conclusion that REM sleep sometimes plays a role in explicit memory consolidation appears to contradict the idea that NREM and REM sleep mechanisms serve consolidation of different types of learning. A partial resolution of these conflicting claims relates to another proposed role for REM sleep, namely, that it is involved in consolidation of memories that have a prominent emotional component. One review even proposed that NREM sleep is involved in both explicit and implicit memory and that REM sleep may be involved *only* in consolidation of emotional memory (Ackermann & Rasch, 2014).

This idea is linked to research showing that people were better at recognizing and remembering emotional stimuli (visual images) than neutral stimuli if they slept after initial exposure to these stimuli (Hu et al., 2006; Nishida et al., 2009). Memory retrieval for these emotional stimuli was correlated with the amount of REM sleep produced after initial exposure (Groch et al., 2013; Menz et al., 2013; Nishida et al., 2009).[8]

There is disagreement, however, about the effects of REM sleep on different aspects of how emotional stimuli are remembered. Some studies examined how well emotion-linked memories are retained relative to neutral memories, which is relevant to the idea that REM sleep is involved in consolidating learning related to one class of events or experiences. Others examined somewhat different, but related, issues like the effects of REM sleep on retention of the emotional valence (positive or negative) or emotional intensity of the memory.

Some studies found that REM sleep helped preserve the emotional and physiological impacts of viewing negative or threatening visual images, and on participants' memory of the stimuli (e.g., images of car wrecks, injuries, weapons) (Baran et al., 2012; Groch et al., 2013; Jones & Spencer, 2019; Menz et al., 2013). Others concluded that REM sleep selectively preserved memory for only the emotional components of an experience (Payne et al., 2012; Wagner et al., 2001). And yet others concluded that REM sleep *reduced* the emotional impact of negative stimuli (and enhanced the impact of positive stimuli) (Gujar et al., 2011; Rosales-Lagarde et al., 2012; Wassing et al., 2019).

[7] This argument may be most relevant to older antidepressant drugs; some currently used antidepressants have only small effects on REM sleep, which may be transient and reversed over a period of weeks (Wilson & Argyropoulos, 2005).

[8] In contrast to results from correlational studies, one study that involved selective REM sleep deprivation found no effect on emotional memory (Morgenthaler et al., 2014).

Different findings related to the role of REM sleep in modifying the impact of emotional stimuli, and affecting memory for these stimuli, likely reflect the use of different kinds of emotional stimuli and the use of correlational versus deprivation methods. The timing of testing after sleep or sleep loss may also be important. When testing occurred 12 h after initial encoding, sleep preserved both the emotional tone and accuracy of memory for neutral and negative stimuli similarly; but after 60 h, memories for both categories declined and negative stimuli were rated as being less negative (Zeng et al., 2021).

Many experimental and analytic differences among studies could affect whether they find a specific role for sleep or REM sleep in memory for emotion-linked stimuli. Three recent reviews summarized the literature related to how sleep (or REM sleep) influences memory for emotional stimuli. A narrative review concluded that, despite some studies showing selective involvement of REM sleep in emotional aspects of memory, there were more studies that failed to show such effects (Davidson et al., 2021). A meta-analysis concluded that across studies there was no specific effect of sleep on emotional memory and that both sleep- and wake-filled periods benefited recall of emotional items more than neutral items. However, studies that used free recall (rather than recognition tests, for example), and that took account of baseline memory immediately after encoding, did show a preferential effect of sleep for retaining memory of emotional items relative to neutral items (Lipinska et al., 2019).

Another meta-analysis also found that there was insufficient evidence to conclude that sleep in general improved retention of emotional over neutral items: only ~40% of publications reviewed showed this effect. However, in a secondary analysis based on studies using split-night designs or deprivation of either REM sleep or SWS, the review concluded that either late-night retention intervals (presumably REM-sleep enriched) or deprivation of SWS favored memory for emotional over neutral items. One interpretation of a lack of a similar effect of overnight sleep in general might be that the benefits of early SWS for retention of neutral items might offset benefits of later REM sleep for emotional items, resulting in an overall lack of selective benefit for emotional over neutral stimuli after overnight sleep (Schäfer et al., 2020).

Although these reviews found that the evidence from human studies is inconsistent, a subset of these studies with specific design and analysis features reported that REM sleep had a larger impact on memory for items with an emotional valence than for neutral items. This possible linkage of REM sleep to memory of emotion-related stimuli suggested a way of resolving other issues related to the role of different sleep stages in consolidating different types of memory.

The suggestion is that many of the results showing involvement of REM sleep in explicit memory actually reflect its role in memory for emotional events (Ackermann & Rasch, 2014; Hutchison & Rathore, 2015). Many studies that demonstrated links between REM sleep amounts and explicit memory in laboratory rodents, for example, involved a learned avoidance response (e.g., avoiding a location where they had experienced a foot shock); extinction of a previously learned fear; or a learned approach response (e.g., to the location of a food or water reward). All of these studies would have involved provoking or modulating intense motivational states.

One study used optogenetic methods in mice to silence GABAergic neurons in the medial septum during REM sleep, which selectively blocked hippocampal theta activity that normally occurs during this stage, without sleep loss. This procedure disrupted contextual memory of an environment in which the mice had undergone fear conditioning, which constitutes explicit (spatial) learning about an emotional event in that location. However, it also disrupted memory in a novel-object, place recognition task that involved no explicit motivational manipulation (Boyce et al., 2016).[9] This finding suggests that features of REM sleep are involved in both emotional and neutral explicit memory consolidation in mice. Similarly, several studies of declarative memory in people that did not involve explicit manipulations of emotional states also linked memory consolidation to REM sleep (Peigneux & Smith, 2017; Rauchs et al., 2004).

Thus, REM sleep may be involved in consolidation of emotional memories under some conditions, which may account for some of the findings related to its role in explicit memory consolidation. However, REM sleep has also been shown to be involved in explicit memory that does not have a clear emotional component in both human and animal studies.

An alternative hypothesis about how REM and NREM sleep interact suggests a possible explanation for mixed evidence for the involvement of both REM and NREM sleep in consolidation of explicit memories. That view is that memory consolidation consists of a series of phases, and that NREM and REM sleep are involved in different ways during these phases, regardless of the type of learning involved. Depending on the methods used in different studies, results favoring a role for one or the other stage might be observed. This idea is discussed further in Sections 17.6 and 17.8.

[9] This example raises the question of whether any study involving people handling and testing small rodents, without any intended manipulation of emotion, is ever free of emotional experiences for the rodents. One study found that handling mice daily for 6 days to habituate them to the experience eliminated the significant increase in levels of corticosterone elicited by handling naïve mice (Vecsey et al., 2013). This finding indicates that well-habituated mice do not show a specific endocrine marker of a stress response during handling, but it remains a matter of speculation whether the experience of being tested in an experiment is free of emotional content for mice.

17.5.1 Summary

Although there have been proposals that REM sleep is specifically involved in consolidation of non-declarative memories, there is also evidence that it plays a role in consolidation of declarative/explicit memories. The evidence, however, has been inconsistent, perhaps depending on the experimental designs and the nature of the stimuli used.

One potential explanation for a role for REM sleep in explicit memory is that it relates specifically to memories that have an emotional component. Some studies reported that REM sleep selectively strengthened explicit memory for stimuli that evoked emotional responses, relative to neutral stimuli, although others have not reported similar effects. Most studies of animal learning used fear or reward to motivate behavior, so REM sleep's role in explicit memory for these events may be attributable to these emotional features. However, disrupting hippocampal theta rhythms during REM sleep in mice reduced consolidation of both emotion-linked memories and those that involved no explicit emotional manipulations. The involvement of emotional components does not seem to account for all findings in which REM sleep played a role in consolidation of explicit memories.

Currently available evidence does not support the idea that REM sleep is involved only in non-explicit memory consolidation and NREM sleep in explicit memories. It also does not support the idea that REM sleep is involved exclusively in memory for emotion-linked memories. One possibility that is discussed in later sections is that REM sleep and NREM sleep are implicated in different phases of the consolidation of memories, regardless of the type of learning involved.

17.6 Sensory/perceptual learning

Sensory/perceptual learning is a form of implicit learning that involves improving skill at detecting a subtle sensory feature, usually visual or auditory. One example illustrating a role for sleep in consolidation of auditory learning comes from a study of starlings (*Sturnus vulgaris*). Birds were trained to discriminate segments of novel starling songs and were then retested after different intervals that either did or not include overnight sleep. Only birds that slept showed improved discrimination performance when they were retested, indicating that sleep strengthened offline consolidation of the new learning (Brawn, Nusbaum, et al., 2010).

A sensory learning test that has been used in human studies is the visual texture discrimination (VTD) task. It involves learning to detect the orientation (vertical vs. horizontal) of an array that is presented very briefly in the periphery of a complex visual display, while the eyes are fixated on the center of the display[10] (Karni & Sagi, 1991; Stickgold, Whidbee, et al., 2000). Performance improved on this task exclusively for stimuli presented in the part of the peripheral visual field that was involved in training and not in other regions. These results indicated that improvement resulted from local neural plasticity in the primary visual cortex (V1), rather than from a nonspecific increase in skill at performing the task (Karni & Sagi, 1991; Walker et al., 2005).[11]

Offline improvement in performance was seen consistently only after participants slept during the period between training and testing, although a few participants improved when tested after 8 h awake (Karni & Sagi, 1993). This impact of sleep was initially attributed to REM sleep because it was prevented by selective REM sleep deprivation and was not affected by selective SWS deprivation (Karni et al., 1994).

A later study found that the degree of overnight improvement was correlated with the total length of sleep, with an apparent minimum requirement of at least 6 h (**Figure 17.5**). Performance improvement in this study was strongly correlated with the amount of SWS shown in the first quarter of the overnight sleep phase, and with the amount of REM sleep shown in the last quarter, suggesting sequential involvement of both SWS and REM sleep (Stickgold, Whidbee, et al., 2000). Another study used a split-night design and found that early sleep alone (with more SWS) produced improvement while late sleep (with more REM sleep) did not, and even produced some decrement in performance (Gais et al., 2000).

These results suggest that early SWS plays the most important role, although it is unclear whether that is reinforced by later REM sleep or not. However, an earlier study found that deprivation of SWS did not interfere with sleep-dependent improvement, while REM sleep loss did (Karni et al., 1994). One interpretation of these studies is that either sleep stage, or both together, may be able to reinforce sensory learning but that neither stage is essential. The results that appear to contradict this conclusion may be related to some subtle aspects of

[10] Because the presentation is very brief, there is not enough time to direct the eyes toward the stimulus and use acute, foveal (central) vision, so peripheral visual receptors (which are poor at resolving details) must be used. In addition, a visually complex masking display is presented with short latency after the target display so that a lingering retinal image of the target cannot be consulted. These features combine to make the VTD a difficult task that requires practice to perform quickly and accurately.

[11] It is possible that mechanisms beyond V1 might contribute to better performance on the VTD after sleep. Performance improvement on a different visual discrimination task that is processed at the level of V1 (depth perception based on binocular disparity) was unaffected by whether participants slept during a retention interval (Klinzing et al., 2021). This result may indicate either that sleep affects one form of plasticity in V1, but not another, or that the effect of sleep on VTD performance is influenced by other parts of the visual system, while plasticity related to binocular disparity is not.

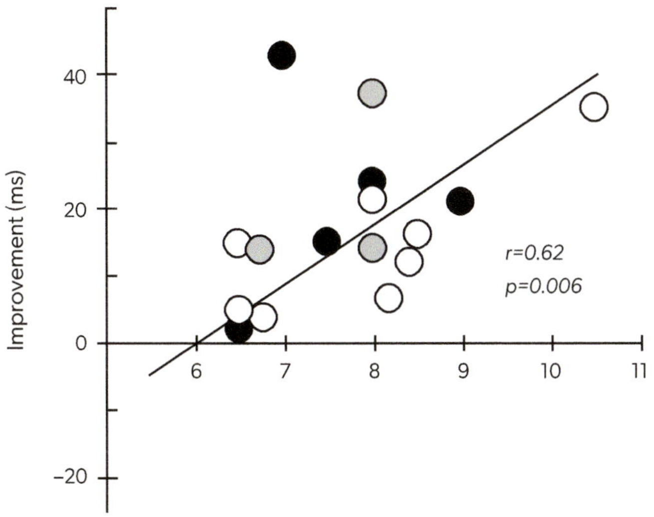

Figure 17.5 A plot of the extent of performance improvement (Y axis) on a visual texture discrimination task as a function of the total length of sleep after training and before retesting (X axis). Higher values indicate better performance during the retest. Different symbols represent different durations from training to testing (13–22.5 h) during which sleep could occur. There was a significant positive correlation between the duration of overnight sleep (from ~6–10.5 h) and off-line performance improvement, with more improvement after longer sleep. Reprinted with permission of the MIT Press from Stickgold, R. et al. (2000) Visual discrimination task improvement: a multi-step process occurring during sleep. *J Cogn Neurosci* 12: 246–254. © 2000 Massachusetts Institute of Technology (2000). doi: 10.1162/089892900562075.

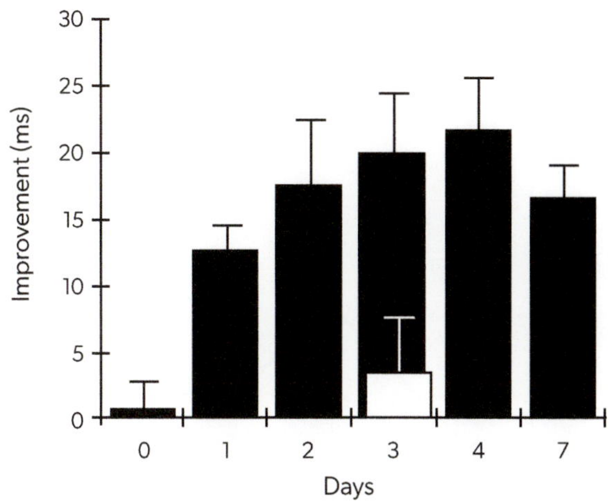

Figure 17.6 Extent of performance improvement on a visual texture display task days after training (higher values indicate greater performance improvement). Some participants were tested 1–7 days after initial training when they were allowed to sleep freely (black columns). Another group was sleep-deprived overnight immediately after training, allowed to sleep freely for the next two nights, and were then tested on day 3 (white column). The lack of performance improvement on day 3 in the sleep-deprived group indicates that sleep immediately after training was needed to produce significant offline improvement. Reprinted with permission from Stickgold, R. et al. (2000) Visual discrimination learning requires sleep after training. *Nat Neurosci* 3:1237–1238. © Springer: Nature (2000). doi: 10.1038/81756.

experimental procedures that are discussed in Section 17.3.1, and the limitations of the designs used.

Deprivation of SWS or REM sleep, for example, required repeatedly waking participants when they started to enter these sleep stages, which could have effects in addition to reducing the amounts of these stages (Karni et al., 1994). However, the use of periods of early and late sleep to define the role of SWS and REM sleep is also complicated because each time window includes a mixture of stages. Both early and late sleep periods included a substantial amount of both SWS and REM sleep, but in different proportions, and both periods included more N2 sleep than either SWS or REM sleep (Gais et al., 2000). These cannot be considered pure tests of the role of either SWS or REM sleep. Thus, it may not be surprising that studies using these different methods reached inconsistent conclusions about the relative importance of these stages for VTD performance improvement.

When participants who slept immediately after training on the VTD were retested several days later, they showed continued offline improvement for up to 3 days. However, if they were kept awake during the night immediately after training, there was no evidence of improvement three days later (i.e., despite two full nights of recovery sleep) (**Figure 17.6**). These results indicate that sleep soon after training is particularly important for reinforcing the neural plasticity involved in enhancing this skill (Stickgold, James, et al., 2000).

Other studies allowed participants short daytime naps after training rather than overnight sleep. When participants were trained on the VTD and were then tested repeatedly while awake during the day, they showed a gradual deterioration of performance that was stabilized after they had a short nap that included SWS. Longer naps that included both SWS and REM sleep not only stabilized but also improved performance (Mednick et al., 2003; Mednick et al., 2002) (**Figure 17.7**). These effects depended on getting sufficient sleep; lying awake in darkness did not prevent deterioration of performance (Mednick et al., 2002; Nissen et al., 2021).

A study of VTD performance changes after naps in patients with different forms of hypersomnia (excessive sleepiness) found that only those who showed NREM sleep followed by REM sleep during the nap improved, and their improvement was related to the production of sleep spindles. A subset of narcolepsy patients (who may show sleep-onset REM episodes; see Section 11.3.2) showed the opposite sequence of REM sleep followed by NREM sleep and did not show nap-related improvement (Strauss et al., 2022).

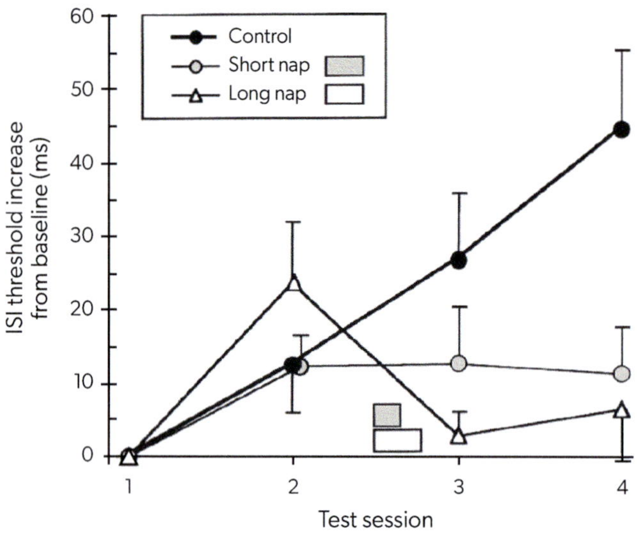

Figure 17.7 Performance on the VTD task after nap opportunities. Higher values on the Y axis in this plot reflect *worse* performance (i.e., requiring longer intervals between presentation of the target stimulus and the mask for similar results). Performance of controls with no nap opportunities deteriorated across repeated test sessions within a single day after initial training (black circles). A short nap after the second test session (gray box at the bottom) stabilized performance and prevented further deterioration in later tests (gray circles), while a longer nap (white box) both reversed deterioration and improved later performance (white triangles). Reprinted with permission from Mednick S. et al. (2002) The restorative effect of naps on perceptual deterioration. *Nat Neurosci* 5:677–681. © Springer: Nature (2002). doi: 10.1038/nn864.

Several lines of evidence in these studies converge on the conclusion that SWS and REM sleep act jointly to improve VTD performance. The amounts of early SWS and late REM sleep correlated with performance improvement during overnight sleep (Stickgold, Whidbee, et al., 2000); early-night sleep was necessary to improve performance, but a full-night's sleep was more effective (Gais et al., 2000); SWS during naps stabilized performance, and the addition of time in REM sleep improved it (Mednick et al., 2003; Mednick et al., 2002); and only a NREM–REM sleep sequence during naps benefited later performance (Strauss et al., 2022).

There were also some inconsistencies among the results of these studies. For example, a few study participants showed improved performance after a period of time spent awake, while most did not (Gais et al., 2000; Karni & Sagi, 1993); but in other studies, participants who stayed awake showed deterioration of performance when tested repeatedly during the day (Mednick et al., 2003; Mednick et al., 2002). Performance on a different sensory discrimination task that is enhanced by sleep after training also showed deterioration as a result of repeated testing (Mednick et al., 2008).

There was also an apparent requirement for ~6 h sleep for overnight improvement in one study, but daytime nap studies demonstrated improvement after much shorter sleep opportunities (Mednick et al., 2003; Mednick et al., 2002; Stickgold, Whidbee, et al., 2000). One potential contributing factor discussed previously is that daytime nap and overnight sleep studies are conducted at different circadian phases. These phases are characterized by different hormonal and neurotransmitter levels, some of which influence neural plasticity and memory consolidation; see Sections 18.13 and 19.2.2.

Later research showed that the amount and type of training and testing contributed to some of the observed differences in results obtained using the VTD task. Depending on the number of training trials and their design, there could be no improvement over either wake or sleep intervals, improvement after both sleep and waking, or improvement only after a sleep period (Censor et al., 2006). More repetitions of training/testing trials while awake was proposed to saturate both relevant and unrelated synaptic connections, which interfered with offline improvements in performance. Sleep was hypothesized to consolidate the relevant synaptic connections and downregulate unrelated connections, thereby enhancing later performance (Censor et al., 2006; Censor & Sagi, 2009). These findings indicate that procedural differences among studies in the pattern of training trials and in the amount of testing after training contributed to whether effects of sleep on memory consolidation could be detected. Other factors that can influence whether memory is affected by sleep after training are discussed in Section 17.9.

17.6.1 Summary

Sleep after training enhanced consolidation of sensory learning in both auditory and visual discrimination tasks and in both people and birds. Enhanced performance on the VTD task occurred offline as a result of changes, apparently in the primary visual cortex, within hours after initial training. Although a few people showed enhanced performance while awake after training, the largest and most consistent improvement followed a period of sleep.

The type of sleep involved in offline enhancement has been controversial. One study found that overnight deprivation of REM sleep disrupted sleep-related enhancement of VTD performance while overnight deprivation of SWS did not. However, other studies found that SWS early in the night and REM sleep late in the night correlated with sleep-related improvement. Similarly, short naps with only SWS sleep stabilized performance while longer naps that included REM sleep improved later performance, and the order of SWS-REM sleep was important. Thus, both sleep stages appear to be involved in a stepwise process that enhances later VTD performance. Different methods of assessing the involvement of different sleep stages have inherent limitations that may have led to some inconsistent conclusions.

There were also apparent discrepancies among studies as to whether or not VTD task performance deteriorates during waking, which are likely attributable to differences in training procedures and in the frequency of testing. When training/testing procedures led to deterioration of performance over a wake interval, periods of SWS combined with REM sleep reversed these effects and enhanced later performance.

17.7 Motor/procedural learning

A common feature of motor/procedural tasks is that they involve learning to perform a motor skill more quickly and/or accurately. Most studies of the involvement of sleep in motor skill memory have been variations on motor sequence learning (MSL): rapidly and repeatedly tapping sequences of keys or producing sequences of thumb-finger touches. Other tasks have included mirror-tracing, which involves learning to trace a complex figure viewed in a mirror, which is therefore left–right reversed (an example of motor adaptation); pursuit-rotor tasks (manually tracking a moving target on a screen); fine-motor skills required for dental repair; juggling balls; and inverse steering (riding a bicycle on which steering in one direction causes it to turn the opposite way) (Bothe et al., 2019; King et al., 2017; Lugassy et al., 2018; Morita et al., 2016; Schönauer et al., 2015; Walker & Stickgold, 2006).

Motor tasks can be either explicit or implicit, as exemplified by MSL tasks. In the explicit version, participants are informed of a specific sequence of key presses that they are instructed to perform as quickly and accurately as possible. In an implicit version (e.g., the Serial Reaction Time Task (SRTT), participants press keys in response to a series of visual prompts but are not told that the series contains a hidden structure, such as an embedded repeating sequence or a grammatical rule related to keystrokes (e.g., C follows A). An embedded sequence or rule can be either deterministic (i.e., fixed, C always follows A immediately) or probabilistic (e.g., C follows A immediately 75% of the time) (Diekelmann et al., 2009; Fischer et al., 2002; Robertson et al., 2004; Song et al., 2007; Walker et al., 2002). In a nominally implicit version, a very simple hidden pattern may be detected by participants, which effectively turns it into an explicit task. But implicit tasks that involve a more complex hidden rule or a probabilistic structure make it difficult for participants to become consciously aware of the patterns involved (Rickard & Pan, 2017; Song et al., 2007).

Among studies that used a MSL task, many reported stable performance after a period awake but improved performance after sleep (Fischer et al., 2002; Walker et al., 2002); for reviews, see (King et al., 2017; Walker & Stickgold, 2006). This sleep benefit appeared for explicit sequences, but performance of implicit sequences was usually not enhanced by later sleep (Fischer et al., 2006; Robertson et al., 2004; Song et al., 2007; van den Berg et al., 2019). However, the explicit/implicit dimension may not fully account for whether sleep benefits memory, which could explain why some studies involving implicit tasks did find benefits (King et al., 2017). Among the other features that may determine whether performance on an implicit task benefits from sleep are the involvement of a contextual dimension in the learning process (Spencer et al., 2006) and the cognitive strategy involved in learning a sequence (van den Berg et al., 2019).

One hypothesis for how motor learning occurs is linked to a model that involves two stages. During an early stage, participants acquire general spatial/sequential information related to the task, and during a later stage they link together specific motor elements to produce the desired pattern. These stages are proposed to involve plasticity in different neural mechanisms, only some of which would benefit from sleep (Doyon et al., 2018; Hikosaka et al., 1999; van den Berg et al., 2019); see Section 18.7. Specifically, the proposal is that sleep influences memory for the more conceptual, spatial/sequential representation component of the task but does not benefit consolidation of the linkages between the specific motor elements involved (Albouy et al., 2013).

There are also mixed results related to mirror-tracing and similar motor adaptation tasks, with some studies observing benefits from sleep after initial learning and others not. One study found a benefit of late-night (REM-enriched) sleep on mirror-tracing skills (Plihal & Born, 1997), and another found that sleep deprivation the night after training impaired later performance (Schönauer et al., 2015). Other studies reported that features of NREM sleep mediated the benefits of sleep for motor adaptation skills (Huber et al., 2004; Tamaki et al., 2008), but some observed no benefit of either daytime naps or overnight sleep on similar tasks (Doyon et al., 2009; Tucker et al., 2006; see King et al., 2017 for additional references).

One interpretation is that in some studies participants can adopt a conscious strategy ("move left when you want the cursor to go right" in a mirror-tracing task), rendering the task partially explicit. This explicit, strategic component of the task may then benefit from later sleep, even if sleep does not affect memory for the specific motor actions involved (King et al., 2017).

The conclusion that sleep after training improves performance of explicit motor sequences has, however, also been challenged. One factor that affects motor performance is that massed training trials increase fatigue and reduce performance quality, a process called "reactive inhibition." As a result, overt performance measured immediately after the end of training is somewhat impaired and does not accurately reflect the full extent of motor skill learning that has occurred (Pan & Rickard, 2015). The adverse effects of intense or repeated training on motor performance resemble the training/testing effects that also complicate interpretation of studies of sensory learning (Censor et al., 2006; Censor & Sagi, 2009); see Section 17.6.

Motor performance improves spontaneously after a 30 min recovery period following a training session, as fatigue is reduced, thereby unmasking the full extent of skill acquired during the training. The apparent degree of benefit from later sleep is calculated by comparing post-sleep performance to a baseline level. However, that baseline can be either the level of performance immediately after training ends (impaired by fatigue effects) or the level after a short recovery period (Pan & Rickard, 2015).

Using post-recovery scores for an explicit motor task as the baseline, performance was found to deteriorate over a lengthy delay interval spent awake. Sleep during the delay interval stabilized performance and prevented deterioration but without producing improvement relative to the post-recovery baseline (Brawn, Fenn, et al., 2010; Nettersheim et al., 2015). Other changes in test procedures (e.g., reducing fatigue buildup using spaced training, or controlling for the circadian phase of testing) also led to the conclusion that sleep after training stabilized performance (i.e., prevented deterioration) but did not improve performance over the (post-recovery) baseline (Cai & Rickard, 2009; Rickard et al., 2008; Rieth et al., 2010).

A review concluded that once variables, such as selection of appropriate baseline values, fatigue effects, and the timing and duration of training and testing, were accounted for, sleep *stabilized* the performance achieved during training but did not *improve* explicit motor memory (Pan & Rickard, 2015). Despite criticisms of some aspects of this analysis, especially in relation to testing children (Adi-Japha & Karni, 2016), adjusting the analysis to address these issues did not change the main conclusion (Rickard & Pan, 2017).

Rather than focusing only on whether post-sleep performance showed improvement relative to performance at the end of training, subsequent reviews have broadened the definition of how sleep affects later performance. These studies assessed whether performance showed a "relative sleep gain" or was "enhanced" after sleep, relative to a similar period spent awake. The concept of "enhancement" of motor memory includes measures of performance stabilization, performance improvement, and resistance to interference relative to performance after a waking interval. Using this broader definition, several reviews concluded that there is an overall enhancement of motor performance among participants who sleep after training, relative to those staying awake. This benefit appeared consistently for explicit MSL tasks but less reliably for mirror-tracing tasks (Doyon et al., 2018; King et al., 2017; Schmid et al., 2020).

Results obtained from research on other skills have been mixed. A study of a complex motor skill (learning to ride an inverse-steering bicycle) found results consistent with the conclusion related to MSL tasks: sleep after initial training stabilized performance, which otherwise deteriorated during waking (Bothe et al., 2019). Skill in performing a complex, fine-motor task did not improve after 12 h that included either sleep or wake but did improve after 24 h involving both states, suggesting a time-dependent consolidation process that was not selectively strengthened by sleep (Lugassy et al., 2018).

Comparisons between different motor tasks indicate that there are differences in how they are affected by sleep or by sleep loss. In one study, after training on two verbal tasks, an MSL task and a mirror-tracing task, participants who were awake during the day or were sleep-deprived overnight before testing showed next-day deficits on both the MSL and the verbal tasks relative to a free-sleep control group. After a night of recovery sleep, however, performance on the MSL and verbal tasks was similarly good for both groups, indicating that either sleep during the next night or the passage of time strengthened consolidation. Performance on the mirror-tracing task after a period of waking, however, was impaired relative to that of a sleep group, and this difference persisted after several days that included recovery sleep. These results indicate that there was a need for sleep shortly after training to prevent performance deterioration of mirror-tracing skills, and that later sleep periods could not compensate for that deficit (Schönauer et al., 2015). A later review concluded that, for MSL tasks, there is no evidence for a specific time window for sleep consolidation after learning (King et al., 2017), while implicit motor tasks, like mirror-tracing, benefit only from sleep immediately after training (Schönauer et al., 2015).

17.7.1 Summary

A variety of tests have been used to assess the role of sleep in consolidating motor learning, but most studies have used MSL tasks involving rapid finger-tapping. These tasks can involve learning sequences that are either explicit or implicit. Most studies found that sleep benefited memory for explicit learning but not for implicit tasks. However, this contrast may not be the only relevant dimension.

An alternative interpretation is that other aspects can affect whether sleep after training benefits later performance, such as the role of contextual factors in learning and the cognitive strategy underlying the performance of the task. One model suggests that motor learning involves two stages and that sleep benefits only the more cognitive, spatial/sequential representation that is involved in learning the task—and not the specific sequence of motor elements that are performed.

The idea that sleep improves performance of learned sequences by strengthening consolidation was challenged by some analyses. One controversial issue identified was the selection of a baseline value against which later performance was assessed. Addressing these issues led to the conclusion that sleep stabilized performance of learned sequences by preventing deterioration during waking but did not improve the skill level achieved by the end of training. Recent reviews have categorized memory improvement, stabilization, and protection from interference together as "memory enhancement." Using this definition, they concluded that sleep after training enhances memory for MSL tasks, and in some cases motor adaptation tasks, compared to waking.

Studies of other forms of motor learning that include very complicated actions, have produced mixed results, with benefits of later sleep being reported for some tasks but not others. Further research is needed to better understand how experimental designs, instructions to participants, the complexity of the actions involved, and data analysis methods influence the identification of effects of sleep on different forms of motor memory.

17.8 Separate or overlapping roles for NREM and REM sleep?

Studies investigating the roles of different sleep stages in memory consolidation have reached different conclusions about which stages are involved with consolidation of different categories of learning. The proposed roles have included the following:

- that declarative learning is consolidated during NREM sleep (Tucker et al., 2006), and motor learning is consolidated during REM sleep (Plihal & Born, 1997);
- that REM sleep is involved specifically in consolidating emotion-related memories, while NREM sleep is responsible for consolidating other explicit and implicit forms of learning (Ackermann & Rasch, 2014; Groch et al., 2013; Nishida et al., 2009; Prehn-Kristensen et al., 2009; Wagner et al., 2001; Walker, 2010; Wassing et al., 2019);
- that REM sleep enhances memory in rats for arbitrary, "unnatural" tasks (e.g., brightness discrimination) but not for tasks that tap into instinctual behaviors (e.g., maze learning) (Pearlman & Becker, 1973);
- that the level of baseline skill at performing a motor task determines whether N2 or REM sleep is involved in consolidating memory for that task (Peters et al., 2007);
- that REM sleep first promotes and then reduces neural plasticity at different time points after an experience (Dumoulin Bridi et al., 2015; Okesenberg et al., 1996);[12] see Section 18.3.

There is mixed evidence related to each of these proposed connections between sleep stages and memory consolidation (Peigneux et al., 2001). One potential explanation for different conclusions among studies is that memory consolidation proceeds through different phases, which may be supported by different sleep features. As a result, multiple sleep stages may be involved in enhancing consolidation of a single type of memory.

One version of a two-phase model proposed that different sleep stages are involved sequentially in first preparing for, and then inducing, the strengthening of a memory or its integration into memory networks (Fogel et al., 2009; Giuditta et al., 1995; Rasch & Born, 2013); see Section 18.3. One example is the finding that NREM sleep alone during a nap stabilized performance on the VTD task, which otherwise deteriorated, but adding REM sleep enhanced performance (Mednick et al., 2003; Mednick et al., 2002); see Section 17.6. Similarly, early acquisition of a cognitive motor skill was related to N2/N3 fast sleep spindles, while later refinement to achieve a highly skilled level depended on REM sleep (Fogel et al., 2015). Consistent with the idea that consolidation can involve multiple sleep stages, substantial overnight deprivation of either REM sleep or SWS impaired memory for an explicit learning task (Casey et al., 2016).

Another hint as to how both sleep stages might be involved comes from a study that used targeted memory reactivation (discussed in Section 18.11). Sound cues that had been uniquely linked to a subset of newly learned words were played during SWS. Participants later recalled more cued than un-cued words, but *only* if the cued-word stimuli presented during SWS triggered significant amounts of subsequent REM sleep. These results might be explained by reactivation and processing of cued memories during SWS followed by their integration into a vocabulary network during REM sleep (Batterink et al., 2017).

The idea that there are unique connections between single sleep stages and specific types of learning and memory is challenged by other evidence. Some models of involvement of SWS in memory consolidation proposed that the hippocampus is involved in explicit learning online and then engages in an interaction with cortical regions during SWS to consolidate a more permanent version of the memory. However, the idea of a unique link between hippocampal activity and explicit learning is not supported by all studies.

For example, in studies of motor sequence learning, acquisition of either an explicit version (which sleep reinforces) or an implicit version (which is not affected by sleep) was associated with increased hippocampal activity (Schendan et al., 2003). In contrast, a presumably "non-hippocampal" task (novel-object recognition) in rats depended on hippocampal activity during later sleep to establish a long-term memory (Sawangjit et al.,

[12] These results relate to early-life, experience-dependent plasticity in the visual system rather than to an explicit learning task.

2018). As discussed in Chapter 18, an alternative interpretation is that different aspects of hippocampal activity are involved in different types of learning and in consolidating the resulting memories during sleep.

17.8.1 Summary

Evidence of dissociations between the effects of different sleep stages on different kinds of memory suggested that single sleep stages may be linked exclusively to different types of memories. This early hypothesis was challenged by evidence for overlapping roles of different sleep stages in studies using a variety of designs. These results suggested that NREM and REM sleep may play complementary or sequential roles in enhancing memories. One model of this dual role includes sequential involvement of NREM sleep in activating or stabilizing a memory trace, followed by a role for REM sleep in strengthening the memory trace or integrating it into existing knowledge networks.

There is evidence that hippocampal activity, which is known to be involved in explicit memory acquisition, is also increased during acquisition and sleep-dependent consolidation of some types of implicit learning. These findings support the conclusion that there is overlap and interaction among sleep mechanisms involved in several kinds of memory consolidation. Because relatively subtle differences in experimental designs and procedures can influence whether effects of sleep on memory are detected, evidence suggesting an apparent lack of involvement of a particular sleep stage in consolidation should be interpreted cautiously (see next section).

17.9 Modulators of sleep effects on memory

In addition to differences related to the types of learning being studied (explicit, semantic, implicit, motor, etc.), a range of other factors have been reported to modify whether and how sleep affects memory. Factors reported to influence whether sleep or a sleep stage play a role include whether a learning task is context-dependent (Spencer et al., 2006); whether a declarative memory task includes an emotional component (Ackermann & Rasch, 2014); whether a memory is related to an established cognitive schema (Hennies et al., 2016); and whether a task involves acquiring a new skill or refining an existing skill (Fogel & Smith, 2011). Other factors affecting how sleep influences memory include the pattern of training used (spaced vs. massed) (see **Box 17.1**) and the intensity of training, which can provoke sensory or motor fatigue that masks the extent of initial learning (see Sections 17.6 and 17.7). The following sections review several other influences on whether and how sleep appears to influence the process of memory consolidation.

17.9.1 Timing of sleep and testing

The length of sleep and the timing of tests after training can influence whether sleep affects memory. A short nap (~10 min) after a verbal learning task marginally improved performance immediately afterward, but memory was unstable and sensitive to later interference from related stimuli. This improvement was also transient; there was no retained benefit of the naps a week later. Those who had longer naps (~60 min) that included N3 sleep showed better performance immediately afterward, were more resistant to interfering stimuli, and still retained a memory benefit a week later (Alger et al., 2012). Similarly, on a test of free recall of a word list, a short (~6 min) nap improved memory performance immediately relative to a wake condition, but there was greater improvement after longer naps (~36 min) (Lahl et al., 2008).

These results raise the question of whether memory consolidation (presumably involving synaptic strengthening; see Section 18.3) is the mechanism involved in facilitating performance immediately after naps lasting only ~6–10 min. Since these naps did not result in stable benefits, it is possible that there was a transient effect because a nap improved alertness, or there were other acute changes in brain function resulting from the state transitions between wake and sleep. Longer naps have larger, more sustained effects that are also resistant to interference. These effects are more likely to imply the involvement of sleep in strengthening the consolidation of plastic changes in the nervous system. For a review of nap effects on cognition, see Lovato & Lack, 2010.

Several studies found that the timing of testing was important for observing effects of sleep on memory. As discussed in Section 17.7, overnight sleep deprivation after training impaired next-day performance on two motor tasks, one explicit and one implicit, and on two explicit semantic memory tasks. But when tested after 3 or 6 days with free sleep, only the implicit motor task (mirror-tracing) still showed deficits in those who were sleep-deprived immediately after training relative to controls who slept. The immediate deficit in performance on the explicit tasks was reversed during the multiday delay with free sleep, so that there were no differences between those sleep-deprived immediately after training and controls who slept.

These effects were attributed to evidence that the two semantic tasks and an explicit motor sequence task depend on the hippocampus for short-term storage. This would make the memory available for delayed systems-level consolidation involving the hippocampus and cortex during sleep periods on the free-sleep days. Memory for the mirror-tracing task, which likely does not depend on the hippocampus for short-term storage, could only be improved by sleep immediately after training, presumably by affecting motor system plasticity directly.

As a result, the deficit observed immediately after sleep deprivation was sustained over days, with no benefit of later recovery sleep (Schönauer et al., 2015). Regardless of whether this interpretation is correct, the evidence shows that the apparent involvement of sleep in enhancing memory depended on both the type of task studied and the delay between training and testing.

Similarly, in the study discussed in **Box 17.1** involving intensive learning of new facts, sleep after learning improved short-term retention, but the benefit of sleep over waking was lost a week later (Cousins et al., 2021). Thus, the timing of testing after initial training would influence whether sleep did or did not appear to benefit memory.

In studies of motor learning, the extent of the apparent benefit attributable to sleep depended on when after the end of training a baseline performance measure was taken. Performance improved spontaneously during a brief period after training ended, so obtaining a baseline measure before that spontaneous improvement could result in artificially inflating the benefit of subsequent sleep for motor skill consolidation (Pan & Rickard, 2015).

17.9.2 Strength of encoding

Baseline performance during training and the opportunity for rehearsal also modify effects of sleep on memory. When participants were pretested on a subset of learned items after initial training, but before a nap opportunity, their memory benefited from the nap only for the items that received extra rehearsal during the pretest. In addition, sleep benefited only participants whose baseline performance quality fell within the top half for the group (Tucker & Fishbein, 2008). Similarly, memory in older participants on a spatial memory task benefited from sleep for those with better baseline performance but not for those with poor baseline performance (Sonni & Spencer, 2015).

There are, however, limits to how strong baseline performance can be in order to benefit from sleep. After intense encoding of word-pair associations, later sleep did not improve performance, but memory for associations encoded with moderate strength was enhanced (Drosopoulos et al., 2007). The accuracy of spatial memories in another study was improved by targeted memory reactivation during sleep for participants with overall good baseline performance, but not for poor learners. Focusing on the specific items that were cued during sleep, there was improved recall of those items that had been learned moderately well at baseline but no benefit for those that had been learned very accurately (Creery et al., 2015).

A possibly related finding is that performance on three relatively easy motor sequence tasks (5-step sequences performed with 1 or 2 hands, and 9-step sequences performed with 1 hand) benefited somewhat from overnight sleep. However, a more difficult task (a 9-step sequence performed with 2 hands), which was performed less efficiently at baseline, benefited even more from the sleep opportunity (Kuriyama et al., 2004).

Following up on evidence that young adults benefited from sleep after learning a motor sequence but children (6–8 years old in one study and 7–11 in another) did not (Fischer et al., 2007; Wilhelm et al., 2008) (**Figure 17.8**), researchers

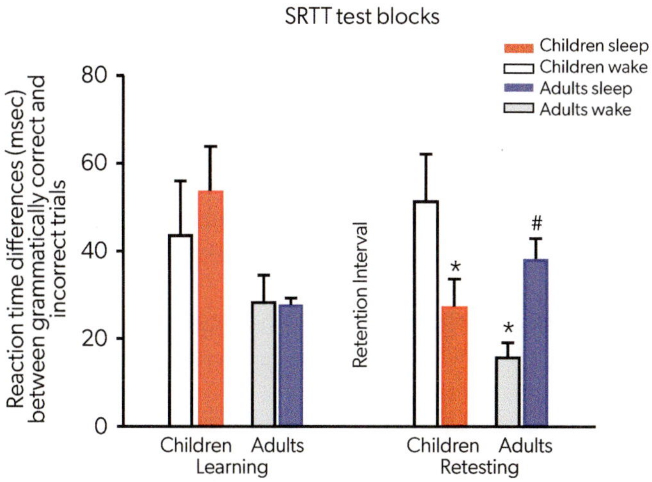

Figure 17.8 **Left:** Performance in children (7–11 years) and adults (20–30 years) at baseline (Learning) on a serial reaction time task (SRTT) that required responding to an apparently random sequence of stimuli that actually included an implicit grammar rule related to letter sequences. The data shown are the *differences* in reaction times (Y axis) to respond to stimuli between the typical, grammatically correct stimuli and the rare, grammatically incorrect stimuli. Large reaction time differences reflect knowledge of the underlying, implicit grammar rule that was being violated. The overall slower average response times of children (~702 ms) as compared to adults (~496 ms) (data not shown) probably account for the resulting larger difference scores in children. The white and gray columns are children and adults assigned to stay awake after training and the red and blue columns are for those assigned to later sleep. **Right:** During retesting following the retention Interval that included either sleep (red) or waking (white), children who slept showed a significant *reduction* in reaction time differences, indicating a loss of implicit knowledge about the grammar rule. However, children who stayed awake during the retention interval showed no significant change in performance (white column, before and after the retention interval). In contrast, adults showed an *increase* in their reaction time differences (blue columns) after sleep, implying consolidation and strengthening of knowledge of the grammar rule, and a *decrease* if they were kept awake (gray columns). *: $p<0.05$ for the comparison to baseline performance; **#:** $p<0.01$ for comparison between sleep and wake conditions. Adapted with permission of The MIT Press from Fischer, S. et al. (2007) Developmental differences in sleep's role for implicit off-line learning: comparing children with adults. *J Cogn Neurosci* 19(2):214–227. © Massachusetts Institute of Technology (2007). doi: 10.1162/jocn.2007.19.2.214.

asked whether the large baseline performance differences between adults and children might be relevant. Children were much slower than adults at baseline in performing this task, reflecting a relatively poor acquisition of the motor skill. The experimenters adjusted training amounts differentially for children (increased) and adults (decreased) to produce a similar range of baseline motor performance in both groups. Both children and adults who achieved very high or low baseline performance did not benefit from a nap opportunity, but those with intermediate baseline performance did benefit, regardless of age (Wilhelm et al., 2012). Thus, the level of baseline performance achieved was a key determinant of whether sleep could enhance memory consolidation; see Section 17.10.1.

Taken together, these studies indicate that very effective learning that results in strong baseline performance does not leave room for further sleep-related enhancement. On the other hand, weak learning resulting in very poor baseline performance apparently does not provide enough substrate for sleep-related processes to act on. Achieving a moderate level of performance before sleep allows the expression of sleep-related enhancement of memory.

There are, however, no standard definitions of "weak" and "strong" learning or what constitutes "very poor" baseline performance across studies. One study operationalized the distinction by presenting word pairs 1, 2, or 4 times. It found that a 2 h nap did not alter the rate of forgetting (relative to a wake control group) over 6 h for participants who had 2 or 4 learning trials. The nap, however, essentially prevented forgetting for the group with 1 trial over 6 or 12 h delays, while the 1-trial wake controls lost >13% and >31% of learned pairings over the two delay intervals (Denis et al., 2021). Based on this outcome, encoding strength after 1 trial would be considered moderate and susceptible to enhancement (in this case, resistance to forgetting) by later sleep, while 2 or 4 learning trials resulted in strong encoding that was not affected by later sleep.

Similarly, participants in a study learned the temporal and spatial arrangements of a set of objects. Those objects for which performance was good at baseline (strong encoding) did not benefit from sleep, apparently because of a ceiling effect. The items that were less well learned at baseline (weaker encoding) showed memory improvement after overnight sleep. Adding retroactive interference to make retrieval of the learned information more difficult resulted in enhanced performance after sleep for items that were both more weakly and strongly encoded. These results indicate that whether an effect of sleep on performance could be detected depended on achieving a moderate strength of initial encoding or having strongly encoded memories weakened by imposed interference (Petzka et al., 2021).

17.9.3 Participants' expectations and motivation

Another variable that influences the involvement of sleep in memory is whether participants anticipate needing to remember the newly learned information. One study used a "directed forgetting" paradigm in which each individual word on a list was tagged as to-be-remembered (R) or to-be-forgotten (F) after initial encoding. Participants recalled both subsets equally well during an immediate recall test. After a nap, however, participants who slept showed better recall of the R words but not of the F words, compared to those kept awake (Saletin et al., 2011).

In a related study, participants were trained on explicit and implicit memory tasks and were then told that they would be retested 9 h later, after a period of either sleep or waking. Those who slept showed better performance when retested, especially on the explicit tasks. Other participants were misled by an instruction that they would be tested on a different task after the 9 h interval. Those who believed (based on a debriefing) the misleading instruction showed no sleep-related benefit when they were instead retested on the original task. Consistent with a critical role for expectations, those who knew or guessed that they would be retested on the original task, showed better performance if they slept after training, but not if they stayed awake. Similar results were obtained with performance on a spatial memory task and a finger-tapping sequence task. Overnight sleep among those expecting to be retested included more SWS and sleep spindles than among those not expecting to be retested (Wilhelm et al., 2011) (**Figure 17.9**).

Participants in another study first learned the spatial locations of images from two different categories (houses and furniture). After training and an initial pretest, participants were misled by being told that only one category of objects would be retested later (e.g., houses). Participants then stayed awake or slept, following which they were retested for *both* categories of objects. Sleep improved memory only for the category that was designated ahead of time as to-be-retested, and the amount of sleep shown correlated with memory enhancement only for that category (van Dongen et al., 2012) (**Figure 17.10**).

Since expectations of retesting were manipulated in these studies either *after* the full learning session or after initial encoding of individual items, instructions about remembering or forgetting could not have influenced the initial learning process. Only the combination of an expectation of future need and intervening sleep improved retention of the learned items. Expecting to be retested, but without a sleep opportunity, did not benefit memory (**Figures 17.9 and 17.10**).

One potential explanation for the effects of expectations is that participants covertly rehearse items that they expect to be retested on before they fall asleep. This rehearsal interpretation

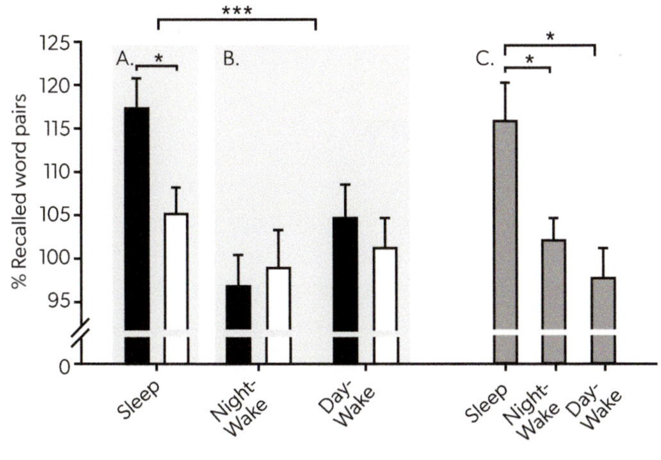

Figure 17.9 How expectations influence participants' later recall of items during a word-pair learning task. Black columns represent participants who were told they would be retested on this task after an interval. White columns represent those who were told they would have a different test after the interval and indicated later that they believed that they would *not* be retested on the original task. **A.** Those who were told they would be retested showed better recall of word-pairs than those who did not think they would be retested, when both groups slept (~7.5 h) before retesting. Note that the % shown on the Y axis represents the difference from baseline performance at the end of training (=100%), so values >100% are possible if recall was better than at baseline testing. **B.** Participants who were told they would be retested (black) or were told they would not be retested (white) did not differ if they stayed awake during the night (night-wake) or the day (day-wake). Those who slept before retesting performed better than those who stayed awake, regardless of their expectations. **C.** Those who were not told they would be retested but reported that they expected to be retested anyway (gray bars), also showed better performance after sleep than after staying awake during either night or day. For those expecting retesting, the quality of performance during retesting was strongly correlated with the number of sleep spindles and with the amount of SWA shown during the sleep period. Reprinted with permission of the Society for Neuroscience from Wilhelm, I. et al. (2011) Sleep selectively enhances memory expected to be of future relevance. *J Neurosci* 31:1563–1569. © The Authors (2011). Licensed under a Creative Commons Attribution License (CC-BY-NC-SA). doi: 10.1523/JNEUROSCI.3575-10.2011.

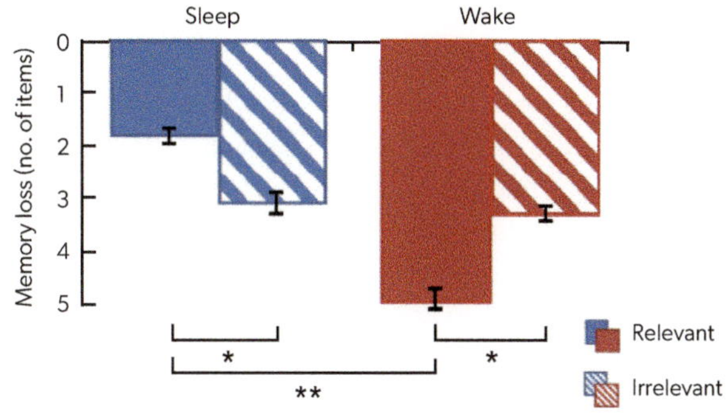

Figure 17.10 Participants in a study of memory for spatial locations were told after training that only one category of stimuli would be retested (Relevant, solid columns) after a period that would be spent either awake (red) or asleep (blue), but instead were retested on both categories of stimuli, including those that they were told would not be retested (Irrelevant; hatched columns). The figure shows results as the extent of memory loss from training to testing (Y axis). Participants showed significantly better memory performance (i.e., less loss) after sleep (left) than after staying awake (right), but only for the items on which they expected to be retested (solid columns). Memory loss for those items on which they expected not to be retested was similar whether they slept or stayed awake (hatched columns). Significant contrasts are shown as * ($p < 0.05$) and ** ($p < 0.005$). Reprinted with permission from van Dongen, E.V. et al. (2012) *PLoS ONE* 7(8): e43426. © van Dongen et al. (2012). This is an open-access article distributed under the terms of a Creative Commons Attribution License. doi:10.1371/journal.pone.0043426.

would be consistent with one model of forgetting, namely, that successful retrieval from memory during rehearsal of some items interferes with later retrieval of other items (Bekinschtein et al., 2018). In the word-pair learning study by (Wilhelm et al., 2011), for example, memory for R items could have been strengthened by covert retrieval and rehearsal before sleep, which would then interfere with retrieval of unrehearsed F items during later testing.

Although rehearsal while awake cannot be ruled out completely, its role in mediating the effects of expectations is unlikely for several reasons. First, lists of words might be relatively easy to rehearse, but it would be more difficult to rehearse expected locations in a spatial memory task or finger-tapping sequence, which were also enhanced by expectations of retesting combined with a sleep opportunity (van Dongen et al., 2012; Wilhelm et al., 2011). Second, those who stayed awake after training and would have had ample opportunity to rehearse did not show a benefit for items on which they expected to be retested. Third, participants in the sleep group of one study played an attention-demanding video game (*Snood*) after training, making it unlikely that they were able to rehearse during the short interval before sleep. Finally, participants who acknowledged during a debriefing that they had actually rehearsed were excluded from the analysis (Wilhelm et al., 2011).

Thus, retrieval and rehearsal of information (internal cueing) during sleep seems the more likely explanation for the effects of expectations. This idea is supported by evidence of changes in sleep (more SWS and sleep spindles) in the group expecting to be retested. It is also supported by evidence that external cueing of specific items during sleep can selectively enhance memory for the cued items (Oudiette et al., 2013); see Section 18.11. Anticipating a future need for new information appears to engage neural processes that enhance memory, perhaps by activating memories of the target information during sleep. Without an expectation of future need, sleep does not improve retention and may even increase forgetting of unneeded information.

Another factor that influences how sleep affects memory consolidation is motivation, including the expectation or experience of reward. Participants in one study were told that improvement during a retest on one of two newly learned finger-tapping sequences would increase payments received. Those who slept after training (but not those who stayed awake) showed selective improvements in performing the sequence linked to an anticipated reward (Fischer & Born, 2009). Another approach was to provide actual rewards for some correct responses during training (in this case, water rewards for thirsty participants) on a version of the VTD task discussed in Section 17.6. The presence of reward during training improved performance during a retest after sleep but not after a period spent awake (Tamaki et al., 2020).

The experience of reward (or its anticipation) for successfully remembering a subset of stimuli must mark these items as the targets of sleep-related processes that enhance memory. One possibility is that during training, participants show increased arousal and attention to stimuli linked to a current reward or to the expectation of a future reward, which "tag" rewarded items for later enhancement during sleep. This process may be one example of how the salience of stimuli in general can facilitate recall, but the nature of the tag and the specific mechanisms involved in enhancing their salience are not known (Oudiette & Paller, 2013). The interpretation that expectations of future need or reward results in more attention to, and better learning of, targeted items cannot, however, explain the effects of labeling one set of items for later retesting only after learning is complete, as in the studies by (van Dongen et al., 2012; Wilhelm et al., 2011).

Despite these convincing demonstrations of effects of manipulating either participants' expectations or the reward value of remembering on the degree to which sleep benefited memory, the full literature on these topics is not consistent. An exhaustive review of published studies concluded that there were at least as many published reports of the absence of such effects as there were of positive findings, and no specific sleep stages were consistently linked to the benefits of sleep, when such benefits occurred (Davidson et al., 2021).

As discussed earlier, one criticism of some studies showing sleep-related memory enhancement is that they involved relatively small numbers of participants, which can increase the risk of finding false-positive results that may not be replicated. Another concern is that attempts to replicate these phenomena often use methods that differ in minor or major ways from the original reports of positive effects. It then becomes difficult to determine whether an apparent lack of confirmation of a phenomenon indicates that the original finding was a spurious result or that detecting the phenomenon is sensitive to some of the altered features of the experimental design or data analytic approach.

17.9.4 Summary

Several procedural differences between studies can determine whether sleep after learning helps preserve or enhance memory. Short naps after learning can improve performance immediately, but this benefit may not persist over days, so later testing may not show any sleep-related benefit. Longer periods of sleep can produce larger enhancements of memory that are more sustained.

Moderate levels of baseline performance after learning allow for strengthening of memory during sleep. Sleep is, however, unlikely to enhance memory for skills or items that are very poorly acquired during learning. In addition, near-perfect performance at baseline after learning may produce a ceiling effect that would not allow detection of a benefit from later sleep.

Participants also show selective enhancement of learned items on which they expect to be retested or for which they anticipate rewards, if they are allowed to sleep after training, relative to periods spent awake. Selective reactivation during sleep of neural traces linked to items targeted for retesting is a likely explanation for how expectations affect sleep-related consolidation. Nevertheless, the evidence that anticipation of retesting or rewards have robust effects on sleep-associated memory consolidation is inconsistent, and the basis for these inconsistencies remains to be determined.

17.10 Sleep effects on memory over the lifespan

17.10.1 Sleep and children's memory

Most studies of the role of sleep in memory have involved young adult participants. Since both sleep and cognitive functions change over the lifespan, it is important to understand whether sleep plays the same or different roles for younger and older people.

Very young infants cannot be tested in the same way as older children or adults. Assessing their memory for an experience often involves measuring systematic changes in infants' gaze, depending on their memory of previously hearing certain language sounds or experiencing pairings of sounds and images. Using these methods, a study of infants ~6 months old showed benefits of a nap compared to a period awake for retaining information about the structure of artificial word segments (Simon et al., 2017). Older infants (9–16 months) also benefited from a nap in retaining and generalizing information about

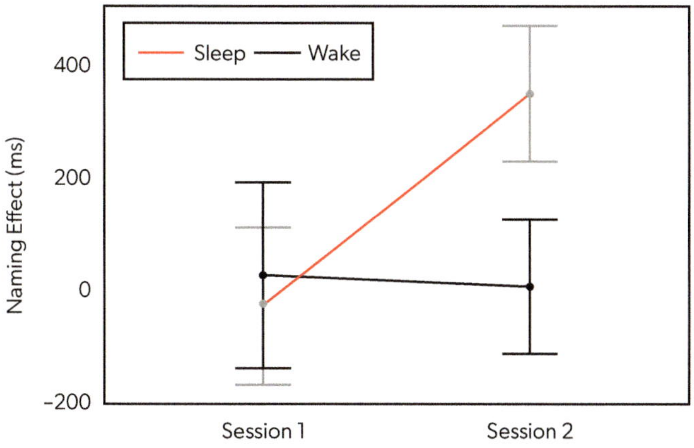

Figure 17.11 Toddlers (~16 months old) were shown images of novel objects with different shapes and colors that were given pseudo-word names. They later slept (red line) for an average of ~1 h or stayed awake (black line) and were tested with two objects shown simultaneously to assess their ability to generalize from training objects to new objects with the same shape and texture but a different color. The measure of knowledge of the correct category names of objects was that infants looked preferentially at an object that had been named. A naming effect (Y axis) of 0 indicates no change in preference for looking at either of the two presented objects as a result of hearing the assigned name of one of the objects. At baseline (Session 1) the two groups showed a similar naming effect. After the sleep or wake opportunity (Session 2), the nap group showed an increase in the time spent looking at the object from the named category after it was named, while those who stayed awake showed no change in behavior. Data shown are means ± standard errors. Reprinted with permission of Oxford University Press from Horváth, K. et al. (2016) A daytime nap facilitates generalization of word meanings in young toddlers. *Sleep* 39:203–207. © Sleep Research Society (2016). doi: 10.5665/sleep.5348.

word categories, language structure, and meaning (Friedrich et al., 2015; Gómez et al., 2006; Horváth et al., 2016; Kurdziel et al., 2013) (**Figure 17.11**).

Studies in older children (3 to 13 years) reported benefits of sleep for declarative, spatial, and emotional declarative memory (Ashworth et al., 2014; Backhaus et al., 2008; Prehn-Kristensen et al., 2009; Wilhelm et al., 2008; Williams & Horst, 2014). Procedural memory, however, did not benefit from sleep in most studies (Prehn-Kristensen et al., 2009; Wilhelm et al., 2008). One exception is a study that used the Tower of Hanoi puzzle,[13] in which memory may have benefited from sleep effects on explicit components of the strategy involved (Ashworth et al., 2014).

As discussed above, studies of implicit and explicit motor memory, which found benefits of sleep among young adults, reported that school-age children not only did not benefit but showed impaired performance if they slept after learning (Fischer et al., 2007; Wilhelm et al., 2008) (see **Figure 17.8**). This result was subsequently shown to depend on differential learning at baseline, with poor skill levels achieved by the children (see left panel of **Figure 17.8**). As discussed in Section 17.9.2, adjusting training to match baseline performance between children (4–6 years) and adults (18–35 years) resulted in similar benefits from sleep among those with intermediate levels of baseline performance (Wilhelm et al., 2012).

A related result was found in a study of effects of sleep on generalization of word learning among toddlers (average age 2.5 years). When tested immediately after training, they showed no evidence of generalization. Those who were tested after a subsequent wake period began to show generalization, while those who had a nap did not. These results indicate that sleep did not benefit, and even impaired the emergence of, generalization of a weakly established semantic skill (Werchan & Gómez, 2014). The evidence that children at different ages showed deterioration rather than improvement after sleep, when initial learning produced relatively poor performance, may be related to findings from a study of song learning in young birds; see **Box 17.2**.

BOX 17.2 Bird Song Learning: Deterioration After Sleep Facilitates Better Final Performance

Interpretation of the effects of sleep on weakly learned skills in children may be informed by the results of a study of juvenile zebra finches (*Taeniopygia guttata*) who were learning to perform their species-typical song. Young finches acquire their songs by imitating the songs of adults. In juvenile finches, sleep after exposure to adult model songs resulted in immediate *deterioration*, rather than improvement, in the juveniles' song performance (i.e., how well it mimicked the adult model song). However, after repeated exposures to a model song, those birds that initially showed the largest performance decrements after sleep eventually developed songs that were closer to the pattern of the model song (Derégnaucourt et al., 2005).

Because several rounds of hearing and mimicking adult songs are needed to perfect performance of the song, an inadequate version could be crystallized early in the learning process if sleep immediately helped to consolidate the first attempted version. Because juveniles' early imitations of the adult song were poor, sleep-related deterioration allowed for the gradual refinement of this partially learned motor skill over several days and eventually contributed to production of a more accurate version.

[13] This strategic puzzle involves moving several different-size rings between pegs to achieve a specific stacking pattern in the fewest moves possible. Learning to perform it efficiently requires both motor/procedural skills and an explicit cognitive strategy.

17.10.2 Sleep and memory in older people

The involvement of sleep in memory consolidation has also been studied in older adults, among whom problems with both sleep and memory are quite common. Although a few studies reported that declarative memory in older people was strengthened by sleep (Aly & Moscovitch, 2010; Wilson et al., 2012), most found reduced or no benefit of sleep for declarative memory consolidation compared to the benefits seen in younger adults (Backhaus et al., 2007; Baran et al., 2016; Mander et al., 2015; Mander et al., 2013; Scullin, 2013; Scullin et al., 2017).

Similarly, older people (and even middle-aged adults) did not benefit from sleep with respect to procedural learning (Spencer et al., 2007; Wilson et al., 2012). For reviews, see (Backhaus et al., 2015; Pace-Schott & Spencer, 2011; Rasch & Born, 2013; Scullin & Bliwise, 2015). One study suggested that reduced fine-motor dexterity in older people contributed to the apparent lack of benefit of sleep for motor tasks (Gudberg et al., 2015). In many studies, however, older and younger people performed equally well after initial training, but older people still did not benefit as much from post-training sleep.

Reduced benefits of sleep for consolidation of declarative memories in older people has been correlated with several brain changes during aging:

- reductions in SWS/SWA (Backhaus et al., 2007; Mander et al., 2015; Mander et al., 2013; Scullin, 2013; Scullin et al., 2017; Westerberg et al., 2012); see Chapter 4);
- loss of frontal lobe gray matter (Mander et al., 2013);
- reductions in sleep spindle numbers (Clawson et al., 2016; Crowley et al., 2002; Seeck-Hirschner et al., 2012);
- disrupted white matter integrity and loss of spindle synchrony with other EEG features (Helfrich et al., 2018; Mander et al., 2017).

Disrupted white-matter integrity (reflecting changes in neural projections) during aging may reduce the efficiency of hippocampal-cortical communication and its timing relative to cortical slow oscillations and sleep spindles. These features play a critical role in the neural plasticity involved in memory consolidation, as discussed in Section 18.6). Thus, changes in sleep physiology appear to underlie aging-related changes in the contribution of sleep to procedural and declarative memory consolidation.

Intentional (or prospective) memory is often the topic of complaints by older people and perhaps less commonly among younger people. It refers to remembering to carry out a planned activity. A typical failure of intentional memory involves forgetting after a delay period to do something that had been scheduled previously (e.g., taking a medication, going to an appointment). Another common form that can occur over very short delays involves a person going to a nearby room or other location with a clear intention that is forgotten by the time they arrive.

In young adults, experimental intentional memory was reported to be better preserved after overnight sleep than after an equivalent duration awake (Scullin & McDaniel, 2010). The benefit was attributed to SWS because 3 h of early sleep (SWS-enriched), rather than 3 h of late sleep (REM sleep-enriched), stabilized intentional memory (Diekelmann et al., 2013). As discussed earlier, split-night studies are not pure measures of the involvement of specific sleep stages, since each half of the night normally includes some amount of both NREM and REM sleep.

Another study compared retention of planned responses to cues that were either logically related to the response (e.g., the cue "clock" paired with the response of setting an alarm) or to cues that involved unrelated pairings (e.g., the cue "mirror" paired with the response of opening a book). Young adults (19–25, average ~22 years) benefited from overnight sleep for retention of the related but not the unrelated pairs. Older adults (57–77, average ~66 years), however, did not benefit from sleep for retention of prospective memories regardless of the type of pairing (Leong et al., 2021). Consistent with this result, a study of adults aged 18–84 years found that retention of intentional memories deteriorated with age. However, NREM sleep measures were not related to memory retention, independently of the effects of age. Instead, memory deterioration was mediated by reduced amounts of overnight REM sleep, regardless of age (Scullin et al., 2019).

These results contrast with most studies of declarative memory, which have associated poorer performance in older people with reduced NREM sleep features (SWS/SWA and/or sleep spindles) (Backhaus et al., 2007; Clawson et al., 2016; Mander et al., 2015; Mander et al., 2013; Scullin, 2013; Scullin et al., 2017; Seeck-Hirschner et al., 2012; Westerberg et al., 2012). There is indirect supportive evidence, however, from a prospective, population-based study, which reported that poorer general cognitive performance in older adults was associated with lower amounts of REM sleep and increased amounts of N1 sleep, while there was no relation to amounts of N2 and N3 sleep (Song et al., 2015).

These different results may reflect complementary roles of NREM and REM sleep in memory enhancement (see Section 17.8) that may be differentially salient, depending on the procedures used in different studies. For example, the study implicating SWS in intentional memory allowed 3 h sleep opportunities at two different times of night (Diekelmann et al., 2013), while the study implicating REM sleep, but not

NREM sleep, assessed the relationship between intentional memory and the total amount of each stage during a full overnight sleep period (Scullin et al., 2019). There is, therefore, agreement that aging reduces the maintenance of intentional memories, but the degree to which this depends on changes in NREM and REM sleep remains to be clarified.

17.10.3 Summary

Sleep consolidates new learning in children, especially declarative and language-related knowledge, starting at a very young age. Children also show benefits of sleep for consolidation of procedural memory if they achieve a moderate level of baseline performance before sleep. Sleep does not improve poorly learned motor or semantic skills in children and may instead contribute to skill deterioration. This role of sleep appears to prevent premature crystallization of an incompletely learned skill.

During aging, the deterioration of frontal cortical anatomy, reduced spindle numbers, altered synchrony of spindles with slow waves, reduced white-matter integrity, and reductions in SWS amounts have been linked to reduced sleep benefits for declarative memories. Consolidation of intentional memory is strengthened by sleep, but there is no agreement as to whether this benefit is related to NREM or REM sleep. Changes in either sleep stage may contribute to the decline in retention of planned behaviors in older people.

17.11 Insight and problem-solving during sleep

17.11.1 Evidence for sleep improving insight

There are well-known anecdotes about people who developed creative solutions to difficult problems during sleep. One example relates to the pharmacologist Otto Loewi, who in 1921 demonstrated the chemical nature of neural signaling, involving release of acetylcholine in the heart, for which he subsequently won a Nobel Prize (1936). He reported that the design for this study, which revolutionized research into neural communication, came to him during a dream.[14]

The chemist Friedrich August Kekulé had been struggling with trying to conceive of a molecular structure that would account for the physicochemical properties of the benzene molecule. He reported that in 1852 he came up with a solution while drowsing by a fire. He had a vision of molecular strings twisting in snake-like fashion and ultimately forming rings. He awoke with the realization that a ring structure could account for the known characteristics of the molecule, which was a turning point in the development of organic and synthetic chemistry.[15]

These and similar dramatic stories have fed the belief that the sleeping brain can develop solutions to problems that the waking brain cannot easily reach. In each case, the individual involved had been trying to solve the problem while awake but attributed a final breakthrough to an idea that appeared during sleep. A possible basis for such creativity might be that the association of incongruous elements that is characteristic of many dreams could lead to novel insights or avenues of thought.

Anecdotes, however, are not objective evidence, and Kekulé himself warned against publishing musings that are not supported by experimental evidence (Rothenberg, 1995). Experimental studies related to whether sleep plays a role in solving more mundane problems have produced mixed results. One issue is the great variety of tasks that can fall under the heading of "problem solving." The role of sleep in this process has been studied using tasks that included detecting hidden regularities in presented stimuli; solving riddles, puzzles, or anagrams; guessing the basis of "magic" tricks; rearranging visual stimuli or objects to produce non-obvious patterns; and restructuring a problem involving logical reasoning. These examples cover a wide range of complexity and of dependence on language, logic, or visual imagery. They undoubtedly involve many different mental processes, but their common element is that the solutions to these problems require a non-obvious insight.

Participants in one study performed a series of simple logic problems (steps) to get to a final numerical answer at the end of step 7 in each series. Each series, however, also contained a hidden structure, such that the final answer at step 7 was always the same as a very early answer, at step 2. Participants who detected this regularity could subsequently provide the correct answer to each series after step 2. After initial experience with a series of these problems, participants were retested following an 8 h period spent either awake or asleep. Of those who remained awake, 23% reached the insightful solution at step 2, but 59% of participants who had a sleep opportunity reached the insightful solution (Wagner et al., 2004) (**Figure 17.12**).

---

[14] Loewi apparently wrote down the design of the experiment after awakening but could not read his scrawled note in the morning. It was only after a second dream involving the design that he undertook the crucial experiment (McCoy & Tan, 2014).

[15] This event is often cited as a prime example of creative insight during sleep, but this interpretation has been seriously questioned. The roots of Kekulé's insights have been traced to much earlier work he performed, and the "dream" report was made many years after the event. It is also not clear that he was claiming to have been asleep, since the German word he used was "Halbschlaf," literally "half-sleep," which has been interpreted as "dozing" (Rothenberg, 1995).

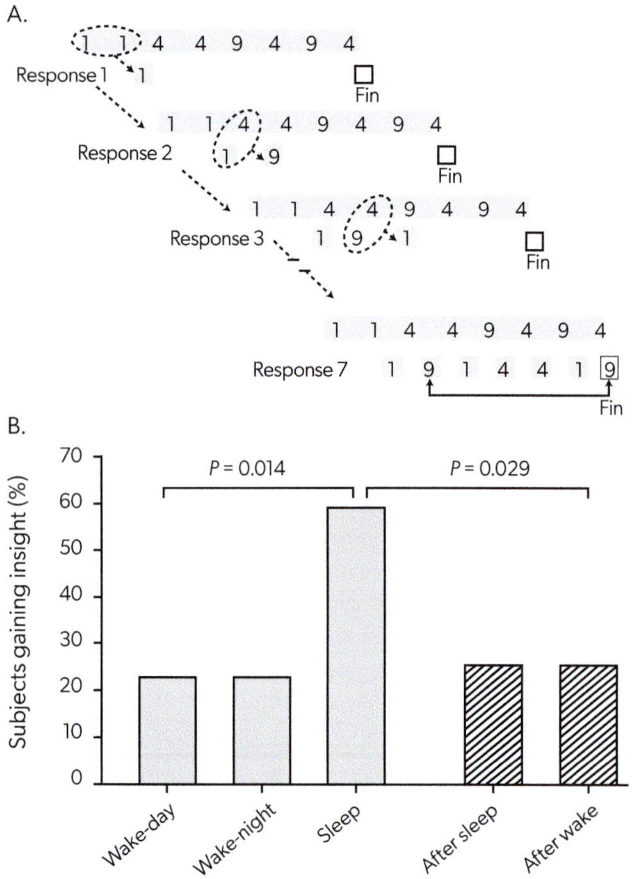

Figure 17.12 **A.** Participants responded with the numbers 1, 4, or 9 to a series of presentations of pairs of these same numbers. The response rule was that if two numbers were the same, the correct response was that number (e.g., Response 1; 1/1→1). If the paired numbers were different, the correct response was the third number (e.g., Response 2; 1/4→9). The overall goal was to provide the "correct" answer to the logic problem (Fin) after the seventh presentation (Response 7). Participants were not informed that the sequence of numbers presented was structured so that the final answer (Response 7) was always the same as Response 2. If participants recognized this structural regularity over several different series of presentations, they could solve a new series after Response 2, rather than going through all seven steps. Thus, providing the final answer at Step 2 indicated that participants had achieved insight into this structural regularity. **B.** Participants who were trained on the task and were then awake either during the day or night (Wake-day; Wake-night) had a ~23% rate of showing the insightful solution (i.e., providing the final answer after Response 2), while those tested after a period of sleep (Sleep) showed a 59% rate of producing the insightful solution. Those who had no prior exposure to the task and were tested for the first time after sleep or wake periods (After sleep and After wake) found the insightful solution about as often as those with earlier experience with the task and no sleep. Reprinted with permission from Wagner, U. et al. (2004) Sleep inspires insight. *Nature* 427:352–355. © Springer: Nature (2004). doi: 10.1038/nature02223.

A subsequent study using the same logic problem allowed participants only a 20 min break, during which they could rest or sleep while being monitored with EEG recordings, before beginning another series of trials. Of participants who reached N1 sleep for at least one 30 sec scoring epoch, but no deeper sleep stage, 80% achieved the insightful solution during the second series. Only 23% of those who did not enter N1 sleep did so. Participants who entered N1 and continued into N2 sleep during the break, did not show an increase in the likelihood of achieving the solution relative to those with no sleep. In addition, the likelihood of finding the insightful solution was highest for those whose EEG during the break showed on average a moderate level of delta-frequency activity and high activity in the alpha range, which are characteristic of N1 sleep (Lacaux et al., 2021).

A very different test, the Remote Associates Task, requires participants to discover a word that forms semantic (i.e., related to meaning) links with several other words that appear superficially to be unrelated (e.g., age, mile, sand).[16] In one study, sleep provided no benefit for solving easy problems of this type, but did facilitate identifying more remote and difficult associations (Sio et al., 2013). In another study, participants generally showed similar success after periods spent either awake or asleep, but there was evidence for a benefit of sleep under one experimental condition. When the key target word was first "primed" by getting participants to use it while engaged in a completely different task, naps that included REM sleep increased the number of successful solutions to the problem (Cai et al., 2009). This result suggests that recent use of a word made it more readily available to be manipulated during later (REM) sleep and to be identified as the solution to the problem.

In a study of insightful solutions to a problem encountered while playing a video game, participants played until they spent 10 min unable to solve a problem at their current level in the game. Following a 90 min waking break or nap opportunity, they were retested at the unsolved level. Among those who slept, 12/14 solved the problem, while among those who stayed awake, only 7/15 were successful. The majority of those who solved the problem after sleep (9/12) had generated SWS and 7/12 had generated REM sleep during their nap (Beijamini et al., 2014).

In a study involving many different puzzles, each was repeatedly linked to a distinctive sound. Participants attempted to solve all puzzles until they had accumulated six unsolved puzzles. They were later exposed during N3 sleep to

[16] The word "stone" forms a compound with each of these apparently unrelated words.

the sounds linked to this subset of unsolved puzzles (an example of targeted memory reactivation; see Section 18.11). The next day, more puzzles that had been cued by linked sounds during N3 sleep were solved (~32%) than those that had not been cued (~21%). These results suggest that reactivating memories of the unsolved puzzles during sleep allowed additional work to be performed on them. It is not known whether this work occurred during exposure to the sounds in N3 sleep or during later sleep stages, once memories had been reactivated (Sanders et al., 2019). There is other evidence, for example, that NREM and REM sleep stages can be involved sequentially in generating novel solutions to problems (Lewis et al., 2018).

For some categories of problems, however, the experimental evidence indicates that sleep does not increase the probability of insightful solutions. For solving riddles and anagrams, solution rates increased similarly after the passage of time regardless of whether it was spent asleep or awake (Brodt et al., 2018). In contrast, neither a break spent awake nor a period of sleep improved solution rates for a problem requiring complex cognitive restructuring (Schönauer et al., 2018).

17.11.2 Potential neural mechanisms

One potential account for why sleep can aid insight for some problems focuses on the involvement of REM sleep. It starts with the observation that there is reduced metabolism in the frontal cortex, as well as functional disconnection of frontal regions from other cortical areas, during REM sleep (Braun et al., 1997; Maquet et al., 1996); see Section 12.5. Frontal cortical regions are involved in executive functions, including judgment, response inhibition, and regulation of attention and emotional expression. Functional disconnection between frontal and other cortical regions has been hypothesized to permit irrational thoughts, bizarre associations among narrative elements, and disinhibited expression of emotions that characterize some dreams.

REM sleep could facilitate solutions to some classes of problems by allowing the spread of memory-related activation more broadly than in NREM sleep (Massimini et al., 2010) (see **Figure 12.7**) and because there is reduced frontal inhibition acting on other brain regions relative to waking. The distinction between tonic and phasic REM sleep may be important. Spread of neural activity across cortical regions in response to sensory input is reduced during deep NREM and phasic REM sleep (see **Figures 12.5 B and 12.6**), but there is a more wake-like spread of activation during tonic REM sleep (see **Figure 12.5 B**) (Wehrle et al., 2007). This result suggests that during tonic REM sleep, internally generated neural activity may also spread more widely among cortical regions. This idea is consistent with evidence that during tonic REM sleep there is a low threshold for external stimuli to trigger arousal, which depends on propagation of signals from primary sensory to other cortical regions (Ermis et al., 2010) (see **Figure 12.5 A**).

Combined with reduced frontal inhibitory connections to other cortical regions, an increased spread of activation across the cortex may allow generation of new functional links. Without the habitual constraints of waking thought patterns, activity during tonic REM sleep may contribute to identifying hidden regularities or increasing the breadth of semantic associations, thereby helping to solve some puzzles and word problems. But these changes may be inadequate to deal with problems that require higher-order mental operations, such as cognitive restructuring, which may depend on the frontal lobes and their connections to other areas (Schönauer et al., 2018).

The evidence that playing puzzle-linked sounds during SWS facilitated later solutions to puzzles (Sanders et al., 2019), combined with the idea that REM sleep may play a role by facilitating novel links among cortical regions, is consistent with other suggestions that SWS and REM sleep may be jointly involved in sleep-related memory processes (Giuditta et al., 1995). Other examples discussed above (Section 17.8) suggest that these stages exert joint effects on memory. These include overlapping roles of SWS and REM sleep in processes like sensory learning (Mednick et al., 2002; Stickgold, Whidbee, et al., 2000; Strauss et al., 2022), vocabulary learning (Batterink et al., 2017), cognitive motor skills (Fogel et al., 2015), and both explicit and implicit memory (Casey et al., 2016).

These lines of evidence suggest potential roles for REM sleep in combination with SWS in facilitating creative cognitions and novel connections among ideas that could permit development of solutions to problems. Reactivation of a memory during SWS may generate replay of neural activity related to the memory and make it available for manipulation, association, or integration during subsequent REM sleep.

This idea, however, cannot explain why very short experiences of N1 sleep were associated with more frequent insight into the structure of a numerical logic problem in one study, nor why adding N2 sleep eliminated this benefit (Lacaux et al., 2021). This finding is, however, consistent with Kekulé dozing by a fire when he solved the benzene ring structure in a state of "half-sleep," which sounds similar to N1. Whether N1 or N3/REM sleep are more useful for solving problems may depend on the type of problem involved and the extent of waking effort already committed to solving it. But it remains to be determined whether different sleep stages are linked to solving different kinds of problems.

The anecdotes about important discoveries made during sleep are intriguing and have helped inspire research showing that some categories of information can be activated, integrated, and reinforced during sleep and that these processes can prompt novel solutions to problems. Another anecdote, however, provides a cautionary tale about insights achieved during different states of consciousness. This one appeared in a lecture delivered in 1870 by the American physician and author, Oliver Wendell Holmes, Sr. He reported that under the influence of a potent dose of ether, he had the feeling of having a profound insight into "all-embracing truth," which he then wrote down. On regaining consciousness, he examined his note and read: "A strong smell of turpentine prevails throughout" (Holmes, 1879).

17.11.3 Summary

There are several frequently cited anecdotes about important insights and solutions to problems that were attributed to mental activity during sleep. The results from experimental studies aimed at demonstrating these benefits of sleep for problem-solving are mixed. Sleep facilitated some creative processes, including identifying an insightful short-cut to the solution of a logic problem, extracting statistical regularities from sets of stimuli, and solving puzzles when related memories were prompted by external stimulation during SWS. Some of these reported sleep-related benefits were, however, quite small. More cognitively complex problem-solving did not seem to benefit from sleep in experimental settings.

During tonic REM sleep, the loss of frontal inhibitory input combined with increased spread of activity across other cortical regions in response to inputs may facilitate interactions that generate both irrational associations among dream elements and the recognition of previously undetected patterns and connections. Both NREM and REM sleep appear to contribute, perhaps sequentially, to generating novel solutions to some simpler problems. However, another finding implied that insight might occur after experiencing only a brief transition phase between waking and sleep, and that other sleep phases could even interfere with that benefit. More research into the involvement of sleep and its stages in providing useful (and in some cases, perhaps misleading) insights into different categories of problems will be needed to clarify the relations among types of problems, sleep stages, and solutions.

Literature cited

Ackermann, S., Hartmann, F., Papassotiropoulos, A., de Quervain, D. J., & Rasch, B. (2015). No associations between interindividual differences in sleep parameters and episodic memory consolidation. *Sleep, 38*(6), 951–959. doi: 10.5665/sleep.4748

Ackermann, S., & Rasch, B. (2014). Differential effects of non-REM and REM sleep on memory consolidation? *Curr Neurol Neurosci Rep, 14*(2), 430. doi: 10.1007/s11910-013-0430-8

Adi-Japha, E., & Karni, A. (2016). Time for considering constraints on procedural memory consolidation processes: comment on Pan and Rickard (2015) with specific reference to developmental changes. *Psychol Bull, 142*(5), 568–571. doi: 10.1037/bul0000048

Albouy, G., Fogel, S., Pottiez, H., Nguyen, V. A., Ray, L., Lungu, O., ... Doyon, J. (2013). Daytime sleep enhances consolidation of the spatial but not motoric representation of motor sequence memory. *PLoS One, 8*(1), e52805. doi:10.1371/journal.pone.0052805

Alger, S. E., Lau, H., & Fishbein, W. (2012). Slow wave sleep during a daytime nap is necessary for protection from subsequent interference and long-term retention. *Neurobiol Learn Mem, 98*(2), 188–196. doi: 10.1016/j.nlm.2012.06.003

Aly, M., & Moscovitch, M. (2010). The effects of sleep on episodic memory in older and younger adults. *Memory, 18*(3), 327–334. doi: 10.1080/09658211003601548

Ashworth, A., Hill, C. M., Karmiloff-Smith, A., & Dimitriou, D. (2014). Sleep enhances memory consolidation in children. *J Sleep Res, 23*(3), 302–308. doi: 10.1111/jsr.12119

Backhaus, J., Born, J., Hoeckesfeld, R., Fokuhl, S., Hohagen, F., & Junghanns, K. (2007). Midlife decline in declarative memory consolidation is correlated with a decline in slow wave sleep. *Learn Mem, 14*(5), 336–341. doi: 10.1101/lm.470507

Backhaus, J., Hoeckesfeld, R., Born, J., Hohagen, F., & Junghanns, K. (2008). Immediate as well as delayed post learning sleep but not wakefulness enhances declarative memory consolidation in children. *Neurobiol Learn Mem, 89*(1), 76–80. doi: 10.1016/j.nlm.2007.08.010

Backhaus, W., Kempe, S., & Hummel, F. C. (2015). The effect of sleep on motor learning in the aging and stroke population - a systematic review. *Restor Neurol Neurosci, 34*(1), 153–164. doi: 10.3233/RNN-150521

Baran, B., Mantua, J., & Spencer, R. M. (2016). Age-related changes in the sleep-dependent reorganization of declarative memories. *J Cogn Neurosci, 28*(6), 792–802. doi: 10.1162/jocn_a_00938

Baran, B., Pace-Schott, E. F., Ericson, C., & Spencer, R. M. (2012). Processing of emotional reactivity and emotional memory over sleep. *J Neurosci, 32*(3), 1035–1042. doi: 10.1523/JNEUROSCI.2532-11.2012

Barham, M. P., Enticott, P. G., Conduit, R., & Lum, J. A. (2016). Transcranial electrical stimulation during sleep enhances declarative (but not procedural) memory consolidation: evidence from a meta-analysis. *Neurosci Biobehav Rev, 63*, 65–77. doi: 10.1016/j.neubiorev.2016.01.009

Barrett, T. E., & Ekstrand, B. R. (1972). Effect of sleep on memory: III. controlling for time-of-day effects. *J Exp Psychol, 96*(2), 321–327.

Batterink, L. J., Westerberg, C. E., & Paller, K. A. (2017). Vocabulary learning benefits from REM after slow-wave sleep. *Neurobiol Learn Mem, 144*, 102–113. doi: 10.1016/j.nlm.2017.07.001

Beijamini, F., Pereira, S. I., Cini, F. A., & Louzada, F. M. (2014). After being challenged by a video game problem, sleep increases the chance to solve it. *PLoS One, 9*(1), e84342. doi:10.1371/journal.pone.0084342

Bekinschtein, P., Weisstaub, N. V., Gallo, F., Renner, M., & Anderson, M. C. (2018). A retrieval-specific mechanism of adaptive forgetting in the mammalian brain. *Nat Commun, 9*(1), 4660. doi: 10.1038/s41467-018-07128-7

Born, J., Rasch, B., & Gais, S. (2006). Sleep to remember. *Neuroscientist, 12*(5), 410–424. doi: 10.1177/1073858406292647

Born, J. A. N., & Wagner, U. (2004). Memory consolidation during sleep: role of cortisol feedback. *Ann NY Acad Sci, 1032*(1), 198–201. doi: 10.1196/annals.1314.020

Bothe, K., Hirschauer, F., Wiesinger, H. P., Edfelder, J. M., Gruber, G., Hoedlmoser, K., & Birklbauer, J. (2019). Gross motor adaptation benefits from sleep after training. *J Sleep Res*, e12961. doi: 10.1111/jsr.12961

Boyce, R., Glasgow, S., Williams, S., & Adamantidis, A. (2016). Causal evidence for the role of REM sleep theta rhythm in contextual memory consolidation. *Science, 352*(6287), 812–816.

Boyce, R., Williams, S., & Adamantidis, A. (2017). REM sleep and memory. *Curr Opin Neurobiol, 44*, 167–177. doi: 10.1016/j.conb.2017.05.001

Braun, A., Balkin, T., Wesensten, N., Carson, R., Varga, M., Baldwin, P., ... Herscovitch, P. (1997). Regional cerebral blood flow throughout the sleep-wake cycle: an $H_2{}^{15}O$ PET study. *Brain, 120*, 1173–1197.

Brawn, T., Nusbaum, H., & Margoliash, D. (2010). Sleep-dependent consolidation of auditory discrimination learning in adult starlings. *J Neurosci, 30*(2), 609–613. doi: 0.1523/JNEUROSCI.4237-09.2010

Brawn, T. P., Fenn, K. M., Nusbaum, H. C., & Margoliash, D. (2010). Consolidating the effects of waking and sleep on motor-sequence learning. *J Neurosci, 30*(42), 13977–13982. doi: 10.1523/JNEUROSCI.3295-10.2010

Brodt, S., Pöhlchen, D., Täumer, E., Gais, S., & Schönauer, M. (2018). Incubation, not sleep, aids problem-solving. *Sleep, 41*(10), zsy155. doi: 10.1093/sleep/zsy155/5065174

Cai, D. J., Mednick, S. A., Harrison, E. M., Kanady, J. C., & Mednick, S. C. (2009). REM, not incubation, improves creativity by priming associative networks. *Proc Natl Acad Sci U S A, 106*(25), 10130–10134. doi: 10.1073/pnas.0900271106

Cai, D. J., & Rickard, T. C. (2009). Reconsidering the role of sleep for motor memory. *Behav Neurosci, 123*(6), 1153–1157. doi: 10.1037/a0017672

Callaway, C. W., Lydic, R., Baghdoyan, H. A., & Hobson, J. A. (1987). Pontogeniculooccipital waves: Spontaneous visual system activity during rapid eye movement sleep. *Cell Mol Neurobiol, 7*, 105–149.

Casey, S. J., Solomons, L. C., Steier, J., Kabra, N., Burnside, A., Pengo, M. F., … Kopelman, M. D. (2016). Slow wave and REM sleep deprivation effects on explicit and implicit memory during sleep. *Neuropsychology, 30*(8), 931–945. doi: 10.1037/neu0000314

Censor, N., Karni, A., & Sagi, D. (2006). A link between perceptual learning, adaptation and sleep. *Vis Res, 46*, 4071–4074. doi: 0.1016/j.visres.2006.07.022

Censor, N., & Sagi, D. (2009). Global resistance to local perceptual adaptation in texture discrimination. *Vis Res, 49*, 2550–2556. doi: 10.1016/j.visres.2009.03.018

Clawson, B. C., Durkin, J., & Aton, S. J. (2016). Form and function of sleep spindles across the lifespan. *Neur Plast, 2016*, 6936381. doi: 10.1155/2016/6936381

Cousins, J. N., Sasmita, K., & Chee, M. W. L. (2018). Memory encoding is impaired after multiple nights of partial sleep restriction. *J Sleep Res, 27*(1), 138–145. doi: 10.1111/jsr.12578

Cousins, J. N., Teo, T. B., Tan, Z. Y., Wong, K. F., & Chee, M. W. L. (2021). Sleep after learning aids the consolidation of factual knowledge, but not relearning. *Sleep, 44*(3), zsaa210. doi: 10.1093/sleep/zsaa210

Cousins, J. N., Wong, K. F., Raghunath, B. L., Look, C., & Chee, M. W. L. (2019). The long-term memory benefits of a daytime nap compared with cramming. *Sleep, 42*(1), zsy207. doi:10.1093/sleep/zsy207/5146032

Creery, J. D., Oudiette, D., Antony, J. W., & Paller, K. A. (2015). Targeted memory reactivation during sleep depends on prior learning. *Sleep, 38*(5), 755–763. doi: 10.5665/sleep.4670

Crowley, K., Trinder, J., Kim, Y., Carrington, M., & Colrain, I. M. (2002). The effects of normal aging on sleep spindle and K-complex production. *Clin Neurophysiol, 113*, 1615–1622.

Dastgheib, M., Kulanayagam, A., & Dringenberg, H. C. (2022). Is the role of sleep in memory consolidation overrated? *Neurosci Biobehav Rev, 140*, 104799. doi: 10.1016/j.neubiorev.2022.104799

Datta, S. (2000). Avoidance task training potentiates phasic pontine-wave density in the rat: a mechanism for sleep-dependent plasticity. *J Neurosci, 20*(22), 8607–8613.

Davidson, P., Jönsson, P., Carlsson, I., & Pace-Schott, E. (2021). Does sleep selectively strengthen certain memories over others based on emotion and perceived future relevance? *Nat Sci Sleep, Volume 13*, 1257–1306. doi: 10.2147/nss.S286701

Deliens, G., Leproult, R., Neu, D., & Peigneux, P. (2013). Rapid eye movement and non-rapid eye movement sleep contributions in memory consolidation and resistance to retroactive interference for verbal material. *Sleep, 36*(12), 1875–1883. doi: 10.5665/sleep.3220

Denis, D., Mylonas, D., Poskanzer, C., Bursal, V., Payne, J. D., & Stickgold, R. (2021). Sleep spindles preferentially consolidate weakly encoded memories. *J Neurosci, 41*(18), 4088–4099. doi: 10.1523/JNEUROSCI.0818-20.2021

Derégnaucourt, S., Mitra, P. P., Fehér, O., Pytte, C., & Tchernichovski, O. (2005). How sleep affects the developmental learning of bird song. *Nature, 433*(7027), 710–716. doi: 10.1038/nature03275

Diekelmann, S., Wilhelm, I., & Born, J. (2009). The whats and whens of sleep-dependent memory consolidation. *Sleep Med Rev, 13*(5), 309–321. doi: 10.1016/j.smrv.2008.08.002

Diekelmann, S., Wilhelm, I., Wagner, U., & Born, J. (2013). Sleep to implement an intention. *Sleep, 36*(1), 149–153. doi: 10.5665/sleep.2322

Doyon, J., Gabitov, E., Vahdat, S., Lungu, O., & Boutin, A. (2018). Current issues related to motor sequence learning in humans. *Curr Opin Behav Sci, 20*, 89–97. doi: 10.1016/j.cobeha.2017.11.012

Doyon, J., Korman, M., Morin, A., Dostie, V., Tahar, A. H., Benali, H., Karni, A., Ungerleider, L. G., & Carrier, J. (2009). Contribution of night and day sleep vs. simple passage of time to the consolidation of motor sequence and visuomotor adaptation learning. *Exp Brain Res, 195*(1), 15–26. doi: 10.1007/s00221-009-1748-y

Drosopoulos, S., Schulze, C., Fischer, S., & Born, J. (2007). Sleep's function in the spontaneous recovery and consolidation of memories. *J Exp Psychol Gen, 136*(2), 169–183. doi: 10.1037/0096-3445.136.2.169

Drummond, S. P. A., Brown, G. G., GIllin, J. C., Stricker, J. L., Wong, E. C., & Buxton, R. B. (2000). Altered brain response to verbal learning following sleep deprivation. *Nature, 403*, 655–657.

Dumoulin Bridi, M. C., Aton, S. J., Seibt, J., Renouard, L., Coleman, T., & Frank, M. G. (2015). Rapid eye movement sleep promotes cortical plasticity in the developing brain. *Sci Adv, 1*(6), e1500105. doi: 10.1126/sciadv.1500105

Ellenbogen, J. M., Hulbert, J. C., Stickgold, R., Dinges, D. F., & Thompson-Schill, S. L. (2006). Interfering with theories of sleep and memory: sleep, declarative memory, and associative interference. *Curr Biol, 16*(13), 1290–1294. doi: 10.1016/j.cub.2006.05.024

Ermis, U., Krakow, K., & Voss, U. (2010). Arousal thresholds during human tonic and phasic REM sleep. *J Sleep Res, 19*(3), 400–406. doi: 10.1111/j.1365-2869.2010.00831.x

Farber, J., Marks, G. A., & Roffwarg, H. P. (1980). Rapid eye movement sleep PGO-type waves are present in the dorsal pons of the albino rat. *Science, 209*(4456), 615–617.

Fischer, S., & Born, J. (2009). Anticipated reward enhances offline learning during sleep. *J Exp Psychol Learn Mem Cogn, 35*(6), 1586–1593. doi: 10.1037/a0017256

Fischer, S., Drosopoulos, S., Tsen, J., & Born, J. (2006). Implicit learning -- explicit knowing: a role for sleep in memory system interaction. *J Cogn Neurosci, 18*(3), 311–319.

Fischer, S., Hallschmid, M., Elsner, A. L., & Born, J. (2002). Sleep forms memory for finger skills. *Proc Natl Acad Sci USA, 99*(18), 11987–11991. doi: 10.1073/pnas.182178199

Fischer, S., Wilhelm, I., & Born, J. (2007). Developmental differences in sleep's role for implicit off-line learning: comparing children with adults. *J Cogn Neurosci, 19*(2), 214–227. doi: 10.1162/jocn.2007.19.2.214

Fogel, S., Smith, C. T., & Cote, K. (2007). Dissociable learning-dependent changes in REM and non-REM sleep in declarative and procedural memory systems. *Behav Brain Res, 180*(1), 48–61. doi: 10.1016/j.bbr.2007.02.037

Fogel, S. M., Ray, L. B., Binnie, L., & Owen, A. M. (2015). How to become an expert: a new perspective on the role of sleep in the mastery of procedural skills. *Neurobiol Learn Mem, 125*, 236–248. doi: 10.1016/j.nlm.2015.10.004

Fogel, S. M., & Smith, C. T. (2011). The function of the sleep spindle: a physiological index of intelligence and a mechanism for sleep-dependent memory consolidation. *Neurosci Biobehav Rev, 35*(5), 1154–1165. doi: 10.1016/j.neubiorev.2010.12.003

Fogel, S. M., Smith, C. T., & Beninger, R. J. (2009). Evidence for 2-stage models of sleep and memory: learning-dependent changes in spindles and theta in rats. *Brain Res Bull, 79*(6), 445–451. doi: 10.1016/j.brainresbull.2009.03.002

Friedrich, M., Wilhelm, I., Born, J., & Friederici, A. D. (2015). Generalization of word meanings during infant sleep. *Nat Commun, 6*, 6004. doi: 10.1038/ncomms7004

Gais, S., & Born, J. (2004). Declarative memory consolidation: mechanisms acting during human sleep. *Learn Mem, 11*(6), 679–685. doi: 10.1101/lm.80504

Gais, S., Plihal, W., Wagner, U., & Born, J. (2000). Early sleep triggers memory for early visual discrimination skills. *Nat Neurosci, 3*(12), 1335–1339. doi: 10.1038/81881

Giuditta, A., Ambrosini, M., Montagnese, P., Mandile, P., Cotugno, M., Grassi Zucconi, G., & Vescia, S. (1995). The sequential hypothesis of the function of sleep. *Behav Brain Res, 69*, 157–166.

Gómez, R. L., Bootzin, R. R., & Nadel, L. (2006). Naps promote abstraction in language-learning infants. *Psychol Sci, 17*(8), 670–674. doi: 10.1111/j.1467-9280.2006.01764.x

Gottselig, J. M., Hofer-Tinguely, G., Borbély, A. A., Regel, S. J., Landolt, H. P., Rétey, J. V., & Achermann, P. (2004). Sleep and rest facilitate auditory learning. *Neuroscience, 127*(3), 557–561. doi: 10.1016/j.neuroscience.2004.05.053

Groch, S., Wilhelm, I., Diekelmann, S., & Born, J. (2013). The role of REM sleep in the processing of emotional memories: evidence from behavior and event-related potentials. *Neurobiol Learn Mem, 99*, 1–9. doi: 10.1016/j.nlm.2012.10.006

Gudberg, C., Wulff, K., & Johansen-Berg, H. (2015). Sleep-dependent motor memory consolidation in older adults depends on task demands. *Neurobiol Aging, 36*(3), 1409–1416. doi: 10.1016/j.neurobiolaging.2014.12.014

Gujar, N., McDonald, S. A., Nishida, M., & Walker, M. P. (2011). A role for REM sleep in recalibrating the sensitivity of the human brain to specific emotions. *Cereb Cortex, 21*(1), 115–123. doi: 10.1093/cercor/bhq064

Helfrich, R. F., Mander, B. A., Jagust, W. J., Knight, R. T., & Walker, M. P. (2018). Old brains come uncoupled in sleep: slow wave-spindle synchrony, brain atrophy, and forgetting. *Neuron, 97*(1), 221–230. doi: 10.1016/j.neuron.2017.11.020

Hennevin, E., & Leconte, P. (1977). Etudes des relations entre le sommeil paradoxal et les processus d'acquisition. *Physiol Behav, 18*, 307–319.

Hennies, N., Lambon Ralph, M. A., Kempkes, M., Cousins, J. N., & Lewis, P. A. (2016). Sleep spindle density predicts the effect of prior knowledge on memory consolidation. *J Neurosci, 36*(13), 3799–3810. doi: 10.1523/JNEUROSCI.3162-15.2016

Hikosaka, O., Nakahara, H., Rand, M. K., Sakai, K., Lu, X., Nakamura, K., … Doya, K. (1999). Parallel neural networks for learning sequential procedures. *Trends Neurosci, 22*(10), 464–471. doi: 10.1016/s0166-2236(99)01439-3

Hoedlmoser, K., Peigneux, P., & Rauchs, G. (2022). Recent advances in memory consolidation and information processing during sleep. *J Sleep Res, 31*(4), e13607. doi:10.1111/jsr.13607

Holmes, O. W. (1879). *Mechanism in Thought and Morals* (5th ed.). Boston: Houghton, Osgood and Company.

Horváth, K., Liu, S., & Plunkett, K. (2016). A daytime nap facilitates generalization of word meanings in young toddlers. *Sleep, 39*(1), 203–207. doi: 10.5665/sleep.5348

Hu, P., Stylos-Allan, M., & Walker, M. P. (2006). Sleep facilitates consolidation of emotional declarative memory. *Psychol Sci, 17*(10), 891–898. doi: 10.1111/j.1467-9280.2006.01799.x

Huang, S., Deshpande, A., Yeo, S. C., Lo, J. C., Chee, M. W., & Gooley, J. J. (2016). Sleep restriction impairs vocabulary learning when adolescents cram for exams: the need for sleep study. *Sleep, 39*(9), 1681–1690. doi: 10.5665/sleep.6092

Huber, R., Ghilardi, M. F., Massimini, M., & Tononi, G. (2004). Local sleep and learning. *Nature, 430*, 78–81. doi: doi:10.1038/nature02663

Hutchison, I. C., & Rathore, S. (2015). The role of REM sleep theta activity in emotional memory. *Front Psychol, 6*, 1439. doi: 10.3389/fpsyg.2015.01439

Ishikawa, A., Kanayama, Y., Matsumura, H., Tsuchimochi, H., Ishida, Y., & Nakamura, S. (2006). Selective rapid eye movement sleep deprivation impairs the maintenance of long-term potentiation in the rat hippocampus. *Eur J Neurosci, 24*(1), 243–248. doi: 10.1111/j.1460-9568.2006.04874.x

Jenkins, J. G., & Dallenbach, K. M. (1924). Obliviscence during sleep and waking. *Am J Psychol, 35*(4), 605–612.

Jones, B. J., & Spencer, R. M. C. (2019). Sleep preserves subjective and sympathetic emotional response of memories. *Neurobiol Learn Mem, 166*, 107096. doi: 10.1016/j.nlm.2019.107096

Karni, A., & Sagi, D. (1991). Where practice makes perfect in texture discrimination: evidence for primary visual cortex plasticity. *Proc Natl Acad Sci USA, 88*, 4966–4970.

Karni, A., & Sagi, D. (1993). The time course of learning a visual skill. *Nature, 365*(6443), 250–252.

Karni, A., Tanne, D., Rubenstein, B. S., Askenasy, J. J. M., & Sagi, D. (1994). Dependence on REM sleep of overnight improvement of a perceptual skill. *Science, 265*, 679–682.

King, B. R., Hoedlmoser, K., Hirschauer, F., Dolfen, N., & Albouy, G. (2017). Sleeping on the motor engram: the multifaceted nature of sleep-related motor memory consolidation. *Neurosci Biobehav Rev, 80*, 1–22. doi: 10.1016/j.neubiorev.2017.04.026

Klinzing, J. G., Nienborg, H., & Rauss, K. (2021). Sleep does not aid the generalisation of binocular disparity-based learning to the other visual hemifield. *J Sleep Res*, e13335. doi: 10.1111/jsr.13335

Korman, M., Doyon, J., Doljansky, J., Carrier, J., Dagan, Y., & Karni, A. (2007). Daytime sleep condenses the time course of motor memory consolidation. *Nat Neurosci, 10*(9), 1206–1213. doi: 10.1038/nn1959

Kurdziel, L., Duclos, K., & Spencer, R. M. (2013). Sleep spindles in midday naps enhance learning in preschool children. *Proc Natl Acad Sci U S A, 110*(43), 17267–17272. doi: 10.1073/pnas.1306418110

Kurinec, C. A., Whitney, P., Hinson, J. M., Hansen, D. A., & Van Dongen, H. P. A. (2021). Sleep deprivation impairs binding of information with its context. *Sleep, 44*(8), zsab113. doi:10.1093/sleep/zsab113

Kuriyama, K., Stickgold, R., & Walker, M. P. (2004). Sleep-dependent learning and motor-skill complexity. *Learn Mem, 11*(6), 705–713. doi: 10.1101/lm.76304

Lacaux, C., Andrillon, T., Bastoul, C., Idir, Y., Fonteix-Galet, A., Arnulf, I., & Oudiette, D. (2021). Sleep onset is a creative sweet spot. *Sci Adv, 7*, 1–9.

Lahl, O., Wispel, C., Willigens, B., & Pietrowsky, R. (2008). An ultra short episode of sleep is sufficient to promote declarative memory performance. *J Sleep Res, 17*(1), 3–10. doi: 10.1111/j.1365-2869.2008.00622.x

Leong, R. L. F., Lo, J. C., & Chee, M. W. L. (2021). Sleep-dependent prospective memory consolidation is impaired with aging. *Sleep*. doi: 10.1093/sleep/zsab069

Lewis, D. J. (1979). Psychobiology of active and inactive memory. *Psychol Bull, 86*(5), 1054–1083.

Lewis, P. A., Knoblich, G., & Poe, G. (2018). How memory replay in sleep boosts creative problem-solving. *Trends Cogn Sci, 22*(6), 491–503. doi: 10.1016/j.tics.2018.03.009

Lim, A., Lozano, A., Moro, E., Hamani, C., Hutchison, W., Dostrovsky, J., … Murray, B. (2007). Characterization of REM-sleep associated ponto-geniculo-occipital waves in the human pons. *Sleep, 30*(7), 823–827.

Lipinska, G., Stuart, B., Thomas, K. G. F., Baldwin, D. S., & Bolinger, E. (2019). Preferential consolidation of emotional memory during sleep: a meta-analysis. *Front Psychol, 10*, 1014. doi: 10.3389/fpsyg.2019.01014

Lovato, N., & Lack, L. (2010). The effects of napping on cognitive functioning. *Prog Brain Res, 185*, 155–166. doi: 10.1016/B978-0-444-53702-7.00009-9

Lugassy, D., Herszage, J., Pilo, R., Brosh, T., & Censor, N. (2018). Consolidation of complex motor skill learning: evidence for a delayed offline process. *Sleep, 41*(9), zsy123. doi:10.1093/sleep/zsy123

Maingret, N., Girardeau, G., Todorova, R., Goutierre, M., & Zugaro, M. (2016). Hippocampo-cortical coupling mediates memory consolidation during sleep. *Nat Neurosci, 19*(7), 959–964. doi: 10.1038/nn.4304

Mander, B. A., Marks, S. M., Vogel, J. W., Rao, V., Lu, B., Saletin, J. M., … Walker, M. P. (2015). Beta-amyloid disrupts human NREM slow waves and related hippocampus-dependent memory consolidation. *Nat Neurosci, 18*(7), 1051–1057. doi: 10.1038/nn.4035

Mander, B. A., Rao, V., Lu, B., Saletin, J. M., Lindquist, J. R., Ancoli-Israel, S., … Walker, M. P. (2013). Prefrontal atrophy, disrupted NREM slow waves and impaired hippocampal-dependent memory in aging. *Nat Neurosci, 16*(3), 357–364. doi: 0.1038/nn.3324

Mander, B. A., Zhu, A. H., Lindquist, J. R., Villeneuve, S., Rao, V., Lu, B., … Walker, M. P. (2017). White matter structure in older adults moderates the benefit of sleep spindles on motor memory consolidation. *J Neurosci, 37*(48), 11675–11687. doi: 10.1523/JNEUROSCI.3033-16.2017

Mantua, J. (2018). Sleep physiology correlations and human memory consolidation: where do we go from here? *Sleep, 41*(2), zsx204. doi: 10.1093/sleep/zsx204

Maquet, P., Péters, J.-M., Aerts, J., Delfiore, G., Degueldre, C., Luxen, A., & Franck, G. (1996). Functional neuroanatomy of human rapid-eye-movement sleep and dreaming. *Nature, 383*, 163–166.

Márquez, G. G. (1970). *One Hundred Years of Solitude* (G. Rabassa, Trans.). New York: Harper & Row.

Massimini, M., Ferrarelli, F., Murphy, M. J., Huber, R., Riedner, B. A., Casarotto, S., & Tononi, G. (2010). Cortical reactivity and effective connectivity during REM sleep in humans. *Cogn Neurosci, 1*(3), 176–183. doi: 10.1080/17588921003731578

McCoy, A. N., & Tan, S. Y. (2014). Otto Loewi (1873–1961): Dreamer and Nobel laureate. *Singapore Med J, 55*(1), 3–4. doi: 10.11622/smedj.2014002

Mednick, S., Nakayama, K., & Stickgold, R. (2003). Sleep-dependent learning: a nap is as good as a night. *Nat Neurosci, 6*(7), 697–698. doi: 10.1038/nn1078

Mednick, S. C., Drummond, S. P. A., Boynton, G. M., Awh, E., & Serences, J. (2008). Sleep-dependent learning and practice-dependent deterioration in an orientation discrimination task. *Behav Neurosci, 122*(2), 267–272. doi: 10.1037/0735-7044.122.2.267

Mednick, S. C., Makovski, T., Cai, D. J., & Jiang, Y. V. (2009). Sleep and rest facilitate implicit memory in a visual search task. *Vision Res, 49*(21), 2557–2565. doi: 10.1016/j.visres.2009.04.011

Mednick, S. C., Nakayama, K., Cantero, J. L., Atienza, M., Levin, A. A., Pathak, N., & Stickgold, R. (2002). The restorative effect of naps on perceptual deterioration. *Nat Neurosci, 5*(7), 877–881. doi: 10.1038/nn864

Menz, M. M., Rihm, J. S., Salari, N., Born, J., Kalisch, R., Pape, H. C., … Buchel, C. (2013). The role of sleep and sleep deprivation in consolidating fear memories. *Neuroimage, 75*, 87–96. doi: 10.1016/j.neuroimage.2013.03.001

Milner, B. (2005). The medial temporal-lobe amnesic syndrome. *Psychiatr Clin N Am, 28*(3), 599–611, 609. doi: 10.1016/j.psc.2005.06.002

Mölle, M., Eschenko, O., Gais, S., Sara, S. J., & Born, J. (2009). The influence of learning on sleep slow oscillations and associated spindles and ripples in humans and rats. *Eur J Neurosci, 29*(5), 1071–1081. doi: 10.1111/j.1460-9568.2009.06654.x

Morgenthaler, J., Wiesner, C. D., Hinze, K., Abels, L. C., Prehn-Kristensen, A., & Goder, R. (2014). Selective REM-sleep deprivation does not diminish emotional memory consolidation in young healthy subjects. *PLoS One, 9*(2), e89849. doi: 10.1371/journal.pone.0089849

Morita, Y., Ogawa, K., & Uchida, S. (2016). Napping after complex motor learning enhances juggling performance. *Sleep Sci, 9*(2), 112–116. doi: 10.1016/j.slsci.2016.04.002

Naiman, R. (2017). Dreamless: the silent epidemic of REM sleep loss. *Ann N Y Acad Sci, 1406*(1), 77–85. doi: 10.1111/nyas.13447

Nettersheim, A., Hallschmid, M., Born, J., & Diekelmann, S. (2015). The role of sleep in motor sequence consolidation: stabilization rather than enhancement. *J Neurosci, 35*(17), 6696–6702. doi: 10.1523/JNEUROSCI.1236-14.2015

Nishida, M., Pearsall, J., Buckner, R. L., & Walker, M. P. (2009). REM sleep, prefrontal theta, and the consolidation of human emotional memory. *Cereb Cortex, 19*(5), 1158–1166. doi: 10.1093/cercor/bhn155

Nissen, C., Piosczyk, H., Holz, J., Maier, J. G., Frase, L., Sterr, A., … Feige, B. (2021). Sleep is more than rest for plasticity in the human cortex. *Sleep, 44*(3), zsaa216. doi:10.1093/sleep/zsaa216

Okesenberg, A., Shaffery, J. P., Marks, G. A., Speciale, S. G., Mihailoff, G., & Roffwarg, H. P. (1996). Rapid eye movement sleep deprivation in kittens amplifies LGN cell-size disparity induced by monocular deprivation. *Dev Brain Res*, *97*, 51–61.

Ong, J. L., Lau, T. Y., Lee, X. K., van Rijn, E., & Chee, M. W. L. (2020). A daytime nap restores hippocampal function and improves declarative learning. *Sleep*, *43*(9), zsaa058. doi: 10.1093/sleep/zsaa058

Oudiette, D., Antony, J. W., Creery, J. D., & Paller, K. A. (2013). The role of memory reactivation during wakefulness and sleep in determining which memories endure. *J Neurosci*, *33*(15), 6672–6678. doi: 10.1523/JNEUROSCI.5497-12.2013

Oudiette, D., & Paller, K. A. (2013). Upgrading the sleeping brain with targeted memory reactivation. *Trends Cogn Sci*, *17*(3), 142–149. doi: 10.1016/j.tics.2013.01.006

Pace-Schott, E. F., & Spencer, R. M. (2011). Age-related changes in the cognitive function of sleep. *Prog Brain Res*, *191*, 75–89. doi: 10.1016/B978-0-444-53752-2.00012-6

Pan, S. C., & Rickard, T. C. (2015). Sleep and motor learning: is there room for consolidation? *Psychol Bull*, *141*(4), 812–834. doi: 10.1037/bul0000009

Payne, J. D., Chambers, A. M., & Kensinger, E. A. (2012). Sleep promotes lasting changes in selective memory for emotional scenes. *Front Integr Neurosci*, *6*, 108. doi: 10.3389/fnint.2012.00108

Pearlman, C., & Becker, M. (1973). Brief posttrial REM sleep deprivation impairs discrimination learning in rats. *Physiol Psychol*, *1*(4), 373–376.

Peigneux, P., Laureys, S., Delbeuck, X., & Maquet, P. (2001). Sleeping brain, learning brain. The role of sleep for memory systems. *NeuroReport*, *12*, A111–A124.

Peigneux, P., & Smith, C. (2017). Memory processing in relation to sleep. In M. H. Kryger, T. Roth, & W. C. Dement (Eds.), *Principles and Practice of Sleep Medicine* (5th ed., pp. 335–347). St. Louis: Elsevier.

Pesonen, A.-K., Ujma, P., Halonen, R., Räikkönen, K., & Kuula, L. (2019). The associations between spindle characteristics and cognitive ability in a large adolescent birth cohort. *Intelligence*, *72*, 13–19. doi: 10.1016/j.intell.2018.11.004

Peters, K. R., Smith, V., & Smith, C. T. (2007). Changes in sleep architecture following motor learning depend on initial skill level. *J Cogn Neurosci*, *19*(5), 817–829. doi: 10.1162/jocn.2007.19.5.817

Petzka, M., Charest, I., Balanos, G. M., & Staresina, B. P. (2021). Does sleep-dependent consolidation favour weak memories? *Cortex*, *134*, 65–75. doi: 10.1016/j.cortex.2020.10.005

Pittaras, E., Colas, D., Chuluun, B., Allocca, G., & Heller, C. (2022). Enhancing sleep after training improves memory in down syndrome model mice. *Sleep*, *45*(4), zsab247. doi:10.1093/sleep/zsab247

Plihal, W., & Born, J. (1997). Effects of early and late nocturnal sleep on declarative and procedural memory. *J Cogn Neurosci*, *9*(4), 534–547.

Plihal, W., & Born, J. (1999). Effects of early and late nocturnal sleep on priming and spatial memory. *Psychophysiology*, *36*, 571–582.

Pöhlchen, D., Pawlizki, A., Gais, S., & Schönauer, M. (2020). Evidence against a large effect of sleep in protecting verbal memories from interference. *J Sleep Res*, e13042. doi: 10.1111/jsr.13042

Prehn-Kristensen, A., Goder, R., Chirobeja, S., Bressmann, I., Ferstl, R., & Baving, L. (2009). Sleep in children enhances preferentially emotional declarative but not procedural memories. *J Exp Child Psychol*, *104*(1), 132–139. doi: 10.1016/j.jecp.2009.01.005

Purcell, S. M., Manoach, D. S., Demanuele, C., Cade, B. E., Mariani, S., Cox, R., … Stickgold, R. (2017). Characterizing sleep spindles in 11,630 individuals from the National Sleep Research Resource. *Nat Commun*, *8*, 15930. doi:10.1038/ncomms15930

Rasch, B., & Born, J. (2013). About sleep's role in memory. *Physiol Rev*, *93*(2), 681–766. doi: 10.1152/physrev.00032.2012

Rauchs, G., F., B., Guillery-Girard, B., Desgranges, B., Kerrouche, N., Denise, P., Foret, J., & Eustache, F. (2004). Consolidation of strictly episodic memories mainly requires rapid eye movement sleep. *Sleep*, *27*(3), 395–401.

Ravassard, P., Hamieh, A. M., Joseph, M. A., Fraize, N., Libourel, P. A., Lebarillier, L., … Salin, P. A. (2016). REM sleep-dependent bidirectional regulation of hippocampal-based emotional memory and LTP. *Cereb Cortex*, *26*(4), 1488–1500. doi: 10.1093/cercor/bhu310

Rickard, T. C., Cai, D. J., Rieth, C. A., Jones, J., & Ard, M. C. (2008). Sleep does not enhance motor sequence learning. *J Exp Psychol Learn Mem Cogn*, *34*(4), 834–842. doi: 10.1037/0278-7393.34.4.834

Rickard, T. C., & Pan, S. C. (2017). Time for considering the possibility that sleep plays no unique role in motor memory consolidation: reply to Adi-Japha and Karni (2016). *Psychol Bull*, *143*(4), 454–458. doi: 10.1037/bul0000094

Rieth, C. A., Cai, D. J., McDevitt, E. A., & Mednick, S. C. (2010). The role of sleep and practice in implicit and explicit motor learning. *Behav Brain Res*, *214*(2), 470–474. doi: 10.1016/j.bbr.2010.05.052

Robertson, E. M., Pascual-Leone, A., & Press, D. Z. (2004). Awareness modifies the skill-learning benefits of sleep. *Curr Biol*, *14*, 208–212. doi: 0.1016/j.cub.2004.01.027

Roediger, H. L. I., & Abel, M. (2022). The double-edged sword of memory retrieval. *Nat Rev Psychol*, *1*, 708–720. doi: 10.1038/s44159-022-00115-2

Rosales-Lagarde, A., Armony, J. L., Del Rio-Portilla, Y., Trejo-Martinez, D., Conde, R., & Corsi-Cabrera, M. (2012). Enhanced emotional reactivity after selective REM sleep deprivation in humans: an fMRI study. *Front Behav Neurosci*, *6*, 25. doi: 10.3389/fnbeh.2012.00025

Rothenberg, A. (1995). Creative cognitive processes in Kekulé's discovery of the structure of the benzene ring. *Am J Psychol*, *108*(3), 419–438.

Sakai, K., & Cespuglio, R. (1974). Evidence for the presence of eye movement potentials during paradoxical sleep in cats. *Electroencephalogr Clin Neurophysiol*, *41*, 37–48.

Saletin, J. M., Goldstein, A. N., & Walker, M. P. (2011). The role of sleep in directed forgetting and remembering of human memories. *Cereb Cortex*, *21*(11), 2534–2541. doi: 10.1093/cercor/bhr034

Sanders, K. E. G., Osburn, S., Paller, K. A., & Beeman, M. (2019). Targeted memory reactivation during sleep improves next-day problem solving. *Psychol Sci*, *30*(11), 1616–1624.

Sara, S. J. (2010). Reactivation, retrieval, replay and reconsolidation in and out of sleep: connecting the dots. *Front Behav Neurosci*, *4*, 185. doi: 10.3389/fnbeh.2010.00185

Sawangjit, A., Oyanedel, C. N., Niethard, N., Salazar, C., Born, J., & Inostroza, M. (2018). The hippocampus is crucial for forming non-hippocampal long-term memory during sleep. *Nature*, *564*, 109–113. doi: 10.1038/s41586-018-0716-8

Schäfer, S. K., Wirth, B. E., Staginnus, M., Becker, N., Michael, T., & Sopp, M. R. (2020). Sleep's impact on emotional recognition memory: a meta-analysis of whole-night, nap, and REM sleep effects. *Sleep Med Rev*, *51*, 101280. doi:10.1016/j.smrv.2020.101280

Schendan, H. E., Searl, M. M., Melrose, R. J., & Stern, C. E. (2003). An fMRI study of the role of the medial temporal lobe in implicit and explicit sequences learning. *Neuron*, *37*, 1013–1025.

Schmid, D., Erlacher, D., Klostermann, A., Kredel, R., & Hossner, E. J. (2020). Sleep-dependent motor memory consolidation in healthy adults: a meta-analysis. *Neurosci Biobehav Rev*, *118*, 270–281. doi: 10.1016/j.neubiorev.2020.07.028

Schönauer, M., Brodt, S., Pöhlchen, D., Bressmer, A., Danek, A. H., & Gais, S. (2018). Sleep does not promote solving classical insight problems and magic tricks. *Front Hum Neurosci*, *12*, 72. doi: 10.3389/fnhum.2018.00072

Schönauer, M., Grätsch, M., & Gais, S. (2015). Evidence for two distinct sleep-related long-term memory consolidation processes. *Cortex*, *63*, 68–78. doi: 10.1016/j.cortex.2014.08.005

Scoville, W. B., & Milner, B. (1957). Loss of recent memory after bilateral hippocampal lesions. *J Neurol Neurosurg Psychiatry*, *20*, 11–21.

Scullin, M. K. (2013). Sleep, memory, and aging: the link between slow-wave sleep and episodic memory changes from younger to older adults. *Psychol Aging*, *28*(1), 105–114. doi: 10.1037/a0028830

Scullin, M. K., & Bliwise, D. L. (2015). Sleep, cognition, and normal aging: integrating a half century of multidisciplinary research. *Perspect Psychol Sci*, *10*(1), 97–137.

Scullin, M. K., Fairley, J., Decker, M. J., & Bliwise, D. L. (2017). The effects of an afternoon nap on episodic memory in young and older adults. *Sleep*, *40*(5). doi: 10.1093/sleep/zsx035

Scullin, M. K., Gao, C., Fillmore, P., Roberts, R. L., Pruett, N., & Bliwise, D. L. (2019). REM sleep mediates age-related decline in prospective memory consolidation. *Sleep*, *42*(6), zsz055. doi:10.1093/sleep/zsz055

Scullin, M. K., & McDaniel, M. A. (2010). Remembering to execute a goal: sleep on it! *Psychol Sci*, *21*(7), 1028–1035.

Seeck-Hirschner, M., Baier, P. C., Weinhold, S. L., Dittmar, M., Heiermann, S., Aldenhoff, J. B., & Goder, R. (2012). Declarative memory performance is associated with the number of sleep spindles in elderly women. *Am J Geriatr Psychiatry*, *20*(9), 782–788. doi: 10.1097/JGP.0b013e31823033da

Siegel, J. M. (2001). The REM sleep-memory consolidation hypothesis. *Science*, *294*(5544), 1058–1063. doi: 10.1126/science.1063049

Simon, K. N. S., Werchan, D., Goldstein, M. R., Sweeney, L., Bootzin, R. R., Nadel, L., & Gomez, R. L. (2017). Sleep confers a benefit for retention of statistical language learning in 6.5 month old infants. *Brain Lang*, *167*, 3–12. doi: 10.1016/j.bandl.2016.05.002

Sio, U. N., Monaghan, P., & Ormerod, T. (2013). Sleep on it, but only if it is difficult: effects of sleep on problem solving. *Mem Cognition*, *41*(2), 159–166. doi: 10.3758/s13421-012-0256-7

Smith, C. (1995). Sleep states and memory processes. *Behav Brain Res*, *69*(1-2), 137–145.

Smith, C. T., Nixon, M. R., & Nader, R. S. (2004). Posttraining increases in REM sleep intensity implicate REM sleep in memory processing and provide a biological marker of learning potential. *Learn Mem, 11*(6), 714–719. doi: 10.1101/lm.74904

Song, S., Howard, J. H., & Howard, D. V. (2007). Sleep does not benefit probabilistic motor sequence learning. *J Neurosci, 27*(46), 12475–12483. doi: 10.1523/jneurosci.2062-07.2007

Song, Y., Blackwell, T., Yaffe, K., Ancoli-Israel, S., Redline, S., Stone, K. L., & Osteoporotic Fractures in Men Study, G. (2015). Relationships between sleep stages and changes in cognitive function in older men: the MrOS Sleep Study. *Sleep, 38*(3), 411–421. doi: 10.5665/sleep.4500

Sonni, A., & Spencer, R. M. C. (2015). Sleep protects memories from interference in older adults. *Neurobiol Aging, 36*(7), 2272–2281. doi: 10.1016/j.neurobiolaging.2015.03.010

Spencer, R. M. C., Gouw, A. M., & Ivry, R. B. (2007). Age-related decline of sleep-dependent consolidation. *Learn Mem, 14*(7), 480–484. doi: 10.1101/lm.569407

Spencer, R. M. C., Sunm, M., & Ivry, R. B. (2006). Sleep-dependent consolidation of contextual learning. *Curr Biol, 16*(10), 1001–1005. doi: 10.1016/j.cub.2006.03.094

Spencer, R. M. C., Walker, M. P., & Stickgold, R. (2017). Sleep and memory consolidation. In M. H. Kryger, A. Roth, & W. C. Dement (Eds.), *Sleep Disorders Medicine* (pp. 205–223). St. Louis: Elsevier.

Stickgold, R., James, L., & Hobson, J. A. (2000). Visual discrimination learning requires sleep after training. *Nat Neurosci, 3*(12), 1237–1238. doi: 10.1038/81756

Stickgold, R., Whidbee, D., Schirmer, B., Patel, V., & Hobson, J. A. (2000). Visual discrimination task improvement: a multi-step process occurring during sleep. *J Cogn Neurosci, 12*(2), 246–254.

Strauss, M., Griffon, L., Van Beers, P., Elbaz, M., Bouziotis, J., Sauvet, F., … Peigneux, P. (2022). Order matters: sleep spindles contribute to memory consolidation only when followed by rapid-eye-movement sleep. *Sleep, 45*(4), zsac022. doi: 10.1093/sleep/zsac022

Tamaki, M., Berard, A. V., Barnes-Diana, T., Siegel, J., Watanabe, T., & Sasaki, Y. (2020). Reward does not facilitate visual perceptual learning until sleep occurs. *Proc Natl Acad Sci U S A, 117*(2), 959–968. doi: 10.1073/pnas.1913079117

Tamaki, M., Matsuoka, T., Nittono, H., & Hori, T. (2008). Fast sleep spindle (13–15 hz) activity correlates with sleep-dependent improvement in visuomotor performance. *Sleep, 31*(2), 204–211.

Tilley, A. J., & Empson, J. A. C. (1978). REM sleep and memory consolidation. *Biol Psychol, 6*, 293–300.

Tucker, M., Hirota, Y., Wamsley, E., Lau, H., Chaklader, A., & Fishbein, W. (2006). A daytime nap containing solely non-REM sleep enhances declarative but not procedural memory. *Neurobiol Learn Mem, 86*(2), 241–247. doi: 10.1016/j.nlm.2006.03.005

Tucker, M. A., & Fishbein, W. (2008). Enhancement of declarative memory performance following a daytime nap is contingent on strength of initial task acquisition. *Sleep, 31*(2), 197–203.

Ujma, P. P., Konrad, B. N., Genzel, L., Bleifuss, A., Simor, P., Potari, A., … Dresler, M. (2014). Sleep spindles and intelligence: evidence for a sexual dimorphism. *J Neurosci, 34*(49), 16358–16368. doi: 10.1523/JNEUROSCI.1857-14.2014

van den Berg, N. H., Al-Kuwatli, J., Paulin, J., Ray, L. B., Owen, A. M., & Fogel, S. M. (2019). Sleep preferentially enhances memory for a cognitive strategy but not the implicit motor skills used to acquire it. *Neurobiol Learn Mem, 161*, 135–142. doi: 10.1016/j.nlm.2019.04.005

van Dongen, E. V., Thielen, J. W., Takashima, A., Barth, M., & Fernandez, G. (2012). Sleep supports selective retention of associative memories based on relevance for future utilization. *PLoS One, 7*(8), e43426. doi: 10.1371/journal.pone.0043426

Vecsey, C. G., Wimmer, M. E., Havekes, R., Park, A. J., Perron, I. J., Meerlo, P., & Abel, T. (2013). Daily acclimation handling does not affect hippocampal long-term potentiation or cause chronic sleep deprivation in mice. *Sleep, 36*(4), 601–607. doi: 10.5665/sleep.2556

Vertes, R. P., & Eastman, K. E. (2000). The case against memory consolidation in REM sleep. *Behav Brain Sci, 23*, 793–1121.

Vorster, A. P., & Born, J. (2015). Sleep and memory in mammals, birds and invertebrates. *Neurosci Biobehav Rev, 50*, 103–119. doi: 10.1016/j.neubiorev.2014.09.020

Wagner, U., Gais, S., & Born, J. (2001). Emotional memory formation is enhanced across sleep intervals with high amounts of rapid eye movement sleep. *Learn Mem, 8*(2), 112–119. doi: 10.1101/lm.36801

Wagner, U., Gais, S., Haider, H., Verleger, R., & Born, J. (2004). Sleep inspires insight. *Nature, 427*(6972), 352–355. doi: 10.1038/nature02223

Walker, M. P. (2010). Sleep, memory, and emotion. In G. A. Kerkhof & H. P. A. Van Dongen (Eds.), *Human Sleep and Cognition* (pp. 49–68). London: Elsevier.

Walker, M. P., Brakefield, T., Seidman, J., Morgan, A., Hobson, J. A., & Stickgold, R. (2002). Sleep and the time course of motor skill learning. *Learn Mem, 10*, 275–284. doi: 10.1101/

Walker, M. P., & Stickgold, R. (2006). Sleep, memory, and plasticity. *Annu Rev Psychol, 57*(1), 139–166. doi: 10.1146/annurev.psych.56.091103.070307

Walker, M. P., Stickgold, R., Jolesz, F. A., & Yoo, S.-S. (2005). The functional anatomy of sleep-dependent visual skill learning. *Cereb Cortex, 15*(11), 1666–1675. doi: 10.1093/cercor/bhi043

Wassing, R., Lakbila-Kamal, O., Ramautar, J. R., Stoffers, D., Schalkwijk, F., & Van Someren, E. J. W. (2019). Restless REM sleep impedes overnight amygdala adaptation. *Curr Biol, 29*(14), 2351–2358 e2354. doi: 10.1016/j.cub.2019.06.034

Wehrle, R., Kaufmann, C., Wetter, T. C., Holsboer, F., Auer, D. P., Pollmacher, T., & Czisch, M. (2007). Functional microstates within human REM sleep: first evidence from fMRI of a thalamocortical network specific for phasic REM periods. *Eur J Neurosci, 25*(3), 863–871. doi: 10.1111/j.1460-9568.2007.05314.x

Werchan, D. M., & Gómez, R. L. (2014). Wakefulness (not sleep) promotes generalization of word learning in 2.5-year-old children. *Child Dev, 85*(2), 429–436.

Westerberg, C. E., Mander, B. A., Florczak, S. M., Weintraub, S., Mesulam, M.-M., Zee, P. C., & Paller, K. A. (2012). Concurrent impairments in sleep and memory in amnestic mild cognitive impairment. *J Int Neuropsych Soc, 18*(3), 490–500. doi: 0.1017/S135561771200001X

Wilhelm, I., Diekelmann, S., & Born, J. (2008). Sleep in children improves memory performance on declarative but not procedural tasks. *Learn Mem, 15*(5), 373–377. doi: 10.1101/lm.803708

Wilhelm, I., Diekelmann, S., Molzow, I., Ayoub, A., Molle, M., & Born, J. (2011). Sleep selectively enhances memory expected to be of future relevance. *J Neurosci, 31*(5), 1563–1569. doi: 10.1523/JNEUROSCI.3575-10.2011

Wilhelm, I., Metzkow-Mészàros, M., Knapp, S., & Born, J. (2012). Sleep-dependent consolidation of procedural motor memories in children and adults: the pre-sleep level of performance matters. *Developmental Sci, 15*(4), 506–515. doi: 10.1111/j.1467-7687.2012.01146.x

Williams, S. E., & Horst, J. S. (2014). Goodnight book: sleep consolidation improves word learning via storybooks. *Front Psychol, 5*, 184. doi:10.3389/fpsyg.2014.00184

Wilson, J. K., Baran, B., Pace-Schott, E. F., Ivry, R. B., & Spencer, R. M. (2012). Sleep modulates word-pair learning but not motor sequence learning in healthy older adults. *Neurobiol Aging, 33*(5), 991–1000. doi: 10.1016/j.neurobiolaging.2011.06.029

Wilson, S., & Argyropoulos, S. (2005). Antidepressants and sleep: a qualitative review of the literature. *Drugs, 65*(7), 927–947.

Yoo, S.-S., Hu, P. T., Gujar, N., Jolesz, F. A., & Walker, M. P. (2007). A deficit in the ability to form new human memories without sleep. *Nat Neurosci, 10*(3), 385–392. doi: 10.1038/nn1851

Zeng, S., Lin, X., Wang, J., & Hu, X. (2021). Sleep's short-term memory preservation and long-term affect depotentiation effect in emotional memory consolidation: behavioral and EEG evidence. *Sleep, 44*(11), zsab155. doi:10.1093/sleep/zsab155

CHAPTER 18

Physiology of Sleep Effects on Memory

18.1 OVERVIEW

One of the most active topics of research on sleep in recent decades has been its role in the regulation of brain plasticity, especially the kind of plasticity involved in consolidating memories. Chapter 17 reviewed primarily behavioral evidence indicating a role for sleep in memory consolidation. This chapter reviews the physiological mechanisms that have been identified as contributing to effects of sleep on memory.

It discusses the role of sleep in model systems of neural plasticity, including the hippocampus and the visual system. It reviews the mechanisms that are involved in the effects of NREM and REM sleep on different kinds of memory. It also reviews how sensory and electrophysiological manipulations during sleep can affect memory, whether one can learn during sleep, and which synaptic mechanisms may be involved in sleep-related plasticity.

18.2 Sleep and neural plasticity: long-term potentiation

The enhancement of memory by sleep for newly learned information or skills depends on its effects on neural plasticity. This term refers to changes in the structure and/or function of neurons and the synapses that connect them as a result of experience. The mechanisms underlying neural plasticity in relation to memory are complex and involve actions at many levels. These include effects on synaptic spines and neurotransmitter receptors, changes in local neural circuits, and interactions among larger systems across the brain. To set the stage for discussing these mechanisms, we will first discuss examples of the involvement of sleep in ostensibly "simpler" forms of plasticity, beginning with long-term potentiation (LTP).

LTP is a phenomenon that is used to investigate the fundamental mechanisms underlying neural plasticity. It has been studied most often in the hippocampus, either in an intact animal or in an in vitro brain slice preparation, but it also occurs in other parts of the brain, including the cortex. A common approach to studying hippocampal LTP is to place a stimulating electrode in the perforant path, which projects from the adjacent entorhinal cortex into the dentate gyrus of the hippocampus (**Figure 18.1**). Perforant path axons are stimulated using a brief, weak electrical stimulus (the test stimulus); for example, a single 1 milliamp (mA), 100 μs duration pulse, as in the study illustrated in **Figure 18.2**).

The response to the test stimulus is measured using an electrode inserted into the granule cell layer of the dentate gyrus and recorded as a population spike, which consists of summed excitatory postsynaptic potentials (EPSPs) from a population of granule cells. The size of the population spike evoked by the test stimulus indicates how strongly granule cells were activated by synaptic input from perforant path axons; stronger stimuli evoke larger population spikes. Similarly, population spikes can be evoked from pyramidal cells in the hippocampal CA1 region by stimulating the Schaffer collaterals, which project to CA1 from the CA3 region (**Figure 18.1**) (Bliss & Collingridge, 1993).

LTP in the granule cell layer is demonstrated by first establishing the baseline population spike evoked by a weak test stimulus in the perforant path and then strongly activating the perforant path with bursts of high-frequency stimulation (tetanizing stimulation). In the study illustrated in **Figure 18.2**, this consists of a high-frequency (400 Hz) burst of 100 pulses of 300 μs duration each, repeated five times over a few minutes. The single test stimulus is then repeated, and it now produces a much larger population spike in the granule cell layer, reflecting a strengthened (potentiated) response. The critical observation is that the experience of a tetanizing stimulation train in an input pathway produces long-lasting changes in the responsiveness of the target neurons. The potentiated response is maintained for many hours or days near maximal level (see

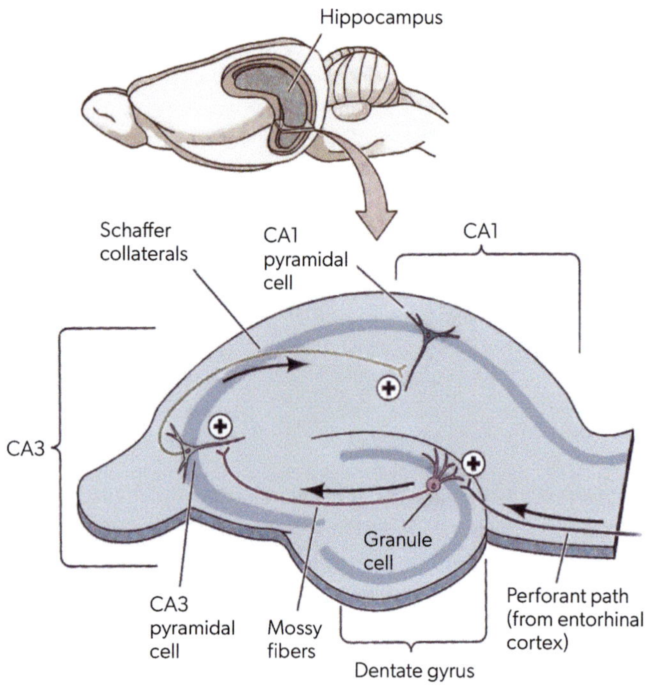

Figure 18.1 The principal circuit elements in the rodent hippocampus. The perforant path is the principal input projection to the hippocampus from the entorhinal cortex, which terminates on granule cells in the dentate gyrus. These neurons project in turn via mossy fibers to pyramidal cells in area CA3. Neurons there, and others from the contralateral hippocampus, project via Schaffer collaterals to pyramidal neurons in the CA1 region. Each of the excitatory synapses indicated by a symbol (+) can undergo long-term potentiation by appropriate stimulation of its afferents. Reprinted with permission of Oxford University Press from *Neuroscience*, 5th edition. Purves, D. et al. (Editors) (2012). Sunderland (MA): Sinauer Associates. © Oxford University Press (2012).

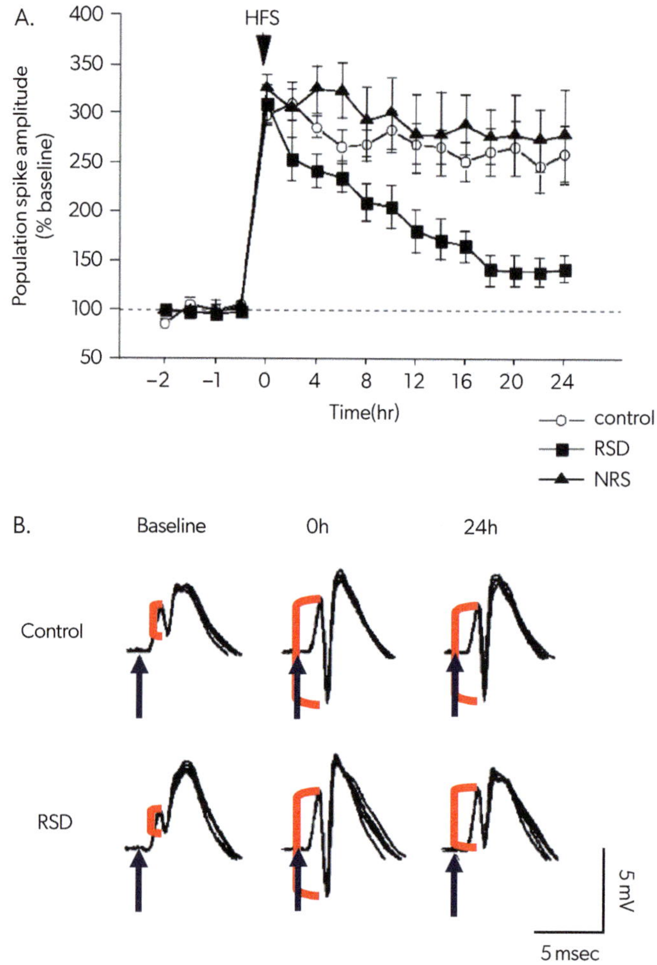

Figure 18.2 **A.** The amplitude of the population spike (Y axis) recorded from granule cells in the dentate gyrus in response to brief, weak stimulation delivered via the perforant path (during the period −2 to 0 h) was dramatically increased by a burst of high-frequency stimulation (HFS) at time 0 h. It was maintained at high amplitude for 24 h in a control group (white circles) and in a group deprived of NREM sleep (NRS; black triangles), but it decreased dramatically in a group deprived of REM sleep during that period (RSD; black squares). **B.** The red brackets illustrate the approximate amplitudes of the population spikes (downward-pointing segments of the traces) at baseline, immediately after LTP (0 h) and 24 h later in control (top) and REM-sleep deprived (RSD) rats (bottom). Arrows show the times at which the test stimuli were applied to evoke population spikes. Adapted with permission of John Wiley and Sons from Ishikawa, A. et al. (2006) Selective rapid eye movement sleep deprivation impairs the maintenance of long-term potentiation in the rat hippocampus. *Eur J Neurosci* 24:243–248. © The Authors (2006). Journal Compilation © Federation of European Neuroscience Societies and Blackwell Publishing. doi: 10.1111/j.1460-9568.2006.04874.x.

Control in **Figure 18.2**), indicating that the excitability of the target neurons to their synaptic input has been chronically increased.[1]

The synaptic plasticity that underlies LTP has been studied for decades as an informative model of the neural circuitry and molecular mechanisms that contribute to learning and memory (Bliss & Collingridge, 1993). In some cases, LTP and its functional opposite, long-term depression (LTD),[2] have been shown to be more than models because they play direct roles in memory. For example, stimulation of auditory nerve input to the amygdala was paired with foot shock in rats to generate a conditioned fear response. Memory of the learned association

[1] This form of plasticity is usually referred to as "Hebbian," after Donald O. Hebb, the Canadian psychologist who proposed a famous "neurophysiological postulate" in 1949. To paraphrase, it stated that memory formation involves the strengthening of synaptic connections that occurs when firing of an afferent projection regularly triggers activation of a target neuron. This idea has been colloquially summarized as "neurons that fire together, wire together" (Cooper, 2005; Hebb, 1949).

[2] LTD in the CA1 region, for example, results from prolonged very low-frequency stimulation (e.g., a 15 min train of 1 Hz pulses) of Schaffer collateral input, which depresses responsiveness of these neurons to input via the same pathway for one or more hours (Dudek & Bear, 1992).

was then erased by producing LTD in the auditory input pathway. Generating LTP later in the same pathway reinstated the conditioned fear response (Nabavi et al., 2014).

Several studies have investigated the involvement of REM sleep in hippocampal LTP both in vivo and in vitro using relatively selective REM sleep deprivation (Davis et al., 2003; Ishikawa et al., 2006; Kim et al., 2005; McDermott et al., 2003). In one study (Ishikawa et al., 2006), the population spike in the hippocampus of rats that was evoked by a test stimulus was measured immediately after induction of LTP by tetanizing stimulation and then repeatedly during the next 24 h. Some rats were selectively deprived of REM sleep during that period using the small-platform ("flowerpot") method (see Section 14.2). The initial potentiation of the population spike (>300% of baseline amplitude) declined during 24 h of selective REM sleep deprivation until it was greatly reduced by the end of the day (to <150% of baseline). Control rats that either slept freely or were deprived selectively of NREM sleep maintained a strongly potentiated population spike (~275% of baseline) throughout the 24 h period (**Figure 18.2**). Other studies used a less stressful form of total sleep deprivation in mice for 6 h or REM sleep deprivation for 4 h *before* inducing LTP. These studies also found reduced amounts of LTP, indicating that loss of sleep, especially of REM sleep, interfered with both generating and maintaining potentiation of the population spike (Florian et al., 2011; Kopp et al., 2006).

The mechanism by which REM sleep deprivation reversed synaptic potentiation was found to involve the reduced availability on hippocampal cell surfaces of a subtype of excitatory glutamate receptors (N-methyl-D-aspartate (NMDA) receptors) (McDermott et al., 2006) (**Figure 18.3**). NMDA receptors have been implicated in acquiring several kinds of memory, especially those that depend on the hippocampus (Morris, 2013). These results indicate that REM sleep deprivation disrupted memory for an experience-dependent change in how neurons respond to excitatory glutamatergic input, implying a role for REM sleep in stabilizing this form of neural plasticity. The same type of REM sleep deprivation that impairs LTP and glutamatergic neurotransmission also impairs formation of hippocampus-dependent spatial memories (McDermott et al., 2003).

18.2.1 Summary

LTP is a model of memory formation that has been studied most often in the hippocampus but also occurs in the cortex and other parts of the nervous system. It involves a long-lasting increase in neural responsiveness (potentiation of the population spike) to a fixed synaptic input as a result of a single experience of high-intensity synaptic activation. It is often considered a model for the neural plasticity underlying memory formation and may be the actual mechanism of memory formation in some preparations.

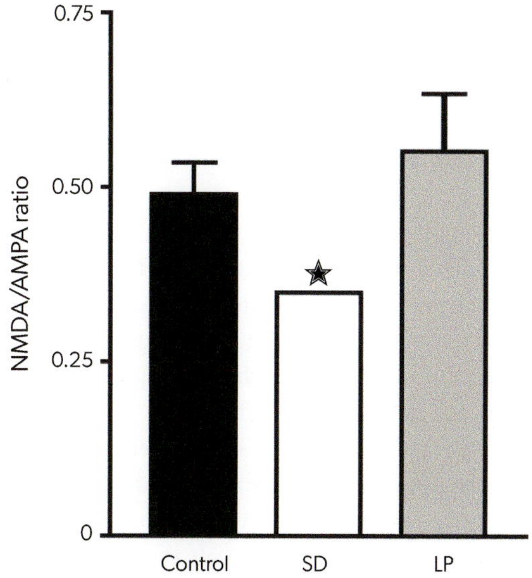

Figure 18.3 Hippocampal slices were prepared from rats that had undergone REM sleep deprivation (SD) for 72 h, using the multi-platform method. Each SD rat was confined to living on platforms that were too small to permit REM sleep but allowed movements among platforms. Control rats slept freely, and other rats were housed on large platforms (LP) that permitted REM sleep without risk of falling from the platform. Hippocampal slices were prepared after 72 h of these housing conditions. Glutamate receptor populations on hippocampal pyramidal neurons were studied in area CA1 after stimulation of Schaffer collaterals in the slice preparation. There was a significant reduction (★) in the ratio of NMDA to AMPA glutamate receptors in SD rats, compared to rats that had not undergone REM sleep deprivation. Reprinted with permission of John Wiley and Sons from McDermott, C.M. et al. (2006) Sleep deprivation-induced alterations in excitatory synaptic transmission in the CA1 region of the rat hippocampus. *J Physiol* 570.3:553–565. © The Authors (2006). Journal compilation © The Physiological Society (2006). doi: 10.1113/jphysiol.2005.093781. Permission conveyed through Copyright Clearance Center, Inc.

Potentiated responses in the rat hippocampus were blocked or strongly attenuated by preventing primarily REM sleep either before or after LTP induction. Reduction of NREM sleep did not prevent the maintenance of potentiation. One effect of REM sleep deprivation that was observed in the hippocampus was reduced availability of NMDA glutamate receptors, which play an important role in synaptic plasticity. Similar REM sleep deprivation impaired the acquisition of hippocampus-dependent spatial memories.

18.3 Sleep and neural plasticity: visual cortex

We previously reviewed the role of sleep in stabilizing and strengthening plasticity in the human visual system as a result of learning to use peripheral vision to detect the orientation of a target (see Section 17.6). The role of sleep in neural plasticity has also been studied in the visual systems of both developing and adult animals, in which the cellular and molecular mechanisms involved can be investigated.

Very young mammals, especially those that are altricial (born at an early developmental stage; see Chapter 4), sleep a great deal (e.g., a full-term, newborn human sleeps for 16–18 h daily). Their brains are maturing and undergoing dramatic changes, many of which are related to their early experiences. These experience-dependent changes make infant mammals a useful system in which to study the underlying mechanisms by which sleep affects neural plasticity.

One approach to this issue used a version of the classic paradigm that demonstrated experience-dependent plasticity in the visual cortex of young kittens (Hubel & Wiesel, 1965).[3] In newborn kittens (and in adult cats that had normal visual experiences during development), most neurons in the primary visual cortex receive largely balanced input from both eyes. A smaller number are driven primarily or exclusively by either the ipsilateral or contralateral eye. Asymmetric postnatal visual experience during a critical period (starting at ~1 month after birth) can reshape this distribution.

Neural plasticity in the visual system was demonstrated by raising kittens in darkness from birth until the critical period. They were then allowed a brief period of visual experience through only one eye, which resulted in the open eye starting to drive a higher proportion of cells in the visual cortex; this is referred to as an ocular dominance shift. The mechanism generating this shift involves long-lasting changes in synaptic function as a result of glutamatergic, cholinergic, and noradrenergic activity in the cortex during the monocular experience (Bear & Singer, 1986; Gu, 2003).

To study the impact of sleep on this form of neural plasticity, dark-reared kittens were then allowed only monocular vision for a period of 6 or 12 h. Cells in their visual cortex were studied immediately afterward to measure the extent of the ocular dominance shift in favor of the open eye. As little as 6 h of visual experience caused a shift toward more neurons in the visual cortex being driven by that eye, and 12 h of visual experience produced even larger shifts in ocular dominance toward the eye with visual experience; see **Figure 18.4**, **MD6** and **MD12** (Frank et al., 2001).

Some kittens that experienced 6 h of monocular vision were then allowed to sleep for 6 h in darkness before assessing the extent of ocular dominance shift. The immediate shift seen after 6 h of monocular vision was increased further after another 6 h spent asleep in total darkness, with no additional

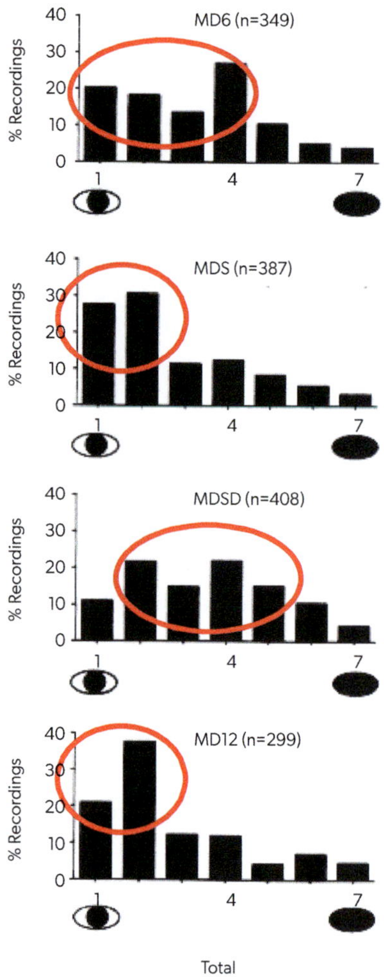

Figure 18.4 Each graph shows the effects of a short period of visual experience for only one eye (illustrated as the open eye below each X axis) in previously dark-reared kittens. The percentage of cells in each ocular dominance category is shown on the Y axis; n is the number of cells studied in each preparation. Most cells in normal kittens are driven equally by both eyes (category 4 on the X axis) and few neurons are driven exclusively or mostly by only one eye (1 or 7). **MD6:** Kittens had 6 h of only monocular visual experience and subsequently showed increased control by the visually experienced eye (ocular dominance shift; red oval). **MDS:** After the 6 h monocular visual experience, kittens were allowed to sleep in the dark for 6 h. They showed a much stronger ocular dominance shift toward the open eye, with most cells falling in categories 1 or 2 (red oval). **MDSD:** After the 6 h monocular visual experience, these kittens were also placed in the dark for 6 h but were sleep-deprived (to varying extents) during that time. Sleep deprivation reversed much of the ocular dominance shift that had been produced by the 6 h visual experience (red oval). **MD12:** Kittens were given 12 h of monocular visual experience and showed a strong ocular dominance shift (red oval) that resembled that shown by the MDS group that had only 6 h of visual experience plus 6 h of sleep. Among kittens in the MDS and MDSD groups, there was a robust positive correlation (r = 0.95) between the amount of shift in ocular dominance and the percentage of the 6 h in darkness spent in NREM sleep. Adapted with permission of Elsevier, Ltd. from Frank, M.G. et al. (2001) Sleep enhances plasticity in the developing visual cortex. *Neuron* 30:275–287. © Elsevier (2001). doi: 10.1016/s0896-6273(01)00279-3.

[3] David H. Hubel and Torsten N. Wiesel won the Nobel Prize in Medicine or Physiology in 1981 for their work on information processing in the visual cortex, an award shared with Roger W. Sperry for his work on functional specialization of the cerebral hemispheres.

visual experience. The extent of the shift approached that caused by 12 h of monocular visual experience (**Figure 18.4, MDS**). This finding showed that during sleep in darkness there was a continuing shift in ocular dominance toward the eye that had received visual experience.

When experimenters tried to keep the kittens awake during the 6 h dark period after 6 h of monocular vision, there was no enhanced shift in ocular dominance. Instead, the kittens lost some of the partial shift already present at the end of the visual experience. The extent of this reversal of the shift was proportional to how successful experimenters were in depriving them of sleep (**Figure 18.4, MDSD**). Thus, sleep both stabilized and further strengthened the plastic changes in the visual cortex that resulted from monocular visual experience. Preventing sleep after monocular experience weakened and even reversed the changes that had already occurred after 6 h (Frank et al., 2001).

This finding raised the question of whether the type of sleep obtained was important to these effects on neural plasticity. The amount of shift retained after the sleep opportunity was positively correlated with the amount of NREM sleep produced during the 6 h in darkness, but it was not possible to evaluate whether there was also a correlation with REM sleep amounts (Frank et al., 2001). Later research found that selective deprivation of REM sleep after monocular visual experience also prevented ocular dominance shifts (Dumoulin Bridi et al., 2015), a finding that echoes the role of REM sleep in hippocampal LTP (Ishikawa et al., 2006).

These results led to the conclusion that both NREM and REM sleep were involved in stabilizing and strengthening the plastic changes induced by monocular vision (Dumoulin Bridi et al., 2015). This interpretation is consistent with evidence that NREM and REM sleep are jointly involved in consolidation of other forms of neural plasticity, including in the visual system (Giuditta et al., 1995; Mednick et al., 2003; Stickgold, Whidbee, et al., 2000); see Sections 17.6 and 17.8.

The effects of sleep on neuronal plasticity in the visual cortex have been attributed to increased production of proteins that strengthen input via the NMDA subtype of glutamate receptors to "principal" neurons in the cortex (Aton, Seibt, Dumoulin, Jha, et al., 2009). The extent to which the firing of these neurons increased during sleep, reflecting stronger glutamatergic input, was correlated with the degree of ocular dominance shift induced by monocular visual input (Aton et al., 2013).

Increasing glutamatergic neurotransmission depended on first transcribing messenger (m)RNAs from the DNA coding for plasticity-related proteins and then translating the mRNAs into functional proteins. The transcription step occurred during the monocular visual experience while awake, but translation from the resulting mRNAs to produce functional proteins occurred during later sleep. These plasticity-related proteins then acted to strengthen synaptic activity related to the waking experience (Seibt et al., 2012). Thus, a neurochemical cascade that was triggered during a waking experience ("online") was completed during later sleep ("offline") in order to selectively strengthen glutamatergic neurotransmission and stabilize the ocular dominance shift. Sleep loss during the period after the visual experience appeared to interfere with this step and reverse some of the initial ocular dominance shift.

Another form of plasticity in the primary visual cortex was produced in adult mice by continuous exposure for a 1 h period to visual gratings (black and white stripes) with a specific orientation. This exposure was followed by a test of visual system sensitivity to these gratings and then by a 6 h period of either sleep or sleep deprivation by distraction/gentle handling.

The firing rates of cortical neurons sensitive to gratings with this orientation were unchanged immediately after the 1 h exposure, but they were selectively increased after the subsequent sleep period. Sleep deprivation after the visual experience prevented the orientation-selective increases in firing rates. Firing-rate increases in response to these gratings after sleep were positively correlated with the amounts of both NREM and REM sleep shown. Increases were also linked to the amount of sleep spindle activity shown during NREM sleep (Aton et al., 2014; Clawson et al., 2018). Similarly, the durations of sleep spindles during a nap after training on a visual texture discrimination task (see Section 17.6) were related to the benefit of sleep for improved performance on this task (Strauss et al., 2022).

Thus, cortical plasticity in relation to orientation selectivity in adult mice was correlated with the amounts of NREM and REM sleep after the plasticity-inducing experience and the amount of sleep spindles produced (Aton et al., 2014; Clawson et al., 2018), which was also the case for plasticity in the kitten visual cortex (Dumoulin Bridi et al., 2015; Frank et al., 2001; Strauss et al., 2022). The plasticity involved in acquiring skill at visual texture discrimination in adult humans was also related to the amounts of both NREM and REM sleep (Mednick et al., 2003; Stickgold, Whidbee, et al., 2000).

18.3.1 Summary

Early asymmetric visual experience during a critical period shifted ocular dominance (control by the left or right eye) of neurons in the primary visual cortex of dark-reared kittens. These shifts in ocular dominance were strengthened by sleep after visual experience and were partially reversed by sleep deprivation. The degree of shift was correlated with the amount of NREM sleep produced during the sleep opportunity. Later studies showed that both NREM and REM sleep, as well as the production of sleep spindles, were involved in stabilizing and strengthening ocular dominance shifts.

Novel visual experience during this early developmental period affected ocular dominance by increasing neural activity of principal cortical neurons via NMDA-type glutamate receptors. The visual experience triggered production of mRNAs, but it was only during later sleep that the transcribed mRNAs were translated into functional, plasticity-related proteins that affected glutamatergic activity.

In adult mice, sustained visual exposure to gratings with a specific orientation did not immediately alter the responsiveness of visual cortex neurons that were tuned to these line orientations. But after a sleep period, these neurons showed a selective increase in responsiveness to the line orientations to which they had been exposed. Both NREM and REM sleep were involved in increasing neuronal responsiveness to the targeted line orientations. These plastic changes in the visual system were prevented by sleep deprivation after the visual experience.

18.4 Neural replay and plasticity

18.4.1 Evidence of replay

As discussed in more detail in Sections 18.5 and 18.6, new declarative memories are represented initially in the hippocampus by changes in synaptic connections and the resulting changes in patterns of neural activity. In this state, memories are relatively unstable and can be disrupted by interference. In order for these memories to become more stable, they must be consolidated and stored in the cortex. The evidence reviewed below indicates that neural activity during sleep is involved in strengthening recently established firing patterns by local rehearsal in the hippocampus and the transfer of the new information to more permanent storage in the cortex.

Neural replay involves the production during sleep of firing sequences among hippocampal neurons that are similar to those that had been generated by these neurons while an animal or person was awake and acquiring new information. A typical example of neural replay involved a rat first learning new spatial information while exploring a novel environment (e.g., a circular runway). Individual pyramidal cells in the hippocampus increased their firing rates consistently and selectively when the rat was in different locations in the runway. These neurons are referred to as place cells because the peak of firing in each neuron codes for a different, specific location in space (O'Keefe & Nadel, 1979).[4]

Recording simultaneously from many hippocampal place cells while a rat explored an environment produced a sequence of increases in firing among these neurons that reflected the path (i.e., sequence of places) traveled by the rat. Neurons in the hippocampus (and also in the cortex and striatum) that fired in a particular sequence while awake and moving through the environment tended to fire in a statistically similar pattern during subsequent sleep or quiet waking. These patterned replays were produced during NREM and REM sleep at an accelerated rate relative to the original timing while awake and sometimes occurred in reverse order from the original pattern (Carr et al., 2011; Euston et al., 2007; Foster & Wilson, 2006; Ji & Wilson, 2007; Louie & Wilson, 2001; Wilson & McNaughton, 1994) (**Figure 18.5**). People may experience a different kind of sensory replay under some conditions; see **Box 18.1**.

There is also evidence that people show memory-related replay of neural patterns acquired during learning tasks. In one study, intracranial electrodes were used to record population firing patterns across the cortex of epilepsy patients. Identified neural firing patterns recorded while awake were reproduced during later sleep (Jiang et al., 2017). Another human study recorded patterns of fMRI activity in the visual cortex of participants while they performed a paired-associate, spatial learning task. These fMRI patterns reappeared spontaneously during both waking and sleep after the learning experience. The frequency with which patterns were repeated after training was positively correlated with the accuracy of retention of the learned pairings (Deuker et al., 2013).

Another study involved recording with implanted microelectrodes in the brain of a patient with quadriplegia as part of a study related to developing brain–computer interfaces. The patient learned to perform a color–sound sequence matching game (similar to the commercial game *Simon*) using a neural–computer interface to move a cursor on a screen. Recordings were made in the motor cortex during performance of the task, and patterns of neural activity were extracted from the recordings.

Similar patterns were later identified more frequently than before training on the task, while the individual was both awake and asleep. These replay events tended to occur at increased speed (1–6 times faster than during task performance), were more common during sleep that included large numbers of slow waves, and often coincided with cortical ripple events (part of slow-wave ripples; see Section 2.3.2) (Rubin et al., 2022). These results recapitulated many of the characteristics of hippocampal replay events in rodents that are hypothesized to be involved in hippocampal-cortical communication related to memory consolidation; see Section 18.6.1.

Quality of hippocampal replay in rats depends on age. Hippocampal recordings were made from young and old rats while they explored a running track and during a later rest/

[4] The discovery of place cells and the related "grid cells" as the mechanisms underlying animals' knowledge of space was the basis for awarding the 2014 Nobel Prize in Physiology or Medicine to John O'Keefe, May-Britt Moser, and Edvard I. Moser.

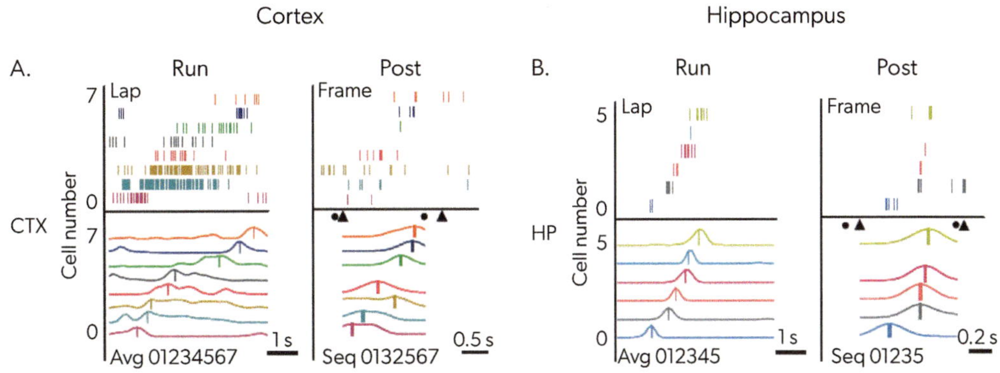

Figure 18.5 **A.** Neural firing sequences in the cortex during exploration of an environment while awake (Run) and during subsequent SWS (Post). The colored vertical marks in the top panels represent the firing of individual neurons, numbered 0-7. 'Lap' refers to the temporal pattern of cell firing during a single run around a track. The bottom panels show the average firing patterns of each neuron across several runs and illustrate the times of peak firing with a vertical line (Avg) for the same cells. Frame refers to a temporal frame within a SWS recording session, and Seq refers to the sequence of firing peaks within the SWS frame. **B.** A similar plot of firing recorded from neurons in the hippocampus during exploration (Run) and during subsequent SWS (Post); note that cell 4 (blue) was silent during the SWS recording. The SWS sequences of firing peaks are not a perfect match to the patterns recorded during exploration. Sequences may have a slightly shifted order (as in the cortex; the timing of firing peaks in cells 2 and 3 (gold and red) was reversed relative to their order during the Run), or one or two neurons may be silent during a Post replay (as in both cortex and hippocampus). The different time scales shown in each panel indicate that the sequences were executed >2X as fast in the cortex and >5X as fast in the hippocampus during sleep, compared to waking. Reprinted with permission from Ji, D. & Wilson, M.A. (2007) Coordinated memory replay in the visual cortex and hippocampus during sleep. *Nat Neurosci* 10: 100-107. © Springer: Nature (2007). doi:10.1038/nn1825.

BOX 18.1 Replay of Game Play

Many people have experienced a phenomenon that is superficially similar to this kind of neural replay when they have engaged in an intense, repetitive activity for hours. In experimental studies, people given sustained practice with engaging video games, like *Alpine Racer* (Wamsley et al., 2010) and *Tetris* (Stickgold, Malia, et al., 2000), reported reexperiencing the visual, and sometimes kinesthetic, experiences of the gameplay during early stages of sleep over several nights. These experiences were reported most frequently during the transition from wake to sleep or early in N1/N2 sleep; they were reported less frequently while awake and during reports of dream recall after morning awakening.

Despite the superficial similarity of this kind of replay to the replay of hippocampal firing-rate patterns that are involved in memory consolidation during sleep, these appear to be different phenomena. The replay of gaming experiences occurred during early, transition stages of sleep rather than during N2, N3, or REM sleep, the stages that are usually reported to be involved in memory consolidation. In addition, these experiences were also observed in people who suffered from severe anterograde amnesia (inability to form new memories) as a result of hippocampal damage (Stickgold, Malia, et al., 2000). The replay during sleep of intensely repeated visual and kinesthetic sensations might reflect activity in cortical sensory and/or motor systems that were intensely engaged while awake but appear to be independent of the mechanisms involved in consolidation of hippocampus-dependent memories.

sleep interval. Both age groups showed replay of waking firing sequences in the hippocampus during rest/sleep. In the older animals, however, the original temporal patterns produced during exploration were less well-preserved during later replay. The quality of replay in individual rats in this study was then found to correlate with their ability to learn a different type of hippocampus-dependent, spatial task. Thus, deficits in replay accuracy during sleep of acquired spatial information in older animals predicted poorer spatial memory performance on a different task (Gerrard et al., 2008). These results may help account for the finding that memory in older people benefits less from consolidation during sleep than in young adults (see discussion in Section 17.10.2).

There have also been reports of the existence of hippocampal "preplay" rather than replay. This evidence suggested that preexisting firing sequences among hippocampal neurons that were recorded in naïve animals could later become linked to sequences of spatial locations during exploration of an environment (Dragoi & Tonegawa, 2011; Dragoi & Tonegawa, 2014). There is, however, also evidence against the existence of preplay and for the gradual evolution of new sequences as learning develops (Lee & Wilson, 2002; Modi et al., 2014; Silva et al., 2015). The issues involved and the potential role of existing memories in providing a framework for the hippocampal representation of new memories are reviewed in a commentary by (Eichenbaum, 2015).

18.4.2 Dendritic plasticity in cortex and hippocampus

Replay has been demonstrated using measures other than neuronal firing rates. Activated neurons can also be identified by increased entry (influx) into dendrites of calcium ions (Ca^{2+}). Learning a new motor skill was associated with an increase in Ca^{2+} influx in a specific set of pyramidal neurons in the motor cortex of mice. The same neurons showed a similar pattern of Ca^{2+} influx during later NREM sleep. Electron microscopic studies showed that Ca^{2+} influx during NREM sleep was associated with the formation of new synaptic spines selectively on the activated neurons, which would reinforce the synaptic connections that had been created or strengthened during motor learning (Yang et al., 2014).

Most of these newly formed synaptic spines were later lost, primarily during REM sleep. This pruning process, however, was selective; those spines that survived were further strengthened (Li et al., 2017). Thus, neural replay during NREM sleep strengthened synaptic connections tied to new learning, but this mechanism interacted with a selective pruning process during REM sleep. The net effect was to stabilize and strengthen neural circuitry directly involved in performing a newly learned motor skill. This conclusion is consistent with other results supporting a joint role for NREM and REM sleep in facilitating other kinds of memory consolidation (see Section 17.8) (Fogel et al., 2009; Giuditta et al., 1995; Mednick et al., 2003; Seibt & Frank, 2019; Stickgold, Whidbee, et al., 2000; Tang & Jadhav, 2018). This role for REM sleep in selectively stabilizing synapses involved in newly acquired motor patterns and eliminating other synapses may explain why infant humans and other species with immature motor systems at birth show large amounts of REM sleep early in the development of their motor systems.

Regulating the survival of dendritic spines in the hippocampus after learning depends on processes involving the key second messenger molecule, cyclic adenosine monophosphate (cAMP). cAMP mediates the effects of many neurotransmitters and hormones and acts through kinases such as the cAMP dependent protein kinase (PKA) to affect gene expression and cellular metabolism in many cells (Nguyen & Woo, 2003). When mice were sleep-deprived after learning an object location task, they showed reduced hippocampal cAMP levels relative to controls who slept, loss of dendritic spines on hippocampal neurons, and impaired performance on a test of memory related to the learning experience. When a pharmacogenetic method was used to increase cAMP levels in the hippocampus during sleep deprivation, synaptic spines were maintained and normal memory performance restored (Havekes et al., 2014; Havekes et al., 2016). Thus, the quality of memory performance and its underlying neural basis in the hippocampus depended on cAMP-mediated plastic changes during sleep.

Findings related to changes in hippocampal dendritic spines as a result of sleep deprivation have, however, not been completely consistent across studies. There are complexities in summarizing these findings because studies used different methods to image and count spines and analyzed multiple subtypes of spines on different branches of dendrites within different dendritic fields.

One study reported decreased spine numbers on dendrites in the hippocampal CA1 region (see **Figure 18.1**) after 5 h of sleep loss (Havekes et al., 2016). A later study reported that similar sleep deprivation resulted in higher densities of spines, especially thin spines, on dendrites in the CA1 region, implying a role for sleep in down-regulating this type of dendritic spine (Gisabella et al., 2020). This apparent contradiction was addressed in a more recent study (Bolsius et al., 2021) that examined changes in spine numbers on different branches of CA1 neuronal dendrites following sleep loss. It observed increases (that were not statistically significant) or stable spine numbers on the same dendritic branches that were reported to show increases after sleep loss in the study by (Gisabella et al., 2020). It also reported decreases of several subtypes of spines on other dendritic branches, and restoration of spine numbers by a 3 h period of recovery sleep (Bolsius et al., 2021).

One potential explanation for varying responses to sleep loss on different dendrites and dendritic branches is that projections to CA1 neurons from the cortex and thalamus, as well as from the hippocampal CA3 region and local interneurons, terminate on different dendrites and on different branches of dendrites (Bolsius et al., 2021). Future studies will be needed to clarify the details of how synaptic spines are regulated by sleep and sleep loss in different regions of the hippocampus and in different dendritic subfields.

18.4.3 Summary

Individual hippocampal place neurons fire at highest rates at specific locations in space. Spatial exploration results in sequences of peak firing rates among hippocampal (and cortical) neurons, and these sequences are replayed in a statistically similar pattern, but usually at a higher speed, during sleep. Older rats that showed less well-preserved firing sequences during neural replay also showed worse memory performance on a separate spatial learning task.

Replay during NREM sleep reinforced memory of a motor skill by increasing the growth of synaptic spines in cortical circuits underlying the behavior. Synaptic spines that were presumably not appropriate were pruned away during later REM sleep, while surviving connections were strengthened. Thus, both NREM and REM sleep were involved in the selective strengthening of learning-related synaptic connections.

Sleep deprivation after learning disrupted formation of dendritic spines in the CA1 region of hippocampus and impaired spatial memory performance. This impairment was mediated by decreasing levels of hippocampal cAMP, a molecule that is critical for synaptic plasticity. Restoring cAMP levels during sleep loss restored memory performance.

Another sleep deprivation study, however, reported increased spine numbers on hippocampal CA1 neurons. A third study found differences in how sleep loss affected spines on different branches of CA1 dendrites. Some branches showed slight (nonsignificant) increases or stable spine numbers, while others showed loss of spines. These differential effects may be linked to different dendritic branches receiving inputs from different classes of afferents.

18.5 An aside on hippocampal neurogenesis, sleep, and depression

Another form of hippocampal plasticity is the process of neurogenesis. Neurogenesis refers to the birth of new neuronal precursor cells and their maturation into neurons. Neurogenesis may seem like an odd topic to introduce into a discussion of sleep and memory, but there is evidence that connects these subjects, and also links them to mood disorders. Neurogenesis has been studied extensively during development, but it also occurs in select brain regions in adult mammals, resulting in the incorporation of some newborn neurons into functional brain circuits (Samuels & Hen, 2011). One brain region that shows adult neurogenesis is the dentate gyrus of the hippocampus, which plays a critical role in forming and consolidating declarative memories.[5]

Neuronal growth factors such as brain-derived neurotrophic factor (BDNF) are involved in promoting neurogenesis, and they also play a role in synaptic plasticity related to learning and to mood regulation (Duman et al., 2016). Both stress and depression reduce neurogenesis in animal models, and they also reduce the size of the hippocampus in people; chronic antidepressant treatment has the opposite effect. Patients with depression show cognitive impairments, including memory problems, beyond what is attributable to their depressed mood (Rock et al., 2014). These and related findings led to the hypothesis that reduced hippocampal neurogenesis contributes to development and/or maintenance of depression and to its associated memory problems, and that successful treatment of depression involves restoring hippocampal neurogenesis (Eisch & Petrik, 2012; Malberg et al., 2000; Samuels & Hen, 2011).

One of the most common symptoms of depression is sleep disruption (see Section 15.3.2), which both results from, and contributes to, the stress and anxiety that often accompany depression. Findings related to the effects of sleep loss provide links between sleep disruption and the symptoms of depression. First, the level of BDNF, which is important for neurogenesis, is reduced by stress, an effect that is mediated by sleep disruption (Giese et al., 2013). Second, hippocampal neuronal proliferation is reduced by lengthy sleep deprivation, chronic sleep fragmentation, or relatively selective REM sleep deprivation (Guzmán-Marín & McGinty, 2006; Guzmán-Marín et al., 2003; Mueller et al., 2008; Sportiche et al., 2010). A review of this topic concluded that sleep is permissive for neuronal proliferation, while sustained wakefulness inhibits the mechanisms involved (Mueller et al., 2013). Thus, chronic sleep disruption adds to (or mediates) the impact of stress that reduces BDNF, inhibits neurogenesis, impairs hippocampal memory function, and prolongs the symptoms of depression.

The impact of sleep disruption on hippocampal neurogenesis and BDNF levels may contribute to the finding that persistent, residual insomnia after successful treatment of major depression is linked to an increased risk of relapsing into depression. This conclusion is supported by evidence that targeted behavioral treatments for sleep problems reduce symptoms of depression and risk of relapse in addition to improving sleep (Blom et al., 2017; Franzen & Buysse, 2008; Wagley et al., 2013; Watanabe et al., 2011); see Figure 15.4 and discussion in Section 15.3.2).

These benefits of treating insomnia could result from both direct effects of better sleep on mood and energy levels and from indirect effects mediated by increased BDNF production (Giese et al., 2013) and a resulting increase in hippocampal neurogenesis. In addition, many studies found that systematic exercise programs reduced symptoms of depression (see Box 10.2 in Section 10.5), and exercise has also been shown to

[5] This interpretation of the role of neurogenesis is one possibility, but there have been many functions attributed to the integration of new neurons into hippocampal circuitry (Lucassen et al., 2019). There is evidence, for example, that high levels of neurogenesis in rodents are associated with more *forgetting* and that preservation of memories is improved by reduced hippocampal neurogenesis, perhaps because integrating newly formed neurons disrupts some existing memory circuits (Akers et al., 2014). However, other evidence indicates that consolidation of new learning depends on activation of newly born hippocampal neurons during REM sleep (Kumar et al., 2020). Much remains to be learned about the role of adult neurogenesis in memory and other brain functions.

increase BDNF levels (Jemni et al., 2023). Since exercise also increases sleep amounts (Youngstedt et al., 1997), it is likely that both exercise and sleep are components of a web of influences that can improve depression symptoms through multiple routes, including effects on BDNF, serotonergic neurotransmission, and hippocampal neurogenesis.

18.5.1 Summary

Adult hippocampal neurogenesis has been proposed to be involved in several functions, including memory. Neurogenesis is promoted by high levels of growth factors, including BDNF and is decreased by sleep deprivation and by depression, resulting in hippocampal cell loss in animals and hippocampal shrinkage in people. Antidepressant drugs have the opposite effect and have been proposed to act in part by restoring neurogenesis. Exercise also increases BDNF levels and reduces depression symptoms; it may act in part by increasing sleep amounts.

Chronic sleep disruption both impairs neurogenesis and makes depression more likely to recur; treating insomnia symptoms can increase the success of treatments for depression. Interventions that increase sleep quality may influence depression symptoms by both reducing stress and improving mood as well as by increasing BDNF levels and hippocampal neurogenesis.

18.6 System-level consolidation in NREM sleep

18.6.1 The role of sharp-wave ripples

Replay of neural activity within the hippocampus strengthens a temporary representation of a new explicit/declarative memory (e.g., new words, life events, spatial locations). Forming a more stable memory, however, requires transferring this information to the cortex via system-level consolidation.[6] This term refers to consolidation processes beyond local reactivation of synaptic connections that were established during learning. It includes the spread of the new information across multiple brain regions and systems to stabilize memory and integrate the information into the framework of existing knowledge.

A frequently discussed model of system-level memory consolidation proposes that newly acquired declarative information is conveyed from temporary storage in the hippocampus to the cortex during sleep (Buzsáki, 1996; Mehta, 2007; Rasch & Born, 2013). **Figure 18.6** illustrates a simplified model of how hippocampal-cortical communication during sleep results in a more stable cortical representation of a new declarative memory (Mehta, 2007).

The three major NREM sleep elements that are involved in system-level consolidation of declarative learning are sharp-wave ripples (SWRs), slow oscillations (SOs), and sleep spindles (see Chapters 2 and 12 for definitions and descriptions). SWRs are generated within the hippocampus. They include sharp waves representing synchronous discharge of a population of hippocampal pyramidal cells, accompanied by bursts of high-frequency neural activity ("ripples") (see Chapter 2 and Figure 2.5). They occur in rats during NREM sleep and during quiet waking when they are stationary or engaged in eating or drinking. Recordings from arrays of individual hippocampal neurons indicate that firing sequences expressed while awake and exploring are often replayed during SWRs.

SWRs during sleep act locally within the hippocampus and are also transmitted to the cortex. Within the hippocampus, SWRs strengthen synaptic connections that were involved in recent learning while selectively reducing the strength of other synapses. Preventing hippocampal SWRs during sleep in mice prevented this selective reduction of synaptic strengths and, as a result, reduced the synaptic capacity for later learning (Norimoto et al., 2018).

SWRs also contribute to system-level consolidation by transmitting memory-related information from the hippocampus to the cortex, and by synchronizing neural activity across multiple cortical regions (Buzsáki, 2015; Carr et al., 2011; Dupret et al., 2010; Wilson & McNaughton, 1994; Ylinen et al., 1995). Disrupting SWRs during post-training rest or sleep impaired later memory retrieval (Ego-Stengel & Wilson, 2010; Girardeau et al., 2009). One study recorded patterns of neural activity from the medial prefrontal cortex (PFC) of rats as they learned to shift their strategy for choosing a potentially rewarded arm of a maze. PFC firing patterns recorded while rats learned to make these choices in the face of altered reward rules were strongly represented during later SWS and were in particular coordinated with the occurrence of SWRs (Peyrache et al., 2009).

A recent review of the molecular mechanisms known to be involved in hippocampal plasticity focused on a two-step hypothesis (Seibt & Frank, 2019). Learning experiences create short-lived plastic changes in hippocampal circuitry by moderately increasing or decreasing synaptic strengths. They also generate chemical "tags" within synapses that do not depend

[6] The concepts of "consolidation" and "stability" in relation to memory have evolved over decades of studying the mechanisms involved. A review of this topic noted that memories can be modified over several time scales and that there is not a single form of consolidation. It concluded that system-level consolidation is best understood as a collection of processes that can transform memories in different ways and may continue to do so as long as the memory remains viable (Dudai et al., 2015).

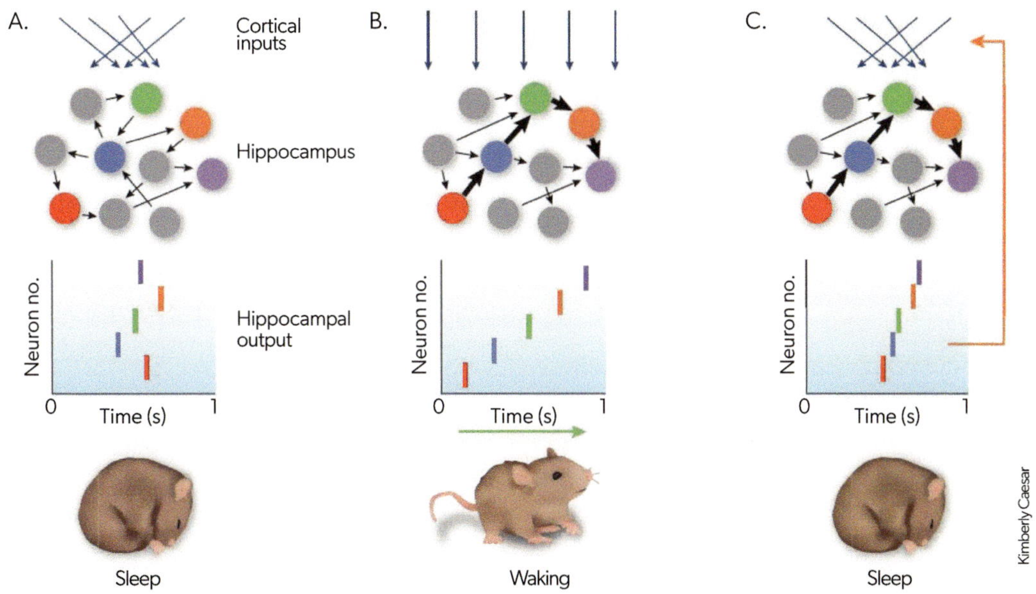

Figure 18.6 A model of the effects of experience on hippocampal cell firing sequences. **A.** There is diffuse, weak connectivity among hippocampal neurons (colored and gray circles) that show no replicable order in their firing patterns while the rodent sleeps; these neurons receive input from cortical neurons (top) that tend to fire synchronously in bursts during slow-wave On states. **B.** When place cells in the hippocampus are activated by sequential sensory input (via the cortex) during waking, they fire in an order that reflects the experienced sequence of places (sequenced cortical inputs) to which each neuron is most responsive. This experience of sequences of peak firing rates strengthens the serial connectivity (thick arrows) among a subset of neurons in the network (red, blue, green, orange, purple), representing the temporal sequence with which these places were experienced. **C.** After this exposure, a similar (speeded-up) sequence of peak firing is more probable during sleep because of this increased connectivity, which persists in the absence of structured environmental input via the cortex. The red arrow indicates that the firing sequence in the hippocampus is played back to and affects the cortex during sleep, resulting in reactivation of the sensory experience and longer-term storage of related memories. This transfer of information occurs during bursts of sharp-wave ripple activity in the hippocampus, which are coordinated with slow oscillations and sleep spindles in the cortex. Reprinted with permission of Springer: Nature from Mehta, M.R. (2007) Cortico-hippocampal interaction during up-down states and memory consolidation. *Nat Neurosci* 10:13–15. © Springer: Nature (2007). doi: 10.1038/nn0107-13.

on new protein synthesis; these tags mark specific synapses for later strengthening or weakening (Frey & Morris, 1997). During hippocampal replay events (including SWRs), the tagged synapses are strengthened (spinogenesis: growth of synaptic spines) or weakened (pruning: loss of synaptic spines) by processes that depend on protein synthesis. The identity of these tags is not certain, but activation of plasticity-related proteins in synapses (e.g., BDNF and Homer1a) has been proposed to be involved (Seibt & Frank, 2019).

SWRs from the hippocampus are produced in coordination with cortical SOs and sleep spindles (Buzsáki, 1998; Buzsáki, 2015; Gonzalez et al., 2018; Siapas & Wilson, 1998; Tang & Jadhav, 2018). (The role of sleep spindles in the triple interactions with SOs and SWRs is discussed below in Section 18.6.2.) Neural activity associated with SWRs is transmitted from the hippocampus via the entorhinal cortex to reach cortical association areas during the depolarized On phase of SOs. The sensitivity of cortical neurons to stimulatory inputs varies with their timing relative to SOs: Cortical neurons are most susceptible to reinforcement of synaptic connections during the On phase of SOs (Timofeev et al., 1996).

The timing of SWRs with respect to SOs therefore facilitates plastic changes in cortical neurons that represent newly acquired memories. This conclusion was supported by evidence from a rat model. Detection of hippocampal SWRs was used to initiate cortical stimulation that triggered time-locked delta waves and sleep spindles. These coordinated events helped consolidate memory for a spatial learning task, while similar cortical stimulation that was not synchronized to SWRs did not (Maingret et al., 2016).

The transfer of information to appropriate cortical regions from its temporary storage in the hippocampus requires precision and specificity in the flow of SWRs from hippocampal to cortical regions. Studies using intracranial recordings in both structures in people who were undergoing surgery related to treatment of epilepsy provided evidence that supports the existence of such specificity. Different hippocampal regions preferentially conveyed SWRs to different cortical regions and did so in characteristic temporal relation to cortical features like slow waves (Jiang et al., 2019).

Functional brain imaging (fMRI) during retrieval of face-image/location pairings immediately after training and 24 h later (including overnight sleep) showed changes in brain connectivity and activation consistent with this model. Successful retrieval after the 24 h interval, compared to immediate retrieval, was accompanied by less hippocampal activation, more neocortical activity, and reduced hippocampal-cortical functional connectivity during the retrieval process (Takashima et al., 2009).

The role of sleep in making memory more dependent on cortical than hippocampal activation was confirmed and extended in an fMRI study that included younger (18–25 years) and older (60–75 years) participants. On two different occasions, they learned word pairs and were tested 5 h later for their memory of the pairings after a period spent awake or including a 2 h nap opportunity. Successful recall was positively correlated with the amount of hippocampal activation during recall testing in all participants and whether they napped or not. The recall performance of the younger adults was also correlated with the amount of SWS/delta-band activity during the nap. However, in this group the amount of hippocampal activation (especially right hippocampus) during successful recall was *negatively* correlated with the percentage SWS and amount of delta-band activity during the nap. These results indicate that more SWA during the nap facilitated consolidation to form a cortically based memory, which made recall less dependent on activation of the hippocampus to retrieve information from temporary storage (Baran et al., 2016).

Older adults undergoing the same procedures showed worse memory recall after the nap condition than the younger group, suggesting that they relied on a less efficient process of memory storage and/or retrieval. Their recall performance was not significantly correlated with the amount of SWS/delta power during the nap, nor did they show a negative correlation between SWS/delta activity during the nap and hippocampal activation during successful recall. During recall testing, older participants showed greater functional connectivity between the hippocampus and frontal cortical regions compared to younger participants. This difference was present only after both groups had a nap opportunity and not after a wake period before testing (Baran et al., 2016).

Older people appeared to be relying more than younger people on continuing hippocampal-cortical communication during memory recall, presumably because there had been less successful SWS-dependent consolidation into a robust cortical form of memory during the nap. When participants stayed awake after learning, the two age groups did not differ in functional connectivity between hippocampus and cortex during later recall testing (Baran et al., 2016). See Sections 17.10 and 18.8 for discussions of how aging alters the role of SWS in memory and the underlying mechanisms involved.

18.6.2 The role of sleep spindles and triple timing

Sleep spindles in adult humans are usually categorized according to their characteristic frequency of oscillation within the sigma-band frequency range: slow spindles (11–13 [or 9–12] Hz) and fast spindles (13–16 Hz).[7] These types of spindles are distributed differently across the adult human cortex, with primarily fast spindles in central and parietal regions and slow spindles in frontal regions (Andrillon et al., 2011; Schabus et al., 2007).

Interactions among sleep spindles, SWRs, and SOs play a critical role in system-level consolidation of memories during sleep, but spindles have also been associated with other functions, which are discussed in later sections. Only a subset of spindles occur in conjunction with SOs in NREM sleep, but the timing of those in young adults is very specific. Fast spindles occur preferentially during the On (depolarized) phase of SOs, while slow spindles tend to occur after the On phase/during the Off (hyperpolarized) phase (Andrillon et al., 2011; Muehlroth et al., 2019; Mölle et al., 2011).

Studies have reported that the number, density, amplitude, timing, or characteristic frequency of spindles shown during NREM sleep correlate with later memory performance. These reported correlations must be interpreted cautiously because spindle features (e.g., number of spindles) have also been correlated in some studies with measures of general intelligence (see Section 18.9). This raises the possibility that the inter-individual correlation of spindle numbers with memory performance may reflect a stable, individual trait (e.g., general learning ability) rather than the involvement of spindles in consolidation of a specific learning experience.

To rule out this interpretation, researchers typically include a night of sleep recording to measure baseline spindle features in the absence of a specific learning experience, followed by a learning session and recordings during a second night of sleep. Finding that the extent to which post-learning features (e.g., spindle numbers) differ from baseline values is correlated with better memory for the newly learned material would more clearly support the involvement of spindles in consolidating the new learning (Gais et al., 2002; Schabus et al., 2008). The changes from baseline that are most commonly reported include increases in the total number of spindles, their density (i.e., number per unit time), their amplitude, and

[7] Sleep spindles are triggered by interactions between the thalamic reticular nucleus (TRN) and corticothalamic and thalamocortical projections. The mechanisms producing spindles are reviewed in Sections 12.2.3 and 12.2.4. The frequency ranges for slow and fast spindles (and for the sigma range) have been defined differently in different publications; see Section 2.3.2.

"spindle activity," a measure that combines spindle amplitude and duration.

In studies that distinguished fast and slow spindles in people, most reported changes in fast sleep spindles after learning that correlated with the strength of memory for motor learning tasks (Barakat et al., 2013; Doyon et al., 2018; Fogel & Smith, 2006; Genzel et al., 2009; Morin et al., 2008; Peters et al., 2008), for declarative learning tasks (Champetier et al., 2023; Genzel et al., 2009; Hahn et al., 2019; Saletin et al., 2011; Schabus et al., 2008), and for cognitively complex procedural learning (Fogel et al., 2015). Changes from baseline in features of slow spindles have generally not been shown to be related to memory consolidation in people. Spindle numbers also increased in rats during NREM sleep; for example, in relation to training on an odor-reward association task (Eschenko et al., 2006).

However, increases in spindles in the 11.25–13.75 Hz range (mostly in the range of slow spindles, but overlapping both types by some definitions) were reported in one study of paired associate learning to be correlated with memory performance for a difficult declarative learning task (one that used less concrete words that are more difficult to form associations with) after a daytime 4 h nap opportunity. Faster spindles (14–16 Hz) were not correlated with memory retention, and neither type of spindle was correlated with retention for an easier task (using more concrete words) (Schmidt, 2006).

It is unclear whether the overlap into what some define as fast spindles, the use of a daytime nap, or the difficulty of the task resulted in this less common result. Another factor to consider is that one study reported circadian variations in the average spindle frequency recorded in young people (Dijk et al., 2000; Wei et al., 1999); see **Figure 8.16**. The observed variation of average spindle frequency across circadian phases ranged between ~12.75 and 13.25 Hz. This range falls close to the typical boundary between slow and fast spindles and overlaps the frequency range of spindles correlated with learning in this study (11.25–13.75 Hz). Thus, circadian variations in spindle frequencies between daytime naps and overnight sleep could affect comparisons between studies that involved sleep at these different phases. It is unclear how this time-of-day variation might affect attributions of different roles to slow and fast spindles.

Changes in fast spindles during sleep after training have been linked to strengthening specific memories rather than to the general experience of having been involved in a learning experiment. This relationship was demonstrated in a study involving tagging a subset of newly learned words before sleep as to-be-remembered (R) and others as to-be-forgotten (F); (for details, see Section 17.9.3). Fast spindle numbers recorded from the left parietal cortex during a later nap opportunity correlated with the ratio of R to F words that were later successfully recalled. This result suggests that the increase in the number of spindles was related to selectively consolidating memory for specific tagged items rather than to the experience of being in a learning study (Saletin et al., 2011). Similarly, using transcranial anodal direct current to selectively activate one region of cortex resulted in localized increases in the number of spindles (12–16 Hz) in that region during a subsequent nap (Thom & Staresina, 2025).

Sleep spindles facilitate consolidation by interacting with other physiological processes to influence synaptic plasticity. For example, after mice experienced prolonged exposure to visual gratings with a specific orientation, synaptic potentiation in the primary visual cortex was linked to the phase-locking of neural firing to sleep spindles (Aton et al., 2014). In other studies, spindle-frequency activity during NREM sleep was correlated with increased Ca^{2+} influx (a marker of both plasticity and cellular activation) in the dendrites of layer 5 cortical pyramidal neurons. In this case, dendritic Ca^{2+} increases did not reflect increased neuronal excitability, as shown by firing rates. Instead, increased Ca^{2+} influx associated with spindles was related to increased synaptic plasticity in dendrites (Seibt et al., 2017).

In an in vitro cortical slice preparation, a pattern of electrical stimulation was applied that was copied from the actual firing pattern of a single neuron involved in a sleep spindle during the On phase of an SO. Stimulating with this firing pattern amplified postsynaptic responses of cortical neurons, resulting in both short- and long-term potentiation of synaptic transmission. Other stimulation patterns, including the reverse of the original spindle pattern, or regular stimulation at the mean firing rate of the neuron during a spindle, did not have similar effects. Triggering increased neural activity in the cortical tissue in the pattern shown by neurons during sleep spindles was uniquely suited to strengthening synaptic connections among targeted neurons (Rosanova & Ulrich, 2005).

In addition to strengthening synaptic transmission on their own, sleep spindles in intact mammalian brains can occur in conjunction with SOs and SWRs, which is critical to their role in memory. Many studies have shown that fast spindles that occur during the On phases of SOs, when principal cortical neurons are maximally depolarized, are involved in memory consolidation, presumably by their effects on synaptic plasticity.[8] SWRs contribute to the process by simultaneously transmitting newly acquired information from the hippocampus to

[8] Fast spindles have also been subtyped as "early" and "late," depending on small differences in their timing relative to the SO On state. Early-fast spindles occurred shortly after the Off state on the depolarizing limb of SOs, and late-fast spindles occurred near the On-state peak. There is evidence for a developmental trend toward increases in late-fast spindles from childhood to midlife and aging (McConnell et al., 2021).

the cortex in synchrony with the occurrence of SO depolarizations and spindles (Gonzalez et al., 2018; Maingret et al., 2016; Siapas & Wilson, 1998; Tang & Jadhav, 2018).

As an example, optogenetic stimulation was applied to the thalamic reticular nucleus in genetically engineered mice to artificially manipulate spindle numbers during sleep. Increasing spindle numbers during the On phases of SOs improved hippocampus-dependent memory; suppressing sleep spindles during the On phases impaired memory. Spindles that were triggered out of phase with the On limb of SOs neither decreased nor increased memory performance (**Figure 18.7**) (Latchoumane et al., 2017).

Another finding related to the impact of reducing spindle activity is based on evidence that inhibition of norepinephrine (NE) release from locus coeruleus neurons is permissive for spindle production. Reduced NE release occurs during REM sleep and in anticipation of each sleep spindle in NREM sleep (Aston-Jones & Bloom, 1981). Preventing this reduction in NE release by optogenetically activating locus coeruleus firing continuously during sleep in rats decreased spindle numbers and delta range activity in NREM sleep (and theta activity in REM sleep). Maintaining stable NE release and reducing spindle numbers prevented improvement in performance of a hippocampus-dependent, spatial learning task (Swift et al., 2018).

During waking activity, sensory and other information reaches the cortex, which then transmits a form of this information to the hippocampus (see **Figure 18.6 B**). During subsequent sleep, the hippocampus is triggered to feed back this information to the cortex at phases of maximal neural plasticity (**Figure 18.6 C**), as part of the process of consolidating memories of the waking events (Qin et al., 1997). Electrophysiological studies of the somatosensory cortex and hippocampus of mice and rats found that bursts of firing in cortical neurons associated with spindle production regularly preceded the onset of SWRs. This finding suggests that spindle activity in the cortex causes it to trigger the hippocampus to transmit information to the cortex via SWRs (Sirota et al., 2003).

Similarly, recordings from rats trained in an auditory-cued task showed that patterned activity in the auditory cortex preceded, and determined the contents of, hippocampal activity during SWRs. Providing auditory cues during sleep biased cortical patterns to select related input from the hippocampus within SWRs (Rothschild et al., 2017).

These results indicate that cortical activity triggers the onset of spindles (via the thalamic reticular nucleus) and SWRs (from the hippocampus) so that both occur during the On phase of slow/delta oscillations and selects the input it is to receive from the hippocampus. This timing may also ensure that hippocampal ripples convey information that biases the selection of the cortical neurons that will participate in plasticity-inducing spindle events (Siapas & Wilson, 1998; Sirota et al., 2003).

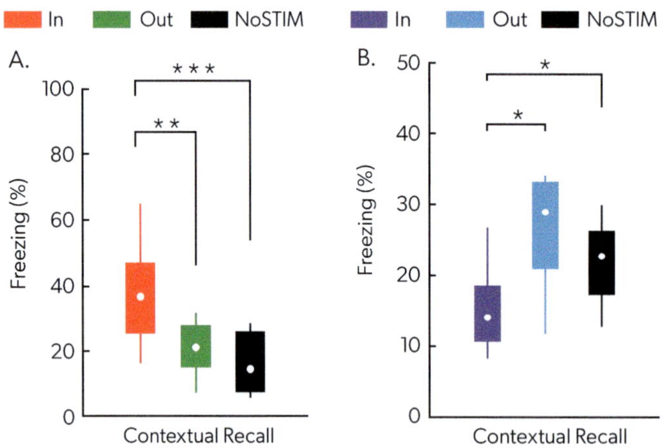

Figure 18.7 **A.** Effects on fear memory (Freezing %; Y axis) in mice of using optogenetic methods to *stimulate* sleep spindle production via the thalamic reticular nucleus in phase (In, red) or out of phase (Out, green) with the depolarized (On) phase of slow oscillations in cortex. In-phase stimulation during sleep improved later memory performance, but the effects of out-of-phase stimulation did not differ from those of no stimulation (NoSTIM, black). **B.** Optogenetic methods were also used to *suppress* spontaneous sleep spindle production either in or out of phase with the On phase of slow oscillations. In-phase inhibition (In, purple) reduced memory performance relative to out-of-phase inhibition (Out, light blue), or no inhibition (black). Data are shown as box and whisker plots, showing the median response (white dot), first to third quartile (colored box) and the full range of data ("whiskers" extending above and below the box); * $p<.05$; **, $p<.01$; *** $p<.001$. Adapted with permission of Elsevier, Ltd. from Latchoumane, C.V. et al. (2017) Thalamic spindles promote memory formation during sleep through triple phase-locking of cortical, thalamic, and hippocampal rhythms. Neuron 95:424–435. © Elsevier (2017). doi: 10.1016/j.neuron.2017.06.025.

The proposed role of cortical activity in initiating the selective cortico-hippocampo-cortical dialogue (Rothschild et al., 2017; Siapas & Wilson, 1998; Sirota et al., 2003) was supported by intracranial recordings in patients undergoing epilepsy-related surgery. One study found that cortical Off states triggered spindles in the thalamus which, as a result of the time constants involved, conveyed the spindle activity to the cortex so that it coincided with the transition to the cortical On state (Mak-McCully et al., 2017). Another study showed that cortical spindles that were synchronized with SOs were likely to trigger input from the hippocampus while spindles not associated with SOs did not. The precise timing relation between SOs and spindles ensured that hippocampal input arrived in relation to the On phase of the SO and near the end of the spindle burst (Helfrich et al., 2019). This timing would ensure arrival of hippocampal input when targeted cortical neurons are most depolarized and susceptible to synaptic strengthening (Rosanova & Ulrich, 2005; Timofeev et al., 1996). During aging, the timing of spindles shifted gradually to earlier in the On phase of SOs, which may reduce their effectiveness in memory consolidation (**Figure 18.8**) (Helfrich et al., 2018; Züst et al., 2023).

The critical role of coordinated timing of SOs and spindles in determining the strength of memory consolidation was confirmed in another human study. It assessed the reactivation during sleep of EEG "signatures" characteristic of different categories of learned information. The findings indicated that memory performance for these categories of information was positively correlated with the precision of temporal coupling between spindles and SOs associated with these signature EEG patterns (Schreiner et al., 2021).

18.6.3 Summary

Increases in the amount of spindle activity (especially fast spindles) during NREM sleep after a learning experience are correlated with the strength of explicit memory consolidation. In vitro models have shown that stimulation of cortical neurons in a pattern characteristic of neural firing during spindles facilitates synaptic plasticity. System-level consolidation of explicit memories during NREM sleep, however, also involves SWRs from the hippocampus and SOs interacting with spindles.

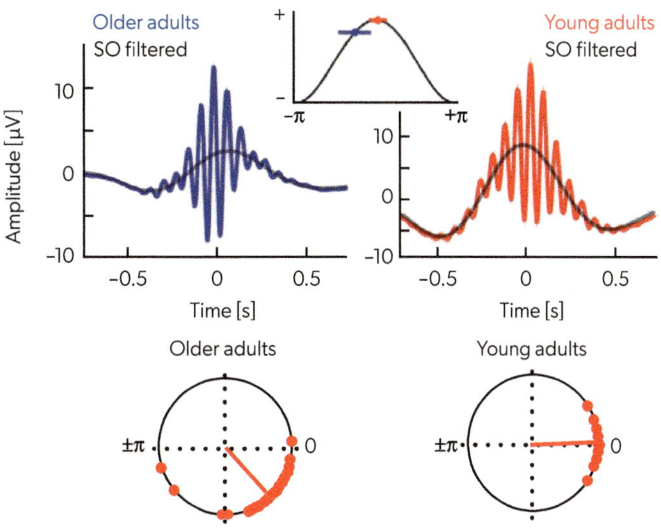

Figure 18.8 **Top:** The average timing of sleep spindles in older adults (~74 years) (blue waveform) and younger adults (~20 years) (red waveform) superimposed on averaged, filtered slow oscillations (black curves), and plotted to show their average timing relative to the peak of the depolarized On phase of the slow oscillation (0 time on the X axis). Note that the average amplitude of slow oscillations is lower in older adults; compare black curves in left and right images. The inset between the two images shows the average (red and blue dots) and standard deviations (horizontal red and blue lines; younger and older people, respectively) of timing of spindles relative to the peak of a sine wave representing a slow oscillation. The labels ± π (pi) refer to pi radians = 180^0 or half a cycle before and after the peak value at phase 0. The average timing of spindles is earlier and shows more variability in older adults. **Bottom:** The average phase of each participant's sleep spindles is plotted as a red dot relative to the peak of the On phase of slow oscillations (phase 0) for older adults (left) and younger adults (right). The average timing of spindles among participants in each group is summarized as a vector (red line), which is slightly shorter for the older adults because of their increased variability. The average vector in older adults also points to an earlier phase relative to phase 0 because spindles tend to occur before the peak On phase of the slow oscillation. Adapted with permission of Elsevier, Ltd. from Helfrich, R.F. et al. (2017) Old brains come uncoupled in sleep: slow wave-spindle synchrony, brain atrophy, and forgetting. *Neuron* 97(1): 221–230. © Elsevier (2017). doi: 10.1016/j.neuron.2017.11.020.

This role of sleep spindles relates to a model of system-level consolidation during NREM sleep in which cortical Off states trigger thalamic spindle production and initiate a transfer of information in the form of SWRs from the hippocampus. These actions are timed so that SWRs arrive in association with sleep spindles and on the positive-going slope (depolarization peak) of SOs. As a result, information from a temporary store in the hippocampus arrives in the cortex when cortical neurons are most depolarized and capable of plastic changes. Enhancing the occurrence of these triple interactions strengthens memory, and preventing the expression of SWRs or spindles at an appropriate phase of SOs impairs memory consolidation. Changes in the timing of spindles during aging may impair memory consolidation in older people.

Memory performance on a paired-associates task was positively correlated with the amount of SWS generated during a nap after training in younger participants. The amount of SWS during the nap was also negatively correlated with the amount of hippocampal activation during successful recall. These results imply that successful transfer of information from hippocampus to cortex during sleep resulted in a primarily cortical locus of information storage and retrieval. In older participants, the amount of SWS shown during the nap did not correlate positively with memory performance, nor was it correlated negatively with hippocampal activation during successful recall. Memory retrieval during testing depended more on continuing hippocampal-cortical communication in older than in younger participants. This difference presumably reflected less effective consolidation of memory in a cortical locus and greater dependence on cortical interrogation of hippocampal representations of memory to recall learned material.

18.7 Neural basis for motor skill learning

Improvement of performance on explicit motor sequence learning (MSL) tasks over a sleep episode is related to activity in several brain regions, including parts of the motor system, especially the striatum and cortical regions rostral to the primary motor area (M1), such as the supplementary motor area (SMA) (Doyon et al., 2018). Patterns of neural activity in M1 and parts of the cerebellum that are related to general motor activity while awake also recur during NREM sleep, when they are expressed during On states in both structures. M1 and the cerebellum also show coherence of spindle frequencies, which may result from indirect cerebellar input to M1 during sleep spindles via the thalamic reticular nucleus (Xu et al., 2021; Xu et al., 2022).

Participants who learned an explicit MSL task and were then tested after a period of either wake or sleep showed better performance of the sequence after sleep. Several brain regions were shown by fMRI to be activated during performance of the motor sequence (motor and sensory cortices, cerebellum, striatum, SMA). However, only the striatum was activated more during performance after a sleep period than after a wake period, suggesting that the striatum is an important target of sleep-dependent consolidation (Debas et al., 2010).

Another study of explicit MSL used fMRI to assess activation patterns during training, sleep, and next-day retesting. Regions of brain activated during task acquisition (striatum, cerebellum, and premotor and parietal cortices) were also activated during next-day retest, with especially strong striatal activation. Several brain regions also showed activations during post-training sleep that were time-locked to the occurrence of NREM sleep spindles (striatum, hippocampus, premotor area, frontal eye fields, thalamus, and cerebellum). Striatal activation (contralateral to the trained hand) that was time-locked to spindles during sleep was also correlated with the degree of overnight performance improvement (Fogel et al., 2017).

During SWS after learning to perform an explicit MSL task, participants showed increased amplitude of both delta-band and fast sigma-band oscillations (equivalent to fast spindles) in the SMA, contralateral to the trained hand (Tamaki et al., 2013). In a similar study, overnight spindle amplitude correlated positively with (left-handed) performance on the MSL task and with the strength of fMRI activation of the right (i.e., contralateral) motor cortex and striatum (especially putamen/globus pallidus) while performing the task the next day (Barakat et al., 2013). These results are consistent with other studies showing that the striatum is involved in motor memory consolidation and that its role involves interactions with sleep spindles and slow-wave activity (SWA) in the cortex (Debas et al., 2010; Fogel et al., 2017).

Implicit learning is sometimes considered to be independent of the hippocampus and other neural systems involved in explicit learning. But there is evidence that "non-hippocampal," implicit motor tasks can include a hippocampal component. The hippocampus (and adjacent cortical structures in the medial temporal lobe) may be involved under several conditions: at an early stage of memory formation; if there is a contextual or strategic aspect to the task; or if the task involves higher-order linkages among temporal and spatial sequences, regardless of whether it is an explicit or implicit learning task (Diekelmann & Born, 2007; Schendan et al., 2003; Spencer et al., 2006; van den Berg et al., 2019).

There is evidence from fMRI studies of motor tasks that both separate and overlapping medial temporal brain regions are involved in explicit and implicit aspects of learning (Schendan et al., 2003). A model of how the hippocampus could be involved in different types of learning proposed that some parts of hippocampal circuitry could, for example, acquire knowledge of explicit events, while other components develop implicit generalizations related to those events (Schapiro et al., 2017). This idea may be related to the finding in patients studied using intracranial recordings that SWRs from different hippocampal regions occurred independently of each other and were directed toward different cortical regions (Jiang et al., 2019). Although not specifically related to motor learning, this model suggests how the hippocampus could be involved simultaneously in acquiring and transmitting both explicit and implicit information related to developing a motor skill.

Taken together, these findings indicate that sleep-related improvement in explicit and, in some cases, implicit aspects of motor skills are related to the co-occurrence of SWRs, sleep spindles, and cortical SWA, as for non-motor types of explicit learning. However, in relation to motor skills, these hippocampal and cortical events occur in conjunction with activation of components of the motor system, in particular, the striatum, cerebellum, and SMA.

18.7.1 Summary

Consolidation of newly learned explicit motor patterns is related to fast sleep spindles in the cortex as well as to activity in the striatum and cerebellum. Learning new motor patterns was associated with increases during sleep in delta-band activity and in fast spindle amplitude in cortical regions. Several structures showed increased activity during both learning and later performance of a motor task, but only the striatum showed larger increases during performance after sleep than after waking. The extent of striatal activation that was time-locked to cortical spindles was correlated with the degree of performance improvement.

Memory for implicit motor tasks may benefit from sleep after training in part because an early stage of implicit learning may involve a hippocampal role especially if the task includes a strategic, higher-order, or context-related component. Both cortical slow waves and sleep spindles are involved in motor learning consolidation, but there are also contributions from activity in the striatum, cerebellum, and cortical motor systems, both during sleep after training and during recall.

18.8 Spindles across the lifespan

As previously discussed, sleep spindles have been implicated in the consolidation of several kinds of memory, although the details of spindle types and their relation to different memory systems are not always consistent across studies. The characteristics of spindles vary over the lifespan, and these differences may have implications for memory functions and cognitive abilities at different ages. Several sleep spindle features have been studied across developmental stages from infancy to late adolescence, and these have been correlated with effects on sleep-related consolidation of new learning (Clawson et al., 2016; Hahn et al., 2019). Spindles have also been linked to measures of general intelligence, which is the topic of Section 18.9.

Studies of the development of spindles in childhood have reported changes in several of their features, based on different methods for spindle detection across different age ranges; the principal trends identified are reviewed here. The characteristic frequency of spindles increased briefly during the first months of infancy, decreased during early childhood (~2 years) and then increased persistently into adolescence (Kwon et al., 2023; Tarokh & Carskadon, 2010; Zhang et al., 2021). The number of spindles produced, reported as either rates or density of spindles, followed a generally similar pattern with an increase in very early infancy, a decrease during the first years of life, and then an increase from about age three into mid-adolescence. Spindle amplitude, however, peaked at about 1 year and declined over the lifespan (Clawson et al., 2016; Kwon et al., 2023; Scholle et al., 2007; Zhang et al., 2021).

Characteristic spindle frequencies also changed across development. Young infants had predominantly fast spindles, but by about 18 months of age, more slow spindles appeared in frontal regions and the average peak frequencies of spindles in frontal regions and central regions diverged, with slower peak frequencies in frontal regions. Spindles in both regions continued to increase in frequency up to ~18 years of age (Kwon et al., 2023).

There is limited information about how sleep spindles relate to cognitive abilities in children. In preschool-age children (averaging 46 months old), immediate recall on a visuospatial memory task was negatively correlated with spindle density (Kurdziel et al., 2013), which is consistent with evidence for a negative correlation with fluid intelligence in older children (average age, 10 years) (Geiger et al., 2011), but seems inconsistent with findings in adults. But the amount of increase in spindle density over a daytime nap after learning was correlated with better retention of visuospatial pairings, which is consistent with findings in adults. Although spindles averaged ~12 Hz, they were recorded at central locations, where fast spindles are more common in adults (Kurdziel et al., 2013). Given the changes in the characteristic frequency of spindles across development, and uncertainty about the functional roles of different spindle frequencies and anatomical locations in different age groups, it is unclear whether 12 Hz spindles in central regions should be considered to be equivalent to adult slow or fast spindles.

Among children aged 9 or 10 at baseline, increases in coherence of sigma-band activity within each hemisphere over a subsequent 1–3 year period was correlated with improved performance on tests of executive functions (Tarokh et al., 2014). Developmental changes in spindle frequency and number, as well as sigma-band power, were also correlated with increased fluid intelligence and performance on speed/accuracy tasks, but not significantly with overall IQ scores[9] (Reynolds et al., 2018).

One group of children was studied during prepuberty (8–11 years) and again during mid-late adolescence (14–18 years). Initially they had more slow than fast spindles across all brain regions, but this shifted after puberty to the adult pattern of more fast spindles at central and parietal sites and slow spindles in frontal regions. At the younger age, an increase in slow spindles overnight after paired-associate learning was related to a *decrease* in memory performance. During adolescence, however, this correlation was lost and there was instead a positive correlation between increases in fast spindles after learning and the extent of overnight memory consolidation (Hahn et al., 2019), as has been reported in adults.

There was also a strong correlation between the memory benefits of sleep and the amount of increase from childhood to adolescence in fast spindle density after learning, implying that maturation of fast spindle mechanisms was closely related to increased effectiveness of sleep for memory enhancement. The importance of the timing of fast spindles was confirmed by evidence that the coupling strength between fast spindles and SOs increased from childhood to adolescence, and the degree of increased coupling was correlated with greater benefits of sleep for memory (Hahn et al., 2020).

Many (but not all) studies of older people found that sleep after learning did not have the benefits for consolidation seen in young adult participants (see Section 17.10.2). This loss of benefit has been linked to characteristic changes in sleep during aging, including more disrupted sleep, reduced SWA (especially in men), and reduced spindle numbers (see Section 4.6) (Crowley et al., 2002; Landolt et al., 1996; Nicolas et al., 2001; Purcell et al., 2017). Consistent with the importance of spindles, the extent of reduction in spindle numbers was positively correlated with deficits in declarative memory performance in older people (Seeck-Hirschner et al., 2012). Similarly, the degree of clustering of fast spindles decreased with age (over 50) and was associated with poorer performance on an explicit spatial memory task (Champetier et al., 2023). Older participants also showed less increase in spindle density than younger participants during sleep after learning a motor task and less performance improvement (Peters et al., 2008).

[9] Overall IQ scores include measures of both fluid intelligence (e.g., general or abstract reasoning ability, not specifically related to previous learning) and crystallized intelligence (e.g., vocabulary, specific facts, grammatical rules).

The timing of spindles relative to cortical slow oscillations (SOs) has been shown to be important for memory consolidation (Latchoumane et al., 2017); see Section 18.6.2. Older adults showed more variable and earlier timing of spindles relative to the peak On phase of frontal SOs. This change in the timing of spindles in relation to SOs was associated with deficits in overnight memory consolidation and with reduced gray matter volume in the medial prefrontal cortex (Helfrich et al., 2018); see **Figure 18.8**.

An analysis of spindles over the lifespan confirmed a gradual reduction in spindle numbers and a shift in spindle timing relative to SOs. After middle age (~50 years), spindles tended to lead the peak phases of SOs rather than coinciding with or following the SO peak (compare to **Figure 18.8**). This change was accompanied by reduced numbers of SO/spindle coupling events, probably because of reductions in sleep duration, SWS, and spindles. Reduced coupling events were also associated with increased blood levels of glial fibrillary acidic protein (GFAP), a marker of astrocytic activation, which could reflect a response to increased inflammation and neuronal damage (Züst et al., 2023).

In addition to their spontaneous occurrence, spindles are also triggered by potentially sleep-disrupting external noises; see discussion in Section 12.4.2. People who generated more spindles in response to noise during sleep were better able to preserve sleep continuity without waking (Dang-Vu et al., 2010). One interpretation is that noise-evoked spindles are a secondary consequence of thalamic suppression of cortical responses to very loud stimuli (Cote et al., 2000).

These findings raise the possibility that sleep spindles and their often associated K complexes play a role in protecting the sleeping brain from external disturbances. Under conditions of external noise, sleep spindles could support memory consolidation in two ways: directly by effects on synaptic plasticity, in interaction with SOs and SWRs, and indirectly by contributing to protection of sleep continuity so sleep-dependent consolidation can proceed. Reduced sleep spindle numbers during aging could impair the benefits of sleep for memory in part by allowing more externally triggered disruption of sleep continuity.

18.8.1 Summary

There are complex changes in spindle features starting in infancy, including initial, transient increases in spindle frequency and density, followed by decreases in toddlers, and then increases from early childhood into adolescence. Across childhood, the dominant frequencies of spindles increase, but a distinction between slow and fast spindles is established by ~18 months. During adolescence, fast spindles become more common in central and parietal regions and slow spindles remain most common in frontal regions.

Although higher spindle density during a daytime nap in young children was associated with better retention of a learned task, older children did not show this benefit for retention of word pairs after overnight sleep. Slow spindle density was actually associated with worse memory performance. The strength of coupling between fast spindles and SOs, as well as the density of fast spindles, increased into adolescence. Post-pubertally, higher density of central fast spindles during sleep was associated with better overnight memory retention, as in adults.

Several changes in sleep among older adults were correlated with reduced benefits of sleep for memory consolidation. These included a reduced number of spindles, reductions in the amount of SWA and in the amplitude of SOs, earlier timing of sleep spindles relative to the peak On phase of SOs, and reduced clustering of spindles.

Spindles, along with K complexes, have also been implicated in inhibiting waking in response to external noises during sleep, thereby helping to preserve sleep continuity. Consolidation in older people could be affected by reductions in spindle numbers both because of reduced neural plasticity and because of increased sensitivity to sleep-disrupting stimuli.

18.9 Sleep spindles and intelligence

Studies in prepubertal children found that slower sleep spindle frequencies were associated with higher scores on several measures related to general intelligence (Geiger et al., 2011; Gruber et al., 2013). In childhood, both spindle activity (a measure combining amplitude and duration) of slow spindles (Hoedlmoser et al., 2014) and increases from childhood to adolescence in the density of slow spindles over frontal regions measured on a baseline night (before a specific learning task), were also correlated with measures of general intelligence (Hahn et al., 2019).

Studies in adults, as in children, reported correlations between features of spindles and measures of general intelligence, but the features identified have been inconsistent across studies. Some studies of adult men and women reported that the density of fast spindles or spindle activity correlated with general intellectual ability (Bódizs et al., 2005; Gais et al., 2002; Schabus et al., 2008) and immediate recall of newly learned material (Gais et al., 2002). Others reported a similar correlation between fast spindle density and intelligence in adult and adolescent females but not in males (Bódizs et al., 2014; Ujma et al., 2014). A study of young men reported instead that only slow spindle durations during a daytime nap correlated with intelligence scores, while other spindle features, including all features of fast spindles examined, did not correlate significantly after adjustment for multiple comparisons (Ujma et al., 2015).

A meta-analysis of studies including children and adults concluded that there was evidence that the amplitude of both fast and slow spindles correlated with intelligence, but that spindle frequency and duration did not. A weak, apparent association of intelligence with the density of slow spindles was ambiguous (Ujma, 2018). Several aspects of spindle physiology change across development, and there are circadian variations in the amount of sigma-band activity (spanning fast and slow spindles) and in the characteristic frequency of spindles (Dijk & Czeisler, 1995; Wei et al., 1999). Thus, the conclusions reached in this analysis may have been affected by the inclusion of studies involving both adults and children and both overnight sleep and daytime nap studies.

Various features of sleep spindles have been correlated with either the strength of memory consolidation or scores on tests of general intelligence. Several factors probably contribute to differences in results among studies. One source of variability relates to the statistical issues that arise from conducting multiple comparisons within a study without controlling for the resulting risk of false positive results.

Different studies have, for example, correlated intelligence scores or memory performance with the "number, density, amplitude, length, power, or peak frequency" (Ujma et al., 2014, p. 16366) of slow spindles, fast spindles, or all spindles. These features have also sometimes been correlated separately for multiple cortical regions and for different segments of a sleep period. Calculating the resulting large number of correlations, especially in small studies, increases the risk of finding one or more statistically significant correlations that are unlikely to be replicated in future studies. Correcting statistically for multiple correlations reduces this risk, but historically such corrections have not always been applied (Ackermann et al., 2015; Mantua, 2018; Pesonen et al., 2019; Ujma et al., 2014).

To illustrate this point, the largest study to date examining the correlation of sleep spindles with intelligence scores (176 older adolescents) found statistically significant ($p < 0.05$) raw correlations between spindle features such as density or duration and intelligence measures in one or both genders. However, none of these correlations remained statistically significant after applying corrections for multiple comparisons (Pesonen et al., 2019).

Another issue is that the various automated systems and software tools that are used to detect spindles in different studies may differ in their ability to detect spindles and to measure different spindle features. Other studies have used measures of sigma-frequency EEG power as an indirect measure of spindle activity rather than counting spindles directly. There is no consensus as to which parameter settings are most appropriate for spindle detection and counting using different automated methods (Adra et al., 2022).

A meta-analysis of 22 studies identified spindle amplitude as the only reliable correlate of intelligence scores. One interpretation of that result is that most measurement tools can assess amplitude more reliably than other spindle features, so amplitude is the most likely feature to be identified consistently across studies as a correlate of intelligence. Variability across studies in measuring other features could obscure any other correlations if they exist (Ujma, 2018).

Another study took a different approach to the measurement issue by assessing which settings for seven variables in one type of spindle detection software (Luna) best predicted scores on tests of crystallized and fluid intelligence using data from 161 adults >18 years of age. The strongest correlations for fluid intelligence were related to fast spindles, with weak or absent correlations for slow spindles, except for a test of working memory that favored slow spindles. The results showed that the strength of these correlations was highly dependent on the settings used to detect spindles. Crystallized intelligence scores were generally not correlated with either spindle type (Adra et al., 2022). A study that examined brain activation patterns time-locked to spindle activity (fast and slow spindles were not distinguished) also found significant correlations with the results of tests of fluid intelligence but not with tests of crystallized knowledge or short-term memory (Fang et al., 2019).

Taken together, these results point to fast spindles in adults as a correlate of fluid intelligence, with some support for the importance of fast spindle amplitude, although contradictory results also exist. Results from studies of children, however, are more consistent with a correlation between intelligence test scores and slow spindles. The evidence indicates that the specific detection parameters and tools used to measure spindle features are critical determinants of the strength of correlations that are observed and the ability to replicate findings across studies.

18.9.1 Summary

Despite a large body of evidence demonstrating that fast sleep spindles are correlated with experience-related plasticity and memory consolidation (Fogel & Smith, 2011; Rasch & Born, 2013), there is less agreement about the connection between sleep spindles and general intelligence, and about which specific spindle features drive these correlations. Different findings among studies probably result from using different methods to measure spindles and applying different statistical analyses to the data. A large study of the relation of spindle features to intelligence found several significant raw correlations, but none remained significant after correcting for multiple comparisons, which was not done consistently across studies.

Frontal, slow spindles have not typically been linked to memory consolidation, but they have been linked to measures of general intelligence in children. Several spindle features have also been correlated with general intelligence in both children and adults. A meta-analysis combining studies of both children and adults concluded that the amplitude of both fast and slow spindles correlated with intelligence test scores. It is unclear whether age-specific effects may have been obscured by including all age groups. It is possible that the strength of correlations of intelligence with spindle amplitude is a consequence of amplitude being measured more consistently than other spindle features using various software tools.

One study showed that adjustments to the settings of several parameters used by a spindle detection algorithm had substantial effects on its outputs. These effects could, in turn, influence which spindle features would be found to correlate with intelligence scores. Regardless of the parameter settings used, the most robust correlations observed in adults were between fast spindles and fluid intelligence, while no significant correlations were observed with crystallized intelligence scores.

18.10 REM sleep and memory consolidation

The sleep features reported to be involved in memory consolidation during NREM sleep, namely, SOs, SWRs, and spindles, are absent in REM sleep. Nevertheless, there is substantial evidence that REM sleep is also involved in some forms of memory consolidation. As discussed in Chapter 17, there is behavioral evidence for the involvement of REM sleep in stabilizing or strengthening memory related to sensory learning, emotion-linked explicit learning, other forms of explicit learning, and some types of implicit learning. Some models of consolidation also propose sequential roles for NREM and REM sleep in consolidation of several types of memory.

Most research addressing the physiological mechanisms by which REM sleep affects memory consolidation has been conducted on laboratory rodents in relation to spatial learning. There is evidence from single-unit recordings in the hippocampus that individual place cells that are activated during waking exploration of an environment by a rat also fire at higher rates later during both REM and NREM sleep (Pavlides & Winson, 1989). Sequences of place cell firing that correspond to the path followed through the environment also get replayed with a statistically higher probability during later NREM sleep and are implicated in place learning (Wilson & McNaughton, 1994); see **Figure 18.5.** But it is not clear whether this kind of ensemble, sequential replay also appears during REM sleep, as this has so far been reported in only one study (Louie & Wilson, 2001).

Studies of the mechanisms of memory consolidation that operate during REM sleep have instead focused primarily on hippocampal theta rhythms in animals. These are oscillating field potentials (4–12 Hz) that are recorded using large (macro) electrodes in the hippocampus. Theta rhythms are produced in the rodent hippocampus during waking locomotor activity and continuously during REM sleep (Kemp & Kaada, 1975; Mizuseki & Miyawaki, 2017; Vanderwolf et al., 1977).[10]

In a study of rats exploring an environment, firing of individual hippocampal place cells (recorded with microelectrodes) occurred near the peak phases of local theta oscillations (recorded with macroelectrodes) during movement through both novel parts of the environment and through familiar, previously explored areas. During subsequent REM sleep, place cells that were activated while exploring and learning about the novel areas maintained peak firing phases near theta rhythm peaks, similar to the pattern shown during waking exploration (**Figure 18.9 B**). However, place cells that were activated while exploring familiar areas (presumably involving minimal new learning) fired at lower rates during later REM sleep. Most critically, they also showed their highest firing rates near theta rhythm troughs, thereby reversing the phase of highest firing rates relative to theta rhythms shown during waking exploration and during REM sleep in relation to novel areas (**Figure 18.9 A**) (Poe et al., 2000).

Firing near theta rhythm peaks is associated with strengthening synaptic connections, so place cells that fired during waking exploration of both familiar and novel places would have strengthened synaptic connections. During later REM sleep, cells that fired in novel areas again fired near theta rhythm peaks, which would reinforce these connections and help to consolidate the new spatial information. Firing near theta rhythm troughs is instead associated with weakening connections, so cells that fired at this phase during REM sleep would be de-potentiating synapses related to old information about a familiar environment. Thus, differences during REM sleep in the timing of firing peaks relative to theta rhythms reflected the selective consolidation of newly acquired spatial information (Poe et al., 2000).

This evidence for selective modification of synaptic strengths during REM sleep is consistent with findings discussed earlier from a study related to motor learning (Section 18.4.2). In that study, some synaptic spines that were formed during motor learning were strengthened during later REM sleep, while others were eliminated (Li et al., 2017).

Another way to test the idea that hippocampal theta rhythms are involved in consolidating explicit spatial learning is to prevent generation of these rhythms. Activity of neurons in the medial septum (which projects to the hippocampus) is required to pace production of hippocampal theta rhythms. Lesions of the medial septum in rats blocked theta rhythm production and interfered with spatial memory performance

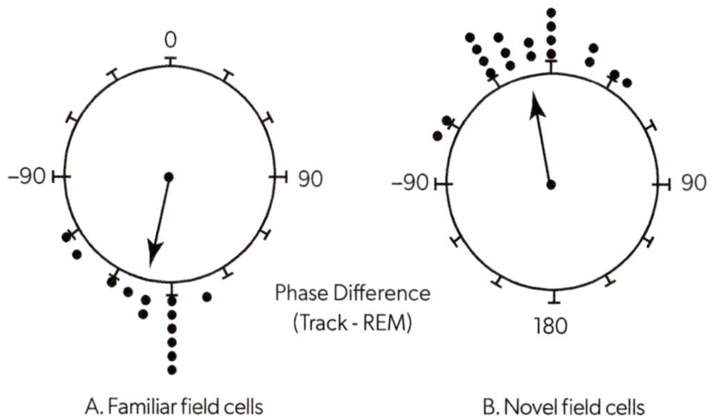

Figure 18.9 Individual hippocampal place cells fired at their highest rates when a rat exploring an environment entered a specific location. A cell's peak firing rate occurred near the peak phase of the ensemble hippocampal theta rhythm (5–10 Hz) during waking exploration (Track). During REM sleep after exploration of an environment, individual place cells fired at different phases of the theta rhythm depending on the familiarity of the location. The circular plots show the *difference* in degrees of a circle between the phase of the highest firing rate and the peak of the theta rhythm (identical phase relation = 0°) between waking exploration and later REM sleep. **A.** Cells coding for a familiar location fired close to the opposite phase (180°) relative to the theta rhythm from their peak firing phase during waking exploration. The average difference in timing of the cells' firing peaks was −168 ± 6° (arrow). **B.** When sleep occurred after first exposure to a new environment, the difference in firing peaks (relative to the theta rhythm) of individual cells between waking and REM sleep was close to 0° (−11 ± 6° [arrow]). Firing of place cells near the theta rhythm peak during REM sleep tends to potentiate synaptic connections related to novel environments, while firing at the opposite phase for familiar locations tends to de-potentiate synaptic connections. Adapted with permission of Elsevier, Ltd. from Poe, G.R. et al. (2000) Experience-dependent phase-reversal of hippocampal neuron firing during REM sleep. *Brain Res* 855:176–180. © Elsevier (2000). doi: 10.1016/s0006-8993(99)02310-0.

(Winson, 1978). This finding is consistent with a role for theta rhythms in spatial memory, but it is also possible that unrelated effects of damage to the septum could have been involved.

A more specific test of the involvement of theta rhythms in memory consolidation used optogenetic methods to block their production. In this study, mice first learned two spatial tasks and a nonspatial control task (classically conditioned fear in response to a sound). Experimenters then optogenetically silenced medial septal neurons during REM sleep and blocked theta rhythm production. Preventing hippocampal theta selectively during REM sleep impaired the mice's memory for both spatial tasks. The nonspatial memory, however, was unaffected, indicating a specific role for REM sleep theta rhythms in consolidation of hippocampus-dependent spatial memories (Boyce et al., 2016).

A different modification of neuronal plasticity during REM sleep has been reported to determine the strength of

[10] These hippocampal rhythms are different from "theta"-band frequencies (typically 4–8 Hz) that are detectable in the human EEG recorded from scalp electrodes, which reflect underlying neocortical activity.

consolidation in mice of a conditioned discrimination between tones signaling danger and safety. Pyramidal cells in the prefrontal cortex of mice showed increased activation of their dendrites, accompanied by suppression of activity in their somata during REM sleep relative to NREM sleep or waking. Within a 4 h window after fear conditioning, two different optogenetic manipulations were then applied to different neurotransmitter systems in the prefrontal cortex, exclusively during REM sleep episodes.

Optogenetic silencing that prevented dendritic activation in pyramidal neurons eliminated the learned discrimination between the safety and danger signals. Optogenetic silencing that prevented the decrease in activation of somata during REM sleep instead enhanced later discrimination performance. These effects were related to evidence from patch-clamp recordings from pyramidal neurons that the treatment that eliminated the discrimination also reduced synaptic plasticity, while the treatment that enhanced discrimination increased synaptic plasticity (Aime et al., 2022).

Another line of research supports the involvement of REM sleep in spatial memory consolidation. Newly born hippocampal neurons in the dentate gyrus of mice (a site of adult neurogenesis) were activated (as indexed by increased Ca^{2+} influx) after mice learned to avoid a location in which they received a foot shock. The same neurons were also activated during REM sleep that occurred within a subsequent 6 h time window, during which memory consolidation is known to occur. Selectively suppressing the activity of these neurons during REM sleep within that time window, but not during waking or NREM sleep, impaired consolidation of the memory and reduced later avoidance of the shock location. It did not impair a nonspatial memory produced by classical conditioning of a fear response to a tone (Kumar et al., 2020).

Suppressing the activity of these neurons during REM sleep also caused reduced expression of plasticity-related genes and changes in synaptic spines that are characteristic of reduced synaptic effectiveness. These results indicate that, during REM sleep, the activity of newly born (but not mature) dentate gyrus neurons promoted anatomical changes in synapses that are involved in consolidation of an explicit spatial memory (Kumar et al., 2020).

It remains to be determined whether the involvement of theta rhythms during REM sleep in explicit, spatial memory in animal models is applicable to people. People generate only transient bursts of theta-frequency rhythms in the hippocampus during REM sleep (Cantero et al., 2004) unlike the continuous theta observed in rodents during that stage. Instead, the human hippocampus generates a slower oscillation (1.5–3 Hz) during REM sleep (Bódizs et al., 2001). This observation may reflect a more general difference in hippocampal rhythms between people and small rodents. For example, "ripple" activity (part of SWRs) in the human hippocampus is also slower than that recorded from rodents (Bragin et al., 1999).

The idea that the slower hippocampal rhythms in people could be functionally similar to those recorded from the rodent hippocampus has some indirect support. A human study using magnetoencephalographic (MEG) recordings found that participants who were acquiring implicit information about spatial context in a visual detection task showed increased "theta" activity (defined as 1–7 Hz) in the right hippocampus. When using this contextual information later in performing the task, participants did not show theta in the hippocampus but did show it in the prefrontal cortex. These results might imply a role for these hippocampal rhythms in the acquisition of implicit spatial information and its transfer to cortical systems (Spaak & de Lange, 2020). These results do not, however, explicitly address whether slow hippocampal oscillations in people are involved in memory consolidation during REM sleep.

18.10.1 Summary

Several experimental approaches have shown that hippocampal theta rhythms produced during REM sleep in rodents are involved in memory consolidation. Firing of hippocampal neurons during the peak depolarized phase of these theta rhythms in rodents strengthens synaptic connectivity, while firing at the opposite phase de-potentiates synapses. Cells coding for familiar locations fired at the trough phase of theta rhythms during REM sleep (weakening recently acquired synaptic strengths), while those linked to novel locations fired at the peak phase (strengthening their connections).

Preventing hippocampal theta rhythms by lesions of the septum (which drives these rhythms) or by optogenetic silencing of septal neurons impaired consolidation of newly learned, explicit spatial information. These manipulations did not interfere with classically conditioned memories, supporting a specific role for hippocampal theta in consolidating spatial memories.

Optogenetic manipulations of neurotransmitter systems in the prefrontal cortex were used to alter the balance of activation between the dendritic fields and somata of pyramidal neurons during REM sleep. These manipulations could either eliminate or enhance classically conditioned fear responses in mice, depending on the direction of change in this balance.

Newly born neurons in the dentate gyrus that were active after spatial learning were also activated during later REM sleep at a time when memory consolidation occurs. Preventing their activity during REM sleep within this time window generated molecular and structural changes in neurons that interfered with consolidation of the spatial memory but did not affect a classically conditioned fear response.

Thus, REM sleep and its characteristic theta rhythms were involved in consolidation of explicit (spatial) learning in rodents. Neurotransmitter-dependent changes in activation of different neuronal compartments in the cortex of mice during REM sleep had a similar role for a classically conditioned memory. The human hippocampus, however, produces slower oscillations with only scattered theta-frequency events during REM sleep. These slower hippocampal rhythms may be important for acquiring and transferring information to the cortex, but their role in memory consolidation during sleep has not been demonstrated.

18.11 Sensory enhancement of memory during sleep

If spontaneous replay of neural patterns during sleep strengthens memories linked to that neural activity, would artificially reinforcing those patterns during sleep also improve memory? One test of this idea involved participants learning the locations of matching pairs of images in a 30-position array (similar to the TV/board game *Concentration*). In addition to this hippocampus-dependent spatial learning task, participants also practiced an MSL (motor) task that was not expected to involve the hippocampus.

During training, one group of participants were exposed to a distinctive novel odor. After training, all participants slept overnight and were exposed either to the same odor or to odorless air selectively during waking, SWS, or REM sleep (**Figure 18.10**). The goal was to use the odor to reactivate hippocampal circuits that had been active while encoding spatial information in the presence of that odor. Unlike other sensory systems, the olfactory system is closely connected to the human hippocampus (Zhou et al., 2021). In a separate brain imaging study, odor presentation during sleep was shown to activate the human hippocampus.

Odor presentation during SWS enhanced later performance on the spatial memory task only for those participants who had also been exposed to that odor during training. Presenting the odor either while participants were still awake or during REM sleep did not affect morning performance on the spatial memory task, regardless of whether they had experienced exposure to the odor during training, nor did odor exposure under any conditions affect performance on the motor task (Rasch et al., 2007). A related study presented a training-linked odor in SWS sleep during a 40 min nap after training; it was also effective in improving spatial memory performance (Diekelmann et al., 2012).

These studies showed that a sensory cue that was present during both a learning experience and later SWS reinforced memory for a hippocampus-dependent, spatial learning task. This kind of memory reactivation has also been shown in other species: presentation of a specific odor to honeybees (*Apis*

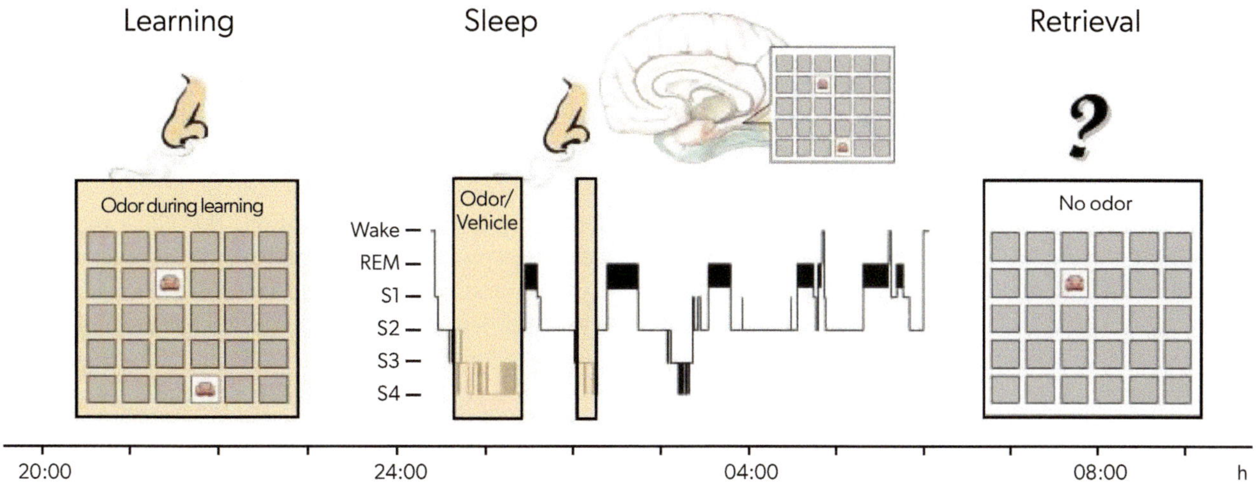

Figure 18.10 Experimental paradigm for a test of the impact of hippocampal reactivation during sleep on later retrieval of newly acquired information. The task involved learning the locations of identical pairs of stimuli in a 30-stimulus array (Learning); some participants were exposed to a novel odor while learning the task. During a later sleep period (Sleep), some participants were exposed to the same odor (or an unscented control vehicle) during SWS (Stages 3/4; as shown by the yellow boxes); others were exposed to the odor while awake just before going to sleep or during REM sleep. The next day (Retrieval), everyone was retested on their ability to retrieve the previously acquired information in the absence of any odor. Only those exposed to the odor during both learning and SWS showed better memory for learned spatial locations than controls. There was no benefit of similar exposure to the odor for a finger-tapping sequence task learned at the same time. Reprinted with permission of AAAS from Rasch, B. et al. (2007) Odor cues during slow-wave sleep prompt declarative memory consolidation. *Science* 315:1426–1429. © AAAS (2007). doi: 10.1126/science.1138581; permission conveyed through Copyright Clearance Center, Inc.

mellifera) while they acquired a learned association and then during a later sleep phase also enhanced their memory for that association (Zwaka et al., 2015).

One human study examined the specificity of memory enhancement by olfactory cuing. A distinctive olfactory context was present while participants learned to associate paired words that were presented as moving to locations within either the left or right visual field. Participants maintained central gaze fixation throughout training in order to lateralize the word-location associations to each hemisphere's visual field (e.g., left visual field pairings seen only by the right hemisphere).

During a later 2 h nap opportunity, the same olfactory stimulation was presented during NREM sleep, but exclusively to one nostril; e.g., the right nostril, which projects ipsilaterally to the right hemisphere that had presumably acquired a memory of the word-location pairings. The lateralized olfactory cuing during sleep maintained baseline recall of word-location pairings processed in the hemisphere targeted by the olfactory input, but there was deterioration of memory for items presented to the other hemisphere. The timing of frontal sleep spindles during NREM sleep relative to slow oscillations (SOs) was affected by unilateral olfactory cuing. Sleep spindles in the cued hemisphere were timed closer to the peak On phase of SOs than spindles in the un-cued hemisphere (Bar et al., 2020).

Olfactory cues during sleep did not improve the speed of performance of an MSL task (Rasch et al., 2007), but motor learning is susceptible to targeted memory reactivation (TMR) using another sensory modality. One study used an implicit serial reaction time task (SRTT) to assess the effects of cued activation using musical tones. Participants used the fingers of one hand to tap an array of buttons in sequences determined by a parallel array of visual cues presented on a screen, with each visual cue accompanied by a unique musical tone. They alternated responding to two different sequences (12 steps each) during training.

The sequence of tones that had accompanied one of these tapping sequences was replayed during later overnight SWS. That resulted in increased speed of performance of the SRTT task the next day for the cued sequence compared to the uncued sequence. Hearing the tone sequences replayed while awake did not provide the same benefit. Performance improvement was also correlated with the number of fast sleep spindles recorded over the relevant motor cortex during TMR (Cousins et al., 2014).

In addition, participants in this study were tested for their explicit knowledge of the sequences the next day and they showed more explicit knowledge of the cued than the uncued sequence. The auditory TMR thus enhanced next-day performance of the cued sequence and promoted the conversion of this implicitly learned motor sequence into a more robust explicit memory of the motor sequence (Cousins et al., 2014).

Other TMR studies have used sounds and words to demonstrate benefits of reactivation during NREM sleep for memory of explicit pairings with spatial information or objects (Oudiette et al., 2013). For example, images on a screen were presented in different locations along with sounds that were inherently linked to the images (e.g., a cat's meow accompanying an image of a cat), and participants were later exposed to a subset of the sounds during NREM sleep. Recall of the spatial locations of the images after a nap period was improved for the subset of images that had their paired sounds presented during sleep, and not for other stimuli. The benefit was correlated with delta power during the nap and with parietal fast spindles during sound presentations (Creery et al., 2015; Rudoy et al., 2009).

In a study in which spoken adjectives were paired with images of either scenes or objects during training, the spoken adjectives were then used as TMR cues during a 90 min nap opportunity. The cues evoked increases (relative to unrelated new adjectives) in central, left-hemisphere fast spindles linked to SOs and improved later recall of the paired objects or scenes. The EEG patterns accompanying evoked fast spindles in response to adjectives linked to either objects or scenes were more similar within these categories than between categories. These observations suggest that the EEG patterns evoked by the TMR cues contained information that represented at least the general categories of the paired words (Cairney et al., 2018).

Participants in another study viewed a screen that displayed two objects on separate sides of the screen, only one of which was appropriately paired with a sound (e.g., "moo"-cow). Participants made a lateralized arm/hand movement (left or right arm) to the side of the display on which the correct sound-related object appeared. During a subsequent nap, the presentation of the sound stimuli evoked neural patterns that could be decoded as reflecting the appropriate lateralization of the correct image location. This effect was specific to cue-object pairings that had been retrieved successfully during a pre-nap test, and it predicted successful performance during a post-nap test. These results indicate that the lateralized EEG patterns evoked by an auditory TMR stimulus were specific to correctly learned information and appeared to contribute to stabilizing the related memory (Wang et al., 2019).

These studies show that sensory stimulation during NREM sleep can evoke neural activity patterns, or at least loci of activation, that echo the activation that occurred during learning in the presence of the same sensory stimulation. The evidence reviewed above indicated that learning-associated stimuli presented during sleep can increase fast spindle activity in the cortex and strengthen the linkage of spindles to the most positive phase of SOs. These altered responses during NREM sleep were also linked to better recall of information learned while awake (Bar et al., 2020).

These results suggest that spindles evoked by learning-linked stimuli during NREM sleep convey information specific to these stimuli and their newly acquired associations. Triggering the memory of a targeted item at a phase of maximal synaptic plasticity may function as a form of covert, neural rehearsal that strengthens the links between the neural representations of the item and of its paired item or location, thereby stabilizing or enhancing the learned association (Bar et al., 2020; Cairney et al., 2018; Wang et al., 2019). A study that used an automated detection system to identify an appropriate sleep phase for presentation of a TMR stimulus found that moderate-intensity stimuli produced the expected enhancement of memory, but louder stimuli did not. This result was attributed to loud stimuli disrupting sleep and therefore the memory enhancement process (Whitmore et al., 2022).

Replay during SWS, however, does not always strengthen memory. A learning paradigm that involved extracting and learning a statistical (i.e., probabilistic, not fixed) pattern from a sequence of sounds produced a different outcome. Replaying the auditory stimulus sequence during SWS interfered with, rather than enhanced, later memory for the abstracted statistical rule (Hennies et al., 2017). An interpretation of that result is that replaying sensory stimuli that evoked learned associations during SWS strengthened those immediate associations, but the resulting reinforcement interfered with the more complicated, secondary task of abstracting and remembering a general, statistical rule based on those specific examples.

Auditory cues in another study were linked to presentation of visual reasoning tasks that required abstraction of a rule. The linked cues were later presented during either SWS or REM sleep. There was no improvement in solving the task for stimuli presented during SWS. TMR during REM sleep, however, did benefit later performance but only when retested a week later, not immediately after the sleep period (Pereira et al., 2023).

These results indicate that activation during SWS using cues linked to a rule abstraction problem did not improve performance. It is not clear whether this result indicates that SWS is not involved in rule abstraction or that the stimulation during SWS interfered with the process. A study that did not involve TMR suggested a possible role for SWS in abstraction of one type. Participants who were exposed to tone sequences with a hidden statistical structure were tested for their ability to recognize elements of the sequences that followed the same statistical rule after a period of wake or sleep. Success in later abstracting the rule based on the sample sequences was improved in the sleep condition and was correlated with the amount of SWS shown (Durrant et al., 2013; Durrant et al., 2011).

18.11.1 Summary

Re-exposure during NREM or SWS to sensory stimuli (smells or sounds) associated with specific items located in different spatial locations stabilized or strengthened memory for the location of these items. The specificity of targeted memory reactivation (TMR) in other studies was shown by enhancing some recently learned associations and not others with selective stimulus-based memory reactivation. TMR in some studies was related to increasing fast spindle activity near the peak of the On phase of SOs, which presumably reinforced the association between the stimulus and, for example, the target item's location. Features of the EEG activity accompanying TMR stimuli could also be decoded as reflecting at least the category or the laterality of a target item (or its linked motor response). These observations imply that future, more refined analyses might identify specific EEG features that represent the process of strengthening associations between a cue and a linked item or its location.

TMR was initially demonstrated for hippocampus-dependent, explicit memories but not for implicit motor learning. Later evidence indicating that TMR could reinforce performance of an implicit motor task (SRTT) was attributed to acquiring explicit knowledge of the sequence information involved, which would effectively render the task explicit. Other evidence supports the idea that some types of implicit learning could involve a hippocampus-dependent step at some stages of memory formation and consolidation, as discussed in Section 17.7.

A different kind of learning; i.e., extraction of a statistical generalization from a series of sample associations, was not reinforced, and was even disrupted, when sensory stimuli linked to these associations were presented during SWS. This result may indicate that reinforcing specific learned associations during SWS can interfere with extracting and retrieving a general rule derived from those associations. However, TMR during REM sleep did support extraction of a general rule, although only during delayed testing a week after training. One study that did not use TMR found that the amount of SWS shown after exposure to tone sequences with hidden statistical structures was correlated with success in recognizing elements that contained that structure. SWS may therefore be involved in abstraction or gist identification based on a set of learned associations, but presenting a series of specific stimuli during SWS may not be appropriate for triggering this function of SWS.

18.12 Manipulating sleep EEG features to enhance memory

A different approach to memory enhancement related to sleep involves using external stimuli to enhance or suppress sleep

EEG features that play a general role in memory consolidation. This approach contrasts to TMR, which uses stimuli that are related to specific learning experiences. As discussed above, the synchronous occurrence of fast spindles with the positive peak of SOs (in combination with SWRs) is correlated with better declarative memory consolidation, so spindles and SOs have been the targets of external manipulations.

As reviewed earlier, optogenetic stimulation via implanted optical fibers in the thalamic reticular nucleus of mice was used to trigger increases in spindle numbers during the On phase of SOs, which improved hippocampus-dependent memory. Suppressing sleep spindles optogenetically during the same SO phase impaired memory. Increasing or decreasing spindles out of phase with the positive limb of SOs had no significant effects on memory (Latchoumane et al., 2017); see **Figure 18.7**. In a rat model, detection of hippocampal SWRs was used to initiate cortical stimulation that triggered time-locked delta waves and sleep spindles. These coordinated events helped consolidate memory for a spatial learning task, while similar cortical stimulation that was not synchronized to SWRs was ineffective (Maingret et al., 2016).

In people, auditory stimuli that were triggered to occur in-phase with SOs amplified SOs, increased the number of sleep spindles, and improved consolidation of memory for word pairs, while out-of-phase stimulation did not (Ngo et al., 2013). Similarly, triggering noise to occur during the positive peak of slow waves improved cued recall of verbal paired-associates the next day, but did not improve performance on other tasks, including a motor memory task (Leminen et al., 2017).

Among the few studies that have used similar methods, results have been mixed. A meta-analysis of these studies found that phase-locked stimulation of SOs in young people produced a significant improvement in memory, but adding studies to the analysis that used non-phase-locked stimulation or older participants diluted the apparent benefits (Wunderlin et al., 2021). This conclusion emphasizes the importance of the phase of SOs at which plasticity-linked events are triggered to occur, as well as the relevance of the age of participants, as reviewed in Section 17.10.2.

An indirect (and surprising) way of promoting increased expression of key memory-enhancing EEG features involves the use of a motorized, slowly rocking bed. Compared to a control night on a stationary bed, people on the rocking bed showed shorter sleep onset latencies, increased and more sustained N3 sleep, more SOs, and more sleep spindles. They also showed better retention of word pairs that had been learned before sleep (Perrault et al., 2019). In a mouse model system, slow rocking increased NREM sleep by effects on the inner-ear vestibular system (Kompotis et al., 2019). Assuming that a similar mechanism operates in people, these findings suggest that the vestibular stimulation associated with slow rocking improved consolidation indirectly by extending N3 sleep and thereby permitting an increased number of SOs and spindles.

A different approach to either improving or disrupting memory in people is altering EEG features during sleep using transcranial stimulation. Studies have used either transcranial electrical stimulation (TES) or transcranial magnetic stimulation (TMS). In most studies, TES was delivered during NREM sleep through scalp electrodes located over the frontal lobes, the presumed site of origin of many SOs, although recent results discussed below suggest an alternative source (Morgan et al., 2021). Stimulation consisted of anodal, transcranial direct current stimulation (tDCS),[11] delivered typically as an oscillating waveform in the SO-frequency range (e.g., 0.75 Hz), which produces neuronal depolarization.

In some studies, 0.75 Hz tDCS increased the number of SOs and amount of N3 sleep, and enhanced declarative memory consolidation (e.g., Cellini et al., 2019; Marshall et al., 2006). Other studies, however, did not observe memory benefits despite using similar stimulation patterns (Bueno-Lopez et al., 2019) or did so only for a subset of participants—those with better baseline memory performance (Koo et al., 2018).

One potential explanation for this variability relates to the observation that the spontaneous strength of SO/fast spindle coupling during a baseline night (before training) predicted the effectiveness of tDCS (delivered during a second night) in improving memory for learned associations (Dehnavi et al., 2021). Thus, both good baseline memory performance (Koo et al., 2018) and more robust baseline spindle/SO coupling (Dehnavi et al., 2021) predicted more benefit from subsequent tDCS treatments. These findings suggest that strong spindle/SO coupling may be a trait marker linked to better memory performance at baseline and to more susceptibility to memory enhancement by tDCS; for reviews see (Barham et al., 2016; Grimaldi et al., 2020). This interpretation is consistent with evidence that altered SO/spindle timing in older participants is associated with reduced sleep-related benefits for memory (Helfrich et al., 2018).

Although most studies using 0.75 Hz tDCS involved adults of different ages, it was also studied in children with attention deficit hyperactivity disorder (ADHD) (9–14 years old). They

[11] "Direct current" (DC) involves current flowing in one direction only. Direct currents can be either fixed or varying over time, which could produce either an oscillation around a mean current value or a sequence of pulses from zero to a higher current value. "Alternating current" (AC) involves continuous switching (alternation) of the direction of current flow.

showed larger memory loss overnight on a declarative learning task (spatial memory using a *Concentration*-type task) than did controls without a diagnosis. When the children with ADHD were treated during NREM sleep with tDCS, they showed increased SO power and improved memory retention, which rose to the level of controls (Prehn-Kristensen et al., 2014).

Other studies have found disruption of memory performance in some participants as a result of tDCS stimulation. In one study, tDCS was applied bilaterally to the temporal lobes, rather than to the frontal lobes, to influence temporal cortical connections to the underlying hippocampus. It resulted in increased SO activity and more nesting of sleep spindles in SOs but did not benefit episodic memory consolidation. In fact, for those with poor initial memory performance, memory deteriorated further after tDCS (Ruch et al., 2021). Higher frequency (5 Hz) tDCS reduced SO numbers and power in the spindle-frequency range and also reduced memory performance, possibly because it disrupted spontaneous SO rhythms by inducing higher frequency EEG oscillations outside the range of slow waves or SOs (Marshall et al., 2011).

A meta-analysis of SO-frequency tDCS presented during naps or nighttime sleep concluded that low-frequency tDCS was (often) effective in enhancing consolidation of declarative learning, but did not affect memory for procedural learning. High-frequency tDCS was instead associated with reduced memory benefit (Barham et al., 2016). Whether the location of tDCS application is critical to its effects remains to be determined.

A different method of delivering TES is transcranial *alternating* current stimulation (tACS). A study that used tACS reported a benefit for motor memory consolidation that was correlated with increases in fast spindle activity but no benefit for a declarative memory task. This stimulation method involved identifying a spontaneous spindle and using it to trigger a period of spindle-frequency stimulation (12 Hz) during NREM sleep, which resulted in generating more spindles (Lustenberger et al., 2016). The implied role for spindles in motor memory consolidation was supported by evidence in mice that post-sleep improvement in a learned motor skill correlated with an increased density of sleep spindles and their stronger coupling to SOs during NREM sleep (Kam et al., 2019).

Another study involving tACS used spontaneous SOs to trigger stimulation that produced sequences of SOs with characteristics similar to those generated spontaneously. This study tested the effects of this "closed-loop" triggering throughout an overnight sleep period on memory related to a visual detection task. While tACS did not improve memory for the specific target stimuli learned during visual detection training, it improved long-term performance based on having acquired a "gist" knowledge of the training stimuli. This effect facilitated later detection of camouflaged versions of the target stimuli, and this improvement was correlated with increased SO activity and coupling of SOs to fast spindle frequencies (Ketz et al., 2018). A related study showed that after training to detect specific targets, generalized detection of targets hidden in complex visual images was improved by overnight closed-loop tACS (Jones et al., 2018).[12]

The mechanism by which tACS improved memory consolidation was assumed to involve increasing and entraining (i.e., synchronizing) SOs and their nested sleep spindles. This idea was challenged by the results of a study of intracranial recordings in patients as part of presurgical assessment for treatment of intractable epilepsy. It found that bursts of sound stimuli evoked synchronous SOs and spindles, but tACS aimed at the dorsolateral frontal cortex did not. These results were interpreted as showing that auditory stimulation can synchronize EEG rhythms by acting through sensory pathways that reach the cortex, but that the mass of the human skull and brain did not allow extracranial tACS to synchronize cortical oscillations (Lafon et al., 2017).

Other studies have, however, shown that tACS delivered to dorsolateral cortical regions had demonstrable effects on EEG activity (Ketz et al., 2018), and that tACS delivered at even lower current intensities and aimed at inferolateral and frontotemporal sites increased N3 sleep and SO activity (Hathaway et al., 2021). The latter result is consistent with the claim that the targeted ventral cortical regions (the so-called limbic cortex) are the principal sources of SOs, rather than the more dorsal, frontal cortical regions that have often been targeted in other studies (Morgan et al., 2021).

Among the studies that have used a form of TES to affect consolidation, there have been variations in many parameters. These included the type of stimulation applied (tDCS, constant or oscillating, or tACS); whether or not EEG features were used to trigger closed-loop stimulation; the timing and duration of stimulation; the number of stimulating electrodes and their positions; and the strength of the current applied. It is not surprising that there have been different conclusions reached as to how TES affects neural activity and the consolidation of different types of memory. Triggering stimulation based on spontaneous production of SOs and/or spindles may have advantages, possibly because the additional SO/spindle activity that is triggered occurs at a phase when the nervous system may already be engaged in memory consolidation. Further research is needed to

[12] In both of these studies, either active or sham tDCS was applied to frontal scalp locations during training while awake, but the presence or absence of tDCS during training did not alter the effects on memory of applying tACS during sleep.

clarify when and how different patterns and modalities of TES can affect sleep features and thereby modify memory.

18.12.1 Summary

The timed expression of fast sleep spindles and SOs plays an important role in offline memory consolidation. In animals, triggering increases in fast sleep spindles during the depolarizing slope or at the peak of SOs using optogenetic or intracranial electrical stimulation improved declarative memory consolidation. Suppressing spindles at those phases impaired memory, but altering the number of fast sleep spindles at other phases of SO rhythms did not influence memory consolidation. Presenting sounds timed to occur in phase with spontaneous SOs in people amplified SOs, increased spindles, and also improved declarative memory retention. Slow rocking during sleep in people also improved memory consolidation, perhaps by vestibular stimulation that increased the amount of N3 sleep and, as a result, the number of SOs and spindles that could be produced.

Transcranial direct current stimulation, especially low-frequency (0.75 Hz) tDCS, also improved memory related to both declarative and motor learning in some studies. There is evidence that tDCS improved memory primarily for those with good baseline memory performance and with large amounts of spontaneous SO/spindle coupling at baseline. Variation in these baseline traits of participants may contribute to variability in results across studies.

Closed-loop tACS improved memory, but its effects were mostly on retention of generalized information ("gist") extracted from pre-sleep learning. Some evidence from intracranial recordings in people suggested that typical extracranial current intensities used in tACS were too weak to affect brain rhythms. Nevertheless, there is evidence that low-current TES increased the number of SOs and the coupling of fast spindles to the On phases of SOs. Recent findings suggest that the dorsofrontal cortical regions that are often the target of TES may not be the source of most SOs, and that targeting ventral, limbic cortical regions may be more effective in increasing SO numbers.

Different electrical manipulations aimed at the brain in several species resulted in increases in the synchronized expression of three key EEG features (SWRs, SOs, and spindles), which were able to strengthen memory consolidation. These effects were not universal, however, and may interact with baseline characteristics of participants, the status of the learned material, and the specific type of stimulation used. The variety of methods and parameters used across TES studies makes it difficult to reach general conclusions about which forms and intensities of stimulation are optimal for reinforcing consolidation and for which types of memory.

18.13 Neurochemical effects on sleep-related consolidation

The studies described earlier in this chapter focused on the involvement in memory consolidation of electrophysiological features of different sleep stages (sleep spindles, SWRs, SOs, and theta rhythms) and patterns of hippocampal-cortical communication. Sleep/wake stages are, however, also characterized by altered activity in several neurotransmitter systems, which can also influence memory consolidation.

One example involves changing levels of acetylcholine (ACh) in the cortex. The flow of information from the hippocampus to the cortex is inhibited at several points by the presence of high ACh levels. These points include connections within the hippocampus, at CA1 projections to the entorhinal cortex, and at entorhinal projections to association cortices (Gais & Born, 2004a; Hasselmo, 2006). ACh levels in the forebrain are high during both waking and REM sleep, but strongly reduced during NREM sleep. The low level of ACh during NREM sleep allows information to flow from the hippocampus to the cortex in order to facilitate memory consolidation, but high levels during waking and REM sleep inhibit this communication (Buzsáki, 1996).

The effects of manipulating ACh levels were studied in participants who learned a word-pair task and stayed awake (with presumably high ACh levels) until they were tested 10 h later. Some participants who stayed awake were treated with two drugs to reduce their cholinergic neurotransmission; they retained more word pairs than waking controls. These results indicate that reducing cholinergic drive while awake (i.e., mimicking the low ACh levels of NREM sleep) facilitated memory consolidation (Rasch et al., 2006) (**Figure 18.11 A**).

In a related study, participants learned word pairs and then slept for 3 h; this early part of sleep would include large amounts of N3 sleep, during which forebrain ACh levels are low. Participants received either a placebo or physostigmine, a cholinesterase inhibitor[13] that would increase cholinergic activity in the brain (mimicking the high ACh levels of waking). Those treated with physostigmine during sleep retained less of what they had learned (**Figure 18.11 B**). These results indicate that artificially elevated ACh levels interfere with consolidation of declarative memories that depends on hippocampal-cortical communication during NREM sleep (Gais & Born, 2004b).

Thus, low ACh levels during a retention interval including either sleep or waking produced better memory retention, and high ACh levels resulted in worse retention regardless of how these changes were produced. These results imply that the

[13] Cholinesterase is an enzyme that breaks down ACh, thereby terminating its synaptic activity. By inhibiting this enzyme, physostigmine prolongs the effects of ACh that is released at synapses.

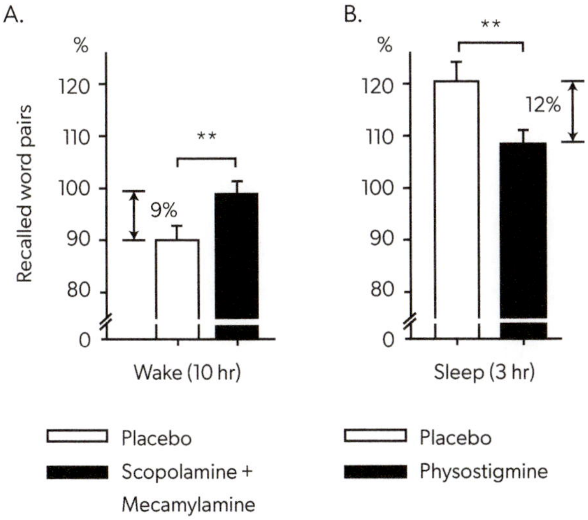

Figure 18.11 **A**. Participants learned a list of word pairs, and their recall performance after a 10 h wake period was compared to their baseline memory at the end of training (=100%). Participants were treated with a combination of muscarinic and nicotinic cholinergic antagonists; respectively, scopolamine and mecamylamine (black column), or a placebo (white column). Participants with suppressed cholinergic activity showed better retention of word pairs than placebo-treated controls who would have had elevated cortical cholinergic activity while awake. **B.** Participants learned word pairs and were then treated with either placebo (white column) or physostigmine (a cholinergic agonist; black column) before a 3 h sleep period (mostly SWS). They were then tested for changes in recall relative to pre-sleep performance. Placebo-treated controls with spontaneously low cholinergic activity during SWS retained more correct pairings than those treated to elevate cholinergic activity. In each case, high levels of cholinergic activity during the retention interval, whether spontaneous while awake or mimicked by physostigmine during sleep, were associated with worse recall performance. Reprinted with permission of The MIT Press from Rasch, B.H. et al. (2006) Combined blockade of cholinergic receptors shifts the brain from stimulus encoding to memory consolidation. *J Cogn Neurosci* 18:793–802. © Massachusetts Institute of Technology (2006). doi: 10.1111/jsr.13731. Based in part on data from Gais, S. & Born, J. (2004) Low acetylcholine during slow-wave sleep is critical for declarative memory consolidation. *PNAS* 101(7):2140-2144. Used with permission of the National Academy of Sciences (USA) © (2004).

benefits of N3 sleep for memory depend in part on a reduction in ACh levels characteristic of that stage, which facilitates hippocampal-cortical communication, in addition to the involvement of specific EEG features in the consolidation process.

The regulation of REM sleep involves interactions among neurotransmitters in several parts of the nervous system. Increased ACh levels in the pons are critical to triggering REM sleep and increased serotonin (5-HT) and norepinephrine (NE) levels act to inhibit REM sleep onset. Either reducing ACh activity or enhancing 5-HT/NE activity will reduce REM sleep amounts (see Sections 10.7.1 and 10.7.2).

Treating healthy people acutely with antidepressants that increase 5-HT and/or NE neurotransmission strongly suppressed the rapid eye movements and atonia that normally occur during REM sleep. Despite the suppression of these REM sleep features, there was no reduction in consolidation of either a motor task (mirror-tracing) or a declarative memory task (word-pair associations). Performance on a motor sequence learning (MSL) task was, in fact, enhanced after sleep in the presence of an antidepressant. The degree of improvement was correlated with the number and density of fast spindles shown, which may have been affected by the drug treatment (Rasch, Pommer, et al., 2009).

Treating people with an antidepressant that has strong anticholinergic effects (amitriptyline) also reduced REM sleep and increased N2 sleep and sleep spindles. Overnight improvement on declarative memory and MSL tasks was unaffected, but performance on a visual texture discrimination (VTD) task was impaired (Goerke et al., 2014).

Blocking both major subtypes of ACh receptors during the second half of the night, when most REM sleep normally occurs, reduced REM sleep amounts by about two-thirds. The treatments did not affect memory for declarative learning, but impaired memory for an MSL task, suggesting a role for either REM sleep or ACh in consolidating this kind of motor learning (Rasch, Gais, et al., 2009).

These results indicate that different drug treatments that all suppress overt signs of REM sleep do not have similar effects on memory consolidation. The PSG signs of REM sleep were suppressed in all or part of the night in these studies, but the effects on memory consolidation were very different. These differences may reflect the different combinations of effects of these treatments on ACh, NE/5-HT, and N2/sleep spindle production (Goerke et al., 2014; Rasch, Gais, et al., 2009; Rasch, Pommer, et al., 2009).

Another example of drugs that affect sleep and neural plasticity relates to benzodiazepines and related GABA agonists that are used as sleep aids and have similar effects on sleep stages, increasing NREM sleep and decreasing REM sleep. Despite similar effects on sleep stages, some of these drugs given after monocular visual experience and before a sleep period strongly reduced ocular dominance shifts related to asymmetric visual experience in young cats (see Section 18.3), but others did not. Among these GABA agonists, those that caused a specific set of changes in $GABA_A$ or 5-HT neurotransmission inhibited ocular dominance shifts, while other agonists without these effects did not (Aton, Seibt, Dumoulin, Coleman, et al., 2009; Seibt et al., 2008). Thus, similar effects of these drugs on sleep stages did not predict similar effects on visual system plasticity.

Taken together, these findings indicate that drugs that influence sleep stage expression can have a variety of effects on neural plasticity and memory that are not predicted solely by their effects on sleep. Systemic treatments with drugs that modify neurotransmission are likely to have multiple effects on receptor populations in different parts of the brain, which could have complex influences on the neural plasticity underlying memory consolidation.

18.13.1 Summary

ACh inhibits neurotransmission at several points on projection paths from the hippocampus to the neocortex. ACh levels in the cortex are low during NREM sleep relative to waking or REM sleep, which facilitates hippocampal-cortical communication that is involved in explicit memory consolidation. Increasing ACh levels during NREM sleep impaired explicit memory consolidation while decreasing normally high ACh levels during waking improved memory. The benefits of NREM sleep for memory consolidation depended in part on its characteristic low levels of ACh.

Drugs that either increase NE/5-HT levels or decrease ACh neurotransmission suppress measurable EEG features of REM sleep. Despite their common effects on REM sleep, they have different effects on consolidation of different types of memory, perhaps because of their effects on expression of N2 sleep and spindles. Similarly, different GABA receptor agonists, all of which suppress REM sleep and increase NREM sleep, have different effects on brain plasticity that are linked to their other neurochemical impacts.

Assessing the involvement of neurotransmitter changes using drug treatments is challenging because most drugs influence several kinds of receptors to varying degrees, and because systemic treatments affect neurotransmission throughout the brain. Findings related to the effects of several classes of neurotransmitters indicate that both the EEG-measurable features of NREM and REM sleep and the patterns of neurotransmission that are linked to these stages may influence memory consolidation during sleep. Changes in the brain's neurochemical profile that are characteristic of different sleep stages should be considered potential factors in determining the involvement of sleep stages in consolidation of different types of memory.

18.14 Learning during sleep

18.14.1 Human studies

There has been a longstanding interest in whether people can learn new information while asleep, in contrast to consolidating already learned information, as reviewed in preceding sections. For example, products have been promoted that promised to teach people new languages in their sleep, but there was no reliable evidence to justify such claims. Early studies that evaluated whether elements of learning can occur during sleep had mixed results. Recent research has developed more convincing evidence that some kinds of learning can occur during sleep, although the results fall short of demonstrating acquisition of a new language.

In one study, participants were classically conditioned by pairing two different tones with either a pleasant or a very unpleasant odor, in response to which people spontaneously produce distinctive breathing patterns. After pairing distinctive tones with each of these odors during sleep, participants showed the predicted respiratory patterns in response to the tones alone, both while still asleep and later after waking up. Conditioning was slightly more successful during REM sleep (Arzi et al., 2012).

In another study, smokers who were trying to quit smoking were exposed to pairings of the smell of cigarette smoke with a very aversive odor during either waking or sleep. Attempted conditioning while awake had no effect on later cigarette use. Those who experienced the pairing during REM sleep, and more so during N2 sleep, showed a significant reduction in cigarette use during the following week (Arzi et al., 2014). Assuming that these results can be replicated, they imply that forms of classical conditioning and implicit learning are possible during sleep.

Other kinds of learning have been studied during sleep. One study involved presentation of bursts of white noise that included a difficult to detect novel sound that was buried within the noise stream. After these sounds were presented repeatedly during light NREM or REM sleep, participants were better able to detect the "hidden" sound while awake. This result can also be seen as an example of implicit learning, in this case, of a sensory discrimination skill. On the other hand, presentation of these stimuli during deep NREM sleep tended to impair later detection of the hidden component while awake (Andrillon et al., 2017).

Another study paired real words that correspond to large or small objects (e.g., elephant vs. key) with pseudowords during NREM sleep. The presentation of the word/pseudoword pairs evoked SOs and increased spindle activity. After repeated pairings, participants were asked while awake to classify the pseudowords as representing either large or small objects. The targeted outcome was whether participants were able to classify pseudowords "correctly", that is, according to the size of the objects represented by the real words that had been paired with them.

Classification of the pseudowords as representing small or large objects was improved by 10% when the pairings occurred so that the pseudoword was heard during the depolarized phase of SOs, compared to when they occurred at other phases (Züst et al., 2019). This outcome may also represent implicit learning based on repeated pairings, since participants received no instruction to remember the word/pseudoword pairings, nor to infer the size of the objects represented by the pseudowords.

However, when participants in this study were subsequently trained while awake to pair these pseudowords with words that were synonyms of those they had learned while asleep, they showed slightly worse performance than for pseudowords that had not been paired during sleep (Ruch et al., 2022). Thus, similarly to the effects of sensory learning (Andrillon et al., 2017), the implicit learning experience during sleep interfered with later acquisition of related information while awake, which might have been expected instead to facilitate learning while awake.

The limited evidence available suggests that implicit learning can occur during both NREM and REM sleep, and one form of implicit learning depended on the precise timing of stimuli during the depolarized phase of evoked SOs during NREM sleep (Züst et al., 2019). Implicit learning during sleep appeared to interfere with subsequent waking acquisition of related information, although it is not clear what the nature of the interference was.

18.14.2 Creating a false memory during sleep

One study of sleep and explicit learning depended on circumventing the limitations of input through sensory systems during sleep. It asked whether mice could acquire a preference for a spatial location while awake or asleep based on pairing that location with electrically stimulated neural activity that did not depend on sensory inputs. This study took advantage of the fact that individual hippocampal place cells increase firing rates selectively whenever a mouse enters a specific location during exploration of an open field (see Section 18.4.1). When mice were allowed to explore an empty open-field apparatus while awake, they showed little or no preference for being in any part of this featureless environment; **Figure 18.12**, PRE).

To determine the effectiveness of the classical conditioning paradigm to be used, researchers electrically activated a single hippocampal place cell in each mouse while it was awake and paired the activation with stimulation of the medial forebrain bundle (MFB) in order to release dopamine. Dopamine is known to be involved in behavioral reinforcement and motivation (Berke, 2018; Berridge, 2007). When returned to the open field later, the mice spent much more time in the location coded for by that place cell. These results indicate that the repeated pairings resulted in classical conditioning of an association between a reward experience and firing of a particular place cell. Spending time in a specific location that triggered firing of that cell had therefore acquired reinforcing properties.

This same experiment was conducted in a different set of mice with paired stimulation of a hippocampal place cell and the MFB confined to sleep, after establishing the lack of a strong place preference. Mice experienced these repeated pairings during a 1 h sleep episode; almost all pairings occurred during SWS, and ~37% occurred during SWRs. The mice were then retested in the open field while awake. The mice were now attracted selectively to the location that the reinforced place cell coded for, an area for which they had no preference before sleep (**Figure 18.12**, **POST**).

This acquired place preference demonstrated that classical conditioning based on a neural reinforcement mechanism was possible during SWS. One interpretation is that the conditioning experience during sleep had created a false memory in the mice that something rewarding had occurred in a specific location, which made it more attractive for them to spend time there (de Lavilléon et al., 2015).

18.14.3 Summary

Several studies in people have shown that classical conditioning and implicit learning can occur during sleep, although some of these effects were quite small. Some studies involved olfactory classical conditioning of either reflex responses or sensory preferences that translated into changes in behavior. Other studies demonstrated implicit learning based on classical conditioning or exposure to sensory inputs while asleep. Implicit learning as a result of pairing words from different size categories with pseudowords produced a small increase in appropriate size categorization of the pseudowords. There is also some evidence that explicit learning experiences while asleep may interfere with later acquisition of related information while awake.

Observations supporting some forms of learning during sleep are consistent with evidence that the brain receives sensory input during sleep to varying degrees, although its effects are strongly modified by brain states, as discussed in Section 12.3. Whether this limited information flow permits learning will depend on the neurochemical environment of the sleeping brain, its current electrophysiological features, and the functional requirements for that type of learning. Effects were reported after manipulations during both NREM and REM sleep, but further research is needed to determine whether different types of conditioning occur more successfully in different sleep stages.

In either waking or sleeping mice, pairing neural reinforcement with increased firing activity of a hippocampal place cell produced a preference for being in the location coded for by that cell, which mice were indifferent to before conditioning. These results show that pairing place-cell firing with neurochemical reinforcement while mice were either awake or asleep created a false memory that something positive had happened in a specific location. Conditioning in this paradigm during

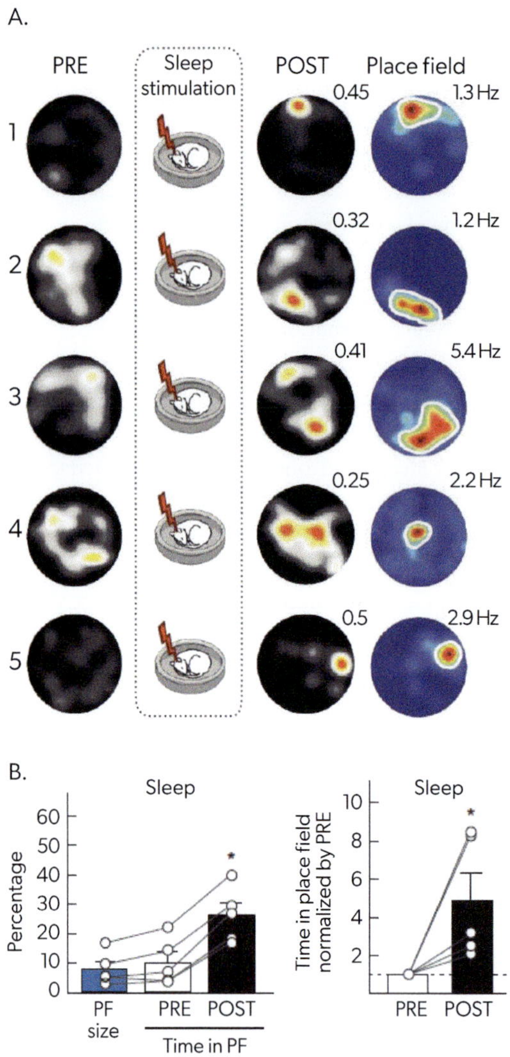

Figure 18.12 **A.** The far left-hand column (PRE) shows the length of time 5 different mice (1–5) spent in different parts of an open field while exploring it at baseline before any manipulation. The time spent is intensity-coded by color, with gray and black regions (mice 1 and 5) indicating no strong preference to be in any location, and white/yellow regions (mice 2, 3, 4) showing a weak preference for one or two broad areas. The far right-hand column shows the locations of place fields triggering highest firing rates of single hippocampal place cells, recorded from these five mice while exploring the open field, and the maximal firing rates (1.2–5.4 Hz) shown by these cells when the mouse was at those locations. The colors, running from dark blue (lowest) to dark red (highest), code the intensity of firing at each location in the open field. During sleep, each mouse received reinforcing medial forebrain bundle (MFB) stimulation paired with stimulation of the hippocampal place cell (Sleep stimulation), whose firing map (place field) is illustrated in the far right-hand column. The column labeled POST, shows the time spent in different locations when exploring the area after the sleep manipulation. The red and orange areas correspond to the locations in which mice spent the longest durations. Mice had developed a preference to be in a location that reflected the place coded for by firing of the reinforced hippocampal neuron (compare PRE to POST). The preferences shown were unrelated to their preexisting weak place preferences (if any). **B.** The left chart shows the percentage of time spent in the targeted place field before the sleep manipulation (PRE) and after receiving paired stimulation of a place cell and the MFB during sleep (POST) for each mouse (circles) and the group average (columns), as well as the size of the targeted place field (PF size). The targeted place fields of the individual neurons averaged ~8% of the entire open field; mice spent ~10% of their time before and ~27% of their time afterward in these fields. The right chart shows the increased time spent POST sleep stimulation in the targeted place field, expressed relative to the baseline time spent there (PRE = 1.0) for each mouse (circles), and averaged for the group (columns). There was an average 5-fold increase in time spent in the targeted place field, including three mice spending 2–3-fold time and 2 spending >8-fold time in the place field relative to baseline durations. Adapted with permission from de Lavilléon, G. et al. (2015) Explicit memory creation during sleep demonstrates a causal role of place cells in navigation. *Nat Neurosci* 18:493–495. © Springer:Nature (2015). doi:10.1038/nn.3970.

sleep produced robust effects, perhaps because it was based on pairing neural events (firing of a place cell and release of dopamine) that did not depend on using sensory input pathways to present the paired stimuli.

18.15 Sleep effects on synaptic strength

18.15.1 Evidence for and against synaptic downscaling

The hypothesis that memory consolidation during sleep is the result of strengthening new synaptic connections, as discussed in previous sections, should be considered in relation to a different model of how sleep affects synaptic strength. The synaptic homeostasis hypothesis (see Section 12.6.3) states that sleep functions to reduce synaptic strength generally (synaptic downscaling) in order to accomplish several goals, including indirectly reinforcing new memories (Tononi & Cirelli, 2006).

This model is based on the idea that waking neural activity triggered by ordinary daily experiences causes incidental strengthening of many synaptic connections across the cortex. Most of these synaptic changes are not relevant to future behavior, and their maintenance imposes a high energy cost. In addition, repeated broad strengthening of cortical synapses will eventually saturate the capacity for synapses to strengthen selectively, which would reduce the adaptive synaptic plasticity needed for learning in the future. Reversing this incidental synaptic strengthening during sleep (downscaling) helps to preserve the capacity for future learning.

Sleep (especially N3 sleep) is proposed to depress synaptic strength broadly in the cortex to achieve the benefits of reduced metabolic costs and increased capacity for future selective synaptic plasticity. In addition, by reducing the background "noise" of incidental increases in synaptic strength, downscaling would also make the strongest synaptic connections that result from specific learning experiences more salient (i.e., it would increase the signal-to-noise ratio at the synaptic level, thereby improving memory).

Several lines of evidence support different aspects of this hypothesis:

- In rats, cortical LTP (a model of learning; see Section 18.2) was induced more easily after periods spent asleep than after periods spent awake. Downscaling of synaptic strength during sleep was proposed to create more capacity for later strengthening in response to LTP (Vyazovskiy et al., 2008).
- In people, cortical EEG responses evoked using transcranial magnetic stimulation (TMS) increased in size progressively during prolonged waking (reflecting increasing synaptic strength) and decreased again after a night of recovery sleep (consistent with downscaling during sleep) (Huber et al., 2012).
- Neurophysiological and molecular markers of synaptic strength were shown to be decreased after sleep and increased after waking (Diering et al., 2017; Liu et al., 2010). These reductions after sleep were observed in small- and medium-sized synapses but not in the largest synapses (de Vivo et al., 2017).
- Extended waking produced an increase in synaptic density and connectivity in the CA1 region of the hippocampus (Spano et al., 2019).
- Blocking ripple activity (part of SWRs) in the mouse hippocampus during sleep prevented downscaling of synaptic strengths and reduced the capacity for later learning (Norimoto et al., 2018).

Despite this supporting evidence, other results from studies of plasticity in sensory and other systems support the idea that learning and other plasticity-inducing experiences are followed by increases in synaptic strength during later sleep:

- When kittens had visual experiences that induced synaptic strengthening, affected neurons did not immediately increase their firing rates while still awake. Instead, firing rates increased (reflecting strengthened synaptic inputs) after later N3 and REM sleep. Increased firing was phase-locked to the occurrence of slow/delta oscillations (0.5–4 Hz) and sleep spindles (Aton et al., 2013; Durkin & Aton, 2016), which are involved in strengthening synaptic connections (Marshall et al., 2006; Rosanova & Ulrich, 2005; Siapas & Wilson, 1998).
- In cat somatosensory cortex, local field potentials that were evoked by stimulating an input pathway while awake were larger, rather than smaller, after a period of SWS, presumably reflecting increased synaptic strength in the afferent pathway (Chauvette et al., 2012).
- Sleep deprivation reduced dendritic spine numbers in the mouse hippocampus and impaired spatial memory, implying that sleep is needed to maintain synaptic connections that are involved in memory (Havekes et al., 2016).
- Hibernating ground squirrels (*Spermophilus* sp.) periodically emerge from hibernation and raise their body temperatures from near-ambient levels (e.g., ~0° C) to normal (euthermic) temperatures. During these euthermic periods, they generate N3 sleep before cooling down again to resume hibernation. In this case, N3 sleep appears to be a mechanism to efficiently restore synaptic connections that were weakened by a lack of neural activity at low body temperatures (Larkin & Heller, 1999; Strijkstra & Daan, 1998); see **Box 5.2** in Chapter 5).

- There is also correlational evidence that is consistent with a link between sleep and synaptic growth rather than pruning. Preadolescent children show long sleep durations with high amounts of N3 sleep. During the same period, there is robust growth in synapse numbers; see **Figure 4.6**. During later childhood and adolescence, N3 and total sleep amounts decrease, and there is broad synaptic pruning, resulting in large reductions in the number of cortical synapses (Huttenlocher, 1990); see Section 4.4.1). These results are consistent with a role for SWS in maintaining or increasing synapse numbers, but these correlations do not establish causality.

18.15.2 Homeostatic scaling

Resolving these apparently contradictory lines of evidence is complicated by the fact that neurons also undergo processes of homeostatic up- and downscaling in response to experience-related changes in functional connectivity (Puentes-Mestril & Aton, 2017; Turrigiano, 1999; Turrigiano, 2017). Neurons whose firing rates were increased or decreased as a result of experimental manipulations (e.g., changes in both functional connectivity and firing rates of visual cortex neurons after early monocular visual experience; see Section 18.3) responded with homeostatic changes over days that gradually restored spontaneous firing rates to near-baseline levels.

This response was hypothesized to maintain neuronal excitability within a middle range that is appropriate for effective information processing (i.e., it allows room for both increases and decreases in firing rates in response to future inputs). These homeostatic changes in firing rates reflect neurons adjusting the strength of their responses to synaptic inputs (Turrigiano, 1999). In visual cortex neurons, this gradual scaling process after a plasticity-inducing visual experience occurred during later periods of waking; neither homeostatic decreases nor increases were observed during sleep (Hengen et al., 2016).

In the absence of specific plasticity-inducing experiences, highly active neurons in rat frontal cortex decreased firing rates during NREM sleep, while low-firing neurons increased their firing rates. During REM sleep, cortical firing rates were generally decreased (Watson et al., 2016). A study of experience-dependent plasticity in the visual cortex of mice found increased firing across sleep by initially sparsely firing, orientation-selective neurons, and decreased firing by less selective, high firing-rate neurons. Most of these changes appeared to be related to REM sleep, with relatively stable firing during NREM sleep (Clawson et al., 2018).

Despite differences related to sleep stages, these studies converge on the conclusion that cortical neurons both increased and decreased firing rates during sleep, and that the direction of change was related to their initial firing rates. These bidirectional homeostatic responses do not support the hypothesis that NREM sleep causes a general reduction in the strength of synapses and consequently of neuronal firing rates. They also complicate attempts to test hypotheses about global, sleep-related changes in synaptic strength.

18.15.3 REM sleep effects on synapses

Synaptic downscaling is usually discussed in relation to SWS, but the role of REM sleep in regulating synaptic strength is also relevant. Several lines of evidence indicate that REM sleep is involved in neural plasticity (Dumoulin Bridi et al., 2015; Ishikawa et al., 2006) and in modulating emotional, spatial, and contextual memories (Boyce et al., 2016; Gujar et al., 2011; Menz et al., 2016; Wagner et al., 2001; Wassing et al., 2019). In addition, consolidation during sleep of some types of learning is jointly affected by both NREM and REM sleep (Giuditta et al., 1995; Li et al., 2017; Mednick et al., 2003; Seibt & Frank, 2019; Stickgold, Whidbee, et al., 2000; Tang & Jadhav, 2018; Yang et al., 2014).

Studies reviewed earlier (see Section 18.4.2) showed that REM sleep can be involved in both selectively pruning and strengthening different subsets of synapses (Li et al., 2017). Similarly, hippocampal place cells were activated at different phases relative to theta rhythms during REM sleep. The result was either strengthening or weakening of memory traces, depending on the novelty of the spatial locations that had been explored while awake (Poe et al., 2000); see Section 18.10).

Hippocampal pyramidal cells recorded from rats in their home cages across sleep episodes throughout a day (without having specific learning experiences) showed an average decrease in firing rates. However, this net decrease was the result of *increases* in firing during periods of NREM sleep along with larger, more rapid, decreases during REM sleep episodes (Grosmark et al., 2012). These observations are consistent with the idea that REM sleep reduces synaptic strengthening that occurs in response to familiar and presumably uninformative waking experiences (Poe et al., 2000). The finding of increased firing during NREM sleep does not support the idea that NREM sleep globally reduces synaptic strengths, at least among principal hippocampal neurons.

18.15.4 Both upscaling and downscaling

There are a number of differences between studies that did and did not report evidence of synaptic downscaling during sleep, including NREM sleep. These include differences in the brain structures, time scales, and species involved. Most importantly, however, synaptic downscaling during (NREM) sleep was typically supported by studies that examined cortical or hippocampal tissue in general rather than focusing specifically on neurons involved in experience-dependent learning or other forms of plasticity (de Vivo et al., 2017; Diering et al., 2017; Huber et al., 2012; Liu et al., 2010; Spano et al., 2019; Vyazovskiy et al., 2008) with some exceptions (Grosmark et al., 2012). Studies supporting a role for sleep in synaptic strengthening (or, at least, not finding evidence of downscaling) instead focused on specific neural circuits or structures that were involved in unique, plasticity-related waking experiences (Areal et al., 2017; Chauvette et al., 2012; Havekes et al., 2016; Hengen et al., 2016; Puentes-Mestril & Aton, 2017).

Taken together, these findings suggest that both synaptic strengthening and weakening occur during sleep (Born & Feld, 2012; Puentes-Mestril & Aton, 2017), an idea that is supported by several lines of evidence:

- Cortical motor neurons involved in acquiring a new motor skill showed increases in synaptic spines during later NREM sleep. These changes were refined during REM sleep by selectively reducing the strength of synapses that were not specifically involved in the skill and not recently activated, while strengthening functionally useful connections (Li et al., 2017; Yang et al., 2014); see Section 18.4.2 These refinements were hypothesized to depend on setting molecular tags during waking to mark synapses differentially for later strengthening or weakening during sleep (Seibt & Frank, 2019).
- There was an overall reduction in firing rates of hippocampal neurons during sleep (in the absence of specific learning experiences), but this depended on increases in firing during NREM sleep and larger decreases during REM sleep (Grosmark et al., 2012).
- Frontal cortical neurons showed both decreasing firing rates (in high-firing neurons) and increasing firing rates (in low-firing neurons) over periods of sleep (Watson et al., 2016).
- In a study of five different classes of synaptic connections in rats, two within the hippocampus and three in projections from the hippocampus to different targets, there were varied changes related to sleep states (Rampon et al., 2023). For example, stimulation of the perforant path projection to the dentate gyrus generated the largest synaptic responses during active waking and progressively smaller responses in quiet waking, NREM, and REM sleep. In contrast, stimulation of Schaffer collateral projections to the CA1 region generated the largest synaptic responses during NREM sleep and progressively smaller responses in quiet waking and active waking/REM sleep. The hippocampal projection via the fornix to the nucleus accumbens showed the largest responses to stimulation during REM sleep and smaller responses during all other states.
- In addition, two synapse classes, that both showed their largest responses during waking, showed opposite changes in response amplitudes after a period of prolonged sleep (Rampon et al., 2023). These synapse-specific differences (and others) demonstrate that, at least in hippocampus-related projections, there is no uniform rule for how synaptic strengths change with sleep-wake states.
- Despite general evidence for molecular, anatomical, and electrophysiological downscaling of synapses over sleep periods (Vyazovskiy et al., 2008), reductions in synaptic sizes were not universal, with the largest class of synapses being preserved after sleep (de Vivo et al., 2017).

The functional roles of the preserved synapses in this last study were not determined. However, the finding that the largest synapses were not reduced in size during sleep is compatible with the idea that both broad downscaling of some synapses and selective reinforcement (or preservation) of recently strengthened synapses occur during sleep in a regionally specific way (for reviews, see Niethard & Born, 2019; Seibt & Frank, 2019). A combination of strengthening and weakening synapses with different histories of involvement in waking activities could produce robust increases in signal-to-noise ratios during sleep. The effect would be to selectively reinforce memory for recently acquired, functionally relevant information while still permitting the benefits of synaptic downscaling in other systems.

18.15.5 Summary

Global synaptic downscaling during sleep, especially during NREM sleep, has been proposed as a mechanism that preserves learning capacity, reduces metabolic costs of synaptic maintenance, and improves memory by increasing signal-to-noise ratios. The extensive evidence supporting this hypothesis is based mostly on studies of large neuronal populations in the absence of specific plasticity-related experiences. Studies of specific tissues involved in learning or neural plasticity, however, tend to find that mechanisms operating during NREM sleep increase or preserve synaptic strengthening that results from waking experiences.

Taken together, these findings indicate that both increases and decreases in synaptic strengths occur during both NREM and REM sleep. These changes appear to function to strengthen connections involved in recent plasticity-related events while weakening other synaptic connections. The net result of this combination of changes is a relative increase in the strength of a subset of neural connections that helps to stabilize and preserve neural changes related to new learning or other plasticity-inducing experiences.

Analysis of how experience-dependent changes in synaptic strengths are affected by later sleep also needs to take account of longer-term homeostatic up- and downscaling of synapses. These changes occur over days and tend to normalize changes in firing rates that were induced initially by experiences while awake. Neurons that had been highly activated gradually reduced firing rates, while the opposite occurred for neurons that had experienced suppression of firing.

The function of these homeostatic responses appears to be to maintain an optimal firing-rate range that allows for adequate responses to both excitatory and inhibitory inputs. These homeostatic processes may overlay and complicate analyses of the processes involved in modulating neural connectivity in relation to consolidation of recent learning and in relation to downscaling to preserve synaptic capacity for future learning.

Literature cited

Ackermann, S., Hartmann, F., Papassotiropoulos, A., de Quervain, D. J., & Rasch, B. (2015). No associations between interindividual differences in sleep parameters and episodic memory consolidation. *Sleep, 38*(6), 951–959. doi: 10.5665/sleep.4748

Adra, N., Sun, H., Ganglberger, W., Ye, E. M., Dümmer, L. W., Tesh, R. A., ... Westover, M. B. (2022). Optimal spindle detection parameters for predicting cognitive performance. *Sleep, 45*(4), zsac001. doi:10.1093/sleep/zsac001

Aime, M., Calcini, N., Borsa, M., Campelo, T., Rusterholz, T., Sattin, A., ... Adamantidis, A. (2022). Paradoxical somatodendritic decoupling supports cortical plasticity during REM sleep *Science, 376*, 724–730.

Akers, K., Martinez-Canabal, A., Restivo, L., Yiu, A., De Cristogaro, A., Hsiang, H.-L. L., ... Frankland, P. (2014). Hippocampal neurogenesis regulates forgetting during adulthood and infancy. *Science, 344*(6184), 598–602.

Andrillon, T., Nir, Y., Staba, R. J., Ferrarelli, F., Cirelli, C., Tononi, G., & Fried, I. (2011). Sleep spindles in humans: insights from intracranial EEG and unit recordings. *J Neurosci, 31*(49), 17821–17834. doi: 10.1523/JNEUROSCI.2604-11.2011

Andrillon, T., Pressnitzer, D., Leger, D., & Kouider, S. (2017). Formation and suppression of acoustic memories during human sleep. *Nat Commun, 8*(1), 179. doi: 10.1038/s41467-017-00071-z

Areal, C. C., Warby, S. C., & Mongrain, V. (2017). Sleep loss and structural plasticity. *Curr Opin Neurobiol, 44*, 1–7. doi: 10.1016/j.conb.2016.12.010

Arzi, A., Holtzman, Y., Samnon, P., Eshel, N., Harel, E., & Sobel, N. (2014). Olfactory aversive conditioning during sleep reduces cigarette-smoking behavior. *J Neurosci, 34*(46), 15382–15393. doi: 10.1523/JNEUROSCI.2291-14.2014

Arzi, A., Shedlesky, L., Ben-Shaul, M., Nasser, K., Oksenberg, A., Hairston, I. S., & Sobel, N. (2012). Humans can learn new information during sleep. *Nat Neurosci, 15*(10), 1460–1465. doi: 10.1038/nn.3193

Aston-Jones, G., & Bloom, F. E. (1981). Activity of norepinephrine-containing locus coeruleus neurons in behaving rats anticipates fluctuations in the sleep-waking cycle. *J Neurosci, 1*, 876–886.

Aton, S. J., Broussard, C., Dumoulin, M., Seibt, J., Watson, A., Coleman, T., & Frank, M. G. (2013). Visual experience and subsequent sleep induce sequential plastic changes in putative inhibitory and excitatory cortical neurons. *Proc Natl Acad Sci USA, 110*(8), 3101–3106. doi: 10.1073/pnas.1208093110

Aton, S. J., Seibt, J., Dumoulin, M., Jha, S. K., Steinmetz, N., Coleman, T., Naidoo, N., & Frank, M. G. (2009). Mechanisms of sleep-dependent consolidation of cortical plasticity. *Neuron, 61*(3), 454–466. doi: 0.1016/j.neuron.2009.01.007

Aton, S. J., Seibt, J., Dumoulin, M. C., Coleman, T., Shiraishi, M., & Frank, M. G. (2009). The sedating antidepressant trazodone impairs sleep-dependent cortical plasticity. *PLoS One, 4*(7), e6078. doi: 10.1371/journal.pone.0006078

Aton, S. J., Suresh, A., Broussard, C., & Frank, M. G. (2014). Sleep promotes cortical response potentiation following visual experience. *Sleep, 37*(7), 1163–1170. doi: 10.5665/sleep.3830

Bar, E., Marmelshtein, A., Arzi, A., Perl, O., Livne, E., Hizmi, E., ... Nir, Y. (2020). Local targeted memory reactivation in human sleep. *Curr Biol, 30*(8), 1435–1446 e1435. doi: 10.1016/j.cub.2020.01.091

Barakat, M., Carrier, J., Debas, K., Lungu, O., Fogel, S., Vandewalle, G., ... Doyon, J. (2013). Sleep spindles predict neural and behavioral changes in motor sequence consolidation. *Hum Brain Mapp, 34*(11), 2918–2928. doi: 10.1002/hbm.22116

Baran, B., Mantua, J., & Spencer, R. M. (2016). Age-related changes in the sleep-dependent reorganization of declarative memories. *J Cogn Neurosci, 28*(6), 792–802. doi: 10.1162/jocn_a_00938

Barham, M. P., Enticott, P. G., Conduit, R., & Lum, J. A. (2016). Transcranial electrical stimulation during sleep enhances declarative (but not procedural) memory consolidation: evidence from a meta-analysis. *Neurosci Biobehav Rev, 63*, 65–77. doi: 10.1016/j.neubiorev.2016.01.009

Bear, M., & Singer, W. (1986). Modulation of visual cortical plasticity by acetylcholine and noradrenaline. *Nature, 320*(6058), 172–176.

Berke, J. D. (2018). What does dopamine mean? *Nat Neurosci, 21*(6), 787–793. doi: 10.1038/s41593-018-0152-y

Berridge, K. C. (2007). The debate over dopamine's role in reward: the case for incentive salience. *Psychopharmacology (Berl), 191*(3), 391–431. doi: 10.1007/s00213-006-0578-x

Bliss, T., & Collingridge, G. L. (1993). A synaptic model of memory: long-term potentiation in the hippocampus. *Nature, 361*, 31–39.

Blom, K., Jernelov, S., Ruck, C., Lindefors, N., & Kaldo, V. (2017). Three-year follow-up comparing cognitive behavioral therapy for depression to cognitive behavioral therapy for insomnia, for patients with both diagnoses. *Sleep, 40*(8), zsx108. doi: 10.1093/sleep/zsx108

Bódizs, R., Gombos, F., Ujma, P. P., & Kovacs, I. (2014). Sleep spindling and fluid intelligence across adolescent development: sex matters. *Front Hum Neurosci, 8*, 952. doi: 10.3389/fnhum.2014.00952

Bódizs, R., Kántor, S., Szabó, G., Szûcs, A., Erõss, L., & Halász, P. (2001). Rhythmic hippocampal slow oscillation characterizes REM sleep in humans. *Hippocampus, 11*(6), 747–753. doi: 10.1002/hipo.1090

Bódizs, R., Kis, T., Lázár, A., Havrán, L., Rigó, P., Clemens, Z., & Halász, P. (2005). Prediction of general mental ability based on neural oscillation measures of sleep. *J Sleep Res, 14*, 285–292.

Bolsius, Y. G., Meerlo, P., Kas, M. J., Abel, T., & Havekes, R. (2021). Sleep deprivation reduces the density of individual spine subtypes in a branch-specific fashion in CA1 neurons. *J Sleep Res, 31*(1), e13438. doi:10.1111/jsr.13438

Born, J., & Feld, G. B. (2012). Sleep to upscale, sleep to downscale: balancing homeostasis and plasticity. *Neuron, 75*(6), 933–935. doi: 10.1016/j.neuron.2012.09.007

Boyce, R., Glasgow, S., Williams, S., & Adamantidis, A. (2016). Causal evidence for the role of REM sleep theta rhythm in contextual memory consolidation. *Science, 352*(6287), 812–816.

Bragin, A., Engel Jr, J., Wilson, C., Fried, I., & Buzsáki, G. (1999). High-frequency oscillations in human brain. *Hippocampus, 9*, 137–142.

Bueno-Lopez, A., Eggert, T., Dorn, H., & Danker-Hopfe, H. (2019). Slow oscillatory transcranial direct current stimulation (so-tDCS) during slow wave sleep has no effects on declarative memory in healthy young subjects. *Brain Stimul, 12*(4), 948–958. doi: 10.1016/j.brs.2019.02.012

Buzsáki, G. (1996). The hippocampo-neocortical dialogue. *Cereb Cortex, 6*, 81–92.

Buzsáki, G. (1998). Memory consolidation during sleep: a neurophysiological perspective. *J Sleep Res, 7*(Supplement 1), 17–23.

Buzsáki, G. (2015). Hippocampal sharp wave-ripple: a cognitive biomarker for episodic memory and planning. *Hippocampus, 25*(1073-1188). doi: 0.1002/hipo.22488

Cairney, S. A., Guttesen, A. A. V., El Marj, N., & Staresina, B. P. (2018). Memory consolidation is linked to spindle-mediated information processing during sleep. *Curr Biol, 28*(6), 948–954 e944. doi: 10.1016/j.cub.2018.01.087

Cantero, J., Atienza, M., Stickgold, R., Kahana, M., Madsen, J., & Kocsis, B. (2004). Sleep-dependent theta oscillations in the human hippocampus and neocortex. *J Neurosci, 23*(34), 10897–10903.

Carr, M. F., Jadhav, S. P., & Frank, L. M. (2011). Hippocampal replay in the awake state: a potential substrate for memory consolidation and retrieval. *Nat Neurosci, 14*(2), 147–153. doi: 10.1038/nn.2732

Cellini, N., Shimizu, R. E., Connolly, P. M., Armstrong, D. M., Hernandez, L. T., Polakiewicz, A. G., ... Simons, S. B. (2019). Short duration repetitive transcranial electrical stimulation during sleep enhances declarative memory of facts. *Front Hum Neurosci, 13*, 123. doi:10.3389/fnhum.2019.00123

Champetier, P., Andre, C., Weber, F. D., Rehel, S., Ourry, V., Laniepce, ... Medit-Ageing Research, G. (2023). Age-related changes in fast spindle clustering during NREM sleep and their relevance for memory consolidation. *Sleep, 46*(5), zsac282. doi:10.1093/sleep/zsac282

Chauvette, S., Seigneur, J., & Timofeev, I. (2012). Sleep oscillations in the thalamocortical system induce long-term neuronal plasticity. *Neuron, 75*(6), 1105–1113. doi: 10.1016/j.neuron.2012.08.034

Clawson, B. C., Durkin, J., & Aton, S. J. (2016). Form and function of sleep spindles across the lifespan. *Neur Plast, 2016*, 6936381. doi: 10.1155/2016/6936381

Clawson, B. C., Durkin, J., Suresh, A. K., Pickup, E. J., Broussard, C. G., & Aton, S. J. (2018). Sleep promotes, and sleep loss inhibits, selective changes in firing rate, response properties and functional connectivity of primary visual cortex neurons. *Front Syst Neurosci, 12*, 40. doi: 10.3389/fnsys.2018.00040

Cooper, S. J. (2005). Donald O. Hebb's synapse and learning rule: a history and commentary. *Neurosci Biobehav Rev, 28*(8), 851–874. doi: 10.1016/j.neubiorev.2004.09.009

Cote, K., Epps, T., & Campbell, K. (2000). The role of the spindle in human information processing of high-intensity stimuli during sleep. *J Sleep Res, 9*, 19–26.

Cousins, J. N., El-Deredy, W., Parkes, L. M., Hennies, N., & Lewis, P. A. (2014). Cued memory reactivation during slow-wave sleep promotes explicit knowledge of a motor sequence. *J Neurosci, 34*(48), 15870–15876. doi: 10.1523/JNEUROSCI.1011-14.2014

Creery, J. D., Oudiette, D., Antony, J. W., & Paller, K. A. (2015). Targeted memory reactivation during sleep depends on prior learning. *Sleep, 38*(5), 755–763. doi: 10.5665/sleep.4670

Crowley, K., Trinder, J., Kim, Y., Carrington, M., & Colrain, I. M. (2002). The effects of normal aging on sleep spindle and K-complex production. *Clin Neurophysiol, 113*, 1615–1622.

Dang-Vu, T. T., McKinney, S. M., Buxton, O. M., Solet, J. M., & Ellenbogen, J. M. (2010). Spontaneous brain rhythms predict sleep stability in the face of noise. *Curr Biol, 20*(15), R626–R627. doi: 10.1016/j.cub.2010.06.032

Davis, C. J., Harding, J. W., & Wright, J. W. (2003). REM sleep deprivation-induced deficits in the latency-to-peak induction and maintenance of long-term potentiation within the CA1 region of the hippocampus. *Brain Res, 973*(2), 293–297. doi: 10.1016/s0006-8993(03)02508-3

Debas, K., Carrier, J., Orban, P., Barakat, M., Lungu, O., Vandewalle, G., ... Doyon, J. (2010). Brain plasticity related to the consolidation of motor sequence learning and motor adaptation. *Proc Natl Acad Sci USA, 107*(41), 17839–17844. doi: 10.1073/pnas.1013176107

Dehnavi, F., Koo-Poeggel, P. C., Ghorbani, M., & Marshall, L. (2021). Spontaneous slow oscillation - slow spindle features predict induced overnight memory retention. *Sleep, 44*(10), zsab127. doi:10.1093/sleep/zsab127

de Lavilléon, G., Lacroix, M. M., Rondi-Reig, L., & Benchenane, K. (2015). Explicit memory creation during sleep demonstrates a causal role of place cells in navigation. *Nat Neurosci, 18*(4), 493–495. doi: 10.1038/nn.3970

de Vivo, L., Bellesi, M., Marshall, W., Bushong, E. A., Ellisman, M. H., Tononi, G., & Cirelli, C. (2017). Ultrastructural evidence for synaptic scaling across the wake/sleep cycle. *Science, 355*(6324), 507–510. doi: 10.1126/science.aah5982

Deuker, L., Olligs, J., Fell, J., Kranz, T. A., Mormann, F., Montag, C., ... Axmacher, N. (2013). Memory consolidation by replay of stimulus-specific neural activity. *J Neurosci, 33*(49), 19373–19383. doi: 10.1523/JNEUROSCI.0414-13.2013

Diekelmann, S., Biggel, S., Rasch, B., & Born, J. (2012). Offline consolidation of memory varies with time in slow wave sleep and can be accelerated by cuing memory reactivations. *Neurobiol Learn Mem, 98*, 103–111. doi: 0.1016/j.nlm.2012.07.002

Diekelmann, S., & Born, J. (2007). One memory, two ways to consolidate? *Nat Neurosci, 10*(9), 1085–1086.

Diering, G., Nirujogi, R., Roth, R., Worley, P., Pandey, A., & Huganir, R. (2017). Homer1a drives homeostatic scaling-down of excitatory synapses during sleep. *Science, 355*(6324), 511–515. doi: doi: 10.1126/science.aai8355

Dijk, D. J., & Czeisler, C. A. (1995). Contribution of the circadian pacemaker and the sleep homeostat to sleep propensity, sleep structure, electroencephalographic slow waves, and sleep spindle activity in humans. *J Neurosci, 15*, 3526–3538.

Dijk, D.-J., Duffy, J. F., & Czeisler, C. A. (2000). Contribution of circadian physiology and sleep homeostasis to age-related changes in human sleep. *Chronobiol Int, 17*(3), 285–311. doi: 10.1081/cbi-100101049

Doyon, J., Gabitov, E., Vahdat, S., Lungu, O., & Boutin, A. (2018). Current issues related to motor sequence learning in humans. *Curr Opin Behav Sci, 20*, 89–97. doi: 10.1016/j.cobeha.2017.11.012

Dragoi, G., & Tonegawa, S. (2011). Preplay of future place cell sequences by hippocampal cellular assemblies. *Nature, 469*(7330), 397–401. doi: 10.1038/nature09633

Dragoi, G., & Tonegawa, S. (2014). Selection of preconfigured cell assemblies for representation of novel spatial experiences. *Phil Trans R Soc Lond B, 369*(1635), 20120522. doi: 10.1098/rstb.2012.0522

Dudai, Y., Karni, A., & Born, J. (2015). The consolidation and transformation of memory. *Neuron, 88*(1), 20–32. doi: 10.1016/j.neuron.2015.09.004

Dudek, S. M., & Bear, M. F. (1992). Homosynaptic long-term depression in area CA1 of hippocampus and effects of N-methyl-D-aspartate receptor blockade. *Proc Natl Acad Sci USA, 89*, 4363–4367.

Duman, R. S., Aghajanian, G. K., Sanacora, G., & Krystal, J. H. (2016). Synaptic plasticity and depression: new insights from stress and rapid-acting antidepressants. *Nat Med, 22*(3), 238–249. doi: 10.1038/nm.4050

Dumoulin Bridi, M. C., Aton, S. J., Seibt, J., Renouard, L., Coleman, T., & Frank, M. G. (2015). Rapid eye movement sleep promotes cortical plasticity in the developing brain. *Sci Adv, 1*(6), e1500105. doi: 10.1126/sciadv.1500105

Dupret, D., O'Neill, J., Pleydell-Bouverie, B., & Csicsvari, J. (2010). The reorganization and reactivation of hippocampal maps predict spatial memory performance. *Nat Neurosci, 13*(8), 995–1002. doi: 0.1038/nn.2599

Durkin, J., & Aton, S. J. (2016). Sleep-dependent potentiation in the visual system is at odds with the synaptic homeostasis hypothesis. *Sleep, 39*(1), 155–159. doi: 10.5665/sleep.5338

Durrant, S. J., Cairney, S. A., & Lewis, P. A. (2013). Overnight consolidation aids the transfer of statistical knowledge from the medial temporal lobe to the striatum. *Cereb Cortex, 23*(10), 2467–2478. doi: 10.1093/cercor/bhs244

Durrant, S. J., Taylor, C., Cairney, S., & Lewis, P. A. (2011). Sleep-dependent consolidation of statistical learning. *Neuropsychologia, 49*(5), 1322–1331. doi: 10.1016/j.neuropsychologia.2011.02.015

Ego-Stengel, V., & Wilson, M. A. (2010). Disruption of ripple-associated hippocampal activity during rest impairs spatial learning in the rat. *Hippocampus, 20*(1), 1–10. doi: 10.1002/hipo.20707

Eichenbaum, H. (2015). Does the hippocampus preplay memories? *Nat Neurosci, 18*(12), 1701–1702. doi: 10.1038/nn.4180

Eisch, A. J., & Petrik, D. (2012). Depression and hippocampal neurogenesis: a road to remission? *Science, 338*(6103), 72–75. doi: 10.1126/science.1222941

Eschenko, O., Molle, M., Born, J., & Sara, S. J. (2006). Elevated sleep spindle density after learning or after retrieval in rats. *J Neurosci, 26*(50), 12914–12920. doi: 10.1523/JNEUROSCI.3175-06.2006

Euston, D. R., Tatsuno, M., & McNaughton, B. L. (2007). Fast-forward playback of recent memory sequences in prefrontal cortex during sleep. *Science, 318*(5853), 1147–1150. doi: 10.1126/science.1148979

Fang, Z., Ray, L. B., Owen, A. M., & Fogel, S. M. (2019). Brain activation time-locked to sleep spindles associated with human cognitive abilities. *Front Neurosci, 13*, 46. doi:10.3389/fnins.2019.00046

Florian, C., Vecsey, C. G., Halassa, M. M., Haydon, P. G., & Abel, T. (2011). Astrocyte-derived adenosine and A1 receptor activity contribute to sleep loss-induced deficits in hippocampal synaptic plasticity and memory in mice. *J Neurosci, 31*(19), 6956–6962. doi: 10.1523/JNEUROSCI.5761-10.2011

Fogel, S., Albouy, G., King, B. R., Lungu, O., Vien, C., Bore, A., ... Doyon, J. (2017). Reactivation or transformation? Motor memory consolidation associated with cerebral activation time-locked to sleep spindles. *PLoS One, 12*(4), e0174755. doi:10.1371/journal.pone.0174755

Fogel, S., Smith, C., & Beninger, R. (2009). Evidence for 2-stage models of sleep and memory: learning-dependent changes in spindles and theta in rats. *Brain Res Bull, 79*(6), 445–451. doi: 10.1016/j.brainresbull.2009.03.002

Fogel, S. M., Ray, L. B., Binnie, L., & Owen, A. M. (2015). How to become an expert: a new perspective on the role of sleep in the mastery of procedural skills. *Neurobiol Learn Mem, 125*, 236–248. doi: 10.1016/j.nlm.2015.10.004

Fogel, S. M., & Smith, C. T. (2006). Learning-dependent changes in sleep spindles and Stage 2 sleep. *J Sleep Res, 15*(3), 250–255. doi: 10.1111/j.1365-2869.2006.00522.x

Fogel, S. M., & Smith, C. T. (2011). The function of the sleep spindle: a physiological index of intelligence and a mechanism for sleep-dependent memory consolidation. *Neurosci Biobehav Rev, 35*(5), 1154–1165. doi: 10.1016/j.neubiorev.2010.12.003

Foster, D., & Wilson, M. (2006). Reverse replay of behavioural sequences in hippocampal place cells during the awake state. *Nature, 440*(7084), 680–683. doi: 10.1038/nature04587

Frank, M. G., Issa, N. P., & Stryker, M. P. (2001). Sleep enhances plasticity in the developing visual cortex. *Neuron, 30*(1), 275–287.

Franzen, P., & Buysse, D. (2008). Sleep disturbances and depression: risk relationships for subsequent depression and therapeutic implications. *Dialogues Clin Neurosci, 10*(4), 473–481.

Frey, U., & Morris, R. G. M. (1997). Synaptic tagging and long-term potentiation. *Nature, 385*, 533–536.

Gais, S., & Born, J. (2004a). Declarative memory consolidation: mechanisms acting during human sleep. *Learn Mem, 11*(6), 679–685. doi: 10.1101/lm.80504

Gais, S., & Born, J. (2004b). Low acetylcholine during slow-wave sleep is critical for declarative memory consolidation. *Proc Natl Acad Sci USA*, *101*(7), 2140–2144. doi: 10.1073/pnas.0305404101

Gais, S., Mölle, M., Helms, K., & Born, J. (2002). Learning-dependent increases in sleep spindle density. *J Neurosci*, *22*(15), 6830–6834. doi: 20026697

Geiger, A., Huber, R., Kurth, S., Ringli, M., Jenni, O., & Achermann, P. (2011). The sleep EEG as a marker of intellectual ability in school age children. *Sleep*, *34*(2), 181–189.

Genzel, L., Dresler, M., Wehrle, F., Grözinger, M., & Steiger, A. (2009). Slow wave sleep and REM sleep awakenings do not affect sleep dependent memory consolidation. *Sleep*, *32*(3), 302–310.

Gerrard, J. L., Burke, S. N., McNaughton, B. L., & Barnes, C. A. (2008). Sequence reactivation in the hippocampus is impaired in aged rats. *J Neurosci*, *28*(31), 7883–7890. doi: 10.1523/jneurosci.1265-08.2008

Giese, M., Unternaehrer, E., Brand, S., Calabrese, P., Holsboer-Trachsler, E., & Eckert, A. (2013). The interplay of stress and sleep impacts BDNF level. *PLoS One*, *8*(10), e76050. doi: 10.1371/journal.pone.0076050

Girardeau, G., Benchenane, K., Wiener, S. I., Buzsáki, G., & Zugaro, M. B. (2009). Selective suppression of hippocampal ripples impairs spatial memory. *Nat Neurosci*, *12*(10), 1222–1223. doi: 10.1038/nn.2384

Gisabella, B., Scammell, T., Bandaru, S. S., & Saper, C. B. (2020). Regulation of hippocampal dendritic spines following sleep deprivation. *J Comp Neurol*, *528*(3), 380–388. doi: 10.1002/cne.24764

Giuditta, A., Ambrosini, M., Montagnese, P., Mandile, P., Cotugno, M., Grassi Zucconi, G., & Vescia, S. (1995). The sequential hypothesis of the function of sleep. *Behav Brain Res*, *69*, 157–166.

Goerke, M., Cohrs, S., Rodenbeck, A., & Kunz, D. (2014). Differential effect of an anticholinergic antidepressant on sleep-dependent memory consolidation. *Sleep*, *37*(5), 977–985. doi: 10.5665/sleep.3674

Gonzalez, C. E., Mak-McCully, R. A., Rosen, B. Q., Cash, S. S., Chauvel, P. Y., Bastuji, H., … Halgren, E. (2018). Theta bursts precede, and spindles follow, cortical and thalamic downstates in human NREM sleep. *J Neurosci*, *38*(46), 9989–10001. doi: 10.1523/JNEUROSCI.0476-18.2018

Grimaldi, D., Papalambros, N. A., Zee, P. C., & Malkani, R. G. (2020). Neurostimulation techniques to enhance sleep and improve cognition in aging. *Neurobiol Dis*, *141*, 104865. doi:10.1016/j.nbd.2020.104865

Grosmark, A. D., Mizuseki, K., Pastalkova, E., Diba, K., & Buzsáki, G. (2012). REM sleep reorganizes hippocampal excitability. *Neuron*, *75*(6), 1001–1007. doi: 10.1016/j.neuron.2012.08.015

Gruber, R., Wise, M. S., Frenette, S., Knaauper, B., Boom, A., Fontil, L., & Carrier, J. (2013). The association between sleep spindles and IQ in healthy school-age children. *Int J Psychophysiol*, *89*(2), 229–240. doi: 10.1016/j.ijpsycho.2013.03.018

Gu, Q. (2003). Contribution of acetylcholine to visual cortex plasticity. *Neurobiol Learn Mem*, *80*(3), 291–301. doi: 10.1016/s1074-7427(03)00073-x

Gujar, N., McDonald, S. A., Nishida, M., & Walker, M. P. (2011). A role for REM sleep in recalibrating the sensitivity of the human brain to specific emotions. *Cereb Cortex*, *21*(1), 115–123. doi: 10.1093/cercor/bhq064

Guzmán-Marín, R., & McGinty, D. (2006). Sleep deprivation suppresses adult neurogenesis: clues to the role of sleep in brain plasticity. *Sleep Biol Rhythms*, *4*(1), 27–34. doi: 10.1111/sbr.2006.4.issue-1

Guzmán-Marín, R., Suntsova, N., Stewart, D. R., Gong, H., Szymusiak, R., & McGinty, D. (2003). Sleep deprivation reduces proliferation of cells in the dentate gyrus of the hippocampus in rats. *J Physiol*, *549*(Pt 2), 563–571. doi: 10.1113/jphysiol.2003.041665

Hahn, M., Joechner, A. K., Roell, J., Schabus, M., Heib, D. P., Gruber, G., … Hoedlmoser, K. (2019). Developmental changes of sleep spindles and their impact on sleep-dependent memory consolidation and general cognitive abilities: a longitudinal approach. *Dev Sci*, *22*(1), e12706. doi: 10.1111/desc.12706

Hahn, M. A., Heib, D., Schabus, M., Hoedlmoser, K., & Helfrich, R. F. (2020). Slow oscillation-spindle coupling predicts enhanced memory formation from childhood to adolescence. *Elife*, *9*, e53730. doi:10.7554/eLife.53730

Hasselmo, M. E. (2006). The role of acetylcholine in learning and memory. *Curr Opin Neurobiol*, *16*(6), 710–715. doi: 10.1016/j.conb.2006.09.002

Hathaway, E., Morgan, K., Carson, M. S., R., Fernandez-Corazza, M., Luu, P., & Tucker, D. M. (2021). Transcranial electrical stimulation targeting limbic cortex increases the duration of human deep sleep. *Sleep Med*, *81*, 350–357. doi: 10.1016/j.sleep.2021.03.001

Havekes, R., Bruinenberg, V. M., Tudor, J. C., Ferri, S. L., Baumann, A., Meerlo, P., & Abel, T. (2014). Transiently increasing cAMP levels selectively in hip pocampal excitatory neurons during sleep deprivation prevents memory deficits caused by sleep loss. *J Neurosci*, *34*(47), 15715–15721. doi: 10.1523/JNEUROSCI.2403-14.2014

Havekes, R., Park, A. J., Tudor, J. C., Luczak, V. G., Hansen, R. T., Ferri, S. L., … Abel, T. (2016). Sleep deprivation causes memory deficits by negatively impacting neuronal connectivity in hippocampal area CA1. *Elife*, *5*, e13424. doi: 10.7554/eLife.13424

Hebb, D. O. (1949). *The Organization of Behavior; A Neuropsychological Theory*. Oxford: Wiley.

Helfrich, R. F., Lendner, J. D., Mander, B. A., Guillen, H., Paff, M., Mnatsakanyan, L., … Knight, R. T. (2019). Bidirectional prefrontal-hippocampal dynamics organize information transfer during sleep in humans. *Nat Commun*, *10*(1), 3572. doi:10.1038/s41467-019-11444-x

Helfrich, R. F., Mander, B. A., Jagust, W. J., Knight, R. T., & Walker, M. P. (2018). Old brains come uncoupled in sleep: slow wave-spindle synchrony, brain atrophy, and forgetting. *Neuron*, *97*(1), 221–230. doi: 10.1016/j.neuron.2017.11.020

Hengen, K. B., Torrado Pacheco, A., McGregor, J. N., Van Hooser, S. D., & Turrigiano, G. G. (2016). Neuronal firing rate homeostasis is inhibited by sleep and promoted by wake. *Cell*, *165*(1), 180–191. doi: 10.1016/j.cell.2016.01.046

Hennies, N., Lambon Ralph, M., Durrant, S., Cousins, J., & Lewis, P. (2017). Cued memory reactivation during SWS abolishes the beneficial effect of sleep on abstraction. *Sleep*, *40*(8), zsx102. doi: 10.1093/sleep/zsx102

Hoedlmoser, K., Heib, D., Roell, J., Peigneux, P., Sadeh, A., Gruber, G., & Schabus, M. (2014). Slow sleep spindle activity, declarative memory, and general cognitive abilities in children. *Sleep*, *37*(9), 1501–1512. doi: 0.5665/sleep.4000

Hubel, D., & Wiesel, T. (1965). Binocular interaction in striate cortex of kittens reared with an artificial squint. *J Neurophysiol*, *28*(6), 1041–1059.

Huber, R., Maki, H., Rosanova, M., Casarotto, S., Canali, P., Casali, A. G., … Massimini, M. (2012). Human cortical excitability increases with time awake. *Cereb Cortex*, *23*(2), 332–338. doi: 10.1093/cercor/bhs014

Huttenlocher, P. R. (1990). Morphometric study of human cerebral cortex development. *Neuropsychologia*, *28*(6), 517–527.

Ishikawa, A., Kanayama, Y., Matsumura, H., Tsuchimochi, H., Ishida, Y., & Nakamura, S. (2006). Selective rapid eye movement sleep deprivation impairs the maintenance of long-term potentiation in the rat hippocampus. *Eur J Neurosci*, *24*(1), 243–248. doi: 10.1111/j.1460-9568.2006.04874.x

Jemni, M., Zaman, R., Carrick, F. R., Clarke, N. D., Marina, M., Bottoms, L., … Konukman, F. (2023). Exercise improves depression through positive modulation of brain-derived neurotrophic factor (BDNF). A review based on 100 manuscripts over 20 years. *Front Physiol*, *14*, 1102526. doi:10.3389/fphys.2023.1102526

Ji, D., & Wilson, M. A. (2007). Coordinated memory replay in the visual cortex and hippocampus during sleep. *Nat Neurosci*, *10*(1), 100–107. doi: 10.1038/nn1825

Jiang, X., Gonzalez-Martinez, J., & Halgren, E. (2019). Coordination of human hippocampal sharpwave-ripples during NREM sleep with cortical theta bursts, spindles, downstates and upstates. *J Neurosci*, *39*(44), 8744–8761. doi: 10.1523/JNEUROSCI.2857-18.2019

Jiang, X., Shamie, I., W, K. D., Friedman, D., Dugan, P., Devinsky, O., … Halgren, E. (2017). Replay of large-scale spatio-temporal patterns from waking during subsequent NREM sleep in human cortex. *Sci Rep*, *7*(1), 17380. doi: 10.1038/s41598-017-17469-w

Jones, A. P., Choe, J., Bryant, N. B., Robinson, C. S. H., Ketz, N. A., Skorheim, S. W., … Pilly, P. K. (2018). Dose-dependent effects of closed-loop tACS delivered during slow-wave oscillations on memory consolidation. *Front Neurosci*, *12*, 867. doi:10.3389/fnins.2018.00867

Kam, K., Pettibone, W. D., Shim, K., Chen, R. K., & Varga, A. W. (2019). Dynamics of sleep spindles and coupling to slow oscillations following motor learning in adult mice. *Neurobiol Learn Mem*, *166*, 107100. doi: 10.1016/j.nlm.2019.107100

Kemp, I., & Kaada, B. (1975). The relation of hippocampal theta activity to arousal, attentive behaviour and somato-motor movements in unrestrained cats. *Brain Res*, *95*(2–3), 323–342.

Ketz, N., Jones, A. P., Bryant, N. B., Clark, V. P., & Pilly, P. K. (2018). Closed-loop slow-wave tACS improves sleep-dependent long-term memory generalization by modulating endogenous oscillations. *J Neurosci*, *38*(33), 7314–7326. doi: 10.1523/JNEUROSCI.0273-18.2018

Kim, E. Y., Mahmoud, G. S., & Grover, L. M. (2005). REM sleep deprivation inhibits LTP in vivo in area CA1 of rat hippocampus. *Neurosci Lett*, *388*(3), 163–167. doi: 10.1016/j.neulet.2005.06.057

Kompotis, K., Hubbard, J., Emmenegger, Y., Perrault, A., Muhlethaler, M., Schwartz, S., … Franken, P. (2019). Rocking promotes sleep in mice through rhythmic stimulation of the vestibular system. *Curr Biol*, *29*(3), 392–401. doi: 10.1016/j.cub.2018.12.007

Koo, P. C., Mölle, M., & Marshall, L. (2018). Efficacy of slow oscillatory-transcranial direct current stimulation on EEG and memory - contribution of an inter-individual factor. *Eur J Neurosci*, *47*(7), 812–823. doi: 10.1111/ejn.13877

Kopp, C., Longordo, F., Nicholson, J. R., & Luthi, A. (2006). Insufficient sleep reversibly alters bidirectional synaptic plasticity and NMDA receptor function. *J Neurosci, 26*(48), 12456–12465. doi: 10.1523/jneurosci.2702-06.2006

Kumar, D., Koyanagi, I., Carrier-Ruiz, A., Vergara, P., Srinivasan, S., Sugaya, Y., ... Sakaguchi, M. (2020). Sparse activity of hippocampal adult-born neurons during REM sleep is necessary for memory consolidation. *Neuron, 107*(3), 552–565. doi: 10.1016/j.neuron.2020.05.008

Kurdziel, L., Duclos, K., & Spencer, R. M. (2013). Sleep spindles in midday naps enhance learning in preschool children. *Proc Natl Acad Sci U S A, 110*(43), 17267–17272. doi: 10.1073/pnas.1306418110

Kwon, H., Walsh, K. G., Berja, E. D., Manoach, D. S., Eden, U. T., Kramer, M. A., & Chu, C. J. (2023). Sleep spindles in the healthy brain from birth through 18 years. *Sleep, 46*(4), zsad017. doi:10.1093/sleep/zsad017

Lafon, B., Henin, S., Huang, Y., Friedman, D., Melloni, L., Thesen, T., ... Liu, A. A. (2017). Low frequency transcranial electrical stimulation does not entrain sleep rhythms measured by human intracranial recordings. *Nat Commun, 8*(1), 1199. doi: 10.1038/s41467-017-01045-x

Landolt, H.-P., Dijk, D.-J., Achermann, P., & Borbély, A. A. (1996). Effect of age on the sleep EEG: slow-wave activity and spindle frequency activity in young and middle-aged men. *Brain Res, 738*, 205–212.

Larkin, J., & Heller, H. (1999). Sleep after arousal from hibernation is not homeostatically regulated. *Am J Physiol, 276*, R522–R529.

Latchoumane, C. V., Ngo, H. V., Born, J., & Shin, H. S. (2017). Thalamic spindles promote memory formation during sleep through triple phase-locking of cortical, thalamic, and hippocampal rhythms. *Neuron, 95*(2), 424–435. doi: 10.1016/j.neuron.2017.06.025

Lee, A., & Wilson, M. (2002). Memory of sequential experience in the hippocampus during slow wave sleep. *Neuron, 36*, 1183–1194.

Leminen, M. M., Virkkala, J., Saure, E., Paajanen, T., Zee, P. C., Santostasi, G., ... Paunio, T. (2017). Enhanced memory consolidation via automatic sound stimulation during non-REM sleep. *Sleep, 40*(3), zsx003. doi: 10.1093/sleep/zsx003

Li, W., Ma, L., Yang, G., & Gan, W. B. (2017). REM sleep selectively prunes and maintains new synapses in development and learning. *Nat Neurosci, 20*(3), 427–437. doi: 10.1038/nn.4479

Liu, Z. W., Faraguna, U., Cirelli, C., Tononi, G., & Gao, X. B. (2010). Direct evidence for wake-related increases and sleep-related decreases in synaptic strength in rodent cortex. *J Neurosci, 30*(25), 8671–8675. doi: 10.1523/jneurosci.1409-10.2010

Louie, K., & Wilson, M. A. (2001). Temporally structured replay of awake hippocampal ensemble activity during rapid eye movement sleep. *Neuron, 29*(1), 145–156.

Lucassen, P. J., Fitzsimons, C. P., Salta, E., & Maletic-Savatic, M. (2019). Adult neurogenesis, human after all (again): classic, optimized, and future approaches. *Behav Brain Res*, 112458. doi: 10.1016/j.bbr.2019.112458

Lustenberger, C., Boyle, M. R., Alagapan, S., Mellin, J. M., Vaughn, B. V., & Fröhlich, F. (2016). Feedback-controlled transcranial alternating current stimulation reveals a functional role of sleep spindles in motor memory consolidation. *Curr Biol, 26*(16), 2127–2136. doi: 10.1016/j.cub.2016.06.044

Maingret, N., Girardeau, G., Todorova, R., Goutierre, M., & Zugaro, M. (2016). Hippocampo-cortical coupling mediates memory consolidation during sleep. *Nat Neurosci, 19*(7), 959–964. doi: 10.1038/nn.4304

Mak-McCully, R. A., Rolland, M., Sargsyan, A., Gonzalez, C., Magnin, M., Chauvel, P., Rey, M., Bastuji, H., & Halgren, E. (2017). Coordination of cortical and thalamic activity during non-REM sleep in humans. *Nat Commun, 8*, 15499. doi:10.1038/ncomms15499

Malberg, J., Eisch, A., Nestler, E., & Duman, R. (2000). Chronic antidepressant treatment increases neurogenesis in adult rat hippocampus. *J Neurosci, 20*(24), 9104–9110.

Mantua, J. (2018). Sleep physiology correlations and human memory consolidation: where do we go from here? *Sleep, 41*(2), zsx204. doi: 10.1093/sleep/zsx204

Marshall, L., Helgadóttir, H., Mölle, M., & Born, J. (2006). Boosting slow oscillations during sleep potentiates memory. *Nature, 444*(7119), 610–613. doi: 10.1038/nature05278

Marshall, L., Kirov, R., Brade, J., Mölle, M., & Born, J. (2011). Transcranial electrical currents to probe EEG brain rhythms and memory consolidation during sleep in humans. *PLoS One, 6*(2), e16905. doi:10.1371/journal.pone.0016905

McConnell, B. V., Kronberg, E., Teale, P. D., Sillau, S. H., Fishback, G. M., Kaplan, R. I., ... Bettcher, B. M. (2021). The aging slow wave: a shifting amalgam of distinct slow wave and spindle coupling subtypes define slow wave sleep across the human lifespan. *Sleep, 44*(10), zsab125. doi: 10.1093/sleep/zsab125

McDermott, C. M., Hardy, M. N., Bazan, N. G., & Magee, J. C. (2006). Sleep deprivation-induced alterations in excitatory synaptic transmission in the CA1 region of the rat hippocampus. *J Physiol, 570*(Pt 3), 553–565. doi: 10.1113/jphysiol.2005.093781

McDermott, C. M., LaHoste, G. J., Chen, C., Musto, A., Bazan, N. G., & Magee, J. C. (2003). Sleep deprivation causes behavioral, synaptic, and membrane excitability alterations in hippocampal neurons. *J Neurosci, 23*(29), 9687–9695.

Mednick, S., Nakayama, K., & Stickgold, R. (2003). Sleep-dependent learning: a nap is as good as a night. *Nat Neurosci, 6*(7), 697–698. doi: 10.1038/nn1078

Mehta, M. R. (2007). Cortico-hippocampal interaction during up-down states and memory consolidation. *Nat Neurosci, 10*(1), 13–15. doi: 10.1038/nn0107-13

Menz, M. M., Rihm, J. S., & Buchel, C. (2016). REM sleep is causal to successful consolidation of dangerous and safety stimuli and reduces return of fear after extinction. *J Neurosci, 36*(7), 2148–2160. doi: 10.1523/JNEUROSCI.3083-15.2016

Mizuseki, K., & Miyawaki, H. (2017). Hippocampal information processing across sleep/wake cycles. *Neurosci Res, 118*, 30–47. doi: 10.1016/j.neures.2017.04.018

Modi, M. N., Dhawale, A. K., & Bhalla, U. S. (2014). CA1 cell activity sequences emerge after reorganization of network correlation structure during associative learning. *Elife, 3*, e01982. doi: 10.7554/eLife.01982

Mölle, M., Bergmann, T. O., Marshall, L., & Born, J. (2011). Fast and slow spindles during the sleep slow oscillation: disparate coalescence and engagement in memory processing. *Sleep, 34*(10), 1411–1421.

Morgan, K. K., Hathaway, E., Carson, M., Fernandez-Corazza, M., Shusterman, R., Luu, P., & Tucker, D. M. (2021). Focal limbic sources create the large slow oscillations of the EEG in human deep sleep. *Sleep Med, 85*, 291–302. doi: 10.1016/j.sleep.2021.07.028

Morin, A., Doyon, J., Dostie, V., Barakat, M., Tahar, A., Korman, M., ... Carrier, J. (2008). Motor sequence learning increases sleep spindles and fast frequencies in post-training sleep. *Sleep, 31*(8), 1149–1156.

Morris, R. G. (2013). NMDA receptors and memory encoding. *Neuropharmacology, 74*, 32–40. doi: 10.1016/j.neuropharm.2013.04.014

Muehlroth, B. E., Sander, M. C., Fandakova, Y., Grandy, T. H., Rasch, B., Shing, Y. L., & Werkle-Bergner, M. (2019). Precise slow oscillation-spindle coupling promotes memory consolidation in younger and older adults. *Sci Rep, 9*(1), 1–15. doi:10.1038/s41598-018-36557-z

Mueller, A. D., Meerlo, P., McGinty, D., & Mistlberger, R. E. (2013). Sleep and adult neurogenesis: implications for cognition and mood. *Curr Top Behav Neurosci, 25*, 151–181. doi: 10.1007/7854_2013_251

Mueller, A. D., Pollock, M. S., Lieblich, S. E., Epp, J. R., Galea, L. A., & Mistlberger, R. E. (2008). Sleep deprivation can inhibit adult hippocampal neurogenesis independent of adrenal stress hormones. *Am J Physiol Regul Integr Comp Physiol, 294*(5), R1693–1703. doi: 10.1152/ajpregu.00858.2007

Nabavi, S., Fox, R., Proulx, C. D., Lin, J. Y., Tsien, R. Y., & Malinow, R. (2014). Engineering a memory with LTD and LTP. *Nature, 511*(7509), 348–352. doi: 10.1038/nature13294

Ngo, H. V., Martinetz, T., Born, J., & Molle, M. (2013). Auditory closed-loop stimulation of the sleep slow oscillation enhances memory. *Neuron, 78*(3), 545–553. doi: 10.1016/j.neuron.2013.03.006

Nguyen, P. V. & Woo, N. H. (2003) Regulation of hippocampal synaptic plasticity by cyclic AMP-dependent protein kinases. *Prog Neurobiol, 71*, 401-437. doi: 10.1016/j.pneurobio.2003.12.003

Nicolas, A., Petit, D., Rompré, S., & Montplaisir, J. (2001). Sleep spindle characteristics in healthy subjects of different age groups. *Clin Neurophysiol, 112*, 521–527.

Niethard, N., & Born, J. (2019). Back to baseline: sleep recalibrates synapses. *Nat Neurosci, 22*(2), 149–151. doi: 10.1038/s41593-018-0327-6

Norimoto, H., Makino, K., Gao, M., Shikano, Y., Okamoto, K., Ishikawa, T., . . . Ikegaya, Y. (2018). Hippocampal ripples down-regulate synapses. *Science, 359*, 1524–15276.

O'Keefe, J., & Nadel, L. (1979). Précis of O'Keefe & Nadel's *The hippocampus as a cognitive map. Behav Brain Sci, 2*, 487–533.

Oudiette, D., Antony, J. W., Creery, J. D., & Paller, K. A. (2013). The role of memory reactivation during wakefulness and sleep in determining which memories endure. *J Neurosci, 33*(15), 6672–6678. doi: 10.1523/JNEUROSCI.5497-12.2013

Pavlides, C., & Winson, J. (1989). Influences of hippocampal place cell firing in the awake state on the activity of these cells during subsequent sleep episodes. *J Neurosci, 9*(8), 2907–2918.

Pereira, S. I. R., Santamaria, L., Andrews, R., Schmidt, E., Van Rossum, M., & Lewis, P. A. (2023). Rule abstraction is facilitated by auditory cueing in REM sleep. *J Neurosci, 43*(32), 3838–3848. doi: 10.1523/JNEUROSCI.1966-21.2022

Perrault, A. A., Khani, A., Quairiaux, C., Kompotis, K., Franken, P., Muhlethaler, M., ... Bayer, L. (2019). Whole-night continuous rocking entrains spontaneous neural oscillations with benefits for sleep and memory. *Curr Biol, 29*(3), 402–411. doi: 10.1016/j.cub.2018.12.028

Pesonen, A.-K., Ujma, P., Halonen, R., Räikkönen, K., & Kuula, L. (2019). The associations between spindle characteristics and cognitive ability in a large adolescent birth cohort. *Intelligence, 72*, 13–19. doi: 10.1016/j.intell.2018.11.004

Peters, K. R., Ray, L., Smith, V., & Smith, C. (2008). Changes in the density of stage 2 sleep spindles following motor learning in young and older adults. *J Sleep Res, 17*(1), 23–33. doi: 10.1111/j.1365-2869.2008.00634.x

Peyrache, A., Khamassi, M., Benchenane, K., Wiener, S., & Battaglia, F. (2009). Replay of rule-learning related neural patterns in the prefrontal cortex during sleep. *Nat Neurosci, 12*(7), 919–926. doi: 10.1038/nn.2337

Poe, G. R., Nitz, D. A., McNaughton, B. L., & Barnes, C. A. (2000). Experience-dependent phase-reversal of hippocampal neuron firing during REM sleep. *Brain Res, 855*, 176–180.

Prehn-Kristensen, A., Munz, M., Goder, R., Wilhelm, I., Korr, K., Vahl, W., Wiesner, C. D., & Baving, L. (2014). Transcranial oscillatory direct current stimulation during sleep improves declarative memory consolidation in children with attention-deficit/hyperactivity disorder to a level comparable to healthy controls. *Brain Stimul, 7*(6), 793–799. doi: 10.1016/j.brs.2014.07.036

Puentes-Mestril, C., & Aton, S. J. (2017). Linking network activity to synaptic plasticity during sleep: hypotheses and recent data. *Front Neural Circuits, 11*, 61. doi: 10.3389/fncir.2017.00061

Purcell, S. M., Manoach, D. S., Demanuele, C., Cade, B. E., Mariani, S., Cox, R., … Stickgold, R. (2017). Characterizing sleep spindles in 11,630 individuals from the National Sleep Research Resource. *Nat Commun, 8*, 15930. doi:10.1038/ncomms15930

Qin, Y.-L., McNaughton, B. L., Skaggs, W. E., & Barnes, C. A. (1997). Memory reprocessing in corticocortical and hippocampocortical neuronal ensembles. *Phil Trans R Soc Lond B, 352*, 1525–1533.

Rampon, M., Carponcy, J., Missaire, M., Bouet, R., Parmentier, R., Comte, J. C., … Salin, P. A. (2023). Synapse-specific modulation of synaptic responses by brain states in hippocampal pathways. *J Neurosci, 43*(7), 1191–1210. doi: 10.1523/JNEUROSCI.0772-22.2022

Rasch, B., & Born, J. (2013). About sleep's role in memory. *Physiol Rev, 93*(2), 681–766. doi: 10.1152/physrev.00032.2012

Rasch, B., Büchel, C., Gais, S., & Born, J. (2007). Odor cues during slow-wave sleep prompt declarative memory consolidation. *Science, 315*(5817), 1426–1429. doi: 10.1126/science.1138581

Rasch, B., Gais, S., & Born, J. (2009). Impaired off-line consolidation of motor memories after combined blockade of cholinergic receptors during REM sleep-rich sleep. *Neuropsychopharmacology, 34*(7), 1843–1853. doi: 10.1038/npp.2009.6

Rasch, B., Pommer, J., Diekelmann, S., & Born, J. (2009). Pharmacological REM sleep suppression paradoxically improves rather than impairs skill memory. *Nat Neurosci, 12*(4), 396–397. doi: 10.1038/nn.2206

Rasch, B. H., Born, J., & Gais, S. (2006). Combined blockade of cholinergic receptors shifts the brain from stimulus encoding to memory consolidation. *J Cogn Neurosci, 18*(5), 793–802. doi: 10.1162/jocn.2006.18.5.793

Reynolds, C. M., Short, M. A., & Gradisar, M. (2018). Sleep spindles and cognitive performance across adolescence: a meta-analytic review. *J Adolesc, 66*, 55–70. doi: 10.1016/j.adolescence.2018.04.003

Rock, P. L., Roiser, J. P., Riedel, W. J., & Blackwell, A. D. (2014). Cognitive impairment in depression: a systematic review and meta-analysis. *Psychol Med, 44*(10), 2029–2040. doi: 10.1017/S0033291713002535

Rosanova, M., & Ulrich, D. (2005). Pattern-specific associative long-term potentiation induced by a sleep spindle-related spike train. *J Neurosci, 25*(41), 9398–9405. doi: 10.1523/jneurosci.2149-05.2005

Rothschild, G., Eban, E., & Frank, L. M. (2017). A cortical-hippocampal-cortical loop of information processing during memory consolidation. *Nat Neurosci, 20*(2), 251–259. doi: 10.1038/nn.4457

Rubin, D. B., Hosman, T., Kelemen, J. N., Kapitonava, A., Willett, F. R., Coughlin, B. F., … Cash, S. S. (2022). Learned motor patterns are replayed in human motor cortex during sleep. *J Neuroscience, 42*(25), 5007–5020. doi: 10.1523/JNEUROSCI.2074-21.2022

Ruch, S., Feher, K., Homan, S., Morishima, Y., Mueller, S. M., Mueller, S. V., … Grieder, M. (2021). Bi-temporal anodal transcranial direct current stimulation during slow-wave sleep boosts slow-wave density but not memory consolidation. *Brain Sci, 11*(4), 410. doi:10.3390/brainsci11040410

Ruch, S., Züst, M. A., & Henke, K. (2022). Sleep-learning impairs subsequent awake-learning. *Neurobiol Learn Mem, 187*, 107569. doi:10.1016/j.nlm.2021.107569

Rudoy, J. D., Voss, J. L., Westerberg, C. E., & Paller, K. A. (2009). Strengthening individual memories by reactivating them during sleep. *Science, 326*(5956), 1079. doi: 10.1126/science.1179013

Saletin, J. M., Goldstein, A. N., & Walker, M. P. (2011). The role of sleep in directed forgetting and remembering of human memories. *Cereb Cortex, 21*(11), 2534–2541. doi: 10.1093/cercor/bhr034

Samuels, B. A., & Hen, R. (2011). Neurogenesis and affective disorders. *Eur J Neurosci, 33*(6), 1152–1159. doi: 10.1111/j.1460-9568.2011.07614.x

Schabus, M., Dang-Vu, T. T., Albouy, G., Balteau, E., Boly, M., Carrier, J., … Maquet, P. (2007). Hemodynamic cerebral correlates of sleep spindles during human non-rapid eye movement sleep. *Proc Natl Acad Sci USA, 104*(32), 13164–13169. doi: 10.1073/pnas.0703084104

Schabus, M., Hoedlmoser, K., Pecherstorfer, T., Anderer, P., Gruber, G., Parapatics, S., … Zeitlhofer, J. (2008). Interindividual sleep spindle differences and their relation to learning-related enhancements. *Brain Res, 1191*, 127–135. doi: 10.1016/j.brainres.2007.10.106

Schapiro, A. C., Turk-Browne, N. B., Botvinick, M. M., & Norman, K. A. (2017). Complementary learning systems within the hippocampus: a neural network modelling approach to reconciling episodic memory with statistical learning. *Phil Trans R Soc Lond B, 372*(1711). doi: 10.1098/rstb.2016.0049

Schendan, H. E., Searl, M. M., Melrose, R. J., & Stern, C. E. (2003). An fMRI study of the role of the medial temporal lobe in implicit and explicit sequences learning. *Neuron, 37*, 1013–1025.

Schmidt, C. (2006). Encoding difficulty promotes postlearning changes in sleep spindle activity during napping. *J Neurosci, 26*(35), 8976–8982. doi: 10.1523/jneurosci.2464-06.2006

Scholle, S., Zwacka, G., & Scholle, H. C. (2007). Sleep spindle evolution from infancy to adolescence. *Clin Neurophysiol, 118*(7), 1525–1531. doi: 10.1016/j.clinph.2007.03.007

Schreiner, T., Petzka, M., Staudigl, T., & Staresina, B. P. (2021). Endogenous memory reactivation during sleep in humans is clocked by slow oscillation-spindle complexes. *Nat Commun, 12*(1), 3112. doi:10.1038/s41467-021-23520-2

Seeck-Hirschner, M., Baier, P. C., Weinhold, S. L., Dittmar, M., Heiermann, S., Aldenhoff, J. B., & Goder, R. (2012). Declarative memory performance is associated with the number of sleep spindles in elderly women. *Am J Geriatr Psychiatry, 20*(9), 782–788. doi: 10.1097/JGP.0b013e31823033da

Seibt, J., Aton, S. J., Jha, S. K., Coleman, T., Dumoulin, M. C., & Frank, M. (2008). The non-benzodiazepine hypnotic zolpidem impairs sleep-dependent cortical plasticity. *Sleep, 31*(10), 1381–1391.

Seibt, J., Dumoulin, M. C., Aton, S. J., Coleman, T., Watson, A., Naidoo, N., & Frank, M. G. (2012). Protein synthesis during sleep consolidates cortical plasticity in vivo. *Curr Biol, 22*(8), 676–682. doi: 10.1016/j.cub.2012.02.016

Seibt, J., & Frank, M. G. (2019). Primed to sleep: the dynamics of synaptic plasticity across brain states. *Front Syst Neurosci, 13*, 2. doi: 10.3389/fnsys.2019.00002

Seibt, J., Richard, C. J., Sigl-Glöckner, J., Takahashi, N., Kaplan, D. I., Doron, G., … Larkum, M. E. (2017). Cortical dendritic activity correlates with spindle-rich oscillations during sleep in rodents. *Nat Commun, 8*(1), 684. doi: 10.1038/s41467-017-00735-w

Siapas, A., & Wilson, M. (1998). Coordinated interactions between hippocampal ripples and cortical spindles during slow-wave sleep. *Neuron, 21*, 1123–1128.

Silva, D., Feng, T., & Foster, D. J. (2015). Trajectory events across hippocampal place cells require previous experience. *Nat Neurosci, 18*(12), 1772–1779. doi: 10.1038/nn.4151

Sirota, A., Csicsvari, J., Buhl, D., & Buzsaki, G. (2003). Communication between neocortex and hippocampus during sleep in rodents. *Proc Natl Acad Sci U S A, 100*(4), 2065–2069. doi: 10.1073/pnas.0437938100

Spano, G. M., Banningh, S. W., Marshall, W., de Vivo, L., Bellesi, M., Loschky, S. S., … Cirelli, C. (2019). Sleep deprivation by exposure to novel objects increases synapse density and axon-spine interface in the hippocampal CA1 region of adolescent mice. *J Neurosci, 39*(34), 6613–6625. doi: 10.1523/JNEUROSCI.0380-19.2019

Spencer, R. M. C., Sunm, M., & Ivry, R. B. (2006). Sleep-dependent consolidation of contextual learning. *Curr Biol, 16*(10), 1001–1005. doi: 10.1016/j.cub.2006.03.094

Sportiche, N., Suntsova, N., Methippara, M., Bashir, T., Mitrani, B., Szymusiak, R., & McGinty, D. (2010). Sustained sleep fragmentation results in delayed changes in hippocampal-dependent cognitive function associated with reduced dentate gyrus neurogenesis. *Neuroscience, 170*(1), 247–258. doi: 10.1016/j.neuroscience.2010.06.038

Spaak, E., & de Lange, F. P. (2020). Hippocampal and prefrontal theta-band mechanisms underpin implicit spatial context learning. *J Neurosci, 40*(1), 191–202. doi: 10.1523/JNEUROSCI.1660-19.2019

Stickgold, R., Malia, A., Maguire, D., Roddenberry, D., & O'Connor, M. (2000). Replaying the game: hypnagogic images in normals and amnesics. *Science, 290*(5940), 350–353.

Stickgold, R., Whidbee, D., Schirmer, B., Patel, V., & Hobson, J. A. (2000). Visual discrimination task improvement: a multi-step process occurring during sleep. *J Cogn Neurosci*, *12*(2), 246–254.

Strauss, M., Griffon, L., Van Beers, P., Elbaz, M., Bouziotis, J., Sauvet, F., ... Peigneux, P. (2022). Order matters: sleep spindles contribute to memory consolidation only when followed by rapid-eye-movement sleep. *Sleep*, *45*(4), zsac022. doi: 10.1093/sleep/zsac022

Strijkstra, A., & Daan, S. (1998). Dissimilarity of slow-wave activity enhancement by torpor and sleep deprivation in a hibernator. *Am J Physiol*, *275*, R1110–R1117.

Swift, K. M., Gross, B. A., Frazer, M. A., Bauer, D. S., Clark, K. J. D., Vazey, E. M., ... Poe, G. R. (2018). Abnormal locus coeruleus sleep activity alters sleep signatures of memory consolidation and impairs place cell stability and spatial memory. *Curr Biol*, *28*(22), 3599–3609 e3594. doi: 10.1016/j.cub.2018.09.054

Takashima, A., Nieuwenhuis, I. L., Jensen, O., Talamini, L. M., Rijpkema, M., & Fernandez, G. (2009). Shift from hippocampal to neocortical centered retrieval network with consolidation. *J Neurosci*, *29*(32), 10087–10093. doi: 10.1523/JNEUROSCI.0799-09.2009

Tamaki, M., Huang, T. R., Yotsumoto, Y., Hamalainen, M., Lin, F. H., Nanez, J. E., Sr., ... Sasaki, Y. (2013). Enhanced spontaneous oscillations in the supplementary motor area are associated with sleep-dependent offline learning of finger-tapping motor-sequence task. *J Neurosci*, *33*(34), 13894–13902. doi: 10.1523/JNEUROSCI.1198-13.2013

Tang, W., & Jadhav, S. P. (2018). Sharp-wave ripples as a signature of hippocampal-prefrontal reactivation for memory during sleep and waking states. *Neurobiol Learn Mem*, *160*, 11–20. doi: 10.1016/j.nlm.2018.01.002

Tarokh, L., & Carskadon, M. A. (2010). Developmental changes in human sleep EEG during early adolescence. *Sleep*, *33*(6), 801–809.

Tarokh, L., Carskadon, M. A., & Achermann, P. (2014). Early adolescent cognitive gains are marked by increased sleep EEG coherence. *PLoS One*, *9*(9), e106847. doi:10.1371/journal.pone.0106847

Thom, J. L., & Staresina, B. P. (2025). Human sleep spindles track experimentally excited brain circuits. *Sleep*, Apr 28, zsaf114. doi:10.1093/sleep/zsaf114

Timofeev, I., Contreras, D., & Steriade, M. (1996). Synaptic responsiveness of cortical and thalamic neurones during various phases of slow sleep oscillation in cat. *J Physiol*, *494*(1), 265–278.

Tononi, G., & Cirelli, C. (2006). Sleep function and synaptic homeostasis. *Sleep Med Rev*, *10*(1), 49–62. doi: 10.1016/j.smrv.2005.05.002

Turrigiano, G. G. (1999). Homeostatic plasticity in neuronal networks: the more things change, the more they stay the same. *Trends Neurosci*, *22*, 221–227.

Turrigiano, G. G. (2017). The dialectic of Hebb and homeostasis. *Phil Trans R Soc Lond B*, *372*(1715), 20160258. doi: 10.1098/rstb.2016.0258

Ujma, P. P. (2018). Sleep spindles and general cognitive ability -a meta-analysis *Sleep Spindles Cort Up Stat*, 1–17. doi:10.1556/2053.2.2018.01

Ujma, P. P., Bodizs, R., Gombos, F., Stintzing, J., Konrad, B. N., Genzel, L., ... Dresler, M. (2015). Nap sleep spindle correlates of intelligence. *Sci Rep*, *5*, 17159. doi:10.1038/srep17159

Ujma, P. P., Konrad, B. N., Genzel, L., Bleifuss, A., Simor, P., Potari, A., ... Dresler, M. (2014). Sleep spindles and intelligence: evidence for a sexual dimorphism. *J Neurosci*, *34*(49), 16358–16368. doi: 10.1523/JNEUROSCI.1857-14.2014

van den Berg, N. H., Al-Kuwatli, J., Paulin, J., Ray, L. B., Owen, A. M., & Fogel, S. M. (2019). Sleep preferentially enhances memory for a cognitive strategy but not the implicit motor skills used to acquire it. *Neurobiol Learn Mem*, *161*, 135–142. doi: 10.1016/j.nlm.2019.04.005

Vanderwolf, C., Kramis, R., & Robinson, T. (1977). Hippocampal electrical activity during waking behaviour and sleep: analyses using centrally acting drugs. *CIBA Found Symp*, *58*, 199–226.

Vyazovskiy, V. V., Cirelli, C., Pfister-Genskow, M., Faraguna, U., & Tononi, G. (2008). Molecular and electrophysiological evidence for net synaptic potentiation in wake and depression in sleep. *Nat Neurosci*, *11*(2), 200–208. doi: 10.1038/nn2035

Wagley, J. N., Rybarczyk, B., Nay, W. T., Danish, S., & Lund, H. G. (2013). Effectiveness of abbreviated CBT for insomnia in psychiatric outpatients: sleep and depression outcomes. *J Clin Psychol*, *69*(10), 1043–1055. doi: 10.1002/jclp.21927

Wagner, U., Gais, S., & Born, J. (2001). Emotional memory formation is enhanced across sleep intervals with high amounts of rapid eye movement sleep. *Learn Mem*, *8*(2), 112–119. doi: 10.1101/lm.36801

Wamsley, E., Perry, K., Djonlagic, I., Reaven, L., & Stickgold, R. (2010). Cognitive replay of visuomotor learning at sleep onset: temporal dynamics and relationship to task performance. *Sleep*, *33*(1), 59–68.

Wang, B., Antony, J. W., Lurie, S., Brooks, P. P., Paller, K. A., & Norman, K. A. (2019). Targeted memory reactivation during sleep elicits neural signals related to learning content. *J Neurosci*, *39*(34), 6728–6736. doi: 10.1523/JNEUROSCI.2798-18.2019

Wassing, R., Lakbila-Kamal, O., Ramautar, J. R., Stoffers, D., Schalkwijk, F., & Van Someren, E. J. W. (2019). Restless REM sleep impedes overnight amygdala adaptation. *Curr Biol*, *29*(14), 2351–2358 e2354. doi: 10.1016/j.cub.2019.06.034

Watanabe, N., Furukawa, T., Shimodera, S., Morokuma, I., Katsuki, F., Fujita, H., ... Perlis, M. (2011). Brief behavioral therapy for refractory insomnia in residual depression: an assessor-blind, randomized control trial. *J Clin Psychiatry*, *72*(12), 1651–1658. doi: 10.4088/JCP.10m06130gry

Watson, B. O., Levenstein, D., Greene, J. P., Gelinas, J. N., & Buzsaki, G. (2016). Network homeostasis and state dynamics of neocortical sleep. *Neuron*, *90*(4), 839–852. doi: 10.1016/j.neuron.2016.03.036

Wei, H. G., Riel, E., Czeisler, C. A., & Dijk, D.-J. (1999). Attenuated amplitude of circadian and sleep-dependent modulation of electroencephalographic sleep spindle characteristics in elderly human subjects. *Neurosci Lett*, *260*, 29–32.

Whitmore, N. W., Harris, J. C., Kovach, T., & Paller, K. A. (2022). Improving memory via automated targeted memory reactivation during sleep. *J Sleep Res*, *31*(6), e13731. doi:10.1111/jsr.13731

Wilson, M. A., & McNaughton, B. L. (1994). Reactivation of hippocampal ensemble memories during sleep. *Science*, *265*, 676–679.

Winson, J. (1978). Loss of hippocampal theta rhythm results in spatial memory deficit in the rat. *Science*, *201*(4351), 160–163.

Wunderlin, M., Züst, M. A., Hertenstein, E., Fehér, K. D., Schneider, C. L., Klöppel, S., & Nissen, C. (2021). Modulating overnight memory consolidation by acoustic stimulation during slow-wave sleep: a systematic review and meta-analysis. *Sleep*, *44*(7), zsaa296. doi: 10.1093/sleep/zsaa296

Xu, W., De Carvalho, F., Clarke, A. K., & Jackson, A. (2021). Communication from the cerebellum to the neocortex during sleep spindles. *Prog Neurobiol*, *199*, 101940. doi:10.1016/j.pneurobio.2020.101940

Xu, W., De Carvalho, F., & Jackson, A. (2022). Conserved population dynamics in the cerebro-cerebellar system between waking and sleep. *J Neurosci*, *42*(50), 9415–9425. doi: 10.1523/JNEUROSCI.0807-22.2022

Yang, G., Lai, C. S., Cichon, J., Ma, L., Li, W., & Gan, W. B. (2014). Sleep promotes branch-specific formation of dendritic spines after learning. *Science*, *344*(6188), 1173–1178. doi: 10.1126/science.1249098

Ylinen, A., Bragin, A., Nádasdy, Z., Jandó, G., Szabó, I., Sik, A., & Buzsáki, G. (1995). Sharp wave-associated high-frequency oscillation (200Hz) in the intact hippocampus: network and intracellular mechanisms. *J Neurosci*, *15*(1), 30–46.

Youngstedt, S. D., O'Connor, P. J., & Dishman, R. K. (1997). The effects of acute exercise on sleep: a quantitative synthesis. *Sleep*, *20*(3), 203–214.

Zhang, Z. Y., Campbell, I. G., Dhayagude, P., Espino, H. C., & Feinberg, I. (2021). Longitudinal analysis of sleep spindle maturation from childhood through late adolescence. *J Neurosci*, *41*(19), 4253–4261. doi: 10.1523/JNEUROSCI.2370-20.2021

Zhou, G., Olofsson, J. K., Koubeissi, M. Z., Menelaou, G., Rosenow, J., Schuele, S. U., ... Zelano, C. (2021). Human hippocampal connectivity is stronger in olfaction than other sensory systems. *Prog Neurobiol*, *201*, 102027. doi:10.1016/j.pneurobio.2021.102027

Züst, M. A., Mikutta, C., Omlin, X., DeStefani, T., Wunderlin, M., Zeller, C. J., Fehér, K. D., Hertenstein, E., ... Nissen, C. (2023). The hierarchy of coupled sleep oscillations reverses with aging in humans. *J Neurosci*, *43*(36), 6268–6279. doi: 10.1523/JNEUROSCI.0586-23.2023

Züst, M. A., Ruch, S., Wiest, R., & Henke, K. (2019). Implicit vocabulary learning during sleep is bound to slow-wave peaks. *Curr Biol*, *29*(4), 541–553 e547. doi: 10.1016/j.cub.2018.12.038

Zwaka, H., Bartels, R., Gora, J., Franck, V., Culo, A., Gotsch, M., & Menzel, R. (2015). Context odor presentation during sleep enhances memory in honeybees. *Curr Biol*, *25*(21), 2869–2874. doi: 10.1016/j.cub.2015.09.069

CHAPTER 19

Neural Plasticity and the Functions of Sleep

19.1 OVERVIEW

This chapter addresses one of the most frequently studied functions of sleep—its role in memory consolidation. It notes some of the inconsistent results in this field and discusses the variables that likely affected the outcomes of these studies. It provides a summary of evidence that sleep in terrestrial mammals plays a role in brain plasticity and memory consolidation and reviews the neural mechanisms that are involved. It discusses the evidence that sleep also plays a role in memory consolidation in animal species other than terrestrial mammals, which must rely to some extent on different sleep-related phenomena. A final section discusses the implications of the role of sleep in memory for the broader issue of the function of sleep.[1]

19.2 The involvement of sleep in neural plasticity and memory

19.2.1 Experimental factors affecting outcomes

Among the several proposed functions of sleep discussed in previous chapters, its role in brain plasticity and memory consolidation has attracted the most experimental attention in recent decades. Summarizing the results of this research is a challenge because of the large number of publications, the variety of experimental methods used, and, in some cases, the different conclusions that have been reached. Inconsistent conclusions do not usually represent failures to replicate (i.e., applying the same methods but finding different results), although those occur. More commonly, methods and analyses in studies aimed at similar questions differed in either small or large ways.

The outcomes of learning and memory studies can be strongly affected by many variables: details of the training and testing procedures; the nature of the instructions given to participants; participants' expectations; the circadian phase of learning and testing, which is usually only partially controlled for (Keisler et al., 2007); the age of participants; and their awareness of the nature of the task (Robertson et al., 2004).

It is therefore especially useful that some studies have experimentally explored the factors that led to different results and conclusions. These studies illustrate how relatively subtle procedural differences can affect the conclusions reached. These include:

- the impact of the number of training and testing trials on the effectiveness of sleep in improving later performance on the VTD task (Censor et al., 2006; Mednick et al., 2008); see Section 17.6;
- the effects of the delay before testing on whether very short sleep episodes facilitated later performance (Alger et al., 2012; Schönauer et al., 2015); see Section 17.9.1;
- how pre-testing altered sleep effects on verbal memory (Tucker & Fishbein, 2008); see Section 17.9.2;
- how the strength of initial encoding of new information altered the degree to which later sleep reinforced memory (Denis et al., 2021; Drosopoulos et al., 2007; Petzka et al., 2021; Tucker & Fishbein, 2008; Wilhelm et al., 2012); see Section 17.9.2;
- the impact of participants' anticipation of how they will be (re)tested, the expectation of reward, and their awareness of other aspects of the study (Fischer & Born, 2009; Robertson et al., 2004; Saletin et al., 2011; van Dongen et al., 2012; Wilhelm et al., 2011); see Section 17.9.3; and
- how baseline characteristics of participants, including amount of spindle/SO coupling, and baseline level of

[1] Because this chapter is a summary of material discussed elsewhere in this volume, it does not include the summaries at the end of each section that were included in preceding chapters.

performance influenced whether transcranial electrical stimulation improved or worsened memory (Dehnavi et al., 2021; Koo et al., 2018; Ruch et al., 2021); see Section 18.12.

Other procedural and analytic differences that could have contributed to varying outcomes in studies of sleep and learning were reviewed in recent publications (e.g., Davidson et al., 2021).

19.2.2 Sleep stages, features, and other correlates

It is unclear whether specific sleep stages are selectively involved in stabilizing or strengthening different categories of learning; see Section 17.8. Some studies that reported memory enhancement by sleep in general did not identify a specific role for any one sleep stage (Ackermann et al., 2015; Debarnot et al., 2011). Other studies reported the selective involvement of NREM or REM sleep in consolidating different categories of learning (e.g., Plihal & Born, 1997; Rasch et al., 2007), while some found that both contributed to consolidation in different ways, such as stabilizing vs. enhancing memory (e.g., Mednick et al., 2003) or facilitating the initial growth vs. later pruning of synapses involved in new learning (Li et al., 2017).

The conclusions reached may also be affected by whether studies correlate performance with spontaneously expressed sleep stage amounts or study the effects of selective sleep stage deprivation. Finding a positive correlation between a change in the amount of one sleep stage (or sleep feature) after learning and later memory performance suggests that the sleep stage/feature may be involved in the consolidation process affecting that memory. However, if studies of selective deprivation of that sleep stage/feature do not cause impairment of consolidation, the opposite conclusion may be reached: that the sleep stage is not involved.

These apparent contradictions may be the result of multiple sleep stages and features either being involved normally in consolidation or being available for recruitment under some conditions. The brain may use a preferred mechanism (characteristic of one sleep stage) to consolidate one kind of new information, leading to a positive correlation between the strength of consolidation and that sleep stage. But it may also achieve the same result in other ways when that sleep stage is unavailable (because of deprivation or temporal restriction of sleep), leading to the conclusion that the missing sleep stage is not involved.

Studies that restrict sleep stage amounts and examine effects on memory and those that correlate spontaneous changes in amounts with memory performance may be asking different questions. Namely, whether changes in a sleep stage/feature are correlated with memory performance and appear therefore to be involved in consolidation vs. how flexibly the system can respond to experimental deprivation or restriction of that stage/feature.

Studies that experimentally manipulate sleep features (e.g., by increasing or decreasing sleep spindle numbers or altering their timing or amplitude) can help resolve whether that feature can influence memory consolidation, but they do not rule out the possibility that other features can serve the same function under different conditions. This argument is similar to that related to neural ablation studies. The results of a neural ablation (or sleep stage restriction) show what the organism is (or is not) capable of in the absence of the ablated structure (or reduced sleep stage). The results cannot, however, demonstrate on their own what its normal function is; see Section 8.2.3.

There is broad support for the idea that three NREM sleep EEG features (slow oscillations/delta waves, spindles, and sharp-wave ripples) are involved in declarative memory consolidation in mammals. These features are modeled as being involved in the transfer of information from the hippocampus to the cortex and helping to stabilize its cortical representation. However, studies have also differed as to whether spindles appear to be involved, where the relevant spindles are located, and which of their characteristics are related to memory consolidation.

One factor contributing to different conclusions is the statistical methods sometimes used to evaluate the role of spindles. Sleep spindles can be characterized along many different dimensions, including amplitude, dominant frequency, density, number, duration, location, etc. The use of uncontrolled multiple correlations to determine whether any of these characteristics are related to later performance has been criticized for increasing the risk of detecting false positive results that may not be replicable (Ackermann et al., 2015; Davidson et al., 2021; Mantua, 2018; Ujma et al., 2014).

Physiological effects of treatments in addition to effects on the expression of typical sleep stages can also affect consolidation and complicate analyses of the role of sleep stages. For example, reducing REM sleep features pharmacologically did not reduce, and even enhanced, consolidation of motor learning that is usually reported to depend on REM sleep (Rasch et al., 2009). Similarly, drug treatments that all reduce REM sleep and increase NREM sleep had different effects on memory, which appeared to be related to other differences in their pharmacological profiles (Aton et al., 2009; Seibt et al., 2008); see Section 18.13).

Endocrine differences can also have important influences on memory consolidation. High cortisol levels during initial encoding of negative stimuli enhanced later consolidation of the related memory during sleep (Bennion et al., 2015). For studies of emotional memory consolidation, the intensity of negative emotional states evoked by stimuli may affect the degree of hypothalamic-pituitary-adrenal activation and lead to different strengths of consolidation during later sleep.

In contrast, increasing cortisol levels early in the night (when levels would normally be low) interfered with consolidation of a previously learned verbal memory task (but not a visuomotor task) (Plihal & Born, 1999), indicating that high cortisol levels during sleep interfere with declarative memory consolidation. Thus, sleep early in the night may be favorable for declarative memory consolidation either because of its high levels of SWS or its low cortisol levels (Born & Wagner, 2004; Payne & Nadel, 2004). The balance of activity in the autonomic nervous system also interacted with sleep in its effects on consolidation of a task involving remote verbal associates (Whitehurst et al., 2016). Processes operating at the levels of individual synapses, circuitry in the CNS, the state of the autonomic system, and levels of endocrine activity can influence the results of studies examining how sleep affects memory.

19.3 Species differences

There is extensive evidence supporting a role for sleep in neural plasticity and memory consolidation in people and other mammals, suggesting that this is one important function served by sleep. But there are also limitations to the generality of this phenomenon as an answer to the question of why animals sleep. Many mammals (and birds) rely on the regular acquisition of new information and skills for their success; humans are probably an extreme example. So, the linkages between memory and daily sleep in these species suggest that facilitating plasticity is a core function of sleep. Other species that sleep, however, may not show a similar reliance on forming new memories. Nor is there a clear correlation between the amounts and types of sleep shown by different species and the apparent prominence of learning in their lives (see Chapter 16).

The evidence that both NREM and REM sleep are involved in neural plasticity in people and in a few mammalian laboratory species does not imply that similar mechanisms serve this role in other species. For example, REM sleep has been shown to be involved in several forms of brain plasticity in people and laboratory mammals (e.g., LTP, motor skills, sensory discrimination learning, emotional memory, and some forms of explicit memory; see Sections 17.4, 17.8 and 18.10). But birds, which show many kinds of behavioral/neural plasticity, including sensorimotor learning, social learning, and extensive spatial learning related to food caching (Brawn et al., 2010; Brawn et al., 2018; Jarvis et al., 2005; Sherry, 1984), generate only brief REM sleep episodes; and marine mammals, who learn readily (Reiss et al., 1997), do not produce REM sleep (Lyamin et al., 2008).

Nevertheless, memory in birds has been shown to benefit from sleep after learning (Brawn et al., 2010; Brawn et al., 2018), suggesting a role for NREM sleep. Since their brains are organized differently from mammalian brains, despite having some homologous features (Jarvis et al., 2005), the mechanisms involved are likely different. Birds have a hippocampus that is homologous to the mammalian hippocampus, and it communicates to the hyperpallium (equivalent to the mammalian neocortex) through a structure that is functionally similar to the entorhinal cortex of mammals (Applegate et al., 2023). Ablation of the hippocampus in black-capped chickadees (*Parus atricapillus*), which can acquire complex spatial memories (Sherry, 1984), disrupted formation of these memories (Sherry & Vaccarino, 1989), as hippocampal damage does in mammals.

Birds also produce slow waves that can be recorded in the hyperpallium; see **Figure 7.11**. In mammalian NREM sleep, cortical slow waves interact with sleep spindles and with sharp-wave ripples originating in the hippocampus to influence memory consolidation; see Section 18.6. However, electrophysiological recordings in birds did not identify sleep spindles in the hyperpallium or the thalamus; nor were there detectable sharp-wave ripples (Rattenborg et al., 2011; van der Meij et al., 2019). Thus, memory consolidation during sleep in birds must rely on mechanisms other than the triplet of NREM features that are proposed to interact in mammals to reinforce synaptic changes after declarative learning.

There is also evidence that sleep affects memory consolidation in bees and fruit flies, which must also rely on other mechanisms, since their nervous systems do not have structures homologous to the hippocampus, thalamus, and cortex of vertebrates (Le Glou et al., 2012; Zwaka et al., 2015); for a review, see Vorster & Born, 2015.

It appears that reinforcing adaptive plasticity is a common function for sleep in some species. The fact that very different nervous systems in diverse phyla have been enlisted to serve this function suggests its importance (Horner, 2014). However, adaptive plasticity as a function for sleep has been demonstrated in only a few species other than mammals, so it remains to be shown that sleep serves this function across a wider range of animal species. Although a few studies have demonstrated physiological links between sleep and brain plasticity in non-mammalian species (e.g., Donlea et al., 2008; Tomita et al., 2011), the mechanisms by which sleep affects memory consolidation in species other than terrestrial mammals remain to be described.

19.4 Epilogue on the functions of sleep

We return now to the general question with which we started the discussion of function in Chapter 16: Which functions are served by sleep that are consistent with its apparently universal presence in the lives of animals? Researchers have proposed a number of different answers to this question. There are (partially overlapping) hypotheses relating to ecological/circadian mechanisms (Meddis, 1975); adaptive inactivity (Siegel, 2009); brain plasticity and connectivity (Horner, 2014; Krueger et al., 2016); synaptic downscaling (Tononi & Cirelli, 2006); (brain) energy restoration or allocation (Benington & Heller, 1995; Schmidt, 2014); and clearance of accumulated toxins (Herculano-Houzel, 2015; Xie et al., 2013).

Some of these hypotheses are tied directly to the consequences of inadequate sleep that were reviewed in Chapters 13–15: cognitive performance deficits, immune system abnormalities, chronic inflammation, metabolic disruption, increased blood-brain barrier permeability, and increased risk of vascular and brain diseases. It is unlikely, however, that the function underlying the evolution and near-universal presence of sleep in animals was prevention of one or more of these negative consequences. Rather, these outcomes of inadequate sleep probably represent the costs of disrupting a fundamental mechanism that is closely integrated into the regulation of animal physiology and adapted to each species' ecological, circadian, and homeostatic constraints.

Each of the more global hypotheses about the function of sleep captures some elements of the available data, and some are better supported than others; see Krueger et al., 2016. Given the evidence supporting some aspects of each of these hypotheses, it appears that sleep currently serves not one but many different functions (Zielinski et al., 2016).

As discussed above, several of the proposed functions of sleep relate to plasticity in the broadest sense, including adjusting behavior and metabolism to meet current adaptive needs; ensuring the capacity for future plasticity; and stabilizing, strengthening, or eliminating neural connections. The role of sleep in consolidating memories provides a useful framework for thinking about other proposed functions of sleep.

Mechanisms that preserve plastic changes in the brain clearly operate in the waking brain; people are quite capable of learning something (e.g., a new PIN number or password) and retrieving that information later during a single waking period. But the existence of sleep created an opportunity to enhance this memory function by taking advantage of unique physiological characteristics of sleep and of the circadian rest phase in which sleep is embedded in some species.

First, stabilizing and strengthening recently acquired information may be more efficient when the brain is not engaged in steering behavior or acquiring additional information, especially information that might interfere with the new memory, as suggested early in the history of sleep research (Jenkins & Dallenbach, 1924). Second, the neurochemical profile of the sleeping brain, along with other sleep-specific features, can facilitate plasticity-related processes in ways that may be unavailable while awake. In fact, these sleep-related features may actually interfere with waking functions, including the acquisition of new information. Examples of some unique features of the sleep state and its circadian phase that can facilitate plasticity include the following:

- The low level of cholinergic activity during NREM sleep facilitates consolidation of hippocampus-dependent memories by allowing more robust hippocampal-cortical communication (Rasch et al., 2009; Rasch et al., 2006); see Section 18.13). But high ACh levels in the cortex while awake are necessary in both motor and sensory systems for the initial encoding of new information based on experience (Bear & Singer, 1986; Conner et al., 2003; Gu, 2003).
- Hippocampal theta during REM sleep promotes both selective deletion of some synapses and strengthening of others that were formed while awake (Li et al., 2017; Poe et al., 2000); see Section 18.10).
- Sharp-wave ripples occur while asleep but also during quiet waking and during some consummatory behaviors in rats; they also co-occur with sleep spindles and slow oscillations during sleep, but not while awake, which may further facilitate cortical plasticity during sleep. The result will be stronger cortical representations of new memories, allowing for more rapid retrieval of information by reducing the extent of cortical-hippocampal interactions during retrieval (see Section 18.6).
- High cortisol levels during learning while awake facilitates later sleep-related consolidation, but increasing the normally low cortisol levels during early-night sleep to high levels interferes with consolidation. The circadian trough of cortisol production early in the night facilitates some forms of memory consolidation (Bennion et al., 2015; Born & Wagner, 2004; Payne & Nadel, 2004; Plihal & Born, 1999).

Parallel arguments can be applied to other functions that have been attributed to sleep. These may also be functions that can be carried out while awake but are enhanced by specific characteristics of sleep and the state of the circadian system. Thus, an animal can rest to conserve energy while awake, but the lower metabolic demands of sleep make conservation more effective. Similarly, an animal can retreat to a safe location and reduce activity to avoid predators while awake, but during sleep, activity levels and awareness of stimuli that could provoke responses are further reduced. This benefit is related to the temporal niche occupied by a species. Foraging, reproduction, and other needs are fulfilled during a circadian active phase, and sleep during the circadian rest phase provides additional benefits for regulating energy balance and reducing risk that are incompatible with these active phase activities. Sleep can thus be seen as providing unique opportunities that have been exploited to enhance both physiological functions and behavioral strategies.

Identifying specific functions of sleep as we observe them today and noting the benefits of sleep for cognitive functions and for both physical and mental health, however, are not equivalent to answering the (perhaps unanswerable) question of why sleep evolved in the first place, presumably very early in the lineage of animals. Evolution operates opportunistically, taking advantage of old mechanisms to increase reproductive success in new ways. Sleep is an ancient mechanism, perhaps linked originally to the cellular circadian cycle or to the cell replication cycle of animals, that has been adapted to serve many different roles in current species, none of which may have been its original function.

Literature cited

Ackermann, S., Hartmann, F., Papassotiropoulos, A., de Quervain, D. J., & Rasch, B. (2015). No associations between interindividual differences in sleep parameters and episodic memory consolidation. *Sleep, 38*(6), 951–959. doi: 10.5665/sleep.4748

Alger, S. E., Lau, H., & Fishbein, W. (2012). Slow wave sleep during a daytime nap is necessary for protection from subsequent interference and long-term retention. *Neurobiol Learn Mem, 98*(2), 188–196. doi: 10.1016/j.nlm.2012.06.003

Applegate, M. C., Gutnichenko, K. S., Mackevicius, E. L., & Aronov, D. (2023). An entorhinal-like region in food-caching birds. *Curr Biol, 33*(12), 2465–2477. doi: 10.1016/j.cub.2023.05.031

Aton, S. J., Seibt, J., Dumoulin, M. C., Coleman, T., Shiraishi, M., & Frank, M. G. (2009). The sedating antidepressant trazodone impairs sleep-dependent cortical plasticity. *PLoS One, 4*(7), e6078. doi: 10.1371/journal.pone.0006078

Bear, M., & Singer, W. (1986). Modulation of visual cortical plasticity by acetylcholine and noradrenaline. *Nature, 320*(6058), 172–176.

Benington, J. H., & Heller, H. C. (1995). Restoration of brain energy metabolism as the function of sleep. *Prog Neurobiol, 45*, 347–360.

Bennion, K. A., Mickley Steinmetz, K. R., Kensinger, E. A., & Payne, J. D. (2015). Sleep and cortisol interact to support memory consolidation. *Cereb Cortex, 25*(3), 646–657. doi: 10.1093/cercor/bht255

Born, J. A. N., & Wagner, U. (2004). Memory consolidation during sleep: role of cortisol feedback. *Ann NY Acad Sci, 1032*(1), 198–201. doi: 10.1196/annals.1314.020

Brawn, T., Nusbaum, H., & Margoliash, D. (2010). Sleep-dependent consolidation of auditory discrimination learning in adult starlings. *J Neurosci, 30*(2), 609–613. doi: 0.1523/JNEUROSCI.4237-09.2010

Brawn, T. P., Nusbaum, H. C., & Margoliash, D. (2018). Sleep-dependent reconsolidation after memory destabilization in starlings. *Nat Commun, 9*(1), 3093. doi: 10.1038/s41467-018-05518-5

Censor, N., Karni, A., & Sagi, D. (2006). A link between perceptual learning, adaptation and sleep. *Vis Res, 46*, 4071–4074. doi: 0.1016/j.visres.2006.07.022

Conner, J., Culberson, A., Packowski, C., Chiba, A., & Tuszynski, M. (2003). Lesions of the basal forebrain cholinergic system impair task acquisition and abolish cortical plasticity associated with motor skill learning. *Neuron, 38*, 819–829.

Davidson, P., Jönsson, P., Carlsson, I., & Pace-Schott, E. (2021). Does sleep selectively strengthen certain memories over others based on emotion and perceived future relevance? *Nat Sci Sleep, Volume 13*, 1257–1306. doi: 10.2147/nss.S286701

Debarnot, U., Castellani, E., Valenza, G., Sebastiani, L., & Guillot, A. (2011). Daytime naps improve motor imagery learning. *Cogn Affect Behav Neurosci, 11*(4), 541–550. doi: 10.3758/s13415-011-0052-z

Dehnavi, F., Koo-Poeggel, P. C., Ghorbani, M., & Marshall, L. (2021). Spontaneous slow oscillation - slow spindle features predict induced overnight memory retention. *Sleep, 44*(10), zsab127. doi:10.1093/sleep/zsab127

Denis, D., Mylonas, D., Poskanzer, C., Bursal, V., Payne, J. D., & Stickgold, R. (2021). Sleep spindles preferentially consolidate weakly encoded memories. *J Neurosci, 41*(18), 4088–4099. doi: 10.1523/JNEUROSCI.0818-20.2021

Donlea, J. M., Ramanan, N., & Shaw, P. J. (2008). Use-dependent plasticity in clock neurons regulates sleep need in *Drosophila*. *Science, 324*, 105–108.

Drosopoulos, S., Schulze, C., Fischer, S., & Born, J. (2007). Sleep's function in the spontaneous recovery and consolidation of memories. *J Exp Psychol Gen, 136*(2), 169–183. doi: 10.1037/0096-3445.136.2.169

Fischer, S., & Born, J. (2009). Anticipated reward enhances offline learning during sleep. *J Exp Psychol Learn Mem Cogn, 35*(6), 1586–1593. doi: 10.1037/a0017256

Gu, Q. (2003). Contribution of acetylcholine to visual cortex plasticity. *Neurobiol Learn Mem, 80*(3), 291–301. doi: 10.1016/s1074-7427(03)00073-x

Herculano-Houzel, S. (2015). Decreasing sleep requirement with increasing numbers of neurons as a driver for bigger brains and bodies in mammalian evolution. *Proc Biol Sci, 282*(1816), 20151853. doi:10.1098/rspb.2015.1853

Horner, R. L. (2014). *The Universal Pastime: Sleep and Rest Explained*. Retrieved from https://store.bookbaby.com/book/the-universal-pastime-sleep-and-rest-explained

Jarvis, E. D., Güntürkün, O., Bruce, L., Csillag, A., Karten, H., Kuenzel, W., ... Consortium, A. B. N. (2005). Avian brains and a new understanding of vertebrate brain evolution. *Nat Rev Neurosci, 6*(2), 151–159. doi: 10.1038/nrn1606

Jenkins, J. G., & Dallenbach, K. M. (1924). Obliviscence during sleep and waking. *Am J Psychol, 35*(4), 605–612.

Keisler, A., Ashe, J., & Willingham, D. T. (2007). Time of day accounts for overnight improvement in sequence learning. *Learn Mem, 14*(10), 669–672. doi: 10.1101/lm.751807

Koo, P. C., Mölle, M., & Marshall, L. (2018). Efficacy of slow oscillatory-transcranial direct current stimulation on EEG and memory - contribution of an interindividual factor. *Eur J Neurosci, 47*(7), 812–823. doi: 10.1111/ejn.13877

Krueger, J. M., Frank, M. G., Wisor, J. P., & Roy, S. (2016). Sleep function: toward elucidating an enigma. *Sleep Med Rev, 28*, 46–54. doi: 10.1016/j.smrv.2015.08.005

Le Glou, E., Seugnet, L., Shaw, P. J., Preat, T., & Goguel, V. (2012). Circadian modulation of consolidated memory retrieval following sleep deprivation in Drosophila. *Sleep, 35*(10), 1377–1384B. doi: 10.5665/sleep.2118

Li, W., Ma, L., Yang, G., & Gan, W. B. (2017). REM sleep selectively prunes and maintains new synapses in development and learning. *Nat Neurosci, 20*(3), 427–437. doi: 10.1038/nn.4479

Lyamin, O. I., Manger, P. R., Ridgway, S. H., Mukhametov, L. M., & Siegel, J. M. (2008). Cetacean sleep: an unusual form of mammalian sleep. *Neurosci Biobehav Rev, 32*(8), 1451–1484. doi: 10.1016/j.neubiorev.2008.05.023

Mantua, J. (2018). Sleep physiology correlations and human memory consolidation: where do we go from here? *Sleep, 41*(2), zsx204. doi: 10.1093/sleep/zsx204

Meddis, R. (1975). On the function of sleep. *Anim Behav, 23*, 676–691.

Mednick, S., Nakayama, K., & Stickgold, R. (2003). Sleep-dependent learning: a nap is as good as a night. *Nat Neurosci, 6*(7), 697–698. doi: 10.1038/nn1078

Mednick, S. C., Drummond, S. P. A., Boynton, G. M., Awh, E., & Serences, J. (2008). Sleep-dependent learning and practice-dependent deterioration in an orientation discrimination task. *Behav Neurosci, 122*(2), 267–272. doi: 10.1037/0735-7044.122.2.267

Payne, J. D., & Nadel, L. (2004). Sleep, dreams, and memory consolidation: The role of the stress hormone cortisol. *Learn Mem, 11*(6), 671–678. doi: 10.1101/lm.77104

Petzka, M., Charest, I., Balanos, G. M., & Staresina, B. P. (2021). Does sleep-dependent consolidation favour weak memories? *Cortex, 134*, 65–75. doi: 10.1016/j.cortex.2020.10.005

Plihal, W., & Born, J. (1997). Effects of early and late nocturnal sleep on declarative and procedural memory. *J Cogn Neurosci, 9*(4), 534–547.

Plihal, W., & Born, J. (1999). Memory consolidation in human sleep depends on inhibition of glucocorticoid release. *NeuroReport, 10*, 2741–2747.

Poe, G. R., Nitz, D. A., McNaughton, B. L., & Barnes, C. A. (2000). Experience-dependent phase-reversal of hippocampal neuron firing during REM sleep. *Brain Res, 855*, 176–180.

Rasch, B., Büchel, C., Gais, S., & Born, J. (2007). Odor cues during slow-wave sleep prompt declarative memory consolidation. *Science, 315*(5817), 1426–1429. doi: 10.1126/science.1138581

Rasch, B., Pommer, J., Diekelmann, S., & Born, J. (2009). Pharmacological REM sleep suppression paradoxically improves rather than impairs skill memory. *Nat Neurosci*, *12*(4), 396–397. doi: 10.1038/nn.2206

Rasch, B. H., Born, J., & Gais, S. (2006). Combined blockade of cholinergic receptors shifts the brain from stimulus encoding to memory consolidation. *J Cogn Neurosci*, *18*(5), 793–802. doi: 10.1162/jocn.2006.18.5.793

Rattenborg, N. C., Martinez-Gonzalez, D., Roth, T. C., 2nd, & Pravosudov, V. V. (2011). Hippocampal memory consolidation during sleep: a comparison of mammals and birds. *Biol Rev Camb Philos Soc*, *86*(3), 658–691. doi: 10.1111/j.1469-185X.2010.00165.x

Reiss, D., McCowan, B., & Marino, L. (1997). Communicative and other cognitive characteristics of bottlenose dolphins. *Trends Cogn Sci*, *1*(4), 140–145.

Robertson, E. M., Pascual-Leone, A., & Press, D. Z. (2004). Awareness modifies the skill-learning benefits of sleep. *Curr Biol*, *14*, 208–212. doi: 0.1016/j.cub.2004.01.027

Ruch, S., Feher, K., Homan, S., Morishima, Y., Mueller, S. M., Mueller, S. V., ... Grieder, M. (2021). Bi-temporal anodal transcranial direct current stimulation during slow-wave sleep boosts slow-wave density but not memory consolidation. *Brain Sci*, *11*(4), 410. doi:10.3390/brainsci11040410

Saletin, J. M., Goldstein, A. N., & Walker, M. P. (2011). The role of sleep in directed forgetting and remembering of human memories. *Cereb Cortex*, *21*(11), 2534–2541. doi: 10.1093/cercor/bhr034

Schmidt, M. H. (2014). The energy allocation function of sleep: a unifying theory of sleep, torpor, and continuous wakefulness. *Neurosci Biobehav Rev*, *47*, 122–153. doi: 0.1016/j.neubiorev.2014.08.001

Schönauer, M., Grätsch, M., & Gais, S. (2015). Evidence for two distinct sleep-related long-term memory consolidation processes. *Cortex*, *63*, 68–78. doi: 10.1016/j.cortex.2014.08.005

Seibt, J., Aton, S. J., Jha, S. K., Coleman, T., Dumoulin, M. C., & Frank, M. (2008). The non-benzodiazepine hypnotic zolpidem impairs sleep-dependent cortical plasticity. *Sleep*, *31*(10), 1381–1391.

Sherry, D. (1984). Food storage by black-capped chickadees: memory for the location and contents of caches. *Anim Behav*, *32*(2), 451–464.

Sherry, D. F., & Vaccarino, A. L. (1989). Hippocampus and memory for food caches in black-capped chickadees. *Behav Neurosci*, *103*(2), 308–319.

Siegel, J. M. (2009). Sleep viewed as a state of adaptive inactivity. *Nat Rev Neurosci*, *10*, 747–753. doi: 0.1038/nrn2697

Tomita, J., Mitsuyoshi, M., Ueno, T., Aso, Y., Tanimoto, H., Nakai, Y., ... Kume, K. (2011). Pan-neuronal knockdown of calcineurin reduces sleep in the fruit fly, *Drosophila melanogaster*. *J Neurosci*, *31*(37), 13137–13146. doi: 10.1523/JNEUROSCI.5860-10.2011

Tononi, G., & Cirelli, C. (2006). Sleep function and synaptic homeostasis. *Sleep Med Rev*, *10*(1), 49–62. doi: 10.1016/j.smrv.2005.05.002

Tucker, M. A., & Fishbein, W. (2008). Enhancement of declarative memory performance following a daytime nap is contingent on strength of initial task acquisition. *Sleep*, *31*(2), 197–203.

Ujma, P. P., Konrad, B. N., Genzel, L., Bleifuss, A., Simor, P., Potari, A., ... Dresler, M. (2014). Sleep spindles and intelligence: evidence for a sexual dimorphism. *J Neurosci*, *34*(49), 16358–16368. doi: 10.1523/JNEUROSCI.1857-14.2014

van der Meij, J., Martinez-Gonzalez, D., Beckers, G. J. L., & Rattenborg, N. C. (2019). Intra-"cortical" activity during avian non-REM and REM sleep: variant and invariant traits between birds and mammals. *Sleep*, *42*(2), 1–13. doi: 10.1093/sleep/zsy230

van Dongen, E. V., Thielen, J. W., Takashima, A., Barth, M., & Fernandez, G. (2012). Sleep supports selective retention of associative memories based on relevance for future utilization. *PLoS One*, *7*(8), e43426. doi: 10.1371/journal.pone.0043426

Vorster, A. P., & Born, J. (2015). Sleep and memory in mammals, birds and invertebrates. *Neurosci Biobehav Rev*, *50*, 103–119. doi: 10.1016/j.neubiorev.2014.09.020

Whitehurst, L. N., Cellini, N., McDevitt, E. A., Duggan, K. A., & Mednick, S. C. (2016). Autonomic activity during sleep predicts memory consolidation in humans. *Proc Natl Acad Sci U S A*, *113*(26), 7272–7277. doi: 10.1073/pnas.1518202113

Wilhelm, I., Diekelmann, S., Molzow, I., Ayoub, A., Molle, M., & Born, J. (2011). Sleep selectively enhances memory expected to be of future relevance. *J Neurosci*, *31*(5), 1563–1569. doi: 10.1523/JNEUROSCI.3575-10.2011

Wilhelm, I., Metzkow-Mészàros, M., Knapp, S., & Born, J. (2012). Sleep-dependent consolidation of procedural motor memories in children and adults: the pre-sleep level of performance matters. *Developmental Sci*, *15*(4), 506–515. doi: 10.1111/j.1467-7687.2012.01146.x

Xie, L., Kang, H., Xu, Q., Chen, M. J., Liao, Y., Thiyagarajan, M., ... Nedergaard, M. (2013). Sleep drives metabolite clearance from the adult brain. *Science*, *342*(6156), 373–377. doi: 10.1126/science.1241224

Zielinski, M. R., McKenna, J. T., & McCarley, R. W. (2016). Functions and mechanisms of sleep. *AIMS Neurosci*, *3*(1), 67–104. doi: 10.3934/Neuroscience.2016.1.67

Zwaka, H., Bartels, R., Gora, J., Franck, V., Culo, A., Gotsch, M., & Menzel, R. (2015). Context odor presentation during sleep enhances memory in honeybees. *Curr Biol*, *25*(21), 2869–2874. doi: 10.1016/j.cub.2015.09.069

APPENDIX A

Dreaming and its Mechanisms in REM and NREM Sleep

A.1 Dreaming in REM and NREM sleep

The discovery of REM sleep and its strong identification with dreaming in the 1950s initiated a new field of research. The identification of an electrophysiologically defined sleep stage with dreaming was seen as opening a window on the physiological basis of dreaming, which had previously been subject only to psychological analysis. Psychiatrists and psychologists were interested in the mechanisms of dreaming in part because of the importance of dreams in Freudian and related psychological theories.

Subsequent research demonstrated that, despite the strong probability of reports of dreams after waking from REM sleep (i.e., from ~75–80% of REM sleep episodes), reports of significant dream-like narratives were also produced by people after waking from NREM sleep, although typically with lower probability (~40–55% of episodes, but this range varied) (Chellappa et al., 2011; Foulkes, 1962; Hobson et al., 2000; Nielsen, 2000). These findings have led to several different interpretations. Some reports of dreams occurring outside REM sleep have been suggested to emerge from REM–NREM transition states or from mixed EEG states that are ambiguous. But other dream reports clearly occur when people wake up from NREM sleep stages (especially lighter sleep stages later in the night) and from transition periods while falling asleep or waking up, which do not include REM sleep. There are fewer dream reports associated with NREM sleep during the early part of the night, which includes more SWS (Antrobus et al., 1995). These findings indicate that some degree of cognitive activity can occur during both REM sleep and lighter NREM sleep stages.

There is controversy about whether the mental activity reported from REM and NREM sleep differs in character. Some researchers suggest that more mundane, less vivid and fantastic cognitive activity is usually recalled out of NREM sleep (Hobson et al., 2000; Takeuchi et al., 2001), while others claim there are only minor differences in the character of dream reports from different sleep stages (Solms, 2000).

One argument is that the typically increased length of dream recall (and perhaps reduced sleep inertia) when waking from REM sleep may permit more elaborate, bizarre content to be reported. An alternative interpretation is that bizarre content requires more words to describe than more mundane material, leading to longer dream reports (Nielsen, 1999). However, after controlling for dream recall length, there was still evidence for more bizarre, emotional, and complex content after waking from REM sleep than from NREM sleep (Nielsen, 2000; Smith et al., 2004).

The finding that dream recall increases across the night is consistent with the increased amount of REM sleep during the second half of the night, but this effect is not specific to REM sleep: dream recall from NREM sleep periods (mostly N2) also increases later in the night (Antrobus et al., 1995; Nielsen, 1999). This observation likely reflects the fact that both N2 and REM sleep are more compatible with reports of mental activity than N3 sleep early in the night.

An alternative interpretation is that there is a circadian factor that increases both the probability of REM sleep and the probability of elaborate dreaming during the late night hours, in particular the daily rhythm of secretion of the adrenal hormone cortisol. Cortisol levels start to rise from a low point near the middle of the night toward a peak level shortly after waking. Higher cortisol levels are known to interfere with episodic memory (i.e., memory for specific events in one's life). As a result, fragmented memories that are incorporated into dreams while cortisol levels are rising might lack the original spatial and temporal contexts that normally frame episodic memories. Attempts by our brains to integrate diverse memory elements that lack spatial and temporal contexts into a single narrative could result in a disjointed, unstable story line, including bizarre linkages, which are typical of many REM sleep-related dreams (Payne, 2010; Payne & Nadel, 2004).

Issues around how sleep stages affect dreaming are difficult to resolve in part because the evidence supporting different views stems from self-reports. There is no independent, objective measure of what the content of a dream is, or during which stage the dream occurred.[1] Characteristics of dream reports on awakening are usually assumed to reflect mental activity during the immediately preceding sleep stage. Differences in the character or content of dreams are therefore usually assumed to reflect differences in the types of mental activity that occur during different sleep stages. However, dream reports could vary across sleep stages for other reasons.

For example, the length and complexity of dream reports could vary because different sleep stages affect the ability to store immediately preceding mental activity in short-term memory and later retrieve it. If REM sleep were more compatible than NREM sleep with generating short-term memories of mental activity, that could lead to more elaborate and detailed dream reports when awakened from REM sleep (Lehmann & Koukkou, 2000), without implying that the content of mental activity is inherently different during REM and NREM sleep stages. Different degrees of success in dream recall among people have also been tied to the resistance of the new memory to interference immediately after waking (Koulack & Goodenough, 1976) and to differences in coherence among components of the brain's default mode network (DMN; see footnote #9 in Section 7.5.3), which could be considered an indicator of the degree of sleep inertia after waking up (Vallat et al., 2020). The involvement of these hypothesized inter-individual factors in dream recall might also apply to differences in dream recall among sleep stages within individuals.

Attributing dreams specifically to NREM sleep after waking from that stage can be complicated for two reasons: brief episodes of "covert" REM sleep may intrude during longer NREM sleep episodes, and reported dream content might be a "residue" of preceding REM sleep episodes that occurred earlier in the night (Nielsen, 2000). When awakened from sleep, individuals report their immediately preceding mental activity, but they may also provide less complete reports of the narrative or emotional content of dreams that they feel occurred earlier in the night. It is not possible, however, to "tag" dream content objectively with respect to when it occurred, only with respect to when it was overtly recalled and reported. Thus, assigning the occurrence of dreams to specific time frames, and to the EEG state at that time, is challenging.

The debate over how tightly dreaming is linked to the REM sleep state can become circular in the absence of an independent marker of the source of a dream. If one assumes a priori that self-reported mental activity during sleep is always a product of REM sleep, then dreams reported on awakening from NREM sleep would necessarily be attributed to REM sleep intrusions, "covert" REM sleep, or residues from previous REM sleep episodes (Nielsen, 1999). This interpretation is supported by evidence that brief intrusions of electrophysiological elements of one sleep stage into another are often observed. If, however, one does not assume that dreaming always occurs in REM sleep, then one can attribute recalled mental activity to the immediately preceding NREM sleep stage. This discussion risks bogging down into a debate in which the conclusions reached are related to initial assumptions rather than to definitive evidence.

One consistent finding is how ephemeral the memories of dreams are. Most people remember only a brief narrative when they wake up from a dream, even if they have been in REM sleep for many minutes. The length of the narrative report may be quite short compared to the amount of mental activity that could, hypothetically, have occurred during a REM sleep episode. If the contents of a dream are not reported immediately, written down, or rehearsed, they are typically lost from memory rapidly and relatively completely. This rapid loss of dream content on waking has been attributed to differences during REM sleep in the function of the hippocampus and other brain regions that are involved in forming explicit memories.

Before drawing strong inferences about memory processes based on this evidence, however, one might ask what kinds of reports one would get from people who have been awake and otherwise idle, if they were asked at irregular intervals to recall every thought they had over the last 10 or 15 min. Most of us would have a difficult time providing a very complete inventory of 10 min of our preceding mental activity unless we experienced particularly striking events or highly organized thought sequences during that time. Perhaps a better analogy to dream recall, however, would be to ask how much coherent detail one could reproduce after watching 10 min of a particularly bizarre movie with a disjointed story line and fantastic features (perhaps directed by David Lynch?).

The mechanisms involved in dream recall are not well understood. Patients with brain damage who suffer from memory problems, even severe amnesia, can still report dream content after waking out of REM sleep (Solms, 2011). It is also unclear what factors contribute to individual differences in skill at dream recall. Many people have noted that the amount of dream recall increases if one starts to keep a dream journal or to report regularly to someone else about one's dreams. This effect may be related to learning to focus attention on the recall of dreams and to rapidly rehearse or record their contents on awakening, before interfering thoughts arise.

[1] One study, however, used fMRI and machine learning to match the patterns of activity in visual cortical regions associated with specific dream content (reported on awakening from early N1/N2 sleep) with the patterns shown while awake in response to a range of visual images. This approach might eventually allow some insight into what someone is dreaming about based on brain activity patterns. The initial matching method, however, still involved linking fMRI activity with self-reports of dream content (Horikawa et al., 2013).

A.1.1 Summary

There is debate about the origins of mental activity experienced as dreams. Dream reports are most common after waking from REM sleep and less common after waking from lighter NREM stages (e.g., during transitions into and out of sleep, as well as late in the night, when N2 sleep dominates). Dream reports are least common after waking from N3 sleep. Reported mental activity after waking from NREM sleep has been attributed by some authors to dreaming during NREM sleep and by others to covert REM sleep, "residues" of earlier REM episodes, or brief intrusions of REM sleep into longer NREM sleep episodes.

There is evidence that dream reports after waking from REM sleep are not only more common, but also more elaborate and bizarre than after waking from NREM sleep. Several factors may contribute to this finding, in addition to differences in the actual dream content. These include the degree of sleep inertia after waking, the EEG state immediately before waking, and the functioning of memory processes during and after the dream process.

A.2 **Neurophysiological basis of dreaming**

The effects of various patterns of brain injury on the expression of REM sleep and the reported experience of dreams have provided additional information about the relation of REM sleep to dreams. A review of this topic concluded that the dream experience and EEG-defined REM sleep are dissociable phenomena (Solms, 2000).

The physiological features of REM sleep depend mainly on the activity of pontine and other brainstem systems (see Chapter 10). The mental experience of dreams (as indicated by self-report) depends on the integrity of a forebrain system, including parts of the hypothalamus, basal forebrain, amygdala (a temporal lobe nucleus critically involved in the regulation of emotions), cortical regions (especially the area at the junction of the temporal, parietal, and occipital lobes: Brodmann's area 40), and on the integrity of brainstem projections to several regions that release the neurotransmitter dopamine. Bilateral damage to ventral prefrontal regions that interrupt some of these dopaminergic pathways greatly reduced dream reports without preventing the physiological signs of REM sleep (Solms, 2000).

Patients who had undergone a prefrontal lobotomy (removal of the prefrontal cortical lobes) or leucotomy (cutting of connections to the prefrontal cortex) as a treatment for intractable schizophrenia during the middle of the 20th century had reduced dream reports after surgery. A well-controlled study compared patients with chronic schizophrenia who had undergone prefrontal lobotomies and were still taking antipsychotic medications with a matched group of unoperated patients taking similar drugs.

Patients with schizophrenia who had undergone lobotomies reported much lower frequencies of dreams than healthy controls, both after spontaneous waking in the morning and after forced awakening from REM sleep. Unoperated schizophrenia patients, however, showed only a relatively small reduction in dream reports, which may have resulted from either their chronic illness or their drug treatments. These differences were not attributable to differences in the EEG patterns or durations of REM sleep, which were very similar between groups, nor to any detectable differences in short-term memory performance (which could affect recall of dreams rather than the act of dreaming) (Jus et al., 1973).

Studies of other patients with either accidental or surgical damage to the prefrontal lobes and their connections to other brain regions are generally consistent in reporting a reduction in the frequency of dream reports. These findings confirm that dream reports (presumably reflecting the experience of dreams) and the electrophysiological signs of REM sleep are independent phenomena. This conclusion is reinforced by evidence that strong suppression (81%) of the electrophysiological signs of REM sleep by administering the antidepressant clomipramine before sleep does not change either the number or complexity of dreams reported. Instead, many more dreams are then reported out of what appears electrophysiologically to be N1 sleep (Oudiette et al., 2012).

The dream experience and the electrophysiological signs of REM sleep may be linked together in intact brains through subcortical (including dopaminergic) projections that reach the ventral prefrontal cortex and other regions, but damage to these pathways or alterations of brain chemistry allows them to be dissociated. The independence of dreaming from the EEG features of REM sleep is also supported by the evidence discussed above that dreams can occur during NREM sleep.

Successful dream recall must depend on encoding a memory during dreaming. One group reported that the extent of dream recall from REM sleep was linked to the amount of theta EEG activity recorded in the frontal lobes just before waking. In contrast, the extent of dream recall from NREM sleep was correlated with a reduction in the intensity of EEG alpha activity in the right temporal lobe before waking. These regions are also areas involved in memory encoding while awake, which suggests that there is continuity in the mechanisms involved in memory formation across states of consciousness (Marzano et al., 2011).

Another study found that reports of dreaming immediately after REM sleep were associated with a reduction of alpha and beta EEG frequencies in frontal cortical regions and an increase in these frequencies in occipital regions, relative to REM sleep that was not accompanied by dream recall. Reports of dreams after NREM sleep were instead associated with decreased low-frequency (delta) activity in frontal regions and decreased spindle activity in central and parietal regions (Chellappa et al., 2011). These results indicate that reported dreaming after REM sleep is facilitated by increased high-frequency activity in occipital regions and reduced high-frequency activity in frontal association cortices. NREM sleep episodes that led to dream reports were instead associated with less frontal delta activity, implying *increased* frontal activation (Braun et al., 1997).

Partially consistent with these results is evidence from another study that the experience of dreaming in either REM or NREM sleep was related to decreasing low-frequency activity in a broad temporo-occipital region of cortex. This pattern was observed when participants reported that they recalled having dreams, regardless of whether they recalled the actual contents of the dreams. Thus, these EEG changes appeared to be related to the *experience* of dreaming but not necessarily to successful encoding of this experience into a (short-term) memory (Siclari et al., 2017).

Note that despite many procedural differences among these studies, dream reports from NREM sleep were commonly associated with reduced low-frequency and increased high-frequency cortical activity. These results suggest that a shift toward a more activated cortex is involved in the production of NREM mental activity. Similarly, a shift toward higher-frequency activity in occipital regions (which includes visual cortical areas) was associated with dream reports linked to REM sleep.

Brain imaging studies of REM sleep and dreaming suggest that dream generation involves activation of parts of the frontal cortex and its connections to occipital cortical regions (responsible for visual experiences) as well as activation of the amygdala and its connections to the cingulate cortex (a deep midline cortical region lying above the corpus callosum) (Maquet et al., 1996; Solms, 2011). Activation of the amygdala and midline cortical regions may add emotional content to the dream narrative while occipital regions contribute visual imagery. These results suggest that the dream experience during REM sleep is a product of cortical activation that links parts of frontal, occipital, midline, and perhaps parietal cortical regions as well as the amygdala.

These physiological results are consistent with the main ideas of the activation-synthesis hypothesis of dream generation during REM sleep (Hobson & McCarley, 1977; Muzur et al., 2002). This model suggests that the activity of brainstem systems during REM sleep results in random (or partially random) activation of forebrain systems that are involved in sensation, movement, memory, and emotion regulation. This model attributes the subjective dream content to attempts by the cortex to synthesize a coherent narrative around these shifting, essentially incoherent, activations of memory traces related to sensory, motor, and emotional experiences. Interacting with this activation pattern are the individual's personal history and memories. Interruption of either the pathways bringing activation to the cortex or those that link cortical regions and permit integration of these different elements would result in a reduced probability of dream generation.

The features of dreaming that are addressed by this model include visual imagery (occipital cortex activation), movement sensations (motor cortex, cerebellum, basal ganglia), emotional experiences (amygdala and cingulate cortex activation), and their integration into a form of narrative (interactions among cortical regions) (Muzur et al., 2002). The cortical activation and integration required is presumably reflected in the high-frequency cortical EEG expressed during REM sleep, triggered by increased cholinergic input to the cortex that characterizes REM sleep, after reduced cholinergic input during NREM sleep.

An alternative to this "bottom-up" view—that sensory and other memories trigger cortical dream activity—is the view that dreams are generated in a more "top-down" manner. This hypothesis proposes that dreaming is closely linked to imagining, in which abstract ideas or wishes are the foundation of narratives that then incorporate a variety of sensory elements, emotions, and memories (Nir & Tononi, 2010).

Other characteristic features of dreaming include the lack of critical evaluation of how bizarre and physically impossible the features of the dream narrative can be and the loss of one's usual sense of self-awareness. This lack of self-reflection and the uncritical acceptance of the apparent reality of even the most impossible dream content has been attributed to reduced activity in the dorsolateral prefrontal cortex during REM sleep and its functional disconnection from other parts of the DMN (Horovitz et al., 2009; Maquet et al., 1996; Muzur et al., 2002).

Although the transition from NREM to REM sleep involves increased activation of most cortical regions, the dorsolateral prefrontal cortex remains metabolically depressed during both NREM and REM sleep. This region has been implicated in the regulation of executive functions, including reasoning, planning, and short-term memory. Low levels of activity in this region and its disconnection from other cortical regions would reduce the capacity for rational reflection about, and insight into, the nature of the dream narrative and perhaps affect the capacity to retain a memory of the dream narrative on waking.

One proposal is that self-awareness during dreams is related to the strength of gamma-band EEG frequencies in the cortex. Synchrony of oscillation in this frequency range has been linked to higher cognitive functions and to integration of information across cortical regions. Some studies indicated that lucid dreaming (a state in which the individual is aware of being asleep and having a dream and may, to some degree, control the dream narrative) was associated with increases in some gamma-range EEG frequencies, especially around 40 Hz. Stimulating fronto-temporal regions at 25–40 Hz was reported to increase reports of some of the characteristics associated with lucid dreaming (Voss et al., 2014). This conclusion was questioned based on evidence that increased 40 Hz activity can be an electrical artifact of extraocular muscle activity, associated with high levels of saccades during REM sleep. This interpretation suggested that lucid dreaming is associated with high-intensity REM activity and increases in both cortical and subcortical activity but not specifically with EEG synchrony in gamma frequency ranges (Baird et al., 2022). A study of lucid dreaming in both healthy controls and patients with narcolepsy, however, identified increased power in the gamma frequency band, decreased delta power, and increases in a measure of neural complexity as markers of lucid, as compared to non-lucid, dreams (Türker et al., 2023).

Findings from a clinical population with a syndrome called auto-activation deficit (AAD) add a further complication to the map of systems involved in dream production. Patients with bilateral brain damage that destroyed large parts of the basal ganglia (caudate/putamen, globus pallidus, and nearby structures) may develop this very rare condition. Patients with AAD fail to initiate behavior spontaneously, but they have relatively intact behavioral and mental functions when prompted to act by someone else. Accompanying this pervasive apathy is a state of "mental emptiness" which varies in degree. This term refers to the fact that when asked about their current or recent thoughts, some of these patients reply with little or no content, in extreme cases denying virtually any ongoing mental activity (Leu-Semenescu et al., 2013).

Most features of sleep organization were found to be relatively normal in a group of 13 patients with AAD, except for reduced sleep spindles during NREM sleep in some patients; see Section 12.2.4. But most patients reported little or no mental activity when awakened from either NREM or REM sleep, suggesting a role for the basal ganglia in dream generation. Remarkably, four patients, including two with very severe loss of spontaneous mental activity when awake, provided dream reports when awakened from REM sleep. Their dream content was limited and lacked the bizarre character of dream reports from intact controls. Nevertheless, reports of any dreams during REM sleep in patients reporting little or no spontaneous, waking mental activity is itself surprising. It may be that in these patients the cortical activation resulting from excitatory input (presumably cholinergic) during REM sleep stimulated mental activity, thereby mimicking the effects of external stimuli that can prompt overt behavior while awake (Leu-Semenescu et al., 2013).

A.2.2 Summary

Dreaming is related to activation of a system involving parts of the hypothalamus; the amygdala; a cortical region (Brodmann's area 40) near the junction of the temporal, parietal, and occipital lobes; and dopaminergic projections reaching several regions, including a ventral prefrontal part of the cortex. Damage to area 40 or to the ventral prefrontal region (e.g., by prefrontal lobotomy) is associated with a large reduction in reports of dreaming. Other characteristic features of REM sleep are preserved after such damage, further confirming that the experience of dreaming and the expression of other REM sleep features are independent and controlled by different mechanisms.

The activation-synthesis hypothesis summarizes the involvement of many brain regions and their contributions to different aspects of dreaming. It proposes that dreams arise from internally generated, random sensory/experiential memories, and the attempt by the cortex to generate a narrative to integrate these disparate elements. An alternative, top-down interpretation links dreaming to imagining. It proposes that thoughts and wishes generate a narrative that then incorporates sensory and other memory elements.

Several different EEG features have been proposed to be correlated with successful recall of dream content. These correlates differ between REM and NREM sleep reports of dreams, but they have in common that dreaming is associated with an activated (high-frequency) EEG pattern. Depressed metabolic activity in the dorsolateral prefrontal cortex is common to both REM and NREM sleep, and this region is also functionally isolated from other components of the DMN during REM sleep; these changes may contribute to the lack of self-awareness and reflection during dreams. Development of self-awareness during lucid dreams has been associated with especially high-intensity REM activity and high levels of cortical and subcortical activation.

Damage to the basal ganglia can lead to reductions in spontaneous, voluntary activity along with "mental emptiness" while awake, a condition in which most patients did not report any spontaneous, ongoing mental activity. Most of these patients did not report dreaming during sleep, suggesting a role for the basal ganglia in dream production. A few patients, however, including some with extreme mental emptiness while awake, reported some relatively simple dream content, which may reflect internal generation of excitatory input to the cortex associated with REM sleep.

Literature cited

Antrobus, J., Kondo, T., Reinsel, R., & Fein, G. (1995). Dreaming in the late morning: summation of REM and diurnal cortical activation. *Conscious Cogn, 4*(3), 275–299.

Baird, B., Tononi, G., & LaBerge, S. (2022). Lucid dreaming occurs in activated REM sleep, not a mixture of sleep and wakefulness. *Sleep, 45*(4), zsab294. doi: 10.1093/sleep/zsab294

Braun, A. R., Balkin, T. J., Wesenten, N. J., Carson, R. E., Varga, M., Baldwin, P., . . . Herscovitch, P. (1997). Regional cerebral blood flow throughout the sleep-wake cycle. An $H2^{15}O$ PET study. *Brain, 120*, 1173–1197.

Chellappa, S. L., Frey, S., Knoblauch, V., & Cajochen, C. (2011). Cortical activation patterns herald successful dream recall after NREM and REM sleep. *Biol Psychol, 87*(2), 251–256. doi: 10.1016/j.biopsycho.2011.03.004

Foulkes, W. D. (1962). Dream reports from different stages of sleep. *J Abnorm Soc Psychol, 65*(1), 14–25.

Hobson, J. A., & McCarley, R. W. (1977). The brain as a dream state generator: an activation-synthesis hypothesis of the dream process. *Am J Psychiatry, 134*, 1335–1348.

Hobson, J. A., Pace-Schott, E. F., & Stickgold, R. (2000). Dreaming and the brain: toward a cognitive neuroscience of conscious states. *Behav Brain Sci, 23*, 793–842.

Horikawa, T., Tamaki, M., Miyawaki, Y., & Kamitani, Y. (2013). Neural decoding of visual imagery during sleep. *Science, 340*(6132), 639–642.

Horovitz, S. G., Braun, A., Carr, W., Picchioni, D., Balkin, T., Fukunaga, M., & Duyn, J. H. (2009). Decoupling of the brain's default mode network during deep sleep. *Proc Natl Acad Sci USA, 106*(27), 11376–11381.

Jus, A., Jus, K., Villeneuve, A., Pires, A., Lachance, R., Fortier, J., & Villeneuve, R. (1973). Studies on dream recall in chronic schizophrenic patients after prefrontal lobotomy. *Biol Psychiatry, 6*(3), 275–293.

Koulack, D., & Goodenough, D. R. (1976). Dream recall and dream recall failure: an arousal-retrieval model. *Psychol Bull, 83*(5), 975–984.

Lehmann, D., & Koukkou, M. (2000). All brain work—including recall—is state-dependent. *Behav Brain Sci, 23*, 964–965.

Leu-Semenescu, S., Uguccioni, G., Golmard, J. L., Czernecki, V., Yelnik, J., Dubois, B., Forgeot d'Arc, B., Grabli, D., . . . Arnulf, I. (2013). Can we still dream when the mind is blank? Sleep and dream mentations in auto-activation deficit. *Brain, 136*(Pt 10), 3076–3084. doi: 10.1093/brain/awt229

Maquet, P., Péters, J.-M., Aerts, J., Delfiore, G., Degueldre, C., Luxen, A., & Franck, G. (1996). Functional neuroanatomy of human rapid-eye-movement sleep and dreaming. *Nature, 383*, 163–166.

Marzano, C., Ferrara, M., Mauro, F., Moroni, F., Gorgoni, M., Tempesta, D., . . . De Gennaro, L. (2011). Recalling and forgetting dreams: theta and alpha oscillations during sleep predict subsequent dream recall. *J Neurosci, 31*(18), 6674–6683. doi: 10.1523/jneurosci.0412-11.2011

Muzur, A., Pace-Schott, E. F., & Hobson, J. A. (2002). The prefrontal cortex in sleep. *Trends Cogn Sci, 6*(11), 475–481.

Nielsen, T. A. (1999). Mentation during sleep: the NREM/REM distinction. In R. Lydic & H. A. Baghdoyan (Eds.), *Handbook of Behavioral State Control: Cellular and Molecular Mechanisms* (pp. 101–128). Boca Raton: CRC Press.

Nielsen, T. A. (2000). A review of mentation in REM and NREM sleep: "Covert" REM sleep as a possible reconciliation of two opposing models. *Behav Brain Sci, 23*(6), 851–866. doi: 10.1017/s0140525x0000399x

Nir, Y., & Tononi, G. (2010). Dreaming and the brain: from phenomenology to neurophysiology. *Trends Cogn Sci, 14*(2), 88–100. doi: 10.1016/j.tics.2009.12.001

Oudiette, D., Dealberto, M. J., Uguccioni, G., Golmard, J. L., Merino-Andreu, M., Tafti, M., . . . Arnulf, I. (2012). Dreaming without REM sleep. *Conscious Cogn, 21*(3), 1129–1140. doi: 10.1016/j.concog.2012.04.010

Payne, J. D. (2010). Memory consolidation, the diurnal rhythm of cortisol, and the nature of dreams. *Int Rev Neurobiol, 92*, 101–134. doi: 10.1016/s0074-7742(10)92006-0

Payne, J. D., & Nadel, L. (2004). Sleep, dreams, and memory consolidation: The role of the stress hormone cortisol. *Learn Mem, 11*(6), 671–678. doi: 10.1101/lm.77104

Siclari, F., Baird, B., Perogamvros, L., Bernardi, G., LaRocque, J. J., Riedner, B., . . . Tononi, G. (2017). The neural correlates of dreaming. *Nat Neurosci, 20*(6), 872–878. doi: 10.1038/nn.4545

Smith, M. R., Antrobus, J. S., Gordon, E., Tucker, M. A., Hirota, Y., Wamsley, E. J., . . . Emery, R. N. (2004). Motivation and affect in REM sleep and the mentation reporting process. *Conscious Cogn, 13*(3), 501–511. doi: 10.1016/j.concog.2004.03.002

Solms, M. (2000). Dreaming and REM sleep are controlled by different brain mechanisms. *Behav Brain Sci, 23*, 843–850.

Solms, M. (2011). Neurobiology and the neurological basis of dreaming. In P. Montagna & S. Chokroverty (Eds.), *Handbook of Clinical Neurology, Sleep Disorders, Part 1* (Vol. **98**, pp. 519–544). Elsevier B.V.

Takeuchi, T., Miyasita, A., Inugami, M., & Yamamoto, Y. (2001). Intrinsic dreams are not produced without REM sleep mechanisms: evidence through elicitation of sleep onset REM periods. *J Sleep Res, 10*, 43–52.

Türker, B., Musat, E. M., Chabani, E., Fonteix-Galet, A., Maranci, J. B., Wattiez, N., . . . Oudiette, D. (2023). Behavioral and brain responses to verbal stimuli reveal transient periods of cognitive integration of the external world during sleep. *Nat Neurosci, 26*(11), 1981–1993. doi:10.1038/s41593-023-01449-7

Vallat, R., Nicolas, A., & Ruby, P. (2020). Brain functional connectivity upon awakening from sleep predicts inter-individual differences in dream recall frequency. *Sleep, 43*(12), zsaa116. doi: 10.1093/sleep/zsaa116

Voss, U., Holzmann, R., Hobson, A., Paulus, W., Koppehele-Gossel, J., Klimke, A., & Nitsche, M. A. (2014). Induction of self awareness in dreams through frontal low current stimulation of gamma activity. *Nat Neurosci, 17*(6), 810–812. doi: 10.1038/nn.3719

APPENDIX B

Obstructive Sleep Apnea

Sleep apnea (literally, "not breathing") is a general term for the most common form of sleep-disordered breathing (SDB). It involves interruption or reduction of airflow, most commonly because of obstruction of the upper airway (obstructive sleep apnea, OSA), and often accompanied by loud snoring (Cao et al., 2011). Other patients have central apneas as a result of a reduced neural drive to breathe during sleep, and there are also mixed conditions involving both types.

Patients with severe OSA may undergo hundreds of episodes of reduced airflow during a night. These include hypopneas (partial obstructions that reduce airflow) and apneas (complete airway obstructions) that can last for seconds or minutes at a time. Apneic episodes usually end with an abrupt awakening and gasping intake of breath, followed by a return to sleep. These repeated respiratory events reduce blood oxygen levels during the episodes as well as disrupting sleep and shortening total sleep time over the course of the night. Typical daytime symptoms include complaints of excessive sleepiness, headaches, unintentional sleep episodes, and cognitive and emotional problems (Cao et al., 2011).

The nighttime symptoms of sleep apnea are often reported by bed partners (loud snoring, breath holding, gasping for air) rather than by those with the condition. These witness reports and patient characteristics (e.g., obesity, large neck circumference, narrow airway, daytime sleepiness) can generate a high degree of suspicion that a person has sleep apnea. A definitive diagnosis, however, usually depends on a laboratory sleep study with monitoring of respiratory air flow (e.g., with a nasal cannula), respiratory effort (using pressure-sensitive bands across the trunk), and blood oxygen saturation (pulse oximetry), sound recordings, and standard EEG, EMG, and EOG recordings. Home-based diagnostic systems have also been used, based primarily on measuring changes in blood oxygen saturation. More recently, home-based systems have been developed that include more comprehensive monitoring abilities that will have to be validated against laboratory-based standards (Collop et al., 2011).

Apnea in adults is typically triggered by the loss of tone in the muscles that normally help keep the trachea open, and it is therefore more common during the atonia of REM sleep. The incidence and severity of apneic episodes are increased by being overweight, by structural features in the throat and/or jaw that reduce airway diameter even while awake, and by sleeping on one's back. Because airway constriction can contribute to snoring, OSA and snoring are often associated, but snoring also occurs in the absence of OSA (Somers et al., 2008). However, the louder and more frequent the snoring, the greater the probability of a diagnosis of sleep apnea (Sowho et al., 2019).

SDB is more common in middle-aged men than women, and risk increases with increased body weight (Young et al., 1997). OSA symptoms, however, including loud snoring, and apneas are also observed in young children, typically because of enlarged tonsils and/or adenoids or structural abnormalities in the jaw or throat that restrict airflow (Marcus, 2001). OSA symptoms in children are associated with poor school performance (Gozal, 1998) and behavioral problems, including hyperactivity and attention difficulties (Bonuck et al., 2012). Some of these children meet criteria for a diagnosis of attention deficit hyperactivity disorder (ADHD). Successful treatment of OSA symptoms can improve sleep and reduce the number of these children that meet ADHD diagnostic criteria (Chervin et al., 1997; Chervin et al., 2006).

Reduced airflow during apneas and hypopneas results in repeated episodes of moderate to severe reductions in levels of oxygen in the blood, and therefore in the brain, during the night. Because of a lack of awareness of the condition among both the public and health practitioners, as well as limited access to treatment resources, it may take years or decades for an individual with OSA to be diagnosed and treated appropriately (Young et al., 1993). Repeated cycles of oxygen desaturation, sleep loss, and daytime sleepiness over years contribute to deficits in a broad range of cognitive functions in OSA patients (Aloia et al., 2004). Some cognitive deficits persist even after successful treatment of the respiratory symptoms. The combination of reduced oxygen levels and chronically disrupted and shortened sleep may be responsible for long-lasting, possibly permanent, injury to the brain (Bédard et al., 1993; Lau et al., 2010; Näegelé et al., 1998; Sforza & Roche, 2012).

The predictable behavioral consequences of reduced and disrupted sleep at night include increased sleepiness and increased risk of falling asleep unintentionally during the day, including while driving (George & Smiley, 1999) or piloting an airplane (http://tinyurl.com/ztvtojh). Physiologically, OSA is associated with increased risk of abnormal glucose regulation, other metabolic conditions, chronically elevated blood pressure (hypertension), lack of blood pressure dipping at night (Dempsey et al., 2010; Hla et al., 2008; Hla et al., 1994), and resulting increased risk of heart disease and stroke (Shahar et al., 2001; Somers et al., 2008); see Chapter 14). Both chronic oxygen desaturation and disruption of sleep probably contribute to these metabolic and vascular effects. But it is uncertain whether the number of apneic episodes or other measures of disease severity best predict metabolic abnormalities and health risks (Pevernagie et al., 2020).

A standard treatment for OSA is a CPAP device (continuous positive airway pressure) that uses air pressure to hold open the obstructed airway, or a related system, BiPAP, that provides different levels of support for inhalation and exhalation. In addition, both oral appliances to help keep airways open and surgical procedures to reduce obstruction or reposition the jaw are also appropriate for some patients (Fleetham et al., 2006; Zaghi et al., 2016). Successful treatments for OSA reduce the incidence of apneas, lower blood pressure (Pepperell et al., 2002), reverse some of its associated metabolic symptoms (Lin et al., 2015), and reduce daytime consequences, such as the elevated rate of transportation accidents that is common among OSA patients (George, 2001).

OSA affects not only the risk of heart attacks but also their timing. In the general population, heart attack risk peaks during the morning hours because of the convergence of several risk factors that are at their worst shortly after waking (e.g., rising blood pressure, increased sympathetic drive, increased tendency toward clot formation); see **Figure 8.1 C** (Muller et al., 1987). Patients with sleep apnea, however, are more likely to have heart attacks and to die from cardiac causes overnight, when most people are at reduced risk for cardiac events. The more severe their apnea, the more likely people are to die suddenly during sleep, presumably because of the stress placed on the vascular system by apneic episodes (Gami et al., 2005; Sert Kuniyoshi et al., 2008).

There is considerable overlap between the physiological symptoms associated with chronic short sleep and those associated with OSA, which itself disrupts and shortens sleep. Thus, as discussed in Chapter 14, it is important to evaluate whether unreported OSA is a confounding variable in studies linking sleep duration to negative health outcomes.

Literature cited

Aloia, M. S., Arnedt, J. T., Davis, J. D., Riggs, R. L., & Byrd, D. (2004). Neuropsychological sequelae of obstructive sleep apnea-hypopnea syndrome: a critical review. *J Int Neuropsych Soc, 10*, 772–785.

Bédard, M.-A., Montplaisir, J., Malo, J., Richer, F., & Rouleau, I. (1993). Persistent neuropsychological deficits and vigilance impairment in sleep apnea syndrome after treatment with continuous positive airway pressure (CPAP). *J Clin Exp Neuropsyc, 15*(2), 330–341. doi: 10.1080/01688639308402567

Bonuck, K., Freeman, K., Chervin, R. D., & Xu, L. (2012). Sleep-disordered breathing in a population-based cohort: behavioral outcomes at 4 and 7 years. *Pediatrics, 129*(4), e857–e865. doi: 10.1542/peds.2011-1402

Cao, M. T., Guilleminault, C., & Kushida, C. A. (2011). Clinical features and evaluation of obstructive sleep apnea and upper airway resistance syndrome. In M. Kryger, T. Roth, & W. C. Dement (Eds.), *Principles and Practice of Sleep Medicine* (5th ed., pp. 1206–1218). St. Louis: Elsevier.

Chervin, R. D., Dillon, J. E., Bassetti, C., Ganoczy, D. A., & Pituch, K. J. (1997). Symptoms of sleep disorders, inattention, and hyperactivity in children. *Sleep, 20*(12), 1185–1192.

Chervin, R. D., Ruzicka, D. L., Giordani, B. J., Weatherly, R. A., Dillon, J. E., Hodges, E. K., . . . Guire, K. E. (2006). Sleep-disordered breathing, behavior, and cognition in children before and after adenotonsillectomy. *Pediatrics, 117*(4), e769–e778.

Collop, N. A., Tracy, S. L., Kapur, V., Mehra, R., Kuhlmann, D., Fleishman, S. A., & Ojile, J. M. (2011). Obstructive sleep apnea devices for out-of-center (OOC) testing: technology evaluation. *J Clin Sleep Med, 7*(5), 531–548. doi: 10.5664/JCSM.1328

Dempsey, J. A., Veasey, S. C., Morgan, B. J., & O'Donnell, C. P. (2010). Pathophysiology of sleep apnea. *Physiol Rev, 90*(1), 47–112. doi: 10.1152/physrev.00043.2008

Fleetham, J., Ayas, N., Bradley, D., Ferguson, K., Fitzpatrick, M., George, C., . . . Tsai, W. (2006). Canadian Thoracic Society guidelines: diagnosis and treatment of sleep disordered breathing in adults. *Can Respir J, 13*(7), 387–392.

Gami, A. S., Howard, D. E., Olson, E. J., & Somers, V. K. (2005). Day-night pattern of sudden death in obstructive sleep apnea. *New Engl J Med, 352*, 1206–1214.

George, C. F. P. (2001). Reduction in motor vehicle collisions following treatment of sleep apnoea with nasal CPAP. *Thorax, 556*, 508–512.

George, C. F. P., & Smiley, A. (1999). Sleep apnea and automobile crashes. *Sleep, 22*(6), 790–795.

Gozal, D. (1998). Sleep-disordered breathing and school performance in children. *Pediatrics, 102*(3), 616–620.

Hla, K. M., Young, T., Finn, L., Peppard, P. E., Szklo-Coxe, M., & Stubbs, M. (2008). Longitudinal association of sleep-disordered breathing and nondipping in nocturnal blood pressure in the Wisconsin Sleep Cohort study. *Sleep, 31*(6), 795–800.

Hla, K. M., Young, T. B., Bidwell, T., Palta, M., Skatrud, J. B., & Dempsey, J. (1994). Sleep apnea and hypertension. A population-based study. *Ann Int Med, 120*, 382–388.

Lau, E. Y. Y., Eskes, G. A., Morrison, D. L., Rajda, M., & Spurr, K. F. (2010). Executive function in patients with obstructive sleep apnea treated with continuous positive airway pressure. *J Int Neuropsych Soc, 16*(06), 1077–1088. doi: 10.1017/s1355617710000901

Lin, M. T., Lin, H. H., Lee, P. L., Weng, P. H., Lee, C. C., Lai, T. C., . . . Chen, C. L. (2015). Beneficial effect of continuous positive airway pressure on lipid profiles in obstructive sleep apnea: a meta-analysis. *Sleep Breath, 19*(3), 809–817. doi: 10.1007/s11325-014-1082-x

Marcus, C. L. (2001). Sleep-disordered breathing in children. *Am J Resp Crit Care Med, 164*, 16–30.

Muller, J. E., Ludmer, P. L., Willich, S. N., Tofler, G. H., Aylmer, G., Klangos, I., & Stone, P. H. (1987). Circadian variation in the frequency of sudden cardiac death. *Circulation, 75*, 131–138.

Näegelé, B., Pepin, J.-L., Levy, P., Bonnet, C., Pellat, J., & Feuerstein, C. (1998). Cognitive executive dysfunction in patients with obstructive sleep apnea syndrome (OSAS) after CPAP treatment. *Sleep, 21*(4), 392–396.

Pepperell, J. C., Ramdassingh-Dow, S., Crosthwaite, N., Mullins, R., Jenkinson, C., Stradling, J. R., & Davies, R. J. (2002). Ambulatory blood pressure after therapeutic and subtherapeutic nasal continuous positive airway pressure for obstructive sleep apnoea: a randomised parallel trial. *Lancet, 359*(9302), 204–210. doi: 10.1016/S0140-6736(02)07445-7

Pevernagie, D. A., Gnidovec-Strazisar, B., Grote, L., Heinzer, R., McNicholas, W. T., Penzel, T., . . . Arnardottir, E. S. (2020). On the rise and fall of the apnea-hypopnea index: a historical review and critical appraisal. *J Sleep Res*, 1–20. doi: 10.1111/jsr.13066

Sert Kuniyoshi, F., Garcia-Touchard, A., Gami, A. S., Romero Corral, A., van der Walt, C., Pusalavidyasagar, S., . . . Somers, V. K. (2008). Day–night variation of acute myocardial infarction in obstructive sleep apnea. *J Am Coll Cardiol, 52*(5), 343–346. doi: 10.1016/j.jacc.2008.04.027

Sforza, E., & Roche, F. (2012). Sleep apnea syndrome and cognition. *Front Neurol, 3*(87). doi: 10.3389/fneur.2012.00087

Shahar, E., Whitney, C. W., Redline, S., T., L. E., Newman, A. B., Nieto, F. J., … Samet, J. M. (2001). Sleep-disordered breathing and cardiovascular disease: cross-sectional results of the Sleep Heart Health Study. *Am J Resp Crit Care Med, 163*(1), 19–25.

Somers, V. K., White, D. P., Amin, R., Abraham, W. T., Costa, F., Culebras, A., … Young, T. (2008). Sleep apnea and cardiovascular disease: an American Heart Association/American College of Cardiology Foundation Scientific Statement from the American Heart Association Council for High Blood Pressure Research Professional Education Committee, Council on Clinical Cardiology, Stroke Council, and Council on Cardiovascular Nursing. *J Am Coll Cardiol, 52*(8), 686–717. doi: 10.1016/j.jacc.2008.05.002

Sowho, M., Sgambati, F., Guzman, M., Schneider, H., & Schwartz, A. (2019). Snoring: a source of noise pollution and sleep apnea predictor. *Sleep, 43*(6), zsz305. doi:10.1093/sleep/zsz305

Young, T., Evans, L., Finn, L., & Palta, M. (1997). Estimation of the clinically diagnosed proportion of sleep apnea syndrome in middle-aged men and women. *Sleep, 20*(9), 705–706.

Young, T., Palta, M., Dempsey, J., Skatrud, J., Weber, S., & Badr, S. (1993). The occurrence of sleep-disordered breathing among middle-aged adults. *New Engl J Med, 328*, 1230–1235.

Zaghi, S., Holty, J. E., Certal, V., Abdullatif, J., Guilleminault, C., Powell, N. B., … Camacho, M. (2016). Maxillomandibular advancement for treatment of obstructive sleep apnea: a meta-analysis. *JAMA Otolaryngol Head Neck Surg, 142*(1), 58–66. doi: 10.1001/jamaoto.2015.2678

APPENDIX C

Methods for Studying Neural Mechanisms Related to Sleep

For readers who are less familiar with neuroscience methods, it would be useful to review the methods commonly used to study neurotransmitter systems involved in the regulation of sleep, and neural features related to the function of sleep, as discussed especially in Chapters 8–12 and 18. If one hypothesizes, for example, that a particular neurotransmitter controls the expression of a sleep stage, which experimental methods can be used to develop evidence to test that hypothesis?

The brief summaries that follow are intended to provide basic information about how some commonly used methods work and to indicate a few of their strengths and weaknesses. It is not meant to be an exhaustive list nor to provide technical details of the methods. Another useful source of information is the review by (Brown et al., 2012), which provides a list of studies that used inactivation of brain regions or neurotransmitter systems to study effects on sleep (their Table 1); these inactivation approaches include methods mentioned in topics C.3–8 below.

C.1 Correlating neurotransmitter levels with sleep stages

The logic underlying this approach is that if a neurotransmitter is hypothesized to act in a brain region specifically to regulate one stage of sleep (e.g., triggering REM sleep), its levels in that region should be elevated during REM sleep but not during NREM sleep and perhaps not during waking. Several variables could affect the measurement of regional levels of a neurotransmitter: rates of release of the neurotransmitter; rates of its metabolism or reuptake (i.e., reabsorption into the releasing membrane); and the number of receptors present that bind the released neurotransmitter, which might make it unavailable for detection using some methods.

A common measurement method involves microdialysis, which uses an implanted probe equipped with a semipermeable membrane that permits small molecules to pass through it. Artificial cerebrospinal fluid is continuously infused into the probe at one end and collected at the other end. Molecules of neurotransmitters in the extracellular space can diffuse through the membrane and into the fluid. The collected fluid can then be analyzed using liquid chromatography to estimate the concentration of neurotransmitters during different stages of sleep.

An alternative family of methods involves electrochemical detection. These methods use specialized electrodes to generate electric currents that trigger chemical reactions specific to different neurotransmitters, followed by measurement of the resulting chemical products. A major advantage of this method is that it can detect the chemical changes corresponding to the presence of different neurotransmitters very quickly. This allows measurement of changes in neurotransmitter levels with finer temporal resolution than is possible with most other methods (Banerjee et al., 2020).

C.2 Measuring neuronal activity during sleep stages

An approach that is used frequently to measure neural activity in relation to neurotransmitter systems is to record the firing rates of populations of neurons or of single neurons in a brain region that produces a particular neurotransmitter. The goal may be to determine the pattern of firing activity across different sleep stages of neurons that produce and presumably release that neurotransmitter. However, recording from a brain nucleus that has been shown anatomically to have a high density of cells that contain that neurotransmitter does not guarantee that the recordings are from that neuronal type. As noted in Chapter 10, a "serotonergic" or "noradrenergic" nucleus that contains a high density of 5-HT- or NE-containing neurons often also includes neurons that use other neurotransmitters. The classic pontine "cholinergic" nuclei, the laterodorsal and pedunculopontine nuclei, as well as forebrain cholinergic nuclei, contain more GABAergic and glutamatergic cells than cholinergic cells (Ford et al., 1995; Kroeger et al., 2017; Luquin et al., 2018; Wang & Morales, 2009). Some neurons that produce a particular neurotransmitter, however, may have a very distinctive firing pattern, so recordings that show that pattern increase confidence that the cell being recorded is the target cell type.

An alternative approach is to use an anatomical marker of cell activation, such as increased levels of a transcription factor like the protein c-Fos or its mRNA. Double-labeling immunocytochemical methods can then be used to detect both the c-Fos protein and a marker of the type of neurotransmitter used by the labeled cell (e.g., serotonin or hypocretin). Using this approach, the c-Fos protein appears in the cell nucleus while the neurotransmitter is stained in the surrounding cytoplasm (see **Figure 11.11**). Expression of the c-Fos mRNA has a rapid onset in response to cell activation, and protein levels accumulate to a peak within 1–2 h. Therefore, the intensity of c-Fos immunocytochemical labeling at the time an animal is killed reflects the degree of cellular activation over the preceding 1–2 h period.

For single-cell electrophysiological studies, chemical phenotyping can also be accomplished by double-labeling the recorded cell immunocytochemically: one label identifies the specific cell that was recorded, and a second label demonstrates immunocytochemical staining of the neurotransmitter of interest. One method to achieve positive identification of the neurotransmitter phenotype of recorded cells is to use intracellular recordings and to inject the cell with a chemical marker that can later be localized histologically inside the cell body. Intracellular recordings, however, are difficult to sustain stably over the durations needed to measure changes associated with sleep–wake cycles and may also influence the functioning of the recorded cell.

An alternative approach is called juxtacellular labeling ("juxta" meaning "next to" in Latin), which uses extracellular recordings that can be sustained more easily over long time periods and are less likely to alter cell function. In this method, after a cell's activity pattern has been recorded and correlated with sleep stages, the cell is forced to take up an intracellular marker (e.g., neurobiotin) by ejecting the marker very close to the cell membrane while an electrical current is applied that causes the cell to fire at a high rate. A double-labeling immunocytochemical method can then be used in histological studies to identify the individual recorded cell (the one labeled with neurobiotin) and to identify its neurotransmitter phenotype (Boucetta et al., 2014).

C.3 Manipulating neural functions chemically or electrically

The involvement of neurotransmitters in sleep regulation can be studied by applying drugs that either enhance or reduce the activity of the target neurotransmitter system and studying the effects on sleep. These drugs include agonists (drugs that have the same effect as the target neurotransmitter), which act by enhancing neurotransmitter release, preventing its reuptake (and therefore leaving it available for longer in the synapse after it is released), reducing its metabolism, or directly mimicking the effect of the neurotransmitter on target receptors.

Other drugs used are antagonists, which function in several ways to reduce the activity of the neurotransmitter. These include occupying receptors for that neurotransmitter without activating them, so that the native neurotransmitter cannot reach the receptors or enhancing neurotransmitter metabolism or reuptake so it is less available to affect its targets. Interpreting the results of these studies depends on knowing the specificity with which chemical agents act on one target neurotransmitter or class of receptors at the concentrations being used. Most drugs have some degree of affinity for multiple receptors or affect multiple neurotransmitter systems, and the specificity of their effects is strongly determined by the dose used and its effective concentration at target synapses.

Neuroactive chemicals can be administered by ingestion, by systemic injections (intravenous or intraperitoneal), or by injections into the cerebrospinal fluid (intraventricular injections). These methods do not allow localization of the site(s) of action. Alternatively, drugs can be administered directly into the target nuclei of interest, which allows a stronger conclusion about the site of action. Drugs can be applied to a localized region by using micropressure to force a tiny volume of fluid into the brain through a micropipette (a fine glass or metal tube inserted into the brain). Other methods involve applying the drug through a micropipette by iontophoresis (using an electrical current to drive molecules out of the micropipette) or by reverse microdialysis (see Section C.1 above) to drive a drug out of a dialysis probe and into the target tissue.

Interpreting the results of these studies depends on the specificity with which stimulation or inhibition can be targeted to individual neurotransmitter systems, without affecting adjacent cells that use different neurotransmitters.

Alternatively, a neurotransmitter system or brain region can be manipulated using electrical currents to activate or suppress the activity of neurons. These can involve implanted electrodes in animals and in some humans during exploratory studies related to clinical interventions. With these methods, as with the application of chemical agonists or antagonists to specific neural targets, physical spread of current to adjacent tissues is a concern that needs to be addressed with appropriate control procedures.

A different approach involves manipulating the neural activity of specific brain regions in people using electrical or magnetic manipulations from outside the skull. These methods can include applying direct or alternating currents or magnetic fields designed to activate, suppress, or alter the timing of sleep-related neural features (e.g., slow waves or sleep spindles); see Section 18.12 for more details.

C.4 Ablation (lesion) methods

Ablation (lesion) methods have been a commonly used tool in behavioral neuroscience research, but the results obtained may be subject to different interpretations. There are several lesion methods that produce different consequences. Coagulating a specific nucleus with heat or electrical current destroys cell bodies, any afferent terminals reaching the region, and any projection pathways passing through it. The effects observed may be related to the loss of any or all of these components.

Excitotoxic lesions can be produced using a chemical agent that kills neurons but spares projection pathways within a region, so the resulting damage can be more reliably attributed to the loss of cells in that region. However, some neurons are resistant to excitotoxic damage. Neurotoxins that are specific to one class of neurotransmitter-expressing cells can produce selective loss of that cell type (e.g., 6-hydroxydopamine destroys dopaminergic neurons). Genetic methods can also produce specific ablations by linking a toxic substance (e.g., ataxin-3) to genetic machinery that is active in only one kind of neurotransmitter-expressing cell. This method was used, for example, to produce selective loss of orexin/hypocretin neurons (Hara et al., 2001).

It is important to recognize that what can be observed after an ablation is the behavior of a system lacking a particular neurotransmitter, cell type, or nucleus. These studies do not directly demonstrate the normal role of that neurotransmitter or cell type in the intact system, but rather the functioning of the brain in its absence. The functional consequences of loss of a regulatory system may not be the logical opposite of the usual function of the missing system. Ablation studies can demonstrate whether or not a structure or neurotransmitter system is *necessary* for a particular function to proceed normally, but they do not unambiguously demonstrate what the normal contribution of the ablated system is to that function.

By way of an analogy, if one damaged an electronic circuit in a smartphone and could no longer play music on it, one would know that the lost circuit is necessary for that function. One might then hypothesize that the missing circuit is involved, for example, in storing the digital files that represent the music. However, the circuit might instead be needed in order to access those files or to receive instructions from the user to play a song, or to activate the speaker, or to perform any number of other steps, each of which is also necessary for the device to respond to a keystroke sequence by generating appropriate music. The absence of music cannot tell us which component process has been compromised. The main use of ablation studies is to generate testable hypotheses based on an observed change in function, which can then be evaluated using different methods.

One example of a classic chemical ablation study related to sleep was the use of para-chlorophenylalanine (PCPA) which prevents the action of a rate-limiting enzyme involved in producing serotonin. The resulting hyperactivity and reduced sleep of animals treated with PCPA, and similar effects of ablation of serotonin-containing raphe neurons, led to the initial hypothesis that serotonin is involved in producing NREM sleep (Jouvet, 1969). A series of later studies using different methods instead suggested a role for serotonin in producing cortical arousal and waking rather than sleep. Other studies suggested that the effects were mediated by altered body temperature regulation. Further research led to several other hypotheses and questioned whether linking serotonin to either waking or NREM sleep adequately describes its complex roles and interactions in the regulation of sleep and waking; see Section 10.5 for details.

C.5 Genetic methods to increase or decrease gene expression

Genetic methods can be used to introduce a variety of changes in neurotransmitter systems. One example would be knocking out or inactivating a gene coding for production of a particular neurotransmitter receptor subtype to assess its role in sleep regulation. A caution in interpreting knockout studies is that the change in neurotransmission introduced by a genetic manipulation is present throughout the development of the organism. As a result, it is possible that compensatory changes occur developmentally in the function of other mechanisms because of the change in the targeted system (e.g., there is a compensatory increase in another receptor subtype when one subtype is lost). The functional consequences that are observed might be the result of a combination of the genetic change that was deliberately introduced and compensatory responses of other mechanisms that might be unobserved and unknown.

A modification of this approach also introduces a genetic change (blocking or augmenting expression of a specific gene) that affects neurotransmission. But the expression of the genetic change is only activated by a manipulation in the adult organism (e.g., introduction or removal of a specific dietary element). As a result, this *conditional* knockout (or knockin) approach avoids the issue of compensatory developmental changes in related systems, so the genetic ablation is less likely to be confounded by other unidentified changes. Allowing for the limitations of any form of ablation study, as discussed above, this approach makes it easier to attribute the resulting changes in sleep to the immediate ("on-line") change in functioning of the particular gene and neurotransmitter system that is being manipulated.

C.6 Optogenetic methods

These methods involve the insertion of a gene that codes for a light-activated molecule (e.g., an enzyme or ion channel) into an organism so that it is expressed in only one type of neuron (e.g., neurons that produce dopamine or hypocretin). A fine fiber-optic or light-emitting diode can then be implanted into the brain (or introduced into a brain slice preparation) to transmit light of an appropriate wavelength to the target neurons that have incorporated the gene. Turning on the light source illuminates the light-sensitive molecule and activates it, causing, for example, the opening or closing of an ion channel, which can increase or decrease the activity of any neuron bearing the engineered gene. This method can be used to selectively and reversibly increase or decrease release of the neurotransmitter in real time in a behaving organism, so one can assess the effects on sleep of very selective and localized changes in that neurotransmitter system's activity; see, for example, Adamantidis et al., 2007; Arrigoni & Saper, 2014.

C.7 Pharmacogenetic methods

This approach is related to the preceding method in that a molecule is inserted via gene transfer so that it is targeted to only one cell type (e.g., cells that produces hypocretin or dopamine). In this case, however, the molecule inserted is an artificial form of G-protein linked receptor. These artificial receptors are engineered so that they trigger a cascade of second messenger effects that either activate or suppress the activity of that class of cells when the receptors are bound by the appropriate ligand.

The important variation is that the artificial receptor is designed to respond to only one kind of ligand, namely, an artificial substance that does not occur in nature. As a result, treatment of an animal with that drug will enhance or suppress the activity of that category of neurons exclusively, without directly affecting any other cell type. Similarly, no naturally occurring substance can act through these receptors and unintentionally affect the animal's physiology since they do not bind any natural molecule.

This method is also referred to as the use of "*d*esigner *r*eceptors *e*xclusively *a*ctivated by *d*esigner *d*rugs" or DREADDs; see, for example, Sasaki et al., 2011. Another advantage of these genetic insertion methods is that they do not require the extensive genetic information needed for other kinds of genetic manipulations. Detailed genetic information is available for only a few species, including the laboratory mouse and fruit fly, but this method permits studies using other species, like the rat, for which more limited genetic information is available.

C.8 Studying clinical populations with neurotransmitter defects

Clinical populations provide useful information, but the lack of experimental control can raise challenges in interpreting results. Brain injuries may affect sleep, but they are rarely, if ever, limited to a single nucleus or to a projection pathway using a specific neurotransmitter. Very rare genetic defects that interfere with production of specific neurotransmitters and generate sleep abnormalities provide an opportunity to study more specific deficits in a clinical population. Interpretation of the results observed is strengthened if it is possible to reverse the loss of the neurotransmitter with medications and show a parallel reversal in sleep-related symptoms.

Similarly, neurodegenerative conditions are unlikely to affect a single neurotransmitter system, but some are at least relatively selective with respect to their impact on sleep, such as the effects of loss of dopaminergic neurons in Parkinson's disease or hypocretin neurons in narcolepsy. As with genetic defects, evidence that sleep-related symptoms can be improved by restoring levels of the affected neurotransmitter strengthens the interpretation of its role; see, for example, Belaid et al., 2014; Leu-Semenescu et al., 2010.

Literature cited

Adamantidis, A. R., Zhang, F., Aravanis, A. M., Deisseroth, K., & de Lecea, L. (2007). Neural substrates of awakening probed with optogenetic control of hypocretin neurons. *Nature, 450*(7168), 420–424. doi: 10.1038/nature06310

Arrigoni, E., & Saper, C. B. (2014). What optogenetic stimulation is telling us (and failing to tell us) about fast neurotransmitters and neuromodulators in brain circuits for wake-sleep regulation. *Curr Opin Neurobiol, 29*, 165–171. doi: 0.1016/j.conb.2014.07.016

Banerjee, S., McCracken, S., Hossain, M. F., & Slaughter, G. (2020). Electrochemical detection of neurotransmitters. *Biosensors (Basel), 10*(8), 1–18. doi: 10.3390/bios10080101

Belaid, H., Adrien, J., Laffrat, E., Tande, D., Karachi, C., Grabli, D., … Francois, C. (2014). Sleep disorders in Parkinsonian macaques: effects of L-dopa treatment and pedunculopontine nucleus lesion. *J Neurosci, 34*(27), 9124–9133. doi: 10.1523/JNEUROSCI.0181-14.2014

Boucetta, S., Cisse, Y., Mainville, L., Morales, M., & Jones, B. E. (2014). Discharge profiles across the sleep-waking cycle of identified cholinergic, GABAergic, and glutamatergic neurons in the pontomesencephalic tegmentum of the rat. *J Neurosci, 34*(13), 4708–4727. doi: 10.1523/JNEUROSCI.2617-13.2014

Brown, R. E., Basheer, R., McKenna, J. T., Strecker, R. E., & McCarley, R. W. (2012). Control of sleep and wakefulness. *Physiol Rev, 92*(3), 1087–1187. doi: 10.1152/physrev.00032.2011

Ford, B., Holmes, C., Mainville, L., & Jones, B. (1995). GABAergic neurons in the rat pontomesencephalic tegmentum: distribution with cholinergic and other tegmental neurons projecting to the posterior lateral hypothalamus. *J Comp Neurol, 363*, 177–196.

Hara, J., Beuckmann, C. T., Nambu, T., Willie, J. T., Chemelli, R. M., Sinton, C. M., … Sakurai, T. (2001). Genetic ablation of orexin neurons in mice results in narcolepsy, hypophagia, and obesity. *Neuron, 30*(2), 345–354. doi: 10.1016/s0896-6273(01)00293-8

Jouvet, M. (1969). Biogenic amines and the states of sleep. *Science, 163*(3862), 32–41.

Kroeger, D., Ferrari, L. L., Petit, G., Mahoney, C. E., Fuller, P. M., Arrigoni, E., & Scammell, T. E. (2017). Cholinergic, glutamatergic, and GABAergic neurons of the pedunculopontine tegmental nucleus have distinct effects on sleep/wake behavior in mice. *J Neurosci*, *37*(5), 1352–1366. doi: 10.1523/JNEUROSCI.1405-16.2016

Leu-Semenescu, S., Arnulf, I., Decaix, C., Moussa, F., Clot, F., Boniol, C., ... Roze, E. (2010). Sleep and rhythm consequences of a genetically induced loss of serotonin. *Sleep*, *33*(3), 307–314.

Luquin, E., Huerta, I., Aymerich, M. S., & Mengual, E. (2018). Stereological estimates of glutamatergic, GABAergic, and cholinergic neurons in the pedunculopontine and laterodorsal tegmental nuclei in the rat. *Front Neuroanat*, *12*, 1–19. doi:10.3389/fnana.2018.00034

Sasaki, K., Suzuki, M., Mieda, M., Tsujino, N., Roth, B., & Sakurai, T. (2011). Pharmacogenetic modulation of orexin neurons alters sleep/wakefulness states in mice. *PLoS One*, *6*(5), e20360. doi: 10.1371/journal.pone.0020360

Wang, H. L., & Morales, M. (2009). Pedunculopontine and laterodorsal tegmental nuclei contain distinct populations of cholinergic, glutamatergic and GABAergic neurons in the rat. *Eur J Neurosci*, *29*(2), 340–358. doi: 10.1111/j.1460-9568.2008.06576.x

APPENDIX D

Narcolepsy, Influenza, and the Immune System

The hypothesis discussed in Section 11.3.3 that narcolepsy is a slowly progressing neurodegenerative disease does not explain what causes the rare occurrence of narcolepsy in children and especially its sudden appearance in otherwise apparently healthy children. There is evidence that over several years there was an increase in the frequency of sudden-onset narcolepsy in children immediately following seasonal peaks in influenza infections. This increase was especially evident after the 2009–2010 H1N1 influenza ("swine flu") pandemic. The peak of influenza infection in China, for example, was followed by the onset of narcolepsy in unusually large numbers of children who had been infected with the H1N1 virus. These findings suggested the possibility that immune system responses to influenza infection triggered the spike in narcolepsy cases in a subset of children who had a genetic susceptibility to the condition (Gool et al., 2023; Han et al., 2011; Wang et al., 2023).

An influenza pandemic in 1918 also preceded the onset of cases of encephalitis lethargica ("sleepy sickness") in Europe that was studied by von Economo in the 1920s (see Chapter 1), and the viral strain involved is related to the H1N1 virus (Taubenberger, 2006). The brain damage and symptoms studied by von Economo may have been the result of the infection and/or of the resulting immune system activation in response to infection.

Not only children who were infected by the 2009–2010 H1N1 virus but also a small proportion of those protected from infection by immunization developed narcolepsy. Because the 2009–2010 pandemic was the first influenza pandemic in 40 years, there was an international campaign to immunize people against the virus to protect them from its potentially lethal effects. Tragically, there is convincing evidence of an increased incidence of narcolepsy among some children who were immunized against the H1N1 virus using one form of the vaccine. This particular vaccine included an adjuvant, a chemical that is added in order to strengthen the immune system response to the viral components in the vaccine.

This outbreak occurred in several countries where a vaccine including this particular adjuvant was used (especially in northern Europe) but not in other countries. In addition, the increased incidence in the countries that were affected was confined almost exclusively to individuals who were positive for the DQB1*06:02 allele (Pellegrino et al., 2015; Tafti et al., 2014). These results indicate that onset of narcolepsy was linked to strong immune system activation in children with this DQB1 allele who were either infected with H1N1 or were vaccinated with this adjuvanted form of the vaccine.

These very rare side effects of vaccination (perhaps 1 case per million vaccinations) appeared to be related to the presence of this one adjuvant, which was not included in other forms of the vaccine (Ahmed et al., 2014; Dauvilliers et al., 2010; Szakács et al., 2013). In addition, the inactivated viral components used to generate this vaccine included a protein with a genetic sequence that cross-reacted with a hypocretin receptor (Ahmed et al., 2015). This finding suggests that the coincidence of this genetic similarity and stimulation of robust immune system activation resulted in damage to the hypocretin system, although the exact mechanisms involved remain uncertain (Gool et al., 2023; Pellegrino et al., 2015).

These factors cannot account for why some genetically susceptible children in China, the vast majority of whom were *not* vaccinated against influenza, also showed an unusually high incidence of narcolepsy onset. These children apparently generated a potent immune system response to infection by the H1N1 influenza virus itself, perhaps in combination with the presence of other upper respiratory tract infections (Han et al., 2011), which resulted in narcolepsy. This influenza virus may be especially potent at triggering intense immune system activity. Thus, a combination of genetic susceptibility and strong immune system activation, in response to either the virus itself or to one specific form of a vaccine, appeared to be involved in all cases.

While some might consider these serious health consequences in a very small number of children as grounds for avoiding influenza vaccines, it is important to note that these rare effects occurred only in children with an existing genetic susceptibility. Those same children would have been at increased risk of developing narcolepsy in response to an H1N1 infection without immunization (as occurred in China), or from other provocative factors later in life. As a result, it is not clear whether it is safer for children with the DQB1*06:02 allele to be vaccinated against influenza or not, since influenza infection alone can provoke narcolepsy, or it can be fatal. These findings suggest that screening for this genotype may be potentially useful, at least with respect to the choice of adjuvants in a vaccine. They also reinforce the conclusion that intense immune system activation in genetically susceptible individuals can lead to development of the classic symptoms of narcolepsy with cataplexy.

Literature cited

Ahmed, S. S., Schur, P. H., MacDonald, N. E., & Steinman, L. (2014). Narcolepsy, 2009 A(H1N1) pandemic influenza, and pandemic influenza vaccinations: what is known and unknown about the neurological disorder, the role for autoimmunity, and vaccine adjuvants. *J Autoimmun*, *50*, 1–11. doi: 10.1016/j.jaut.2014.01.033

Ahmed, S. S., Volkmuth, W., Duca, J., Corti, L., Pallaoro, M., Pezzicoli, A., ... Steinman, L. (2015). Antibodies to influenza nucleoprotein cross-react with human hypocretin receptor 2. *Sci Transl Med*, *7*(294), 294ra105. doi: 10.1126/scitranslmed.aab2354

Dauvilliers, Y., Montplaisir, J., Cochen, V., Desautels, A., Einen, M., Lin, L., ... Mignot, E. (2010). Post-H1N1 narcolepsy-cataplexy. *Sleep*, *33*(11), 1428–1429.

Gool, J., Schinkelshoek, M. S., & Fronczek, R. (2023). What triggered narcolepsy: H1N1 vaccination, virus or both? Important lessons learned from China. *Sleep*, *46*(3), zsad005. doi:10.1093/sleep/zsad005

Han, F., Lin, L., Warby, S. C., Faraco, J., Li, J., Dong, S. X., ... Mignot, E. (2011). Narcolepsy onset is seasonal and increased following the 2009 H1N1 pandemic in China. *Ann Neurol*, *70*(3), 410–417. doi: 10.1002/ana.22587

Pellegrino, P., Clementi, E., & Radice, S. (2015). On vaccine's adjuvants and autoimmunity: current evidence and future perspectives. *Autoimmun Rev*, *14*(10), 880–888. doi: 10.1016/j.autrev.2015.05.014

Szakács, A., Darin, N., & Hallböök, T. (2013). Increased childhood incidence of narcolepsy in western Sweden after H1N1 influenza vaccination. *Neurology*, *80*, 1315–1321.

Tafti, M., Hor, H., Dauvilliers, Y., Lammers, G. J., Overeem, S., Mayer, G., ... Kutalik, Z. (2014). DQB1 locus alone explains most of the risk and protection in narcolepsy with cataplexy in Europe. *Sleep*, *37*(1), 19–25. doi: 10.5665/sleep.3300

Taubenberger, J. K. (2006). The origin and virulence of the 1918 "Spanish" influenza virus. *Proc Am Philosoph Soc*, *150*(1), 86–112.

Wang, X., Xiao, F., Wang, Y., Deng, X., Chen, Z., Dong, X., ... Yu, H. (2023). Changed epidemiology of narcolepsy before, during, and after the 2009 H1N1 pandemic: a nationwide narcolepsy surveillance network study in mainland China, 1990–2017. *Sleep*, *46*(3), zsac325. doi:10.1093/sleep/zsac325

Index

For the benefit of digital users, indexed terms that span two pages (e.g., 52–53) may, on occasion, appear on only one of those pages.

Tables, figures, and boxes are indicated by an italic *t*, *f*, and *b* following the page number.

K

L

M

N

Q

R

T

U

V